646.72
M59
2004

P9-ARS-792
3 5674 04011228 7

MILADY'S STANDARD Cosmetology

Arlene Alpert
Margrit Altenburg
Diane Bailey
Letha Barnes
Lisha Barnes
Debbie Beatty
Mary Brunetti
Jane Crawford
Aly Evirs
Catherine M. Frangie
John Halal
Colleen Hennessey
Mary Beth Janssen
Toni Love
Vivienne Mackinder
Carey Nash
Ruth Roche
Teresa Sammarco
Sue Sansom
Sue Schultes

THOMSON
DELMAR LEARNING™
Australia Canada Mexico Singapore Spain United Kingdom United States

WILDER BRANCH LIBRARY
7140 E. SEVEN MILE RD.
DETROIT, MI 48234
JUN -- 2005

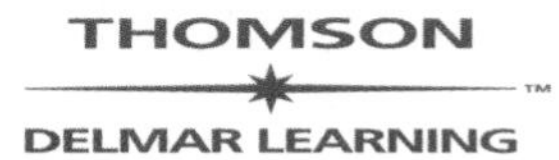

Milady's Standard: Cosmetology

MILADY STAFF:

President:
Susan L. Simpfenderfer

Acquisitions Editor:
Pamela B. Lappies

Executive Production Manager:
Wendy A. Troeger

Production Editor:
Eileen M. Clawson

Composition:
ThomasTech Solutions

Executive Marketing Manager:
Donna J. Lewis

Channel Manager:
Stephen G. Smith

Cover and Text Design:
Spiral Design Studio

COPYRIGHT © 2004 by Milady, an imprint of Delmar, a division of Thomson Learning, Inc. Thomson Learning™ is a trademark used herein under license

Printed in the United States of America
5 6 7 8 9 10 XXX 06 05 04

For more information contact Milady,
Executive Woods, 5 Maxwell Drive
Clifton Park, New York 12065-2919

Or find us on the World Wide Web at http://www.milady.com

All rights reserved. No part of this work covered by the copyright hereon may be reproduced or used in any form or by any means—graphic, electronic, or mechanical, including photocopying, recording, taping, Web distribution or information storage and retrieval systems—without written permission of the publisher.

For permission to use material from this text or product, contact us by
Tel (800) 730-2214
Fax (800) 730-2215
www.thomsonrights.com

Library of Congress Cataloging-in-Publication Data

Milady's standard: cosmetology / Arlene Alpert ... [et al.].
p. cm.
Rev. ed. of: Milady's standard textbook of cosmetology,
Includes index.
ISBN 1-56253-880-2 (softcover)
ISBN 1-56253-879-9 (hardcover)
1. Beauty culture. I. Alpert, Arlene. II. Milady Publishing Company.
III. Title: Milady's standard textbook of cosmetology.

TT957 .M5518 2002
646.7'2--dc21 2002074216

NOTICE TO THE READER

Publisher does not warrant or guarantee any of the products described herein or perform any independent analysis in connection with any of the product information contained herein. Publisher does not assume, and expressly disclaims, any obligation to obtain and include information other than that provided to it by the manufacturer.

The reader is expressly warned to consider and adopt all safety precautions that might be indicated by the activities herein and to avoid all potential hazards. By following the instructions contained herein, the reader willingly assumes all risks in connection with such instructions.

The Publisher makes no representation or warranties of any kind, including but not limited to, the warranties of fitness for particular purpose or merchantability, nor are any such representations implied with respect to the material set forth herein, and the publisher takes no responsibility with respect to such material. The publisher shall not be liable for any special, consequential, or exemplary damages resulting, in whole or part, from the readers' use of, or reliance upon, this material.

PART 1

ORIENTATION

PART 2

COSMETOLOGY SCIENCES

PART 3

HAIR CARE

PART 4

SKIN CARE

PART 5

NAIL CARE

PART 6

THE BUSINESS OF COSMETOLOGY

PART 1

ORIENTATION

PART 2

COSMETOLOGY SCIENCES

PART 3

HAIR CARE

PROCEDURES

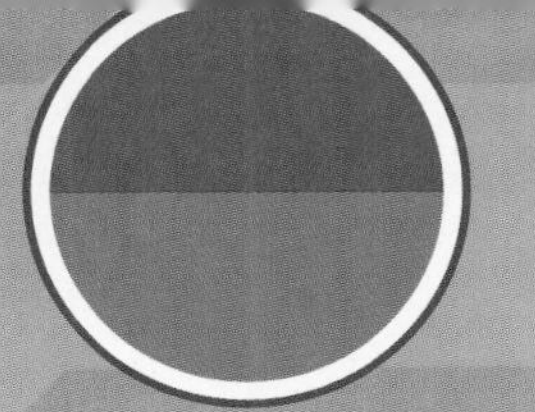

PROCEDURES (Continued)

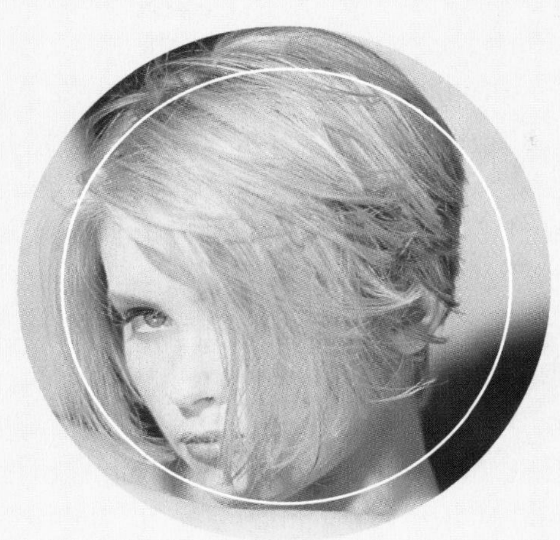

Milady's Standard Cosmetology

Preface

Congratulations! You are about to start on a journey that can take you in many directions and holds the potential to make you a confident, successful professional in cosmetology. As a cosmetologist, you will become a trusted professional, the person your clients rely on to provide them with ongoing service, enabling them to look and feel their best. You will become as personally involved in your clients' lives as their physicians or dentists are, and with study and practice, you can be as much in demand as a well-regarded medical provider.

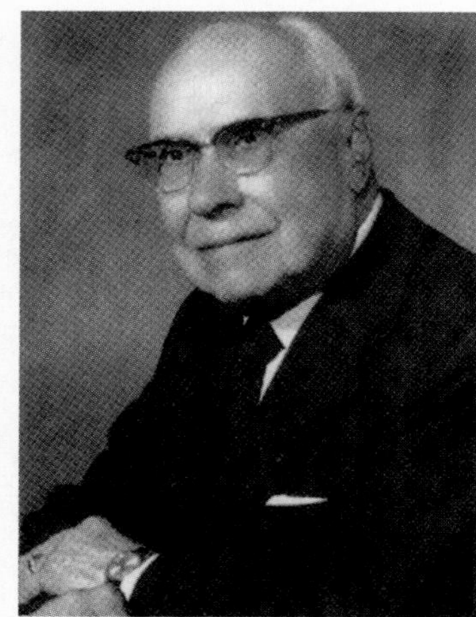

Milady's Standard Textbook of Cosmetology* was the creation of Nicholas F. Cimaglia, founder of Milady Publishing Company, which he established in 1927. He began his career in the beauty business as a salesman for a beauty supply distributor, selling his book, the *New York State Barbering Exam*, along with hair tonics and razors, door to door to barber shops in New York City. In 1938, Nick Cimaglia published the first edition of *Milady's Standard Textbook of Cosmetology*, and it has been the textbook of choice for cosmetology education ever since and has undergone many revisions. Throughout its lifetime, it has consistently been the most-used cosmetology textbook in the world. With the many changes in the field of cosmetology, new editions of the text are needed periodically, and Milady is committed to making it the best cosmetology education available.

THE INDUSTRY STANDARD

This edition of *Milady's Standard Cosmetology* provides you with the information you will need to pass the licensure exams as well as the most contemporary techniques to ensure your success once you are on the job. Before beginning this revision, Milady surveyed 600 educators and professionals, held two focus groups, and received in-depth comments from dozens of reviewers to learn what needed to be changed, added, or deleted. Next we consulted with educational experts to learn the best way to present the material, so that all types of learners could understand it and remember it. Then we went to twenty experts in various cosmetology-related fields to write or revise the chapters. Finally, we sent the finished manuscripts to yet more subject experts to ensure the accuracy and thoroughness of the material. What you hold in your hands is the result.

Milady's Standard Cosmetology contains new information on many subjects, including sanitation and infection control, braiding, haircutting, and haircoloring. In addition, there is a greater emphasis on personal skills in the many new chapters, such as "Life Skills," "Communicating for Success," and "Seeking Employment."

As a part of your cosmetology education, this book will serve as a valuable guide, and you'll refer to it again and again throughout your career.

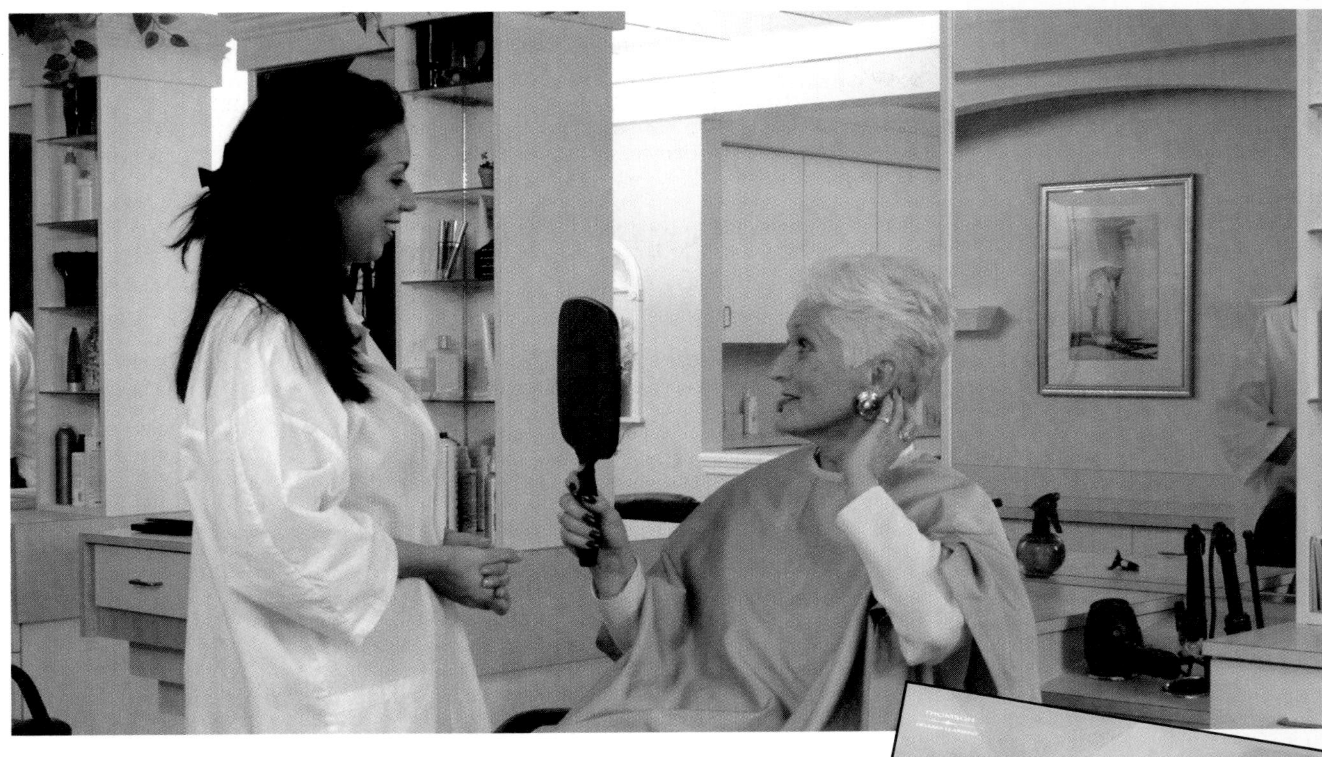

FEATURES OF THIS EDITION

In response to the suggestions of the cosmetology educators and professionals who reviewed the *Standard* and to those submitted by the students who use this text, this edition includes dramatic changes, including many new chapters. Milady has also changed the design of the textbook and included new photography and illustrations to bring you the most valuable, effective educational material available.

To get the most out of the time you will spend studying, take a few minutes first to learn about the textbook and how to use it before you begin. Use the Preface information that follows as a guide to lead you through the special features the textbook provides to help you learn, understand, and retain the important information within.

Contents in Brief

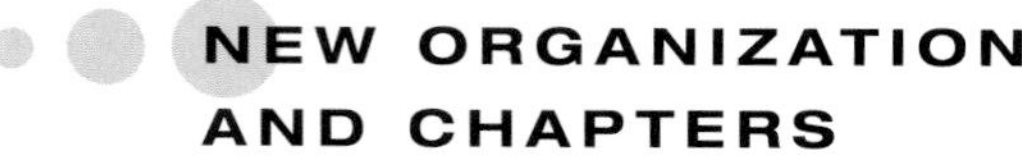

NEW ORGANIZATION AND CHAPTERS

By learning and using the tools in this text along with your teachers' instruction, you will develop the abilities you need to build a loyal and satisfied clientele. To help you locate information more easily, the chapters are now grouped in six main parts.

Part 1: Orientation consists of four chapters that cover the field of cosmetology and the personal skills you will need to become successful. The first chapter, "Cosmetology: The History and Opportunities" outlines where cosmetology came from and where it can take you. In "Life Skills," the second chapter, the ability to set goals and maintain a good attitude are emphasized along with the psychology of success. "Your Professional Image" stresses the importance of inward beauty and health as well as outward appearance, and "Communicating for Success" describes the important process of building client relationships based on trust and effective communication.

Part 2: Cosmetology Sciences includes important information you need to know to keep yourself and your clients safe and healthy. "Infection Control: Principles and Practice" offers the most current, vital facts about Hepatitis, HIV, and other infectious viruses and bacteria and tells how to prevent their spread in the salon. "Basics of Anatomy and Physiology" and "Basics of Chemistry and Electricity" provide essential information that will affect how you work with clients and tools.

Part 3: Hair Care offers almost all new material on every aspect of hair. "Properties of the Hair and Scalp" presents the basics of the physical composition of hair, while "Principles of Hair Design" explores the ways it can be sculpted to enhance a client's facial shape. The foundation on which almost every hair service is built is covered in "Shampooing, Rinsing, and Conditioning," followed by a totally new "Haircutting" chapter, complete with step-by-step procedures for core cuts. Step-by-step procedures are also found in "Hairstyling," along with information on new tools and techniques. A totally new chapter is included on "Braiding and Braid Extensions," followed by "Wigs and Hair Enhancements." Both "Chemical Texture Services" and "Haircoloring" reflect the most recent advances in these areas.

Part 4: Skin Care focuses on another area in which new advances have altered the way students must be trained. The basics about skin are presented in "Histology of the Skin." The popular topic of "Hair Removal" covers waxing, tweezing, and popular methods. "Facials" and "Facial Makeup" offer the critical information you'll need for these increasingly requested services in the expanding field of esthetics. Procedures are included for many of the services needed in salons and day spas.

Part 5: Nail Care contains the revised chapters "Nail Structure and Growth" and "Manicuring and Pedicuring," which includes procedures for a Basic Manicure, a Basic Pedicure, and a French Manicure. New to this edition is the chapter "Advanced Nail Techniques," which covers nail tips, acrylics, gels, and wraps. Nail art is depicted in the text and the photographs.

Part 6: The Business of Cosmetology opens with the updated chapter "The Salon Business," in which students are exposed to the numerous types of salons and salon ownerships available to them. A new chapter, "Seeking Employment," prepares students for licensure exams as well as for job interviews and explains how to create a résumé and portfolio. What you will be expected to know and do as a newly licensed cosmetologist is described in "On the Job," another new chapter. It offers tips on how to make the most of your first job, and how to learn the most from it, too.

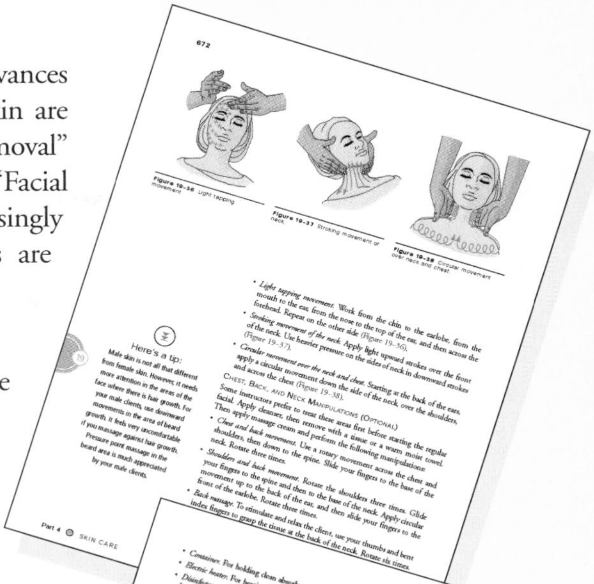

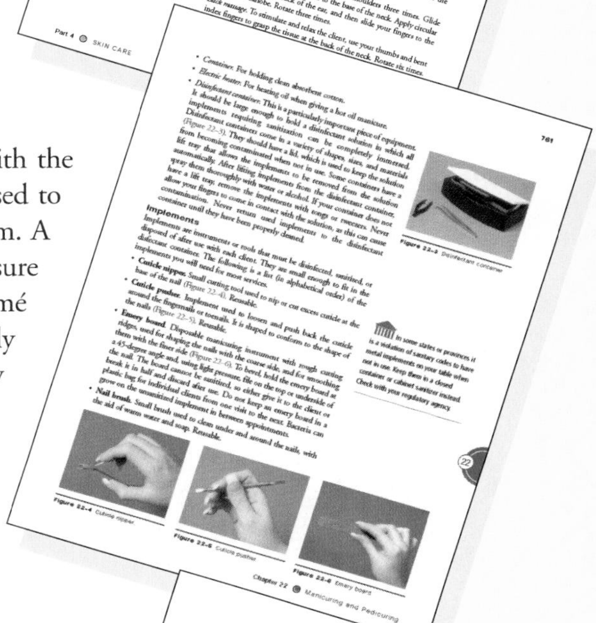

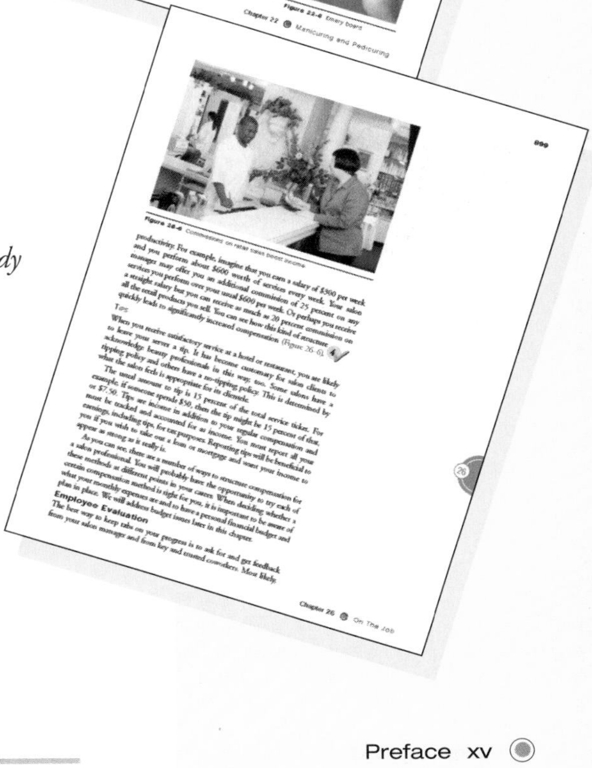

A special Closing, written by Robert Cromeans, one of the most widely recognized personalities in today's professional hair industry, provides a message to students who have completed their course of study and are ready to enter the professional world. Robert's message will motivate and encourage you and send you off to what can be one of the most lucrative and fun careers available today.

ELEMENTS NEW TO THIS EDITION

As part of the comprehensive revision of this edition, many new features have been added to help you master key concepts and techniques.

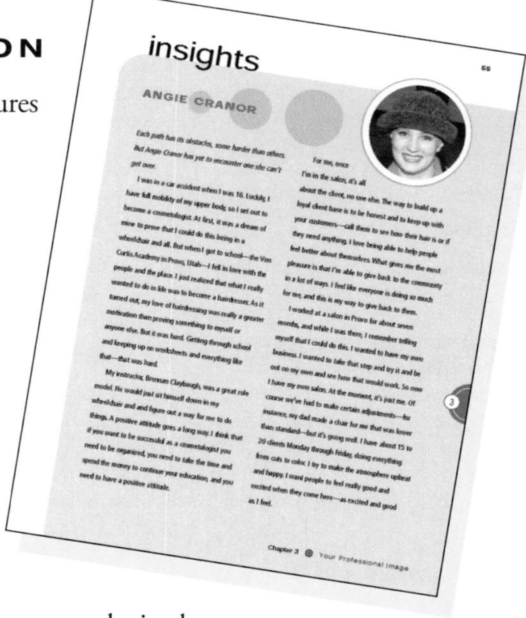

insights These personal stories told by licensed cosmetologists provide a glimpse into the variety of paths they have traveled. Their stories range from tragic to transcendent, illustrating the very different journeys a cosmetologist may take.

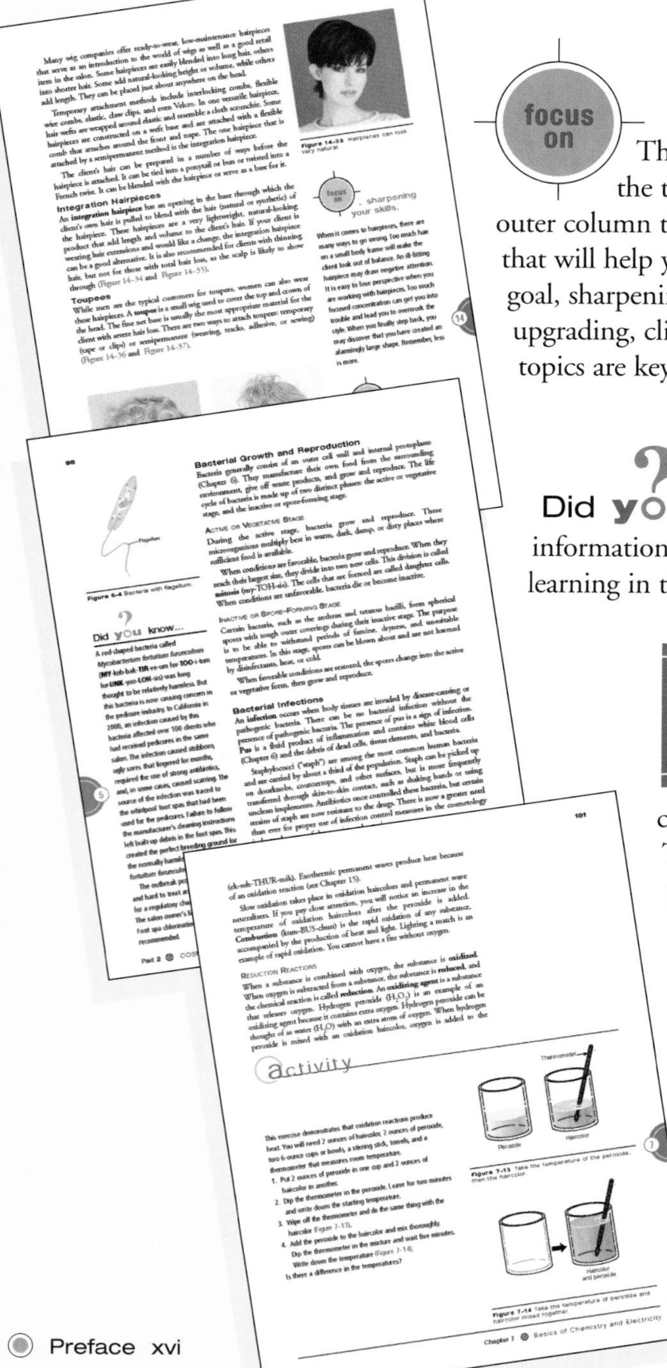

focus on Throughout the text are short paragraphs in the outer column that draw attention to various skills and concepts that will help you reach your goal. The "Focus On . . ." pieces target the goal, sharpening technical skills, sharpening personal skills, ticket upgrading, client consultation, and building your client base. These topics are key to your success as a student and as a professional.

Did you know... These features provide interesting information that will enhance your understanding of what you are learning in the text and call attention to a special point.

5 Each page contains its chapter number, located in a semicircle using the main color for that part. For instance, Chapter 5 is in Part 2, which is the color for all three chapters contained within that part. This color-coding will help you locate topics without going to the table of contents or index.

activity The "Activity" boxes describe classroom exercises that will help you understand firsthand the concepts being explained in the text.

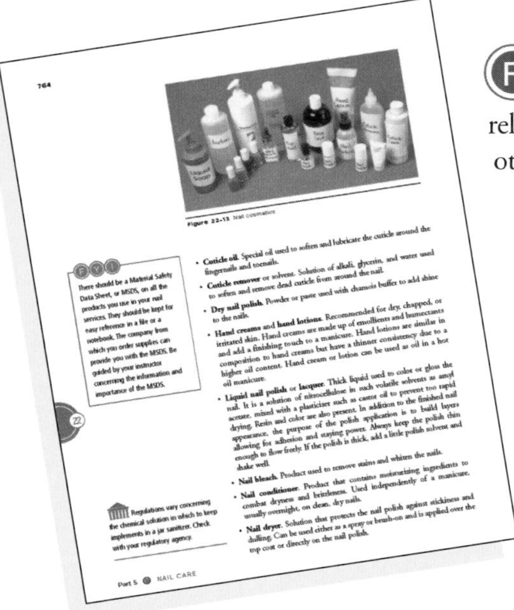

FYI These features offer important, interesting information related to the content. Often "FYI" boxes direct you to a Web site or other resource for further information.

Laws differ from region to region, so it is important to contact state boards and provincial regulatory agencies to learn what is allowed and not allowed where you are studying. In this text you will find the "Check with Your Regulatory Agency" feature next to procedures or practices that are regulated differently from state to state, alerting you to check the laws in your region. Your instructor will provide you with contact information.

Here's a tip: These helpful hints draw attention to situations that might arise or quick ways of doing things. Look for these tips in procedures and throughout the text.

Key Terms The words you will need to know in a chapter are given at the beginning, in a list of "Key Terms." The first time a word is used and defined in the text, the word appears in boldface. If the word is difficult to pronounce, a phonetic pronunciation appears after it in parentheses.

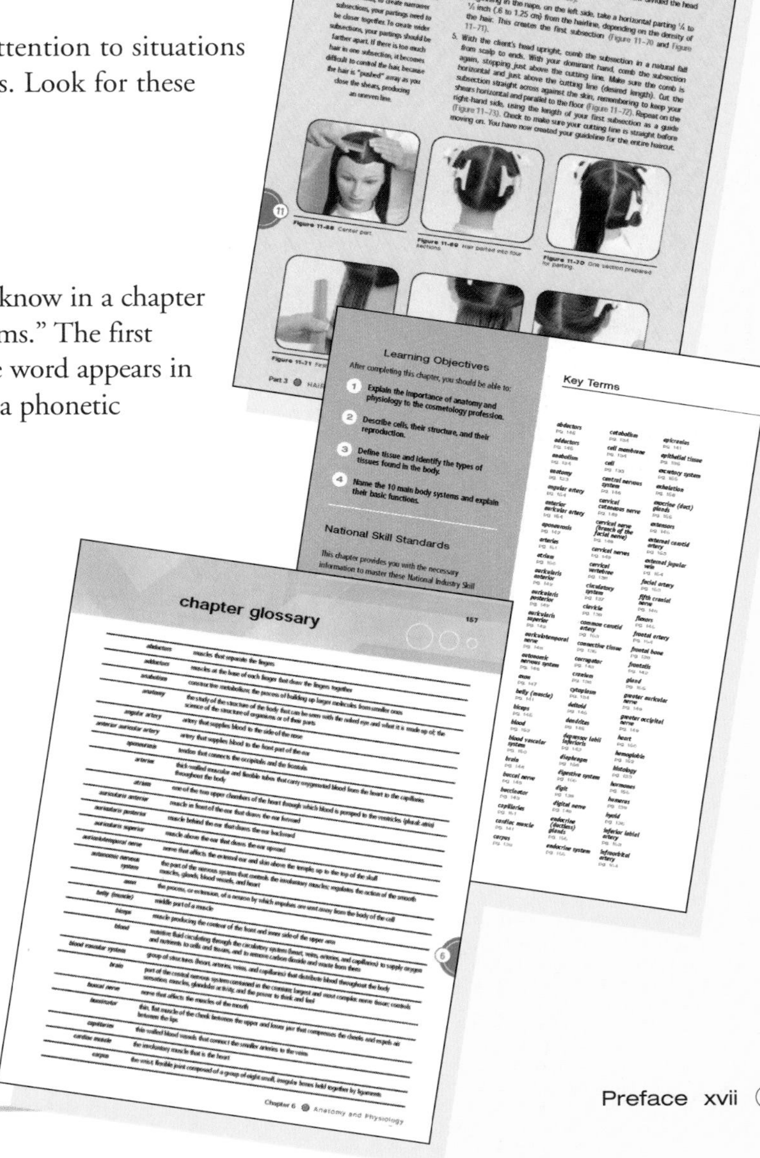

chapter glossary

All key terms and all their definitions are included in the "Chapter Glossary" at the end of the chapter, as well as in the Glossary/Index at the end of the text.

OTHER ELEMENTS

Many features from previous editions of *Milady's Standard* have been retained in this new edition.

Learning Objectives

At the beginning of each chapter is a list of learning objectives that will tell you what important information you will be expected to know from the chapter. Icons placed at the end of the section indicate that a learning objective has been completed at that point.

National Skill Standards

The "National Industry Skill Standards for Entry-Level Cosmetologists" were developed by the Cosmetology Advancement Foundation to help newly licensed cosmetologists know what will help them be successful. These standards include some skills that cannot be measured on licensure exams but are extremely important to your professional success. They are not intended to replace or refute the requirements for licensure. Rather, they are guidelines for success in the cosmetology field. The opening of each chapter lists the skills that are addressed in that chapter. (You may find the same skill listed at the start of several chapters.) Use them to identify your areas of strength and weakness so you will know what improvements you can make.

Some information is so critical for your safety and the safety of your clients that it deserves special attention. The text directs you to this information in the "Caution" boxes found in the margins.

review questions

Each chapter ends with questions designed to test your understanding of the information in it. Your instructor may ask you to write the answers to these questions as an assignment or to answer them orally in class. If you have trouble answering a question, go back to the chapter to review the material and try again. The answers to the "Review Questions" are in your instructor's *Course Management Guide*.

PROCEDURE

Sixty-four new step-by-step procedures offer clear, easy-to-understand directions and multiple photographs for learning the techniques. Step-by-step instructions occur in Parts 2, 3, 4, and 5 of the text. A list of the needed implements and materials appears at the start, along with any preparation that must be completed before the procedure, and the finished result appears at the end. Clear, precise instructions make following the procedure easy. Specific steps for cleanup and sanitation appear at the end of the procedure.

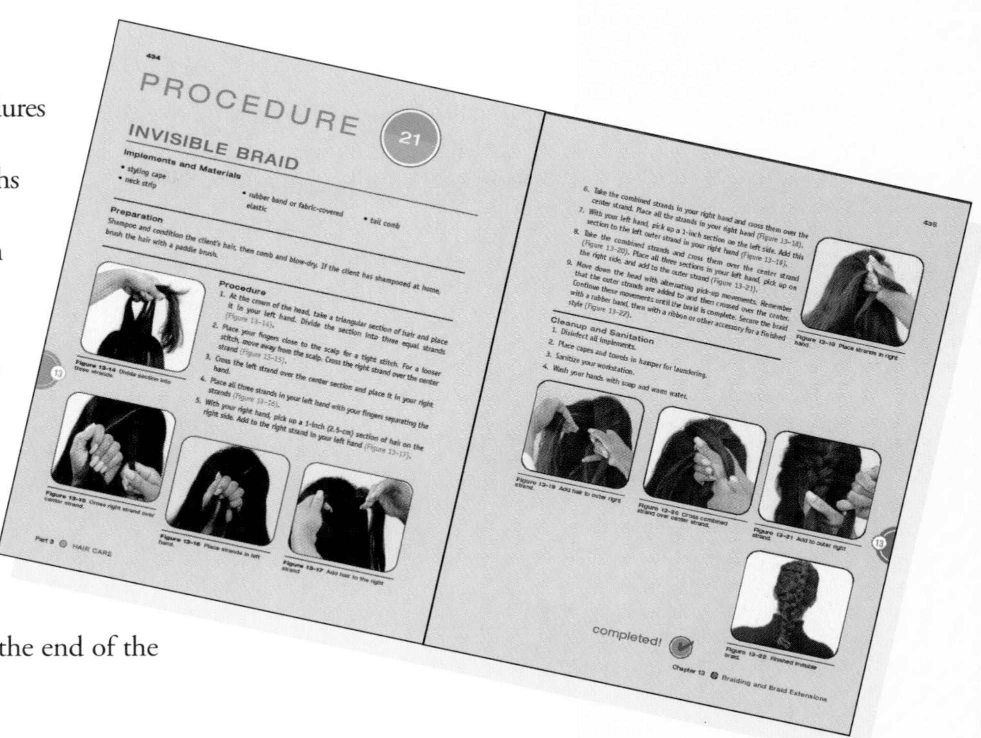

FRESH NEW DESIGN

The changes in this edition of *Milady's Standard Cosmetology* go far beyond the new content and features. New art and photographs—over fourteen hundred—enhance this book, along with a totally new text design that incorporates an easy-to-read type and easy-to-follow layout.

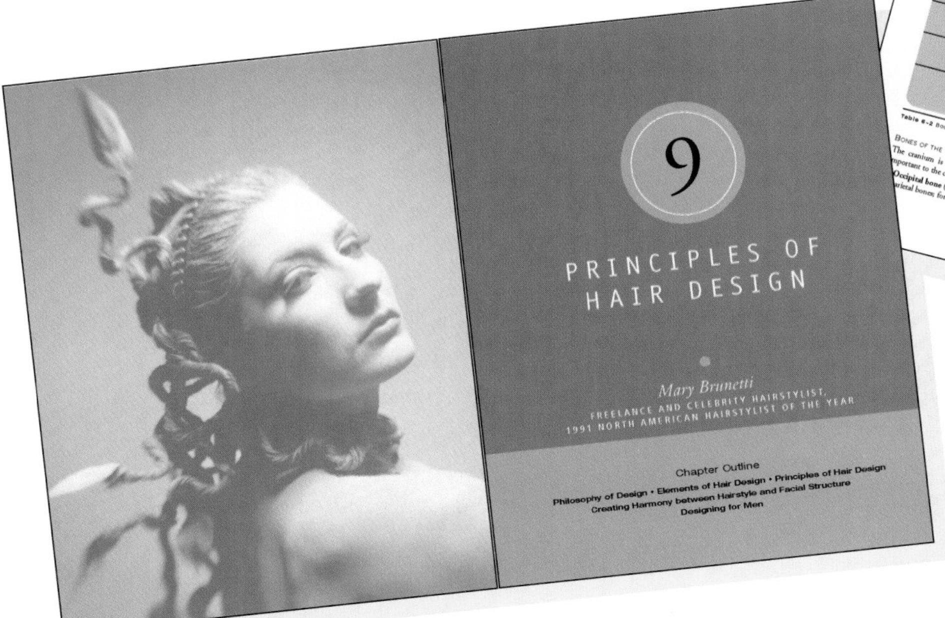

FRESH NEW ART

More than a thousand new photographs and three-hundred and fifty illustrations were created for this edition to complement the new text design. Photographs using mannequins and live models are included to illustrate styles and procedures. New structure graphics developed from 3-D animated figures are used to show lines, forms, reference points, and more, ensuring comprehension of theory.

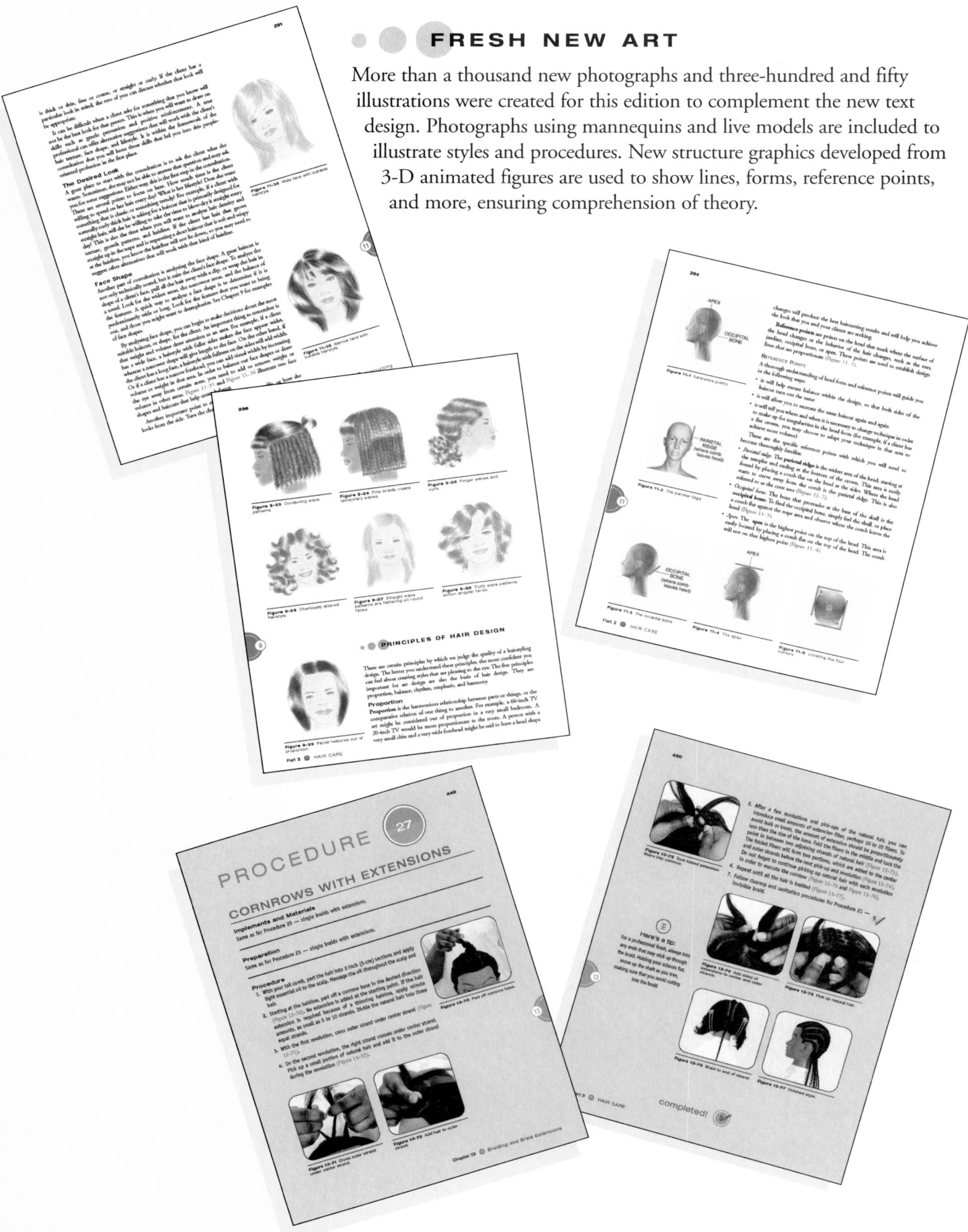

EXTENSIVE LEARNING/TEACHING PACKAGE

While *Milady's Standard Cosmetology* is the center of the curriculum, students and educators have a wide range of supplements from which to choose. All supplements have been revised and updated to complement the new edition of the textbook, and several new supplements are being offered for the first time with this edition.

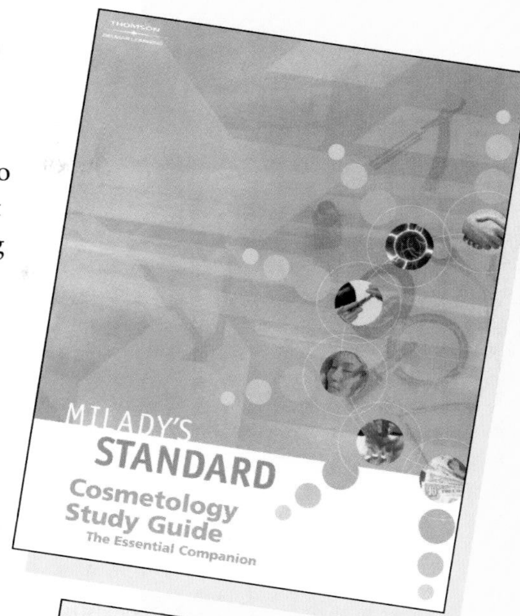

Student Supplements

In addition to the textbook, Milady has created many supplements to meet every student's needs. All supplements have been revised, and two new ones have been added, *Preparing for the Practical Exam* and *Milady's Standard Cosmetology Study Summaries.*

Milady's Standard Cosmetology Study Guide: The Essential Companion

Milady's Standard Cosmetology Study Guide: The Essential Companion is a colorful new study guide to help students recognize, understand, and retain the key concepts presented in each chapter of *Milady's Standard Cosmetology*. The student-led exercises require minimal educator assistance. *The Essential Companion* provides five easy-to-follow features for each chapter—Essential Objectives, Essential Subjects, Essential Concepts, Essential Review, and Essential Notes. Each one presents the key content in a different manner to help all students comprehend and remember it. The attractive color design will engage all types of students so they can learn the important theory and practical aspects necessary for licensure and professional success. Answers are supplied in *Milady's Standard Cosmetology Study Guide: The Essential Companion Answer Key.*

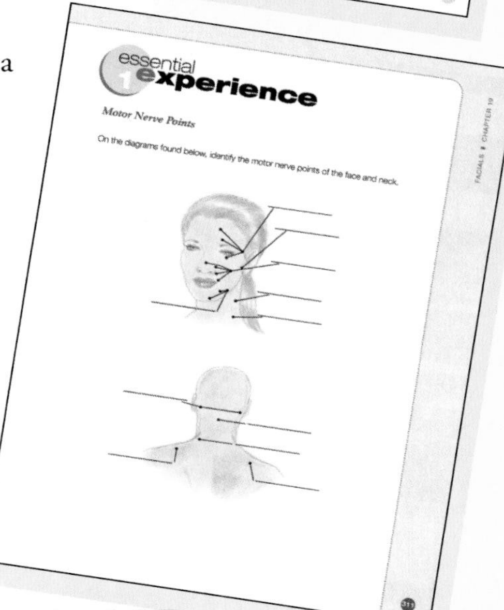

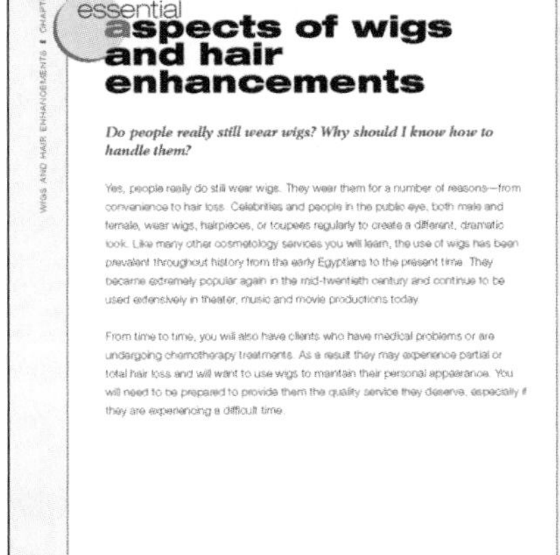

essential aspects of wigs and hair enhancements

Do people really still wear wigs? Why should I know how to handle them?

Yes, people really do still wear wigs. They wear them for a number of reasons—from convenience to hair loss. Celebrities and people in the public eye, both male and female, wear wigs, hairpieces, or toupees regularly to create a different, dramatic look. Like many other cosmetology services you will learn, the use of wigs has been prevalent throughout history from the early Egyptians to the present time. They became extremely popular again in the mid-twentieth century and continue to be used extensively in theater, music and movie productions today.

From time to time, you will also have clients who have medical problems or are undergoing chemotherapy treatments. As a result they may experience partial or total hair loss and will want to use wigs to maintain their personal appearance. You will need to be prepared to provide them the quality service they deserve, especially if they are experiencing a difficult time.

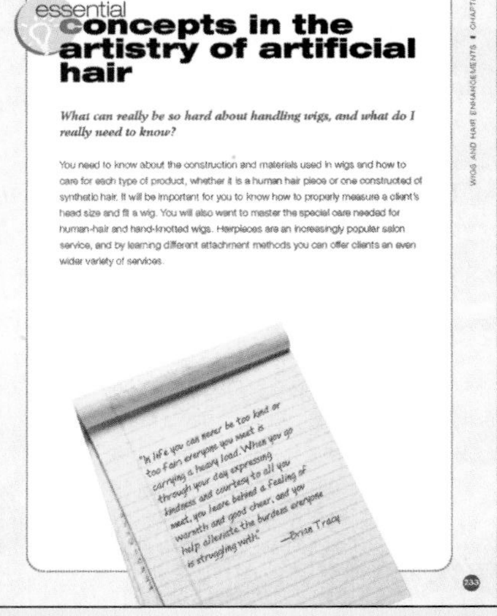

essential concepts in the artistry of artificial hair

What can really be so hard about handling wigs, and what do I really need to know?

You need to know about the construction and materials used in wigs and how to care for each type of product, whether it is a human hair piece or one constructed of synthetic hair. It will be important for you to know how to properly measure a client's head size and fit a wig. You will also want to master the special care needed for human-hair and hand-knotted wigs. Hairpieces are an increasingly popular salon service, and by learning different attachment methods you can offer clients an even wider variety of services.

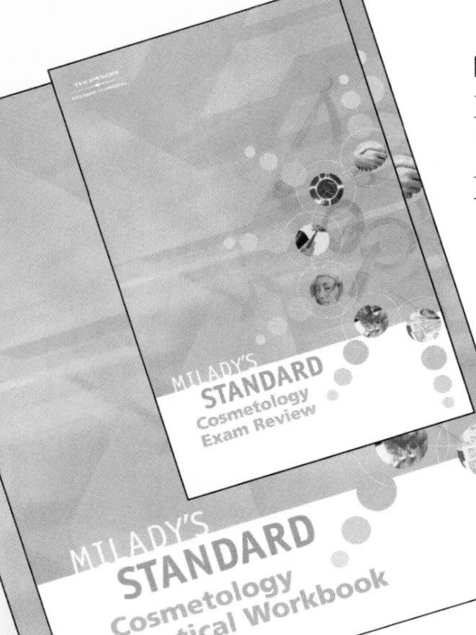

Milady's Standard Cosmetology Theory Workbook

Designed to reinforce classroom and textbook learning, the *Theory Workbook* contains chapter-by-chapter exercises on theory subjects. Included are fill-in-the-blank, multiple-choice, matching, and labeling exercises, all coordinated with material from the text. Final review examinations at the end of the workbook prepare students for testing.

Milady's Standard Cosmetology Practical Workbook

The *Practical Workbook* helps students master the techniques, procedures, and product usage needed for licensure as covered in the textbook. Using fill-in-the-blank, matching, multiple-choice, and labeling exercises, students will benefit from the reinforcement of practical applications.

Milady's Standard Cosmetology Exam Review

The *Exam Review* contains chapter-by-chapter questions in a multiple-choice format to help students prepare for the licensure exam. While not intended to be the only form of review offered to students, it aids in overall classroom preparation. The *Exam Review* has been revised to meet the most stringent test-development guidelines. The questions in the *Exam Review* are for study purposes only and are not the exact questions students will see on the licensure exams.

Preparing for the Practical Exam: Cosmetology

NEW

A new supplement, *Preparing for the Practical Exam: Cosmetology* provides step-by-step information for students who are required to take practical exams. Because procedures vary from region to region, options for certain procedures are given, making this a book that students from every state can use.

Milady's Standard Cosmetology Study Summaries: Vietnamese, Korean, and Chinese

NEW

Students whose native language is Vietnamese, Korean, or Chinese now have study guides that help them with coursework and licensure exams. Each *Standard Cosmetology Study Summary* contains the main topic heads from the text along with procedures and the complete *Exam Review*, all in Vietnamese, Korean, or Chinese. Each *Standard Cosmetology Study Summary* should be used along with the text for maximum effectiveness.

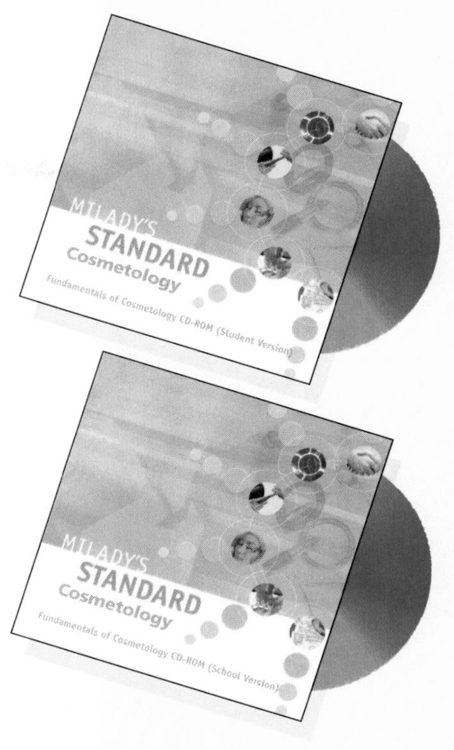

Milady's Fundamentals of Cosmetology CD-ROM

Milady's Fundamentals of Cosmetology CD-ROM is an interactive student product designed to reinforce classroom learning, stimulate the imagination, and aid in preparation for board exams. Featuring more than 100 helpful video clips and graphical animations to demonstrate practices and procedures, this exciting educational tool also contains a test bank with 1,300 chapter-by-chapter or randomly accessed multiple-choice and matching questions to help students study for the exam. Another feature is the game bank, which offers games to strengthen knowledge of terminology, and a glossary that pronounces and defines each term.

The content follows and enhances *Milady's Standard Cosmetology*. The technology of the program is interactive, allowing the learner to be surrounded or "pulled into" the content, and it tracks the student's progress through the program. The CD-ROM is also available as a networkable product for schools.

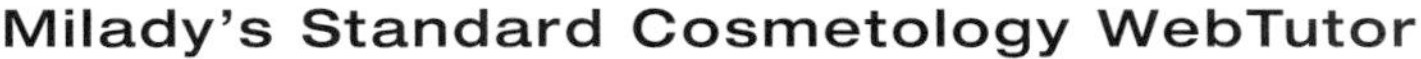

Milady's Standard Cosmetology WebTutor

The *WebTutor* is a content-rich, Web-based learning aid that reinforces and clarifies complex concepts in the textbook. *WebTutor* presents information in a new and different way, making it easier to understand material as well as allowing easier management of time, progress checks, exam preparation, and organization of notes. Available on either the WebCT or Blackboard platform, *WebTutor* is fully customizable and includes a course calendar, chat, e-mail, threaded discussions, and many more features custom-designed to your individual course.

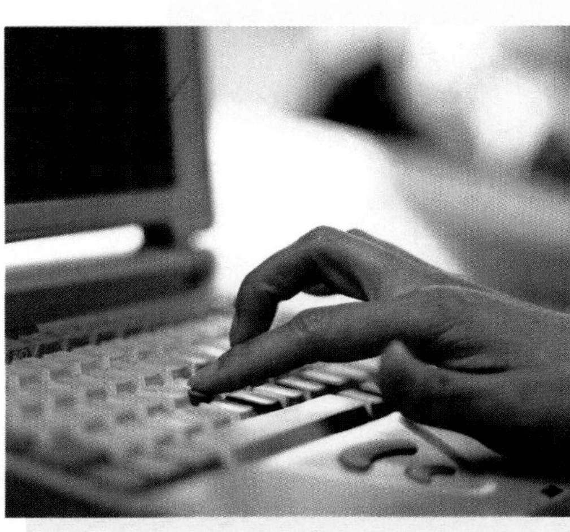

Features:

- Chapter Learning Objectives
- National Skill Standards
- Online Course Preparation
- Study Sheets
- Online Chapter Quizzes
  - Fill-in-the-Blank
  - Multiple Choice
  - True/False
  - Matching
- Flashcards
- Discussion Topics
- Web Links
- FAQs
- Glossary

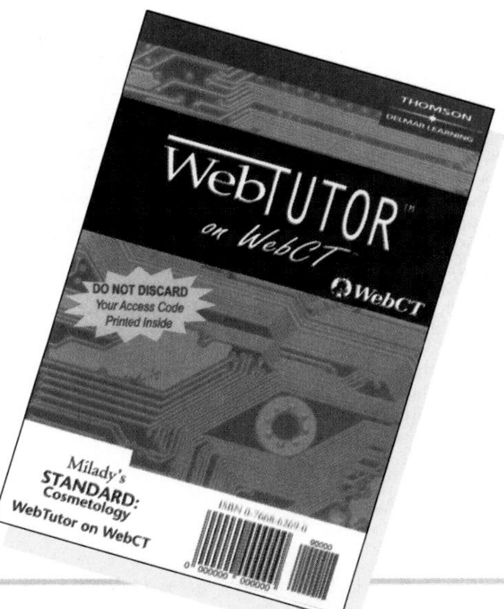

Milady's Online Licensing Preparation: Cosmetology

Milady's Online Licensing Preparation: Cosmetology provides students with a technology study alternative to better prepare them for licensure exams, whether taken on a computer or on paper. Over 1,300 multiple-choice questions for cosmetology appear with rationales for correct and incorrect choices, and the correct answer links to the portion of *Milady's Standard Cosmetology* in which the information is given. Students have the flexibility to study from any computer, whether at home or at school. Because exam review preparation is available to students at any time of day or night, class time can be used for other activities. Students gain familiarity with a computerized test environment as they prepare for licensure.

Educator Supplements

Milady offers a full range of products created especially for cosmetology educators to make classroom preparation and presentation simple, effective, and enjoyable.

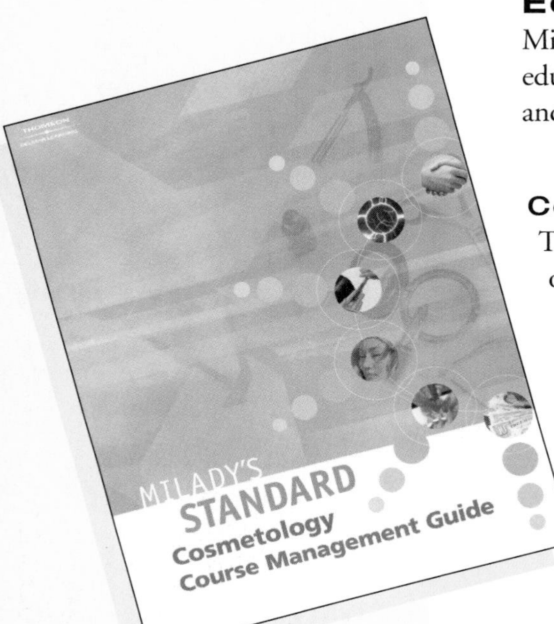

Course Management Guide

The *Course Management Guide* contains all the materials educators need in one package. This innovative instructional guide is written with cosmetology educators in mind and is designed to make exceptional teaching easy. With formatting that provides easy-to-use material for use in the classroom, it will transform classroom management and dramatically increase student interest and understanding. Included in the three-ring binder are: Lesson Plans, Chapter Tests, Transparencies, the complete text of the National Skill Standards, and Resources. The binder is accompanied by the answer key to the *Theory* and *Practical* workbooks.

Added features you will find on the Course Management Guide CD-ROM version:

- Every page from the *Course Management Guide* can be printed to appear exactly like the page from the print product.
- A Computerized Testbank contains new multiple-choice questions that instructors can use to create random tests from a single chapter or the whole book. In this new edition, Computerized Testbank questions are not the same questions in the *Exam Review*. Answer keys are automatically created. A gradebook feature to track students' progress is also included.
- An Image Library of 500 photos and illustrations from *Milady's Standard Cosmetology* can be added to PowerPoint presentations or printed onto paper or acetate for overheads. They can even be imported into other documents.

DVD Series

For the first time Milady has produced a DVD series, complete with five hours of almost all-new video content. This three-DVD set offers interactive content with features for classroom use that provide instructors with easy-search features, easy-to-use student assessment exercises, and optional Spanish subtitles. More than just video on DVD, this series creates the option of viewing a procedure from several camera angles.

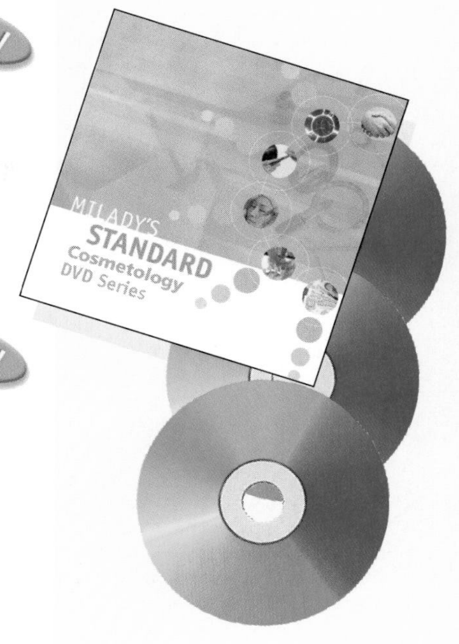

PowerPoint Presentations

The new PowerPoint Presentations to accompany the *Standard Cosmetology* make lesson plans simple yet incredibly effective. Complete with photos and art, this chapter-by-chapter CD-ROM has ready-to-use presentations that will help engage students' attention and keep their interest through its varied color schemes and styles. Instructors can use it as is or adapt it to their own classrooms by importing photos they have taken, changing the graphics, or adding slides.

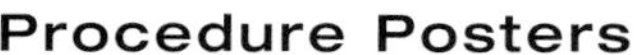

Procedure Posters

The clear and appealing photographs in *Milady's Standard Cosmetology* can now be seen in a new poster series. The posters feature key procedures, including haircuts, haircoloring, permanent waves, manicures, and skin care techniques to use for repeated reference on the clinic floor. Large in size, each poster contains photos and text in a step-by-step format. The design coordinates with the textbook.

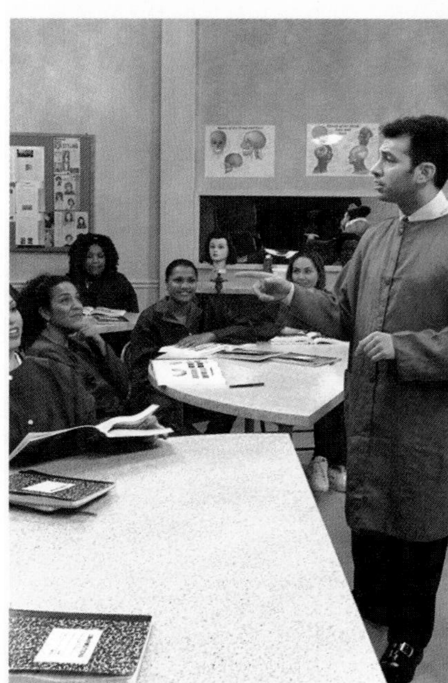

Wall Charts

Milady's Wall Charts have been revised in a new size and format. Now 26.5" by 36", the *Wall Charts* include a transparent overlay with labels, directional lines, and other information. Each wall chart has two metal grommets for hanging. *Wall Charts* are available for the following topics:

Revised Charts:

- Anatomy of the Hand and Arm
- Bones of the Head and Face
- Circulation of the Blood
- Histology of the Hair, Follicles
- Histology of the Skin, Hair, Glands
- Motor Points of the Face
- Muscles of the Head, Face, and Neck
- Nerves of the Head, Face, and Neck
- Foot and Ankle Massage

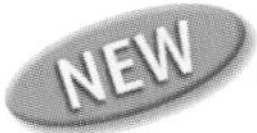

Charts

- Foot Reflexology
- Lymphatic System
- Anatomy of the Nail
- Facial Movements and Manipulations
- Face Shapes
- Facial Areas for Product Application
- Anatomy of the Foot and Ankles
- Hand and Arm Massage

CONTRIBUTING AUTHORS

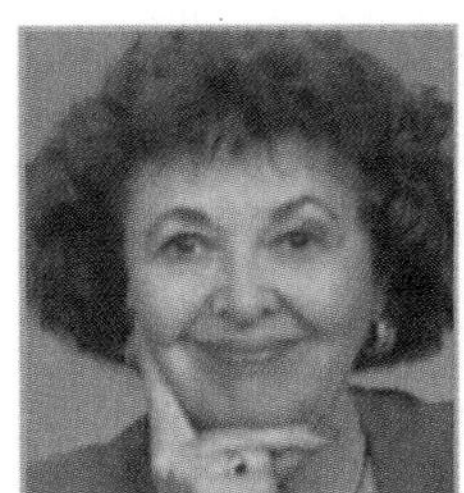

Arlene Alpert

Arlene Alpert, MS, LMHC, is President/CEO of Jupiter Consulting & Training Institute. She has been a licensed psychotherapist for 25 years, business relationships consultant, coach, educator, professional speaker, and past president of the Florida Speakers Association. Ms. Alpert has advanced degrees in psychology and counseling and is considered an authority on "The Business of Relationships." Her latest book is *Traveling Beyond Life's Roadblocks: Creating a Life of Choice.* Ms. Alpert is also a continuing education provider. She has given workshops in the United States, Canada, and Europe. Her coaching and consulting practice is focused on advancing personal and professional development, increasing self-esteem and confidence, and clearing up any "trouble spots" that may prevent individuals from having remarkable relationships and being effective communicators and decision-makers.

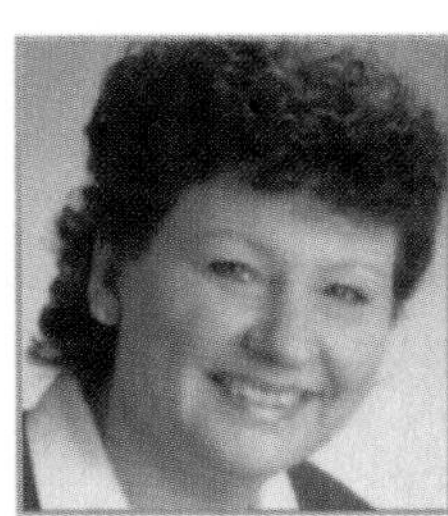

Margrit Altenburg

Educated and licensed in Switzerland, Margrit Altenburg has been working in the beauty industry since 1976. She owned her own skin care clinic for 17 years and obtained her Master's in Skin and Body Care in 1990. Altenburg received her CIDESCO international board certification in 1991, and served as General Secretary from 1992 to 1998. She spent the early 1990s working in a Swiss dermatologist's clinic and moved to Houston in 1999 to accept the esthetics department head teacher position at the first CIDESCO-accredited school in the US – the Institute of Cosmetology & Esthetics – where she became the director a year later. Altenburg is active organizing educational workshops in Switzerland and Germany, has taught several classes for the National Cosmetology Association in the U.S., and is a CIDESCO international examiner worldwide.

Diane Carol Bailey

At 21, Diane Carol Bailey graduated from Hunter College and entered beauty school, but her calling first began at age nine, when she started experimenting with her own hair. She began braiding at home and was frustrated by the bias and lack of education for the care and treatment of natural hair. Bailey became involved in the natural hair care movement in 1987, and helped found the International Braiders Network (IBN) in 1992, whose members drafted and adopted the first natural hair care license in July 1994. Today, as President of IBN, she works to promote and establish professional standards, procedures, and training for natural hair care stylists and braiders.

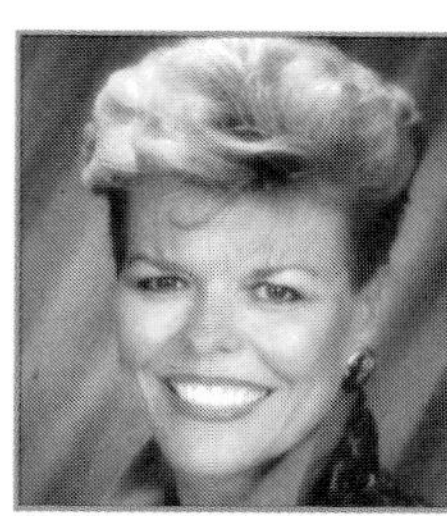

Letha Barnes

Commitment toward cosmetology education is what Letha Barnes is all about. In her 34 years of industry experience, she served as President of AACS, where she helped revive and expand the mission of their educational committee, Cosmetology Educators of America (CEA). She also gained recognition for her service as Chairman of the Accreditation committee and has been teaching accreditation workshops for years. She founded and is the past president of Olympus, Inc., which operates four cosmetology schools in New Mexico, and became the Director of Milady's Career Institute in January 2000. In her spare time, she authored *Milady's Standard Cosmetology Course Management Guide*, *Milady's Master Educator*, and the *Milady's Standard Cosmetology Study Guide - The Essential Companion*, all receiving positive feedback from educators in the industry.

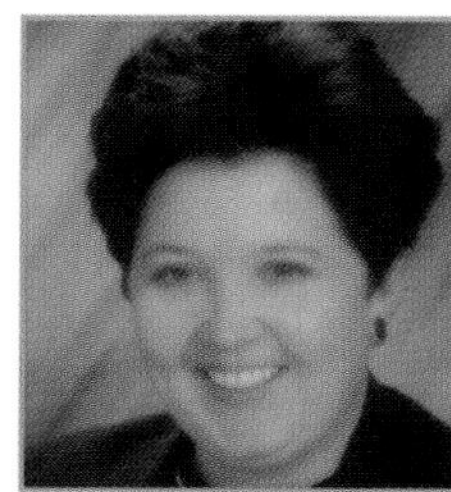

Lisha Barnes

A licensed cosmetologist, instructor, and barber, Lisha Barnes is committed to improving the quality of cosmetology education. She received a B.S. in Communications from Eastern New Mexico University in 1990, and completed her cosmetology training at Olympian University of Cosmetology, where she has served as Field Administrator for four campuses and oversees educational practices. Barnes is a member of Cosmetology Educators of America and has worked on numerous projects for Milady and The Career Institute, where her experience in education, communications, and administration add insight to her presentations.

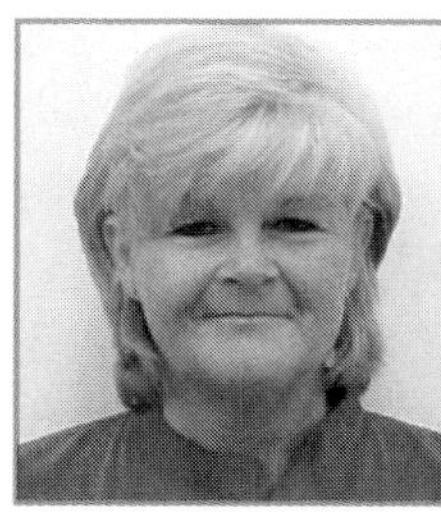

Deborah Beatty

"Education must have value but must also be interesting, fun, motivational, and realistic," says Deborah Beatty. She derived this philosophy from 32 years in the cosmetology industry, of which 14 were spent in the educational sector. She is a licensed cosmetology instructor, master cosmetologist, and master barber. She's also a licensed nurse and holds her teaching certificate from the Professional Standards Commission. Beatty is a regular contributor and reviewer of Milady products and has enlightened countless cosmetologists, instructors, and students in the classroom and through her motivational seminars.

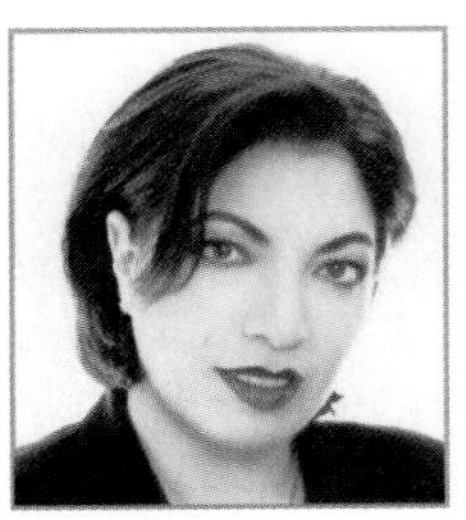

Mary Brunetti

Twenty focused years of shutter speeds have made Mary Brunetti an expert behind the lens. This accomplished session stylist divides her time between photography studios and location shoots for top fashion magazines, including *Elle*, *Vogue*, *Bridal Guide*, and *Town & Country*. A two-time recipient of the Editor's Choice Award, she was also the first woman awarded the prestigious title of North American Hairstylist of the Year in 1991. Brunetti has since served as judge and consultant for the North American Hairstylist Awards (NAHA) and authored a book, *The Inside Track to NAHA*, where she shares her expertise. She was part of the Trevor Sorbie National Artistic Team and she educates regularly for the International Beauty Shows.

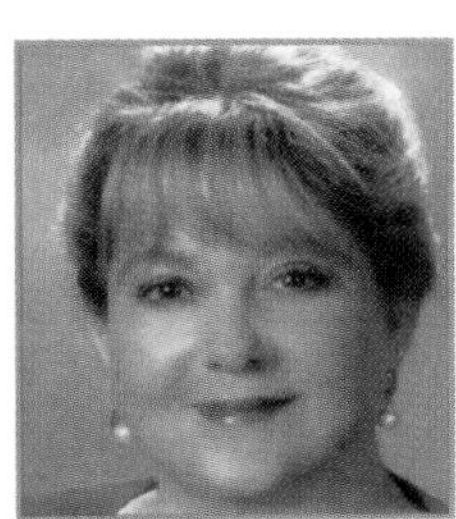

Jane Crawford

As CEO of Jane Crawford Associates, this entrepreneur earned the title of "America's Foremost Medi-Spa Consultant" by growing her own business from the ground up. Basing her expertise on her own medical spa in South Carolina – which she established, built, and later sold – Crawford successfully addressed the challenges in skin care clinic/spa site selection, building and design, selection of services, quality assurance, state inspections, staff selection, and management of revenue and expenses. Having received her medical esthetician's training from the University of South Carolina, she regularly presents post-graduate and advanced courses in esthetics and the medical industry. Crawford lectures internationally on medi-spa practices and sits on the board of the American Aestheticians Education Association.

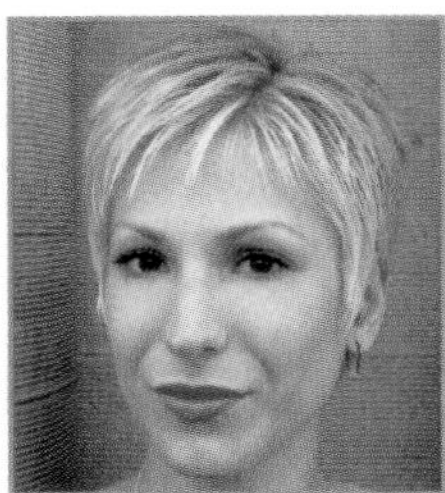

Aly Evirs

Upon receiving her esthetics instructor's license from the Institute of Beauty and Wellness in Milwaukee, Wisconsin, Aly Evirs worked as a full-time esthetician and makeup artist for the Skin Institute and Day Spa. Three years later, she returned to her alma mater where she has been Esthetics Instructor, Education Department Team Leader, Wisconsin Spa and Salon Network Coordinator, and Post Graduate Education Coordinator. Evirs balances teaching the esthetics portion of the program with her freelance work and attending advanced education seminars around the country.

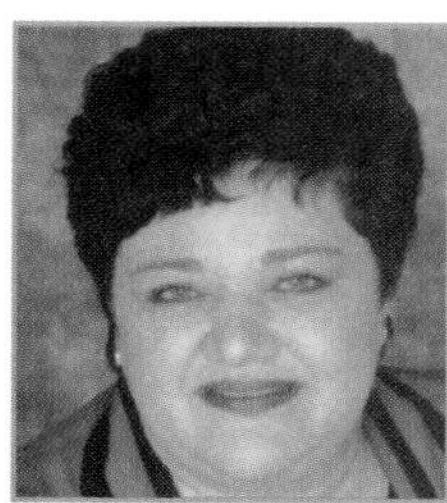

Catherine Frangie

For 20 years, Catherine Frangie has demonstrated her dedication and passion towards the beauty industry as a licensed cosmetologist, salon owner, and beauty school instructor. As VP of Marketing and Communication for Joico Laboratories, she spearheaded re-imaging campaigns and numerous product launches, including the Kpak Collection, Joico's most successful line extension. Frangie spent 10 years as VP of Milady, where she served as textbook editor and international spokesperson, and launched *SalonOvations Magazine*, the official publication of the National Cosmetology Association from 1997 to1998. She has lectured at the International Beauty Show in NYC and was named Beauty Industry Role Model by the Cosmetology Advancement Foundation in 1990.

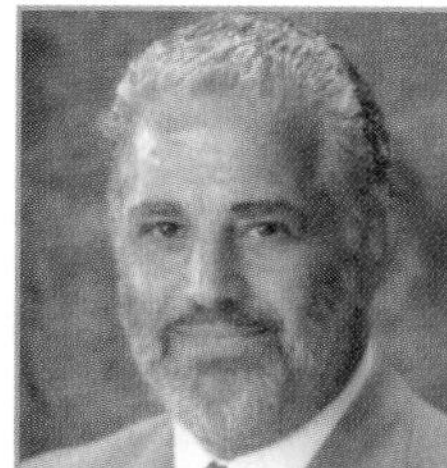

John Halal

Thirty years in hairstyling have taught John Halal a trick or two about the salon industry. He owns and operates International Concepts Beauty Supply and Honors Beauty College, Inc., along with John & Friends, Inc., his two award-winning salons in suburban Indianapolis. He is an active member of the National Cosmetology Association (NCA), the Salon Association (TSA), the Indiana Cosmetology Educators Association (ICEA), the American Association of Cosmetology Schools (AACS), the Beauty & Barber Supply Institute (BBSI), and the Society of Cosmetic Chemists (SCC). Halal has published numerous articles, received an Outstanding Call for Presentation Papers award by the BBSI, and received an award for Outstanding Educational Program from the Indiana State Cosmetologists Association.

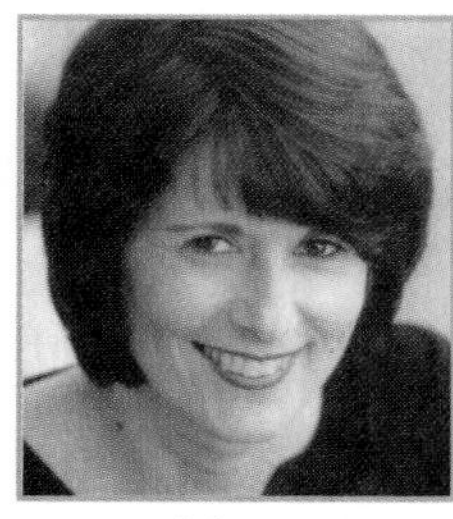

Colleen Hennessey

Educator and creative artist. This rare combination of skills describes Colleen Hennessey, the Master Colorist and Education Coordinator at the renowned Adam Broderick Image Group. As a former Exclusive Color Designer and Senior Manager of Clairol Professional's Education division, she has gained national recognition as a master haircolorist, platform artist, and educator. Hennessey shares her artistry and passion for easy color techniques throughout the U.S. as an active salon educator and established platform artist performing at the industry's mega-trade shows: Haircolor USA, Long Beach, IBS, and Midwest.

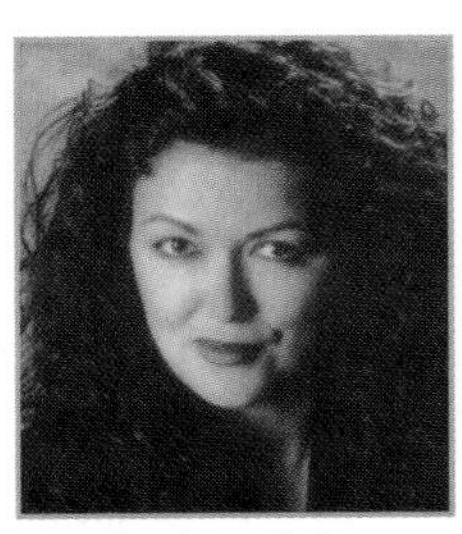

Mary Beth Janssen

Mary Beth Janssen is an internationally acclaimed educator and designer with over 25 years as a licensed cosmetologist and teacher. She's produced and directed numerous projects for the beauty industry and her expertise has graced magazine editorials, television shows, and commercials. She's a regular beauty industry speaker and has authored several books on beauty and wellness. Janssen currently oversees and directs all activities of The Janssen Source, Inc., a Chicago-based company integrating Janssen's message of beauty and wellness. Because Janssen believes "real beauty begins with health – and true wellness is directly related to how we nurture our mind, body, and spirit," she inspires cosmetologists and clients alike to tap into their higher consciousness through educational seminars, on-site visits, and one-on-one consultations. Janssen was the 1996 recipient of the Rocco Bellino Award for outstanding contributions in education, and is also a certified herbalist, aromatherapist, massage therapist, and yoga teacher.

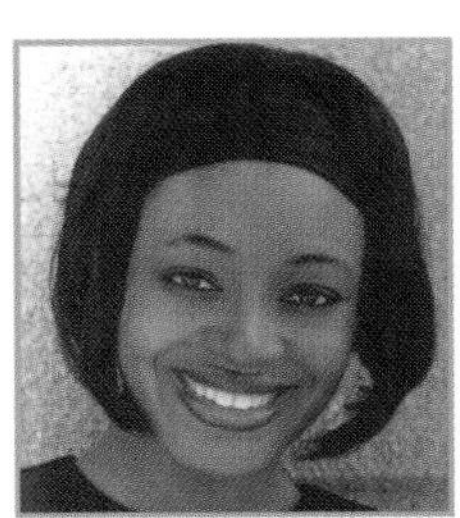

Toni Love

As the daughter of a beautician and niece to a barber, Toni Love was a natural for the field of cosmetology. She began working in her mother's salon at age 14, and after completing basic training for the U.S. Army Reserves, she attended a private cosmetology school. Love obtained a Bachelor's degree in Business Administration and a Master's in Continuing Education and began teaching cosmetology at Greensboro Public School in Alabama. After three years, she moved on to the collegiate level, teaching cosmetology at Shelton State Community College in Tuscaloosa. Today, she teaches at hair shows and seminars around the world and has self-published her first book, *Tips to Pass the Cosmetology State Board Exam*.

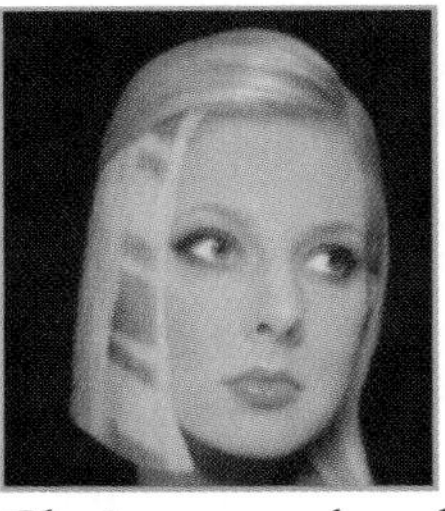

Vivienne Mackinder

This London native has placed her worldwide stamp on the beauty, fashion, and hairstyling industries. Vivienne Mackinder developed her expertise for precision cutting and eye for classic to avant-garde design through her work as Artistic Director for Vidal Sassoon and Trevor Sorbie. The recipient of four NAHA and three Editor's Choice awards, she continues to impact the industry through her internationally published books, her new video collection, her Web-based educational forum, and her work with fashion designers on the runways of Paris, London, and New York.

Carey Nash

Carey Nash received her cosmetology license in 1958, and a year later received her instructor's license at the age of 20. She worked full- and part-time in a salon for 6 years and was an instructor at the Bartmore Beauty Colleges until 1970. At that time, she joined the Marinello Schools of Beauty and has held various titles, including: Instructor, Assistant Supervisor, Supervisor, Registrar, Manager, Accreditation Specialist, Director of Education, and her current title, Director of Compliance. She has also served as an expert witness and test analyst, where she helped validate the written examination for the California State Board of Cosmetology.

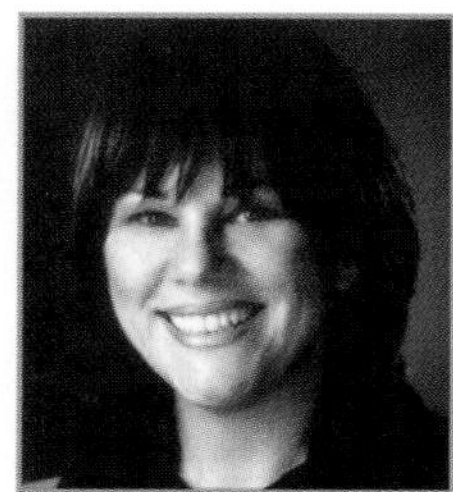

Ruth Roche

When it comes to hairdressing, Ruth Roche has done it all. With 15 years as a salon, platform, and session stylist, she has developed successful hair styling products; traveled extensively demonstrating advanced techniques worldwide; performed live makeover and beauty segments on national television; and had her work featured in leading trade and consumer magazines, including *Modern Salon*, *Salon News*, *Cosmopolitan*, *Harper's Bazaar*, and *New Woman*, to name a few. She was the Global Artistic Director of Design for Redken and National Artistic Director for Trevor Sorbie. In addition to being voted Top Rising Star in 1995, she was named one of the Top 75 Educators of the Century and has received numerous Editor's Choice and NAHA awards.

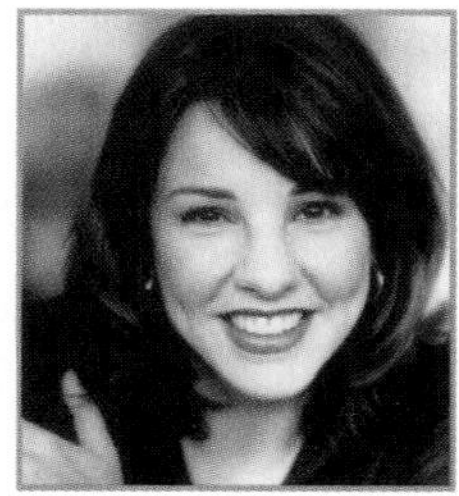

Teresa Sammarco

The last decade has provided makeup artist Teresa Sammarco with a strong foundation in the industry. As a dual makeup artist and hairstylist, she has created looks for top fashion designers, photographers, print advertisements, television commercials, and theater productions. She's even known to frequently appear in front of the camera herself. Sammarco is a regular on the lecture circuit, providing both tips and techniques, and she freelances nationwide, performing makeup and hairstyling looks and consultations.

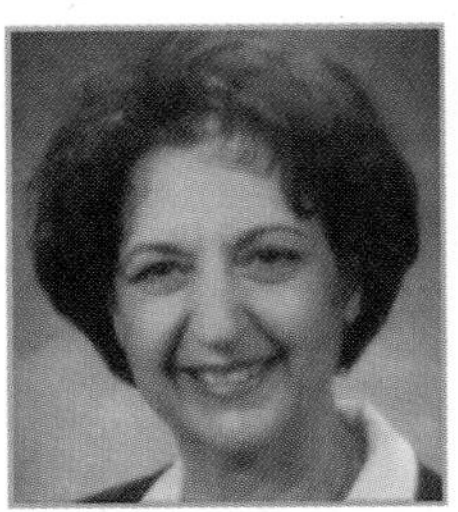

Sue Sansom

When Sue Sansom received a high school scholarship to attend beauty school in 1963, she saw it as a way to help pay for law school. After a year in a salon, however, she discovered a love for cosmetology that led her to become Arizona's youngest licensed cosmetology instructor at age 19. Rather than pursue a law degree, Sue instead applied her passion for administrative law to the cosmetology field, and became the first Executive Director of the Arizona State Board of Cosmetology in 1984. A member of the Arizona Regulatory Licensing Board of Directors, she has spent 17 years involved with the National Interstate Council of Cosmetology Boards (NIC), actively promoting both education and regulation with respect to health and safety in the cosmetology industry.

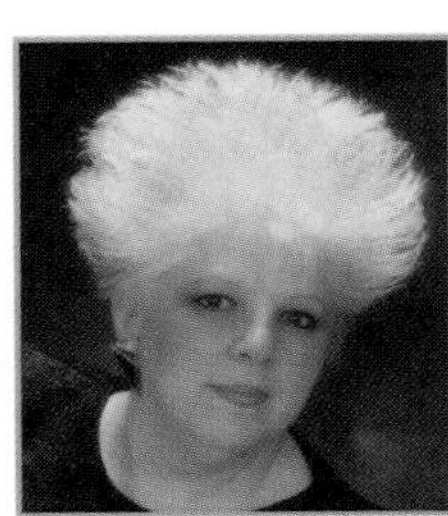

Sue Ellen Schultes

Sue Schultes is an award-winning nail artist and salon owner whose salon has been recognized as one of the top 100 nail salons in the country by *Nails* magazine ten years running. Sue is recognized as one of the leading authorities in nail art technology in the U.S. and teaches extensively throughout the United States, conducting workshops and seminars. Sue currently serves as Competition Judge for various trade shows, both nationally and internationally. She was invited this year to serve as judge for the nail competition at the Brighton Beauty Show in Brighton, England. Besides acting as series editor and contributing author for *Milady's Standard Nail Technology*, Sue also contributes special interest articles to *Nails* magazine, *NailPro*, the *Beauty News*, *Nail Shows* magazine, and several newspapers. Sue was commissioned by the Smithsonian Institute's National Museum of American History to create a full set of nails commemorating the United States Presidents' Inaugurations.

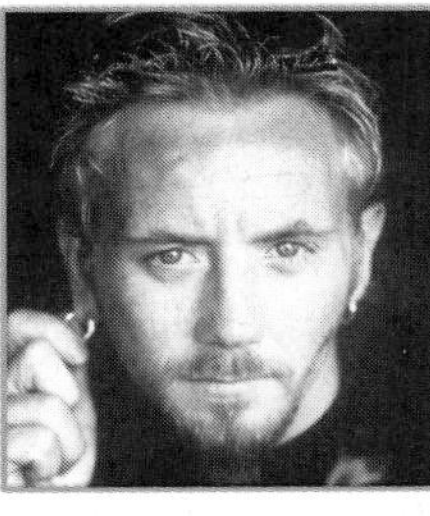

Robert Cromeans

Robert Cromeans is the artistic director for John Paul Mitchell Systems and the owner of four successful salons. As a hairdresser, he is known for his daring and innovative designs. He has made guest appearances on national and international television an radio shows and has appeared in numerous publications such as *Vogue, Bazaar,* and *Glamour,* and beauty industry magazines. Cromeans was named Platform Artist of the Year for *behindthechair.com's* Stylists Choice Awards. Known for his wit, wisdom, and great sense of personal sytle, Robert Cromeans is widely respected and in demand globally as an educator, motivator, and hairdresser.

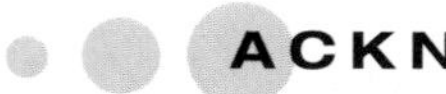

ACKNOWLEDGMENTS

Many cosmetologists and educators have contributed to the development of this book over the years since its initial publication in 1938. *Milady's Standard Textbook of Cosmetology* owes its creation to the lifetime dedication of Nicholas F. Cimaglia, founder of Milady Publishing Company. Mr. Cimaglia was also one of the founders of the National Association of Accredited Cosmetology Schools and the Teachers' Education Council, and helped form the National Accrediting Commission for Cosmetology Art and Sciences.

The standard set by Mr. Cimaglia has been carried on in the beauty education industry by his son, Thomas Severance, and by two gentlemen whose tireless efforts have established the success of *Milady's Standard:* Jacob Yahm, the father of accreditation in our industry and a driving force behind the National Interstate Council of State Boards of Cosmetology; and Arnold DeMille, founding editor of the *National Beauty School Journal* and continuing education specialist.

Milady recognizes with gratitude and respect the many professionals who have offered their time to contribute to this edition of the *Standard.* Milady wishes to extend enormous thanks to the following people who have played a part in this edition.

Elizabeth Tinsley
Developmental Editor
Chatham, NY

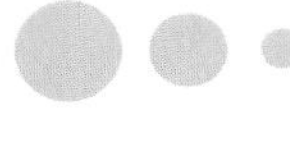

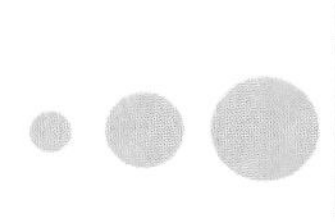

Dorothy McKinley-Soressi
Content Editor
New York International Beauty School
New York, NY

Alan Gelb
Developmental Writer
Levine-Gelb Communications
East Chatham, NY

Special Thanks:

Dawn Ahern, Executive Assistant to Robert Cromeans, San Diego, CA
Dr. Robert Bangert-Drowns, State University of New York, Albany, NY
Ada De Jesus Boddie, New York International Beauty School, New York, NY
A'Lelia Bundles, author, *On Her Own Ground* (Scribner, 2001)
Celebrity Signatures International, Inc., Kansas City, MO, for supplying hair additions from the Raquel Welch Signature Collection and the Put On Pieces Collection
Gerri Cevetillo, Ultronics, Mahwah, NJ
Elizabeth Graham, Makeup Artist, Schenectady, NY
Joyce Hainley, Celebrity Signatures International, Kansas City, MO
Elizabeth Hitchcock-Agostino, Clairol, Inc., Stamford, CT
Elma Jordan, New York International Beauty School, New York, NY
Michael Kleinman, Eva Gabor International, Elkins Park, PA
Mary E. Nicholson, owner of Personal Enhancement Center and Day Spa, Clifton Park, NY
Valerie Parker, owner of C'est la Vie, Clifton Park, NY
Steve Royster, New York International Beauty School, New York, NY
Janine Smalls, New York International Beauty School, New York, NY
David Stanko, Redken Fifth Avenue, New York, NY
Pallavi Wagle, L'Oreal Professionnel USA, New York, NY

Standard Revision Focus Groups:

Letha Barnes, Director, The Career Institute, Santa Teresa, NM
Lisha Barnes, Olympian University of Cosmetology, Alamogordo, NM
Cindy Lee Davidson, Northwest College of Hair Design, Hillsboro, OR
Sue Derosier, Rob Roy Academy, Worcester, MA
Deborah Fitzpatrick, Artistic Group, Phoenix, AZ
Wadad Frangie, Capital District Educational Opportunity Center, Troy, NY
Dennis James, Von Curtis Academy of Hair Design, Provo, UT
Wendy James, Supercuts, New York, NY
Toni Love, Dudley Products, Kernersville, NC
Sharon MacGregor, Middletown Beauty School, Middletown, NY
Dorothy McKinley-Soressi, New York International Beauty School, New York, NY
Jimmy Montan, Aveda Institute, Minneapolis, MN
Peggy Moon, Practical Exam Developer, Lavonia, GA
Regina Pelayo, Skyline Community College, San Bruno, CA
Ollie Pendley, Cosmetology Educator/Consultant, Lithia Springs, GA
Cindy Wadsworth, Aveda Institute, Minneapolis, MN

Reviewers:

Rae Ann Amacher, Orleans-Niagara BOCES, Sanborn, NY
Pearl Bailey-Anderson, La Pearl Beauty Emporium, Philadelphia, PA
Frances Archer, The Nail Clinic School of Manicuring, Columbia, SC
Letha Barnes, The Career Institute, Santa Teresa, NM
Lisha Barnes, Olympian University, Alamogordo, NM
Barbara Bealer, Allentown School of Cosmetology, Allentown, PA
Deborah Beatty, Columbus Technical College, Fortson, GA
Laurie Biagi, Skyline Community College, San Bruno, CA
Linzi Biesinger, Altoona Beauty School, Inc., Altoona, PA
Linda Bostjancic, Raymond Salons Ltd., Vancouver, BC, Canada
Ross Briggs, Champion Beauty College, Houston, TX
George Campbell, former school and salon owner, Roanoke Rapids, NC
Chiquita Carter, CC's Cosmetology College, Tulsa, OK
Jerry Kelon Carter, CC's Cosmetology College, Tulsa, OK
Melissa Chapman, York County School of Technology, York, PA
Brennan Claybaugh, Paul Mitchell The School, Costa Mesa, CA
Elizabeth Crilley, Middle Bucks Institute of Technology, Richboro, PA
Kathy Earl, Apollo Career Center, Lima, OH
Debbie Fitzpatrick, Artistic Beauty Colleges, Phoenix, AZ
Wadad Frangie, Capital District Educational Opportunity Center, Troy, NY
Kathy Gotter, Meridian Technology Center, Stillwater, OK
John Halal, Honors Beauty College, Indianapolis, IN
Stacy Heatherly, Image Enhancers, Papillion, NE
Jan Heil, Bayshire Beauty Academy, Bay City, MI
Judith Holmes, Maricopa Beauty College, Avondale, AZ
Caryl Ann Johnson, International Academy of Hair Design, Tempe, AZ
Toni Love, Dudley Products, Kernersville, NC
Sharon MacGregor, Beauty School of Middletown, Middletown, NY
Dorothy McKinley-Soressi, New York International Beauty School, New York, NY
Ollie Pendley, Cosmetology Educator/Consultant, Lithia Springs, GA

Roseanne Perea, Supercuts, Novato, CA
Kathy Phelps, Moore Norman Tech Center, Norman, OK
Martha Phillips, Ford Beauty Academy, Boardman, OH
Sue Saulter, Ultima College of Cosmetology, Westminster, CO
Phyllis Sippel, Midwest College of Cosmetology, Normal, IL
Charlotte Snelgrove, Kingston, Ontario, Canada
David Stanko, Redken Fifth Avenue, New York, NY
Margie Wagner, Empire Beauty School, Pottsville, PA
Bobbie Whitehall, Future #1 College of Cosmetology, La Grande, OR
Linda Zimmerle, Lake Land Community College, Mattoon, IL

Photography Credits:

Chapter 1: chapter opener, courtesy of Tony Kendall, French Lick Hair Museum, French Lick, Indiana. Figs. 1-2 and 1-3, Corbis. Figs. 1-4 and 1-6, Delmar Learning. Photos of Madam C. J. Walker and Madam Walker's Wonderful Hair Grower, A'Lelia Bundles/Walker Family Collection. Fig. 1-5, Michael Dzaman. Figs. 1-7 and 1-8, Larry Hamill. Fig. 1-10, Ed Hille.

Chapter 2: chapter opener and Fig. 2-3, Getty Images. Figs. 2-2 and 2-7, Corbis. Fig. 2-9, Ed Hille.

Chapter 3: Fig. 3-6, Food Guide Pyramid courtesy of USDA and DHHS, 1992, Leaflet no. 572, Washington, DC.

Chapter 4: Fig. 4-6, Getty Images.

Chapter 5: Figs. 5-5 and 5-6, Delmar Learning. Fig. 5-7, courtesy of Robert A. Silverman, MD, Clinical Associate Professor, Department of Pediatrics, Georgetown University. Fig. 5-8, Kimberley's...A Day Spa, Latham, NY. Figs. 5-9 and 5-12, Ultronics, Mahwah, NJ. Figs. 5-20 and 5-21, Michael Dzaman. Fig. 5-22, Larry Hamill.

Chapter 6: chapter opener, Getty Images.

Chapter 7: chapter opener, Getty Images. Figs. 7-23 and 7-24, Larry Hamill.

Chapter 8: chapter opener, Getty Images. Fig. 8-2, reprinted with permission of Clairol, Inc. Figs. 8-4, 8-8, 8-9, 8-10, 8-12, 8-13, and 8-14, courtesy Gillette Company Research Institute, Rockville, MD. Figs. 8-17, 8-18, and 8-19, courtesy of Pharmacia & Upjohn Company. Figs. 8-20 and 8-24, courtesy of Robert A. Silverman, MD, Clinical Associate Professor, Department of Pediatrics, Georgetown University. Figs. 8-21, 8-22, 8-23, and 8-25, Delmar Learning. Fig. 8-26, courtesy of Hogil Pharmaceutical Corporation.

Chapter 9: chapter opener, Getty Images. Fig. 9-2, Scruples Professional Salon Products, Inc.

Chapter 11: Figs. 11-11, 11-12, 11-13, 11-21, 11-24, 11-28, 11-32, 11-87, 11-89, 11-124, 11-153, 11-157, 11-165, and 11-167, photos used with the permission of the authors, Martin Gannon and Richard Thompson, as featured in their book, Mahogany: Steps to Cutting, Colouring and Finishing Hair. Copyright © Martin Gannon and Richard Thompson, 1997. Fig. 11-20, John Paul Mitchell Systems, hair by John Chadwick, photo by Alberto Tolot. Figs. 11-23 and 11-169, John Paul Mitchell Systems, The Relaxer Workshop, photo by Sean Cokes. Figs. 11-26 and 11-86, Gebhart International, hair by Dennis & Sylvia Gebhart, makeup by Rose Marie, production by Purely Visual, photo by Winterhalter. Fig. 11-30, John Paul Mitchell Systems, hair by People & Schumacher, photo by Andreas Elsner. Fig. 11-34, Mario Tricoci Hair Salons & Day Spas, hair by Mario Tricoci, makeup by Shawn Miselli. Figs. 11-88 and 11-158, Getty Images. Fig. 11-91, hair by Brian & Sandra Smith, makeup by Rose Marie, wardrobe by Victor Paul, photo by Taggart/Winterhalter, production by Purely Visual. Figs. 11-155, 11-160, and 11-163, Delmar Learning. Fig. 11-159, John Paul Mitchell Systems, hair by Jeanne Braa, photo by Alberto Tolot.

Chapter 12: chapter opener, Getty Images. Fig. 12-1, Sculpt Salon, hair by George Alderete, makeup by Rose Marie, production by Purely Visual, photo by Taggart/Winterhalter.

Chapter 14: Figs. 14-33, 14-34, and 14-35, photography from the Gabor Collection, supplied by Eva Gabor International. Figs. 14-36 and 14-37, photography from American Hairlines, supplied by Eva Gabor International. Fig. 14-62, photography from Great Lengths USA, supplied by Eva Gabor International.

Chapter 15: chapter opener, Image State. Fig. 15-1, photo used with the permission of the authors, Martin Gannon and Richard Thompson, as featured in their book, Mahogany: Steps to Cutting, Colouring and Finishing Hair. Copyright © Martin Gannon and Richard Thompson, 1997. Fig. 15-95, hair by Geri Mataya, makeup by Mary Klimek, photo by Jack Cutler.

Chapter 16: Figs. 16-1 and 16-87, photos used with the permission of the authors, Martin Gannon and Richard Thompson, as featured in their book, Mahogany: Steps to Cutting, Colouring and Finishing Hair. Copyright © Martin Gannon and Richard Thompson, 1997. Fig. 16-8, reprinted with permission of Clairol, Inc. Figs. 16-66, 16-83, 16-85, and 16-86, Delmar Learning.

Chapter 17: chapter opener, Corbis. Figs. 17-7, 17-8, 17-11, 17-12, 17-13, 17-15, 17-17, 17-18, 17-19, 17-20, 17-22, 17-23, 17-24, and 17-25, reprinted with permission from the American Academy of Dermatology. All rights reserved. Fig. 17-9, courtesy of Timothy Berger, MD, Associate Clinical Professor, University of California San Francisco. Fig. 17-16, courtesy of Centers for Disease Control and Prevention (CDC). Fig. 17-21, T. Fitzgerald, Color Atlas and Synopsis of Clinical Dermatology, 3e, 1996. Reprinted with permission of The McGraw-Hill Companies. Fig. 17-26, Getty Images.

Chapter 18: Fig. 18-1, Larry Hamill.

Chapter 19: chapter opener, Corbis. Fig. 19-69, Michael Dzaman. All other photos, Larry Hamill.

Chapter 20: chapter opener, Stockbyte. Fig. 20-1, Stephen Ciuccoli. Figs. 20-2 through 20-10, 20-16 through 20-18, and 20-76 through 20-81, Larry Hamill.

Chapter 21: chapter opener, Image State. Figs. 21-2, 21-7, 21-8, 21-12, 21-13, 21-15, 21-16, 21-19 and 21-22, courtesy of Godfrey F. Mix, DPM, Sacramento, CA. Figs. 21-4a, 21-4b, 21-5, 21-6, 21-9, 21-10a, 21-10b, 21-11, 21-14, 21-17, 21-24, and 21-29, Delmar Learning. Fig. 21-18, Michael Dzaman. Fig. 21-21, courtesy of Orville J. Stone, MD, Dermatology Medical Group, Huntington Beach, CA.

Chapter 22: Fig. 22-3, Ultronics, Mahwah, NJ. All other photos, Michael Dzaman.

Chapter 23: Figs. 23-1 through 23-7, 23-9 through 23-27, 23-40, 23-43, and 23-51 through 23-53, Michael Dzaman. Figs. 23-29, 23-30, 23-31, 23-34 through 23-38, 23-39, and 23-44 through 23-49, courtesy of Nail Systems International (NSI). All rights reserved.

Chapter 24: chapter opener and Fig. 24-4, Getty Images. Fig. 24-2, Personal Enhancement Center, Clifton Park, NY. Fig. 24-7, Delmar Learning. Fig. 24-9, Tom Stock. Fig. 24-13, Stephen Ciuccoli.

Chapter 25: chapter opener, Corbis. Fig. 25-2, Getty Images. Fig. 25-5, Jerry Kelon Carter, CC's Cosmetology College, Tulsa, OK. Fig. 25-7, Ed Hille.

All other photos by Paul Castle, Castle Photography, Inc., Troy, NY.

part 1

ORIENTATION

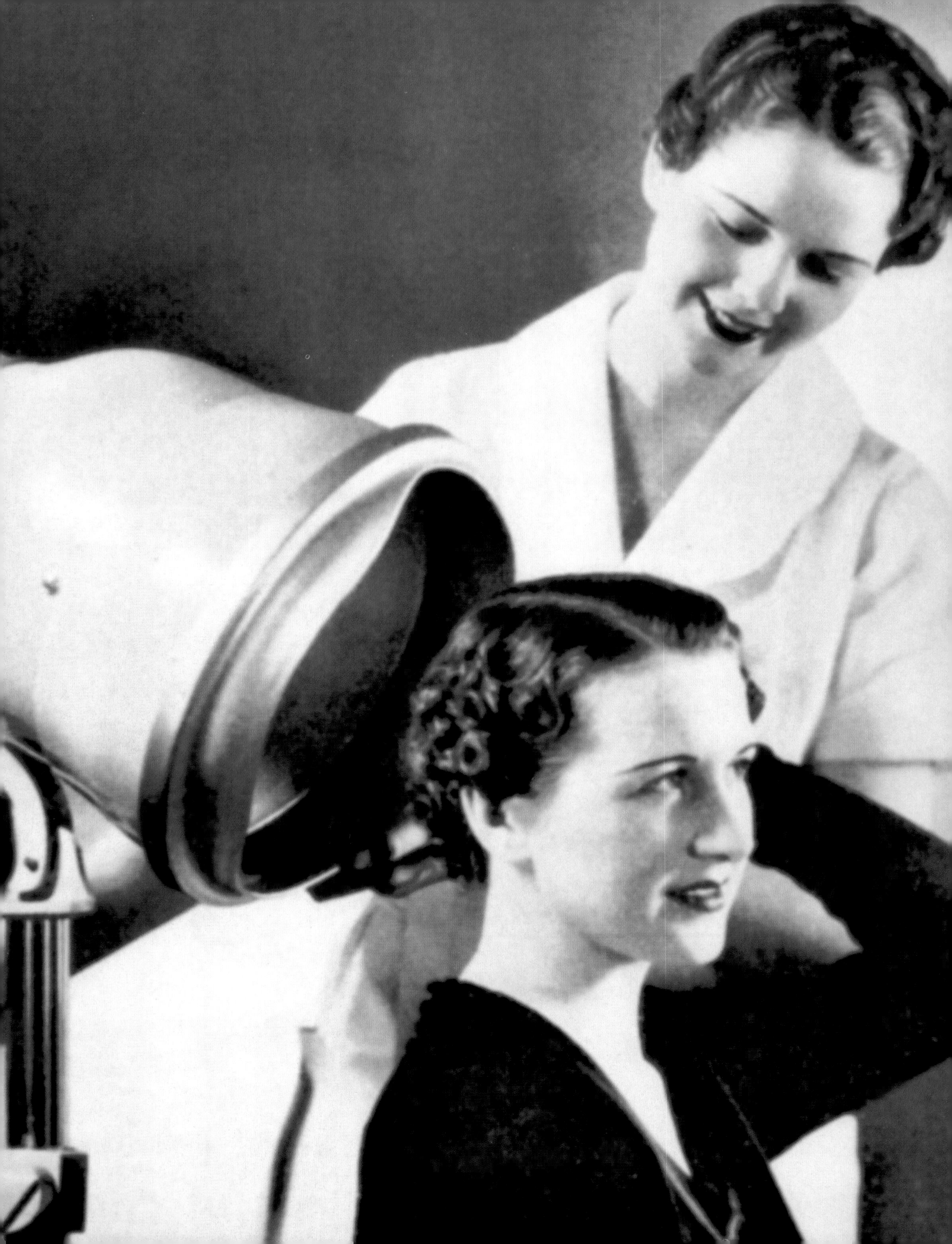

COSMETOLOGY: THE HISTORY AND OPPORTUNITIES

Lisha Barnes
FIELD ADMINISTRATOR, OLYMPIAN UNIVERSITY OF COSMETOLOGY

Chapter Outline

Reaching Your Goals • Early History • The Twentieth Century
Career Opportunities • A Bright Future Ahead

Learning Objectives

After completing this chapter, you should be able to:

1. **Describe the origins of hairstyling and barbering.**
2. **Name some of the pioneers of modern cosmetology and discuss their roles in its development.**
3. **Describe the advancements made in cosmetology during the nineteenth and twentieth centuries.**
4. **List the career opportunities available to a licensed cosmetologist.**

National Skill Standards

This chapter provides you with the necessary information to master this National Industry Skill Standard for Entry-Level Cosmetologists.

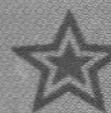

Participating in lifelong learning to stay current with trends, technology, and techniques pertaining to the cosmetology industry.

Key Terms

Page number indicates where in the chapter the term is used.

barba
pg. 7

cosmetology
pg. 7

kosmetikos
pg. 7

First, we would like to say welcome. Here you are, beginning a journey down a road that has been beckoning you for a long time. You are excited, nervous, and perhaps even amazed that you are finally here. For whatever reason—creative impulse, a desire to help people look their best and feel good about themselves, a wish for financial security, or any and all of the above—you have decided that this is the route that best suits you. You will work long and hard, you will have your successes and your failures, you will encounter problems, and you will find solutions. But, ultimately, you will be rewarded.

After graduation, you will be facing a diversity of job possibilities including hairstylist, colorist, nail technician, educator, platform artist, or makeup artist (Figure 1–1). You may choose to work in an independent salon, a day spa, a national franchise, an independent chain, or you may even choose to open your own salon at some point. Will you specialize in salon management or haircolor? Will you choose to be an educator or a product demonstrator? The future truly is limitless. Who knows? You may even team up with chemists to develop and market your own product line.

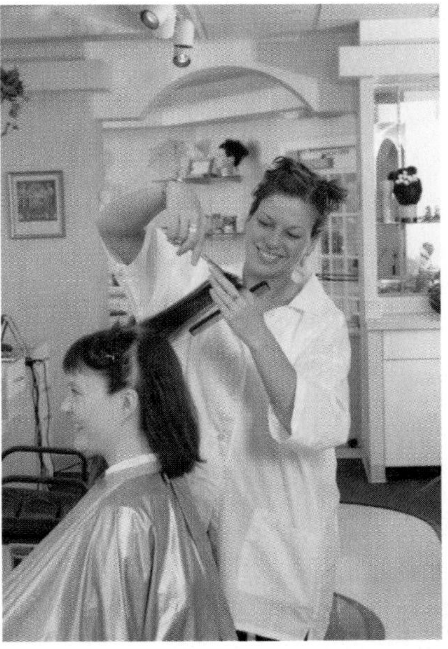

Figure 1–1 Cutting hair in a salon is one of the many choices open to you.

Whatever path you choose, you will play an important role in the lives of your clients. They will come to you for your advice, your professional expertise, and your artistic vision. And you will share these with them in an environment that you will do your best to make soothing and relaxing. Your goal as a cosmetologist is to become a trusted professional. For many of the people who will seek your services in the years ahead, you will be the one to make them look their best and, consequently, to feel their best.

You are entering a career that will demand a lot of you. You must be a talented hairstylist, and to some degree or other, a personal services expert, a businessperson, a self-promoter, and a poised and well-groomed salesperson. You must understand and practice sanitation and safety precautions. You must come to recognize physical conditions that could keep you from performing a service on a client. You must consult, advise, and listen to your clients, and you must consider the unique needs and lifestyles of each one. In addition, your clients will expect you to have a current knowledge of styles, techniques, and products, which means that you will need to continue your education through trade shows, seminars, advanced training classes, and the regular reading of professional magazines. You will be asked to do much more than your counterparts had to do at the beginning of the twentieth century.

REACHING YOUR GOALS

To be successful, you must take ownership of your education. While your instructors can create motivational circumstances and an environment that will facilitate the learning process, the ultimate responsibility for learning is yours. To get the greatest benefits from your education, commit yourself to the following "rules" that will take you a long way down the road to success.

- Attend all classes.
- Arrive for class early.
- Have all necessary materials ready.
- Listen attentively to your instructor.
- Highlight important points.
- Take notes for later review.
- Pay close attention during summary and review sessions.
- Ask, ask, ask when something is not clear.
- Seek further education continually and never stop learning. The cosmetology industry always is changing. There always are new trends, techniques, products, and information. Read industry magazines and books, and attend trade shows and advanced educational classes throughout your career.

Most of all, feel a love and a passion for what you do. If you have that love and passion, there will be no limits to the possibilities that await you.

EARLY HISTORY

From its humble beginnings, hairstyling and barbering has evolved over centuries as one of the oldest professions in the world. An overview of the history of hairstyling will make you appreciate the accomplishments attained by the early practitioners. The cultural, esthetic, and technical breakthroughs of these pioneers formed the basis for the prestige and respect the profession enjoys today.

Cosmetology, the art and science of beautifying and improving the skin, nails, and hair, and the study of cosmetics and their application, is a term that comes from the Greek word **kosmetikos**, meaning "skilled in the use of cosmetics." The term barber is derived from the Latin word **barba**, meaning "the beard or the hair of the beard."

Archeological studies reveal that haircutting and hairstyling were practiced in some form as early as the glacial age. The simple but effective implements used at the dawn of history were shaped from sharpened flints, oyster shells, or bone. Animal sinew or strips of hide were used to tie the hair back, or as adornment.

The Egyptians were the first to cultivate beauty in an extravagant fashion, and became well-versed in the art of makeup and hairdressing. Ancient written records tell us that barbers serviced the nobility and priesthood of Egypt over 6,000 years ago. The ancient Egyptians also were the first to use cosmetics as part of their personal beautification habits, and in religious ceremonies and when preparing the deceased for burial (Figure 1–2).

Ancient records also show that coloring matter made from berries, the bark of trees, minerals, insects, nuts, herbs, leaves, and other materials were used on the hair, skin, and nails. Although eye paint was the most popular of all cosmetics, henna (a dye extracted from the leaves of an ornamental shrub) was used extensively to impart a reddish tint to the hair and still is used today. The first recorded use of henna as a hair coloring agent was in 1500 B.C. Excavations from Egyptian tombs also have revealed relics such as combs, brushes, mirrors, cosmetics, and razors made of tempered copper and bronze.

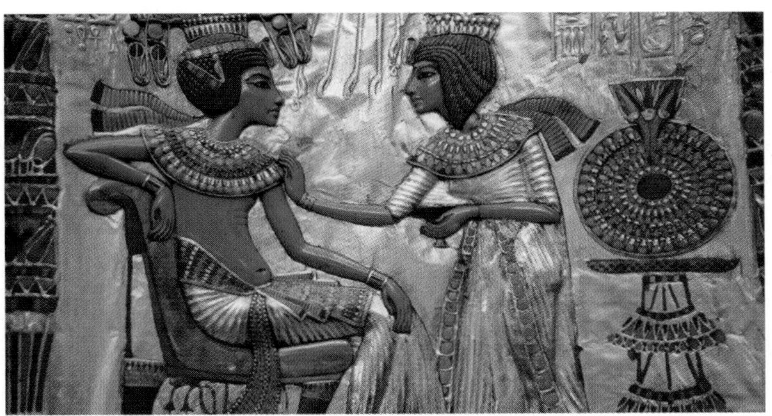

Figure 1–2 The Egyptians wore elaborate hairdos and cosmetics.

?

Did you know...

The barber pole, symbol of the barber-surgeon, has its roots in the medical procedure known as bloodletting. The pole is thought to represent the staff that the patient would hold tightly in order for the veins in the arm to stand out during the procedure. The bottom end cap represents the basin used to catch the blood. The white bandages used to stop the bleeding were hung on the staff to dry. The stained bandages would then twist around the pole in the breeze, forming a red and white pattern. One interpretation of the colors of the barber's pole was that red represented the blood, blue the veins, and white the bandages. Modern barber-stylists have retained this symbol (Figure 1–3).

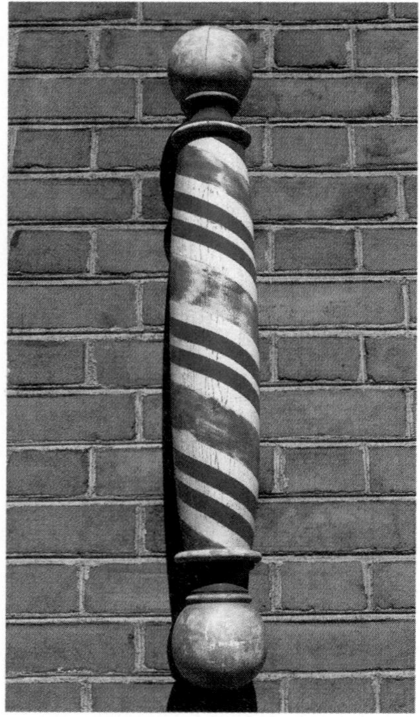

Figure 1-3 A traditional barber pole.

Hairdressing was an art for the Egyptians who wore elaborate wigs and headdresses. Egyptian women, and the Roman women who followed them, were known to apply a mixture of soil and water to their hair. The hair then was wrapped on crudely made wooden rollers to bake in the sun, creating a temporary wave. In Africa, at approximately the same point in history, hair was groomed with intricately carved combs and adorned with beads, clay, and colored bands. Masai warriors used braiding extensively with intricate patterns that denoted status within the tribe.

The first evidence of nail care recorded in history was prior to 3,000 B.C. in Egypt and China. Ancient Egyptian men and women of high social rank stained their nails with red-orange henna. The color of a person's nails was a sign of rank. Kings and queens wore deep red, while people of lower rank wore only pale colors. Meanwhile, at roughly the same time in China, nails were painted black and red.

Beauty and elements of grooming took on great symbolic significance in many cultures. Military commanders in Egypt, Babylon, and early Rome would spend hours before a battle, having their hair lacquered and curled, and their nails painted the same shade as their lips. The ancient Britons brightened their blonde hair with washes made of tallow, lime, and the extracts of certain vegetables. They dressed their hair for adornment and beautification, and for ornamentation during battle.

During the Golden Age of Greece (500 B.C.), hairstyling became a highly developed art. Hairstyling services were introduced in Rome around 300 B.C. Women used haircolor to indicate their class in society. Noblewomen tinted their hair red, middle-class women colored their hair blonde, and poor women colored their hair black.

Hairstyling and barbering continued to grow in importance, and eventually became identified with the world of medicine. Barbers figured prominently in the development of surgery as a recognized branch of medical practice. During medieval times, cosmetology and medicine were taught as combined subjects in English universities. When Pope Alexander III forbade the clergy to shed blood, barbers were enlisted to assist monks and priests during surgery. Barbers regularly performed bloodletting and minor surgery, administered herbs, and later pulled teeth. In fact, for centuries, dentistry was performed only by barbers and for more than a thousand years, they were known as barber-surgeons. 1 ✓

The fourteenth century marked the transition in Western civilization from medieval times to modern history. During the Renaissance, particular emphasis was placed on physical appearance. The hair was dressed carefully, and ornaments and headdresses were worn.

Around this time, in 1450, a law was enacted that separated the practices of barbering and surgery. With the exception of dentistry, barbers no longer could perform surgery, and surgeons were forbidden to act as barbers. In 1541, however, Henry VIII reunited the barbers and surgeons of London by granting a charter to the Company of Barber Surgeons. This reunion was short-lived, however, as the advancement of medicine made the ancient practice of bloodletting obsolete. Although their role in medical practice dwindled in importance, barber-surgeons still were relied on for dispensing medicinal herbs and pulling teeth. Finally, during the late sixteenth century, a law was passed that officially separated the barbers from the surgeons and hairstyling began to emerge as an independent profession. Many Europeans, however, had become so dependent on the services of their barber-surgeons that the settlers brought barbers with them to America.

The nineteenth century, an era marked by research and innovation, saw many changes in the field of hair care. In 1875, a Frenchman named Marcel Grateau developed the technique of using irons for waving and curling the hair.

This practice developed into the art of thermal waving, still known today as marcel waving. In 1892, another Frenchman named Alexandre F. Godefroy invented a hot-blast hair dryer. In 1890, the first hairdressing academy was opened in Chicago by Brisbois and Federmeyer.

THE TWENTIETH CENTURY

Before the twentieth century, hairstyling typically was limited to the upper class. Hairstyles and makeup were used to mark social status, religious beliefs, political status, military rank, and simply fashion. Beginning with the twentieth century, hairstyling began to follow trends, and soon became available to all classes of people who could choose their styles based on their own needs and desires.

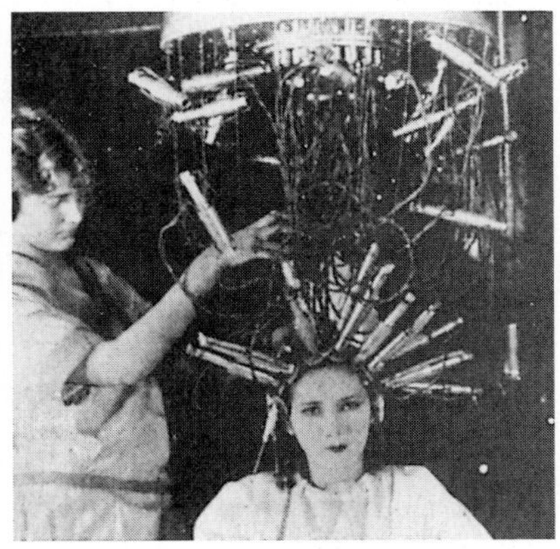

Figure 1–4 Machine permanent wave in the early twentieth century.

History of Permanent Waving

In 1905, Charles Nessler invented a heavily wired machine that supplied electrical current to metal rods around which hair strands were wrapped. These heavy units were heated during the waving process. They were kept away from the scalp by a complex system of counterbalancing weights, suspended from an overhead chandelier mounted on a stand (Figure 1–4).

Two methods were used to wind hair strands around the metal units. Long hair was wound from the scalp to the ends in a technique called spiral wrapping. After World War I, when women cut their hair into the short bobbed style, the croquignole wrapping technique was introduced. In this method, shorter hair was wound from the ends toward the scalp. The hair was then styled into deep waves with loose end curls.

insights

Madam C. J. Walker

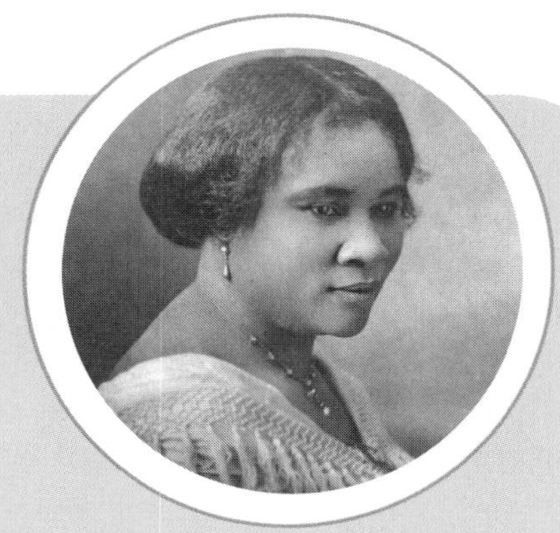

One of the most notable success stories of the cosmetology industry, if not American history in general, is that of Madam C. J. Walker. Madam Walker was the daughter of former slaves, and transformed herself from an uneducated washerwoman into one of the twentieth century's most successful entrepreneurs.

Born Sarah Breedlove in 1867, Madam Walker was orphaned at the age of seven and went to work in the cotton fields of the Mississippi delta. To escape an abusive brother-in-law with whom she was living, Sarah got married at the age of 14, became a mother at 17, and was widowed by the age of 20. She went to St. Louis to join her four brothers who were working as barbers, and managed to eke out a living and find the funds necessary to educate her daughter.

During the 1890s, Sarah suffered from a scalp condition and began to lose her hair. She started to experiment with store-bought products and homemade remedies.

In 1906, Sarah married her third husband, C. J. Walker, and became known as Madam C. J. Walker. She began to sell her scalp conditioning and healing treatment, "Madam Walker's Wonderful Hair Grower," the formula for which came to her in a dream, she always claimed. Devising sophisticated sales and marketing strategies, she traveled extensively throughout the South and Southeast, giving product demonstrations door-to-door, and in church basements and lodges. In 1910, she moved her company to Indianapolis where she built a factory, hair salon, and training school. As she developed new products, her empire grew. She acquired a townhouse in Harlem that was regarded as one of the most fabulous private residences in all of New York. She also devoted much time and money to a variety of causes including the National Association for the Advancement of Colored People (NAACP) and the YMCA in Indianapolis, and lobbied in Washington for antilynching legislation. In 1917, she organized a convention for her Madam C. J. Walker Hair Culturists Union of America. This was one of the first national meetings for businesswomen ever held.

By the time of her death, she had established herself as a pioneer of the modern black hair care and cosmetics industry. She always traced her success to tenacity and perserverance, to faith in herself and in God, to the quality of her products, and to her honesty in business dealings. "There is no royal flower-strewn path to success," she commented. "If I have accomplished anything in life it is because I have been willing to work hard."

In 1998, the U.S. Postal Service issued the Madam C. J. Walker commemorative stamp, the 21st in the Black Heritage Series.

Read more about Madam Walker in *On Her Own Ground: The Life and Times of Madam C. J. Walker* by A'Lelia Bundles (Scribner, 2001).

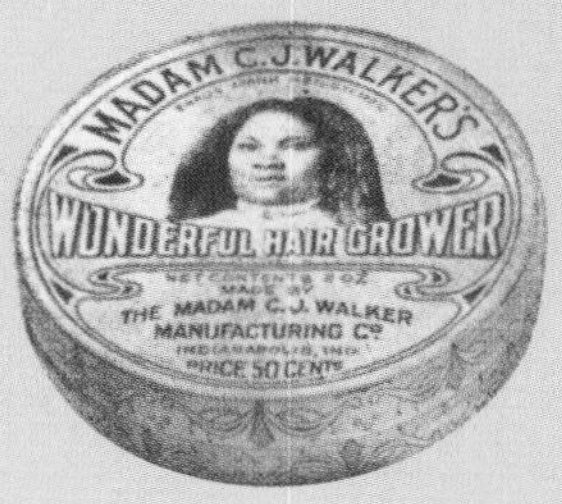

The client's fear of being "tied" to an electrical contraption with the possibility of receiving a shock or burn led to the development of alternative methods of waving hair. In 1931, the preheat method was introduced. Hair was wrapped using the croquignole method. Then clamps, preheated by a separate electrical unit, were placed over the wound curls. An alternative to the machine perm was introduced in 1932 when chemists Ralph L. Evans and Everett G. McDonough pioneered a method that used external heat generated by chemical reaction. Small, flexible pads containing a chemical mixture were wound around hair strands. When the pads were moistened with water, a chemical heat was released that created long-lasting curls. Thus, the first machineless permanent wave was born. Salon clients were no longer subjected to the dangers and discomforts of the Nessler machine. 2✓

In 1941, scientists developed another method of permanent waving that used waving lotion. Because this perm did not use heat, it was called a cold wave. Cold waves replaced virtually all predecessors and competitors, and the terms cold waving and permanent waving became almost synonymous. Modern versions of cold waves, usually referred to as alkaline perms, are very popular today. The term texture services is used today to refer to the variety of permanent wave services available for different hair types and conditions.

During the latter half of the twentieth century, the cosmetology industry has seen growth and expansion unrivaled by any other time in history. Advancements in technology and innovative techniques in haircutting, chemical services, esthetics, and nail extensions have freed stylists to pursue new avenues of creativity and service for their clients.

Along with hair texture services, haircoloring has also evolved dramatically. What began with the use of henna and vegetable extracts has become a multibillion-dollar industry of professional products. These products can create colors from the lightest blondes to the darkest blacks, and everything in between. The public's interest in the health and beauty of skin has also grown, allowing salons to add facials, makeup, corrective and therapeutic skin care, and hair removal to their list of services. Manicuring, pedicuring, and nail extensions have also developed into some of the salon's most popular services (Figure 1–5).

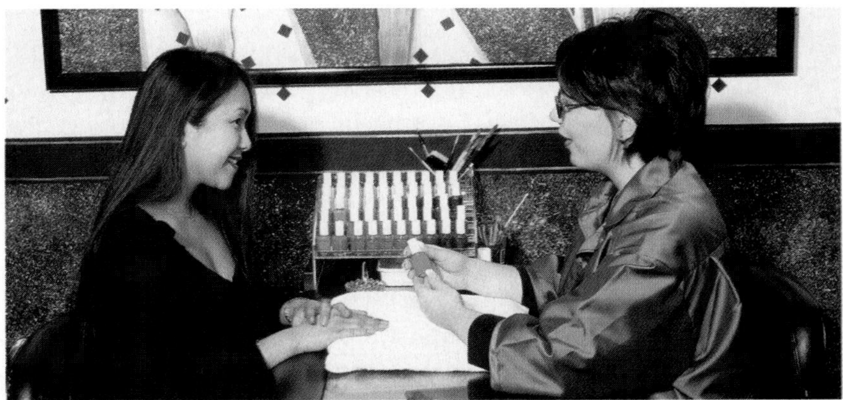

Figure 1-5 Performing nail services.

The huge growth in day spas has also been a significant development. These spas, which have been opening all over the country, offer hair and esthetic services as well as specialized services such as aromatherapy, hydrotherapy, massage treatments, and nutritional counseling. What was once a luxury service for the wealthy has become a routine service for many.

The domain of cosmetology has changed dramatically over the course of time. All the new services and skills have transformed and expanded the role of cosmetologists, requiring them to know more than ever and to make continuing education a necessity. 3✓

CAREER OPPORTUNITIES

At this point in your journey, you may not know whether you prefer working with hair, skin, or nails. Even if you do have something in mind, it is best in the beginning to leave yourself open to other possibilities. Let your learning guide you. Enter each classroom with an open mind and a wholehearted desire to learn as much as you can. Some of the best-known people in the beauty industry changed vocational direction in the course of their studies. You have many career possibilities ahead so let us take a look at some of them.

Salon Stylist

As an entry-level cosmetologist, you may be expected to perform all the services offered in the salon. These will vary depending on the type of salon you choose to work in. In addition, you may be asked to handle reception desk duties such as meeting and greeting clients, answering the telephone, making appointments, calling clients to remind them of upcoming appointments, and selling retail products to clients. You will also need to focus on refining your practical skills, building a clientele, and referring clients to other specialists in the salon. You will keep your record cards updated, practice good customer relation skills and consumer safety, and be dependable and on time for your appointments. You will be responsible for keeping your work area clean and sanitary, as well as helping with sanitation duties in the salon.

As you advance in your career, your responsibilities may grow to include being a mentor to a younger stylist or student. You may decide to specialize in a specific area such as haircolor or nail art. You may become a salon manager in charge of keeping product inventory, ordering supplies, providing job evaluations for employees, and handling customer complaints. For a cosmetologist with good skills and a winning attitude, the possibilities are unlimited.

Haircolor Specialist

If you have an eye for color, you may want to pursue this vocational direction. A color technician or haircolorist selects the best color, formulates it, and processes it to enhance a client's hair. This is an extremely creative area of the industry. You may want to specialize at a salon, become a color trainer, work for a color manufacturer, or become a platform artist demonstrating your techniques. As a haircolorist, it is imperative that you continue your education by attending advanced haircolor classes. This will give you a creative edge and provide you with special and highly marketable skills. In addition, the art of color correction is a very lucrative business and requires extensive knowledge of haircolor and related products (Figure 1–6).

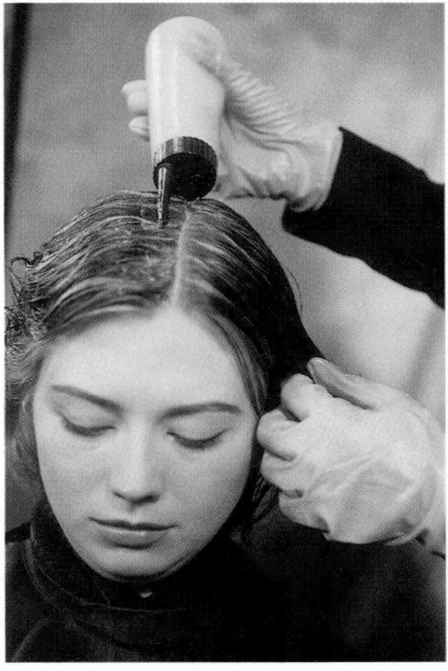

Figure 1–6 Haircolor specialists are in great demand.

Texture Service Specialist

If you enjoy creating an entirely new look for your clients, consider becoming a texture service specialist. All hair has a natural look, or movement or wave pattern, but many clients choose to change these aspects of their hair. By specializing in chemical texture services, you can give clients the look they want simply by adding or removing curl in varying degrees. Or perhaps you will want to get involved in product research and development. Whichever area you choose, rest assured that these, too, are very lucrative parts of the cosmetology profession.

Wig or Extensions Specialist

As a specialist in hair extensions or wig services, you can work with clients to create subtle or dramatic changes in their hair length, texture, and color by adding extensions through braiding, weaving, bonding, gluing, or sewing. Or you may enjoy working with cancer patients who are experiencing hair loss as a result of chemotherapy or radiation treatments. Assisting them with wig selection and fittings can make a real difference in the quality of their lives. Another possibility is to become a men's hair replacement specialist. You can specialize in treating men with hair loss through various nonsurgical procedures such as hair weaves, hairpieces, and other hair replacement methods.

Retail Specialist

If you communicate well, have a flair for selling, and enjoy working with people, you may want to consider becoming a retail specialist. You can work in a salon, spa, or department store handling the merchandise or inventory. Retail specialists also work as trainers, representing product manufacturers at general sales seminars all over the country. If this area interests you, it is important that you understand how to work with products and how to articulate the merits of a specific product line. And, of course, you can be both a stylist and a retail specialist. In fact, at least half of a stylist's income comes from retail sales.

Skin Care Specialist/Esthetician

An esthetician offers treatments to perfect the look and health of the skin. Among the options available to estheticians are working in a salon or spa, teaching, giving demonstrations at cosmetology shows, or becoming a consultant for a cosmetics company. With specialized training in esthetics, you may choose to work in a dermatology clinic and provide various treatments for problematic skin under the supervision of a dermatologist.

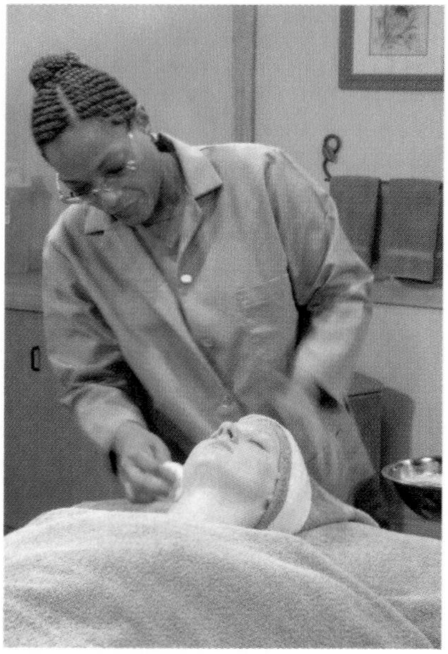

The opportunities in this area of the industry are excellent, due to growing public demand and the ever-expanding older population. Many skin care specialists even wind up owning their own businesses (Figure 1–7).

Figure 1-7 Skin care services are growing more popular.

Makeup Artist

A makeup artist applies cosmetics to enhance a client's appearance. It is an area best suited to those who are artistically inclined and creative. A makeup artist will blend, shade, and create any image a client requires. As a makeup artist, you may establish yourself in a salon with a private clientele, become makeup director for a prestigious department store, represent a line of cosmetics, work in TV or film production, find a position in a fashion magazine doing makeup for photo shoots, or work behind the scenes in theater production. You can operate as an independent freelancer, which allows you to create your own schedule, or you can find full-time employment with one company.

Nail Technician/Manicurist

If you choose to specialize in nails, you will be joining one of the fastest growing areas of the cosmetology profession. You can work in a full-service salon and provide your clients with manicures and pedicures, or you may choose to work in a nail-care-only salon that offers a variety of artificial nail services. This avenue allows you to practice creative nail art and to enjoy one of the most rewarding careers in cosmetology today. In fact, this area of cosmetology is seeing so much growth that many nail care specialists wind up owning their own businesses.

Day Spa Stylist or Technician

Today, many clients choose to visit a day spa to escape the stress and rush of everyday life. The central theme of the day spa is no longer hair. Instead, it is seen as a one-stop, full-service facility, concentrating on the overall appearance of the individual, and on the health of the skin and body. A full range of services is available at day spas including haircuts, styling, texture services, haircolor, manicures and pedicures, facial treatments, body massage, body wraps, and hydrotherapy services. Clients may also opt for a day of luxury that includes a combination of all these services. Working in a day spa will involve teamwork with other employees specializing in different areas. If you enjoy working with clients to improve and maintain their appearance, and you enjoy networking with different stylists and massage therapists, a day spa may be the ideal professional environment for you (Figure 1–8).

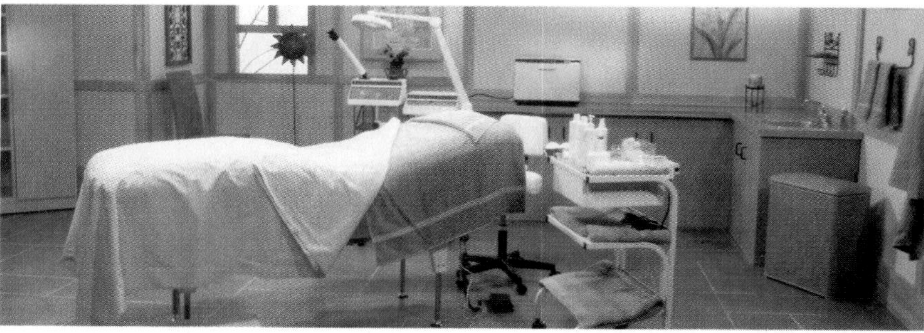

Figure 1-8 Facial and body treatments are two of the services offered by day spas.

Salon Manager

If you feel you are good at supervising people, have a natural ability to deal with clients, and still enjoy working behind the chair as a stylist, salon management may be for you. The salon manager leads by example, and is responsible for helping team members achieve their goals through training and development, counseling, and coaching. You must possess styling skills (although not all managers are stylists) in addition to sound business skills including purchasing, personnel development, advertising, sales, budgeting, and people skills.

Salon Owner

As a salon owner, you will take on a variety of responsibilities and challenges. You will enjoy exercising your creativity, versatility, and independence, as long as you do not mind making hard decisions and working long hours. Running your own salon allows you to set a standard for the quality of service you bring to the workplace. You can choose the products and services and determine the level of skill you demand from your staff. Owning a salon means assuming responsibility for paying bills, payroll, and taxes. Contact your local small business bureau and obtain literature about businesses in your area if the idea of owning a business interests you.

Product Educator

As a product educator-distributor, you will need to possess good communication skills, people skills, and a dynamic image. Product educators must be poised and good at listening, observing, and speaking to groups. They are based out of local supply houses and travel to specific regional territories selling professional products to licensed professionals and establishment owners. In addition, they are required to provide product knowledge classes and if licensed, to present product demonstrations at area salons and schools. If you enjoy traveling, meeting new people, and sharing your knowledge, this may be the perfect position for you.

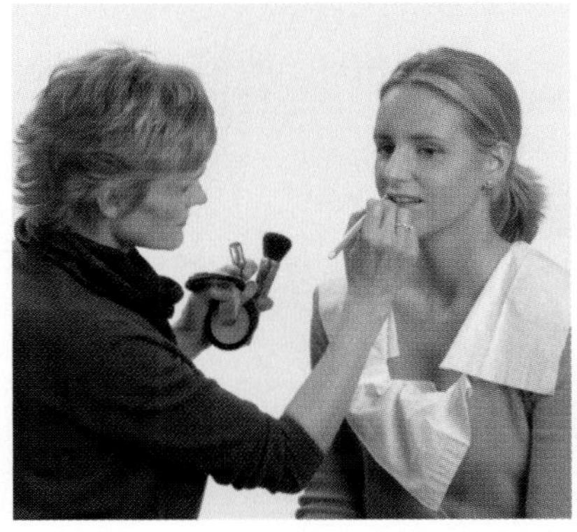

Figure 1–9 A session stylist often works with models.

Cosmetic Chemist

A cosmetic chemist meets the cosmetology industry's expanding needs by creating new products through research and experimentation. As a cosmetic chemist, you can work for a cosmetics manufacturer or become a consultant to several companies. You may want to consider applying for an internship with a cosmetic company where you might work on a panel that studies new products. It is important to have a good understanding of chemistry and additional education may be required to meet the demands of this position.

Session Stylist

A session stylist works to style hair and makeup for models being photographed for magazines and books. You may work as a freelancer or on the staff of a specific magazine. If you have excellent hairstyling and makeup skills, and enjoy fashion and photography, this may be a good opportunity for you (Figure 1–9).

Hairstylist for TV, Movies, or Theater

If you like the idea of working with celebrities, you may want to consider this career option. You can choose to style hair for a weekly TV show, be a makeup artist for the latest theatrical production, or even create the newest alien race as part of a special-effects team for a science fiction movie. Working in this area will allow you to color hair, add texture, use hair extensions, work with wigs, or simply style hair. Who knows? There may even be an Academy Award in your future.

Styles Director/Artistic Director

If you are good at meeting deadlines, working within a budget, managing people, have an artistic or creative bent, and are able to forecast trends, you may enjoy becoming a styles director. You will work with videographers, fashion magazines, publishing companies, product manufacturers, and education companies to help create just the right fashion look for magazine and book layouts, and video shoots. Many large corporations are also hiring artistic directors to attend to their esthetic needs.

Design Team Member

If you like fashion, drama, and excitement, consider becoming a member of a design team that works with the artistic director. Individuals join together to create presentations for fashion shows, runway work, convention luncheons, gala banquets, or hair shows. These presentations often have themes ranging from spring weddings to futuristic scenes, or to the Roaring Twenties. This provides you the opportunity to show off your most innovative and dramatic ideas. In addition, you might join a national association that develops the latest in trend releases, allowing you to be on the cutting edge of fashion and design.

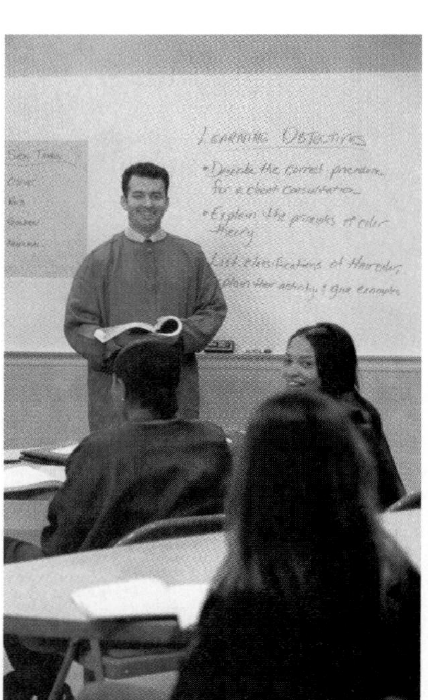

Figure 1-10 An educator enjoys sharing his knowledge with students.

Platform Artist

A platform artist should enjoy being on stage, performing for people, sharing knowledge, and traveling. As a platform artist, you will most likely work out of a salon during the week. But on weekends, you will travel to local or national hair shows to demonstrate the most current trends and techniques, or to represent products for professional product companies. Salon experience is a must, as well as excellent communication skills and stage presence.

Competition Champion

Competition champions compete for prizes and prestige in various cosmetology world championships. Here, "the best" display their individual talents and techniques. You must have dedication, good work habits, and, above all, skills to enter this honored realm that holds so many rewards. Competition champions often establish their own salons. Their reputations as distinguished artists attract a following and add to the prosperity of their business endeavors. Champions can also work as trainers, coaching the next generation of competitors.

Educator

There are numerous teaching opportunities in the field of cosmetology. You may choose to work as an educational consultant for a product manufacturer; become a continuing education provider to other licensees; or work as an educator, school director, or school manager for a cosmetology school. An educator enjoys teaching and sharing knowledge with others.

Educators should have patience, people skills, communication skills, and energy. If you have a passion for the cosmetology industry and enjoy seeing others benefit from your ideas, teaching may be just the career for you. Keep in mind that additional training, experience, and continuing education may be required (Figure 1–10).

Writer

With a cosmetology background, you can write articles, books, brochures, columns, educational textbooks, and even produce videos. As a writer with a cosmetology license, you can work for a publishing company, as a freelancer, review new textbooks and products, or develop a lifestyle that combines them all. Fine-tune your writing skills by taking writing courses and reading as much as possible. It is essential to keep current with what is going on in the industry by attending seminars and hair shows.

State Board Member

A way to serve your industry, and contribute to its growth and improvement, is to serve on one of the various regulatory agencies in your state or province such as the Board of Cosmetologists. This will allow you to take a proactive role in the regulatory issues affecting the cosmetology industry. By becoming actively involved on a state, province, or even federal level, you can play an important role in maintaining and improving standards within the industry. If this opportunity appeals to you, check with your state on the specific guidelines for becoming a member of the regulatory agency in your area. Another possibility for serving your industry would be to become a state board examiner or state board inspector. 4 ✓

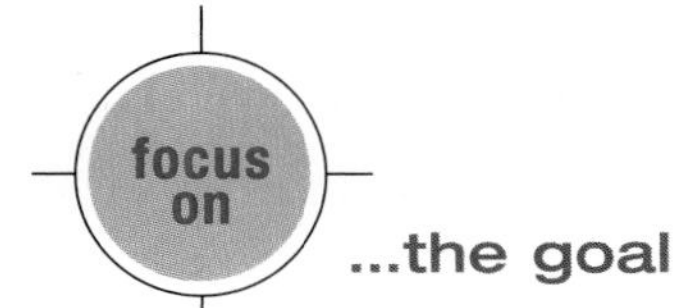

Make this commitment to yourself: I have taken my first steps on my journey to success. I have given myself the courage to enroll in school. By taking this step, I have made the conscious decision that I want more for my life and for those for whom I am responsible. This decision will allow me to accomplish my dreams. No one can take this dream away from me unless I allow it. I am my own greatest resource. I will complete my education. I can only fail if I give up.

A BRIGHT FUTURE AHEAD

As you can see, the world of cosmetology offers vast opportunities. The salon industry grosses approximately $50 billion a year in revenue. If you are dependable, ambitious, and committed, have excellent people skills, technical skills, and a strong work ethic, you can look forward to a career that offers glamour, excitement, creative expression, and outstanding monetary rewards.

Today, you stand at the threshold of opportunity. If you apply yourself, there will be no limit to the possibilities. To get the most out of your career, you must make the most of your education. Every lesson has something to teach if you can maintain an open mind and a positive attitude. Subscribe to professional publications to supplement your education, maintain membership in relevant trade associations, and continue your education by attending events presented by those organizations. Your license will unlock countless doors, but it is your education and personal desire for success that will really launch your career.

This is the beginning of an exciting journey that we hope will lead you where you want to go. We wish you luck and best wishes for your success. And we hope that you will love what you do. As the great German poet Goethe once wrote, “We don’t get to know anything but what we love.”

chapter glossary

barba	Latin word meaning the beard or the hair of the beard
cosmetology	the art and science of beautifying and improving the skin, nails, and hair, and the study of cosmetics and their applications
kosmetikos	Greek word meaning skilled in the use of cosmetics and from which the word "cosmetology" is derived

1

review questions

1. What is the meaning of the Greek word kosmetikos?
2. From what Latin word is the term barber derived?
3. How did ancient Egyptian and Roman women temporarily wave their hair?
4. Explain the significance of hairstyles in early cultures.
5. What was the historical relationship of barbers to medicine?
6. Describe the evolution of the barber pole.
7. Who was Madam C. J. Walker?
8. When and where was the first hairdressing academy opened?
9. Describe the early development of permanent waving. Who developed the permanent wave machine?
10. Explain how salon services have expanded in the twentieth century.
11. List career opportunities available to licensed cosmetologists in salons.
12. List career opportunities available to licensed cosmetologists outside of the salon.

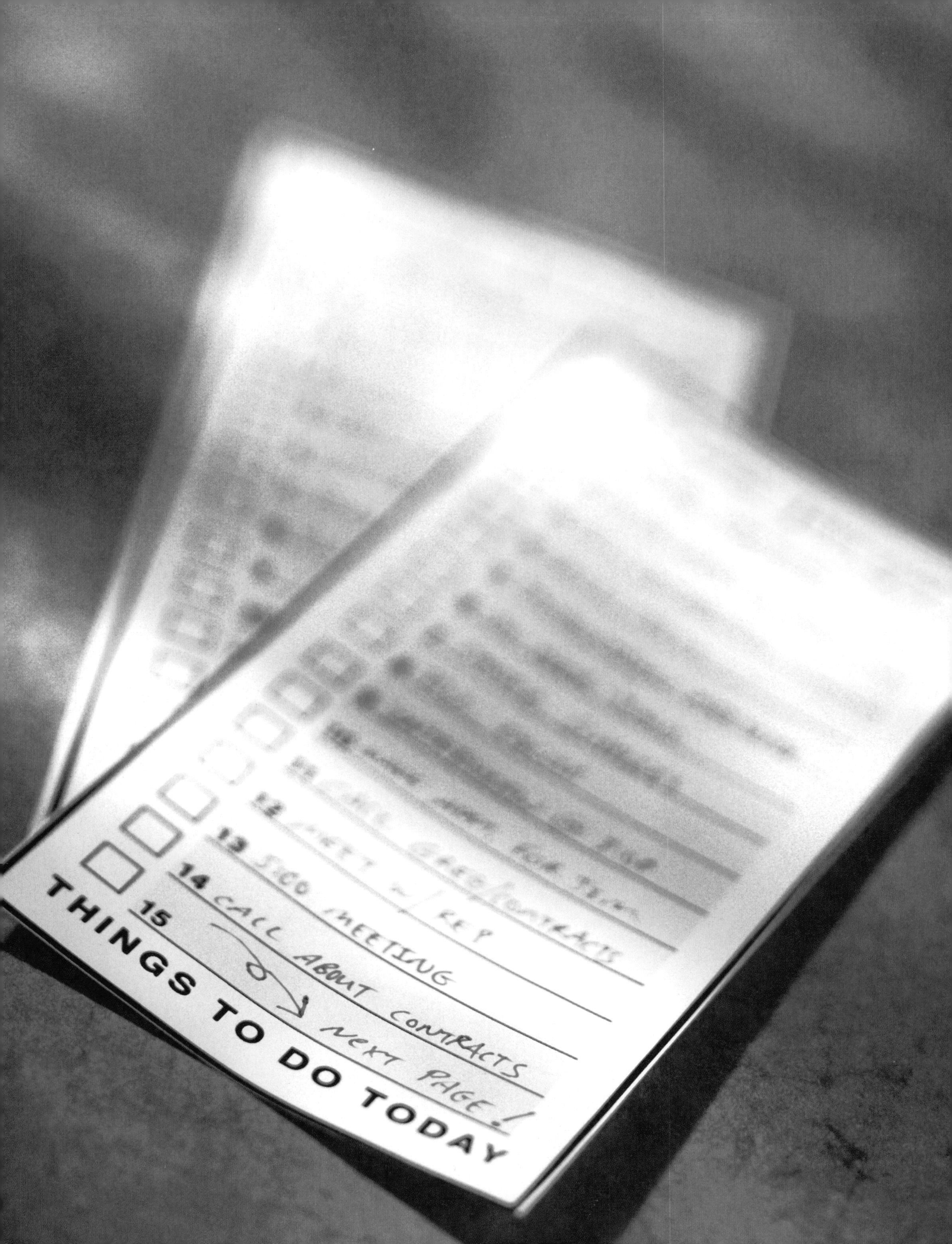

THINGS TO DO TODAY
14 CALL ABOUT CONTRACTS
15
NEXT PAGE!

LIFE SKILLS

Arlene Alpert
MS, LMHC
BUSINESS RELATIONSHIPS CONSULTANT
JUPITER CONSULTING & TRAINING INSTITUTE

Chapter Outline

The Psychology of Success • Motivation and Self-Management
Managing Your Career • Goal Setting • Time Management • Study Skills
Ethics • Personality Development and Attitude • Human Relations

Learning Objectives

After completing this chapter, you should be able to:

1. **List the principles that contribute to personal and professional success.**
2. **Explain the concept of self-management.**
3. **Create a personal mission statement.**
4. **Explain how to set long- and short-term goals.**
5. **Discuss the most effective ways to manage time.**
6. **Describe good study habits.**
7. **Define ethics.**
8. **List the characteristics of a healthy, positive attitude.**

National Skill Standards

This chapter provides you with the necessary information to master these National Industry Skill Standards for Entry-Level Cosmetologists.

Consulting with clients to determine their needs and preferences.

Interacting effectively with coworkers as part of a team.

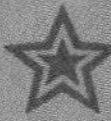

Effectively managing your time in order to provide efficient client service.

Using appropriate methods to ensure personal health and well-being.

Key Terms

Page number indicates where in the chapter the term is used

compartmentalization
pg. 25

ethics
pg. 35

game plan
pg. 26

goal-setting
pg. 30

mission statement
pg. 29

perfectionism
pg. 26

prioritize
pg. 31

procrastination
pg. 26

All the technical skills that you are now acquiring in school are vastly important. But these technical skills need to rest on a solid foundation of "life skills." Life skills are a set of tools and guidelines that prepare you for living as a mature adult in a complicated world. With these tools, you can construct a framework that will be useful in all situations.

For example, think of a house. There may be all kinds of decorations around a house that make it special: shutters, window boxes, awnings, and such. But if a storm comes along—and life, as we know, is full of storms—the decorations are likely to blow away. If the house has a strong frame and a good foundation, it will continue to stand. Life skills are your foundation. They will help you construct a worthwhile and substantial life and keep you standing in the storm.

There are a great many life skills that lead to a more satisfying and productive existence. Some of the most important are:

- being genuinely caring and helpful to other people.
- successfully adapting to different situations.
- sticking to a goal and seeing a job to completion.
- developing a deep reservoir of common sense.
- making good friends and feeling good about yourself.
- maintaining a cooperative attitude in all situations.
- defining "courage" for yourself and living courageously within your definition.
- approaching all your work and personal matters with a strong sense of responsibility.
- learning techniques that will help you become more organized.
- having a sense of humor to bring you through difficult situations.
- acquiring that great virtue known as "patience."
- consistently making an effort in all projects you undertake and always striving for excellence.

- dedicating yourself to becoming an honest and trustworthy individual.

Many people believe that when they attain success, all their problems will be solved. In fact, success often comes with its own set of problems. The best solution to these problems is to have a sturdy set of life skills in place. The way you act toward others and handle yourself will determine whether you can sustain success. Acquiring life skills empowers you. Without them, you will wind up being ordinary at best. With life skills, there is no telling how good you can get.

THE PSYCHOLOGY OF SUCCESS

Everyone defines success in different ways. For some, success depends on how much money they make. For others, what matters is career satisfaction or the feeling of being able to help others. How do you define success?

We think of real success as the coming together of various elements that make a person truly multidimensional. The most successful people live according to disciplined habits they have learned from teachers, books, family, friends, and associates whom they admire. A common characteristic shared by most successful people is that they love what they do.

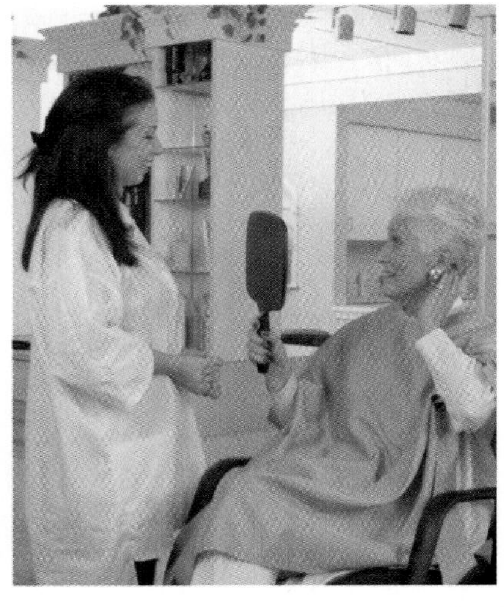

Figure 2–1 Loving your work is critical to your success.

Can you see yourself loving what you have set out to do? Here you are in school, learning the skills you will need for a career in cosmetology. It is hard work. But this hard work is much easier when you put that extra amount of effort, enthusiasm, and excitement into your studies. You can have all the talent in the world and still not be successful if your talent is not fueled by the passion for your work that will sustain you over the course of your career (Figure 2–1).

Guidelines for Success

As we have said, defining success is a very personal thing. There are some basic principles, however, that form the foundation of personal and business success. You can begin your journey to success right now by examining and putting into practice these principles.

- *Build self-esteem.* Self-esteem is based on inner strength and begins with trusting your ability to reach your goals. No one sustains success without feeling good about himself, both personally and professionally. Therefore, it is essential that you begin now, while you are still a student, to work on increasing your self-esteem.
- *Visualize.* Imagine a movie screen. Picture yourself on this screen as a person of confidence, competence, and maturity. See yourself as well-

dressed and conducting yourself in a professional manner that earns the respect and trust of your clients. The more you visualize, the more easily you can turn the possibilities in your life into realities.

- *Build on your strengths.* Practice doing whatever it is that helps you maintain a positive self-image. If you are good at something (playing the guitar, running, cooking, gardening, or singing), the time you invest in that activity will allow you to feel good about yourself (Figure 2–2). And the things you are good at do not have to be things you can see. You could be good at listening to others, helping someone less fortunate than yourself, or being a caring and considerate friend.
- *Be kind to yourself.* Put a stop to self-critical and negative thoughts that can work against you. The unfortunate truth is that there are lots of people in the world who are ready to be rude and insensitive to you; you do not have to be rude and insensitive to yourself. If you make a mistake, tell yourself that it is okay and you will do your best next time.
- *Define success for yourself.* Be a success in your own eyes. Do not depend on other people's definitions of success. What is right for your father, your sister, or your best friend may not be right for you.
- *Practice new behaviors.* Because creating success is a skill, you can help to develop it by practicing other new behaviors such as speaking with confidence, standing tall, using good grammar when you speak, and sounding proud when you list your achievements.
- *Keep your personal life separate from your work.* People who talk about themselves or others at work promote second-rate team spirit that makes the whole salon suffer. The same is true in the classroom. If you find it difficult to keep your personal life out of the classroom, try this exercise. Imagine that you have two file cabinets; one is labeled Personal, the other Professional. See yourself locking the Personal file cabinet before leaving for school and opening the Professional one when you get to class. This is called **compartmentalization**—storing things away in the different compartments of the mind—and it works.
- *Keep your energy up.* Get enough rest. Successful people know how to pace themselves. They do not run themselves ragged, and they do not eat, sleep, and drink business. They take time to meet their human needs like spending time with family and friends, exercising, and eating a good nutritious diet. They know that success means having a clear head, a fit body, and the ability to refuel and recharge.
- *Respect others.* Make a point of relating to everyone you know with a conscious feeling of respect. Exercise good manners with others: use words like please, thank you, and excuse me. Avoid interrupting and do not discuss your personal life with a neighboring stylist, even if you think clients cannot hear you (they can and do). As your awareness grows, this kind of respect will become a way of life. And the act of respecting others comes with a gift for you. When you treat people well, they will respect you, and their respect helps build that precious self-esteem discussed above.

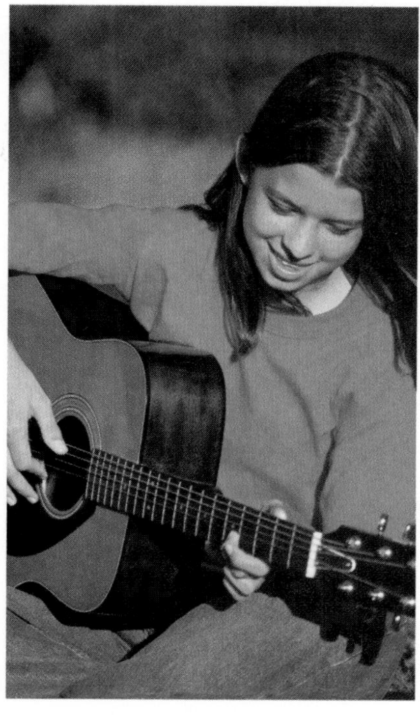

Figure 2–2 Spend time on the things you do well.

- *Stay productive.* There are three habits that can keep you from maintaining peak performance: procrastination, perfectionism, and the lack of a game plan. You will see an almost instant improvement when you work on eliminating these troublesome habits.

Procrastination is putting off until tomorrow what you can do today. This dangerous but widespread habit robs you of self-esteem. Most people do not like themselves when they do not complete what they have set out to do. It is also the hallmark of poor study habits ("I'll study tomorrow") and may be a symptom of taking on too much in the first place, which, in turn, is a symptom of faulty organization.

Perfectionism is a compulsion to do things perfectly, and it is unhealthy. Success is not simply a matter of always doing things right. No one does it right every time. In fact, someone who never makes a mistake may not be trying hard enough in the first place to stretch himself. A better definition of success is to not give up, even when things get really tough. It took Thomas Edison a thousand tries to discover how to create a light bulb, but he never felt like a failure because his self-esteem convinced him that one day he would get it right.

Invest in yourself by coming up with a **game plan**, the conscious act of planning your life instead of just letting things happen. You may think it is easier to just coast along from day to day, but the road to success is best reached with a clear game plan that will lead you where you want to go. Game plans are often structured in large chunks of time, (five or ten years ahead), but it is just as important to set daily, monthly, and yearly goals for yourself. Begin by asking where you want to be in five years. Or ten years, or ten months, or ten days. What kind of resources and training will you need to get there? It may seem harder at first to approach life in this way, but you will find it brings greater rewards. Winners are people who decide what they want to do, set a goal, and stick to it. 1

2

MOTIVATION AND SELF-MANAGEMENT

Motivation is the ignition for success. Self-management is the fuel that will keep you going on the long ride to your destination.

While motivation propels you to do something and can come from inside you in a way that is very instinctive, self-management is a well-thought-out process for the long term. For example, when you are hungry, you are motivated to eat. But it is self-management that helps you decide what you will do to get food.

It is important to feel motivated, especially when you are a student. A motivated student finds it much easier to learn. The best motivation for learning comes from an inner desire to know. This is usually linked to an interest in your subject matter. If you have always been interested in the world of beauty, then you are likely to be interested in the material you will be studying in cosmetology school. If your motivation has come from some external source—your parents, friends, or some glamorous ad—you may not make it to graduation. To make a career for yourself, you need more than a push from others. You need to feel a sense of excitement and a good reason for staying the course. No one should have to motivate you to study other than yourself. You are the one in charge of managing your own life and learning.

As you go through school, you will be faced with a large amount of new information. At some point, you may ask yourself, "Why do I need to know this? How is this material going to help me in my career?" While you may not understand completely why you need to learn certain concepts and techniques, especially if you cannot see how you will apply them in the job you hope to get one day, you must boost your motivation by looking ahead. Remind yourself that this is the career you want. Then take it on faith that what you are being asked to learn will be helpful to you at some point in your working life.

Although motivation is not a life skill, self-management is. It is a skill that will help point you where you want to go. Through the skills of self-management, you will learn to rely on yourself. You can do that by taking care of yourself through meeting the five basic human needs and by stimulating your creative capability. 2

Satisfying Your Basic Human Needs

The needs of all human beings are interrelated and must be met before an individual can achieve real happiness. In fact, these needs are arranged in a kind of ladder. Only when you achieve one set of needs can you move on to the next. For most people, these basic human needs are arranged as follows.

1. *Physical.* No one can be happy on an empty stomach. That does not mean you have to have a giant burrito three times a day to put a smile on your face, but you do need to have basic nutrition, along with adequate sleep and exercise. Going without any of these is a sure way to get yourself stalled in your pursuit of happiness.
2. *Emotional.* We all want to feel good about ourselves. We want to feel self-love and self-acceptance. Unfortunately, we may have to resist the pull of the larger culture to achieve this. For example, if we are surrounded by visual images of thin models and actors, and our genes dictate that we will never look that way, we have to work hard at rejecting such stereotypes. Happiness can come only when we can look in a mirror, and love and accept ourselves for who we are.
3. *Social.* Most people are not happy living isolated lives. Relationships with family, friends, and even pets are critical to most human beings. It is the rare individual who does not seek some feeling of belonging to something larger than himself (Figure 2–3).
4. *Mental.* People want to do good work. We want to use our brains and our abilities to contribute to the world. We want feedback telling us that we are doing just that.

2

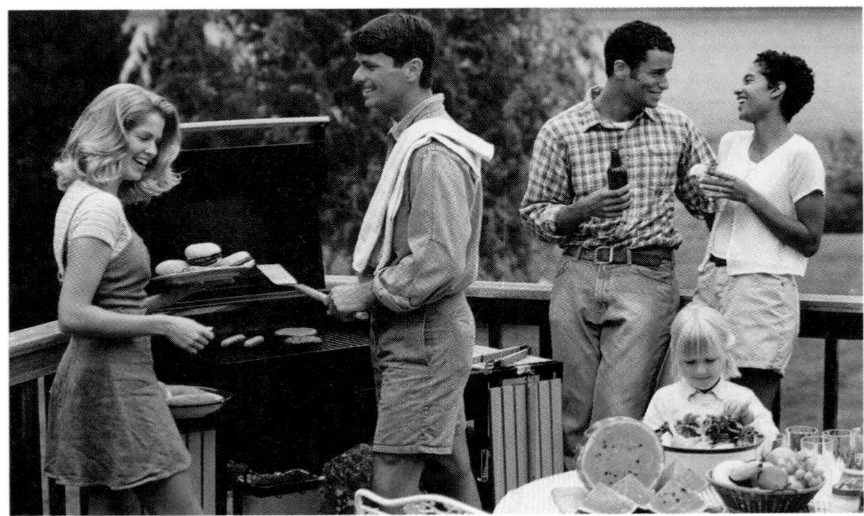

Figure 2–3 Build strong relationships.

5. *Spiritual.* Most people are able to address this final need only when they have experienced a sense of satisfaction about the other four. The spiritual need is the feeling that there is a higher truth, a pattern that gives life meaning. It may take people their entire lives to get to the point where they can begin to address this need. Better late than never, we say.

Accessing Your Creative Capability

Another self-management skill we can draw on is creativity. Creativity means having a talent like painting or acting, or having a way with hair. Creativity is also an unlimited inner resource of ideas and solutions for the many challenges we face in our lives. Creativity is not just for geniuses like Beethoven, Michelangelo, or Walt Disney. Creativity is available to the average individual who can look inward to find new ways of thinking and problem-solving. To enhance the skill of creativity, keep these guidelines in mind.

- *Stop criticizing yourself.* Criticism blocks the creative mind from exploring ideas and discovering solutions to challenges.
- *Stop asking others what to do.* This can be a way of hoping that others will motivate you instead of finding the motivation from within. This does not rule out the importance of mentors, but in the long run, being able to tap into your own creativity will be your best way to manage your own success.
- *Change your vocabulary.* Build a positive vocabulary of active problem-solving words like "explore," "analyze," "determine," "judge," "assess," and so on.
- *Do not try to go it alone.* Being creative does not mean doing everything alone. The best self-managers ask for help. They have caring family and friends, peers, a coach, or a mentor. In today's hectic and pressured world, we may find that our creativity is stimulated best in an environment in which people work together and pool ideas.

MANAGING YOUR CAREER

No matter how creative, talented, or motivated you are, as you navigate your career, you will come up against shallow spots, rocks, swift currents, and even an occasional iceberg. Knowing how to manage your career will make all the difference in staying afloat. Your career should be like a trim and sturdy boat, flexible and built for the long run.

Design a Mission Statement

Every successful business has a business plan. An essential part of this plan is the **mission statement**, that sets forth the values the business plans to live by and that establishes future goals. Individuals can have mission statements, too. If you are to succeed in life and in your work, you need a sense of purpose and a reason for being. These can be validated in a written statement. At a later point when you have secured employment, you may want to write a statement that reflects your standards of customer service. For now, however, try to prepare a mission statement in one or two sentences that communicates who you are and what you want for your life. Writing such a statement can go a long way toward helping you take command of your life.

You can write your mission statement on a 3 x 5 card on which you briefly state your commitment to do the best you can as you go through life. An example of a simple yet thoughtful statement is, "I am dedicated to pursuing a successful life with dignity, honesty, and integrity." Whatever you want for your future will be based on the mission statement you make now. It will point you in a solid direction and help you feel secure when things are not working out as you hoped they would. For reinforcement, keep a copy of your mission statement in your wallet, another in your car, one in a small frame on your desk, and still another pinned up on your wall or on your night table (Figure 2–4). You need to be able to see it every day.

When you get that first job, and think about the standards you set for your professional life, you will need a career mission statement that will define your vision. Write one that you can place on the wall or in a frame at your station that will clearly express to your clients how important your career is to you, and your service is to them. 3

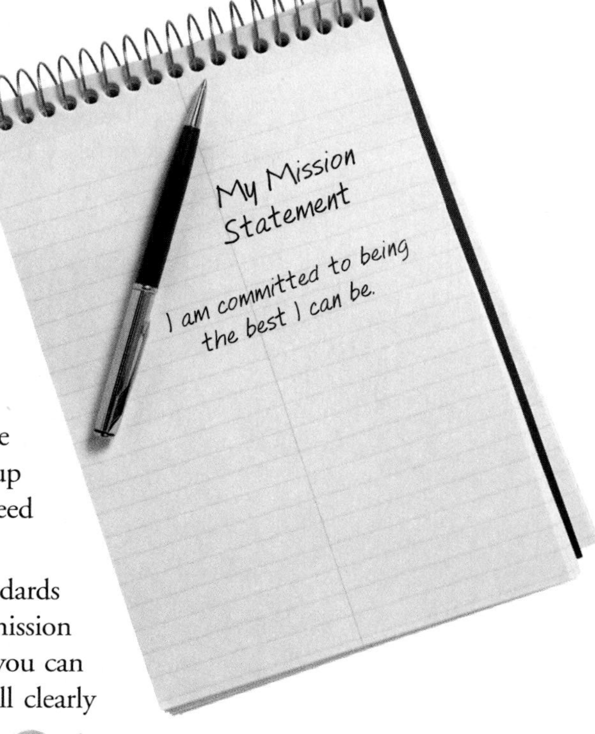

Figure 2–4 An example of a personal mission statement.

GOAL SETTING

What are you working toward at this time in your life? Can you picture your goal in your mind? Is it a little rose-covered cottage with you, your spouse, and lots of children, dogs, and cats? Is it a glamorous job in a big city with expensive cars and closets full of beautiful clothes? Is it something in between?

Some people never fix a goal in their minds. They go through life one day at a time without really deciding what it is they want, where they can find it, or how they are going to live their lives once they get it. They have no motivation, no desire, and no plan. They drift from one activity to the next with no direction. They attend classes, sometimes less than they should, and they daydream the time away. Is that you? Or are you the kind of person who has drive, desire, and a dream? If so, do you have a reasonable idea of how to go about meeting your goal?

If you were traveling to some destination you had never been to before, chances are you would arm yourself with a map. In fact, you are traveling to a place you have never been to before—the future—so why would you set out on this very important journey without some kind of map, chart, or compass to guide your way?

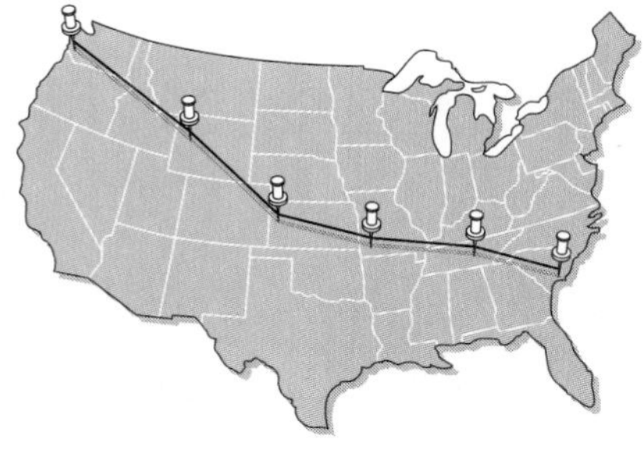

Figure 2-5 Lay out a "map" to get you to your goal.

Setting goals is like bringing along a map or a compass on a road trip. **Goal setting** helps you decide what you want out of your life. When you know what that is, then you can start to make your map. You can draw a circle around your destination and chart the best route to get you there. When you map out your goal, you will see where you need to focus your attention and what you need to learn in order to fulfill your dreams (Figure 2–5).

How Goal Setting Works

There are two types of goals: short term and long term. An example of a short-term goal is to get through a midterm exam successfully. Another short-term goal could be your graduation from cosmetology school. Short-term goals are usually those you wish to accomplish in a year at the most.

Long-term goals, on the other hand, are measured in larger sections of time such as five years, ten years, or even longer. An example of a long-term goal is telling yourself that in five years you will be a manager of a salon, or within ten years you will own a salon. Another kind of long-term goal might be to marry, have children, or live abroad.

Once you have organized your thinking around your goals, and have written some of them down in "short-term" or "long-term" columns, divide each set of goals into workable segments. In this way, reaching the goal will not seem out of sight or overwhelming. Let us use as an example the license toward which you are working. At first, the prospect of getting a license may seem to require a huge amount of time and effort. When you separate this goal into short-term goals, however, (such as going to class on time, completing homework assignments, mastering the techniques, and passing tests), you begin to see how you can accomplish each one without too much

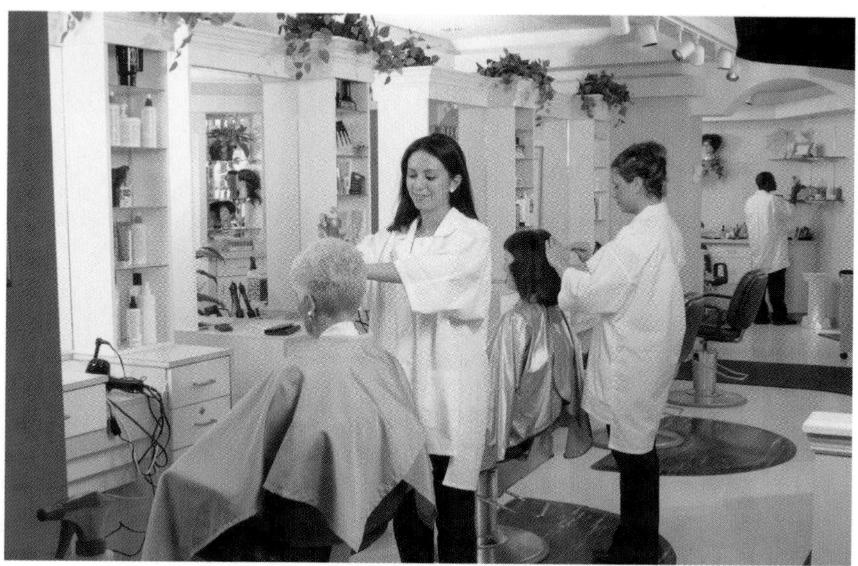

Figure 2-6 The goal.

difficulty. And off in the distance is that long-term goal you have set for yourself: acquiring a license to practice (Figure 2–6).

The important thing to remember about goal setting is to have a plan and reexamine it often to make sure you are staying on track. The most successful professionals continue to set goals for themselves, even after they have accumulated fame, fortune, and respect. They adjust their goals and action plans as they go along but never lose sight of the fact that their goals are what keep them going. 4

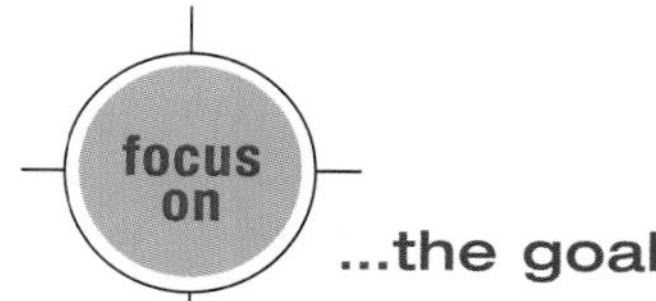

focus on ...the goal

Determine whether your goal-setting plan is a good one by asking yourself these questions:

- Are there specific skills I will need to learn in order to meet my goals?
- Is the information I need to reach my goals readily available?
- Am I comfortable asking for help?
- Would I be willing to seek out a mentor or a coach to enhance my learning?
- What is the best method or approach that will allow me to accomplish my goals?
- Am I always open to finding better ways of putting my plan into practice?

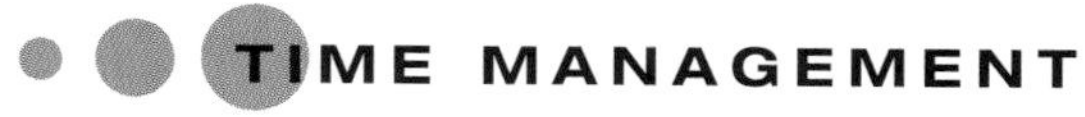

TIME MANAGEMENT

If you are familiar with racing, then you know the importance of pacing yourself. Think of reaching your goal as reaching a finish line. Pacing is so important. You must realize that it will take you time to get to that finish line, or goal, and you need to use your energy wisely. One way to do that is by managing your time as efficiently as you can.

Many experts have researched how to make time more manageable. One thing they all have noted is that every one of us has an inner organizer. When we pay attention to our natural rhythm, we can learn how to manage our time more efficiently. Here are some tips from the experts.

- Learn to **prioritize**, by making a list of tasks that need to be done in the order of most to least important.
- When you design your own time management system, make sure it will work for you. For example, if you are a person who needs a fair amount of flexibility, schedule in some blocks of unstructured time.

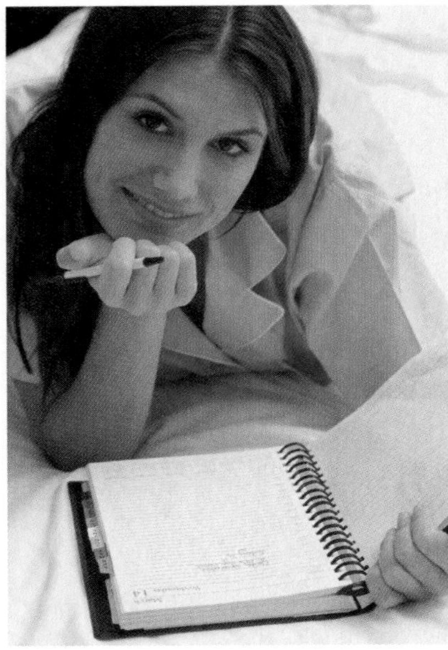

Figure 2–7 Keep a schedule for yourself and be sure to refer to it.

- Stress is counterproductive to time management. In fact, stress eats up time. For tips on how to reduce your stress, refer to Chapter 3.
- Never take on more than you can handle. Learn to say "no" firmly but kindly, and mean it. You will find it easier to complete your tasks if you limit your activities and do not spread yourself too thin.
- Learn problem-solving techniques that will save you time by uncovering solutions.
- Give yourself a time-out whenever you are frustrated, overwhelmed, irritated, worried, or feeling guilty about something. You lose valuable time and energy when you stew in your own juices. Make the time-out something that feels good: a long walk, a few moments listening to a favorite song, throwing a ball to your dog, chatting on the telephone with a friend. Whatever works. However, there may be situations, like being in the classroom, when you simply cannot get up and walk away. Handling these times can be difficult unless you learn the amazing technique of deep breathing. Just fill your lungs as much as you can and exhale slowly. You can do this without anyone noticing. After about 5 to 10 breaths, you will find you have calmed down and that your energy has been restored.
- Carry 3 x 5 cards or a memo pad with you. You never know when a good idea might strike. How often have you forgotten what you were thinking and then wasted precious time trying to remember?
- Make daily, weekly, and monthly schedules for study and exam times, and any other regular commitments. Plan at least one-hour time slots to study, then schedule greater amounts of time as needed for larger undertakings (Figure 2–7).
- Identify those times of day when you are highly energetic and those times when you just want to relax. Then plan accordingly.
- Reward yourself with a special treat for work well done and time managed efficiently. Your reward might be a fruit smoothie, a movie with friends, a nap, or any other enjoyable activity.
- Do not neglect physical activity. Remember that exercise and recreation stimulate clear thinking and planning.
- Schedule at least one block of free time a day. This will be your hedge against events that come up unexpectedly like car trouble, baby-sitting problems, and so on.
- Understand the value of to-do lists for the day or week. They can help you prioritize your tasks and activities, which is key to organizing your time efficiently (Figure 2–8).
- Make time management a habit.

To do today:
Laundry
Work out - lift weights today?
Call Marcy - set up a time to study
Ask teacher about the chemistry project!!!
Do homework 3 - 5:30
Movie tonight with Sharon and Joey

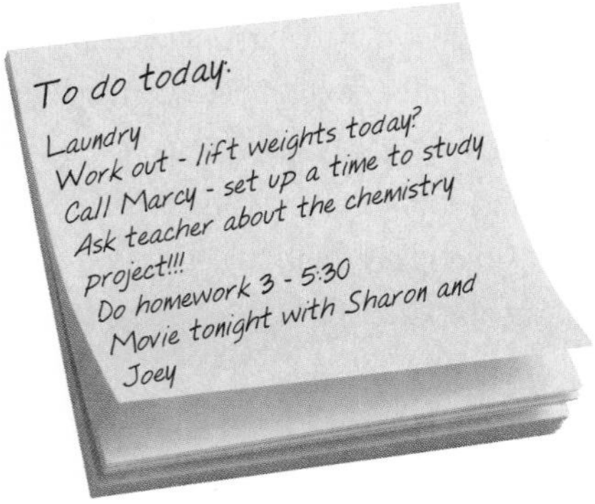

Figure 2–8 An example of a to-do list.

STUDY SKILLS

Good study skills are taught from the beginning of our schooling all the way through to the end. Some of us learn these study skills early on and have a relatively smooth time soaking up the information we are taught. Others of us, however, may never develop these skills and will always struggle with learning situations, overwhelmed by material that has to be memorized, practiced, and mastered for our future. You may be such a person, and you may be struggling right now as you try to digest and absorb this book. Nevertheless, it is vitally important to be able to apply what you have been taught, and there is no way to do that except by bringing a sense of discipline to your studies.

If you have a low tolerance for studying or paying attention in class, you need to get to the bottom of it. Perhaps you really do not think highly enough of yourself in the first place to visualize ever getting a license. Maybe you fear that you are not smart enough to get through your courses and tests. If that is the case, the first step you need to take is to focus on small tasks at a time. It's the "baby steps" approach. By building up your skills little by little, you soon will be walking.

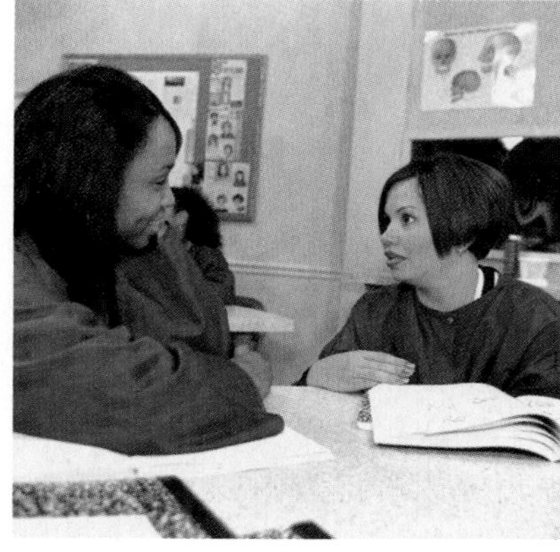

Figure 2–9 Studying with a friend is effective and fun.

For example, instead of trying to study for three hours at a stretch and suffer a personal defeat when you fold after forty minutes, set the bar lower. Tell yourself you will study for thirty minutes or even for fifteen minutes. When you achieve that goal, you will be able to pat yourself on the back instead of berating yourself.

What if you are the sort of student whose mind wanders in class? Do you find yourself thinking about dinner or Saturday night or that blouse you like over at the mall? If this sounds familiar, try writing down key words or phrases as your instructor discusses them. Then, if your mind wanders, stay after class and ask questions that are cued by what you have written down. This is not the best way to be an efficient student, but it is reasonable to think that you will get beyond this stage in time and that your mind will wander less.

Another way to get a better handle on studying is to find other students who are open to being helpful and supportive. See if you can study with them. Talk to them about the lessons you learned in class. Find out if they have any good study habits and hints that might make your life easier. Can you remember back to your summer camp days when you had a "buddy" at the pool or lakefront? The buddy was there to make sure you stayed afloat. Having a "study buddy" is another way you can make sure you stay afloat (Figure 2–9). Also, the more you discuss new material with others, the more comfortable you are liable to become with it and the more successful you will be.

Remember that every effort you make to follow through on your education is an investment in your future. The progress you make with your learning will increase your confidence and self-esteem across the board. In fact, when you have mastered a range of information and techniques, your self-esteem will soar as will your grades.

Learning Styles

One way to become better at studying is to recognize that we all have different learning styles and that it helps to know what kind of learner you are. There are four basic styles of learning. Which style feels like yours?

1. *Interactive learners.* These learners (also known as imaginative learners) do best when they can ask "Why?" They learn by watching, listening, and sharing ideas. They appreciate instructors who can involve them in the learning experience and who are supportive, sympathetic, and friendly. They like to have discussions with other students and study well with a group of people.
2. *Reader/listener learners.* These individuals (also called analytical learners) ask "What?" They learn best by reading and hearing new ideas, then mulling over information in their minds. They are eager to find the reasons for things, and are excellent at remembering facts and details. They work well with instructors who answer their questions freely and who keep them focused on the subject matter.
3. *Systematic learners.* When these learners (also called common-sense learners) sit down to study, they get more out of the information when they can connect what they are studying to real-life situations. They tend to ask "How?" They study best by themselves because they can concentrate better. Their favorite instructors are those who challenge them to "check things out," and who are down-to-earth and fair.
4. *Intuitive learners.* These learners (also known as dynamic learners) ask "What if…" They like to learn through trial and error. When they are studying, they actually want to try out what they are reading about. They appreciate instructors who understand their need to be stimulated with new ideas and who do not insist on just one way of doing something.

As you recognize your particular learning style, you can begin to apply it to your own study habits so that you can maximize your effectiveness as a student.

Setting Good Study Habits

Part of developing good, consistent study habits is knowing where, when, and how to study. Keep these pointers in mind.

When

- Start out by estimating how many hours of study you need.
- Study when you feel most energetic and motivated.
- Find odd "down" times to study like while you are waiting to see the dentist.

WHERE

- Select a quiet location where you will not be disturbed.
- Study sitting in a chair instead of lying down. Your head will stay clearer.
- Maintain a routine by studying in the same place.

HOW

- Stay focused on your reason for studying (in other words, keep your goals in mind).
- Resist distractions during those times you have set aside to study.
- Be persistent and disciplined.
- Think about tackling the tougher chapters first.
- Study in briefer time spans and give yourself short breaks in between. This keeps you fresh and you won't waste time.
- Study habits work better when you take time out to "play." Do not deprive yourself of being with friends and family.
- Remember that sleep, good nutrition, and exercise keep the brain and body in good working order.

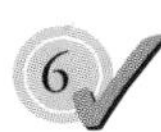

ETHICS

Ethics are the principles of good character, proper conduct, and moral judgment expressed through personality, human relation skills, and professional image. In other words, ethics are the moral principles by which we live and work. In different professions, codes of ethics are classified by boards or by commissions. In cosmetology, for example, each state board sets the ethical standards that all cosmetologists who work in that state must follow. Another way that ethics enters into your professional life is in the role you assume with your clients and fellow employees. When your actions show you are respectful, courteous, and helpful, you are behaving in a professionally ethical manner. 7

Some ethical characteristics to which you will want to aspire include honesty, compassion, attentiveness, punctuality, cooperativeness, and a pleasant and agreeable personality.

Various characteristics, principles, and values contribute to the development of a high standard of professionalism, and it can be a challenge to keep those ethics in place year after year. The one trait that is absolutely essential in order to reach and remain at the highest level of professionalism is commitment. The most ethical people make a commitment to cultivate the character traits outlined above as part of their personal and professional growth. Such people often embody the following qualities as well.

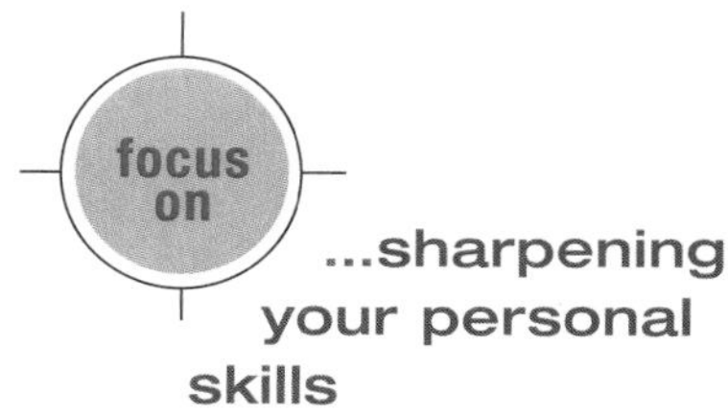

...sharpening your personal skills

Here are five ways to show that you are an ethical person:

1. Provide skilled and competent services with regard and respect for your clients.
2. Be honest, courteous, and sincere with clients.
3. Never share with others what they have told you privately.
4. Participate in ongoing education and stay on track with new information, techniques, and skills. Ethically and professionally, you have a responsibility to stay informed.
5. Always give correct information to clients about treatments and any products they may want to purchase.

2

- *Self-care.* As a cosmetologist, you will be seen as a kind of a caregiver. It is well-known that many caregivers suffer from stress and eventual burnout, largely because they focus their energy and time on their clients, often at the expense of their own needs. If you are to be truly helpful to others, it is essential that you take care of yourself. Try the Self-Care Test to see how you rate (Figure 2–10).
- *Integrity.* Maintain your integrity by making sure your behavior and actions match your values. For example, if you believe it is unethical to sell products you do not really believe in just to turn a profit, then do not do so. On the other hand, if you feel that a client needs products and additional services for healthy skin maintenance, it would be unethical *not* to give the client that information. A sense of integrity also involves not talking poorly about the client's last haircut, not "stealing" clients, and not borrowing another person's equipment or supplies. It does include endorsing your employer's price structure and other policies.
- *Discretion.* Do not share your personal problems with your clients. Nor should you *ever breach their confidentiality* by telling other people the concerns they may have shared with you. Maintain your professional boundaries and standards by standing firm in the conviction that you are a cosmetologist, not a counselor.
- *Communication.* Your responsibility and ethical behavior extend to your communication with your customers and the other people with whom

The Self-Care Test

Some people know intuitively when they need to stop, take a break, or even take a day off. Other people forget when to eat. You can judge how well you take care of yourself by noting how you feel physically, emotionally, and mentally. Here are some questions to ask yourself to see how you rate on the self-care scale.

1. Do you wait until you are exhausted before you stop working?
2. Do you forget to eat nutritious food and substitute junk food on the fly?
3. Do you say you will exercise and then put off starting a program?
4. Do you have poor sleep habits?
5. Are you constantly nagging yourself about not being good enough?
6. Are your relationships with people filled with conflict?
7. When you think about the future are you unclear about the direction you will take?
8. Do you spend most of your spare time watching TV?
9. Have you been told you are too stressed and yet you ignore these concerns?
10. Do you waste time and then get angry with yourself?

Score 5 points for each yes. A score of 0-15 says that you take pretty good care of yourself, but you would be wise to examine those questions you answered yes to. A score of 15-30 indicates that you need to rethink your priorities. A score of 30-50 is a strong statement that you are neglecting yourself and may be headed for high stress and burnout. Reviewing the suggestions in these chapters will help you get back on track.

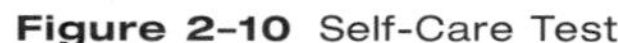

Figure 2–10 Self-Care Test.

you work. Your interactions must be clear and direct, not passive and withholding. Creating a clear line of communication with all those in your working world will serve you well.

Many people begin a career with a strong desire to fulfill their dreams and a dedication to being the best. They may be sidetracked by any number of factors, however, such as friction on the job, being overlooked for promotions, feeling undervalued or underpaid, or personal problems at home. This is called life, and it intrudes on the aspirations of us all. If you remain committed to the highest ethical principles of your profession, however, you can ride through the hard times. The respect you get from your clients and peers, and most important, from yourself, will help you stay the course.

PERSONALITY DEVELOPMENT AND ATTITUDE

Some occupations require less interaction with people than others. For example, if you are a computer programmer, you may not be exposed to all different sorts of people every day. As a cosmetologist, however, dealing with people is a major aspect of your work. It is useful, therefore, to have some sense of how personalities work.

Your personality defines who you are. It is the way you walk and talk; the way you hold your head. It includes whether you understand things quickly or need time to absorb information. Your personality is the sum total of who you are and it is what distinguishes you from other people. You can get an idea of the nature of inborn personality characteristics by watching newborn babies. One baby may be resting calmly, another may be restless, and a third crying. The very same stimulus may set off entirely different reactions from child to child based on the personality traits of each.

How do we define attitude? It can be defined as one's outlook. Attitude stems from what we believe and it can be influenced by our parents, teachers, friends, and even books and movies. We may not be able to change a characteristic with which we were born but we can change our attitude. We can tell a person's attitude by what they think, by their emotions, and by what they do. For example, Charlie, a cosmetology student, has the attitude that studying is boring. He feels frustrated when he has too much homework and sometimes goes to the movies instead. Charlie would find it easier to study if he changed his attitude. Instead of thinking that studying is boring, he could experiment by giving it another label. He could call it "challenging" and see how that impacts on his work.

You may not be able to alter your inborn characteristics but you certainly can work on your attitude. This is a process that continues throughout your life. And since no one is perfect—or ever can be—it makes no sense to strive

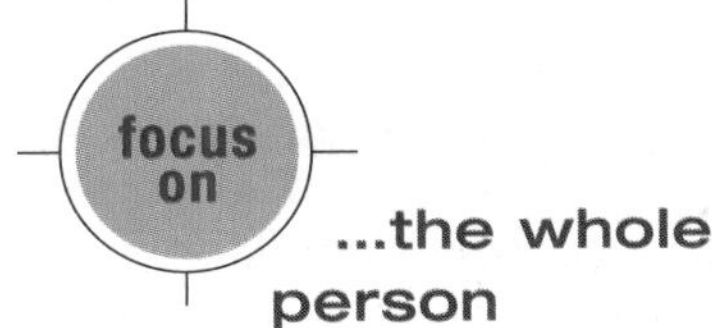

Some say that attitude is everything and that with a winning attitude, you cannot miss being a success. So ask yourself: "Am I a winner? Do I have faith in my success?" If you can answer "yes," then you may be able to create the life you want. If the answer is "no," then you have more work to do on the attitude front.

insights

Harry Comp, Jr.

There are many professional directions one can take in the world of cosmetology. Educator Harry Comp, owner of a cosmetology school in New Jersey, has chosen the right one for him.

I was born in the color room dispensary of a beauty salon. Maybe not literally, but close enough. My mom and dad were both top cosmetologists. So 44 years ago they got together and made a baby cosmetologist.

You might think I would have played the cards I was dealt and gone right into cosmetology, but I resisted it. After growing up in a household that revolved around the business, I wanted to do something else. So I went to college and focused on accounting courses. But my accounting professor didn't feel I belonged in accounting. He said I wasn't regimented enough. I was more of a people person, artistic and creative. He told me I should be an entrepreneur. At that time, I didn't know what the word "entrepreneur" meant. My professor said, "You've got to be kidding. It's a businessman." I said, "Oh, my parents are in business, but they're not entrepreneurs. They're hairdressers." He said, "If they own their own business, then they're entrepreneurs." Well, he certainly had that right.

My parents were unbelievable role models for me. They really were the top in their field. My father was a grand-prize award winner and a distributor, my mother was published, and they had a business that was like one of today's day spas.

I became a licensed hairdresser, but I wasn't behind the chair very long. Maybe three years. I wasn't very good at the technical end of it, and I didn't dedicate myself to getting better. It was always hard for me, hairdressing—it never came naturally. My hands just don't work that way. But what I really loved was the part that had to do with working with people. To get the client to come back—it excited me to have the power to do that. Every tip that you get, every referral, is just a great honor. I found I could get that kind of satisfaction, too, from working with other professionals in the field.

I might not have been such a great hairdresser, but I am really good at motivating people. My job is all about students. I love exposing future salon professionals to great ideas and great mentors. I love working with people. That inspires me the most.

for perfection. You only have to do your best. In business and in your personal life, a pleasing attitude gains more associates, clients, and friends. Refer often to the following ingredients of a healthy, well-developed attitude to see if they match your recipe.

- *Diplomacy.* Being assertive is a good thing. It helps people know where you are coming from. It is a short step, however, from behaving in an assertive manner to being aggressive and even bullying. Take your attitude temperature to see how well you practice the art of tact. Being tactful means being straightforward but not critical. That is the art of diplomacy.
- *Tone of voice.* Here is a good example of an inborn personality trait you can modify. If you happen to have a deep, gravelly voice, it is probably due to the way your vocal cords are placed. You cannot change that physical trait. However, you can soften the sounds you make. You can speak clearly. Also, if you have a positive attitude, you can deliver your words pleasantly.
- *Emotional stability.* Our emotional life is important. It is essential to have feelings and express them appropriately. But some people have no control over their feelings, and may express themselves excessively or inappropriately. When they are happy they get almost frantic, and when they are angry they fly into a rage. People feel uncomfortable around them. Learning how to handle a confrontation as well as letting people know how you feel without going overboard are life skills, and important indicators of maturity.
- *Sensitivity.* Your personality shines the most when you show concern for the feelings of others. Sensitivity is a combination of understanding, empathy, and acceptance. When you are sensitive, you are aware of how damaging criticism can be and you always offer your criticisms constructively. A person who has a sensitive personality is not a doormat. Being sensitive does not mean you have to let people take advantage of you. Being sensitive means being compassionate and responsive to other people. It is strength, not weakness.
- *Values and goals.* Neither values nor goals are inborn characteristics. We acquire these as we move through life. It is important that we do acquire them, however, as they guide us on our journey through the world. They show us how to behave and what to aim toward.
- *Receptivity.* Some people are more open and sharing than others. Some people give more freely of themselves than others do. To be receptive means to be interested in other people, and to be responsive to their opinions, feelings, and ideas. Receptivity involves taking the time to really listen instead of pretending to do so (Figure 2–11).
- *Communication skills.* A person with a warm, caring personality has an easy time talking about herself and listening to what others have to say. When such a person wants something, she can ask for it clearly and directly. When she sees that a person needs help, she can offer that help without strings attached. 8

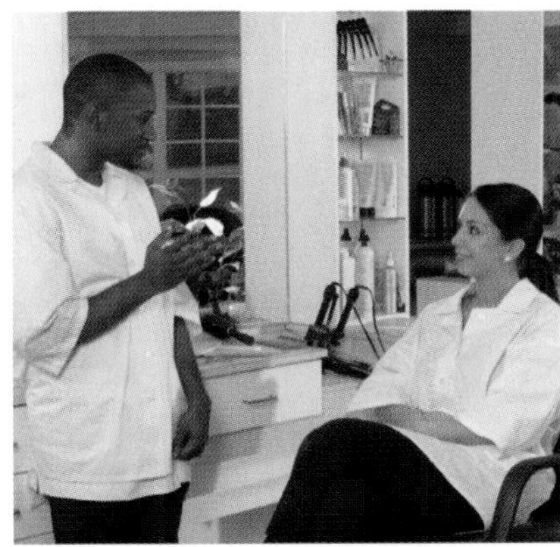

Figure 2–11 Being receptive is a good personal skill.

HUMAN RELATIONS

No matter where you work, you will not get along with everyone all the time. It is not possible to always understand what people need, even when you know them well. Even if you do think you understand what people want, you cannot always be sure that you will satisfy them. This can lead to tension and misunderstanding.

The ability to understand people is the key to operating effectively in many professions. It is especially important in cosmetology where customer service is central to success. Most of your interactions will depend on your ability to communicate successfully with a wide range of people such as your boss, your coworkers, your clients, and the different vendors who come into the salon to sell products. When you clearly understand the motives and needs of others, you are in a better position to do your job professionally and easily.

The best way to understand others is to begin with a firm understanding of yourself. When you know what makes you tick, it is easier to appreciate others and help them get what they need. Basically, we all have the same needs. When we are treated with respect and people listen to us, we feel good about them and about ourselves. When we create an atmosphere where customers and staff have confidence in us, we will get the respect we deserve. Good relationships are built on mutual respect and understanding. The next section contains a brief look at the basics of human relations, followed by some practical tips for dealing with situations you are likely to encounter.

A fundamental factor in human relations has to do with how secure we feel. When we feel secure, we are happy, calm, and confident, and we act in a cooperative and trusting manner. When we feel insecure, we become worried, anxious, overwhelmed, perhaps angry, and suspicious, and usually do not behave very well. We might be uncooperative, hostile, or withdrawn.

Human beings are social animals. When we feel secure, we like to interact with other people. We enjoy giving our opinion, we take pleasure from having people help us, and we take pride in our ability to help others. When people feel secure with us, they are a joy to be with. You can help people feel secure around you by being respectful, trustworthy, and honest.

However, no matter how secure you are, there will be times when you will be faced with people and situations that are difficult to handle. You already may have had such experiences. There are always some people who create conflict wherever they go. They can be rude, insensitive, or so full of themselves that being considerate simply does not enter their minds. Even though you may wonder how anyone could be so unfeeling, try to remember that this person at this particular time feels insecure or he wouldn't be acting this way.

To become skilled in human relations, learn to make the best of situations that could otherwise drain both your time and your energy. Here are some good ways to handle the ups and downs of human relations.

Respond instead of reacting. A fellow was asked why he didn't get angry when a driver cut him off. "Why should I let someone else dictate my emotions?" he replied. A wise fellow, don't you think? He might have even saved his own life by not reacting with "an eye for an eye" mentality. This person knows there are three ways to deal with emotions: 1) you can hold them in, 2) you can blow up, or 3) you can express them. He discovered that when he put a lid on his feelings, he got a headache. Yet when he boiled over, a fight would start. Learning that he could state calmly how he felt has made all the difference to him. One way he stays calm is to take deep breaths and tell himself that he does not have to take it personally.

Believe in yourself. When you do, you trust your judgment, uphold your own values, and stick to what you believe is right. It is easy to believe in yourself when you have a strong sense of self-worth. It comes with the knowledge that you are a good person and deserve to be successful. Believing in yourself makes you feel strong enough to handle almost any situation in a calm, helpful manner. Imagine, for example, that a client makes an unreasonable demand. When you feel secure about who you are, you do not retaliate. Instead, you quietly ask what is wrong and then try, with the client's help, to correct the problem. This does not mean that you let people walk all over you. It means that you have a strong belief in your own high standards and can relate to others appropriately.

Talk less, listen more. There is an old saying that we were given two ears and one mouth for a reason. You get a gold star in human relations when you listen more than you talk. When you are a good listener, you are fully attentive to what the other person is saying. If there is something you do not understand, ask a question to gain understanding.

Be attentive. Each client is different. Some are clear about what they want, others are aggressively demanding, and still others may be hesitant. If you have an aggressive client, instead of trying to handle it by yourself, ask your manager for advice. You will likely be told that what usually calms difficult clients down is agreeing with them, then asking what you can do to make the service more to their liking. This approach is virtually guaranteed to work (Figure 2–12).

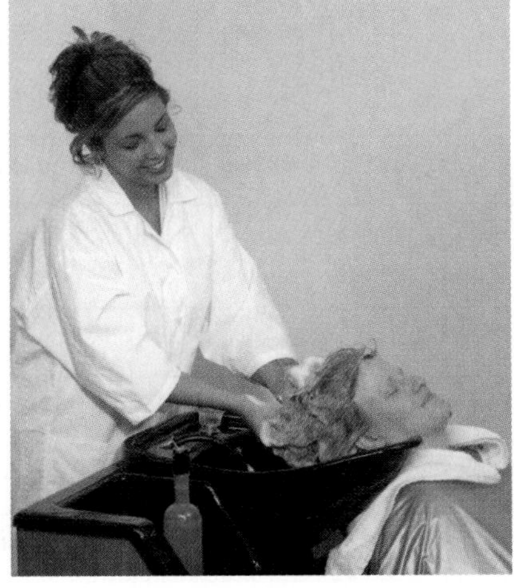

Figure 2–12 Be attentive to your client's needs.

Take your own temperature. If you are tired or upset about a personal problem, or have had an argument with a fellow student, you may be feeling down about yourself and wish you were anywhere but in school. If this feeling lasts a short time, you will be able to get back on track easily enough and there is no cause for alarm. If, however, you begin to notice certain chronic behaviors about yourself once you are in a job, pay careful attention to what is happening. Your clients may pick up your negative feelings and think you are upset with them. An important part of being in a service profession is taking care of yourself first, and resolving whatever conflicts are going on so that you can take care of your client. Trust can be lost in a second without your even knowing it. And once lost, trust is almost impossible to regain.

To conclude, human relations can be rewarding or demoralizing. It all depends on how willing you are to give.

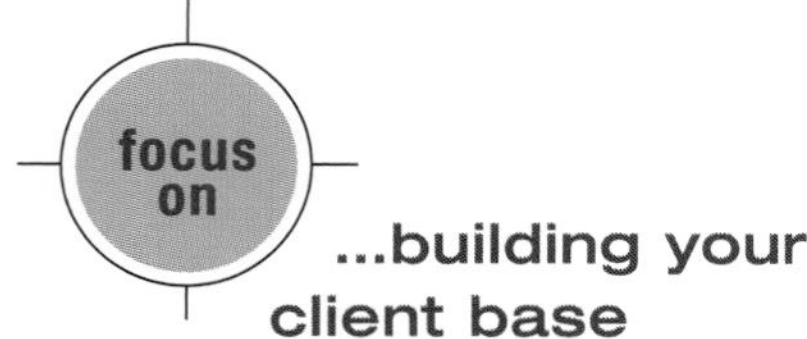

...building your client base

It is a good idea to keep track of what your clients like and dislike, and of important events in their lives. Your awareness of these details will make them feel important. Make notations on client cards about the following:

- client's birthday
- new baby
- upcoming wedding
- jobs held and job promotions

. . . or whatever else you think matters to them.

The Golden Rules of Human Relations

Keep the following guidelines in mind for a crash course in human relations that will always keep you in line and where you should be.

- Communicate from your heart; problem-solve from your head.
- A smile is worth a million times more than a sneer.
- It is easy to make an enemy; it is harder to keep a friend.
- See what happens when you ask for help instead of just reacting.
- Show people you care by listening to them and try to understand their point of view.
- Tell people how great they are (even when they are not acting so great).
- Being right is different from acting righteous.
- For every service you do for others, do something for yourself.
- Laugh often.
- Show patience with other people's flaws.
- Build shared goals; be a team player and a partner to your clients.
- Always remember that listening is the best relationship builder.

chapter glossary

compartmentalization	the capacity to keep different aspects of your mental activity separate so you can achieve greater self-control
ethics	principles of good character, proper conduct, and moral judgment, expressed through personality, human relation skills, and professional image
game plan	the conscious act of planning your life rather than just letting things happen
goal-setting	the identification of long- and short-term goals
mission statement	a statement that sets forth the values that an individual or institution lives by and that establishes future goals
perfectionism	a compulsion to do things perfectly
prioritize	to make a list of tasks that need to be done in the order of most to least important
procrastination	putting off until tomorrow what you can do today

review questions

1. How do you personally define success?
2. List and explain ten basic guidelines for personal and professional success.
3. What are three common habits that can prevent people from being productive?
4. Explain the difference between motivation and self-management.
5. What are the five basic human needs?
6. List at least three steps you can take to enhance your creativity.
7. In three to five sentences, write a mission statement for yourself.
8. List three short-term and three long-term goals you have set for yourself.
9. Why is it so important to learn how to manage your time?
10. Name and describe the different learning styles.
11. List the qualities and characteristics of professional ethics.
12. Explain the difference between personality and attitude.
13. Explain the best way to deal with an unhappy client.

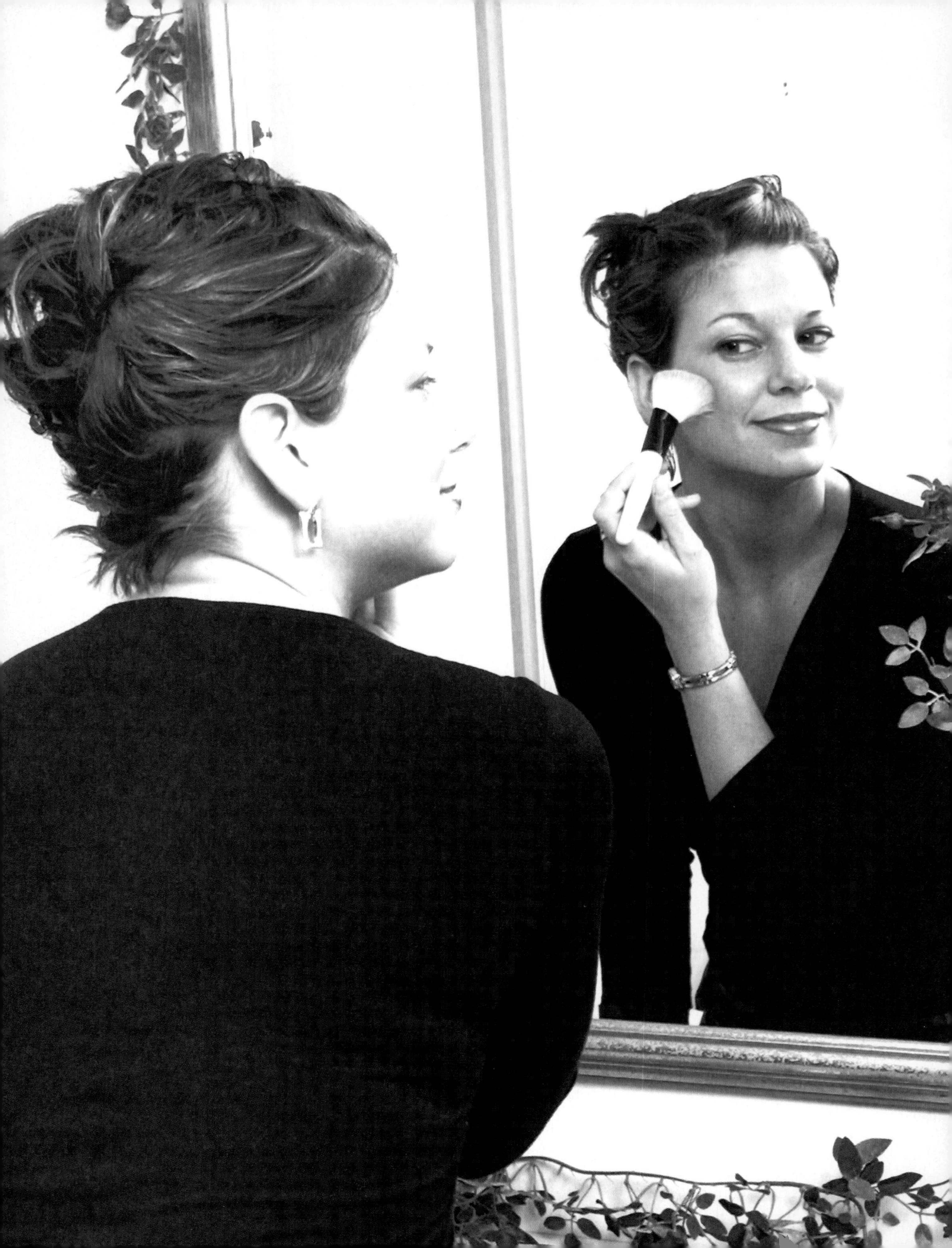

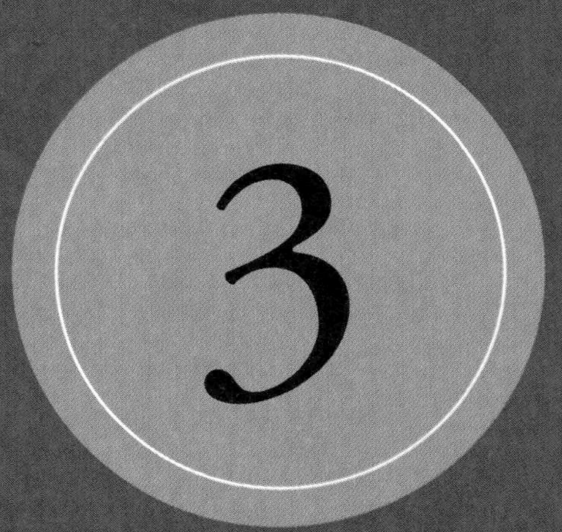

YOUR PROFESSIONAL IMAGE

Mary Beth Janssen

PRESIDENT OF THE JANSSEN SOURCE, INC., A COMPANY DEVOTED TO THE HEALING ARTS

Chapter Outline

Learning Objectives

After completing this chapter, you should be able to:

1. Explain the concept of wellness as it relates to image.
2. List the basic habits of daily personal hygiene.
3. Explain the concept of dressing for success.
4. Describe methods for reducing stress.
5. Identify the basic principles of sound nutrition and exercise.
6. Demonstrate ways to improve posture, both standing and sitting.
7. Demonstrate an understanding of ergonomic principles and ergonomically correct postures and movement.

National Skill Standards

This chapter provides you with the necessary information to master this National Industry Skill Standard for Entry-Level Cosmetologists.

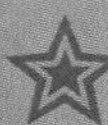

Using appropriate methods to ensure personal health and well-being.

Key Terms

Page number indicates where in the chapter the term is used

ergonomics
pg. 61

personal hygiene
pg. 49

physical presentation
pg. 58

professional image
pg. 47

stress
pg. 53

You have probably heard the expression "Image is everything." It is this belief that has traditionally driven the beauty and fashion industries, although this is now changing. Today, we are beginning to view "image" as the combination of our external appearance—how we look to the world—with who we are deep inside or how we look to ourselves.

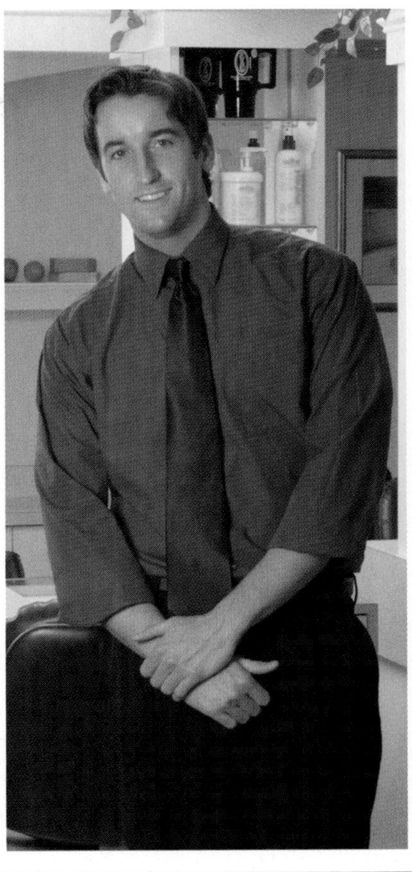

Figure 3–1 Project a professional image.

Every one of us has an image, but the problem is that our images are not necessarily the ones we hope to project. You might wish to be thought of as glamorous and sophisticated, while others actually think of you as wholesome and rather innocent. Think about the ways that people describe you. This will clue you in to your image.

Your personal image may not necessarily be the same as your professional image, but in this chapter, we are concerned with the latter. Your **professional image** is the impression you project as a person engaged in the profession of cosmetology, and consists of your outward appearance and the conduct you exhibit in the workplace. This image is extremely important. Your appearance, attitude, abilities, and energy create a mental picture in the minds of your clients and associates. You want that image to conjure up respect, trust, and eagerness for your knowledge, creativity, technical skills, and sense of style.

Your professional image is also tied into your role as a model for your clients. Do not forget that your work in the area of beauty not only helps your clients to look their best but also touches on wellness as you advise clients how to care for their hair, skin, and nails, and as you alert them to lifestyle decisions that can have an impact on their beauty concerns. That means you will need to look your best and express lifestyle choices that signify a real sense of responsibility for your own health (Figure 3–1). Keep in mind that people are coming to you so that you can make them look good. If you do not look good, your clients may assume that you cannot make them look good.

Your professional image is not one single thing. Rather, it emerges from the interaction between the external and the internal. You should strive for a holistic image, one that reflects the whole person. Your professional and personal lives need not be entirely separate from each other. If you truly know who you are and are comfortable with yourself, you will always present your authentic self at both work and play. Of course, you will probably dress and groom yourself in a more structured way at work than you would at home, and communicate with your clientele and fellow beauty professionals differently from the way you would with your mother, spouse, or best friend. Yet the person you present to the world should reflect the real you.

Most people start to develop an image by focusing on the surface. The way you dress and groom yourself is very important. However, your external appearance should reflect your authentic self. If you are essentially an informal sort of person, it might take you a while to feel comfortable in a situation that requires you to dress up and make up all the time. Your surface image also has to do with the graciousness of your speech, how pleasing your voice is, how you stand and carry yourself, and the facial expressions you show to the world. Your surface is just a reflection of what you carry inside yourself. How you feel about people and the world is reflected on your surface. Do you like people? Do you have an optimistic approach to life? When you feel whole in body, mind, and spirit, then you can present your best self to the world.

BEAUTY AND WELLNESS

With the growth of the spa culture in our profession, you will be called on more than ever before to integrate beauty and wellness. You will be providing services that make others look good and feel good. Think of yourself as a professional "toucher." That means you should have a caring and healing quality that you can transmit to others. As a cosmetologist and a beauty and wellness consultant, you are also a caregiver. As such, your first concern is to take care of yourself so that you can go on to take care of others. To do this, you must start by paying attention to your health.

Defining Health

The word "health" comes from the Old English *hal*, meaning "whole." We are at our best when all the dimensions of our selves—body, mind, and spirit—come together as a whole. When you are in good health—when body, mind, and spirit are all working together and cooperatively—you will be able to enjoy the pleasures of life and work creatively and productively. Optimal health will increase your feelings of self-worth and will add to your value in the eyes of your clients, associates, employer, and the beauty and wellness community in general. In this chapter, we will be looking at specific ways you can promote health and well-being.

Creating Balance

Real beauty begins with health, and real beauty stays grounded in health. Good health greatly impacts your energy level, your attitude, and, ultimately, your appearance. One of the most important factors in promoting and maintaining health is balance.

Balance can be hard to achieve in this day and age. For many of us, it can be a challenge to manage stress. But when in balance, we are able to make the right choices for ourselves. If you consistently undermine your well-being with poor choices, you may be leading a highly unbalanced lifestyle and putting yourself at risk for disease. Eating poorly, smoking, drinking excessively, taking drugs, skipping exercise, holding on to toxic emotions, and lacking a sense of purpose are just some of the ways in which we create a disconnect between the mind and body.

Every thought you have sets off a molecular change in your body. It is up to you to make those choices that are most life-affirming. Achieving balance in your life—between what you want for yourself and what others want for you, between work and play, between self-interest and a sensitivity to others—is the key to leading a happy and productive life.

Looking Your Best

You are probably familiar with the proverb "Clothes make the man." Wearing clothing that expresses your personal style and is also appropriate for your surroundings is key to looking your best. Your clothing is your packaging. Anybody who has ever tried to sell something knows packaging counts for a lot.

Before we get into the issue of clothing, however, let us focus on grooming, which begins with personal hygiene.

Personal Hygiene

Personal hygiene is the daily maintenance of cleanliness and healthfulness through certain sanitary practices. It is customary to learn many of these principles as a child. "Wash your hands before you sit down at the table" and "Cover your face when you sneeze" are examples. Today, as an adult, sticking to these principles will help you maintain and project your best image.

The basics of personal hygiene include:

- daily bathing or showering, shaving for men, and freshening up throughout the day as necessary (Figure 3–2).

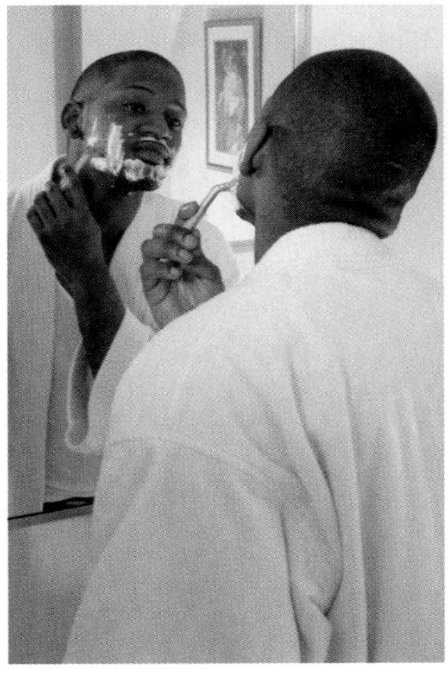

Figure 3-2 Practice personal hygiene every day.

- washing your hands throughout the day as required, such as when beginning a service with a new client or after visiting the bathroom.
- using underarm deodorant or antiperspirant.
- brushing and flossing your teeth, as well as using a mouthwash or breath mints throughout the day as needed.

Remember that offensive odors can be quite a turnoff for your clients. It can even keep them from returning. We all have different body chemistries, so while garlic on a pizza may be quickly neutralized in one person, it may linger unpleasantly in another. Similarly, one person may sweat profusely in stressful circumstances while another remains as cool as a cucumber. Be mindful of your personal hygiene. This means doing self-checks periodically during the day to make sure that everything is as it should be. If it is not, freshen up.

CAUTION

One word here concerning perfume. More and more salons and spas are establishing a no-fragrance policy on their premises. Many individuals today are sensitive or allergic to a variety of chemicals, including some of the ingredients in fragrances. Be careful in your use of perfume. Do not let it overpower you. You may enjoy your perfume selection, but your client may not.

Skin, the body's largest organ, is responsible for eliminating toxins from the system through perspiration. In order to perform its many jobs properly, the skin deserves special daily care to keep bacteria in check. Cleanse, moisturize, exfoliate, and protect your bodily and facial skin with a regular skin care regimen.

Naturally, in the line of work you have chosen, a supremely important element of your image is well-groomed hair that will serve as an advertisement for your hairstyling skills. After all, if you cannot make yourself look good, your clients may wonder how you can service them. When it comes to hair, well groomed means more than its being brushed and combed. We travel through polluted environments every day, and hair serves as a magnet for dust and dirt. If you tend to have an oily scalp, the need for scrupulous grooming is even more pressing. Dirty, greasy hair is truly unattractive, especially when it is seen on a salon professional. Shampoo and condition your hair and scalp as required to keep it fresh and clean. For most of us, this means every day. Use styling aids appropriate for your hair type and the style you are trying to achieve.

Then there are your nails. Remember to keep them clean, trimmed, and filed, both fingernails and toenails. Be meticulous about your manicure and pedicure. Nails that are uneven, chipped, or dirty project an "I don't care" attitude. Take care of hangnails immediately. Keep your hands and feet moisturized, so they will not become dry, rough, and chapped. 2

Personal Grooming

As a stylist, your poised and attractive appearance will ensure that your clients think of you as a professional. Many salon owners and managers consider appearance, personality, and poise to be just as important for success as technical knowledge and skills. So it is a good idea to take the issue of grooming quite seriously.

One of the most important aspects of good personal grooming is the careful maintenance of your wardrobe. First and foremost, your clothes must be clean, not simply free of the dirt you can see, but clean in the sense that they smell fresh. Press any clothes that require it. Periodically bleach or whiten your white items or replace them when they are yellowed or dingy. Shoes should be cleaned and polished and kept in good repair, with well-tended heels. Clothing that is torn or ripped should be mended, if possible, or reserved for some use outside the salon.

Personal Sense of Style

While we all have our own personal sense of style, it is important to note that every salon or spa has its own image and energy. The salon may be chic and glamorous, or it may be a casual and diverse neighborhood salon that is an integral part of the community. Perhaps it has a young and hip environment, attracting the teenage to twenty-something crowd. Or perhaps it is a spa that is primarily wellness-oriented.

When you are interviewing for a position, you will want to visit many salons to get a feel for their energy and image, and to determine if that energy and image are consistent with the ones you wish to project. You will also get a sense of the dress code and grooming policy of each establishment. When you interview with a given salon, inquire into their dress code and grooming policy. If a salon requires uniforms and you are simply not a uniform sort of person, you may want to look elsewhere for work. You should understand, however, that a professional image may not allow for the kind of self-expression you are used to. The workplace requires some compromise, or give-and-take, both on your part and on your employer's.

Dress for Success

At the salon, strive to have your hair, makeup, and clothing style blend harmoniously with the surroundings. Although your self-expression may be a big part of who you are, it is not always wise to have your attire become the topic of conversation with your clients or your fellow beauty professionals. If you want to go out on the weekend and wear something wild, outrageous, and/or sexy, that is your choice. But while you are employed at a place of business, you will want to consider whether your wardrobe selection expresses a professional image that is consistent with the image of the salon.

A few ideas out of the many possibilities of classic wardrobe selections could include these. For women, it might be an A-line skirt in simple muted colors with no patterns, coupled with a white or black silk T-shirt. Men can adopt a comfortable, dignified, all-purpose look by wearing a shirt and tie every day with clean, tailored khakis. These "uniforms" project the kind of professional appearance and attitude that may allow you to charge more for your services. Extremely short dresses or skirts, bare legs, exposed underarms, torn blue jeans, or faded T-shirts for men or women may be acceptable in some types of salons, but are generally not considered proper attire when you are trying to present a professional image.

To some degree, your clothing can reflect the fashions of the season with current colors, textures, skirt lengths, and so forth. Depending on your place of work, it may be allowed or even appropriate to wear "new-looking" blue jeans or T-shirts that are clean and simple. You may find yourself in a salon that caters to the art world or to young professionals. Such an environment projects a hip, modern energy, and so individualized and fashionable clothing may be worn by each individual in the salon. Just remember to "tune in" to your salon's energy and clientele so that you can make the most appropriate clothing selections (Figure 3–3).

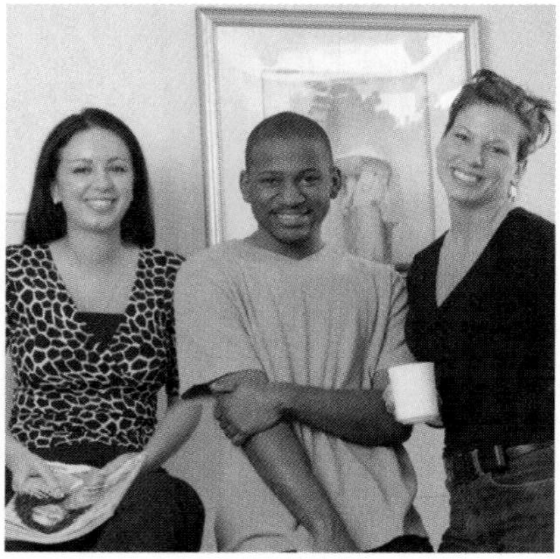

Figure 3–3 Be guided by your salon's dress code.

You should always be guided by your salon's or spa's dress code with regard to these matters, but the following guidelines are generally appropriate.

- Make sure your clothing is clean, fresh, and in proportion to your height, weight, and body shape.
- Choose clothing that is functional as well as aesthetically pleasing. It must be comfortable enough to get you through a long day, and it should be able to move with the physical demands of your job.
- Wear clean undergarments every day and keep them out of view. Underwear elastic peeking out of your pants, exposed bra straps, or the glimpse of a slip are inconsistent with the professional image you are doing your best to cultivate.
- Accessories are best kept simple and attractive, whether hair ornamentation, scarves, jewelry, belts, or ties.
- Socks or hosiery need to be free of runs, and you will want them to harmonize with your attire.
- Keep shoes clean and comfortable, and with good support. Complicated, faddish shoes and any with high heels may not be appropriate in a work setting where you may be required to stand all day.
- Because feet perspire quite heavily over the course of a day, it is a good idea to use a natural foot powder in your shoes and to alternate pairs of shoes from one day to the next, so that one pair can air out in between.

Hair Care

Just as your clothing can reflect who you really are, so can your hair and makeup choices. As with your clothing, one of your first considerations should be comfort and utility. You will want your haircut to work with your own texture and wave pattern (natural or artificial), and be easy to maintain.

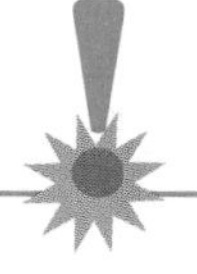

CAUTION

Always discard any unused makeup every six months and start anew. Makeup is a breeding ground for bacteria, so it is best to keep your makeup as fresh as possible. Do not share it with anyone else. Conjunctivitis, sties, and herpes are just a few of the diseases you may encounter if you share makeup.

With this in mind, trim your hair every six to eight weeks (as often as every four weeks for men), so that the line and shape of the cut looks fresh and defined. Stay abreast of hairstyles that are in fashion, both for yourself and your client. Use liquid styling tools to achieve the effect you are looking for in textural definition, volume enhancement, or contoured closeness. Light-hold gels and foams will give the hair a polished and defined edge, while keeping the hair fluid and touchable. Medium- to firmer-hold products will help you maintain your style throughout the day. Of course, your product selection will depend in large part on your hair type and condition.

Haircolor and texture services can be an important part of your personal hairstyle statement and image as well. Dimensional coloring, blonding, highlights, and gray hair coverage are enhancements you might wish to consider. Using these services on yourself will also work as an excellent advertisement to help sell these services to your clients.

A note on personal grooming for male cosmetologists: if you wear any form of facial hair, you will want to keep your beard, goatee, and/or mustache regularly trimmed.

The Art of Makeup

Makeup is an exciting realm for beauty professionals. It helps you promote your professional image and is an area where some of your most lucrative sales can be made. You will be learning the basics of makeup application while in school, but the most important point to keep in mind is that your makeup should accentuate your best features and mask your less flattering ones.

A clean, natural approach in makeup is key to presenting yourself professionally. Unless you are working in a rock and roll, punk, or Goth-oriented salon, heavily blackened eyes, blue lips, or green nail polish are generally best left to the nightlife scene. Let the salon's image guide you in how you present yourself (Figure 3–4).

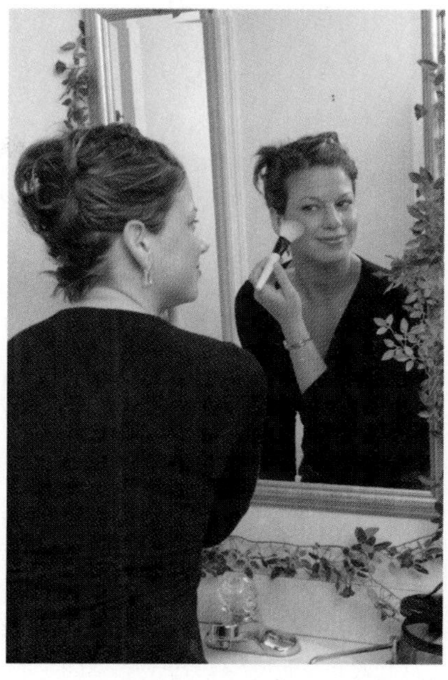

Figure 3–4 Well-applied makeup is part of a professional image.

HEALTHY MIND AND BODY

Having focused on your external appearance, let us now look at the very important issues of how to protect and sustain the inner person. The goal is to achieve and maintain optimal health so that you can be the best you can be.

Reduce Stress

Stress is so present in our lives today that the World Health Organization (WHO) has classified it as a worldwide epidemic. Stress is defined as the inability to cope with a threat, real or imagined, to our well-being that results in a series of responses and adaptations by our minds and bodies. Stress can also be thought of as any situation that causes tension. Some experts believe that up to 80 percent of visits to doctors are related to mind and/or body stress.

As you work in a salon environment (or even a spa environment whose very purpose is to reduce stress), you may often feel that you have selected a particularly stressful arena in which to work. In some ways it is true: you have. As a beauty professional, you have to deal with the high expectations of your clientele and your employer. You have to handle a wide range of personalities among clients and colleagues. You may be asked to work faster than you wish and standing on your feet all day does not help matters either.

Some individuals actually thrive on this kind of pressure whereas others may suffer. It all depends on your personality type, temperament, physical health, and on your coping skills.

For example, some of us may tend toward anxiety in a stressful situation, others may become angry, and still others may become withdrawn. Think about your own coping style when you are under pressure. Remember, in addition to the stress that comes with the workplace, there are other stressful

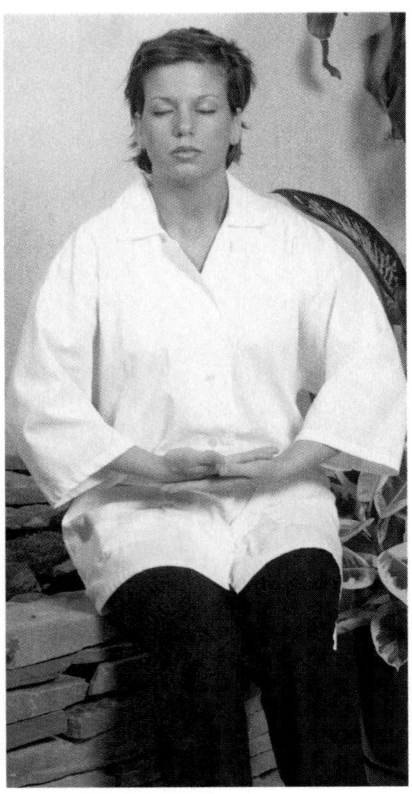

Figure 3-5 Take a few minutes to relax during the workday.

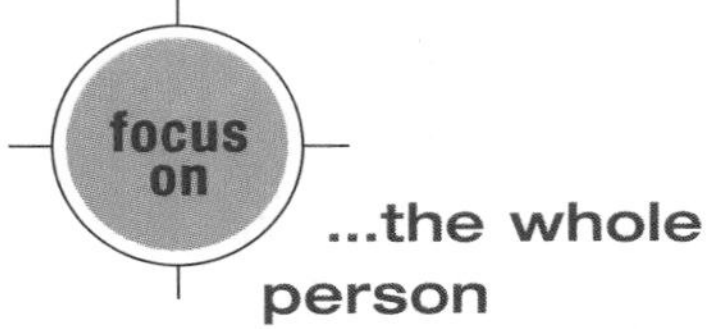

focus on ...the whole person

3 Deep breathing is a simple but very effective practice. Breathe deeply into the lungs through the nose. Your abdomen should extend outward as you inhale. When you fully exhale, the abdomen will contract inward. Try to integrate deep breathing into your day as often as possible. Deep breathing calms and energizes simultaneously. It can also lower blood pressure and is a true stress-buster!

factors that may affect your personal life, including exposure to chronically negative emotions, unhealthy relationships, and environmental toxins.

The long-term effects of chronic stress can be very damaging to the body. One way to alleviate stress is to carve out a small amount of time every day to go inward and connect with your spiritual side. Meditation, prayer, yoga, walks in nature, and positive affirmations are methods by which you can quiet the mind. Deep breathing is another technique that will help you calm down and reduce the flow of stress hormones that may be circulating through your body (Figure 3–5).

Try to establish a daily routine. This helps promote balance and stability that can give great comfort in stressful times. Try to go to bed and wake up at the same time every day if possible. Eat your meals at regular times. Try not to take on more than you can handle. Connect with nature daily. Live a life of moderation, which means eating in moderation, working in moderation, sleeping in moderation, playing in moderation, watching TV in moderation, and so on. Such practices can bring balance and harmony into your life that will be reflected in your outer appearance.

Rest and Relaxation (R and R)

One critical way to manage stress and gain wellness is to get a nurturing amount of rest every day and to build relaxation and leisure-time activities into your daily routine.

Adequate sleep is essential. Without it, you cannot expect to function efficiently. The body should be allowed to recover from the fatigue of the day's activities and replenish with a good night's sleep. During sleep, tissues and organs are rebuilt and renewed. The amount of sleep needed to feel refreshed varies from person to person. However, medical professionals recommend at least seven to eight hours of sleep every night. For those who are particularly stressed, going to bed before 10 P.M. will normalize levels of stress hormones.

In addition to sleep, renew yourself with relaxation. Relaxation represents a very important change of pace from your day-to-day routine. Taking in a movie, going to a museum, reading a book, seeing friends and family, biking or walking, dancing, and even watching a bit of TV (not too much, though) are all ways for you to "get away from it all." When you return to work, you will feel refreshed and eager to face the work at hand. Taking a few long weekends and yearly vacations is essential as well. This is 4
part of living a balanced, joyful life.

Nutrition

Like stress reduction, good nutrition is a vital factor in your overall health picture. Food serves as fuel for our body by providing energy. It also provides the raw material that renews and repairs our body's tissues and organs. The Surgeon General has said that 70 percent of all disease is related to deficiencies in our diet, and the National Academy of Sciences tells us that 30 percent of all cancer is diet-related. Every day, researchers discover chemical constituents in whole, nutritious foods that can help stave off a wide variety of illnesses.

insights

ANGIE CRANOR

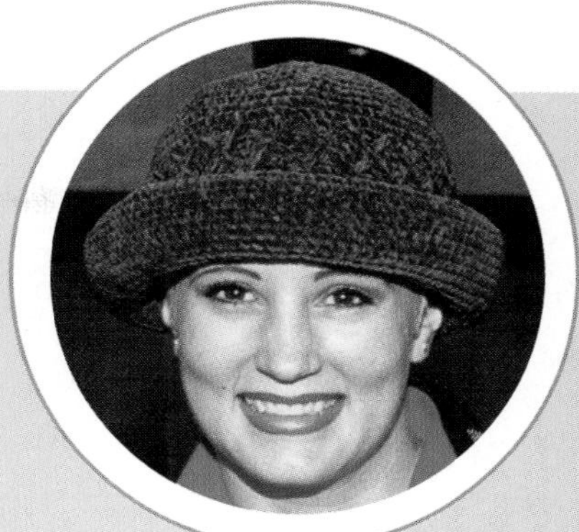

Each path has its obstacles, some harder than others. But Angie Cranor has yet to encounter one she can't get over.

I was in a car accident when I was 16. Luckily, I have full mobility of my upper body, so I set out to become a cosmetologist. At first, it was a dream of mine to prove that I could do this being in a wheelchair and all. But when I got to school—the Von Curtis Academy in Provo, Utah—I fell in love with the people and the place. I just realized that what I really wanted to do in life was to become a hairdresser. As it turned out, my love of hairdressing was really a greater motivation than proving something to myself or anyone else. But it was hard. Getting through school and keeping up on worksheets and everything like that—that was hard.

My instructor, Brennan Claybaugh, was a great role model. He would just sit himself down in my wheelchair and figure out a way for me to do things. A positive attitude goes a long way. I think that if you want to be successful as a cosmetologist you need to be organized, you need to take the time and spend the money to continue your education, and you need to have a positive attitude.

For me, once I'm in the salon, it's all about the client, no one else. The way to build up a loyal client base is to be honest and to keep up with your customers—call them to see how their hair is or if they need anything. I love being able to help people feel better about themselves. What gives me the most pleasure is that I'm able to give back to the community in a lot of ways. I feel like everyone is doing so much for me, and this is my way to give back to them.

I worked at a salon in Provo for about seven months, and while I was there, I remember telling myself that I could do this. I wanted to have my own business. I wanted to take that step and try it and be out on my own and see how that would work. So now I have my own salon. At the moment, it's just me. Of course we've had to make certain adjustments—for instance, my dad made a chair for me that was lower than standard—but it's going well. I have about 15 to 20 clients Monday through Friday, doing everything from cuts to color. I try to make the atmosphere upbeat and happy. I want people to feel really good and excited when they come here—as excited and good as I feel.

There is great truth in the old adage "We are what we eat." There are 40 specific nutrients in our food that fall into the categories of carbohydrates, proteins, fats, vitamins, minerals, and water. All of these are part of a healthy diet. People vary, however, in the way they use these nutrients according to their height and weight, level of activity, and metabolism.

Some basic guidelines for good nutrition include:

- eating a diet of nutrient-packed, whole (preferably organic) foods whenever possible. That means plenty of fruits and vegetables, beans, and whole grains.
- eating a wide variety of foods to optimize your nutritional intake. Broaden your food horizons. Experiment. And, whatever you do, try not to make fast foods a habit. They tend to be packed with salt, sugars, and fat. Use sugar, salt or sodium, and alcohol only in moderation.
- maintaining a healthy weight. Eat sensible portions, take your meals in a calm environment if possible, and chew each bite of food thoroughly. Do not eat when you are not hungry. Too many of us try to relieve stress by turning to food. Excessive eating at such times and the guilt that can result from such eating often aggravate our stress.
- staying hydrated. This is very important. Drink plenty of water every day, eight 8-ounce glasses at minimum. Take a large container of water with you to work if necessary. Our bodies are made up of 60 to 70 percent water, that is responsible for a wide variety of metabolic functions. It also oxygenates your blood and gives you energy.

Did you know...

When you smile, a number of physiological changes take place. Laughter can rev up your immune system, lower your blood pressure, and help you sleep better. Laughing is good for the soul, whether at work or at play.

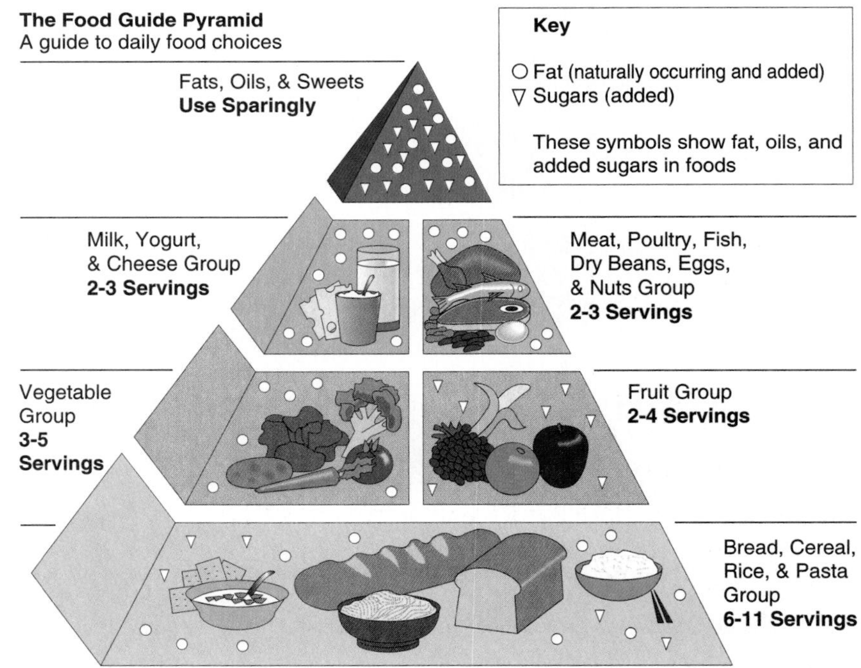

Figure 3-6 Food Guide Pyramid.

The Food Guide Pyramid, developed by the U.S. Department of Agriculture (USDA), is an efficient guide to selecting nutritious foods. The pyramid is divided into tiers, or levels. The bottom tier consists of bread, cereal, rice, and pasta (6 to 11 servings are recommended per day). Tier two is fruits and vegetables (3 to 5 servings of vegetables and 2 to 4 servings of fruits per day). Tier three includes meat, poultry, fish, dry beans, eggs, and nuts (2 to 3 servings per day), as well as milk, yogurt, and cheese (2 to 3 servings daily). The fats, oils, and sweets at the top of the pyramid should make up only a small part of a healthy diet (Figure 3–6).

The best way to take charge of your diet and ensure proper nutrition is by preparing your own meals, including those you have during the workday. Try bringing healthful lunches and snacks to work. You will save money and you will be getting wholesome and energizing food as well. The following discussion of the various food groups will help us understand what our bodies need.

- *Fats.* It is important to understand that there are good fats and bad fats. Saturated and hydrogenated fats, found in junk foods as well as red meats, whole-milk dairy, butter, and processed foods should be restricted in any diet. Fats from nuts, seeds, grains, fish, and liquid oils (olive, canola, peanut, and other vegetable oils) are a healthier choice. A no-fat or extremely low-fat diet can be detrimental to your health. Instead, try to make sure your fat calories come from healthy sources and comprise no more than 30 percent of your diet.
- *Carbohydrates.* The USDA Food Pyramid advises 6 to 11 servings of grain-based carbohydrates a day. Whole-grain foods are considered more desirable in a healthy diet than refined foods. Whole-grain foods are digested more slowly, promote long-term health, and may provide some protection from diabetes, heart disease, certain cancers, and gastrointestinal problems. Excellent sources include brown rice, whole-grain breads, oatmeal, kasha and buckwheat, barley, and more.
- *Protein.* Although the USDA Food Pyramid advocates a daily protein intake, some of the recommended protein sources are now considered undesirable when consumed in large quantities, specifically red meats. Healthy alternative protein sources include beans and nuts, fish, poultry, and eggs.
- A diet rich in fruits and vegetables can help lower blood pressure, decrease chances of having heart disease or stroke, provide protection against certain types of cancer and gastrointestinal problems, and reduce the severity of age-related problems such as cataracts.

Get Up and Go

While good nutrition is vital to our overall well-being, the importance of regular physical activity cannot be overemphasized. If nothing else, the physical aspect of salon work can be intense, and you will need to be in shape to meets these demands. Therefore, it is essential that you begin a fitness program of some sort.

?

Did you know...

Most of us have heard of the USDA Food Guide Pyramid, but did you know there are other food pyramids you may find more appealing? Some of these alternatives reflect healthful eating habits from cultures around the world (Asian, Mediterranean, or Latin American). Some pyramids emphasize seafood whereas others are based on a vegetarian diet. Still others address specific health problems. Whatever pyramid you decide to "climb" depends largely on your nutritional goals, your lifestyle, and your taste buds.

An adequate amount of physical activity ensures the proper functioning of organs such as the heart and lungs, strengthens muscles and bones, enhances immune function, and improves circulation. Improved cardiovascular and respiratory functioning will result in the enhanced transport of oxygen and nutrients to every cell in the body and facilitates the movement of carbon dioxide and waste products from body tissues into the bloodstream and on into the excretory organs.

Did you know...

Physical exercise is a great way to relieve stress. Going for a vigorous walk or a run on a track or treadmill, biking or swimming, or doing aerobic dancing is valuable personal time during which you can put aside the demands of your work. This is one reason it is relaxing. It has beneficial physiological effects. One exercise session can generate up to two hours of the relaxation response, or what is called the "endorphin high."

A Sound Fitness Program

The optimal fitness program includes three main areas of activity.

1. Aerobic activity that includes brisk walking, jogging, swimming, biking, cross-country skiing, and dancing. This activity pays off in cardiovascular health, increased immune system function, greater endurance, stress reduction, and overall improved quality of life. Start your program with a brisk 20-minute walk before work or in the middle of the day and see the difference it makes in your energy level.
2. Stretching activities to enhance flexibility. Stretching movements (no bouncing!) ease physical tension, improve range of bodily motion and agility, and act as a warm-up or cool-down from aerobic activity. Stretching activities may include yoga or tai chi, forms of movement that connect the mind-body with its energy source. Try to build stretching movements into the workday, even after every client. All it takes is a few stretches done in less than a minute, and the payoff can be immense (Figure 3–7).
3. Weight-bearing activities to build strength and endurance. In building muscle, you develop a leaner, fat-burning body, and help to prevent osteoporosis. Consider a program that includes the use of free weights or weight machines. Brisk walking and yoga can also provide weight-bearing benefits.

A good, attainable goal is to have no fewer than three 30-minute sessions of aerobic activity a week. Ideally, though, it is best to make exercise a part of your daily routine. Long walks, stretching, and light weightlifting will do wonders. If you have been sedentary, consult your doctor before beginning a regular physical activity program. 5

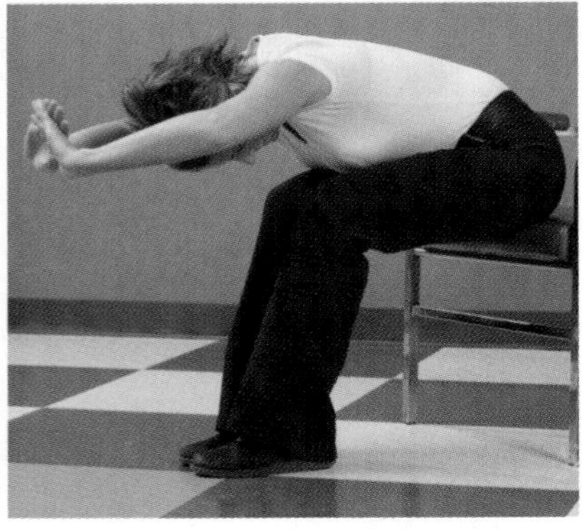

Figure 3–7 Stretching is good for muscles and joints.

YOUR PHYSICAL PRESENTATION

Another important aspect of professional image is what is called **physical presentation.** To a large degree, your physical presentation is made up of your posture, walk, and movements. Do you stand straight or do you slouch? Do you walk confidently with your head held high or do you scuffle along, stooped over, dragging your feet? Your physical presentation enhances or detracts from your attractiveness and is also an important part of your well-being. Unhealthy or defective body postures can cause a number of physical problems, particularly when these postures become habit.

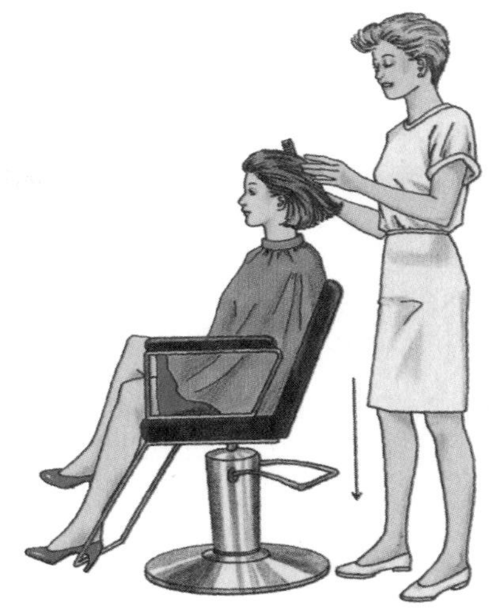

Figure 3–8 Good physical presentation.

Posture

Good posture is a very important part of your physical presentation. It shows off your figure to its best advantage and conveys an image of confidence. It can also prevent fatigue and many other physical problems. When you work as a professional cosmetologist, you spend a large amount of your time on your feet, and good posture will prove to be one of your best aids to get you through the day.

Good posture should be developed as early in your lifetime as possible, then reinforced through self-awareness and regular physical activity. Yoga is particularly helpful in creating and maintaining correct bodily alignment. Any type of accident, even a small one, should be addressed with appropriate physical or movement therapies. If accidents and traumas are not addressed, the resulting "incorrect" bodily adaptation can lead to chronic physical alignment problems.

Some guidelines for achieving and maintaining good standing posture are:

- keeping your head up and chin level with the floor.
- keeping the neck elongated and balanced directly above the shoulders.
- lifting your upper body so that your chest is out and up (do not slouch).
- holding your shoulders level and relaxed, not scrunched up.
- standing with your spine straight, not curved laterally or swayed from front to back.
- pulling your abdomen in so that it is flat.
- keeping your hips level (horizontally), making sure they do not protrude forward or back.
- flexing your knees slightly and positioning them over your feet (Figure 3–8).

Correct Sitting Posture

To sit down comfortably and attractively, use your thigh muscles and support from your hands and arms to lower your body smoothly into a chair. Do not fall or flop into the chair. This can worsen an already sloppy posture. When lowering your body, keep your back straight. Do not bend at the waist or reach with the buttocks. When seated, slide to the back of the chair by placing both hands on the front edge of the chair at the sides of your hips. Raise your body slightly and slide back. Do not wiggle or inch back (Figure 3–9).

3

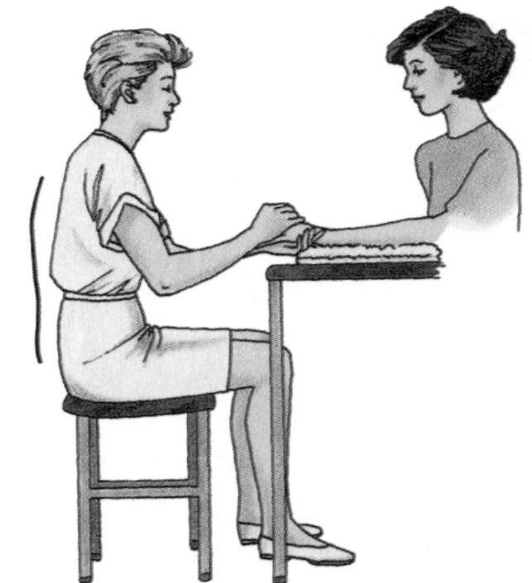

Figure 3–9 Proper sitting posture.

When giving a manicure or a facial, sit with the lower back against the chair, leaning slightly forward. If a stool is used, sit on the entire stool. Keep your chest up and rest your body weight on the full length of your thighs.

Some tips for a proper sitting position include:

- keeping your back straight.
- keeping the soles of the feet entirely on the floor.

- not crossing your legs or your feet at the ankles.
- not bending forward from the waist or stooping forward from the shoulder. Bend from the hips, or sit on a chair or wedge-shaped cushion that tilts forward. 6

Care of the Feet

On average, your feet will carry you more than 115,000 miles in your lifetime. Such faithful servants deserve to be treated with care and attention. But the fact is that most people do not spend a lot of time thinking about their feet until they begin to hurt. The human foot is a complex creation. It contains 26 bones, 20 muscles, and 114 ligaments. Therein lies the potential for many foot problems.

As a cosmetologist, you will no doubt be spending a great deal of time on your feet. Proper foot care will help you maintain good posture and a cheerful attitude. Sore feet and/or ill-fitting shoes can cause great discomfort that will, in turn, affect your posture and well-being.

Shoes

Foot and leg problems generally stem from wearing improper shoes and standing for long periods, particularly on hard floors. High heels are particularly bad for you, whether they are chunky or narrow. Scientists have found that both types of heels apply pressure to the knees. High heels throw off your center of gravity, creating or aggravating a variety of musculoskeletal problems, including back and knee pain and arthritis (Figure 3–10).

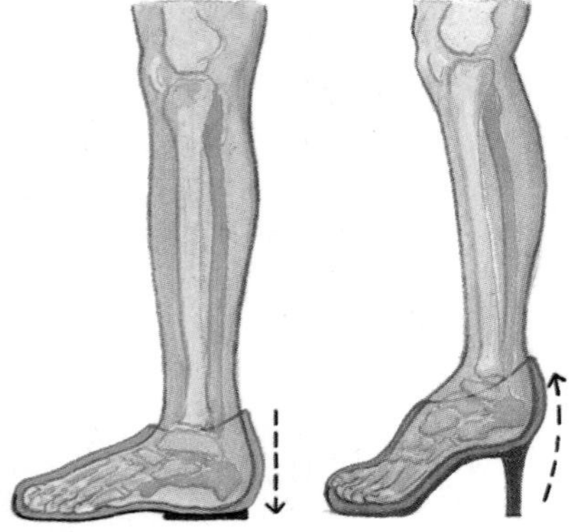

Figure 3–10 Working in high heels can throw off the body's balance.

For your work, wear low-heeled, wider shoes that spread shock absorption on the foot and give the toes more room. These shoes will give you the support and balance that will help maintain good posture and offset fatigue. Carpeted or cushioned surfaces also help alleviate stress to the foot. Cushioned mats made specifically for the purpose of reducing fatigue are available for use in salons.

Daily Foot Care

Exercise, massage, and comfortable, well-fitting shoes encourage healthy blood circulation to the feet. Give your feet some tender loving care by massaging them for a few minutes with oil or lotion before showering. Afterwards, thoroughly dry the feet, especially between the toes, and apply an antiseptic foot lotion or a natural foot powder. Try massaging your feet with a moisturizing lotion or oil before going to bed at night. Slip on cotton socks to preserve the moisturizing effect.

Regular pedicures are well worth the investment. A pedicure that includes cleansing, removal of callused skin, massage, and toenail trims will keep your feet at their best. Also, make an effort to put your feet up at intervals throughout the day. This will give the vascular system in the legs a much-needed rest, however brief, and may help prevent varicose veins.

Ergonomics

Each year, hundreds of workers, including cosmetologists, report musculoskeletal disorders (MSDs), including carpal tunnel syndrome, tendonitis, and back injuries. Beauty professionals expose their bodies to potential injury on a daily basis. They have to stand all day and hold their bodies in unnatural positions for long periods of time. They are particularly susceptible to problems of the hands, wrists, shoulders, neck, back (the entire spinal column), feet, and legs. If not attended to, these problems may become serious, sometimes so much so that a person can no longer work.

Prevention is the key to alleviating these problems. It is very important that you fit your work to your body and not your body to your work. An awareness of your body posture and movements, coupled with better work habits and proper tools and equipment, will enhance your health and comfort. An understanding of ergonomics is useful as well. **Ergonomics** is the study of human characteristics for the specific work environment. It attempts to "fit the job to the person." The principles of ergonomics are being applied in more and more workplaces.

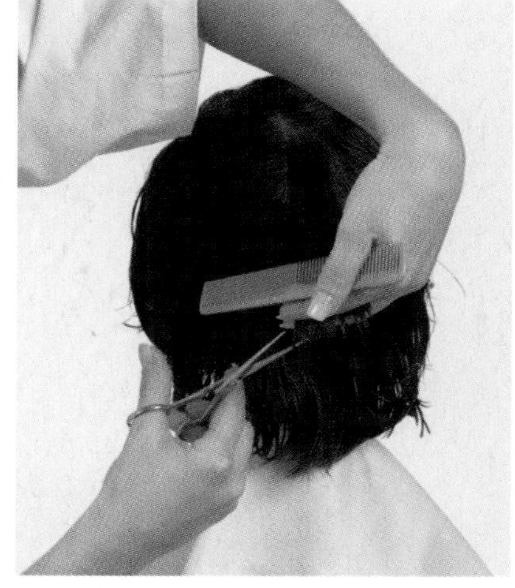

Figure 3–11 Improper haircutting position.

Monitor yourself as you work to see if you are:

- gripping or squeezing implements too tightly.
- bending the wrist up or down constantly when cutting the hair, using a blow-dryer, or using a round brush.
- holding your arms away from your body as you work, or holding your elbows above a 60-degree angle outward from your body for extended periods of time (Figure 3–11).
- bending forward and/or twisting your body to get closer to your client or to reach for something, a position that results in neck or back strain.
- standing for long periods of time in ill-fitting shoes that can lead to leg and back fatigue.

Try these measures to avoid some of the problems discussed above.

- Adjust the height of the client's chair so that the client's head is at a comfortable working level. Swivel the chair as often as necessary to maintain a comfortable arm and back position.
- Gently tilt the client's head as necessary during any hair services.
- During haircutting and other hair services, keep your wrists in a straight or neutral position as much as possible (Figure 3–12).
- Keep your shears sharpened and lubricated.
- Try holding the blow-dryer sideways to avoid raising your arms above shoulder level.
- Use your fingers rather than your wrist when handling the round brush. Use curling irons with a revolving base.
- Keep your back straight. Bend at the hips or knees, especially when picking up an object. Bending over at the waist leads to back strain and possible back injury.
- Try placing one foot on a small stool if you must stand for long periods of time. Alternate feet as necessary. Standing on a cushioned mat also helps prevent muscle fatigue.

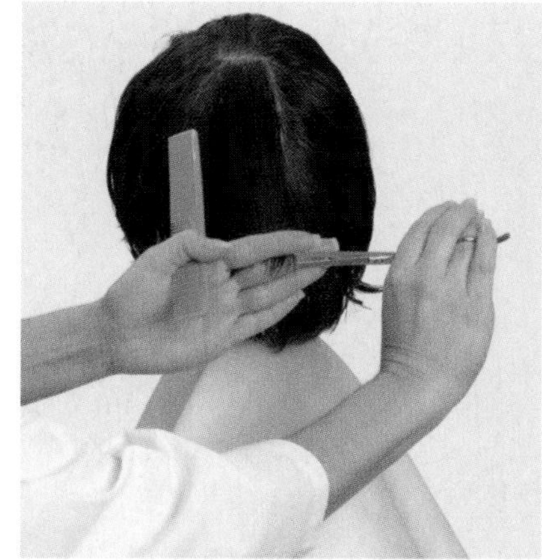

Figure 3–12 Correct wrist and hand position for haircutting.

- If possible, use a cutting stool and adjust as needed.
- Wear comfortable, well-fitting, low-heeled shoes with good arch supports. If you have flat feet or overly high arches, try wearing orthopedic inserts (available at most drugstores).
- When giving a manicure, avoid reaching across the manicure table and gripping the client's hand. Instead, have the client extend his or her hand across the table to you (Figure 3–13).
- When giving a pedicure, keep your back straight, whether you are sitting on a low stool or kneeling on the floor. Keep your wrists in a neutral position as much as possible.

Your work environment would likely benefit from an ergonomic assessment. Evaluate your workstation according to these criteria.

- Workstations should have adequate space between them so that you and your coworkers do not have to worry about bumping into each other.
- Cabinets should be easy to reach. A "rollabout" is a good place to keep implements close at hand.
- There are cutting shears and other implements available that make it easier to maintain a relatively neutral hand and wrist position for a variety of cutting elevations.
- Free-standing shampoo bowls are an excellent investment for a salon or spa. The shampoo is done from behind the client instead of from the side, which is a safer position and which can help stylists avoid back problems.

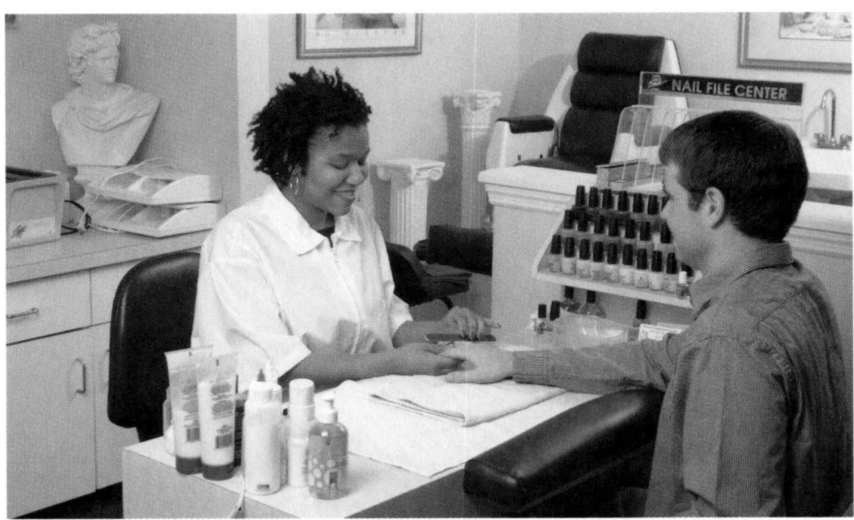

Figure 3–13 Follow proper ergonomic technique when giving nail services.

- Hydraulic chairs that can be raised or lowered at least five inches are highly recommended.
- Manicure tables with armrests for the wrists allow you to keep your knuckles below your wrists as you work.
- Facial chairs should be adjustable for height.

If you work in an environment that has any physical discomfort built into it, as most of us do, try to counter the problem by including regular stretching intervals in your schedule to break up the repetitiveness of the motions you use. 7

IMAGINE THIS

Imagine an image. It is your image. You are committed to your personal wellness. You are consistently well groomed and suitably dressed for your work. You eat well, know how to handle stress, and have an ongoing program to keep yourself fit. You know the tricks of the trade to prevent repetitive work motions from taking their toll.

An impossible fantasy? Hardly. Everything we have asked you to imagine is within your reach. Your image is yours to create and define, and once you move into it, you will see your professional life grow and flourish.

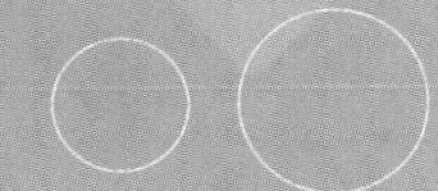

chapter glossary

ergonomics	the study of human characteristics related to the specific work environment
personal hygiene	daily maintenance of cleanliness and healthfulness through certain sanitary practices
physical presentation	a person's physical posture, walk, and movements
professional image	the impression projected by a person engaged in any profession, consisting of outward appearance and conduct exhibited in the workplace
stress	the inability to cope with a threat, real or imagined, to our well-being, which results in a series of responses and adaptations by our minds and bodies; a situation that causes tension

review questions

1. Define image. List the elements of professional image.
2. How does balance relate to good health?
3. List and describe three basic habits of personal hygiene.
4. List the general guidelines of dressing for success.
5. What are some methods the cosmetologist can use to reduce stress?
6. List basic guidelines for a sound nutritional program.
7. Why are adequate rest and sleep important for good health?
8. What are the benefits of regular exercise?
9. Name the three different kinds of exercise that should be part of your exercise program.
10. What is the role of posture in good health?
11. Assess your own standing and sitting posture. How can it be improved?
12. List ergonomic guidelines for hair and nail services.

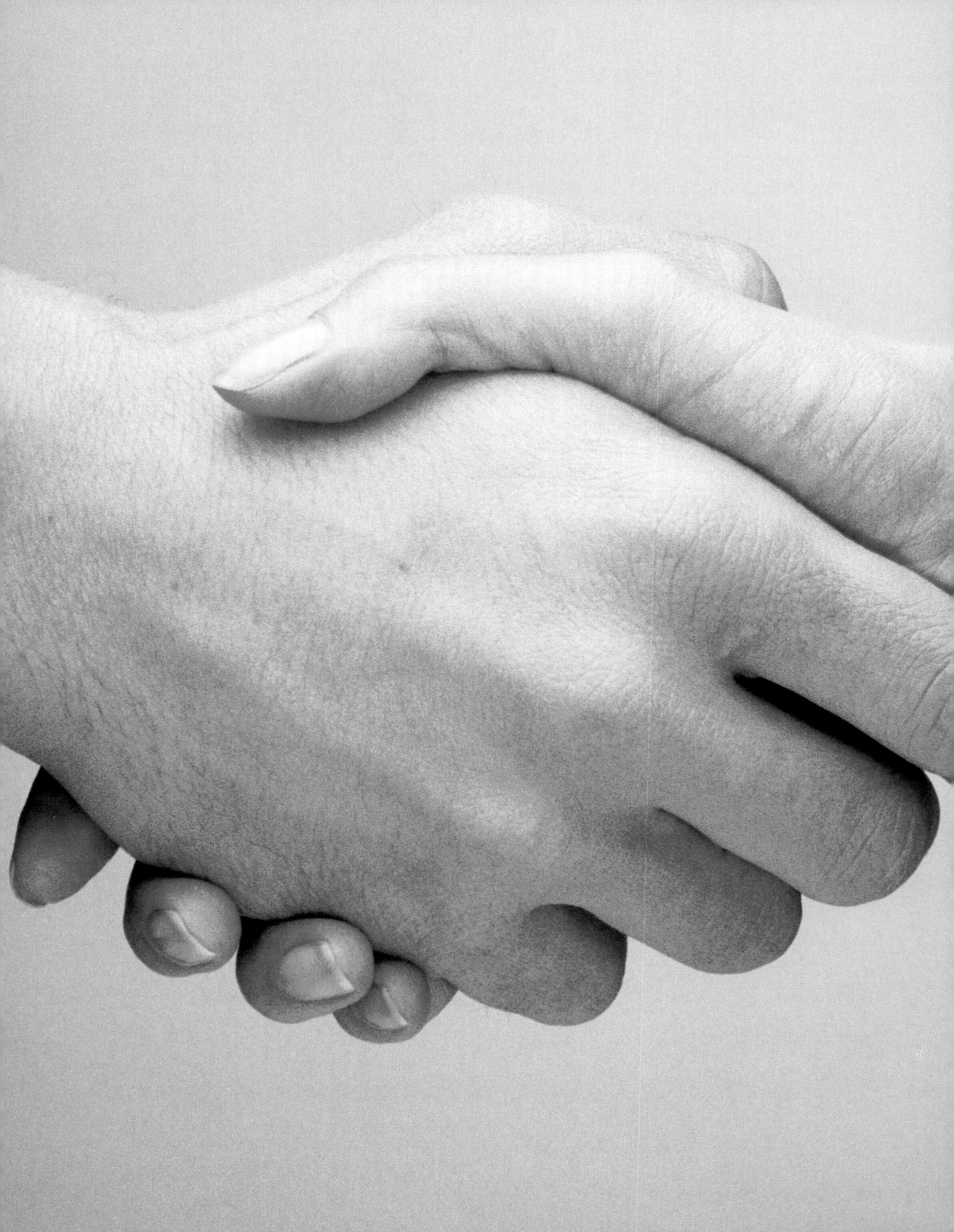

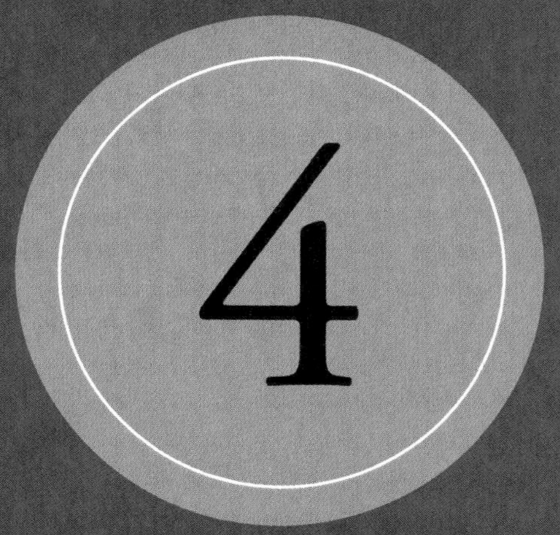

COMMUNICATING FOR SUCCESS

Catherine Frangie
BEAUTY INDUSTRY CONSULTANT

Chapter Outline

Communication Basics • The Client Consultation
Special Issues in Communication • In-Salon Communication

Learning Objectives

After completing this chapter, you should be able to:

1. Explain the basic processes of effective communication.
2. Assess a client's needs based on the "total look" concept.
3. Conduct a successful client consultation.
4. Handle delicate communication with your clients.
5. Build open lines of communication with coworkers and salon managers.

National Skill Standards

This chapter provides you with the necessary information to master these National Industry Skill Standards for Entry-Level Cosmetologists:

Consulting with clients to determine their needs and preferences as they relate to cosmetology services.

Interacting effectively with coworkers as part of a team.

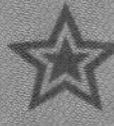
Taking the necessary steps to develop and retain clients.

Key Terms

Page number indicates where in the chapter the term is used

articulate
pg. 70

clarify
pg. 70

client consultation
pg. 72

communication
pg. 69

reflective listening
pg. 71

Are you very gifted when it comes to the technical skills that are such an important part of cosmetology? Do you possess a creative flair that sets you apart from your peers? If the answer to either of these two questions is yes, then we congratulate you. You should realize, however, that your skills and flair will only take you so far in this business. Your ability to form satisfying relationships with your customers is the key factor that will determine if cosmetology will be just a job or a fulfilling career. And this ability depends, in large part, on how well you develop your powers of communication.

Communication is your way of ensuring that you understand perfectly the needs, wants, and desires of the people around you. And since communication is a two-way street, it also ensures that your clients will understand your ideas and suggestions as well. Good communicators get and keep good jobs. Good communicators get and keep clients, too. Clients can go virtually anywhere and get good service, but they stay with stylists who create the best atmosphere, treat them with respect, and have honed their interpersonal skills. That is the way it is in this business, as in most businesses, and it is important to know that from the beginning.

COMMUNICATION BASICS

Cosmetologists need to become familiar with many processes, including cutting, perming, tinting, and so on. Another equally important process is the process of communication. **Communication** is the act or instance of transmitting information in the form of symbols, gestures, or behaviors, in order to express an idea or concept so that it is satisfactorily understood. When you communicate, you engage in sending messages, receiving messages, and establishing relationships (Figure 4–1).

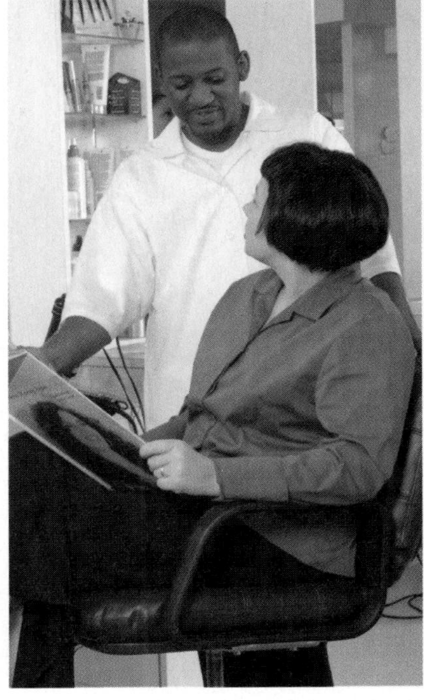

Figure 4–1 Communication is part of building relationships.

Organizing Your Thoughts

The first step in the communication process is to collect your thoughts and feelings—what you want others to understand. This can be a simple task if you are truly in touch with your thoughts and feelings. However, it can require more time if you need to more fully explore your thoughts or form opinions on certain topics.

4

Collecting thoughts and feelings is something clients have to do as well. For example, when your client comes to you for a color service and tells you she wants to go blonde but does not know just what shade of blonde she wants, she has not completed the process of collecting her thoughts. She has made the decision to color her hair, but she has not yet gone on to the next level of decision-making: that is, will she be an ash blonde, a honey blonde, a platinum blonde, or a strawberry blonde? This is where you come in; to help her get organized. But you have to be able to organize your own thoughts before you can help other people organize theirs.

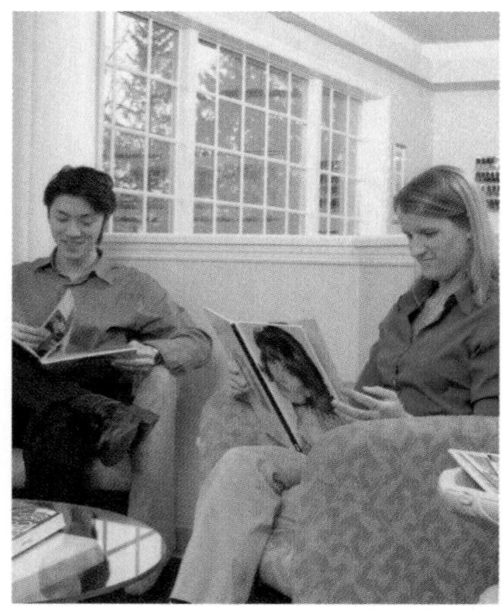

Figure 4–2 Style magazines can help clients communicate their wishes.

Sending Messages

Communication has always been about sending symbols. Whether it is smoke signals, flag-waving, facial expressions, or language itself, we rely on symbols to get our messages across. So after you have organized your thoughts, your next step in the communication process is to translate those thoughts and feelings into symbols that can be easily understood by others.

If you have a client sitting in your chair who says she wants to become a blonde, you have to assess if you have enough information to go on. Has the client given you enough symbols to adequately tell you what she is hoping to achieve? Are there questions in your mind about what she thinks "blonde" is? Does the blonde shade she is thinking of have a warm base color or is it a light platinum color with a violet base? Does she want her whole head colored with this shade or only a few strands? You may need to help your clients **articulate**, or clearly express, their true wants and desires by providing them with symbols they can adopt as their own.

Where are you going to get these symbols? The good news is that they are all over the place. We use any number of symbols every day to represent our thoughts and feelings, such as photographs, drawings, color palettes, music preferences, the kind of car we drive, the style of clothes we wear, the language or vocabulary we use, and the words we write.

4

In the example of your client who yearns to be a blonde, a color swatch chart or color samples would be helpful, as would magazines or books with photos of haircolor in them (Figure 4–2). Or perhaps she has come in armed with some "beginner" symbol—a photo, let's say, of a popular singer—and together you will refine that symbol until you have a clear message of what she desires.

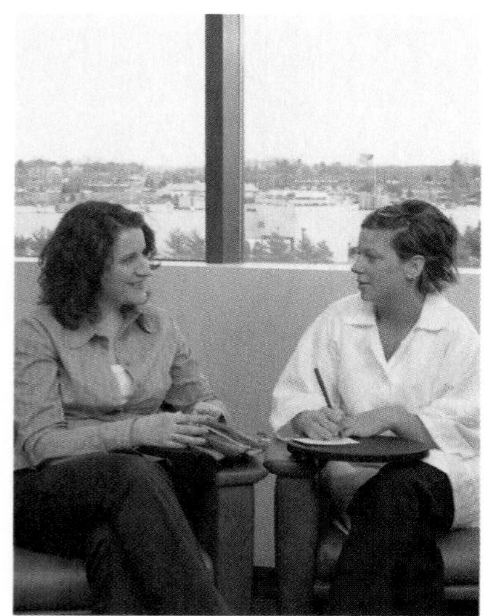

Figure 4–3 A quiet space is essential for your initial client consultation.

Interpreting Messages

When dealing with clients, your first step will be to **clarify**, or make clear, the client's meaning. Begin by eliminating clutter, which is any type of distraction that can keep you from focusing on your conversation. It is difficult to focus on the main point of conversation if there is a lot of loud music playing in the salon or if people are interrupting you or your client. Take your client to a quiet place in the salon that has been dedicated—to the best of the salon's ability—to privacy and peace (Figure 4–3).

Once you have the client's undivided attention, seek out all the specifics you can. Show her all the options for blonde shades, using symbols of your own (photos and color charts). Allow her to consider each shade for as long as she needs to. Ask her for her thoughts as she looks at each one. Ask why she likes one shade more than another. You want her to be as specific as possible so that you can begin to build the same picture in your mind that she has in hers.

Next, repeat back to the client, in your own words, what you think she is telling you. This is called **reflective listening**, and it will determine whether the two of you are on the same page. Reflective listening is a good exercise because as you describe to your client what you think she has said to you, she can make the necessary corrections or adjustments. Remember, this is her picture, not yours. Your job is not to put a different picture in her head. Your job is to bring her picture of herself to life. This will be impossible if you are hanging on to your own picture of what *you* think she should want.

After clarifying and reflecting, the next step involves an intake of the client's particular situation and lifestyle needs. Find out how she normally cares for her hair each day. Explain the maintenance regimen she must follow after her hair is colored and styled so she will know exactly what is required in terms of cleansing, conditioning, and styling. Alert her to styling products available. At this point, your discussion should be highly specific to your client and not couched in general terms.

The final step in the interpretation process consists of reading all the clues and symbols the client is putting out. Observe her gestures and facial expressions during the conversation. What are they saying to you about how she feels? Is she at ease? Is she uncomfortable or unsure of herself? Is she concerned about something you have mentioned? Now is the time to address any questions that could have an impact on the final service. Why does your client think she wants blonde hair? Is it because she believes it will make her more attractive to her husband? Does she think it will make her look younger? Does she feel like doing something totally different? Or is it that she has always wanted to be a platinum blonde and now feels ready for that kind of dramatic change? The answers to these questions are very important in getting to the heart of the client's request.

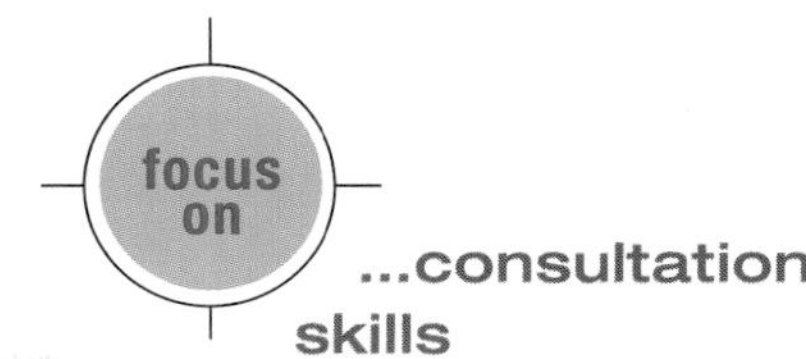

In the relationship between stylist and client, there must be a balance between what the client is asking for and what the professional knows is in the client's best interest. After all, one reason clients patronize professionals is to be advised of what is best for them. This is a delicate communication but one that is vital to satisfying the client. If it appears she does not fully realize that her choice will not benefit her, it is your obligation to find a way to sensitively let her know. Use whatever symbols are available to you to get your point across. Tell her that you can, of course, perform any service, but that in your professional opinion certain services or shades will be more complementary to her skin tone, eye color, or lifestyle than others.

Objectivity in Communication

The interpretation process outlined above is just one phase in what will hopefully be a long and important process of relationship-building with your client. Over time, she may share important and personal material with you about her feelings, her preferences, her health issues, her grooming concerns, her self-image, and more. You may come to know this person very well and find yourself participating in her quest to become the person she wants to be.

At times, your client may even tell you things that seem too personal. Sometimes, when a client forms a bond of trust with her stylist, she may have a hard time differentiating between a professional and a personal relationship. That will be *her* problem, but you must not make it *your* problem. Your job is to handle your client relationships tactfully and sensitively. You cannot become your clients' counselor, career guide, parental sounding board, or motivational coach. Your job and your relationship with your clients are very specific: the goal is to advise and service clients in their hair and other esthetic needs, and nothing more. 1

focus on ...professionalism

A long-time client reveals to you one day that she and her husband are going through a messy divorce. You care for her and try to be understanding as she reveals increasingly personal details. Other stylists and their clients are soon listening to every word of this conversation. You want to be helpful and supportive, but this is not the right time or place. What can you do?

Try this. Bring her a beverage. Tell her you understand the situation is very difficult, but while she is in the salon you want to do everything in your power to give her a break from it. Suggest that she relax in another room of the salon, listen to some soft music, sip her beverage, and have some quiet time. Let her know that while she is in your care, you should both concentrate on her enjoyment of the services and not on the things that are stressing her. She will appreciate the suggestion, and you will have put her back on the track of her real reason for coming to see you.

THE CLIENT CONSULTATION

Although you will be communicating with your client during your time together, there is a specific and prescribed period of time that is dedicated to communication with a very focused purpose. The **client consultation** is the verbal communication with a client to determine desired results. Some professionals skip the client consultation altogether, regarding it as a waste of time, or they make time for it only on a client's first visit to the salon. It is our belief that these professionals are making a serious mistake. The client consultation is the most important communication you will have with your client, and it should be performed, on some level, as part of every single service and salon visit.

Preparing for the Client Consultation

In order for your time to be well spent during the client consultation, it is important that you be prepared for it, because most likely your clients will not be. Since they may never have had the kind of thorough communication they are about to have with you, they will not expect to be answering the types of questions you will be asking. To help them, you should have certain important items on hand.

Styling Books

Have a variety of styling books for your hair service clients to look through. There should be at least one that depicts short hair, one for medium-length hair, and one with longer styles in it, as well as an assortment of photos representing all the different haircolor possibilities, such as blondes, reds, and darker colors.

In addition, it is always a good idea to have a portfolio of your own work on hand. Keep a camera at your station (a disposable or Polaroid camera is fine) and take photos of whatever cuts, colors, perms, and other types of chemical or styling work you perform. A portfolio will help put new clients at ease about your abilities and will help them decide what they want to have done. As you show the photos, explain why you performed the various services the way you did. This will help new clients understand why certain things can or cannot be achieved and will also reassure them that you are knowledgeable and serious about their needs.

HAIR SWATCHES

A handy tool for discussing haircolor is swatches. These are provided by the companies that manufacture haircolor and are generally packaged in a ring, book, or paper chart. Swatches are bundles of hair dyed to the exact color of the tube or bottle color. Usually made from a synthetic material, swatches are very durable and easy to use in consultations. If the swatch is long enough, it can be held up to the client's face or integrated into her own hair to see how it looks. Swatches are perfect "symbols" to help stylist and client reach a working level of communication on the subject of haircolor (Figure 4–4).

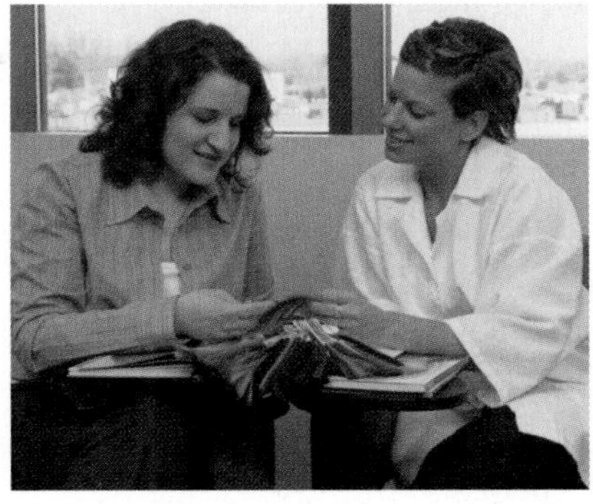

Figure 4–4 Color swatches and other tools help clients make styling choices.

Many times, you will find yourself consulting with a client who asks for a specific cutting technique or color that she may have heard about from a friend or a previous stylist. You know that not every technique or color will work for every client, and just because her friend was happy with the results does not mean that she will be. (And guess who will catch the blame?) In this situation, it may be time to take her through the process, step by step, explaining why or why not this particular style, cut, or color will or will not work for her.

Understanding the Total Look Concept

While the health and styling of hair will always be your primary concern as a cosmetology professional, it is important to remember that the hair adorns the head, which is attached to the body, which, in turn, is reflective of an entire lifestyle. How can you help a client make choices that reflect her own sense of style? Start the process by doing a little research. Go to your local library, find a couple of books that describe fashion styles, and become familiar with them (we are talking about general styles, not individual designers or designs). This exercise is useful for developing a profile of the broad fashion categories that you can refer to when consulting with clients.

For example, a person may be categorized as having a classic style if she prefers simple and sophisticated clothing, in monochromatic colors, with no bright patterns. A person who prefers a classic styling in her clothing will likely want a simple, elegant, and sophisticated hairstyle rather than one that is overly complex or wildly colored (Figure 4–5).

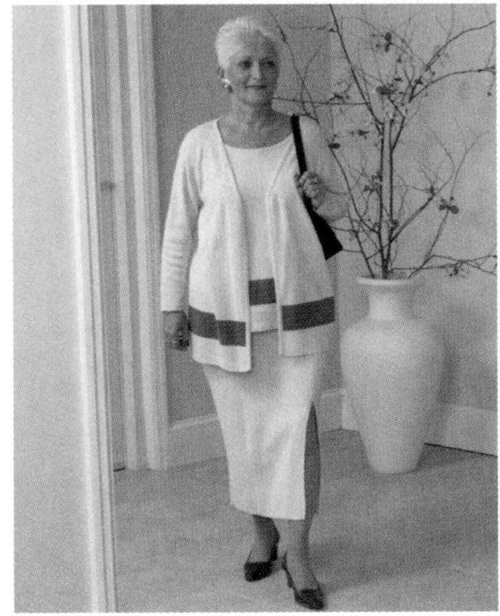

Figure 4–5 A "classic" look.

Conversely, someone who prefers a more dramatic look will choose clothing, hairstyles, and accessories that demand greater attention and allow for more options. This person will likely wear ornate clothes and may enjoy accessories like scarves, jewelry, and belts. She may ask for more daring haircolors and hairstyles. She may be more willing to try a variety of new products and is more likely to spend time having additional services, such as perms, coloring, or other specialized treatments that will help her achieve her desired look (Figure 4–6).

Getting an idea of the client's lifestyle will give you a good indication of how committed she will be to certain styling and grooming requirements. For example, your client may be a businesswoman running a department with many employees. She styles her hair and applies her makeup early in the morning. Then, throughout the day, she devotes as little time as possible

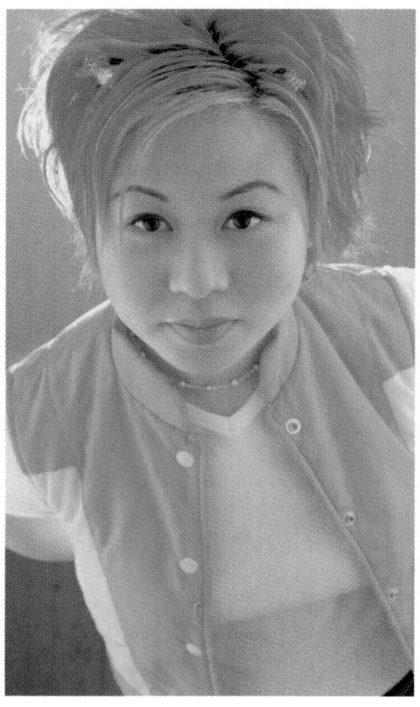

Figure 4-6 A "dramatic" look.

to making the necessary adjustments. This client requires a style that is both professional and easy to maintain. While she is willing to spend time on herself and her appearance, she probably will not stray too far from her current styling and coloring if they suit her needs and lifestyle. She will be a steady customer and will likely remain loyal to her current look.

Another client, a woman with small children, does not work outside the home. She needs a hairstyle that is easy to style and care for. She may be eager to change her style, even drastically, if she can find a low-maintenance style. She may be willing to go from a medium-length blunt cut to a very short, cropped style or a curly perm if she thinks it will make her life easier.

During a conversation about the total look concept, you will also want to ask the client how she wears her hair or what her style is when she is casual or when she is dressed up and going out. These alternative styling preferences will be indicators of how to dress her hair so that it works well within the total look concept. You will also want to talk about the client's skin care and makeup preferences as well as her nail care and foot care grooming habits.

Putting the wrong look on a client can be a big mistake, not only for the client but also for you. No matter how gorgeous a client looks when she leaves your chair, if she cannot maintain the look once she is back in her own environment, you will probably take the blame and lose her as a client. Determining what will work for her total look will earn her loyalty. 2

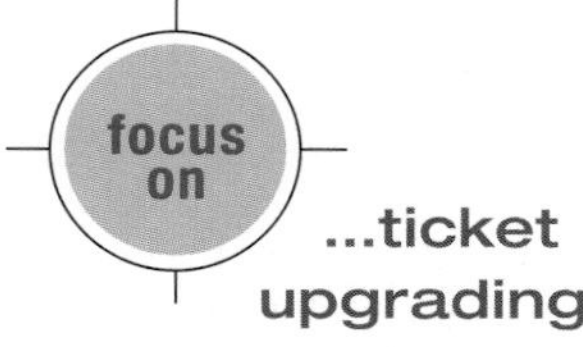

...ticket upgrading

While you are going through hairstyle books and discussing your client's particular needs, take the opportunity to direct her attention to other services available at the salon. Let her know that in addition to a new haircut, she might also want to consider some of the salon's offerings in the areas of skin and nail care. Use the photos in the styling books to offer examples of these services as well.

A Nail Consultation

A consultation prior to a nail service is best done at the manicure table, as long as it is a comfortable place to talk. Ask how often your client attends to her nails, what she prefers to use on them (some clients may prefer one type of overlay to another), and if she has had any negative experiences with manicures or pedicures. Ask a few questions about her lifestyle to assess how long her nails should be and the types of polish designs that are appropriate.

In general, the nail consultation is brief, but long enough for you to obtain the information you need relevant to servicing this client's needs and total look.

A Skin Care Consultation

A consultation prior to a skin care service will be more in-depth than the consultation for a nail care service and may require a tailored version of the consultation card. This consultation should take place in a private room because you will want to speak candidly with your client about any issues she may have with her skin care. She may also need to remove makeup, so privacy is best. As with the hair service consultation, you will need detailed information on your client's history. Be patient and schedule at least one-half hour for the first visit.

insights

Dennis James

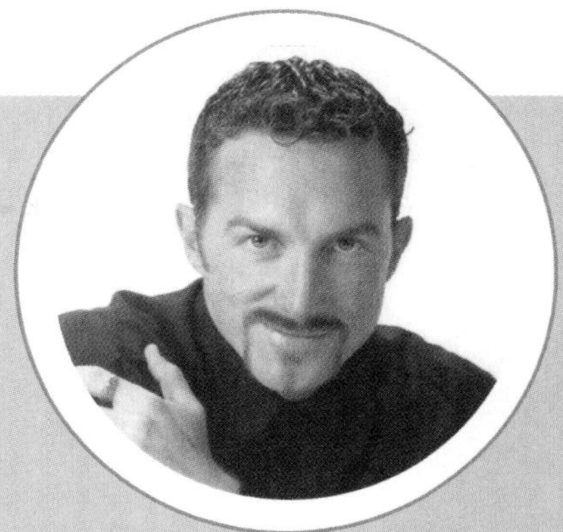

Dennis James is director of education for Paul Mitchell—The School and Partner Programs. He believes in always keeping a values list.

I came into the industry in a kind of roundabout way. My mother was in the industry, but I never really thought of it as a career choice. I thought it was just something mothers did to survive, particularly if you had seven boys and you had to learn how to cut their hair. My brothers and I were in the entertainment business. We had a family act—I was the baby—and we played venues like Disneyland, the Sea Worlds, and the Vegas circuits. Then, when my older brothers got married and had kids, they decided it was time to get "real" jobs, and so the act split up. I was 18 and drifted until I was 21.

I was living in Oregon, and a friend of mine, a woman named Lois, had this salon in a beautiful health club where I used to hang out. I saw how well she could provide for her family and what a great time she was having doing this thing called work. So I went to school. But I wasn't your model student. In fact, I was the worst one in my class. It took me two days to do my first haircut. But I really admired my teachers—they were young and hip—and six months into my career I said teaching is something I can do.

I loved being with a group of learners; I love moving people emotionally and helping them to connect to the learning process. And I make continuing education a part of my own life, too.

I've always believed in keeping a values list, including professional, personal, spiritual, intellectual, and physical values. On the professional side, my goal is to never stop learning. There are always new ways of doing things, new ways of communicating, new ways of operating your business. If you're going to succeed in this profession, I think you have to keep three things in mind. You need to be happy. Even if it's a bad day, you have to fake it. The second rule I got from my mom: "If it's not fatal, don't fret it." I used to take everything personally—if a client didn't like her hair, if a student didn't show up—but that was just my ego talking. And then you have to learn the skills of communication.

As for keeping your creative side fresh and alive, don't just look to your job for that. Live creativity every day. When you get home, you have to paint, you have to play music, you have to dance. Anything that's creative—that's the key to stretching and growing your creative side.

The Consultation Card

Many professionals who service the public keep a consultation or record card for their clients. For example, when you arrive at a new doctor's or dentist's office, you are generally asked to fill out a fairly lengthy document that asks you for information about yourself, your current health situation, and your history.

Whether in the salon or in school, a consultation form or record card can be useful to you in much the same way that the doctor's form is useful. Some cards ask for a lot of detailed information, and some do not. In cosmetology school, the consultation card may be accompanied by a release statement in which the client acknowledges that the service is being provided by a student who is still learning. This protects the school and the student from any legal action by a client who may be unhappy with the service. Whatever type of form is used, be sure to fill it out faithfully and make it a part of each service. The consultation card gives you an opportunity to build an excellent relationship with your clients (Figure 4–7).

Consultation cards can be obtained from a number of sources. You can buy preprinted cards, often from your salon's distributor, or you can make your own card to request exactly the kind of information you want. With your own customized card, you are free to make changes as you see fit.

Also, depending on the service you are providing at the time, whether hair, skin, or nail care, you can tailor the consultation accordingly. For example, getting a client's hair history will probably be considerably more involved than getting the nail history.

How to Use the Consultation Card

The client card can be used from the moment a new client calls the salon to make an appointment. Schedule the appointment for 20 or 30 minutes earlier than she has requested to allow for consultation time. Let her know at the start that you and the salon will require some information before you can begin the service, and that it is important for her to arrive early enough to fill out a consultation card. In many salons, the receptionist calls to remind clients about their appointment the day before it is scheduled. This is a good time to remind the client that she will need to fill out a consultation card. It will probably take her five to 10 minutes to fill out the card and then another 15 or 20 minutes for the first consultation. Don't rush through either step of this process. It is time well spent.

When the client arrives at the salon at the appointed time, she should be greeted by the receptionist, who will ask for her name and will give her a client card, a pen, and a clipboard. After the client completes the form and returns it to the receptionist, you are ready to begin the consultation. Take a moment to scan the information before you greet the client. Make sure you have something to write with, and if you need it, grab a clipboard, too.

Make note of her first and last names. Then, with consultation card in hand, approach your new client. Remember, she has never been in the salon before. Approach her with your hand extended and greet her pleasantly,

Client Consultation Card

Dear Client,

Our sincerest hope is to serve you with best hair care services you've ever received! We not only want you to be happy with today's visit but we also want to build a long-lasting relationship with you—we want to be your hair care salon. In order for us to do so, we would like to learn more about you, your hair care needs and your preferences. Please take a moment now to answer the questions below as completely and as accurately as possible.

Thank you, and we look forward to building a "beautiful" relationship!

Name: ______________________________

Address: ______________________________

Address: ______________________________

Phone Number: (day) __________ (evening) __________

Sex: _____ Male _____ Female Age:_____

How did you hear about our salon?

If you were referred, who referred you?

Please answer the following questions in the space provided. Thanks!

1. Approximately when was your last salon visit?
2. In the past year have you had any of the following services either in or out of a salon? (Please indicate the date on which you had it.)
   - ____ Haircut
   - ____ Hair color
   - ____ Permanent Wave or Texturizing Treatment
   - ____ Chemical Relaxing or Straightening Treatment
   - ____ Highlighting or Lowlighting
   - ____ Full head lightening
   - ____ Haircolor correction
   - ____ Waxing (what type?)
   - ____ Manicure
   - ____ Artificial nail services (please describe)
   - ____ Pedicure
   - ____ Facial/Skin Treatment
   - ____ Other (please any other services you've enjoyed at a salon that may not be listed here).
3. Are you currently taking any medications? (Please list.)
4. What is your natural hair color shade?
5. How would you describe your hair's texture?
6. How would you describe your hair's condition?
7. How would you describe the condition of your scalp?
8. What type of skin do you have? ____ Dry ____ Oily ____ Normal ___ Combination
9. What type of skin care regimen do you follow? (Please explain) ________________

   ____
10. How would you characterize your nails? ____ normal ____ brittle ____ flexible
11. Do you have any of the following nail services? (Check all that apply) ____ Silk wraps ____ Porcelain ____ Acrylic wraps ____ Glue manicure ____ Natural manicure ____ Paraffin hand treatments
12. Do you have any of the following foot services? (Check all that apply) ____ Basic Pedicure ____ Spa Pedicure ____ Paraffin foot treatments
13. Do you ever experience dry, itchy skin? ____ Scalp? If so, how often?
14. Do you notice your ability to manage your hair, skin, or nail regimens change with the change in climate? How so?

Figure 4-7 A typical client consultation card.

4

15. How often do you shampoo your hair?
16. How often do you condition your hair?
17. Once cleansed and conditioned, how do you style your hair?
18. Please list all of the products that you use on your hair, skin, and nails regularly.
19. On average, how much time do you spend each day styling your hair?
20. Are you now or have you ever been allergic to any of the products, treatments or chemicals you've received during any salon service—hair, nails or skin? (Please explain)
21. What is your biggest complaint concerning your hair?
22. What is your biggest complaint concerning your skin?
23. What is your biggest complaint concerning your nails?
24. What do you like about your hair?
25. What do you like about your complexion?
26. What do you like about your nails?
27. Please describe the best hairstyle you ever had and explain why you felt it was the best.
28. What is the one thing that you want your stylist to know about you/your beauty regimens?

NOTE: If this card were used in a beauty school setting, it would include a release form at the bottom such as the one below.

Statement of Release: I hereby understand that cosmetology students render these services for the sole purpose of practice and learning and that, by signing this form, I recognize and agree not to hold the school, its employees or the student liable for my satisfaction or the service outcome.

Client signature ______________________________ Date ______________________

Service Notes

Today's Date:
Today's Services:
Notes:

Today's Date:
Today's Services:
Notes:

Today's Date:
Today's Services:
Notes:

Today's Date:
Today's Services:
Notes:

Today's Date:
Today's Services:
Notes:

Figure 4-7 *(continued)*

"Hello, Ms. Hansen. I'm Michelle, and I'd like to welcome you to our salon today. I'm eager to get started, so will you follow me to our consultation area?" (Figure 4–8).

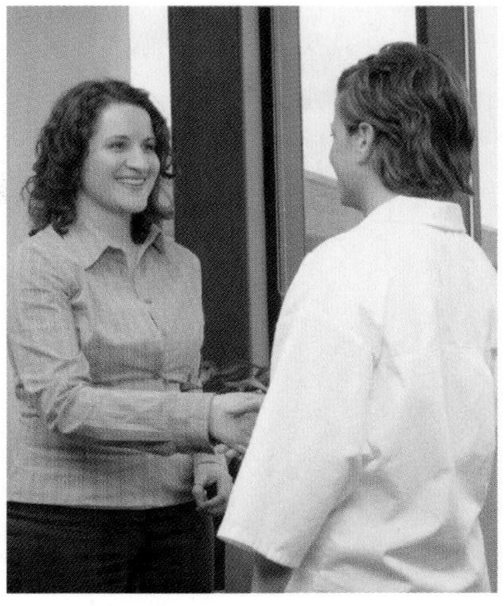

Figure 4-8 Welcome your client to the salon.

The Consultation Area

Although many salons do not have enough space to devote an entire room to consultations, others may set aside a makeshift area for this purpose. Whatever your particular situation, it is important that the area be big enough for you and the client to sit in comfortably and quiet enough that you will not be interrupted or distracted by other activities in the salon.

The space should also be equipped with all the things you will need to complete the consultation, such as style books, haircolor swatches, and a mannequin. You will appear to be unprepared if you have to go looking for any of these once you have begun the consultation. Be sure the area is set up and tidy *before* you bring the client in, and that the consultation materials are in acceptable shape. Handing a new client a book or magazine that is torn or is missing information looks tacky and amateurish. You and your coworkers must make every effort to keep this area of the salon neat and attractive. Presentation counts for a lot in a business that is concerned with style and appearances.

Once you have brought the client into the consultation area, make sure she is comfortable. You and she are about to begin an important conversation that will clue you in to her needs and preferences. This is the first of what will hopefully be many conversations, so comfort counts.

Begin by looking over and reviewing the consultation card. Take the time to read her answers to your questions carefully. Feel free to comment or ask questions. This bit of friendly conversation will serve two purposes: it will put you and your new client at ease, and it will give you an overview of her "hair history." Note how often she gets her hair cut. This is a good indication of her grooming and hair growth patterns, how long she expects a certain style or cut to last, and how often she is willing to invest in her look (Figure 4–9).

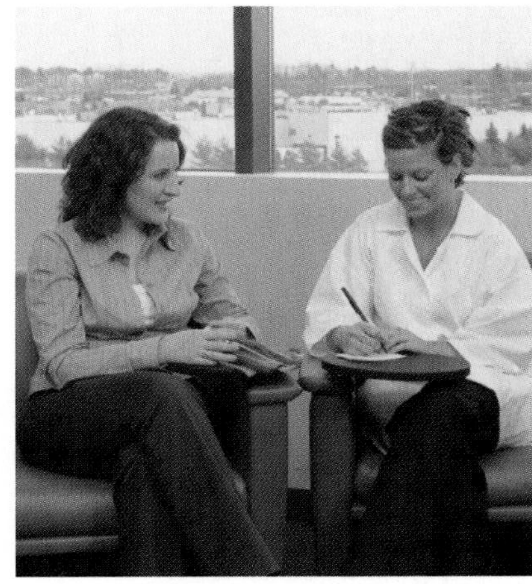

Figure 4-9 Discuss the information on the consultation card with your client.

Ask her about the kinds of chemical services she uses. If she used to perm her hair but has not done so for a while, find out why. If she colors, ask her where she has the color done and how often. Do not be shocked if she explains that she colors, perms, or straightens her own hair. Many clients feel they can perform these services perfectly well at home. The purpose of the consultation is not to lecture the client about the merits of patronizing salon professionals, but to gather information. Ask her how often she performs the procedure, how she determines which formula or strength of product to use, and how satisfied she is with the results. The answers to these questions will help you assess the condition of her hair.

Ask her to describe her styling regimen. Check her responses against what she has written on the card. Ask her why she uses certain products and whether or not she is satisfied with them.

Take ample time to discuss the client's answers to questions 5, 6, 11, and 12 on the card (Figure 4–7). Let her describe her hair and its characteristics as best she can. See if she has brought along any photos of herself in hairstyles she really liked. While it may seem that you are spending too much time on this client's hair history, it is time well spent. In our culture today, hair has become a symbol of one's personality, and has great significance in the person's overall self-esteem and self-image. The more you know about how the client sees herself, the better able you will be to serve her and ultimately retain her as a client.

Developing Listening and Observational Skills

While you are conversing with your client, you must listen to what she is saying and observe how she says it. If, for example, she is having a hard time explaining the look she desires, this is a clear indication that she needs help. Start by clarifying. You could ask, "Do you prefer to wear your hair chin length?" "Do you want bangs?" "Are you happy with the highlighted look?" Give her time to digest the questions and compose her answers. Although it is true that these questions can all be answered by a simple yes or no, it benefits you to have her elaborate as long as she does not lose focus. Go back and confirm what you heard her answer to be. Say, "Oh, so you *do not* like your hair as short as chin length. You *prefer* it shoulder length." Wait for confirmation. Once she confirms what you have just said, move on to the next point for clarification.

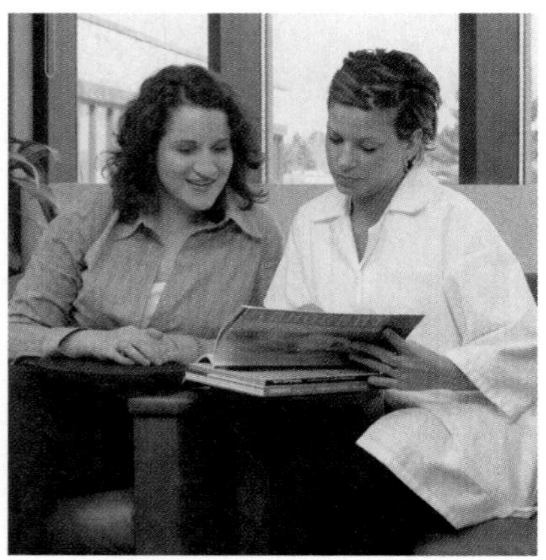

Figure 4–10 Use a styling book to help confirm your client's choice.

During this time of receiving, interpreting, and confirming messages, turn to your aids to help with the process. First, there is the mirror. Every consultation area should have a mirror in which you and the client can look at the client's hair together. Once you have used the mirror to clarify some of the basic points (she likes her hair medium length with reddish highlights), you can go on to the other props.

Pick up the style book that shows various styles in a medium length and look through it with her. Start by showing her a style that is similar to the one she is currently wearing and use it to confirm her style: "Ms. Hansen, here's a photo of the style you are wearing. The hair comes down to just about shoulder level; it is blunt cut and there are no bangs. She even has the same soft strawberry highlights you have." Give her a moment to absorb the hairstyle she is looking at. Let her look in the mirror to confirm that hers is, in fact, the same style. She may be unaware of the resemblance. As far as she is concerned, her hair is shorter or darker, or both. Ask her if she sees what you see. If she does not, take a moment to explain why you believe that the looks are similar. Use layman's terms. Remember, as a cosmetologist you are used to technical terms, but she most likely will not be. You are the teacher; help her to see what you see (Figure 4–10).

If you use the techniques described above in your consultations, you and your client should be able to achieve the same, or close to the same, visions. You should both keep in mind, however, that every person is different. While you will do your best to achieve a look exactly as it appears in a photo or duplicate a color exactly as it appears on a swatch, it will never be a perfect match. Never tell a client that you can make her "look exactly like the picture," because it is simply impossible. Clients need to understand that and to appreciate your honesty.

Throughout the consultation and especially once a course of action is decided on, make notes on the consultation card. Record any formulations or products that you use, including the strength, and include any specific techniques you follow or goals you are working toward so that you can remember them for future visits.

Once the service is finished and the client has let you know whether or not she is satisfied, take a few more minutes to record the results on the record card. Ask for her reactions and record them, too. Note anything you did that you might want to do again as well as anything that does not bear repetition. Also, make note of the condition of the client's hair after the service, and any retail products that you recommended for her purchase. Be sure to date your notes and file them in the proper place. Now give yourself a nice pat on the back because you have completed one of the most important aspects of your job.

The more you consult, the better your consultations will become. Be sure to have some sort of consultation whenever a client comes to you for service. You may never need to spend as much time as you do the first time around, but touching base with your clients during the consultation is a valuable tool that you should never neglect. 3

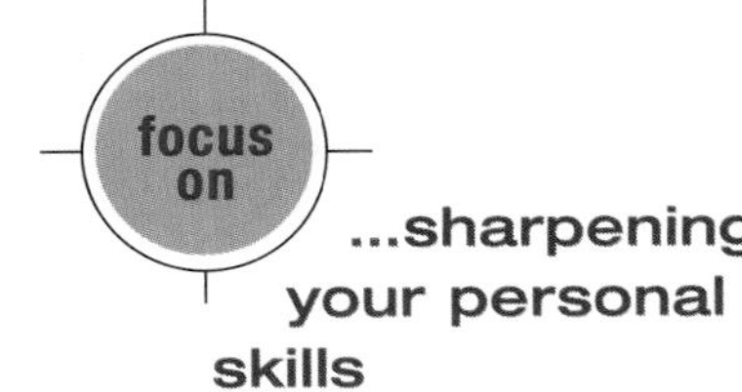

To become and remain successful in your professional life, follow these reminders every day.

- Smile and be courteous to clients and coworkers and remember that the client is always right.
- Count to ten (or, if necessary, twenty) before you reply to or become engaged in a difficult situation or conversation.
- Be honest and ethical at all times, even when it is easier not to be.
- Do not jump to conclusions. Give others the benefit of the doubt and remain professional at all times.

SPECIAL ISSUES IN COMMUNICATION

Although you may do everything in your power to communicate well and effectively, you will sometimes encounter situations that are beyond your control. The solution is not to try to control the circumstances but to communicate past the issue. Your reactions to situations and your ability to communicate in the face of problems will be the measure of whether or not you are successful in a "people" profession such as the beauty industry.

Meeting and Greeting New Clients

One of the most important communications you will have with a client is the first time you meet that person. Be polite, friendly, and inviting (which you will continue to be in all your encounters), and remember that your clients are coming to you for services for which they are paying hard-earned cash. That means you need to court them every time they come to see you; otherwise you may lose them to another stylist.

To earn their trust and loyalty, you need to remember a few basic things.

- Always approach a new client with a smile on your face. Even if you are having a difficult day or have a problem of some sort, keep it to yourself. The time you are with your client is for your client and her needs, not yours.

- Always introduce yourself. Names are powerful, and they are meant to be used. Many clients have had the experience of being greeted by the receptionist, ushered back to the shampoo area, then led to the stylist's chair, and when the service has been performed and the appointment is over, they have not learned the name of a single person.
- Set aside a few minutes to take the client on a quick tour of the salon. Introduce her to the receptionist and anyone else you might run into along the way. This helps her to feel comfortable and at home.
- Be yourself. Don't try to trick your clients into thinking you are someone or something that you are not. Just be who you are. You will be surprised at how well that will work for you.

Handling Tardy Clients

Tardy clients are a fact of life in every service industry. Because the cosmetologist is so dependent on appointments and scheduling to maximize working hours, a client who is very late for an appointment or one who is habitually late can cause problems. One tardy client can make you late for every other client you service that day, and the pressure involved in making up for lost time can take its toll. You also inconvenience the rest of your clients who are prompt for their appointments. Here are a few guidelines for handling late clients.

- Know and abide by the salon's tardy or late policy. Many salons set a limited amount of time they allow a client to be late before they require them to reschedule. Generally, if clients are more than 15 minutes late, they should be asked to reschedule. Most will accept responsibility and be understanding about the rule, but you may come across a few clients who insist on being serviced immediately. Explain that you have other appointments and are responsible to those clients as well. Explain also that rushing through the service is unacceptable to you. Make another, more convenient appointment.
- If your tardy client arrives and you have the time to take her without jeopardizing another client's appointment, let her know why you are taking her even though she is late. You can deliver this information and still remain pleasant and upbeat. Say, "Oh, Ms. Lee, we're in luck! Even though you're a bit late, I can still take you because my next appointment isn't for two hours. Isn't it great that it worked out?" This lets her know that being late is not acceptable under normal circumstances but that if you can accommodate her, you will.
- As you get to know your clients, you will learn who is habitually late. You may want to schedule such clients for the last appointment of the day or ask them to arrive earlier than their actual appointments. In other words, if a client is always one-half hour late, schedule her for 2:30 but tell her to arrive at 2:00!
- Imagine this scenario. In spite of your best efforts, you are running late. You realize that no matter what has happened in the salon that day, your clients want and deserve your promptness. If you have your clients'

telephone numbers, call them and let them know about the delays. Give them the opportunity to reschedule or to come a little later than their scheduled appointments. If you cannot reach them beforehand, be sure to approach them when they come into the salon and let them know that you are delayed. Tell them how long you think the wait will be and give them the option of changing their appointment. Apologize for the inconvenience and show a little extra attention by getting them coffee or mineral water. Even if these clients are not happy about the delay or the need to change their appointment, at least they will feel informed and respected.

Handling Scheduling Mix-Ups

We are all human, and we all make mistakes. Chances are, you have gone to an appointment on a certain day at a certain time only to discover that you are in the wrong place at the wrong time. The way you are treated at that moment will determine if you ever patronize that business again. The number one thing to remember when you, as a professional, get involved with a scheduling mix-up is to be polite and never argue the point of who is correct. Being right may sound good, but this kind of situation is not about being right. It is about preserving your relationship with your client. If you handle the matter poorly, you run the risk of never seeing that client again. Even if you know for sure that she is mistaken, tell yourself that the client is always right. Assume the blame if it helps keep her happy. *Do not, under any circumstances, argue the point with the client.*

Once you have the chance to consult your appointment book, you can say, "Oh, Mrs. Montez, I have you in my appointment book for 10:00, and unfortunately I have already scheduled other clients for 11:00 and 12:00. I'm so sorry about the mix-up. Can I reschedule you for tomorrow at 10:00?" Even though the client may be fuming, you need to stay disengaged. Your focus is to move the conversation away from who is at fault and squarely in the direction of resolving the confusion. Make another appointment for the client and be sure to get her telephone number so that you can call and confirm the details of the appointment in advance (Figure 4–11).

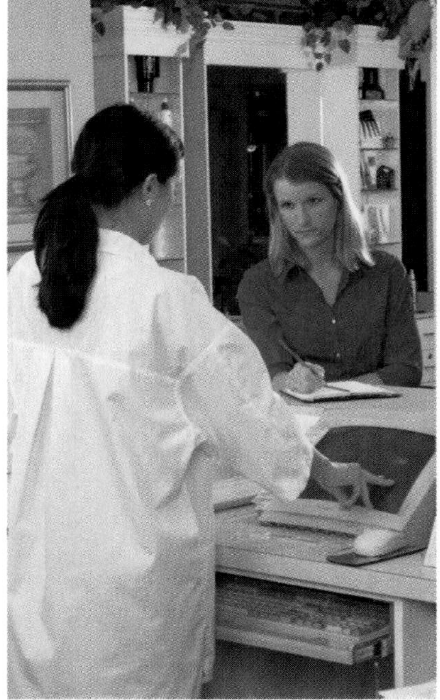

Figure 4–11 Accommodate an unhappy client promptly and calmly.

Handling Unhappy Clients

No matter how hard you try to provide excellent service to your clients, once in a while you will encounter a client who is dissatisfied with the service. The way you and the salon handle this difficult situation will have lasting effects on you, the client, and the salon, so you need to know how best to proceed. Once again, it is important to remember the ultimate goal: to make the client happy enough to pay for the service and return for more of the same.

Here are some guidelines to follow.

- Try to find out why the client is unhappy. Ask for specifics. If she has a difficult time articulating it, break the service down for her piece by piece. Ask, "Are you happy with the length at the nape?" "Do you like the shape around the ears?" "Would you prefer layers at the temple area?" Keep going until you get warm.

focus on ...communication

You will no doubt be in a position at some time in your career when a client is unhappy about something that was done either during the service or in scheduling. No matter how well you communicate, handling a situation like this can be hard. The best way to prepare is to practice. Role-play with a classmate, taking turns being the client and the stylist. Role-playing both sides of the issue will give you a better understanding of the entire situation.

- If it is possible to change what she dislikes, do so immediately. If she is unhappy with the cut or the color and you can determine how to repair the damage, look at your schedule to see how soon you can do it. You may need to enlist the help of the receptionist in rescheduling your other appointments. If the client is open to it, ask her to return to the salon at a time when you are free. If this is not possible, explain that you will begin her service but will need to take your next client and will be relying on help from another stylist. Do whatever you have to do to make her happy, and explain along the way who will be working with her and what that other stylist will be doing.
- If you cannot change what the client does not like because it might damage her hair or it is simply impossible to change ("It's too short!"), you must honestly and tactfully explain the reason why you cannot make any changes. She will not be happy, but you can offer any options that may be available, such as conditioning treatments, styling options, and the like.
- Again, never argue with the client or try to force your opinion on her. Telling her how great she looks in the cut or color that is making her unhappy will not help her feel better, even if, in your opinion, she does look better than when she walked in. As a matter of fact, telling her that will just fuel the fire.
- Do not hesitate to call on a more experienced stylist or your salon manager for help. They have probably encountered a similar situation at some point in their careers (maybe even yesterday), and they may have insights that can help you.
- If, after you have tried everything, you are unable to satisfy the client, defer to your manager's advice on how to proceed. The client may be too upset to handle the situation maturely, and it may be easier for her to deal with someone else. This does not mean that you have failed; it simply means that another approach is needed.
- Confer with your salon manager after the experience. If you have a good salon manager, this incident will not be held against you but viewed instead as an inevitable fact of life from which you can learn. Follow your manager's advice and move on to your next client. Use whatever you may have learned from the experience to perform future client consultations and services better. 4

IN-SALON COMMUNICATION

While you are in the salon, you will be communicating and building relationships with your clients, coworkers, and managers. These relationships are critical because your colleagues can help you, teach you, and give you lots of valuable advice, if you know how to seek out and accept such communications.

Behaving in a professional manner is the first step in making this meaningful communication possible. Unfortunately, many beauty professionals act immaturely and get overly involved in the salon rumor mill. The salon community is usually a close-knit one in which people spend long hours side by side. You will work together and in a sense "live" together, sharing professional and personal experiences. For this reason, it is important to maintain boundaries around what you will and will not do or say at the salon. Remember, the salon is your place of business, and as such, must be treated respectfully and carefully.

Communicating with Coworkers

As with all communication, there are basic principles that must guide your interactions. In a work environment, you will not have the opportunity to handpick your colleagues. There will always be people you like or relate to better than others, and people whose behaviors or opinions you find yourself in conflict with. These people can try your patience and your nerves, but they are your colleagues and are deserving of your respect.

Here are some guidelines to keep in mind as you interact and communicate with fellow staffers.

- *Treat everyone with respect.* Regardless of whether or not you like someone, your colleagues are professionals who service clients who bring revenue into the salon. And, as practicing professionals, they have information they can offer you. Look at these people as having something to teach you, and hone in on their talents and their techniques.
- *Remain objective.* Different types of personalities working side by side over long and intense hours are likely to breed some degree of dissension and disagreement. In order to learn and grow, you must make every effort to remain objective and resist being pulled into spats and cliques. When one or two people in the salon behave disrespectfully toward one another, the entire team suffers because the atmosphere changes. Not only will this be unpleasant for you but also will be felt by the clients, who may decide to take their business elsewhere if they find the atmosphere in your salon too tense.
- *Be honest and be sensitive.* Many people use the excuse of being honest as license to say anything to anyone. While honesty is always the best policy, using unkind words or actions with regard to your colleagues is never a good idea. Be sensitive. Put yourself in the other person's place and think through what you want to say before you say it. That way, any negative or hurtful words can be suppressed.
- *Remain neutral.* Undoubtedly, there will come a time when you are called on to make a statement or to "pick a side." Do whatever you can not to get drawn into the conflict. If you have a problem with your colleagues, the best way to resolve it is to speak with them directly and privately. Speaking to or gossiping with others about someone never resolves a problem. It only makes it worse and is often as damaging to you as it is to the object of your gossip.
- *Seek help from someone you respect.* If you find yourself in a position where you are at odds with a coworker, you may want to seek out a third party—

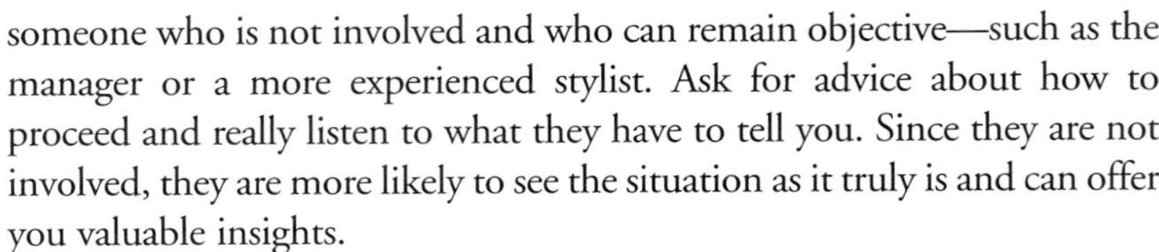

someone who is not involved and who can remain objective—such as the manager or a more experienced stylist. Ask for advice about how to proceed and really listen to what they have to tell you. Since they are not involved, they are more likely to see the situation as it truly is and can offer you valuable insights.

- *Do not take things personally.* This is often easier said than done. How many times have you had a bad day or been thinking about something totally unrelated when a person asks you what's wrong or wonders if you are mad at them? Probably lots of times. Just because someone is behaving in a certain manner and you happen to be there, do not interpret the words or behaviors as being meant for you. If you are confused or concerned by someone's actions, find a quiet and private place to ask the person about it. The person may not even realize she was giving off any signals.
- *Keep your private life private.* There is a time and a place for everything, but the salon is never the place to discuss your personal life and relationships. It may be tempting to engage in that kind of conversation, especially if others in the salon are doing so, and to solicit advice and opinions, but that is why you have friends. Coworkers can become friends, but those whom you selectively turn into friends are different from the ones whose chairs happen to be next to yours.

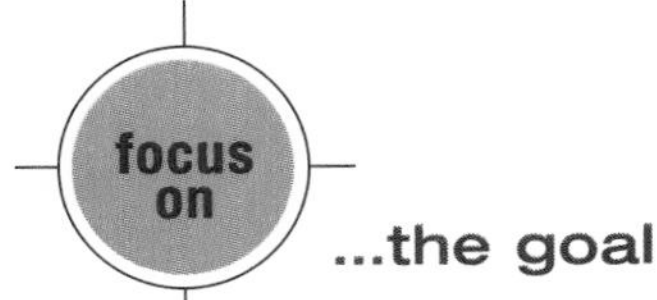

...the goal

Too much time spent on your personal life means time away from the task of perfecting your skills and artistry and building up the business for yourself and the salon.

Communicating with Managers

Another very important relationship for you within the salon is the one you will build with your manager. The salon manager is generally the person who has the most responsibility for how well the salon is run, in terms of daily maintenance and operations and client service. The manager's job is a very demanding one. Often, in addition to running a hectic salon, she also has a clientele that she personally services.

Your manager is likely to be the one who hired you and is responsible for your training and for how well you move into the salon culture. Therefore, your manager has a vested interest in your success. As a salon employee, you will see the manager as a powerful and influential person, but it is also important to remember that she is a human being. She isn't perfect, and she will not be able to do everything you think should be done in every instance. Whether she personally likes you or not, her job is to look beyond her personal feelings and make decisions that are best for the salon as a whole. The best thing you can do is to try to understand the decisions and rules that she makes whether you agree with them or not.

Many salon professionals utilize their salon managers in inappropriate ways, by asking them to solve personal issues between staff members. Inexperienced managers, hoping to keep everything flowing smoothly, may make the mistake of getting involved in petty issues. You and your manager must both understand that her job is to make sure the business is running smoothly, not to baby-sit temperamental stylists.

Here are some guidelines for interacting and communicating with your salon manager.

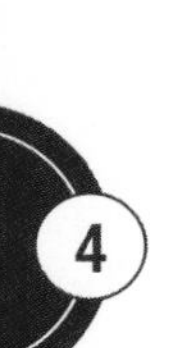

- *Be a problem-solver.* When you need to speak with your manager about some issue or problem, think up some possible solutions beforehand. This will indicate that you are working in the salon's best interest and are trying to help, not make things worse.
- *Get your facts straight.* Make sure that all your facts and information are accurate before you speak to your salon manager. This way you will avoid wasting time solving a "problem" that really does not exist.
- *Be open and honest.* When you find yourself in a situation you do not understand or do not have the experience to deal with, tell your salon manager immediately and be willing to learn.
- *Do not gossip or complain about colleagues.* Going to your manager with gossip or to "tattle" on a coworker tells your manager that you are a troublemaker. If you are having a legitimate problem with someone and have tried everything in your power to handle the problem yourself, then it is appropriate to go to your manager. But you must approach her with a true desire to solve the problem, not just to vent.
- *Check your attitude.* The salon environment, although fun and friendly, can also be stressful, so it is important to take a moment between clients to "take your temperature." Ask yourself how you are feeling. Do you need an attitude adjustment? Be honest with yourself.
- *Be open to constructive criticism.* It is never easy to hear that you need improvement in any area, but keep in mind that part of your manager's job is to help you achieve your professional goals. She is supposed to evaluate your skills and offer suggestions on how to increase them. Keep an open mind and do not take her criticism personally.

Communicating During an Employee Evaluation

Salons that are well run will make it a priority to conduct frequent and thorough employee evaluations. Sometime in the course of your first few days of work, your salon manager will tell you when you can expect your first evaluation. If she does not mention it, you might ask her about it and request a copy of the form she will use or the criteria on which you will be evaluated. Take some time to look over this document. Be mindful that the behaviors and/or activities most important to the salon are likely to be the ones on which you will be evaluated. This is very useful information. You can begin to watch and rate yourself in the weeks and months ahead so you can assess how you are doing. Remember, everything you are being evaluated on is there for the purpose of helping you improve. Make the decision to approach these communications positively.

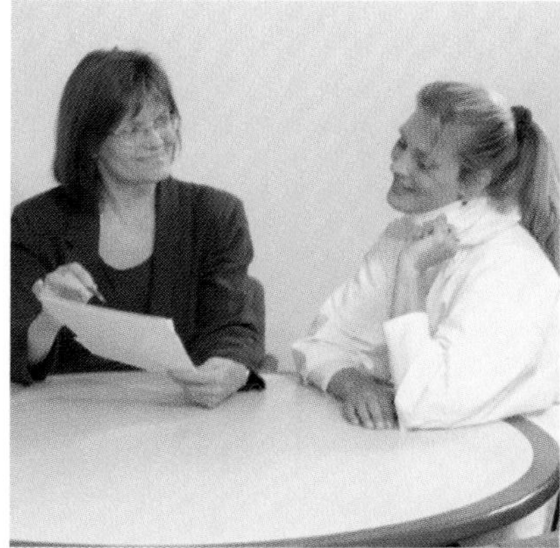

Figure 4–12 Your employee evaluation is a good time to discuss your progress with your manager.

As the time draws near for the evaluation, try filling out the form yourself. In other words, give yourself an evaluation, even if the salon has not asked you to do so. Be objective, and carefully think out your comments. Then, when you meet with the manager, show her your evaluation and tell her you are serious about your improvement and growth. She will appreciate your input and your desire. And, if you are being honest with yourself, there should be no surprises (Figure 4–12).

Before your evaluation meeting, write down any thoughts or questions you may have so you can share them with your manager. Do not be shy. If you want to know when you can take on more services, when your pay scale will be increased, or when you might be considered for promotion, this meeting is the appropriate time and place to ask. Many beauty professionals never take advantage of this crucial communication opportunity to discuss their future because they are too nervous, intimidated, or unprepared. Do not let that happen to you. Participate proactively in your career and in your success by communicating your desires and interests.

At the end of the meeting, thank your manager for taking the time to do an evaluation and for the feedback and guidance she has given you. 5 ✓

4

chapter glossary

articulate	to express clearly
clarify	to make clear
client consultation	verbal communication with a client to determine desired results
communication	act or instance of transmitting information, in the form of symbols, gestures, or behaviors, in order to express an idea or concept so that it is satisfactorily understood
reflective listening	listening to the client and then repeating, in your own words, what you think the client is telling you

review questions

1. Define communication.
2. What are the basic processes of communication?
3. How should you prepare for a client consultation?
4. What is the "total look" concept?
5. List and describe the elements of a successful client consultation.
6. Name some types of information that should go on a client consultation card.
7. How should you handle tardy clients?
8. How should you handle a scheduling mix-up?
9. How should you handle an unhappy client?
10. List at least five things to remember when communicating with your coworkers.
11. List at least four guidelines for communicating with salon managers.

COSMETOLOGY SCIENCES

part 2

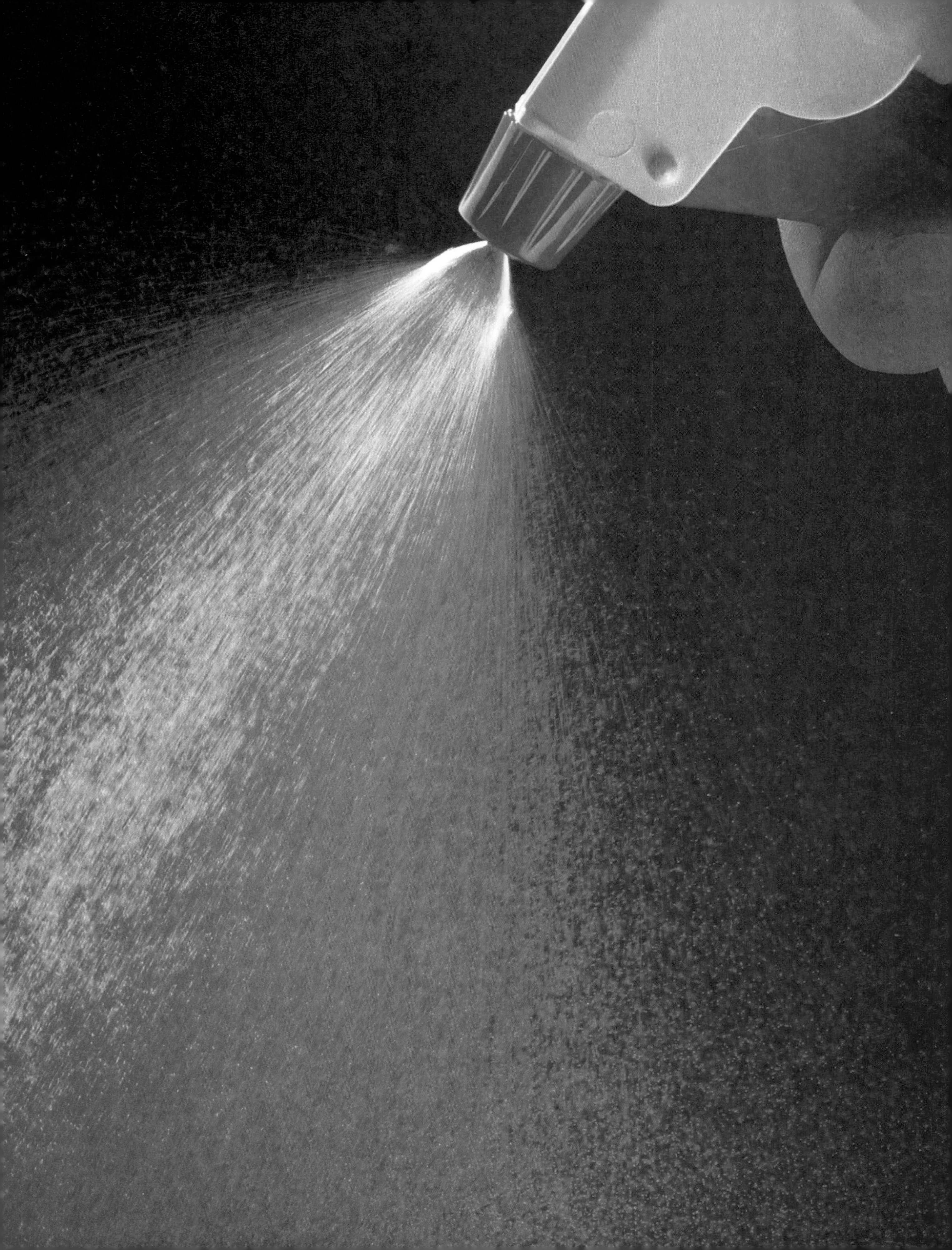

INFECTION CONTROL: PRINCIPLES AND PRACTICE

Sue Ellen Sansom
EXECUTIVE DIRECTOR, ARIZONA STATE BOARD OF COSMETOLOGY
Mary Darlene Hudson
OFFICE MANAGER, ARIZONA STATE BOARD OF COSMETOLOGY

Chapter Outline

Learning Objectives

After completing this chapter, you should be able to:

1. **List the types and classifications of bacteria.**
2. **Define hepatitis and AIDS and explain how they are transmitted.**
3. **Describe vegetable and animal parasites that may be seen in the salon.**
4. **Discuss the different types of disinfectants and how they are used.**
5. **Describe how to safely sanitize and disinfect various salon tools and surfaces.**
6. **Explain the differences between sterilization, disinfection, and sanitation.**
7. **Discuss Universal Precautions and your responsibilities as a salon professional.**

National Skill Standards

This chapter provides you with the necessary information to master these National Industry Skill Standards for Entry-Level Cosmetologists.

Conducting services in a safe environment and taking measures to prevent the spread of infectious and contagious disease.

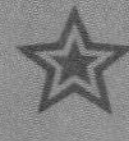

Safely using a variety of salon products while providing client services.

Key Terms

acquired immunity pg 104
acute disease pg 99
AIDS pg 101
allergy pg 99
antiseptics pg 118
asymptomatic pg 118
bacilli pg 97
bacteria pg 95
bactericidal pg 110
bacteriology pg 96
bloodborne pathogens pg 103
chronic disease pg 99
cilia pg 97
cocci pg 96
congenital disease pg 99
contagious disease pg 98
contaminants pg 105
contraindication pg 99
decontamination pg 105
diagnosis pg 99
diplococci pg 97
disease pg 99
disinfectants pg 106
disinfection pg 106
efficacy pg 110
epidemic pg 99
etiology pg 99
flagella pg 97
fungi pg 103
fungicidal pg 110
general infection pg 98
hepatitis pg 101
HIV pg 101
immunity pg 104
infection pg 98
infectious pg 96
infectious disease pg 99
inflammation pg 99
local infection pg 98
microbiology pg 96
microorganism pg 96
mildew pg 117
mitosis pg 98
mold pg 117
motility pg 97
MSDS pg 106
natural immunity pg 104
nonpathogenic pg 95
objective symptoms pg 99
occupational disease pg 100
-ology pg 96
parasite pg 96
parasitic disease pg 100
pathogenic pg 96
pathogenic disease pg 100
pathology pg 100
pediculosis capitis pg 104
phenol pg 111
porous pg 106
prognosis pg 100
pseudomonacidal pg 110
pus pg 98
quaternary ammonium compounds (quats) pg 111
sanitation or sanitizing pg 116
saprophytes pg 96
scabies pg 104
seasonal disease pg 100
sodium hypochlorite pg 112
spirilla pg 97
staphylococci pg 97
sterilization pg 105
streptococci pg 97
subjective symptoms pg 100
systemic disease pg 100
toxins pg 96
tuberculocidal pg 110
Universal Precautions pg 118
venereal disease pg 100
virology pg 96
virucidal pg 110
virus pg 100

Every year, the cosmetology industry serves hundreds of thousands of clients. That means billions on billions of germs, viruses, and bacteria are coming along for the ride. To combat this army of invaders, regulatory agencies and governmental departments of health require that any business that serves the public, such as a salon, must follow certain prescribed sanitary precautions. As a practitioner, it is your duty to ensure that your clients receive their services in the safest possible environment. This chapter will help you understand the need for preventing infection and will introduce you to practices that will allow you to perform your work in a safe manner that protects individual and public health.

In this chapter, we will learn the nature of various organisms, how they relate to disease, and how their spread can be prevented in the salon and at school. Let us begin with bacteria.

BACTERIA

Bacteria are one-celled microorganisms (my-kroh-OR-gah-niz-ums) with both plant and animal characteristics. Also known as germs or microbes, bacteria can exist almost anywhere: on the skin, in water, air, decayed matter, secretions of body openings, on clothing, and beneath the nails.

Bacteria can only be seen with the aid of a microscope. Fifteen hundred rod-shaped bacteria will fit comfortably on the head of a pin.

Types of Bacteria

There are hundreds of different kinds of bacteria. However, bacteria are classified into two main types, depending on whether they are beneficial or harmful.

- Most bacteria are **nonpathogenic** organisms (helpful or harmless; not disease-producing), which perform many useful functions, such as decomposing garbage and improving soil fertility. In the human body, nonpathogenic bacteria help metabolize food, protect against infectious microorganisms, and stimulate immune response. Some bacteria cultures

Term	Definition
bacteria (singular: bacterium)	one-celled microorganisms with both plant and animal characteristics; some are harmful, some harmless; also known as microbes or germs
bacteriology	the science that deals with the study of microorganisms called bacteria
infectious	communicable by infection from one person to another person or from one infected body part to another
microbes/germs	synonyms for disease-producing bacteria
microbiology	the science that deals with microorganisms and their effects on other forms of life
microorganism	microscopic plant or animal cell
-ology	suffix meaning "scientific study of" (example: microbiology)
parasite	a vegetable or animal organism that lives on or in another organism and draws its nourishment from that organism
toxin	any of various poisonous substances produced by some microorganisms
virology	the study of viruses and viral diseases
virus (plural: viruses)	a submicroscopic structure capable of infesting almost all plants and animals, including bacteria; infectious agent that lives only by penetrating cells and becoming part of them

Table 5-1 Definitions Relating to Causes of Disease

are used to produce penicillin, acidophilus yogurt, and a special type of milk used for gastrointestinal disorders. **Saprophytes** (SAH-pruh-fyts), a type of nonpathogenic bacteria, lives on dead matter.

- **Pathogenic** (path-uh-JEN-ik) bacteria (microbes or germs) are harmful and, although in the minority, cause disease when they invade plant or animal tissue. To this group belong the **parasites**, which require living matter for their growth. It is because of pathogenic bacteria that salons and cosmetology schools must maintain certain sanitary standards.

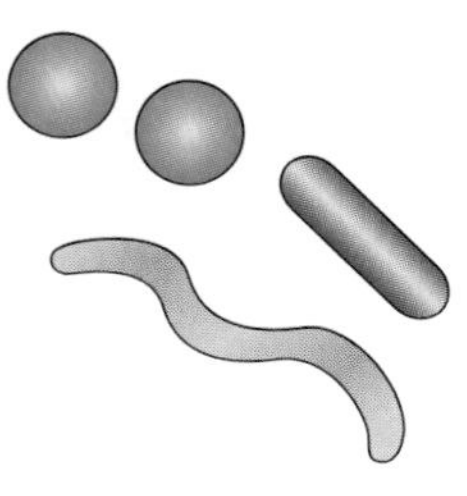

Figure 5-1 General forms of bacteria.

Classifications of Pathogenic Bacteria

Bacteria have distinct shapes that help to identify them. Pathogenic bacteria are classified as follows (Figure 5–1).

1. **Cocci** are round-shaped bacteria that appear singly (alone) or in the following groups (Figure 5–2):

- **Staphylococci**—Pus-forming bacteria that grow in clusters like a bunch of grapes. They cause abscesses, pustules, and boils.
- **Streptococci**—Pus-forming bacteria arranged in curved lines resembling a string of beads. They cause infections such as strep throat and blood poisoning.
- **Diplococci**—Spherical bacteria that grow in pairs and cause diseases such as pneumonia.

2. **Bacilli** are short, rod-shaped bacteria. They are the most common bacteria and produce diseases such as tetanus (lockjaw), typhoid fever, tuberculosis, and diphtheria (Figure 5–3).
3. **Spirilla** are spiral or corkscrew-shaped bacteria. They are subdivided into subgroups, such as *Treponema pallida*, which causes syphilis, a sexually transmitted disease (STD) or *Borrelia burgdorferi*, which causes Lyme disease. 1

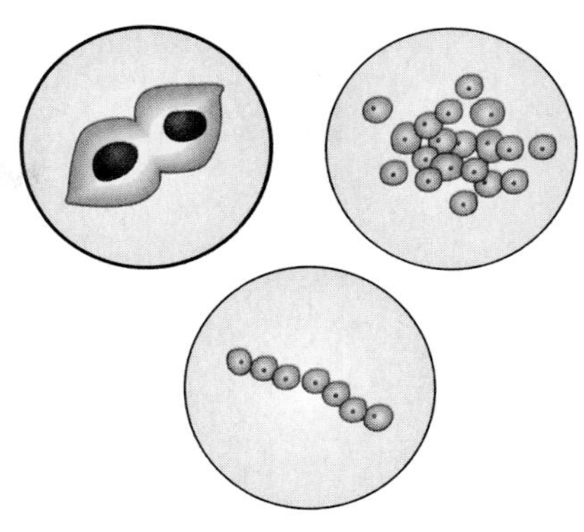

Figure 5–2 Different forms of cocci.

Movement of Bacteria

Different bacteria move in different ways. Cocci rarely show active **motility** (self-movement). They are transmitted in the air, in dust, or within the substance in which they settle. Bacilli and spirilla are both motile and use slender, hairlike extensions, known as **flagella** (fluh-JEL-uh; singular: flagellum) or **cilia** (SIL-ee-uh), for locomotion (moving about). A whiplike motion of these hairs moves the bacteria in liquid (Figure 5–4).

Bacilli (rod)

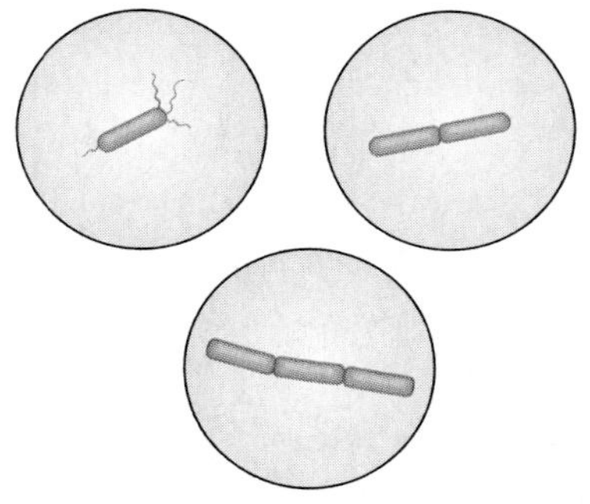

Spirilla (spiral)

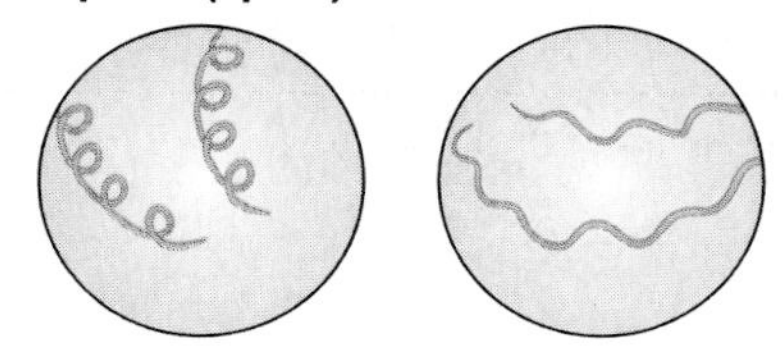

Figure 5–3 Forms of bacilli and spirilla.

Singular	Plural
coccus (KO K-us)	cocci (KOK-sy)
bacillus (bah-SIL-us)	bacilli (bah-SIL-ee)
spirillum (spy-RIL-um)	spirilla (spy-RIL-ah)
staphylococcus (staf-uh-loh-KOK-us)	staphylococci (staf-uh-loh-KOK-sy)
streptococcus (strep-toh-KOK-us)	streptococci (strep-toh-KOK-eye)
diplococcus (dip-loh-KOK-us)	diplococci (dip-lo-KOK-sy)

Table 5–2 Pronunciations of Terms Relating to Pathogenic Bacteria

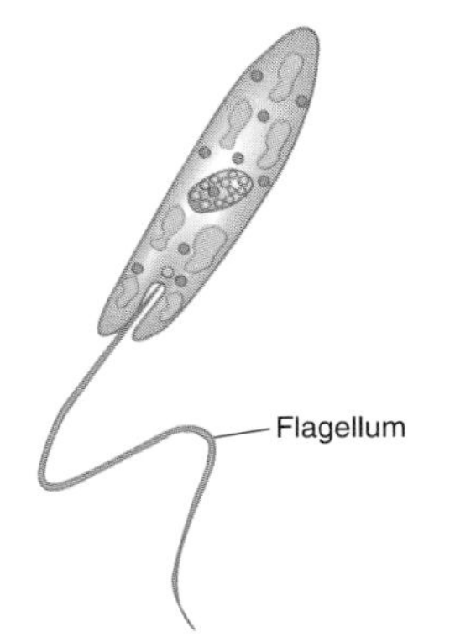

Figure 5–4 Bacteria with flagellum.

Did you know...

A rod-shaped bacteria called *Mycobacterium fortuitum furunculosis* (**MY**-koh-bak-**TIR**-ee-um for-**TOO**-i-tum fur-**UNK**-yoo-**LOH**-sis) was long thought to be relatively harmless. But this bacteria is now causing concern in the pedicure industry. In California in 2000, an infection caused by this bacteria affected over 100 clients who had received pedicures in the same salon. The infection caused stubborn, ugly sores that lingered for months, required the use of strong antibiotics, and, in some cases, caused scarring. The source of the infection was traced to the whirlpool foot spas that had been used for the pedicures. Failure to follow the manufacturer's cleaning instructions left built-up debris in the foot spas. This created the perfect breeding ground for the normally harmless *Mycobacterium fortuitum furunculosis.*

The outbreak proved to be expensive and hard to treat and created a need for a regulatory change in the industry. The salon owner's license was revoked. Foot spa chlorination is now recommended.

Bacterial Growth and Reproduction

Bacteria generally consist of an outer cell wall and internal protoplasm (Chapter 6). They manufacture their own food from the surrounding environment, give off waste products, and grow and reproduce. The life cycle of bacteria is made up of two distinct phases: the active or vegetative stage, and the inactive or spore-forming stage.

Active or Vegetative Stage

During the active stage, bacteria grow and reproduce. These microorganisms multiply best in warm, dark, damp, or dirty places where sufficient food is available.

When conditions are favorable, bacteria grow and reproduce. When they reach their largest size, they divide into two new cells. This division is called **mitosis** (my-TOH-sis). The cells that are formed are called daughter cells. When conditions are unfavorable, bacteria die or become inactive.

Inactive or Spore-Forming Stage

Certain bacteria, such as the anthrax and tetanus bacilli, form spherical spores with tough outer coverings during their inactive stage. The purpose is to be able to withstand periods of famine, dryness, and unsuitable temperatures. In this stage, spores can be blown about and are not harmed by disinfectants, heat, or cold.

When favorable conditions are restored, the spores change into the active or vegetative form, then grow and reproduce.

Bacterial Infections

An **infection** occurs when body tissues are invaded by disease-causing or pathogenic bacteria. There can be no bacterial infection without the presence of pathogenic bacteria. The presence of pus is a sign of infection. **Pus** is a fluid product of inflammation and contains white blood cells (Chapter 6) and the debris of dead cells, tissue elements, and bacteria.

Staphylococci ("staph") are among the most common human bacteria and are carried by about a third of the population. Staph can be picked up on doorknobs, countertops, and other surfaces, but is more frequently transferred through skin-to-skin contact, such as shaking hands or using unclean implements. Antibiotics once controlled these bacteria, but certain strains of staph are now resistant to the drugs. There is now a greater need than ever for proper use of infection control measures in the cosmetology industry because of these resistant bacteria.

A **local infection**, such as a pimple or abscess, is one that is confined to a particular part of the body and is indicated by a lesion containing pus. A **general infection** results when the bloodstream carries the bacteria or virus and their toxins (poisons) to all parts of the body. Syphilis is an example.

When a disease spreads from one person to another by contact, it is said to be **contagious** (kon-TAY-jus) or communicable (kuh-MYOO-nih-kuh-bul). Some of the more common contagious diseases that will prevent a cosmetologist from servicing a client are tuberculosis, common cold, ringworm, scabies, and viral infections. The chief sources of contagion are unclean hands and implements, open sores, pus, mouth and nose discharges, and shared drinking cups and towels. Uncovered coughing or sneezing and spitting in public also spread germs.

Table 5–3 lists general terms and definitions that are important for an understanding of disease in general.

Term	Definition
acute disease	disease having a rapid onset, severe symptoms, and a short course or duration
allergy	reaction due to extreme sensitivity to certain foods, chemicals, or other normally harmless substances
chronic disease	disease of long duration, usually mild but recurring
congenital disease	disease that exists at birth
contagious disease	disease that is communicable or transmittable by contact
contraindication	any condition or disease that makes an indicated treatment or medication inadvisable
diagnosis	determination of the nature of a disease from its symptoms
disease	abnormal condition of all or part of the body, organ, or mind that makes it incapable of carrying on normal function
epidemic	appearance of a disease that simultaneously attacks a large number of persons living in a particular locality
etiology	study of the causes of disease and their mode of operation
infectious disease	disease caused by pathogenic microorganisms or viruses that are easily spread
inflammation	condition of some part of the body as a protective response to injury, irritation, or infection, characterized by redness, heat, pain, and swelling
objective symptoms	symptoms that are visible, such as pimples, pustules, or inflammation

(continued)

Table 5-3 General Terms Relating to Disease

5

Term	Definition
occupational disease	illness resulting from conditions associated with employment, such as coming in contact with certain chemicals or tints
parasitic disease	disease caused by vegetable or animal parasites, such as pediculosis and ringworm
pathogenic disease	disease produced by disease-causing bacteria, such as staphylococcus and streptococcus (pus-forming bacteria), or viruses
pathology	science that investigates modifications of the functions and changes in structure caused by disease
prognosis	foretelling of the probable course of a disease
seasonal disease	disease influenced by the weather
subjective symptoms	symptoms that can be felt, such as itching, burning, or pain
systemic disease	disease that affects the body generally, often due to under- or overfunctioning of the internal glands
venereal disease	contagious disease commonly acquired by contact with an infected person during sexual intercourse, characterized by sores and rashes on the skin

Table 5-3 *(continued)*

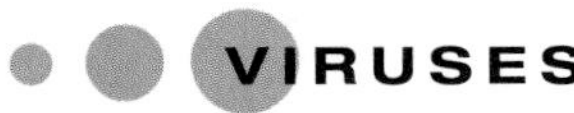

VIRUSES

A **virus** (VY-rus) is a submicroscopic structure capable of infesting almost all plants and animals, including bacteria. They are so small that they can even pass through the pores of a porcelain filter. They cause common colds and other respiratory and gastrointestinal (digestive tract) infections. Other viruses that plague humans are measles, mumps, chicken pox, smallpox, rabies, yellow fever, hepatitis, polio, influenza, and HIV which causes (AIDS).

One difference between viruses and bacteria is that a virus lives only by penetrating cells and becoming part of them, while bacteria are organisms that can live on their own. It is for this reason that bacterial infections can usually be treated with specific antibiotics while viruses are hard to kill without harming the body in the process. Generally, viruses are resistant to antibiotics. Vaccination prevents viruses from penetrating cells, but vaccinations are not available for all viruses.

Hepatitis

Hepatitis, a disease marked by inflammation of the liver, is caused by a bloodborne virus similar to HIV in transmission. It is more easily contracted than HIV, however, as it is present in all body fluids. Three types of hepatitis are of concern to the cosmetologist.

1. *Hepatitis A.* The illness usually lasts about three weeks. Symptoms are similar to those of the flu. Adults often have yellowing of the skin or the eyes. The disease is spread through close household contact, such as common bathroom use; poor sanitation; poor personal hygiene; contaminated food, milk, water, and shellfish; infected food handlers; and sexual contact. A vaccine is available.
2. *Hepatitis B (HBV) Standard.* This illness can cause long-term hepatitis, cirrhosis, and/or liver cancer. About half the people with the disease do not have symptoms, although the disease can mirror the flu. The disease is primarily transferred through sexual contact or parenteral exposure (piercing mucous membranes or skin barrier) to blood or blood products. A vaccine is available.
3. *Hepatitis C (HCV).* The illness can progress slowly, and about one-third of those with the illness do not have symptoms, though symptoms can include fatigue and stomach pain. The disease is transferred through parenteral contact and sexual activity with infected partners. No vaccine is available.

HIV/AIDS

HIV (Human Immunodeficiency Virus) is the virus that causes **AIDS** (Acquired Immune Deficiency Syndrome). AIDS, the disease, breaks down the body's immune system. HIV is passed from person to person through blood and other body fluids, such as semen and vaginal secretions. A person can be infected with HIV for up to 11 years without having symptoms. Sometimes, people who are HIV-positive have never been tested and do not know they are infecting other people.

The HIV virus is transmitted through unprotected sexual contact, the sharing of needles by intravenous (IV) drug users, and accidents with needles in health-care settings. It can enter the bloodstream through cuts and sores and can be transmitted in the salon by a sharp implement. It is *not* transmitted by holding hands, hugging, kissing, sharing food or household items like the telephone, or even toilet seats. There are no documented cases of the virus being transmitted by food handlers, insects, or casual contact.

2

insights

Kirby Morris

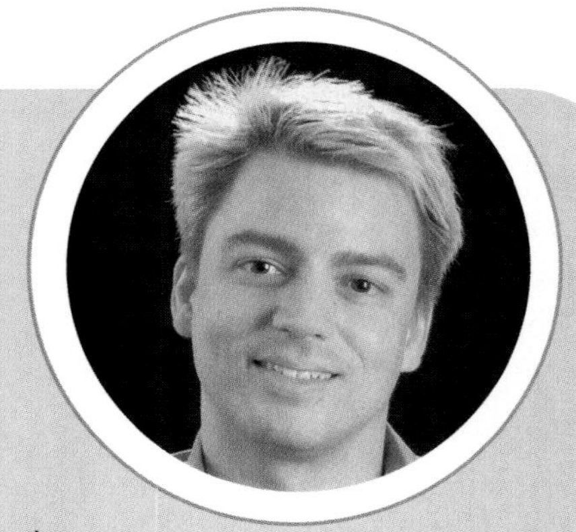

Wyoming-based salon owner Kirby Morris is active on his state board and functions as an inspector and examiner.

I got into this business by virtue of family tradition. After ten years as a grocery store manager, I decided I could make more money doing hair. I'd watched my aunt and my grandmother run salons, and my father, too. I'm glad to say that this field has really been the right one for me. I love the hands-on contact with the clientele. People will tell a cosmetologist more than they'll tell a psychiatrist!

I always advise those who are starting out in the field that the one thing they need to offer their clients, above anything else, is consistency. You have to make sure that your clients feel comfortable and that they'll get what they expect, whether that means you're never late for their appointments or that you'll always give them the same good cut. Also, you have to check your attitude in the parking lot. I always tell the new kids that when they decided to become cosmetologists, they gave up their right to have a bad day at work. All of your days have to be good ones because clients are paying for your time. In a service industry, you can't afford to have an "off" day.

Consistency is also important when it comes to sanitation. Every state has standards—for basic sanitation, wet disinfectants, blood spill procedures, and other things—that are posted in the salon. My suggestion to salon owners is to make everyone who's licensed in the salon read and sign that document on the back, like a contract. I make sure mine do that, and that they're provided with all the sanitation things they need. I was educated about sanitation in beauty school, but cosmetologists tend to forget those procedures and stop doing them. Then I was reeducated and found out how serious it was. My reeducation occurred during an inspection—I felt I had the cleanest salon in town, but the inspector—Diane Pennington, later my mentor—found a few things I wasn't doing right. I was actually embarrassed.

Many consumers know about sanitation issues. So, for example, you need to make sure there's always a neck strip or towel between their skin and the cape. You don't want that cape to touch one person and then another—you can actually spread disease, rashes, or irritations that way. If you don't put a neck strip on, the consumer knows you are not following the rules, and if you are breaking that one, you could be breaking many more. When I started doing everything properly, I realized it's just as easy to do it right. You feel much better when you know you're protecting your clients. And that leads right back to their feeling comfortable.

HOW PATHOGENS ENTER THE BODY

Pathogenic bacteria or viruses can enter the body through:

- a break in the skin, such as a cut, pimple, or scratch.
- the mouth (contaminated water or food).
- the nose (air).
- the eyes or ears.
- unprotected sex

The body fights infection by means of:

- unbroken skin, which is the body's first line of defense.
- body secretions, such as perspiration and digestive juices.
- white cells within the blood that destroy bacteria.
- antitoxins that counteract the toxins produced by bacteria and viruses.

Bloodborne Pathogens

Disease-causing bacteria or viruses that are carried through body in the blood or body fluids, such as hepatitis and HIV, are called **bloodborne pathogens.** If you accidentally cut a client who is HIV-positive or is infected with hepatitis and you continue to use the implement without cleaning and disinfecting it, you risk puncturing your skin or cutting another client with a contaminated tool. Similarly, if you are shaving a client's face or neck with a razor or clipper blades and pick up body fluid from a blemish or open sore, transmission is possible. Risks are also present when waxing and tweezing.

PARASITES

Parasites are vegetable or animal organisms that live in or on another living organism and draw their nourishment from that organism (referred to as a host). They are not capable of sustaining their own life without a host.

Vegetable (plant) parasites or **fungi** (FUN-jy), which include molds, mildews, and yeasts, can produce contagious diseases, such as ringworm and favus (FAY-vus), both skin diseases. Nail fungus can be contracted through implements that have not been disinfected properly or by moisture trapped under nail enhancements. Nail fungus is chronic and usually localized but can be spread to other nails and from client to client if implements are not disinfected before and after each client. Treatment is generally applied directly to the affected area. In serious cases, however, a physician's care is required (Figure 5–5).

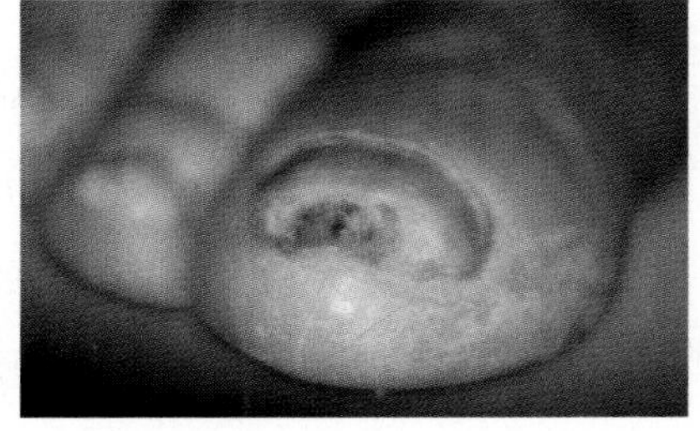

Figure 5–5 Nail fungus.

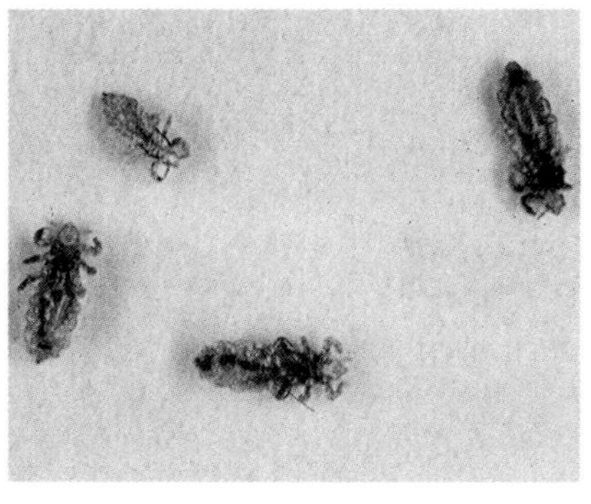

Figure 5–6 Head lice.

Animal parasites, such as head lice, are responsible for contagious diseases and conditions (Figure 5–6). A skin disease caused by an infestation of head lice is called **pediculosis capitis** (puh-dik-yuh-LOH-sis). **Scabies** (SKAY-beez) is another contagious skin disease and is caused by the itch mite, which burrows under the skin (Figure 5–7).

Contagious diseases and conditions caused by parasites should never be treated in a cosmetology school or salon. Clients should be referred to a physician. Contaminated countertops should be cleaned with a pesticide or insecticide according to manufacturer's directions. 3

IMMUNITY

Immunity is the ability of the body to destroy any bacteria that have gained entrance and to resist infection in general. Immunity against disease can be natural or acquired and is a sign of good health. **Natural immunity** is partly inherited and partly developed through hygienic living. **Acquired immunity** is immunity that the body develops after it overcomes a disease, or through inoculation (such as vaccination).

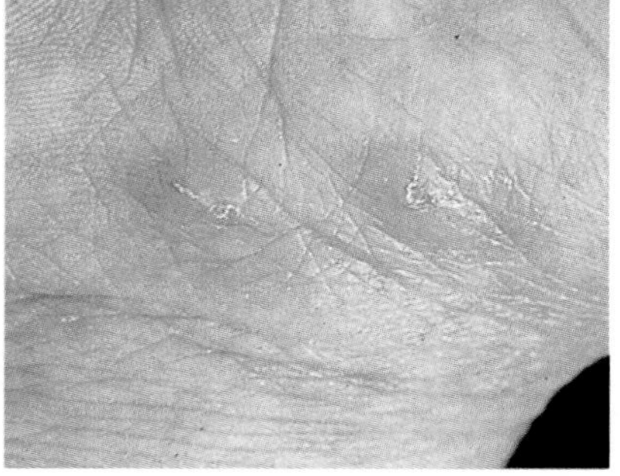

Figure 5–7 Scabies.

PRINCIPLES OF PREVENTION

There is no better way for a salon to make a good first impression than to maintain the highest level of cleanliness. This makes a positive statement that fills clients with confidence (Figure 5–8).

There is more to a clean salon, however, than a well-swept floor or vacuumed rugs. Proper care must be taken to meet rigorous health standards. Otherwise, the salon could be contributing to the spread of disease.

Controlling infection and disease is a vitally important aspect of the salon industry. Clients depend on you to ensure their safety. One careless action could cause injury or serious illness. Being a salon professional can be fun and rewarding, but it is also a great responsibility. Fortunately, preventing the spread of dangerous diseases is not hard to do if you know how to do it and, more important yet, if you practice what you know.

Decontamination

Take a look around you. What do you see? No doubt, wherever you are, you are looking at some sort of surface. It could be a table, the wall, the floor, the doorknob, or your hand. Almost everything presents a surface of some kind. These surfaces may seem clean to you, even sparkling, but no matter how clean they appear to the naked eye, chances are they are contaminated.

Surfaces of tools or other objects that are not free from dirt, oils, and microbes are covered with **contaminants**, which are any substances that can cause contamination. Many things can be contaminants, such as hair left in a comb, makeup on a towel or brush, or nail dust on a file.

Tools and other surfaces in the salon can also be contaminated with bacteria, viruses, and fungi. Even tools that appear to be clean are usually covered with these microorganisms.

Of course, a salon can never be completely free from all contamination, and it would not make sense to attempt such a goal. However, it is your responsibility as a salon professional to be on constant alert for disease-causing contaminants.

The removal of pathogens and other substances from tools and surfaces is called **decontamination**. Decontamination involves the use of physical or chemical means to remove, inactivate, or destroy pathogens so that the object is rendered safe for handling, use, or disposal. There are three main levels of decontamination: sterilization, disinfection, and sanitation. Only disinfection and sanitation are required in the salon.

STERILIZATION

Sterilization is the highest level of decontamination. It completely destroys every organism on a surface, whether beneficial or harmful. Sterilization even kills bacterial spores, the most resistant form of life on Earth. Methods of sterilization include the steam autoclave and dry heat (a form of extreme heat.)

Sterilization is a process used by dentists and surgeons, whose tools are designed to break and penetrate the skin barrier. Estheticians also use needles and probes that lance the skin, so they must follow the same

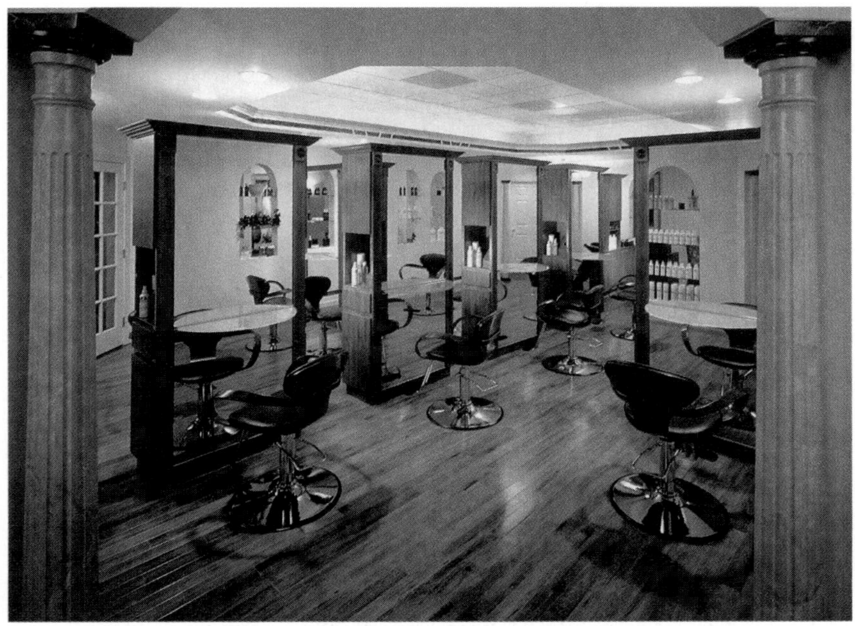

Figure 5-8 A sparkling clean salon gains your clients' confidence.

sterilization procedures. Presterilized disposable lancets or needles are a simpler solution to the issue of sterilization.

The word "sterilize" is often used incorrectly. For example, some practitioners tell clients that they are "sterilizing the nail plate or skin." This is impossible. Sterilizing the skin would quickly kill it and would destroy the nail plate as well. We can only sterilize surfaces that are not **porous** (having pores or openings that permit liquids or gases to pass through). Metal implements are nonporous and can be sterilized, but wood surfaces, which are porous, cannot. In short, sterilization is impractical and unnecessary in salons.

Some states and provinces prohibit the use of invasive procedures in the salon, including those requiring needles, lancets, and probes. Check with your regulatory agency.

Disinfection

Disinfection is a higher level of decontamination than sanitation. It is second only to sterilization. Disinfection controls microorganisms on hard, nonporous surfaces such as cuticle nippers and other salon implements.

Disinfection provides the level of protection required by the salon to kill most organisms, with one exception. Disinfection does not kill bacterial spores, but this is not necessary in the salon environment. It is important only in hospitals and other health-care facilities where instruments are used to penetrate or cut the skin. Lancets and other metal implements used in advanced facial treatments should be sterilized, or disposable implements should be used.

Disinfectants are chemical agents used to destroy most bacteria and some viruses and to disinfect implements and surfaces. *Disinfectants are not for use on human skin, hair, or nails.* Never use disinfectants as hand cleaners. Any substance powerful enough to quickly and efficiently destroy pathogens can also damage skin.

Read Carefully Before Using

Manufacturers take great care to develop safe and highly effective systems. However, just because something is safe does not mean that it cannot be dangerous if used improperly. Any professional salon product can be dangerous if used incorrectly. Like all tools, disinfectants must always be used in strict accordance with manufacturer's instructions.

All disinfectants must be approved by the Environmental Protection Agency (EPA) and each individual state. The disinfectant's label must also have an EPA registration number. Look for this number when choosing a disinfectant. It is the only way to ensure that the EPA has the necessary test data on file and that the product has been proven effective against certain organisms. The product label will also tell you exactly which organisms the disinfectant has been tested for, such as HIV-1 or the Hepatitis B virus. The law requires testing for specific organisms, or it should not appear on the label (Figure 5–9).

Besides the EPA registration number, federal law requires manufacturers to provide you with important information in the form of a Material Safety Data Sheet (**MSDS**) (Figure 5–10), along with other important information, such as directions for proper use, safety precautions, and a list of active ingredients. The MSDS provides all pertinent information on products, ranging from content and associated hazards to combustion levels and storage requirements. These sheets should be available for every product used in the

Thoroughly pre-clean. Completely immerse brushes, combs, scissors, clipper blades, razors, tweezers, manicure implements, and other non-porous instruments for 10 minutes (or as required by local authorities). Wipe dry before use. Fresh solution should be prepared daily or more often when the solution becomes diluted or soiled.
*For Complete Instructions For Hepatitis B Virus (HBV) and Human Immunodeficiency Virus (HIV-1) DISINFECTION Refer To Enclosed Hang Tag.
Statement of Practical Treatment:
In case of contact, immediately flush eyes or skin with plenty of water for at least 15 minutes. For eye contacts, call a physician. If swallowed, drink egg whites, gelatin solution or if these are not available, drink large quantities of water. Avoid alcohol. Call a physician Immediately.
Note to Physician: Probable mucosal damage may contraindicate the use of gastric lavage.
Note: Avoid shipping or storing below freezing.
If product freezes, thaw at room temperature and shake gently to remix components.

Figure 5-9 An efficacy label.

cosmetology school or salon, and may be obtained from the product's distributor and/or manufacturer. Operating without an MSDS poses a health risk to anyone in a salon who comes into contact with hazardous materials.

Take the time to read all of this vital information. Only then will you be certain that you are protecting yourself and your clients to the best of your ability.

CAUTION

Mixing chemicals stronger than recommended by the manufacturer counteracts their effectiveness. The use of goggles or glasses and gloves is usually recommended.

OSHA

The Occupational Safety and Health Administration (OSHA) was created as part of the U.S. Department of Labor to regulate and enforce safety and health standards in the workplace. Regulating employee exposure to toxic substances and informing employees about the dangers of materials used in the workplace are key points of the Occupational Safety and Health Act of 1970. This act established the Hazard Communication Rule, which requires that chemical manufacturers and importers assess the hazards associated with their products. Material Safety Data Sheets and product labeling are two important results of this law.

The standards set by OSHA are particularly relevant to the cosmetology industry because of the nature of the chemicals used. Issues having to do with the mixing, storing, and disposal of chemicals; the general safety of the workplace; and, most important, the right of the cosmetologist to know what is contained in the products she uses all are regulated by OSHA standards.

Choosing a Disinfectant

Disinfectants are chemicals. To use a disinfectant properly, you must read and follow the manufacturer's instructions. Such variables as mixing precautions and exposure times demand particular attention. The product

Material Safety Data Sheet
May be used to comply with
OSHA's Hazard Communication Standard,
29 CFR 1910.1200. Standard must be
consulted for specific requirements.

U.S. Department of Labor
Occupational Safety and Health Administration
(Non-Mandatory Form)
Form Approved
OMB No. 1218-0072

IDENTITY *(As Used on Label and List)*	*Note: Blank spaces are not permitted. If any item is not applicable or no information is available, the space must be marked to indicate that.*

Section I

Manufacturer's Name	Emergency Telephone Number
Address *(Number, Street, City, State, and ZIP Code)*	Telephone Number for information
	Date Prepared
	Signature of Preparer *(optional)*

Section II — Hazardous Ingredients/Identity Information

Hazardous Components (Specific Chemical Identity; Common Names(s))	OSHA PEL	ACGIH TLV	Other Limits Recommended	% *(optional)*

Section III — Physical/Chemical Characteristics

Boiling Point		Specific Gravity (H_2O - 1)	
Vapor Pressure (mm Hg.)		Melting Point	
Vapor Density (Air - 1))		Evaporation Rate (Butyl Acetate - 1)	
Solubility in Water			
Appearance and Odor			

Section IV — Fire and Explosion Hazard Data

Flash Point (Method Used)	Flammable Limits	LEL	UEL
Extinguishing Media			
Special Fire Fighting Procedures			
Unusual Fire and Explosion Hazards			

(Reproduce locally) OSHA 174, Sept. 1985

Figure 5-10 A sample MSDS.

5

Material Safety Data Sheet (MSDS)

Section V — Reactivity Data

Stability	Unstable		Conditions to Avoid
	Stable		

Incompatibility (Materials to Avoid)

Hazardous Decomposition or Byproducts

Hazardous Polymerization	May Occur		Conditions to Avoid
	Will Not Occur		

Section VI — Health Hazard Data

Route(s) of Entry:	Inhalation?	Skin?	Ingestion?

Health Hazards *(Acute and Chronic)*

Carcenogenicity:	NTP?	IARC Monographs	OSHA Regulated?

Signs and Symptoms of Exposure

Medical Conditions
Generally Aggravated by Exposure

Emergency and First Aid Program

Section VII — Precautions for Safe Handling and Use

Steps to Be Taken in Case Material is Released or Spilled

Waste Disposal Method

Precautions to Be Taken in Handling and Storing

Other Precautions

Section VIII — Control Measures

Respiratory Protection (Specify Type)

Ventilation	Local Exhaust	Special
	Mechanical (General)	Other

Protective Gloves	Eye Protection

Other Protective Clothing or Equipment

Work/Hygienic Practices

Page 2

Figure 5-10 *(continued)*

5

label will explain what the disinfectant has been tested for. To meet salon requirements, a disinfectant must have the correct **efficacy** (effectiveness) to be used against bacteria, fungi, and viruses. A disinfectant that is "Formulated for Hospitals and Health Care Facilities," or a "Hospital Disinfectant," must be **pseudomonacidal** (SOO-dum-ohn-uh-SIDE-ul) (effective against the bacteria *Pseudomonas* described in Chapter 21), in addition to being **bactericidal** (back-teer-uh-SYD-ul), **fungicidal** (fun-jih-SYD-ul), and **virucidal** (vy-rus-SYD-ul). If a disinfectant has been tested for additional organisms such as HIV-1, it will be stated on the label. Check for the label number and efficacy standard on the label (see Figure 5–9).

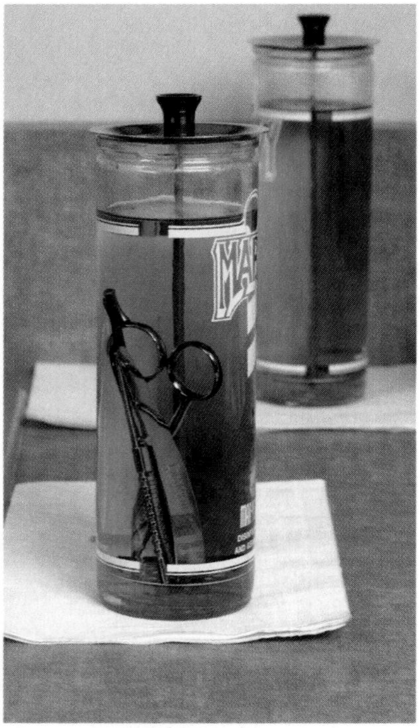

For bloodborne pathogens, OSHA issued a policy in 1997 stating that, in order to comply with OSHA's Bloodborne Pathogens Standard, the use of an EPA-registered **tuberculocidal** (tuh-bur-kyoo-loh-SYD-ul) disinfectant or an EPA-registered disinfectant labeled as effective against HIV and HBV is required. For this reason, when salon implements accidentally come into contact with blood or body fluids, they should be cleaned and completely immersed in an EPA-registered disinfectant that kills HIV-1 and Hepatitis B virus, or in a tuberculocidal disinfectant. The National Interstate Council of State Cosmetology Boards (NICS) follows this standard for examinations as well.

Figure 5–11 Submerge implements completely in disinfectant.

Proper Use of Disinfectants

Any item that is used on a client must be disinfected or discarded after each use. Items that do not have the capacity to be disinfected, such as orangewood sticks, must be discarded. Combs, brushes, scissors, razors, clipper blades, nippers, electrodes, and other commonly used, nonporous tools must be disinfected.

Even the best disinfectants will not work well if mixed or used incorrectly. All implements should be thoroughly cleaned before soaking to avoid contaminating the disinfecting solution. Hair, nail filings, creams, oils, and makeup will lessen the effectiveness of the solution. Besides, a dirty jar of disinfectant would not fill your clients with confidence. Implements must be completely submerged for proper disinfection (Figure 5–11).

Ultrasonic cleaners use high-frequency sound waves to create powerful, cleansing bubbles in the liquid. This cleansing action is an effective way to clean tiny crevices that are impossible to reach with a brush. Without an effective disinfectant solution, however, these devices only sanitize implements.

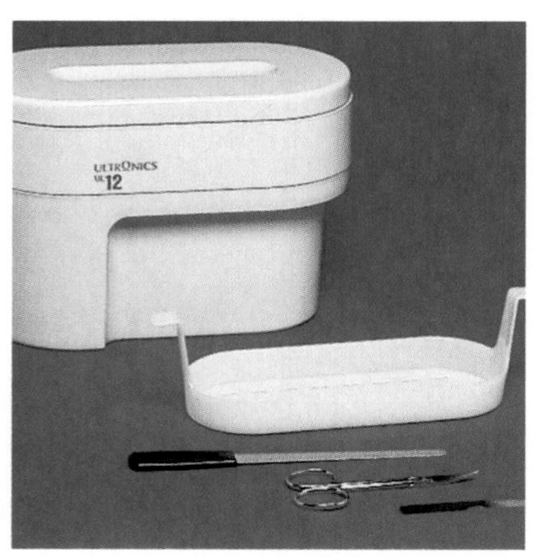
Figure 5–12 Ultrasonic bath.

Ultrasonic cleaners are a useful addition to your disinfection process, but are not required. Many systems disinfect with great effectiveness without relying on such devices. However, some salons feel that this added cleansing benefit is well worth the extra expense. It also saves time by eliminating cleaning by hand (Figure 5–12).

Types of Disinfectants

There are a variety of disinfectants that the salon can choose from.

Quats

Quaternary ammonium compounds (KWAT-ur-nayr-ree uh-MOH-nee-um), commonly called quats, are a type of disinfectant considered non-toxic, odorless, and fast-acting. Older formulas were not very effective, but the newer products, called dual quat formulas, are dramatically more effective.

Most quat solutions disinfect implements in 10 to 15 minutes. Leaving some tools in the solution for too long may damage them. Keep in mind that long-term exposure to any water solution or disinfectant may damage fine steel. With today's modern formulas, however, corrosion of metal surfaces can be easily avoided, especially if you keep implements separated while disinfecting. Metal implements such as scissors and nail clippers should be oiled regularly to keep them in perfect working order.

Quats are also very effective for cleaning tables and countertops.

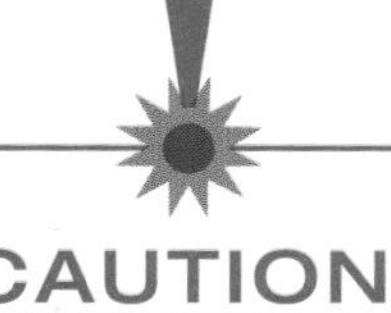

CAUTION

In the past, formalin, a solution of formaldehyde in water, *was* recommended as a disinfectant and fumigant in dry cabinet sanitizers. However, formalin is not safe for salon use. Formaldehyde (for-MAL-duh-hyd), a pungent gas, is a suspected cancer-causing agent. It is poisonous when inhaled and is extremely irritating to the eyes, nose, throat, and lungs. It can also cause skin allergies, irritation, dryness, and rash. After long-term use, formaldehyde vapors can cause symptoms similar to chronic bronchitis or asthma. These symptoms usually worsen over time with continued exposure.

Phenols

Like quats, phenolic (fi-NOH-lik) disinfectants, or phenols (FEE-nohlz), have been used reliably over the years to disinfect implements. **Phenol** is a caustic poison, but it can be safe and extremely effective if used according to instructions. One disadvantage is that most rubber and plastic materials may be softened or discolored by phenols. Phenols in 5 percent solution are used mostly for metal implements.

Extra care should be taken to avoid skin contact with phenols. Phenolic disinfectants can cause skin irritation, and concentrated phenols can seriously burn the skin and eyes. Some are poisonous if accidentally ingested.

Alcohol and Bleach

The word alcohol is often misunderstood. There are many chemical compounds that may be classified as alcohol. The three most widely used are methyl (METH-ul) alcohol (methanol), ethyl (ETH-ul) alcohol (ethanol or grain alcohol), and isopropyl (eye-soh-PROH-pul) alcohol (isopropanol or rubbing alcohol).

In the salon, ethyl and isopropyl alcohol are sometimes used to disinfect implements. To be effective, the strength of ethyl alcohol must be no less than 70 percent, and the strength of isopropyl alcohol must be 99 percent. Since alcohol is not an EPA-registered disinfectant, it is not permitted for use with implements in states requiring hospital disinfection. This means it is not legal to use alcohol as a disinfectant in most states.

There are many disadvantages to using alcohols. They are extremely flammable, evaporate quickly, and are slow-acting and less effective when compared to other recommended disinfectants. Alcohols corrode tools and cause sharp edges to become dull. They also discolor and damage the surface of floors and countertops. The vapors formed on evaporation can cause headaches and nausea when inhaled in high concentrations or after prolonged exposure.

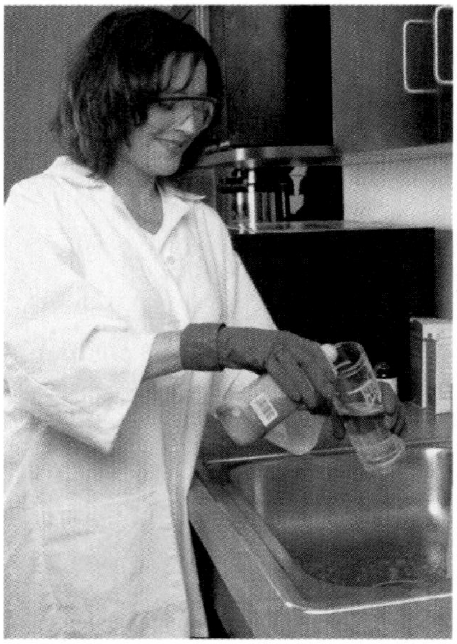

Figure 5–13 Wear gloves and safety goggles while handling disinfectants.

Household bleach (**sodium hypochlorite**) (SOH-dee-um hy-puh-KLOR-ite) is an effective disinfectant, but shares some of the same drawbacks as alcohols. Neither bleach nor alcohols are professionally designed and tested for disinfection of salon implements. Bleach and alcohol may have been used extensively in the past, but have since been replaced by more advanced and effective technologies. Bleach is, however, a very effective laundering additive.

Although quats are perfectly suitable for cleaning any surface (unless otherwise specified in the manufacturer's directions), you may wish to clean floors, bathrooms, sinks, and waste receptacles with a commercial cleaner such as Lysol or Pine-Sol. Both are very effective disinfectants, but should not be used on salon implements. They are general "household level" disinfectants and are not designed for professional tools.

Disinfectant Safety

Disinfectants are powerful, professional-strength tools that can be hazardous if used incorrectly. Disinfectants can be poisonous if ingested and can cause serious skin and eye damage, especially in a concentrated form. A good rule to remember is *use caution*! In addition, you should:

- always wear gloves and safety glasses when mixing chemicals with water (Figure 5–13).
- always add disinfectant to water, not water to disinfectant.
- use tongs, gloves, or a draining basket to remove implements from disinfectants.
- always keep disinfectants away from children.
- never pour quats, phenols, formalin, alcohol (not legal in most states), or any other disinfectant over your hands. This hazardous practice can cause skin irritation and increase the chance of infection. Wash your hands with soap and warm water and dry them thoroughly.
- carefully weigh and measure all products to ensure that they perform at their peak efficiency.
- never place any disinfectant or other product in an unmarked container (Figure 5–14). Disinfectants come in different forms such as ready-to-use sprays (for surface cleaning), liquid concentrate, and powders. Some disinfectants appear clear while others are a little cloudy.
- always follow manufacturer's recommendations for mixing and using, and check the efficacy to make sure you are using the right disinfectant.
- avoid overexposure. Disinfectants are chemicals, and overuse is detrimental to the environment.

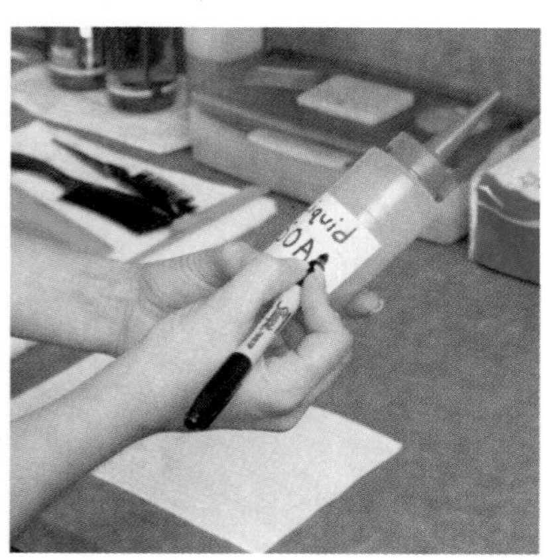

Figure 5–14 All containers should be labeled.

Jars or containers used to disinfect implements are often incorrectly called wet sanitizers. Of course, the purpose of these containers is not to sanitize but to disinfect. The disinfecting soak solution must be changed daily and kept free from debris unless otherwise directed by the manufacturer's instructions. Strict adherence to the principles of good hygiene and disinfection must be maintained.

Disinfection Procedures

Always disinfect your tools or other implements according to the guidelines listed for EPA wet disinfectants. This means complete immersion for the required amount of time. The following are guidelines for specific salon materials.

Disinfecting Implements

Most tools and implements can be disinfected. These include combs, brushes, rollers, picks, styling tools, scissors, tweezers, nail clippers, and some nail files.

1. Pre-clean to remove hair, filings, and other such loose matter by scrubbing with soap and water (Figure 5–15).
2. Rinse thoroughly and pat dry with a clean towel.
3. Put on gloves, goggles, or safety glasses.
4. Mix disinfectant according to manufacturer's directions, always adding disinfectant to the water (Figure 5–16).
5. Using gloves or tongs, completely immerse implements or tools and leave for the required amount of time, as per manufacturer's instructions (Figure 5–17).
6. Remove implements with tongs, basket, or gloves so as not to contaminate the disinfectant (Figure 5–18).
7. Rinse thoroughly and dry.
8. Place disinfected implements in a clean, closed, dry, disinfected container (such as a plastic container with a lid).

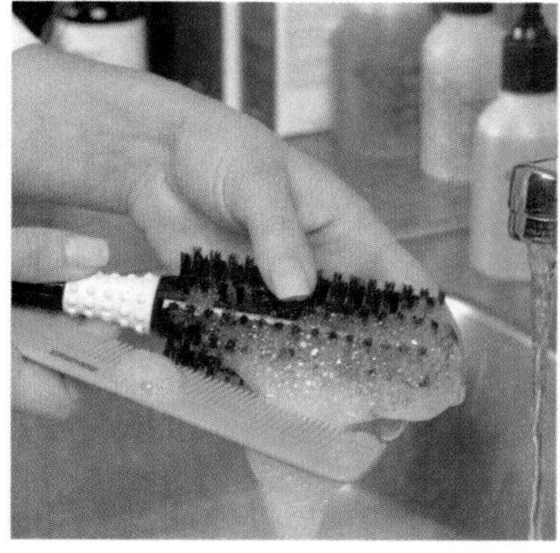

Figure 5–15 Remove hair from brushes and combs before disinfecting.

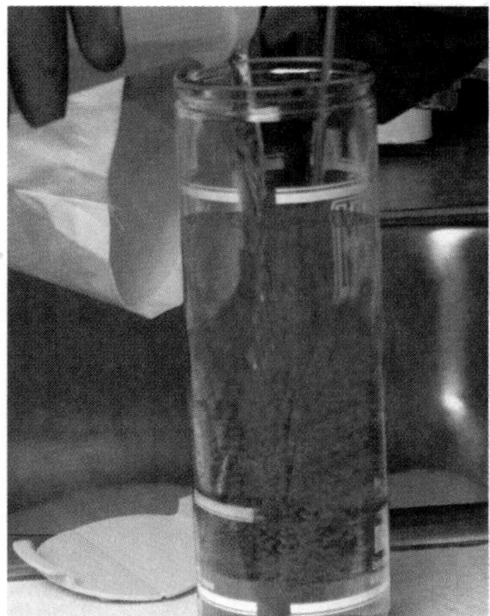

Figure 5–16 Carefully pour disinfectant into the water when preparing wet disinfectant solution.

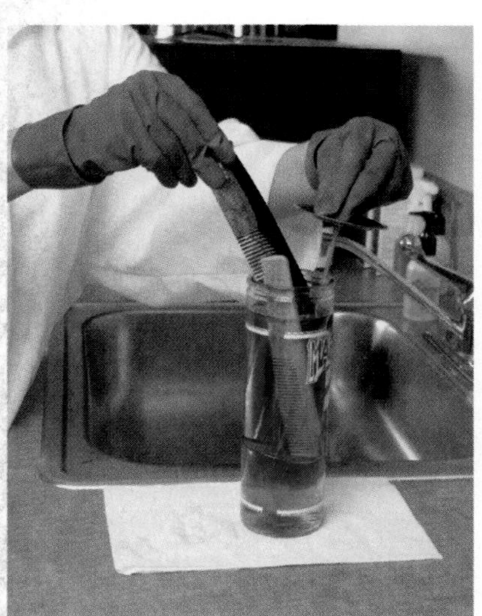

Figure 5–17 Submerge combs and brushes in disinfectant solution.

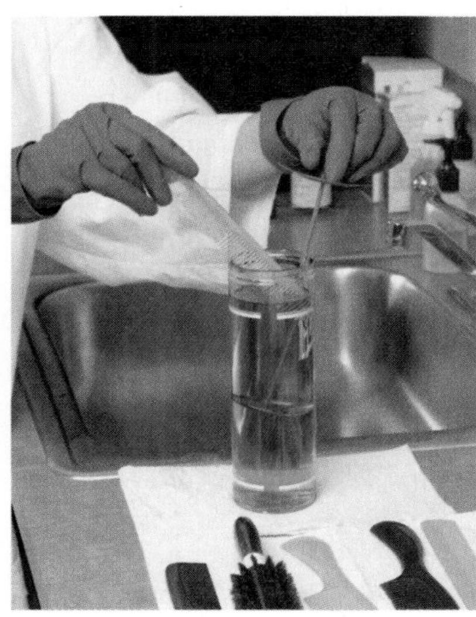

Figure 5–18 Remove implements with tongs, gloves, or a draining basket.

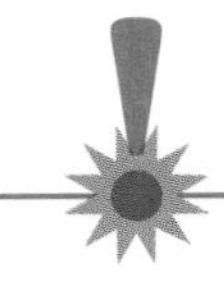

CAUTION

Electric or bead "sterilizers" *do not* sterilize implements. They do not even properly disinfect tools. Only the tip of the implement can be inserted into the hot glass beads, and the handles remain contaminated. They only give users a false sense of security. These devices represent a dangerous gamble with your client's health.

Disinfecting Linens and Capes

All linens should be used once and then laundered with bleach according to label directions. Capes or drapes that come into contact with a client's skin should be laundered in the same manner.

Disinfecting Electrical Equipment

The contact points of equipment that cannot be immersed in liquid, such as hair clippers, electrotherapy tools, and nail drills, should be wiped or sprayed with an EPA-registered, hospital-grade disinfectant created especially for electrical equipment (Figure 5–19). Electrical equipment must be kept in good repair.

Disinfecting Work Surfaces

Before and after each client, an EPA-registered, hospital-grade disinfectant should be used on the work surface (manicure table, workstation, esthetic bed, and the like). The disinfectant should be left on the surface the full amount of time prescribed by the manufacturer's directions. Remember to disinfect all surfaces. This includes doorknobs, handles, and so on (Figure 5–20).

The shampoo bowl should be cleaned and the drain cleared of all hair after each client. The neck of the bowl should be disinfected the same as other work surfaces.

Disinfecting Whirlpool Pedicure Foot Spas

When using whirlpool pedicure foot spas, you must follow proper disinfection procedures to ensure proper maintenance of the equipment and to prevent the spread of bacterial or parasitic disease. Take time to carefully read the manufacturer's cleaning instructions and ask your manufacturer and/or distributor for a demonstration as well. Improperly disinfected equipment can harbor bacteria that may spread disease or infection to clients, cosmetologists, or nail technicians who come into contact with it.

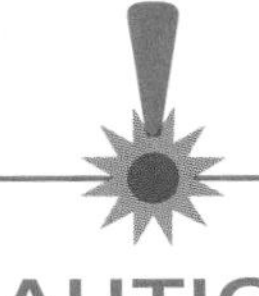

CAUTION

Ultraviolet (UV) sanitizers are useful storage containers. However, they will not disinfect salon implements. Never use these devices to disinfect.

5

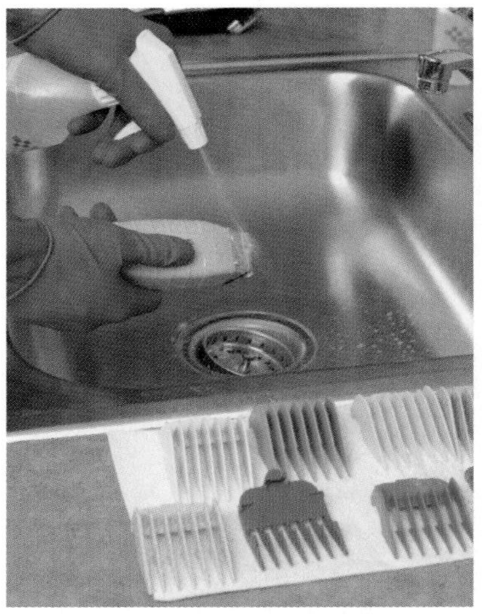

Figure 5–19 Spray clippers with disinfectant.

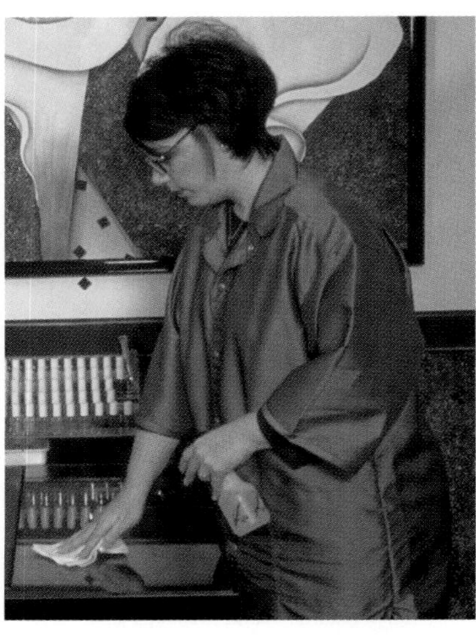

Figure 5–20 Apply disinfectant on manicure tables.

PROCEDURE

DISINFECTING FOOT SPAS

After each customer:

1. Drain all water and remove all foreign matter from the foot spa.
2. Clean the surfaces and walls of the foot spa with soap or detergent and rinse with clean, clear water.
3. Disinfect with an EPA-registered disinfectant with bactericidal, fungicidal, virucidal (and in some states tuberculocidal) efficacy, according to manufacturers' instructions (Figure 5–21).
4. Rinse and wipe dry with a clean towel.

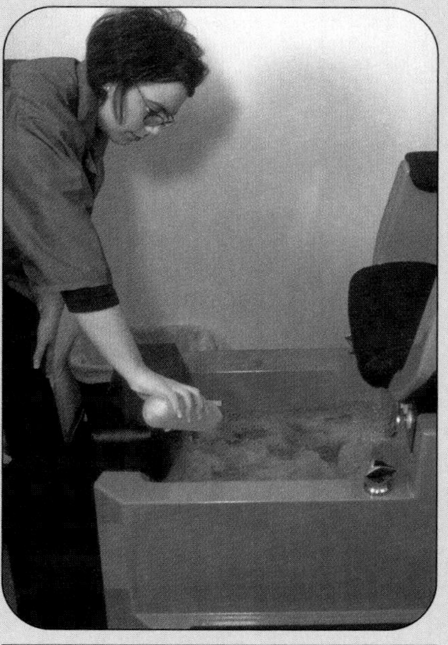

Figure 5–21 Disinfecting a foot spa.

At the end of each day:

1. Remove the screen and clean all debris trapped behind the screen of each foot spa.
2. Wash the screen and inlet with soap or detergent and a chlorine solution (5 percent chlorine bleach to 1 gallon of water), or wash the screen with soap or detergent and clean, clear water. Then totally immerse in an EPA-registered disinfectant with bactericidal, fungicidal, virucidal (and in some states tuberculocidal) efficacy, according to manufacturers' instructions.
3. Flush the system with low-sudsing soap and warm water for ten minutes. Then rinse, drain, and let air-dry.

Every two weeks:

1. After following the recommended daily cleaning procedure described above, fill the foot spa tub (5 gallons) with water and four teaspoons of 5 percent bleach solution (a dose of 50 parts per thousand).
2. Circulate the solution through the foot spa system for 5 to 10 minutes.
3. Let the solution sit overnight (at least 6 to 10 hours).
4. The following morning, in advance of the first customer, drain and flush the system.

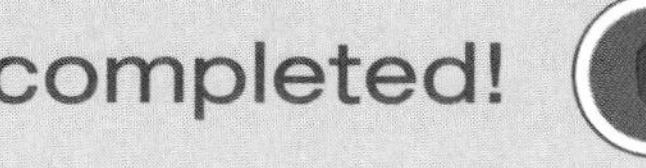

Blood Spill Disinfection

Blood spills occur when you or a client are accidentally cut with a sharp instrument. If a blood spill should occur during a procedure, proper steps must be taken for the safety of both people.

1. If a cut is sustained, stop the service and clean the injured area.
2. Use a finger guard or gloves as appropriate.
3. Apply antiseptic and/or liquid or spray styptic without contaminating the container.
4. Cover the injury with a Band-Aid or other appropriate dressing.
5. Clean client and workstation as necessary.
6. Discard all disposable contaminated objects such as wipes or cotton balls by double-bagging (place the waste in a plastic bag and then in a trash bag). Use a biohazard sticker (red or orange) or a container for contaminated waste. Deposit sharp disposables in a sharps box (Figure 5–22).
7. Remove your gloves. Wash your hands with soap and warm water before returning to the service.
8. All tools and implements that have come into contact with blood or body fluids must be disinfected by complete immersion in a EPA-registered, hospital-grade disinfectant that kills HIV-1 and Hepatitis B Virus or in a tuberculocidal disinfectant. Be sure to mix and use the disinfectant according to the manufacturers' directions.

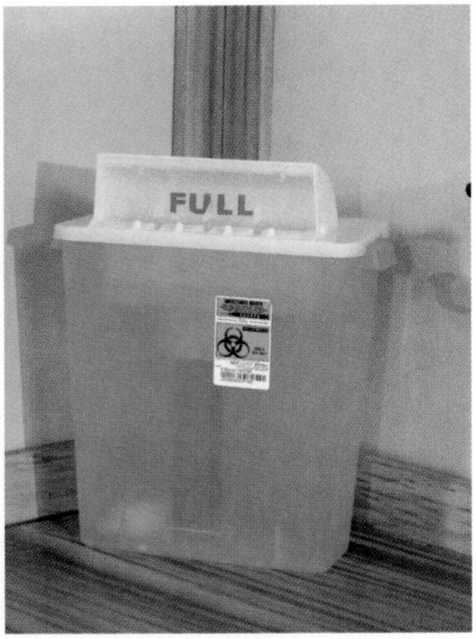

Figure 5-22 A sharps box.

Because blood can carry many pathogens, you should never touch a client's open sore or wound.

Dispensary

The dispensary must be kept clean and orderly, with all containers marked clearly as to content. An MSDS on every chemical in stock should be kept readily available to all those working in the salon or school. The MSDS should also indicate the appropriate disinfectant to be used with each chemical.

Handling Disposable Supplies

To prevent the spread of disease, all disposable supplies, such as orangewood sticks, emery boards, cotton, gauze, neck strips, and the like, should be thrown away. Anything exposed to blood, including microdermabrasion debris, must be double-bagged and marked with a biohazard sticker or marked and disposed of according to OSHA standards (separated from other waste and disposed of according to federal, state, and local regulations). Puncture-proof containers should be used in the disposal of all sharps. *Remember: Disinfect or Discard.*

Sanitation

The third, or lowest, level of decontamination is called **sanitation** or **sanitizing**. These words are often frequently misused and misunderstood. To sanitize means "to significantly reduce the number of pathogens or disease-producing organisms found on a surface." Cleaning with soaps or detergents will sanitize salon tools and other surfaces.

Sanitized surfaces may still harbor pathogens or other organisms. Removing hair from a brush and washing the brush with detergent is considered sanitation. Putting antiseptics designed for hands or feet on your skin or washing your hands is another example of sanitation. Your hands may appear very clean when you are finished but will still harbor pathogens found in the tap water and on the towel.

An emerging health concern is the growth of mold and mildew in buildings. **Mold** is a fungus growth that usually grows in dark, damp places. **Mildew** is a moldy coating produced by fungi that can appear on walls, fabrics, and the like, and also occurs in damp areas. Mold spores carry **toxins** that can cause allergic reactions and sickness in some people. These spores are almost always present in outdoor and indoor air and on most furnishings and construction materials. Dirt on surfaces provides nutrients for mold. Practicing proper sanitation provides protection against the growth of mildew and mold in the salon.

CAUTION

Avoid using bar soaps in the salon. Bar soap can actually grow bacteria. It is a better practice to provide pump-type liquid soaps.

Washing the Hands

Hand-washing is one of the most important actions that can be taken to prevent the transfer of microorganisms from one person to another. Hand-washing removes microorganisms from the folds and grooves of the skin by lifting and rinsing them from the skin surface.

In the salon, hands should be thoroughly washed before and after each service. When washing your hands in a public rest room, avoid touching items such as bar soap, a towel dispenser, or a doorknob after washing and before leaving the restroom. Use a paper towel to turn the doorknob when leaving the rest room. This way you avoid contaminating your clean hand with any microorganisms. At the end of the day, wash your hands to prevent carrying microorganisms outside of the salon.

Soap and warm water are generally sufficient for hand-washing, although some antibacterial soaps can kill microorganisms in deeper layers of the skin than plain soap or detergents do. When overused, however, the relatively harsh, drying action of antibacterial soaps may actually leave the skin vulnerable to skin problems such as eczema. Alcohol-based no-rinse products designed for use without water are also very drying to the skin.

The correct procedure for washing the hands consists of these steps:

1. Wet your hands with warm water.
2. Using liquid soap, scrub your hands together and work up a good lather for 15 to 20 seconds. Give particular attention to the areas between the fingers, the nails, both sides of the hands, and the exposed portions of the arms (Figure 5–23).
3. Rinse your hands well with warm water.
4. Dry your hands using a disposable paper towel or air blower. Do not use cloth towels unless they are dispensed one to a person.

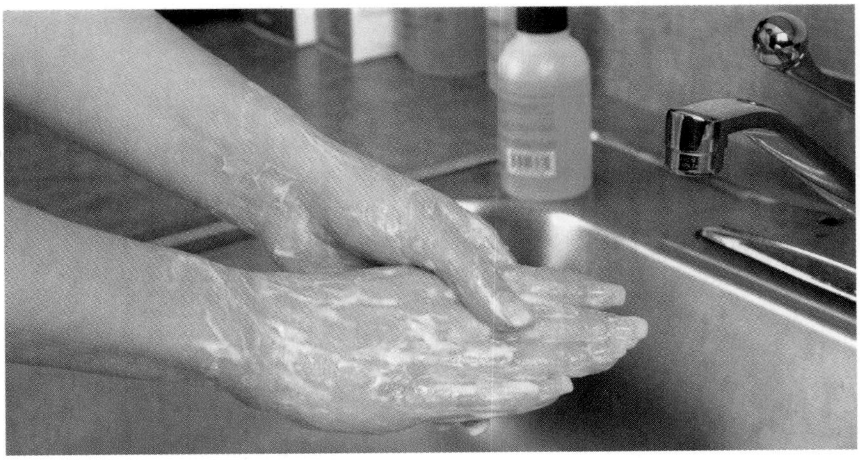

Figure 5-23 Proper hand-washing technique.

Antiseptics (ant-ih-SEP-tiks) can kill, retard, or prevent the growth of bacteria, but they are not classified as disinfectants. Antiseptics such as 3 percent solutions of hydrogen peroxide are weaker than disinfectants and are safe for application to skin (usually used prior to a manicure or pedicure). They are considered sanitizers and are not adequate for use on instruments and surfaces. 6 ✓

UNIVERSAL PRECAUTIONS

Many infectious diseases do not present visible symptoms on the infected person. Because you will not necessarily be able to identify clients with infectious diseases, the same infection control practices should be used with all clients.

OSHA sets the standard that must be used in the industry for dealing with bloodborne pathogens. The standard prescribes the use of Universal Precautions as the approach to infection control. **Universal Precautions** are a set of guidelines and controls, published by the Centers for Disease Control and Prevention (CDC), that require the employer and the employee to assume that all human blood and specified human body fluids are infectious for HIV, HBV, and other bloodborne pathogens. Precautions include hand-washing; gloving; personal protective equipment such as goggles; injury prevention; and proper handling and disposal of needles, other sharp instruments, and products that have been contaminated by blood or other body fluids.

In most instances, clients who are infected with Hepatitis B Virus or other bloodborne pathogens are **asymptomatic**, which means that they show no symptoms or signs of infection. Many individuals who have a minor, nonspecific symptom may not even know they are infected. Exposure to blood in the salon setting presents a risk of exposure to various diseases, including hepatitis and AIDS. Therefore, the blood of all clients should be treated as if infected.

Item	Level of Decontamination	Procedure
Lancets or other facial tools and implements used to puncture or break the skin, or anything that comes in contact with pus or oozing.	Sterilization	Steam autoclave (high pressure and heat) and dry heat. Dispose of all sharps in a puncture-proof container.
Nonporous tools and implements such as combs, brushes, razors, haircutting shears, clipper attachments, picks, bobby pins, rollers, Velcro rollers, nippers, tweezers, immersible nail files, attachments, and so on, that have *not* come in contact with body fluids or blood.	Disinfection	Complete immersion in EPA-registered, hospital-grade,bactericidal, pseudo-monacidal, fungicidal, and virucidal disinfectant for amount of time specified by the manufacturer.
Nonporous hair-care tools and implements that have come in contact with parasites such as head lice.	Disinfection	Complete immersion in a Lysol solution (2 tablespoons in 1 quart of water) for one hour.
Nonporous tools and implements such as nippers, razors, or haircutting shears that have accidentally come in contact with blood or body fluids.	Disinfection	Complete immersion in an EPA-registered, disinfectant with demonstrated efficacy against HIV-1/HBV or tuberculosis for the amount of time specified by the manufacturer.
Electrotherapy tools, electric clippers, electric files.	Disinfection	Spraying or wiping with an EPA-registered, hospital-grade disinfectant specifically made for electrical equipment.

(Continued)

Table 5-4 Infection Prevention Guidelines

5

Item	Level of Decontamination	Procedure
Countertops, shampoo bowls, sinks, floors, toilets, doorknobs, mirrors, magnifying lamps, dispensary.	Sanitation	Use an EPA-registered cleaning product designed for surfaces. The efficacy label states what is appropriate for such surfaces as floors, countertops, toilets, towels, sinks, and the like.
Towels, linens, capes, headbands.	Sanitation	Laundering in hot water and detergent, with bleach or Lysol added to rinse water.
Your hands prior to each service.	Sanitation	Washing with liquid soap and warm water.
Your hands, client's hands, and/or feet before each manicure or pedicure service.	Sanitation	Soap and warm water or antiseptic designed for use on hands and/or feet.

Table 5–4 *(continued)*

5

THE PROFESSIONAL IMAGE

Overall health, safety, and cleanliness should be an integral part of your normal routine and the routines of all those who work with you. In this way, you and your coworkers can project a steadfast professional image (Figure 5–24). Following are some simple guidelines that will help keep the salon looking its best and being its best.

1. Sweep floors clean after each client service, especially after every haircut.
2. Deposit all waste materials in a waste receptacle with a self-closing lid.
3. Mop floors and vacuum carpets daily.
4. Control all types of dust.
5. Keep windows, screens, and curtains clean.
6. Regularly clean fans, ventilation systems, and humidifiers.
7. Keep all work areas well lit.
8. Keep rest rooms clean and tidy. Remember to clean bathroom door handles.
9. Provide toilet tissue, paper towels, and pump-type liquid soap in the rest room.
10. Clean sinks and drinking fountains regularly.
11. Provide disposable drinking cups.
12. Keep the salon free from insects and rodents.
13. Do not allow the salon to be used for cooking or living quarters.
14. Never place food in refrigerators used to store salon products.
15. Prohibit eating, drinking, and smoking in areas where services are performed.
16. Empty waste receptacles regularly throughout the day.
17. Wear clean, freshly laundered clothing.
18. Make sure all containers are properly marked, tightly closed, and properly stored.
19. Keep the outside of all containers clean.
20. Do not place any tools, combs, rollers, or hairpins in your mouth or pockets.
21. If you drop an implement on the floor, disinfect it before using it again. Properly clean and disinfect all tools and implements after each use and store them in a clean, covered container.
22. Avoid touching your face, mouth, or eye areas during services.
23. Do not allow any pets or animals in the salon except for trained service animals.
24. Clean and disinfect all work surfaces, including manicure tables, aesthetic beds, workstations, and chairs, between client services. Clean shampoo bowls and disinfect the neck of the bowl after each client.
25. Use only freshly laundered or new disposable linens on clients. Use separate closed containers for soiled linens. Use disposable towels or tissues whenever possible. Use neck strips or towels to ensure that there is no skin contact with cutting or shampoo capes. Disinfect all linens during the wash cycle with detergent and bleach.
26. Monitor air quality in the salon. Four to ten air changes per hour are recommended for public buildings. Air changes remove suspended particles such as hair spray, nail filings, and microscopic particles

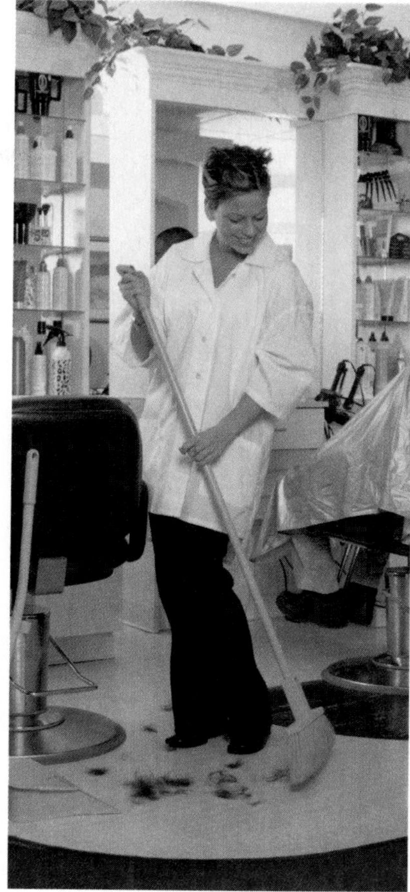

Figure 5-24 Proper sanitation is part of a professional image.

loosened when brushing the scalp. An air purification system or an EPA-registered air cleaner are effective in removing these particles.

These are only a few of the things professionals must do in order to safeguard themselves and their clients. Contact your local state board of cosmetology or health department for a complete list of regulations.

Your Professional Responsibility

You have many responsibilities as a salon professional. None is more important than your responsibility to protect your clients' health and safety as well as your own. Never take shortcuts when it comes to sanitation and disinfection. Remember, this is a hands-on profession. The beauty of it is that you come into close contact with all sorts of people. This is why a "people" person like yourself has chosen this field. But you must be wise and careful about this contact. If you are to be an effective practitioner, you must learn the rules—every one of them—and you must always follow them to the letter of the law. This is how you, your colleagues, and your clients can maintain a sense of trust and respect for each other. 7

chapter glossary

acquired immunity	immunity that the body develops after it overcomes a disease, or through inoculation (such as vaccination)
acute disease	disease having a rapid onset, severe symptoms, and a short course or duration
AIDS	Acquired immunodeficiency syndrome; a disease caused by the HIV virus that breaks down the body's immune system
allergy	reaction due to extreme sensitivity to certain foods, chemicals, or other normally harmless substances
antiseptics	chemical agents that may kill, retard, or prevent the growth of bacteria; not classified as disinfectants
asymptomatic	showing no symptoms or signs of infection
bacilli (singular: bacillus)	short, rod-shaped bacteria; the most common bacteria; produce diseases such as tetanus (lockjaw), typhoid fever, tuberculosis, and diphtheria
bacteria	one-celled microorganisms with both plant and animal characteristics; some are harmful, some harmless; also known as microbes or germs
bactericidal	capable of destroying bacteria
bacteriology	the science that deals with the study of microorganisms called bacteria
bloodborne pathogens	Disease-causing bacteria or viruses that are carried through the body in the blood or body fluids
chronic disease	disease of long duration, usually mild but recurring
cilia	slender, hair-like extensions that permit locomotion in certain bacteria; whip-like motion moves them in liquid
cocci	round-shaped bacteria that appear singly (alone) or in groups
congenital disease	disease that exists at birth
contagious disease	disease that is communicable or transmittable by contact
contaminants	substances that can cause contamination
contraindication	any condition or disease that makes an indicated treatment or medication inadvisable
decontamination	removal of pathogens and other substances from tools and surfaces
diagnosis	determination of the nature of a disease from its signs and symptoms
diplococci	spherical bacteria that grow in pairs and cause diseases such as pneumonia
disease	abnormal condition of all or part of the body, organ, or mind that makes it incapable of carrying on normal function
disinfectants	chemical agents used to destroy most bacteria and some viruses and to disinfect implements and surfaces
disinfection	second highest level of decontamination, nearly as effective as sterilization but does not kill bacterial spores; used on hard, nonporous surfaces
efficacy	effectiveness
epidemic	appearance of a disease that simultaneously attacks a large number of persons living in a particular locality

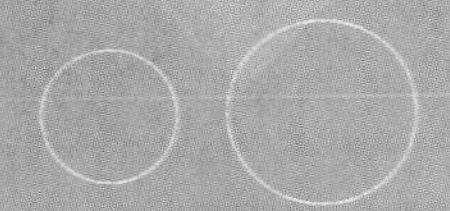

chapter glossary *(continued)*

etiology	study of the causes of disease and their modes of operation
flagella (singular: flagellum)	slender, hair-like extensions that permit locomotion in certain bacteria; their whip-like motion moves bacteria in liquid
fungi (singular: fungus)	vegetable (plant) parasites, including molds, mildews, and yeasts
fungicidal	capable of destroying fungi
general infection	infection that results when the bloodstream carries bacteria or viruses and their toxins (poisons) to all parts of the body
hepatitis	disease marked by inflammation of the liver and caused by a bloodborne virus
HIV	human immunodeficiency virus; virus that causes AIDS
immunity	ability of the body to destroy any bacteria that have gained entrance to the body and to resist infection in general
infection	the invasion of body tissues by disease-causing bacteria; having evidence of pus
infectious	communicable by infection from one person to another person or from one infected body part to another
infectious disease	disease caused by pathogenic microorganisms or viruses that are easily spread
inflammation	condition of some part of the body as a protective response to injury, irritation, or infection, characterized by redness, heat, pain, and swelling
local infection	infection that is confined to a particular part of the body and is indicated by a lesion containing pus
microbiology	the science that deals with microorganisms and their effects on other forms of life
microorganism	microscopic plant or animal cell
mildew	moldy coating produced by fungi that can appear on walls, fabrics, and the like, and usually occurs in damp areas
mitosis	cells dividing into two new cells (daughter cells)
mold	fungus growth that usually grows in dark, damp places
motility	self-movement
MSDS	Material Safety Data Sheet; information compiled by a manufacturer about its product, ranging from ingredient content and associated hazards to combustion levels and storage requirements
natural immunity	natural resistance to disease, partly inherited and partly developed through hygienic living
nonpathogenic	not harmful; not disease-producing; organisms that perform useful functions
objective symptoms	symptoms that are visible, such as pimples, pustules, or inflammation
occupational disease	illness resulting from conditions associated with employment, such as coming in contact with certain chemicals or tints

-ology	suffix meaning "scientific study of " (example: microbiology)
parasite	organism that lives in or on another organism and draws its nourishment from that organism
parasitic disease	disease caused by vegetable or animal parasites, such as pediculosis and ringworm
pathogenic	causing disease; harmful
pathogenic disease	disease produced by disease-causing bacteria, such as staphylococcus and streptococcus (pus-forming bacteria), or viruses
pathology	science that investigates modifications of the functions and changes in structure caused by disease
pediculosis capitis	skin disease caused by infestation of head lice
phenol	carbolic acid; caustic poison; in 5 percent dilute solution is used to sanitize metallic implements
porous	having pores or openings that permit liquids or gases to pass through
prognosis	foretelling of the probable course of a disease
pseudomonacidal	capable of destroying *Pseudomonas* bacteria
pus	fluid product of inflammation that contains white blood cells and the debris of dead cells, tissue elements, and bacteria
quaternary ammonium compounds (quats)	disinfectant that is considered nontoxic, odorless, and fast-acting
sanitation or sanitizing	third level of decontamination; significantly reducing the number of pathogens or disease-producing organisms found on a surface
saprophytes	nonpathogenic bacteria that normally grow on dead matter
scabies	contagious skin disease caused by an itch mite burrowing under the skin
seasonal disease	disease influenced by the weather
sodium hypochlorite	common household bleach; disinfectant used to sanitize implements
spirilla	spiral or corkscrew-shaped bacteria, such as *Treponema pallida*, which causes syphilis, and *Borrelia burgdorferi*, which causes Lyme disease
staphylococci	pus-forming bacteria that grow in clusters like a bunch of grapes; cause abscesses, pustules, and boils
sterilization	highest level of decontamination; completely destroys every organism on a nonporous surface, whether beneficial or harmful
streptococci	pus-forming bacteria arranged in curved lines resembling a string of beads; cause infections such as strep throat and blood poisoning
subjective symptoms	symptoms that can be felt, such as itching, burning, or pain
systemic disease	disease that affects the body generally, often due to under- or overfunctioning of the internal glands
toxins	any of various poisonous substances produced by some microorganisms

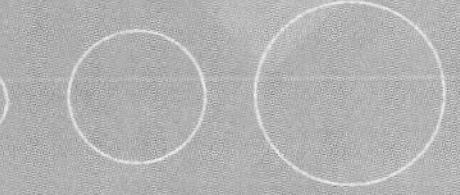

chapter glossary *(continued)*

tuberculocidal	capable of destroying the bacteria that causes tuberculosis
Universal Precautions	set of guidelines and controls, published by the Centers for Disease Control and Prevention (CDC), that require the employer and the employee to assume that all human blood and specified human body fluids are infectious for HIV, HBV, and other bloodborne pathogens
venereal disease	contagious disease commonly acquired by contact with an infected person during sexual intercourse, characterized by sores and rashes on the skin
virology	the study of viruses and viral diseases
virucidal	capable of destroying viruses
virus	a submicroscopic structure capable of infesting almost all plants and animals, including bacteria; infectious agent that lives only by penetrating cells and becoming part of them

review questions

1. What are bacteria?
2. Name and describe the two main classifications of bacteria.
3. What are some of the beneficial functions performed by nonpathogenic bacteria?
4. Name and describe the three forms of pathogenic bacteria.
5. What is the difference between local and general infection?
6. How are viruses different from bacteria?
7. How does AIDS affect the body? How is it transmitted? How is it not transmitted?
8. What is a contagious or communicable disease?
9. Define immunity and name the two types.
10. Describe the procedure for taking care of a blood spill in the salon.
11. What is decontamination? Explain the three levels of decontamination.
12. What is efficacy and why is it important?
13. What is an MSDS?
14. List and describe three types of salon disinfectants.
15. Explain how to disinfect the following: implements for haircutting and styling; metal nail implements; linens and capes; electrical tools that cannot be immersed; work surfaces.
16. List at least six precautions to follow when using disinfectants.
17. What are Universal Precautions?

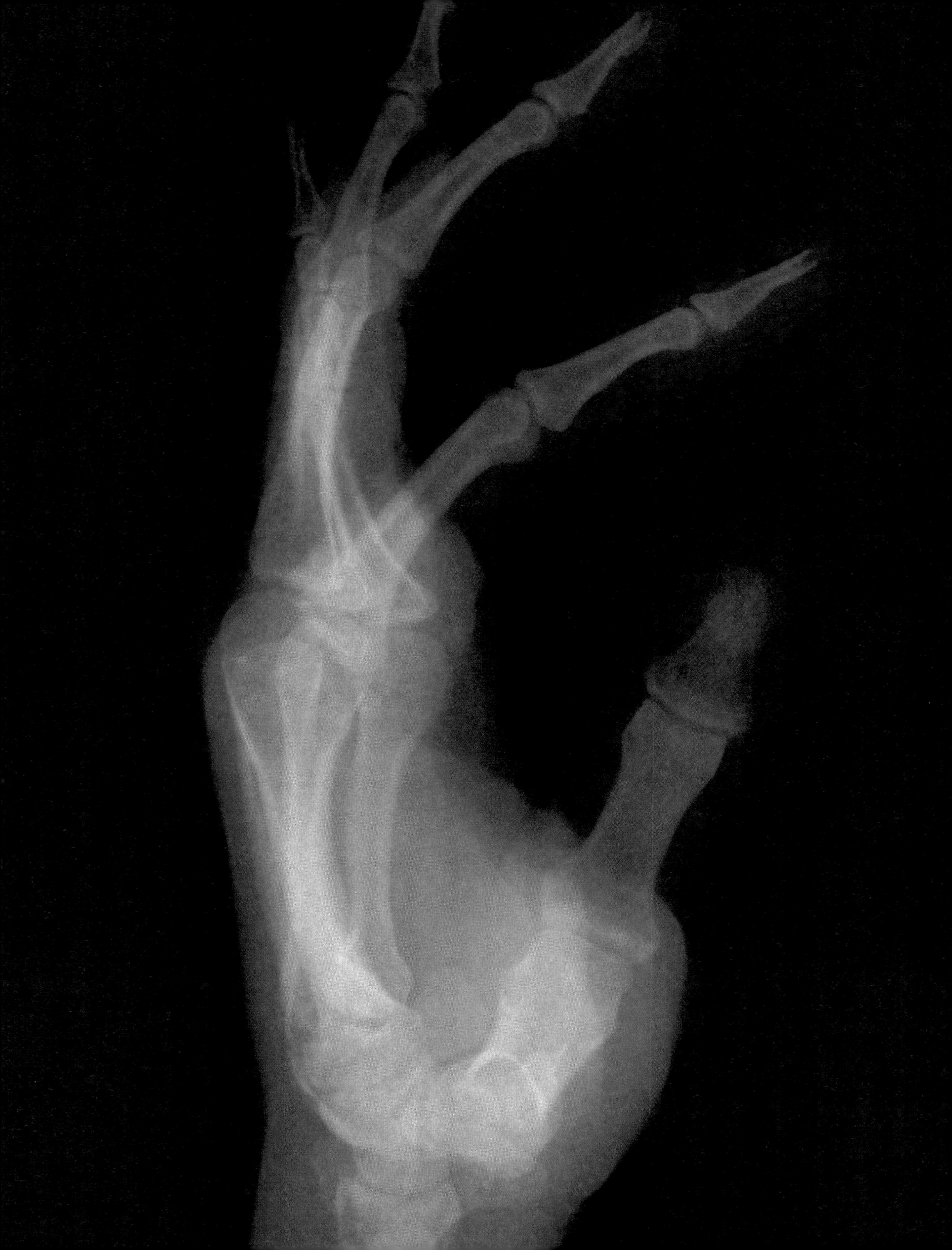

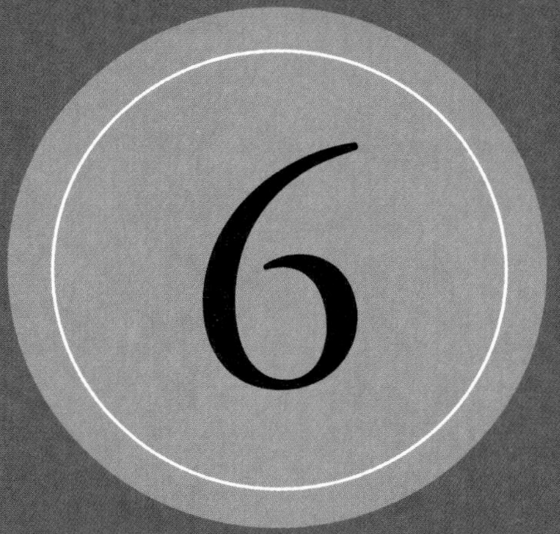

ANATOMY AND PHYSIOLOGY

Deborah Beatty
COSMETOLOGY EDUCATOR AND WRITER

Chapter Outline

Learning Objectives

After completing this chapter, you should be able to:

1. Explain the importance of anatomy and physiology to the cosmetology profession.
2. Describe cells, their structure, and their reproduction.
3. Define tissue and identify the types of tissues found in the body.
4. Name the 10 main body systems and explain their basic functions.

National Skill Standards

This chapter provides you with the necessary information to master these National Industry Skill Standards for Entry-Level Cosmetologists.

 **Providing basic skin care services.**

 **Providing basic manicures and pedicures.**

Key Terms

abductors pg. 145
adductors pg. 145
anabolism pg. 134
anatomy pg. 133
angular artery pg. 154
anterior auricular artery pg. 154
aponeurosis pg. 142
arteries pg. 151
atrium pg. 150
auricularis anterior pg. 142
auricularis posterior pg. 142
auricularis superior pg. 142
auriculotemporal nerve pg. 148
autonomic nervous system pg. 146
axon pg. 147
belly (muscle) pg. 141
biceps pg. 145
blood pg. 152
blood vascular system pg. 150
brain pg. 146
buccal nerve pg. 149
buccinator pg. 143
capillaries pg. 151
cardiac muscle pg. 141
carpus pg. 139
catabolism pg. 134
cell membrane pg. 134
cell pg. 133
central nervous system pg. 146
cervical cutaneous nerve pg. 149
cervical nerve (branch of the facial nerve) pg. 149
cervical nerves pg. 149
cervical vertebrae pg. 138
circulatory system pg. 137
clavicle pg. 139
common carotid artery pg. 153
connective tissue pg. 135
corrugator pg. 143
cranium pg. 136
cytoplasm pg. 134
deltoid pg. 145
dendrites pg. 145
depressor labii inferioris pg. 143
diaphragm pg. 156
digestive system pg. 155
digit pg. 139
digital nerve pg. 149
endocrine (ductless) glands pg. 155
endocrine system pg. 155
epicranius pg. 141
epithelial tissue pg. 135
excretory system pg. 155
exhalation pg. 156
exocrine (duct) glands pg. 155
extensors pg. 145
external carotid artery pg. 153
external jugular vein pg. 154
facial artery pg. 153
fifth cranial nerve pg. 148
flexors pg. 145
frontal artery pg. 154
frontal bone pg. 138
frontalis pg. 142
gland pg. 155
greater auricular nerve pg. 149
greater occipital nerve pg. 149
heart pg. 150
hemoglobin pg. 152
histology pg. 133
hormones pg. 155
humerus pg. 139
hyoid pg. 138
inferior labial artery pg. 153
infraorbital artery pg. 154

As you get deeper into your study of cosmetology, you may be asking yourself what drew you to this field. Was it because your high school guidance counselor thought it would be good for you? Were your friends doing it? Does someone in your family own a salon? Any of these reasons may have contributed to your choice of career. But another reason may be that you have a deep and long-held interest in the human form.

You have probably always been interested in the human form and the human body, because these subjects are fascinating. All of us should, of course, be familiar with how our bodies work. But for cosmetology professionals, knowing how the body works is essential.

WHY STUDY ANATOMY?

As a professional in this field, an overview of human anatomy and physiology will enable you to:

- understand how the human body functions as an integrated whole.
- recognize changes from the norm.
- determine a scientific basis for the proper application of services and products.
- perform a professional makeup application that might otherwise be difficult without a knowledge of facial bones and muscle structure.
- provide shampoos, scalp manipulations, haircuts, and style designs aided by your knowledge of head contours, bones, and muscle structure.
- create a style, based on your knowledge of facial bones and muscle structure that will enhance your client's facial structure.
- recognize the facial bones, nerves, and muscle structure when performing a facial.
- perform manipulations involving the face, hands, arms, shoulders, neck, feet, and lower legs safely and effectively as a result of your understanding of bones, muscles, nerves, and circulation. 1

As a professional cosmetologist, you will seldom hear actual medical terminology being used for the bones, muscles, arteries, veins, and nerves. But an understanding of anatomy and physiology will help you become more proficient at performing professional salon services. In addition, you should also have a working knowledge of histology. Let us look at the following definitions.

- **Anatomy** is the study of the structures of the human body that can be seen with the naked eye, and what they are made up of; the science of the structure of organisms or of their parts.
- **Physiology** (fiz-ih-OL-oh-jee) is the study of the functions and activities performed by the body structures.
- **Histology** (his-TAHL-uh-jee) is the study of the science of the minute structures of organic tissues; microscopic anatomy.

CELLS

Any discussion of anatomy and physiology must begin with **cells**, the basic unit of all living things, from bacteria to plants to animals to human beings. Without cells, life does not exist. As a basic functional unit, the cell is responsible for carrying on all life processes. There are trillions of cells in the human body, and they vary widely in size, shape, and purpose.

Basic Construction of the Cell

The cells of all living things are composed of a substance called **protoplasm** (PROH-toh-plaz-um), a colorless jellylike substance in which food elements such as proteins, fats, carbohydrates, mineral salts, and water are present. You can visualize the protoplasm of a cell as being similar to the white of a raw egg.

In addition to protoplasm, most cells also include the following (Figure 6–1).

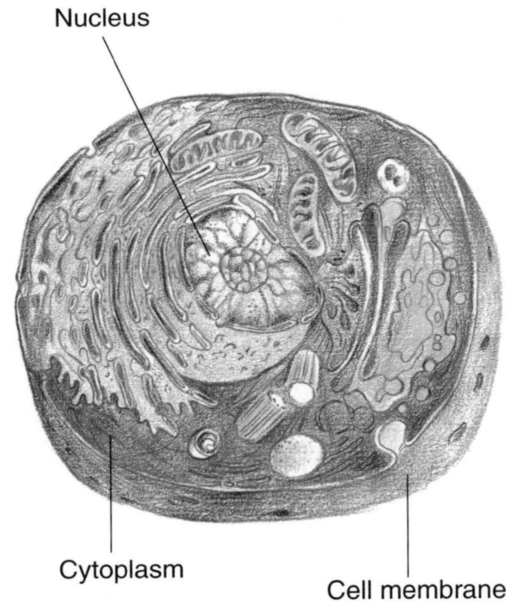

Figure 6–1 Anatomy of the cell.

- The **nucleus** (NOO-klee-us) is the dense, active protoplasm found in the center of the cell. It plays an important part in cell reproduction and metabolism. You can visualize the nucleus as the yolk of a raw egg.
- The **cytoplasm** (sy-toh-PLAZ-um) is all the protoplasm of a cell except that which is in the nucleus; the watery fluid that contains food material necessary for growth, reproduction, and self-repair of the cell.
- The **cell membrane** encloses the protoplasm and permits soluble substances to enter and leave the cell.

Cell Reproduction and Division

Cells have the ability to reproduce, thus providing new cells for the growth and replacement of worn or injured ones. Most cells reproduce by dividing into two identical cells called daughter cells. This reproduction process is known as **mitosis** (my-TOH-sis). As long as conditions are favorable, the cell will grow and reproduce. Favorable conditions include an adequate supply of food, oxygen, and water; suitable temperatures; and the ability to eliminate waste products. If conditions become unfavorable, the cell will become impaired or may be destroyed. Unfavorable conditions include toxins (poison) and disease. 2

Cell Metabolism

Metabolism (muh-TAB-uh-liz-um) is a chemical process that takes place in living organisms, whereby the cells are nourished and carry out their activities. Metabolism has two phases.

1. **Anabolism** (uh-NAB-uh-liz-um) is constructive metabolism, the process of building up larger molecules from smaller ones. During this process, the body stores water, food, and oxygen for the time when these substances will be needed for cell growth and repair.
2. **Catabolism** (kuh-TAB-uh-liz-um) is the phase of metabolism that involves the breaking down of complex compounds within the cells into smaller ones. This process releases energy that is stored by special molecules to be used in muscle contractions, body secretions, or heat production.

Anabolism and catabolism are carried out simultaneously and continually within the cells.

TISSUES

A **tissue** (TISH-oo) is a collection of similar cells that perform a particular function. Each tissue has a specific function and can be recognized by its characteristic appearance. Body tissues are composed of 60 to 90 percent water, along with various other substances. There are five types of tissue in the body.

1. **Connective tissue** serves to support, protect, and bind together other tissues of the body. Examples of connective tissue are bone, cartilage, ligaments, tendons, fascia (which separates muscles), and fat or adipose tissue.
2. **Epithelial tissue** (ep-ih-THEE-lee-ul) is a protective covering on body surfaces. Skin, mucous membranes, and the lining of the heart, digestive, and respiratory organs, and glands are all examples of epithelial tissue.
3. **Liquid tissue**, such as blood and lymph, carries food, waste products, and hormones through the body.
4. **Muscular tissue** contracts and moves the various parts of the body.
5. **Nerve tissue** carries messages to and from the brain and controls and coordinates all bodily functions. Nerve tissue is composed of special cells known as neurons, which make up the nerves, brain, and spinal cord. 3✓

ORGANS

Organs are groups of tissues designed to perform a specific function. Table 6–1 lists some of the most important organs of the body.

BODY SYSTEMS

Systems are group of bodily organs acting together to perform one or more functions. The human body is composed of ten major systems (Table 6–2).

6

THE SKELETAL SYSTEM

The **skeletal system** is the physical foundation of the body. It is composed of 206 bones that vary in size and shape and are connected by movable and immovable joints. **Osteology** (ahs-tee-AHL-oh-jee) is the science of the anatomy, structure, and function of the bones. *Os* means "bone" and is used as a prefix in many medical terms, such as osteoarthritis, a joint disease.

Except for the tissue that forms the major part of the teeth, bone is the hardest tissue in the body. It is composed of connective tissue consisting of

Organ	Function
brain	controls the body
eyes	control vision
heart	circulates the blood
kidneys	excrete water and waste products
lungs	supply oxygen to the blood
liver	removes toxic products of digestion
skin	forms external protective covering of the body
stomach and intestines	digest food

Table 6–1 Some Major Body Organs and Their Functions

about one-third animal matter, such as cells and blood, and two-thirds mineral matter, mainly calcium carbonate and calcium phosphate.

The primary functions of the skeletal system are to:

- give shape and support to the body.
- protect various internal structures and organs.
- serve as attachments for muscles and act as levers to produce body movement.
- help produce both white and red blood cells (one of the functions of bone marrow).
- store most of the body's calcium supply as well as phosphorus, magnesium, and sodium.

A **joint** is the connection between two or more bones of the skeleton. There are two types of joints: movable, such as elbows, knees, and hips; and immovable, such as the pelvis or skull, which allows little or no movement.

Bones of the Skull

The skull is the skeleton of the head and is divided into two parts: the **cranium** (KRAY-nee-um), an oval, bony case that protects the brain; and the facial skeleton, which is made up of 14 bones (Figure 6–2).

System	Function
circulatory	controls the steady circulation of the blood through the body by means of the heart and blood vessels
digestive	changes food into nutrients and wastes; consists of mouth, stomach, intestines, salivary and gastric glands, and other organs
endocrine	affects the growth, development, sexual activities, and health of the entire body; consists of specialized glands
excretory	purifies the body by the elimination of waste matter; consists of kidneys, liver, skin, intestines, and lungs
integumentary	serves as a protective covering and helps in regulating the body's temperature; consists of skin, accessory organs such as oil and sweat glands, sensory receptors, hair, and nails
muscular	covers, shapes, and supports the skeleton tissue; also contracts and moves various parts of the body; consists of muscles
nervous	controls and coordinates all other systems and makes them work harmoniously and efficiently; consists of brain, spinal cord, and nerves
reproductive	responsible for processes by which plants and animals produce offspring
respiratory	enables breathing, supplying the body with oxygen, and eliminating carbon dioxide as a waste product; consists of lungs and air passages
skeletal	physical foundation of the body; consists of the bones and movable and immovable joints

Table 6–2 Body Systems and Their Functions

6

Bones of the Cranium

The cranium is made up of eight bones. Of those, the following are important to the cosmetologist.

- **Occipital bone** (ahk-SIP-ih-tul)—hindmost bone of the skull, below the parietal bones; forms the back of the skull above the nape.

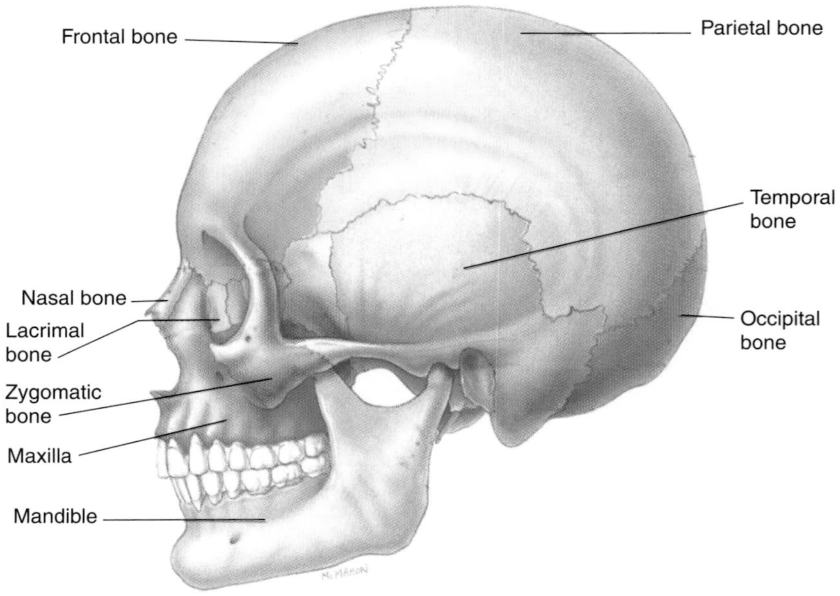

Frontal bone
Parietal bone
Temporal bone
Nasal bone
Lacrimal bone
Occipital bone
Zygomatic bone
Maxilla
Mandible

Figure 6–2 Bones of the cranium, face, and neck.

- Two **parietal bones** (puh-RY-uh-tul)—form the sides and crown (top) of the cranium.
- **Frontal bone** (FRUNT-ul)—forms the forehead.
- Two **temporal bones** (TEM-puh-rul)—form the sides of the head in the ear region.

Bones of the Face

The bones of the face involved in facial massage include:

- two **nasal bones** (NAY-zul). They form the bridge of the nose.
- two **lacrimal bones** (LAK-ruh-mul). Small, thin bones located at the front inner wall of the orbits (eye sockets).
- two **zygomatic or malar bones** (zy-goh-MAT-ik). Form the prominence of the cheeks; cheekbones.
- two **maxillae** (mak-SIL-ee). Bones of the upper jaw (singular: maxilla).
- **mandible** (MAN-duh-bul). Lower jawbone; largest and strongest bone of the face.

Bones of the Neck

The main bones of the neck are the:

- **hyoid bone** (HY-oyd). U-shaped bone at the base of the tongue that supports the tongue and its muscles; also called "Adam's apple."
- **cervical vertebrae** (SUR-vih-kul VURT-uh-bray). The seven bones of the top part of the vertebral column located in the neck region (Figure 6–3).

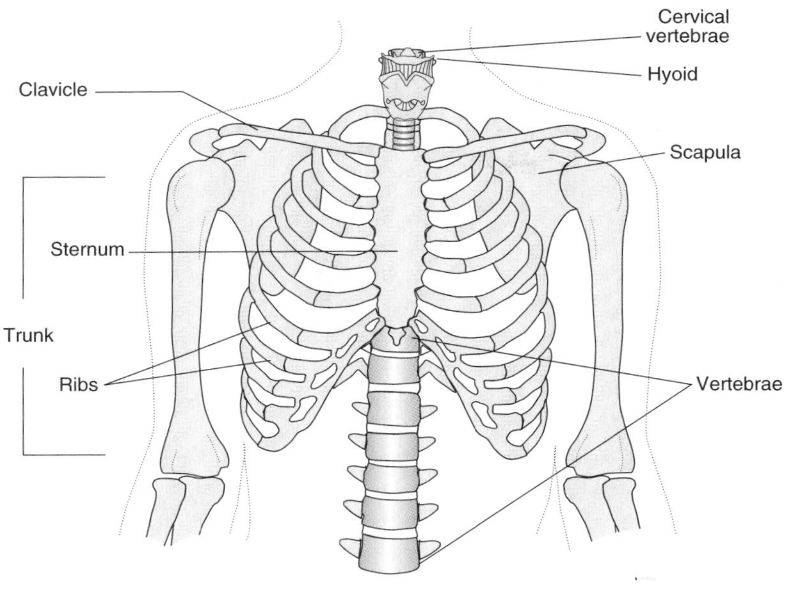

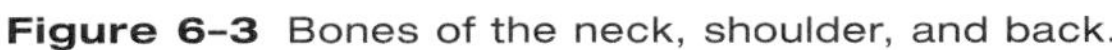

Figure 6–3 Bones of the neck, shoulder, and back.

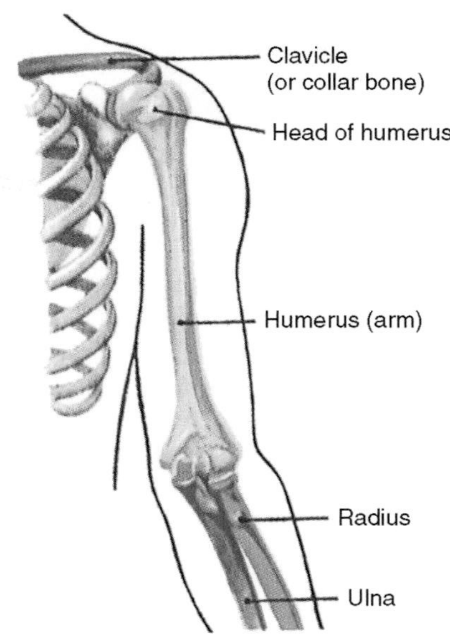

Figure 6–4 Bones of the arm.

Bones of the Chest, Shoulder, and Back

The bones of the trunk or torso (Figure 6–3) consist of the:

- **thorax** (THOR-aks). The chest; elastic, bony cage that serves as a protective framework for the heart, lungs, and other internal organs.
- **ribs**. Twelve pairs of bones forming the wall of the thorax.
- **scapula** (SKAP-yuh-luh). One of a pair of shoulder blades; a large, flat, triangular bone of the shoulder.
- **sternum** (STUR-num). Breastbone; flat bone that forms the ventral (front) support of the ribs.
- **clavicle.** Collarbone; bone that joins the sternum and scapula.

Bones of the Arms and Hands

The important bones of the shoulder, arms, and hands that you should know about (Figure 6–4 and Figure 6–5) include the:

- **humerus** (HYOO-muh-rus). Uppermost and largest bone of the arm, extending from the elbow to the shoulder.
- **ulna** (UL-nuh). Inner and larger bone of the forearm (lower arm), attached to the wrist and located on the side of the little finger.
- **radius** (RAY-dee-us). Smaller bone in the forearm (lower arm) on the same side as the thumb.
- **carpus** (KAR-pus). The wrist; flexible joint composed of a group of eight small, irregular bones (carpals) held together by ligaments.
- **metacarpus** (met-uh-KAR-pus). Bones of the palm of the hand; parts of the hand containing five bones between the carpus and phalanges.
- **phalanges** (fuh-LAN-jeez). Bones in the fingers, or **digits** (also the toes), consisting of three in each finger and two in each thumb, totaling fourteen bones.

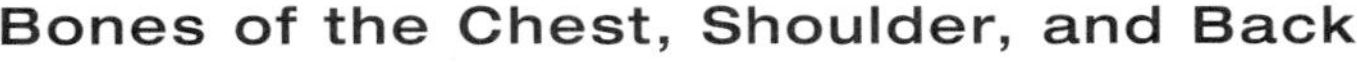

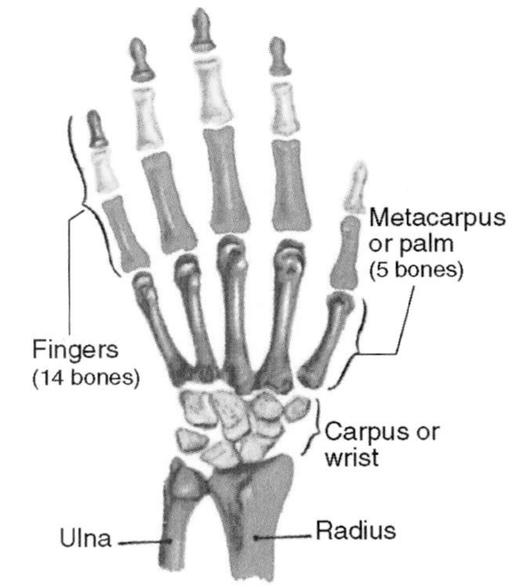

Figure 6–5 Bones of the hand.

insights

Ray Beckfield

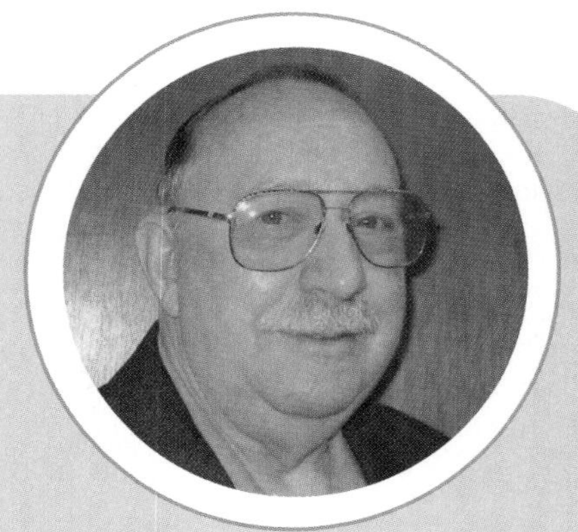

After almost a half-century in the field, Ray Beckfield, an educator with the Minneapolis Community College Cosmetology program, believes your education should never stop.

I first started cutting hair while I was in the service. I was stationed aboard a ship and they were looking for somebody to cut hair. Having been raised on a farm, I'd done a little of that, so I told them I knew how. I was planning to be a men's barber, but when I got out of the service in 1959, the barber schools were all filled up. I had a cousin who was a cosmetologist, so I decided to go that route.

Fortunately, I had a perfect instructor. Her name was Edie, and she was really good with hair. She motivated me and was a great role model. I've been in this business a long time, but I think continuing education is a must. I still take classes on different things. At least four times a year, I go to hairdressing and product shows. To me, education is all about learning how to become goal-oriented and focused on what you want to do. Education for a cosmetologist is not just about learning about hair. You really have to learn the inner skills. Don't forget, your job is to deal with people.

Everyone has an inner beauty, and you'll want to help your clients enhance what they have by finding out what they want and making suggestions. I think the most challenging aspect of our work is to deal with customers who are afraid of change. It's a challenge, too, to work with customers who are crabby and mad at the world. I tell my students that they have to change their personalities to suit each client.

If I were a young stylist starting out today, I'd look for a salon that offered training, not just in hair but also in human relations. A cosmetologist should have good communication skills and should develop loyalty to the clients. It also helps to learn how to sell. And look for a salon that is going to help you continue your education. Think about me: I've been doing this so long, but I still work in a salon, or at least try to, on Friday afternoons. It's all I can manage with my teaching responsibilities, but it's mainly to keep up my skills so that I can take it and teach it. You've got to be really committed to make it in this field.

THE MUSCULAR SYSTEM

The **muscular system** is the body system that covers, shapes, and supports the skeleton tissue. It contracts and moves various parts of the body. **Myology** (my-AHL-uh-jee) is the science of the nature, structure, function, and diseases of the muscles. The human body has over 600 muscles, which are responsible for approximately 40 percent of the body's weight. Muscles are fibrous tissues that have the ability to stretch and contract according to the demands of the body's movements.

There are three types of muscular tissue.

1. **Striated muscles** (STRY-ayt-ed), also called skeletal or voluntary muscles, are attached to the bones and are controlled by the will. Striated (skeletal) muscles create heat and energy for the body during muscle contractions, assist in maintaining the body's posture, and protect some internal organs (Figure 6–6).
2. **Nonstriated muscles**, also called involuntary, visceral, or smooth muscles, function automatically, without conscious will. These muscles are found in the internal organs of the body, such as the digestive or respiratory systems. They function without conscious thought or control (Figure 6–7).
3. **Cardiac muscle** is the involuntary muscle that is the heart. This type of muscle is not found in any other part of the body (Figure 6–8).

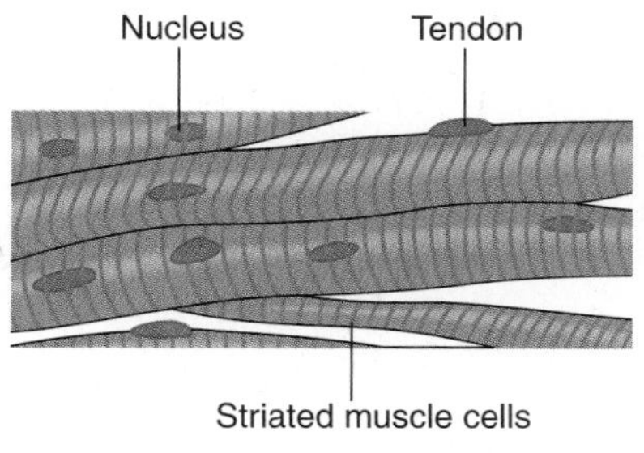

Figure 6–6 Striated muscle cells.

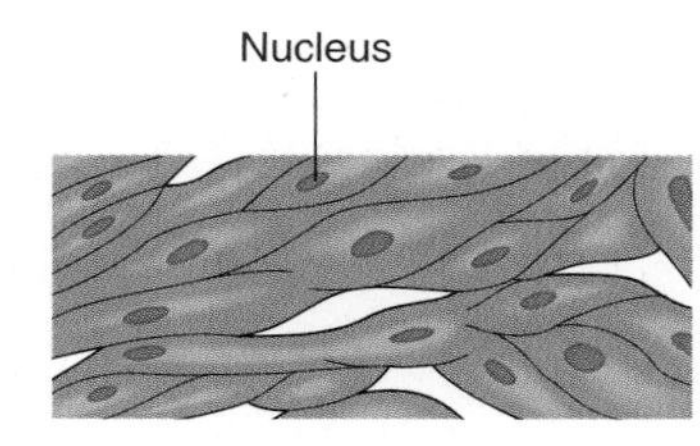

Figure 6–7 Nonstriated muscle cells.

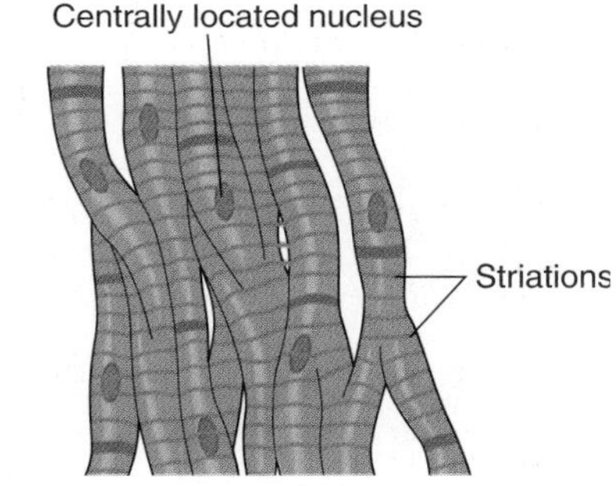

Figure 6–8 Cardiac muscle cells.

A muscle has three parts. The **origin**, is the part that does not move; it is attached to the skeleton and is usually part of a skeletal muscle. The **insertion** is the part of the muscle at the more movable attachment to the skeleton. The **belly** is the middle part of the muscle. Pressure in massage is usually directed from the insertion to the origin.

Muscular tissue can be stimulated by:

- massage (hand or electric vibrator).
- electrical current (high frequency or faradic current).
- light rays (infrared rays or ultraviolet rays).
- heat rays (heating lamps or heating caps).
- moist heat (steamers or moderately warm steam towels).
- nerve impulses (through the nervous system).
- chemicals (certain acids and salts).

Muscles

The cosmetologist must be concerned with the voluntary muscles of the head, face, neck, arms, and hands. It is essential to know where these muscles are located and what they control.

Muscles of the Scalp

- **epicranius** (ep-ih-KRAY-nee-us) or occipito-frontalis (ahk-SIP-ih-toh-frun-TAY-lus). The broad muscle that covers the top of the skull; consists of two parts: occipitalis and frontalis.

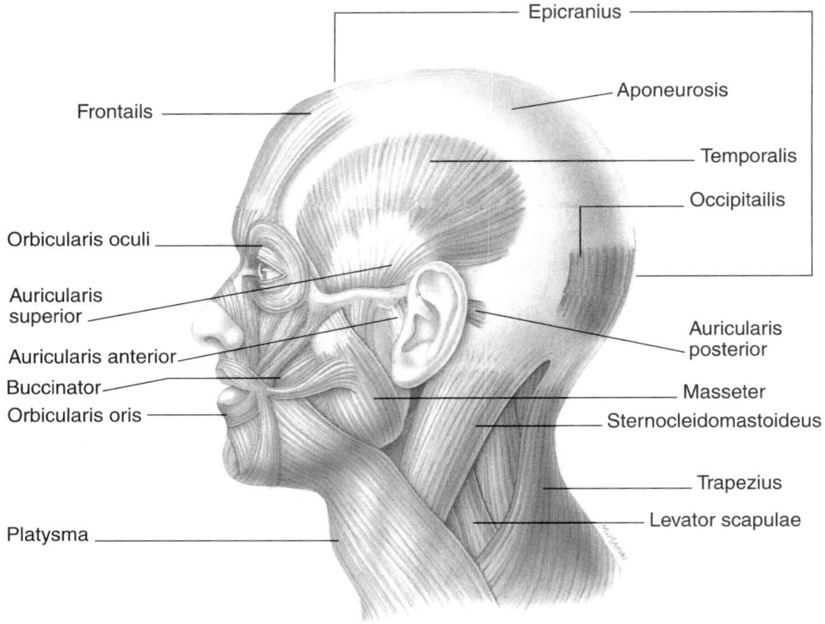

Figure 6–9 Muscles of the head, face, and neck.

- **occipitalis** (ahk-SIP-i-tahl-is). Back of the epicranius; muscle that draws the scalp backward.
- **frontalis** (frun-TAY-lus). Anterior (front) portion of the epicranius; muscle of the scalp that raises the eyebrows, draws the scalp forward, and causes wrinkles across the forehead.
- **aponeurosis** (ap-uh-noo-ROH-sus). Tendon that connects the occipitalis and the frontalis (Figure 6–9).

Muscles of the Ear

Three muscles of the ear have no function (although some people can contract them to move the ears). They include the:

- **auricularis superior** (aw-rik-yuh-LAIR-is). Muscle above the ear that draws the ear upward.
- **auricularis anterior**. Muscle in front of the ear that draws the ear forward.
- **auricularis posterior.** Muscle behind the ear that draws the ear backward.

Muscles of Mastication (Chewing)

The **masseter** (muh-SEE-tur) and the **temporalis** (tem-poh-RAY-lis) muscles coordinate in opening and closing the mouth and are sometimes referred to as chewing muscles.

Muscles of the Neck

Muscles of the neck include the:

- **platysma** (plah-TIZ-muh). Broad muscle extending from the chest and shoulder muscles to the side of the chin; responsible for lowering the lower jaw and lip.

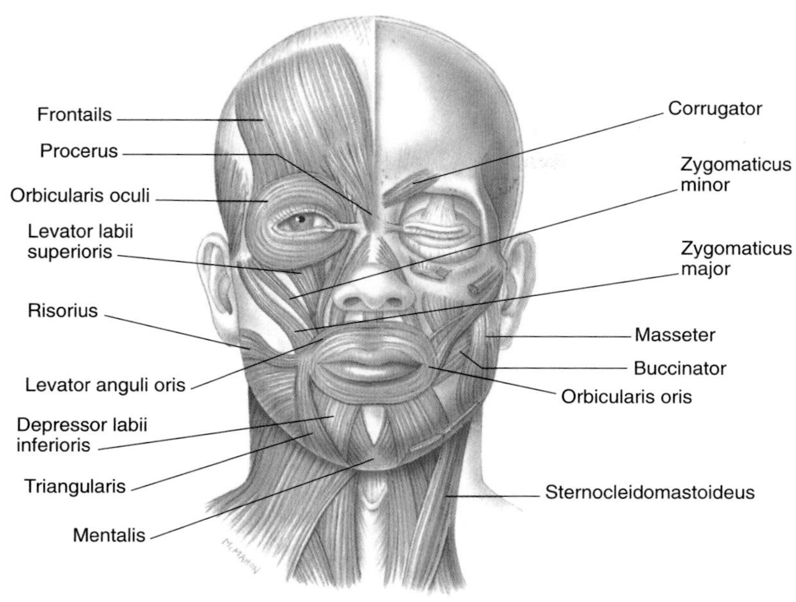

Figure 6–10 Muscles of the face.

- **sternocleidomastoideus** (STUR-noh-KLEE-ih-doh-mas-TOYD-ee-us). Muscle of the neck that lowers and rotates the head.

Muscles of the Eyebrow

These include the:

- **corrugator muscle** (KOR-oo-gay-tohr). Muscle located beneath the frontalis and orbicularis oculi that draws the eyebrow down and wrinkles the forehead vertically (Figure 6–10).
- **orbicularis oculi** (or-bik-yuh-LAIR-is AHK-yuh-lye). Ring muscle of the eye socket; enables you to close your eyes.

Muscles of the Nose

These include the:

- **procerus** (proh-SEE-rus). Covers the bridge of the nose, lowers the eyebrows, and causes wrinkles across the bridge of the nose.
- other nasal muscles that contract and expand the openings of the nostrils.

Muscles of the Mouth

Important ones to know include the:

- **buccinator** (BUK-sih-nay-tur). Thin, flat muscle of the cheek between the upper and lower jaw that compresses the cheeks and expels air between the lips.
- **depressor labii inferioris** (dee-PRES-ur LAY-bee-eye in-FEER-ee-or-us). Also known as quadratus labii inferioris, a muscle surrounding the lower lip; lowers the lower lip and draws it to one side, as in expressing sarcasm.
- **levator anguli oris** (lih-VAYT-ur ANG-yoo-ly OH-ris). Also known as caninus (kay-NY-nus), a muscle that raises the angle of the mouth and draws it inward.

6

- **levator labii superioris** (lih-VAYT-ur LAY-bee-eye soo-peer-ee-OR-is). Also known as quadratus (kwah-DRA-tus) labii superioris, a muscle surrounding the upper lip; elevates the upper lip and dilates the nostrils, as in expressing distaste.
- **mentalis** (men-TAY-lis). Muscle that elevates the lower lip and raises and wrinkles the skin of the chin.
- **orbicularis oris** (or-bik-yuh-LAIR-is OH-ris). Flat band around the upper and lower lips that compresses, contracts, puckers, and wrinkles the lips.
- **risorius** (rih-ZOR-ee-us). Muscle of the mouth that draws the corner of the mouth out and back, as in grinning.
- **triangularis** (try-ang-gyuh-LAY-rus). Muscle extending alongside the chin that pulls down the corner of the mouth.
- **zygomaticus** (zy-goh-MAT-ih-kus) major and minor. Muscles extending from the zygomatic bone to the angle of the mouth; elevate the lip, as in laughing.

Muscles that Attach the Arms to the Body

These include the:

- **latissimus dorsi** (lah-TIS-ih-mus DOR-see). Broad, flat superficial muscle covering the back of the neck and upper and middle region of the back, controlling the shoulder blade and the swinging movements of the arm (Figure 6–11).
- **pectoralis major** (pek-tor-AL-is) and **pectoralis minor**. Muscles of the chest that assist the swinging movements of the arm.
- **serratus anterior** (ser-RAT-us an-TEER-ee-or). Muscle of the chest that assists in breathing and in raising the arm (Figure 6–12).
- **trapezius** (trah-PEE-zee-us). Muscle that covers the back of the neck and upper and middle region of the back; rotates and controls swinging movements of the arm.

6

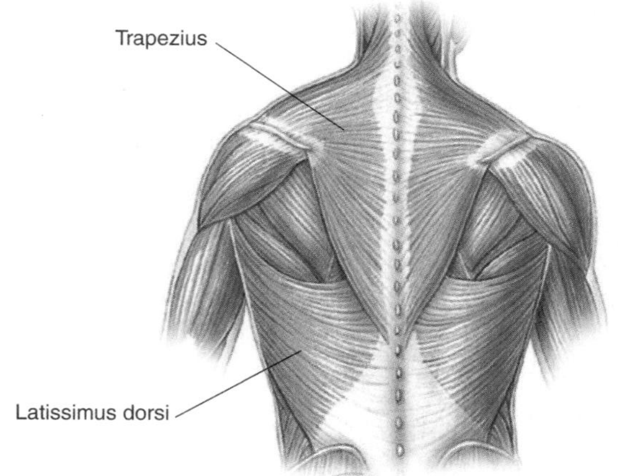

Figure 6–11 Muscles of the back and neck.

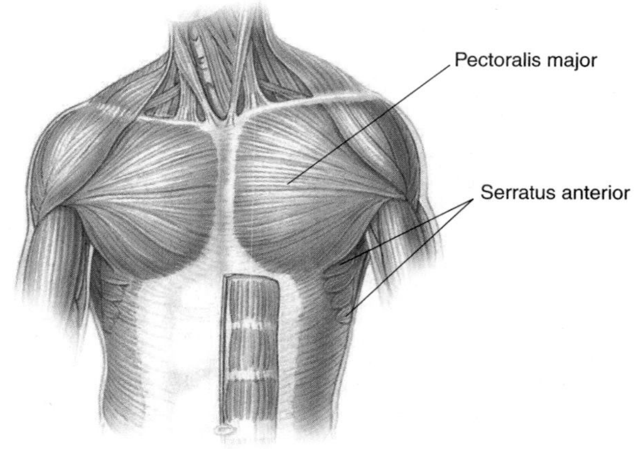

Figure 6–12 Muscles of the chest.

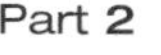

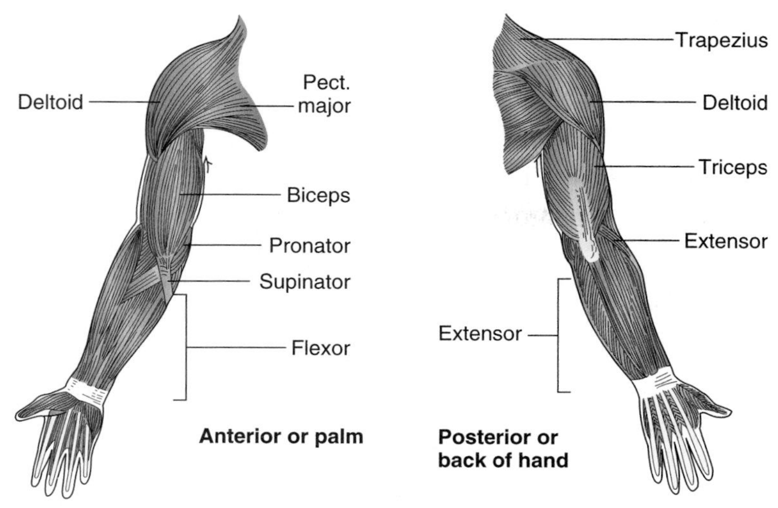

Figure 6–13 Muscles of the shoulder and arm.

Muscles of the Shoulder and Arm

There are three principal muscles of the shoulders and upper arms (Figure 6–13). They include the:

- **biceps** (BY-seps). Muscle producing the contour of the front and inner side of the upper arm; they lift the forearm, flex the elbow, and turn the palms outward.
- **deltoid** (DEL-toyd). Large, triangular muscle covering the shoulder joint that allows the arm to extend outward and to the side of the body.
- **triceps** (TRY-seps). Large muscle that covers the entire back of the upper arm and extends the forearm.

The forearm is made up of a series of muscles and strong tendons. As a cosmetologist, you will be concerned with:

- **extensors** (ik-STEN-surs). Muscles that straighten the wrist, hand, and fingers to form a straight line.
- **flexors** (FLEK-surs). Extensor muscles of the wrist, involved in bending the wrist.
- **pronators** (proh-NAY-tohr). Muscle that turn the hand inward so that the palm faces downward.
- **supinator** (SOO-puh-nayt-ur). Muscle of the forearm that rotates the radius outward and the palm upward

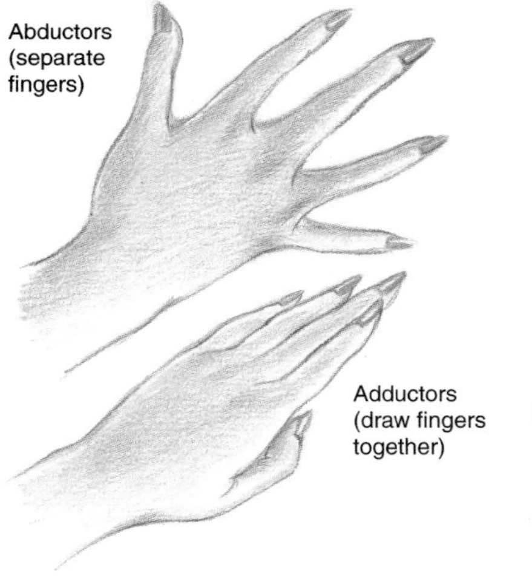

Figure 6–14 Muscles of the hand.

Muscles of the Hand

The hand is one of the most complex parts of the body, with many small muscles that overlap from joint to joint, providing flexibility and strength to open and close the hand and fingers. Important muscles to know include the:

- **abductors** (ab-DUK-turz). Muscles that separate the fingers (Figure 6–14).
- **adductors** (ah-DUK-turz). Muscles at the base of each finger that draw the fingers together.
- **opponent muscles** (uh-POH-nent). Muscles in the palm that act to bring the thumb toward the fingers.

THE NERVOUS SYSTEM

The **nervous system** is an exceptionally well-organized system that is responsible for coordinating all the many activities that are performed both inside and outside of the body. Every square inch of the human body is supplied with fine fibers known as nerves; there are over 100 billion nerve cells, known as neurons, in the body. The science of the structure, function, and pathology of the nervous system is known as **neurology** (nuh-RAHL-uh-jee).

An understanding of how nerves work will help you perform services in a more proficient manner when administering massages or shampoos. It will also help you understand the effects that these treatments have on the body as a whole.

Divisions of the Nervous System

The principal components of the nervous system are the brain, spinal cord, and the nerves themselves (Figure 6–15). The nervous system as a whole is divided into three main subdivisions.

1. The **central nervous** or cerebrospinal (ser-ree-bro-SPY-nahl) system consists of the brain, spinal cord, spinal nerves, and cranial nerves. It controls consciousness and all mental activities, voluntary functions of the five senses (seeing, hearing, feeling, smelling, and tasting), and voluntary muscle actions, including all body movements and facial expressions.
2. The **peripheral nervous system** (puh-RIF-uh-rul) is a system of nerves that connect the peripheral (outer) parts of the body to the central nervous system; it has both sensory and motor nerves. Its function is to carry impulses, or messages, to and from the central nervous system.
3. The **autonomic nervous system** (aw-toh-NAHM-ik) is the part of the nervous system that controls the involuntary muscles; it regulates the action of the smooth muscles, glands, blood vessels, and heart.

The Brain and Spinal Cord

The **brain** is the largest and most complex nerve tissue in the body. The brain is contained in the cranium and weighs an average of 44 to 48 ounces. It controls sensation, muscles, glandular activity, and the power to think and feel. It sends and receives telegraphic messages through 12 pairs of cranial nerves that originate in the brain and reach various parts of the head, face, and neck.

The **spinal cord** is the portion of the central nervous system that originates in the brain, extends down to the lower extremity of the trunk, and is protected by the spinal column. Thirty-one pairs of spinal nerves extending from the spinal cord are distributed to the muscles and skin of the trunk and limbs.

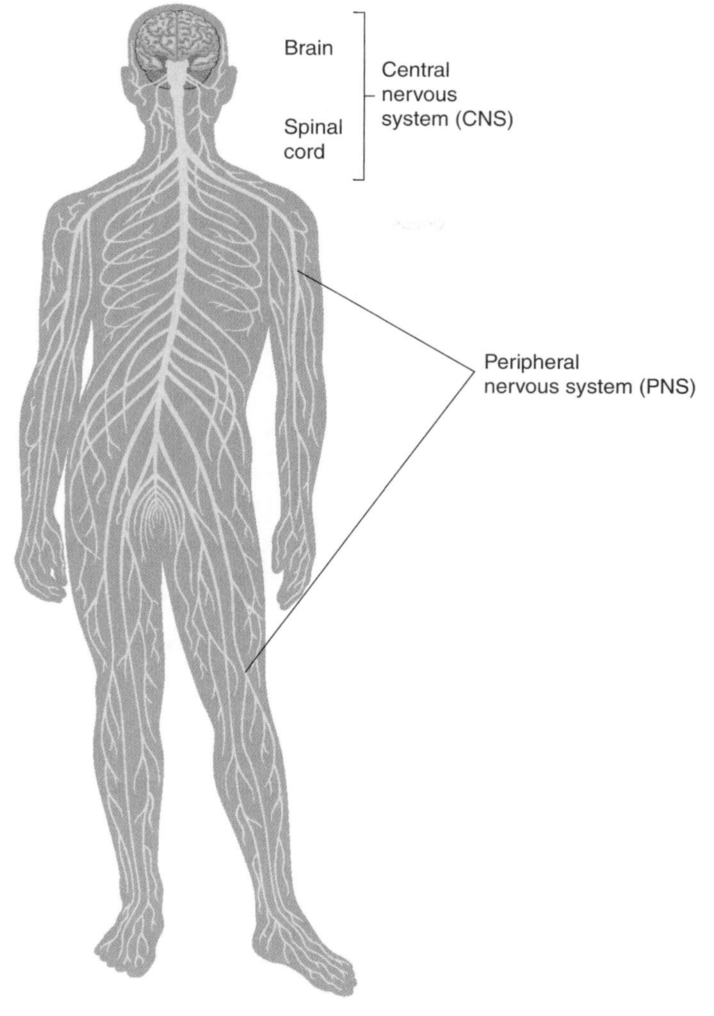

Figure 6–15 Principal parts of the nervous system.

Nerve Cell Structure and Function

A **neuron** (NOO-rahn), or nerve cell, is the primary structural unit of the nervous system (Figure 6–16). It is composed of:

- cell body and nucleus.
- **dendrites** (DEN-dryts), a tree-like branching of nerve fibers extending from the nerve cell that receive impulses from other neurons.
- **axon** (AK-sahn) and axon terminal send impulses away from the cell body to other neurons, glands, or muscles.

Nerves are whitish cords made up of bundles of nerve fibers held together by connective tissue, through which impulses are transmitted. Nerves have their origin in the brain and spinal cord and send their branches to all parts of the body.

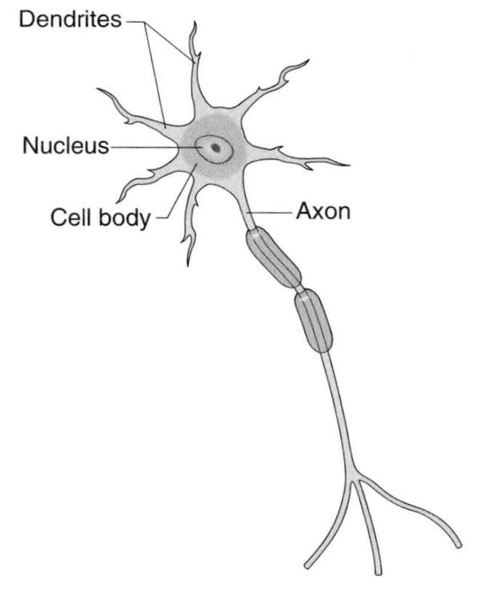

Figure 6–16 A neuron or nerve cell.

Types of Nerves

Sensory nerves, also called **afferent nerves** (AF-feer-ent), carry impulses or messages from the sense organs to the brain, where sensations of touch, cold, heat, sight, hearing, taste, smell, pain, and pressure are experienced. Sensory nerve endings called receptors are located close to the surface of the skin. As impulses pass from the sensory nerves to the brain and back through the motor nerves to the muscles, a complete circuit is established, resulting in movement of the muscles.

Motor nerves, or **efferent nerves** (EF-fuh-rent), carry impulses from the brain to the muscles. The transmitted impulses produce movement.

Mixed nerves contain both sensory and motor fibers and have the ability to send and receive messages.

A **reflex** (REE-fleks) is an automatic nerve reaction to a stimulus that involves the movement of an impulse from a sensory receptor along the afferent nerve to the spinal cord, and a responsive impulse along an efferent neuron to a muscle, causing a reaction (for example, the quick removal of the hand from a hot object). Reflexes do not have to be learned.

Nerves of the Head, Face, and Neck

The largest of the cranial nerves is the **fifth cranial nerve**, also known as the trifacial (try-FAY-shul) or trigeminal (try-JEM-un-ul) nerve. It is the chief sensory nerve of the face, and serves as the motor nerve of the muscles that control chewing. It consists of three branches: **ophthalmic** (ahf-THAL-mik), **mandibular** (man-DIB-yuh-lur), and **maxillary** (MAK-suh-lair-ee) (Figure 6–17).

The following are the branches of the fifth cranial nerve that are affected by massage.

- **auriculotemporal nerve** (aw-RIK-yuh-loh-TEM-puh-rul) affects the external ear and skin above the temple, up to the top of the skull
- **infraorbital nerve** (in-fruh-OR-bih-tul) affects the skin of the lower eyelid, side of the nose, upper lip, and mouth

6

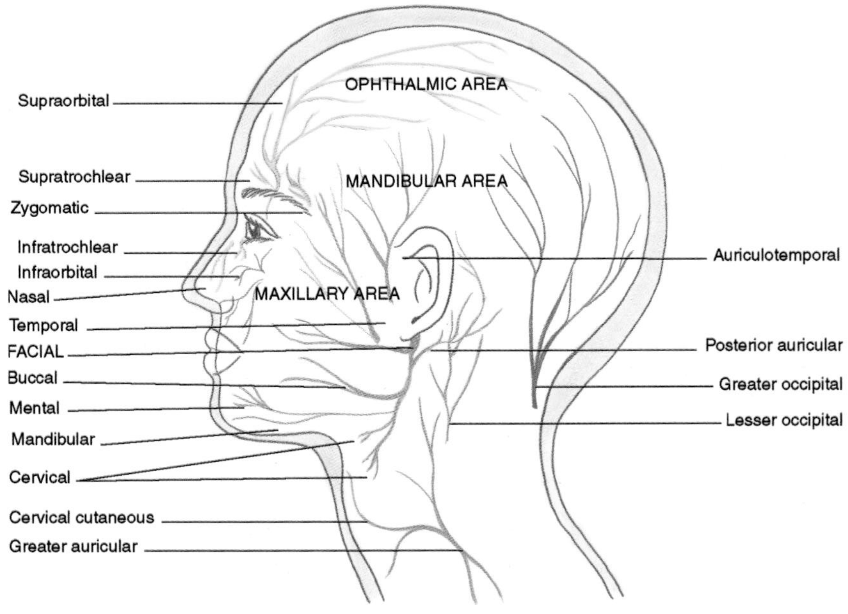

Figure 6–17 Nerves of the head, face, and neck.

- **infratrochlear nerve** (in-frah-TRAHK-lee-ur) affects the membrane and skin of the nose
- **mental nerve** affects the skin of the lower lip and chin
- **nasal nerve** (NAY-zul) affects the point and lower side of the nose
- **supraorbital nerve** (soo-pruh-OR-bih-tul) affects the skin of the forehead, scalp, eyebrow, and upper eyelid
- **supratrochlear nerve** (soo-pruh-TRAHK-lee-ur) affects the skin between the eyes and upper side of the nose
- **zygomatic nerve** (zy-goh-MAT-ik) affects the muscles of the upper part of the cheek

The **seventh (facial) cranial nerve** is the chief motor nerve of the face. It emerges near the lower part of the ear and extends to the muscles of the neck. Its divisions and their branches supply and control all the muscles of facial expression. The following are the most important branches of the facial nerve:

- **posterior auricular nerve** affects the muscles behind the ear at the base of the skull
- **temporal nerve** affects the muscles of the temple, side of the forehead, eyebrow, eyelid, and upper part of the cheek
- **zygomatic nerve** (upper and lower) affects the muscles of the upper part of the cheek
- **buccal nerve** (BUK-ul) affects the muscles of the mouth
- **mandibular nerve** affects the muscles of the chin and lower lip.
- **cervical nerves** (SUR-vih-kul) (branches of the facial nerve) affect the side of the neck and the platysma muscle

Cervical nerves originate at the spinal cord, and their branches supply the muscles and scalp at the back of the head and neck, as follows:

- **greater occipital nerve**, located in the back of the head, affects the scalp as far up as the top of the head
- **smaller (lesser) occipital nerve**, located at the base of the skull, affects the scalp and muscles behind the ear
- **greater auricular nerve**, located at the side of the neck, affects the face, ears, neck, and parotid gland
- **cervical cutaneous nerve** (kyoo-TAY-nee-us), located at the side of the neck, affects the front and sides of the neck as far down as the breastbone

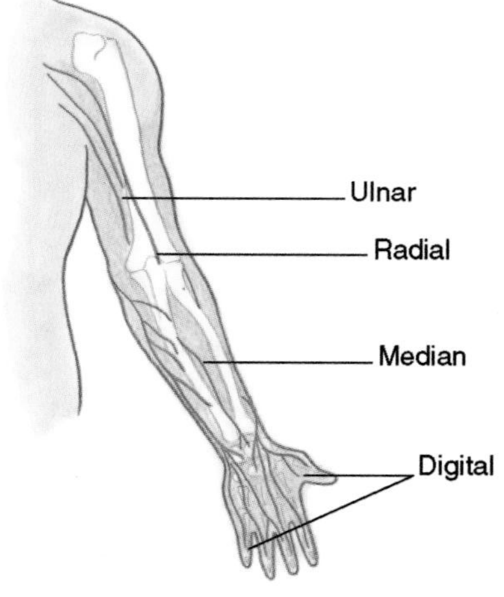

Figure 6–18 Nerves of the arm and hand.

Nerves of the Arm and Hand

The principal nerves supplying the superficial parts of the arm and hand are as follows (Figure 6–18):

- **digital nerve** (DIJ-ut-tul) (sensory-motor), with its branches, supplies the fingers
- **radial nerve** (RAY-dee-ul) (sensory-motor), with its branches, supplies the thumb side of the arm and back of the hand

- **median nerve** (MEE-dee-un) (sensory-motor), smaller nerve than the ulnar and radial nerves that, with its branches, supplies the arm and hand
- **ulnar nerve** (UL-nur) (sensory-motor), with its branches, affects the little finger side of the arm and palm of the hand

THE CIRCULATORY SYSTEM

The **circulatory system**, also referred to as the cardiovascular or vascular system, controls the steady circulation of the blood through the body by means of the heart and blood vessels. The circulatory system is made up of two divisions.

1. The **blood vascular system** that consists of the heart, arteries, veins, and capillaries for the distribution of blood throughout the body.
2. The **lymph vascular system** (LIMF VAS-kyoo-lur) or lymphatic system that acts as an aid to the blood system and consists of the lymph, lymphatics (lymph vessels), lymph nodes, and other structures. **Lymph** is a clear yellowish fluid that circulates in the lymphatics of the body. It carries waste and impurities away from the cells.

The Heart

The **heart** is often referred to as the body's pump. It is a muscular cone-shaped organ that keeps the blood moving within the circulatory system. It is enclosed by a membrane known as the **pericardium** (payr-ih-KAR-dee-um). The heart is the approximate size of a closed fist, weighs approximately 9 ounces, and is located in the chest cavity. The heartbeat is regulated by the vagus (tenth cranial) nerve and other nerves in the autonomic nervous system. In a normal resting state, the heart beats 72 to 80 times per minute.

The interior of the heart contains four chambers and four valves. The upper, thin-walled chambers are the right **atrium** (AY-tree-um) and left atrium. The lower, thick-walled chambers are the right **ventricle** (VEN-truh-kul) and left ventricle. **Valves** between the chambers allow the blood to flow in only one direction. With each contraction and relaxation of the heart, the blood flows in, travels from the atria (plural of atrium) to the ventricles, and is then driven out, to be distributed all over the body (Figure 6–19).

The blood is in constant and continuous circulation from the time it leaves the heart until it returns to the heart. Two systems attend to this circulation. **Pulmonary circulation** sends the blood from the heart to the lungs to be purified. **Systemic circulation** or general circulation carries the blood from the heart throughout the body and back to the heart. The following is an overview of how these systems work.

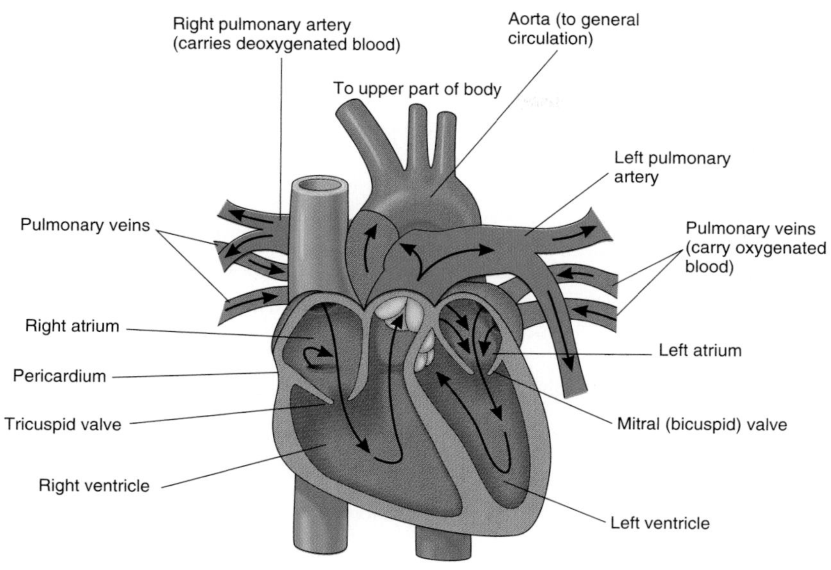

Figure 6-19 Anatomy of the heart.

1. Blood flows from the body into the right atrium.
2. From the right atrium, it flows through the tricuspid valve into the right ventricle.
3. The right ventricle pumps the blood to the lungs, where it releases waste gases and receives oxygen. The blood is then considered to be oxygen rich.
4. The oxygen-rich blood returns to the heart, entering the left atrium.
5. From the left atrium, the blood flows through the mitral valve into the left ventricle.
6. The blood then leaves the left ventricle and travels to all parts of the body.

Blood Vessels

The blood vessels are tubelike structures that include the arteries, capillaries, and veins. The function of these vessels is to transport blood to and from the heart, and then on to various tissues of the body.

Arteries are thick-walled, muscular, flexible tubes that carry oxygenated blood away from the heart to the capillaries. The largest artery in the body is the aorta.

Capillaries are minute, thin-walled blood vessels that connect the smaller arteries to the veins. They bring nutrients to the cells and carry away waste materials.

Veins are thin-walled blood vessels that are less elastic than arteries. They contain cuplike valves that prevent backflow and carry blood containing waste products from the various capillaries back to the heart. Veins are located closer to the outer skin surface of the body than arteries (Figure 6–20).

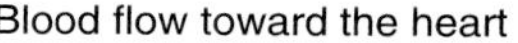

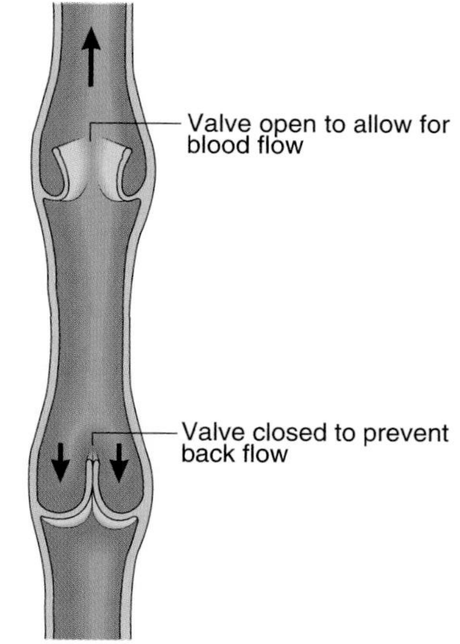

Figure 6-20 Valves in the veins.

The Blood

Blood is a nutritive fluid circulating through the circulatory system. There are approximately 8 to 10 pints of blood in the human body, which contribute about one-twentieth of the body's weight. Blood is approximately 80 percent water. It is sticky and salty, with a normal temperature of 98.6° Fahrenheit (36° Celsius). It is bright red in the arteries (except for the pulmonary artery) and dark red in the veins. The color change occurs with the exchange of carbon dioxide for oxygen as the blood passes through the lungs and the exchange of oxygen for carbon dioxide as the blood circulates throughout the body.

Composition of the Blood

The blood is composed of red and white corpuscles, platelets, plasma, and hemoglobin.

Red blood cells, also called red corpuscles (KOR-pus-uls) or erythrocytes (ih-RITH-ruh-syts), are produced in the red bone marrow. They contain **hemoglobin** (HEE-muh-gloh-bun), a complex iron protein that gives the blood its bright red color. The function of red blood cells is to carry oxygen to the body cells.

White blood cells, also called white corpuscles or leukocytes (LOO-koh-syts) perform the function of destroying disease-causing germs.

Platelets, also called thrombocytes (THRAHM-buh-syts), are much smaller than red blood cells. They contribute to the blood-clotting process, which stops bleeding.

Plasma (PLAZ-muh) is the fluid part of the blood in which the red and white blood cells and blood platelets flow. It is about 90 percent water and contains proteins, sugars, and oxygen. The main function of plasma is to carry food and secretions to the cells and to take carbon dioxide away from the cells.

Chief Functions of the Blood

Blood performs the following critical functions.

- It carries water, oxygen, food, and secretions to all cells of the body.
- It carries away carbon dioxide and waste products to be eliminated through the lungs, skin, kidneys, and large intestines.
- It helps to equalize the body's temperature, thus protecting the body from extreme heat and cold.
- It aids in protecting the body from harmful bacteria and infections through the action of the white blood cells.
- It closes injured minute blood vessels by forming clots, thus preventing blood loss.

The Lymph Vascular System

The lymph vascular system, also known as the lymphatic system, acts as an aid to the blood system. Lymph is circulated through the lymphatic vessels and filtered by the **lymph nodes**, which are gland-like bodies in the lymphatic vessels. This filtering process helps to fight infection.

The primary functions of the lymph vascular system are to:

- carry nourishment from the blood to the body cells.
- act as a defense against invading bacteria and toxins.
- remove waste material from the body cells to the blood.
- provide a suitable fluid environment for the cells.

Arteries of the Head, Face, and Neck

The **common carotid arteries** (kuh-RAHT-ud) are the main sources of blood supply to the head, face, and neck. They are located on either side of the neck, and each one is divided into an internal and external branch.

The **internal carotid artery** supplies blood to the brain, eyes, eyelids, forehead, nose, and internal ear. The **external carotid artery** supplies blood to the anterior (front) parts of the scalp, ear, face, neck, and side of the head (Figure 6–21).

The external carotid artery subdivides into a number of branches. Of particular interest to the cosmetologist are the following arteries.

The **facial artery** or external maxillary artery supplies blood to the lower region of the face, mouth, and nose. Some of its branches are the:

- **submental artery** (sub-MEN-tul) that supplies blood to the chin and lower lip.
- **inferior labial artery** (LAY-bee-ul) that supplies blood to the lower lip.

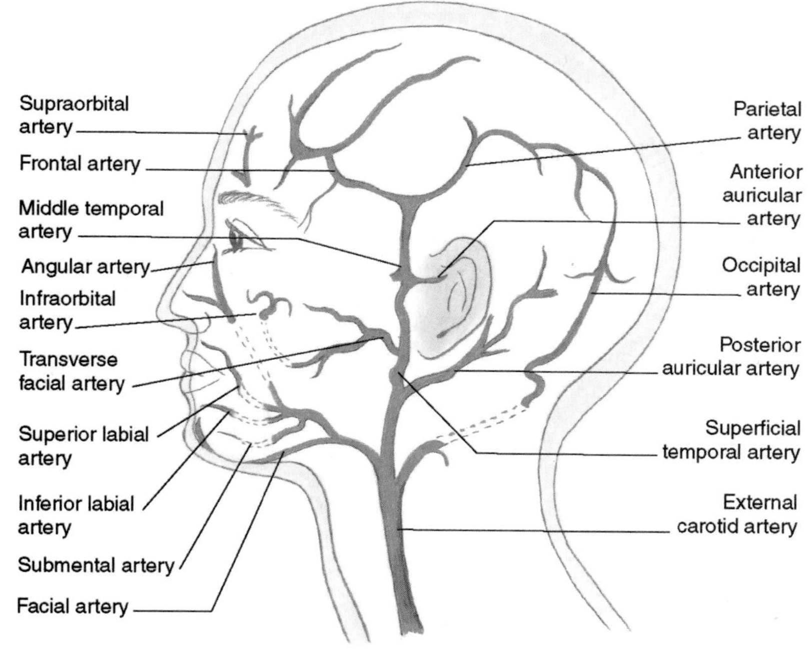

Figure 6–21 Arteries of the head, face, and neck.

- **angular artery** (ANG-gyoo-lur) that supplies blood to the side of the nose.
- **superior labial artery** that supplies blood to the upper lip and region of the nose.

The **superficial temporal artery** is a continuation of the external carotid artery and supplies blood to the muscles of the front, side, and top of the head. Some of its important branches include the:

- **frontal artery** that supplies blood to the forehead and upper eyelids.
- **parietal artery** that supplies blood to the side and crown of the head.
- **transverse facial artery** (tranz-VURS) that supplies blood to the skin and masseter.
- **middle temporal artery** that supplies blood to the temples.
- **anterior auricular artery** that supplies blood to the front part of the ear.

Two other arteries that branch from the external carotid artery are the:

- **occipital artery** that supplies blood to the skin and muscles of the scalp and back of the head up to the crown.
- **posterior auricular artery** that supplies the scalp, the area behind and above the ear, and the skin behind the ear.

Two branches of the internal carotid artery are important to know are the:

- **supraorbital artery** (soo-pruh-OR-bih-tul) that supplies blood to the upper eyelid and forehead.
- **infraorbital artery** (in-frah-OR-bih-tul) that supplies blood to the muscles of the eye.

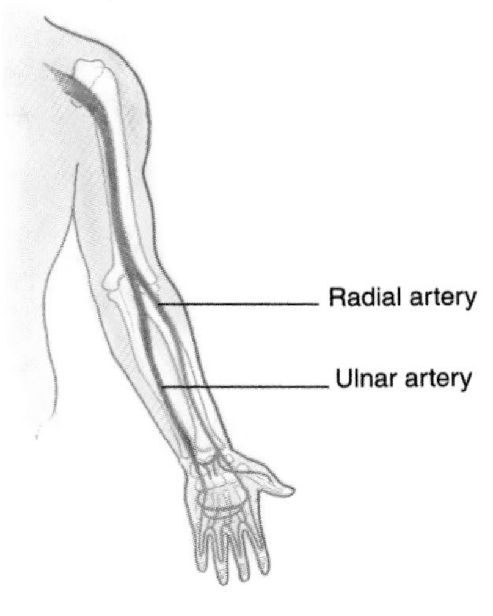

Figure 6–22 Arteries of the arm and hand.

Veins of the Head, Face, and Neck

The blood returning to the heart from the head, face, and neck flows on each side of the neck in two principal veins: the **internal jugular** (JUG-yuh-lur) and **external jugular**. The most important veins of the face and neck are parallel to the arteries and take the same names as the arteries.

Blood Supply of the Arm and Hand

The ulnar and radial arteries are the main blood supply of the arms and hands (Figure 6–22). The **ulnar artery** and its numerous branches supply the little-finger side of the arm and palm of the hand. The **radial artery** and its branches supply the thumb side of the arm and the back of the hand.

The important veins are located almost parallel with the arteries and take the same names as the arteries. While the arteries are found deep in the tissues, the veins lie nearer to the surface of the arms and hands.

THE ENDOCRINE SYSTEM

The **endocrine system** (EN-duh-krin) is made up of a group of specialized glands that affect the growth, development, sexual activities, and health of the entire body. **Glands** are specialized organs that remove certain elements from the blood to convert them into new compounds.

There are two main types of glands.

- **Exocrine glands**(EK-suh-krin) or duct glands produce a substance that travels through small tube-like ducts. Sweat and oil glands of the skin and intestinal glands belong to this group.
- **Endocrine glands** or ductless glands release secretions called **hormones** directly into the bloodstream, which in turn influence the welfare of the entire body. Hormones, such as insulin, adrenaline, and estrogen, stimulate functional activity or secretion in other parts of the body.

THE DIGESTIVE SYSTEM

The **digestive system**, also called the gastrointestinal (gas-troh-in-TES-tun-ul) system, is responsible for changing food into nutrients and waste. Digestive enzymes (EN-zymz) are chemicals that change certain kinds of food into a form that can be used by the body. The food, now in soluble form, is transported by the bloodstream and used by the body's cells and tissues. The entire digestive process takes about nine hours to complete.

THE EXCRETORY SYSTEM

The **excretory system** (EK-skre-tor-ee) is responsible for purifying the body by eliminating waste matter. The metabolism of body cells forms various toxic substances that, if retained, could poison the body.

Each of the following organs plays a crucial role in the excretory system.

- The kidneys excrete urine.
- The liver discharges bile.
- The skin eliminates perspiration.
- The large intestine eliminates decomposed and undigested food.
- The lungs exhale carbon dioxide.

THE RESPIRATORY SYSTEM

Did you know...

Have you ever wondered why someone has green eyes instead of brown, or red hair instead of blonde? It is because of the genetic information enclosed within the fusing cells during conception. As a cosmetologist, working with all sorts of people, you will become aware of how a person's genetic code will largely determine appearance. No matter how many services you provide, you will not make curly hair straight forever!

The **respiratory system** enables breathing (**respiration**) and consists of the lungs and air passages. The **lungs** are spongy tissues composed of microscopic cells in which inhaled air is exchanged for carbon dioxide during one breathing cycle. The respiratory system is located within the chest cavity and is protected on both sides by the ribs. The **diaphragm** is a muscular wall that separates the thorax from the abdominal region and helps control breathing (Figure 6–23).

With each breathing cycle, an exchange of gases takes place. During **inhalation** (in-huh-LAY-shun), or breathing in, oxygen is absorbed into the blood. During **exhalation** (eks-huh-LAY-shun), or breathing outward, carbon dioxide is expelled from the lungs.

Oxygen is more essential than either food or water. Although people may survive for more than 60 days without food, and a few days without water, if they are deprived of oxygen, they will die in a few minutes.

THE INTEGUMENTARY SYSTEM

The **integumentary system** is made up of the skin and its various accessory organs, such as the oil and sweat glands, sensory receptors, hair, and nails. (Skin anatomy and physiology are discussed in detail in Chapter 17.) 4

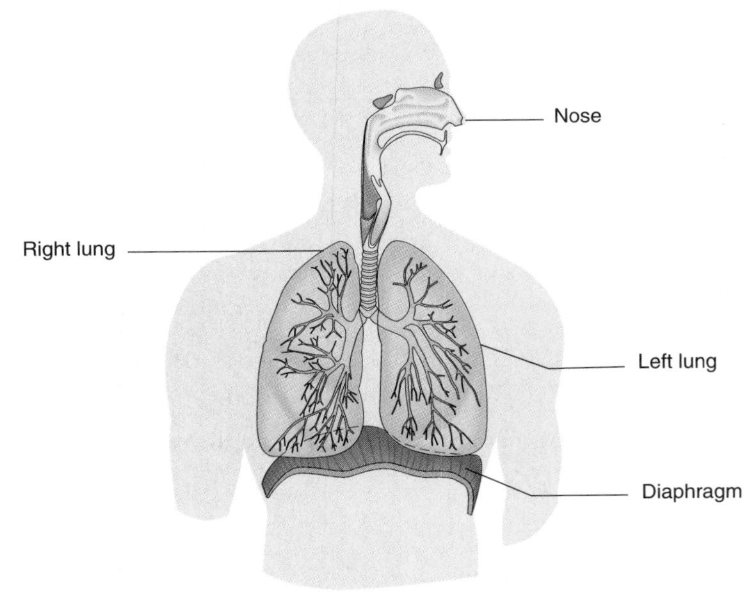

Figure 6–23 The respiratory system.

chapter glossary

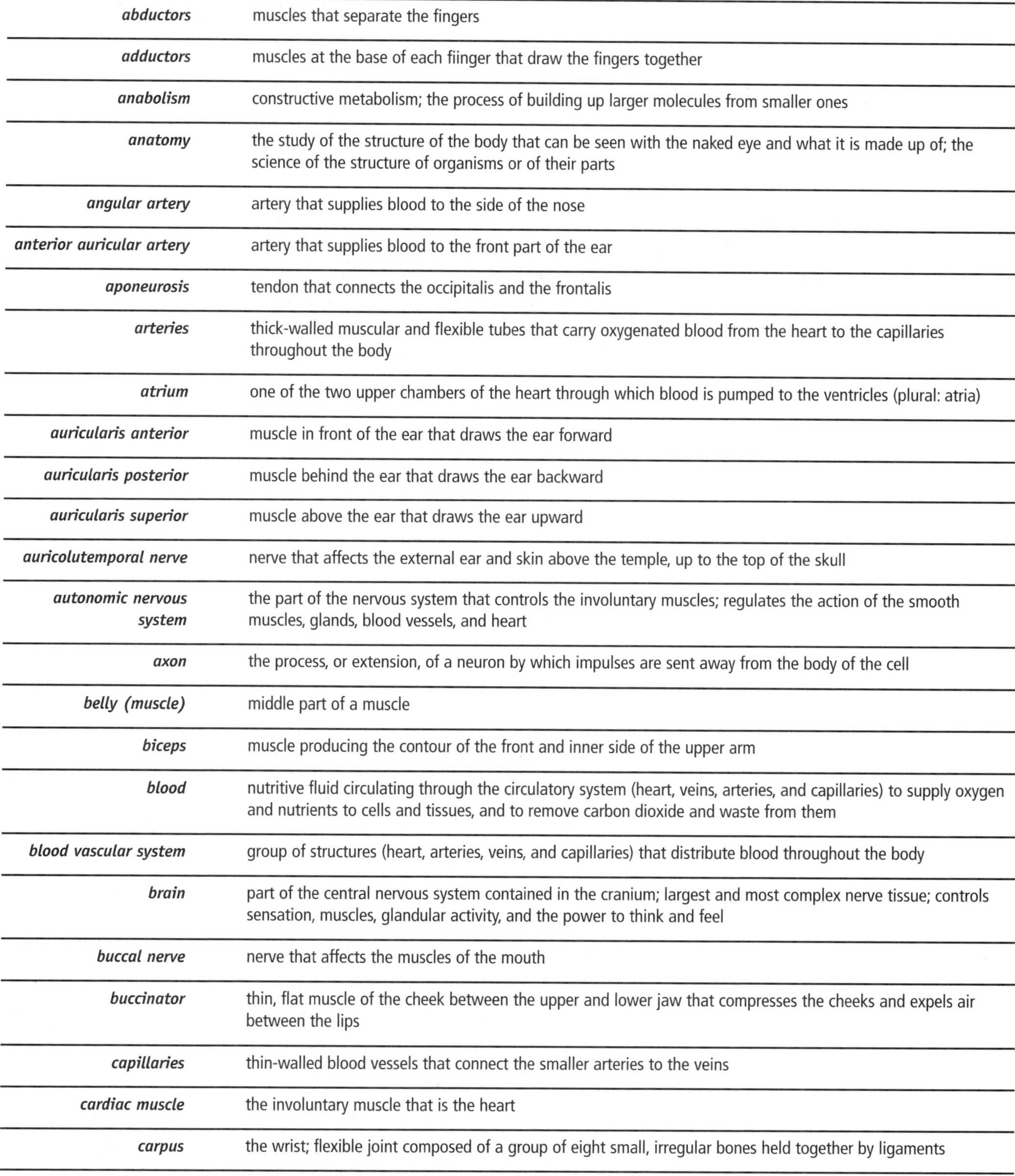

abductors	muscles that separate the fingers
adductors	muscles at the base of each fiinger that draw the fingers together
anabolism	constructive metabolism; the process of building up larger molecules from smaller ones
anatomy	the study of the structure of the body that can be seen with the naked eye and what it is made up of; the science of the structure of organisms or of their parts
angular artery	artery that supplies blood to the side of the nose
anterior auricular artery	artery that supplies blood to the front part of the ear
aponeurosis	tendon that connects the occipitalis and the frontalis
arteries	thick-walled muscular and flexible tubes that carry oxygenated blood from the heart to the capillaries throughout the body
atrium	one of the two upper chambers of the heart through which blood is pumped to the ventricles (plural: atria)
auricularis anterior	muscle in front of the ear that draws the ear forward
auricularis posterior	muscle behind the ear that draws the ear backward
auricularis superior	muscle above the ear that draws the ear upward
auricolutemporal nerve	nerve that affects the external ear and skin above the temple, up to the top of the skull
autonomic nervous system	the part of the nervous system that controls the involuntary muscles; regulates the action of the smooth muscles, glands, blood vessels, and heart
axon	the process, or extension, of a neuron by which impulses are sent away from the body of the cell
belly (muscle)	middle part of a muscle
biceps	muscle producing the contour of the front and inner side of the upper arm
blood	nutritive fluid circulating through the circulatory system (heart, veins, arteries, and capillaries) to supply oxygen and nutrients to cells and tissues, and to remove carbon dioxide and waste from them
blood vascular system	group of structures (heart, arteries, veins, and capillaries) that distribute blood throughout the body
brain	part of the central nervous system contained in the cranium; largest and most complex nerve tissue; controls sensation, muscles, glandular activity, and the power to think and feel
buccal nerve	nerve that affects the muscles of the mouth
buccinator	thin, flat muscle of the cheek between the upper and lower jaw that compresses the cheeks and expels air between the lips
capillaries	thin-walled blood vessels that connect the smaller arteries to the veins
cardiac muscle	the involuntary muscle that is the heart
carpus	the wrist; flexible joint composed of a group of eight small, irregular bones held together by ligaments

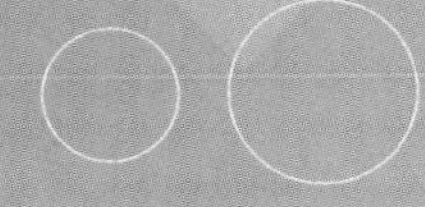

chapter glossary *(continued)*

catabolism	the phase of metabolism that involves the breaking down of complex compounds within the cells into smaller ones, often resulting in the release of energy to perform functions such as muscular efforts, secretions, or digestion
cell membrane	part of the cell that encloses the protoplasm and permits soluble substances to enter and leave the cell
cells	basic units of all living things; minute masses of protoplasm capable of performing all the fundamental functions of life
central nervous system	cerebrospinal nervous system; consists of the brain, spinal cord, spinal nerves, and cranial nerves
cervical cutaneous nerve	nerve located at the side of the neck that affects the front and sides of the neck as far down as the breastbone
cervical nerve (branch of the facial nerve)	nerve that affects the side of the neck and the platysma muscle
cervical nerves	nerves that originate at the spinal cord, whose branches supply the muscles and scalp at the back of the head and neck
cervical vertebrae	the seven bones of the top part of the vertebral column, located in the neck region
circulatory system	system that controls the steady circulation of the blood through the body by means of the heart and blood vessels
clavicle	collarbone; bone joining the sternum and scapula
common carotid arteries	arteries that supply blood to the face, head, and neck
connective tissue	fibrous tissue that binds together, protects, and supports the various parts of the body such as bone, cartilage, and tendons
corrugator	facial muscle that draws eyebrows down and wrinkles the forehead vertically
cranium	oval, bony case that protects the brain
cytoplasm	all the protoplasm of a cell except that which is in the nucleus; the watery fluid that contains food material necessary for growth, reproduction, and self-repair of the cell
deltoid	large, triangular muscle covering the shoulder joint that allows the arm to extend outward and to the side of the body
dendrites	tree-like branching of nerve fibers extending from a nerve cell; short nerve fibers that carry impulses toward the cell
depressor labii inferioris	muscle surrounding the lower lip; depresses the lower lip and draws it to one side; also known as quadratus labii inferioris
diaphragm	muscular wall that separates the thorax from the abdominal region and helps control breathing
digestive system	the mouth, stomach, intestines, and salivary and gastric glands that change food into nutrients and wastes
digit	a finger or toe
digital nerve	nerve that, with its branches, supplies the fingers and toes

endocrine (ductless) glands	glands (such as the thyroid, pituitary, and suprarenal glands) that release hormonal secretions directly into the bloodstream
endocrine system	group of specialized glands that affect the growth, development, sexual activities, and health of the entire body
epicranius	broad muscle that covers the top of the skull; also called occipito-frontalis
epithelial tissue	protective covering on body surfaces, such as the skin, mucous membranes, and the lining of the heart, digestive and respiratory organs, and glands
excretory system	group of organs including the kidneys, liver, skin, large intestine, and lungs that purify the body by the elimination of waste matter
exhalation	the act of breathing outward, expelling carbon dioxide from the lungs
exocrine (duct) glands	glands that produce a substance that travels through small tubelike ducts, such as the sudoriferous (sweat) glands and the sebaceous (oil) glands
extensors	muscles that straighten the wrist, hand, and fingers to form a straight line
external carotid artery	artery that supplies blood to the anterior parts of the scalp, ear, face, neck, and side of the head
external jugular vein	vein located on the side of the neck that carries blood returning to the heart from the head, face, and neck
facial artery	artery that supplies blood to the lower region of the face, mouth, and nose; also called external maxillary artery
fifth cranial nerve	chief sensory nerve of the face; controls chewing; also known as trifacial or trigeminal nerve
flexors	extensor muscles of the wrist, involved in flexing the wrist
frontal artery	artery that supplies blood to the forehead and upper eyelids
frontal bone	bone forming the forehead
frontalis	anterior or front portion of the epicranium; muscle of the scalp
glands	specialized organs that remove certain constituents from the blood to convert them into new compounds
greater auricular nerve	nerve at the sides of the neck affecting the face, ears, neck, and parotid gland
greater occipital nerve	nerve located in the back of the head, affecting the scalp
heart	muscular cone-shaped organ that keeps the blood moving within the circulatory system
hemoglobin	coloring matter of the blood; the oxygen-carrying pigment in the blood and iron-containing protein in red blood cells
histology	science of the minute structures of organic tissues; microscopic anatomy
hormones	secretion produced by one of the endocrine glands and carried by the bloodstream or body fluid to another part of the body or a body organ to stimulate functional activity or secretion
humerus	uppermost and largest bone in the arm, extending from the elbow to the shoulder
hyoid	U-shaped bone at the base of the tongue that supports the tongue and its muscles; also called "Adam's apple"

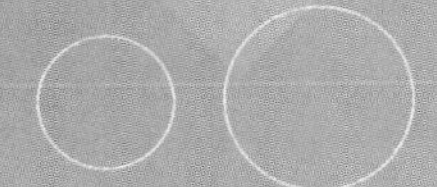

chapter glossary *(continued)*

inferior labial artery	artery that supplies blood to the lower lip
infraorbital artery	artery that originates from the internal maxillary artery and supplies blood to the muscles of the eye
infraorbital nerve	nerve that affects the skin of the lower eyelid, side of the nose, upper lip, and mouth
infratrochlear nerve	nerve that affects the membrane and skin of the nose
inhalation	the breathing in of air
insertion	parts of the muscle at the more movable attachment to the skeleton
integumentary system	the skin and its accessory organs, such as the oil and sweat glands, sensory receptors, hair, and nails
internal carotid artery	artery that supplies blood to the brain, eyes, eyelids, forehead, nose, and internal ear
internal jugular vein	vein located at the side of the neck to collect blood from the brain and parts of the face and neck
joint	connection between two or more bones of the skeleton
lacrimal bones	small, thin bones located in the anterior medial wall of the orbits (eye sockets)
latissimus dorsi	broad, flat superficial muscle covering the back of the neck and upper and middle region of the back, controlling the shoulder blade and the swinging movements of the arm
levator anguli oris	muscle that raises the angle of the mouth and draws it inward; also known as caninus
levator labii superioris	muscle surrounding the upper lip; elevates the upper lip and dilates the nostrils, as in expressing distaste; also known as quadratus labii superioris
liquid tissue	body tissue that carries food, waste products, and hormones by means of blood and lymph
lungs	organs of respiration; spongy tissues composed of microscopic cells in which inhaled air is exchanged for carbon dioxide during one respiratory cycle
lymph	clear yellowish fluid that circulates in the lymph spaces (lymphatic) of the body; carries waste and impurities away from the cells
lymph nodes	glandlike bodies in the lymphatic vessels that filter lymph
lymph vascular system	body system that acts as an aid to the blood system and consists of the lymph spaces, lymph vessels, and lymph glands
mandible	lower jawbone; largest and strongest bone of the face
mandibular nerve	branch of the fifth cranial nerve that supplies the muscles and skin of the lower part of the face; also, nerve that affects the muscles of the chin and lower lip
masseter	one of the muscles of the jaw used in mastication (chewing)
maxillae	bones of the upper jaw
maxillary nerve	branch of the fifth cranial nerve that supplies the upper part of the face

median nerve	nerve, smaller than the ulnar and radial nerves, that supplies the arm and hand
mentalis	muscle that elevates the lower lip and raises and wrinkles the skin of the chin
mental nerve	nerve that affects the skin of the lower lip and chin
metabolism	chemical process taking place in living organisms whereby the cells are nourished and carry out their activities
metacarpus	bones of the palm of the hand; parts of the hand containing five bones between the carpus and phalanges
middle temporal artery	artery that supplies blood to the temples
mitosis	cells dividing into two new cells (daughter cells); the usual process of cell reproduction of human tissues
mixed nerves	nerves that contain both sensory and motor fibers and have the ability to send and receive messages
motor (efferent) nerves	nerves that carry impulses from the brain to the muscles
muscular system	body system that covers, shapes, and supports the skeleton tissue; contracts and moves various parts of the body
muscular tissue	tissue that contracts and moves various parts of the body
myology	science of the nature, structure, function, and diseases of the muscles
nasal bones	bones that form the bridge of the nose
nasal nerve	nerve that affects the point and lower sides of the nose
nerve	whitish cord made up of bundles of nerve fibers held together by connective tissue, through which impulses are transmitted
nerve tissue	tissue that controls and coordinates all body functions
nervous system	body system composed of the brain, spinal cord, and nerves; controls and coordinates all other systems and makes them work harmoniously and efficiently
neuron	nerve cell; basic unit of the nervous system, consisting of a cell body, nucleus, dendrites, and axon
neurology	science of the structure, function, and pathology of the nervous system
nonstriated muscles	also called involuntary, visceral, or smooth muscles, muscles that function automatically, without conscious will
nucleus	dense, active protoplasm found in the center of the cell; plays an important part in cell reproduction and metabolism
occipital artery	artery that supplies blood to the skin and muscles of the scalp and back of the head up to the crown
occipital bone	hindmost bone of the skull, located below the parietal bones
occipitalis	back of the epicranius; muscle that draws the scalp backward
ophthalmic nerve	branch of the fifth cranial nerve that supplies the skin of the forehead, upper eyelids, and interior portion of the scalp, orbit, eyeball, and nasal passage

chapter glossary *(continued)*

opponent muscles	muscles in the palm that act to bring the thumb toward the fingers
orbicularis oculi	the ring muscle of the eye socket; closes the eyelid
orbicularis oris	flat band around the upper and lower lips that compresses, contracts, puckers, and wrinkles the lips
organs	in plants and animals, structures composed of specialized tissues and performing specific functions
origin	part of the muscle that does not move; it is attached to the skeleton and is usually part of a skeletal muscle
os	bone
osteology	science of the anatomy, structure, and function of the bones
parietal artery	artery that supplies blood to the side and crown of the head
parietal bones	bones that form the sides and top of the cranium
pectoralis major and minor	muscles of the chest that assist the swinging movements of the arm
pericardium	double-layered membranous sac enclosing the heart
peripheral nervous system	system of nerves and ganglia that connects the peripheral parts of the body to the central nervous system; has both sensory and motor nerves
phalanges	bones of the fingers or toes (singular: phalanx)
physiology	study of the functions or activities performed by the body's structures
plasma	fluid part of the blood and lymph that carries food and secretions to the cells and carbon dioxide from the cells
platelets	blood cells that aid in the forming of clots
platysma	broad muscle extending from the chest and shoulder muscles to the side of the chin; responsible for depressing the lower jaw and lip
posterior auricular artery	artery that supplies blood to the scalp, behind and above the ear
posterior auricular nerve	nerve that affects the muscles behind the ear at the base of the skull
procerus	muscle that covers the bridge of the nose, depresses the eyebrows, and causes wrinkles across the bridge of the nose
pronators	muscles that turn the hand inward so that the palm faces downward
protoplasm	colorless jelly-like substance in cells in which food elements such as protein, fats, carbohydrates, mineral salts, and water are present
pulmonary circulation	blood circulation from heart to lungs and back to heart
radial artery	artery that supplies blood to the thumb side of the arm and the back of the hand; supplies the muscles of the skin, hands and fingers, wrist, elbow, and forearm

radial nerve	nerve that, with its branches, supplies the thumb side of the arm and back of the hand
radius	smaller bone in the forearm on the same side as the thumb
red blood cells	also called red corpuscles or erythrocytes, blood cells that carry oxygen from the lungs to the body cells and transport carbon dioxide from the cells back to the lungs
reflex	automatic nerve reaction to a stimulus that involves the movement of an impulse from a sensory receptor along the afferent nerve to the spinal cord, and a responsive impulse along an efferent neuron to a muscle, causing a reaction
reproductive system	body system responsible for processes by which plants and animals produce offspring
respiration	act of breathing; the exchange of carbon dioxide and oxygen that takes place in the lungs between the blood and cells, and within the cell
respiratory system	body system consisting of the lungs and air passages; enables breathing, supplying the body with oxygen and eliminating carbon dioxide as a waste product
ribs	the 12 pairs of bones forming the wall of the thorax
risorius	muscle of the mouth that draws the corner of the mouth out and back, as in grinning
scapula	one of a pair of shoulder blades; large, flat triangular bone of the shoulder
sensory (afferent) nerves	nerves that carry impulses or messages from the sense organs to the brain, where sensations of touch, cold, heat, sight, hearing, taste, smell, pain, and pressure are experienced
serratus anterior	muscle of the chest that assists in breathing and in raising the arm
seventh (facial) cranial nerve	chief motor nerve of the face, emerging near the lower part of the ear
skeletal system	physical foundation of the body, composed of the bones and movable and immovable joints
smaller (lesser) occipital nerve	nerve located at the base of the skull, affecting the scalp and muscles behind the ear
spinal cord	portion of the central nervous system that originates in the brain, extends down to the lower extremity of the trunk, and is protected by the spinal column
sternocleidomastoideus	muscle of the neck that depresses and rotates the head
sternum	the flat bone or breastbone that forms the ventral support of the ribs
striated muscles	also called voluntary or skeletal muscles; muscles that are controlled by the will
submental artery	artery that supplies blood to the chin and lower lip
superficial temporal artery	artery that supplies blood to the muscles of the front, side, and top of the head
superior labial artery	artery that supplies blood to the upper lip and region of the nose
supraorbital artery	artery that supplies blood to the upper eyelid and forehead

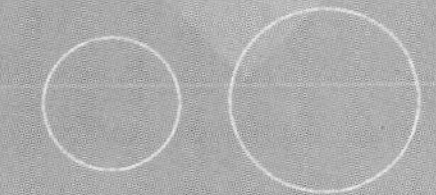

chapter glossary *(continued)*

supraorbital nerve	nerve that affects the skin of the forehead, scalp, eyebrow, and upper eyelid
supratrochlear nerve	nerve that affects the skin between the eyes and upper side of the nose
supinator	muscle of the forearm that rotates the radius outward and the palm upward
systems	comprised of a group of bodily organs acting together to perform one or more functions
systemic circulation	circulation of blood from the heart throughout the body and back again to the heart; also called general circulation
temporal bones	bones forming the sides of the head in the ear region
temporal nerve	nerve that affects the muscles of the temple, side of the forehead, eyebrow, eyelid, and upper part of the cheek
temporalis	temporal muscle; one of the muscles involved in mastication (chewing)
thorax	the chest; elastic, bony cage that serves as a protective framework for the heart, lungs, and other internal organs
tissue	collection of similar cells that perform a particular function
transverse facial artery	artery that supplies blood to the skin and the masseter
trapezius	muscle that covers the back of the neck and upper and middle region of the back; rotates and controls swinging movements of the arm
triangularis	muscle extending alongside the chin that pulls down the corner of the mouth
triceps	large muscle that covers the entire back of the upper arm and extends the forearm
ulna	inner and larger bone of the forearm, attached to the wrist and located on the side of the little finger
ulnar artery	artery that supplies blood to the muscle of the little finger side of the arm and palm of the hand
ulnar nerve	nerve that affects the little finger side of the arm and palm of the hand
valve	structures that temporarily close a passage, or permit flow in one direction only
veins	thin-walled blood vessels that are less elastic than arteries; they contain cup-like valves to prevent backflow and carry impure blood from the various capillaries back to the heart and lungs
ventricle	one of the two lower chambers of the heart
white blood cells	blood cells that perform the function of destroying disease-causing germs; also called white corpuscles or leukocytes
zygomatic or malar bones	bones that form the prominence of the cheeks; the cheekbones
zygomatic nerve	nerve that affects the skin of the temple, side of the forehead, and upper part of the cheek
zygomaticus	muscle extending from the zygomatic bone to the angle of the mouth; elevates the lip, as in laughing

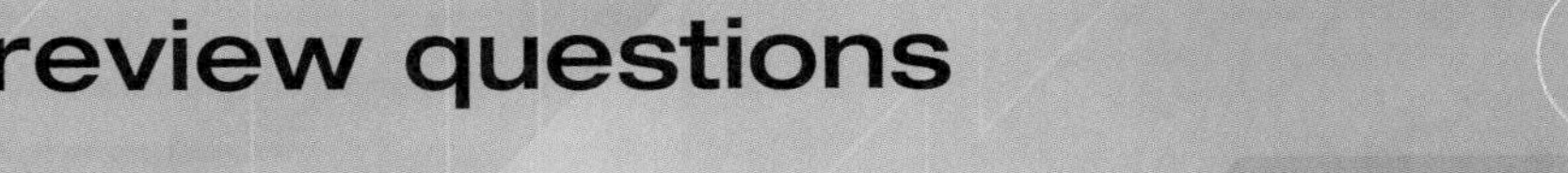

review questions

1. Define anatomy, physiology, and histology.
2. Why is the study of anatomy, physiology, and histology important to the cosmetologist?
3. Name and describe the basic structures of a cell.
4. Explain cell metabolism and its purpose.
5. List and describe the functions of the five types of tissue found in the human body.
6. What are organs?
7. List and describe the functions of the main organs found in the body.
8. Name the 10 body systems and their main functions.
9. List the primary functions of the bones.
10. Name and describe the three types of muscular tissue found in the body.
11. Name and describe the three types of nerves found in the body.
12. Name and briefly describe the three type of blood vessels found in the body.
13. List and describe the components of blood.
14. Name and discuss the two types of glands found in the human body.
15. List the organs of the excretory system and their function.

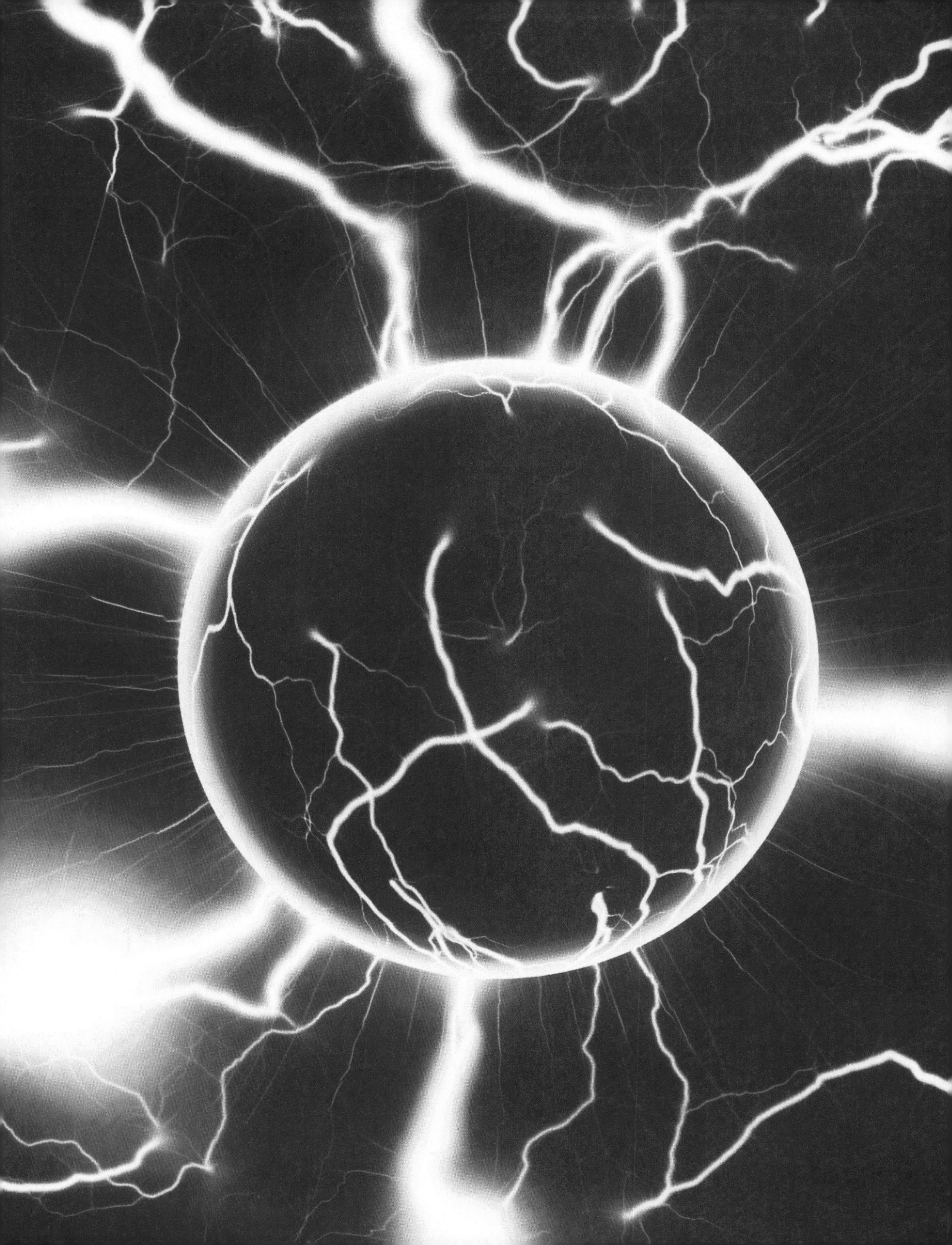

BASICS OF CHEMISTRY AND ELECTRICITY

John Halal
PRESIDENT, HONORS BEAUTY COLLEGE, INC., INDIANAPOLIS, IN

Chapter Outline

Learning Objectives

After completing this chapter, you should be able to:

1. Explain the difference between organic and inorganic chemistry.
2. Discuss the different forms of matter: elements, compounds, and mixtures.
3. Explain pH and the pH scale.
4. Describe oxidation and reduction (redox) reactions.
5. Define the nature of electricity and the two types of electric current.
6. Describe the four types of electrotherapy and their uses.
7. Explain electromagnetic radiation and the visible spectrum of light.
8. Describe the five types of light therapy and their benefits.

National Skill Standards

This chapter provides you with the necessary information to master these National Industry Skill Standards for Entry-Level Cosmetologists.

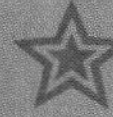 Marketing professional salon products.

 Using a variety of salon products while providing client services.

 Using appropriate methods to ensure personal health and well-being.

 Providing basic skin care services.

Key Terms

Page number indicates where in the chapter the term is used.

acid pg. 179

active electrode pg. 187

alcohol pg. 178

alkali pg. 179

alkanolamines pg. 178

alternating current (AC) pg. 183

ammonia pg. 178

amp pg. 184

anaphoresis pg. 187

anion pg. 178

anode pg. 187

atom pg. 171

blue light pg. 192

cataphoresis pg. 187

cathode pg. 187

cation pg. 178

chemical change pg. 173

chemical compounds pg. 174

chemical properties pg. 172

chemistry pg. 170

circuit breaker pg. 184

combustion pg. 181

complete circuit pg. 183

compound molecules pg. 171

conductor pg. 182

converter pg. 183

direct current (DC) pg. 183

desincrustation pg. 187

electric current pg. 182

electricity pg. 182

electrode pg. 187

electromagnetic radiation pg. 191

electrotherapy pg. 187

element pg. 171

elemental molecules
pg. 171

emulsion
pg. 175

exothermic
pg. 180

faradic current
pg. 188

fuse
pg. 184

galvanic current
pg. 187

glycerin
pg. 178

hydrophilic
pg. 175

immiscible
pg. 175

inactive electrode
pg. 187

infrared rays
pg. 192

inorganic chemistry
pg. 170

insulator or nonconductor
pg. 183

ion
pg. 178

ionization
pg. 178

iontophoresis
pg. 187

kilowatt
pg. 184

lipophilic
pg. 175

matter
pg. 171

milliampere
pg. 184

miscible
pg. 175

modalities
pg. 186

molecule
pg. 171

ohm
pg.184

oil-in-water (O/W) emulsion
pg. 176

organic chemistry
pg. 170

oxidation
pg. 180

oxidize
pg. 181

oxidizing agent
pg. 181

pH
pg. 179

physical change
pg. 173

physical mixture
pg. 174

physical properties
pg. 172

polarity
pg. 187

pure substance
pg. 173

rectifier
pg. 183

red light
pg. 192

redox
pg. 182

reduce
pg. 181

reduction
pg. 181

silicones
pg. 178

sinusoidal current
pg. 188

solute
pg. 175

solution
pg. 175

solvent
pg. 175

surfactants
pg. 175

suspension
pg. 175

Tesla high-frequency current
pg. 188

therapeutic lamps
pg. 191

ultraviolet (UV) rays
pg. 192

visible light
pg. 191

volatile
pg. 178

volatile organic compounds (VOCs)
pg. 178

volt
pg. 184

wall plate
pg. 186

water-in-oil (W/O) emulsion
pg. 177

watt
pg. 184

wavelength
pg. 191

white light
pg.192

You might be wondering why you are reading a chapter with the words "chemistry" and "electricity" in the title. After all, didn't you leave those subjects behind in high school? The fact is, a large part of a cosmetologist's work has to do with chemicals and electricity. Today's salon services would not be possible without them. Permanent waving, chemical hair relaxing, haircoloring, wet setting, and thermal styling all rely on the use of chemicals and electricity. To use chemicals and electricity effectively and safely, you need to have a basic working knowledge of these sciences. This chapter will provide you with the overview you need.

CHEMISTRY

Chemistry is the science that deals with the composition, structures, and properties of matter and how matter changes under different chemical conditions.

Organic chemistry is the study of substances that contain carbon. All living things, whether they are plants or animals, are made up of compounds that contain carbon. Although the term "organic" is often used to mean "natural" because of its association with living things, the term also applies to anything that has ever been alive. Cow manure, for instance, is an organic fertilizer.

You may also be surprised to learn that gasoline, motor oil, plastics, synthetic fabrics, pesticides, and fertilizers are also organic substances. These products are all manufactured from natural gas and oil, which are the remains of plants and animals that died millions of years ago. Organic compounds will burn.

The majority of products that are used in a modern salon are organic (again, in the sense of being derived from plants or animals, not in the sense of being "natural" or "healthful"). All haircoloring products, chemical hair texturizers, shampoos, conditioners, and styling aids are made with organic compounds from either natural or synthetic sources.

Inorganic chemistry is the branch of chemistry dealing with compounds lacking carbon. Inorganic substances are not, and never were, alive. Metals, minerals, pure water, and clean air are examples of inorganic substances. Inorganic substances do not burn. 1

Matter

Matter is any substance that occupies space, has physical and chemical properties, and exists in the form of a solid, liquid, or gas. Although matter has physical properties that we can touch, taste, smell, or see, not everything that we can see is necessarily matter. For instance, we can see visible light and electric sparks, but these are forms of energy, and energy is not matter. Energy does not occupy space or have physical properties, like weight. We will discuss energy later in this chapter.

Elements

An **element** is the simplest form of matter and cannot be broken down into a simpler substance without loss of identity. There are about 90 naturally occurring elements, each with its own distinctive physical and chemical properties. All matter in the universe is made up of one or more of these 90 different elements.

Each element is identified by a letter symbol, such as O for oxygen, C for carbon, and H for hydrogen. You can look up these symbols in the Periodic Table of Elements, found in any chemistry textbook.

Atoms

Atoms are the structural units that make up the elements. Atoms are the particles from which all matter is composed. An **atom** is the smallest particle of an element that still retains the properties of that element. Atoms cannot be divided into simpler substances by ordinary chemical means.

Molecules

A **molecule** is formed by joining two or more atoms chemically. The two types of molecules are elemental molecules and compound molecules.

Elemental molecules contain two or more atoms of the same element that are united chemically. Atmospheric oxygen, in the air we breathe, is the elemental molecule O_2. The ozone in the atmosphere, which protects us from ultraviolet radiation, is the elemental molecule O_3 (Figure 7–1).

Compound molecules are chemical combinations of two or more atoms of different elements (Figure 7–2). Sodium chloride (NaCl), or common table salt, is a compound molecule that is a chemical combination of one atom of sodium (Na) and one atom of chlorine (Cl).

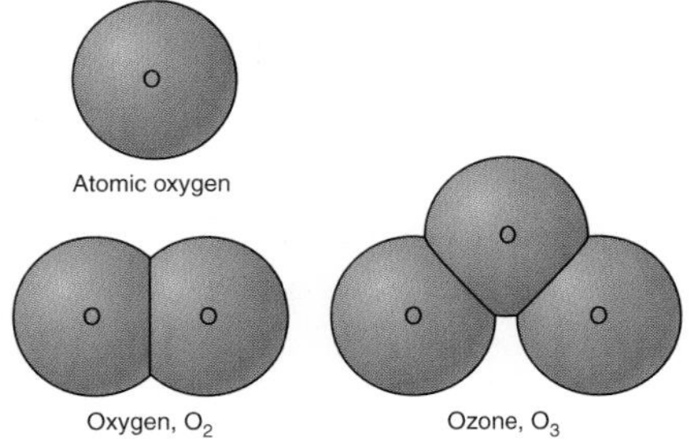

Figure 7-1 Elemental molecules.

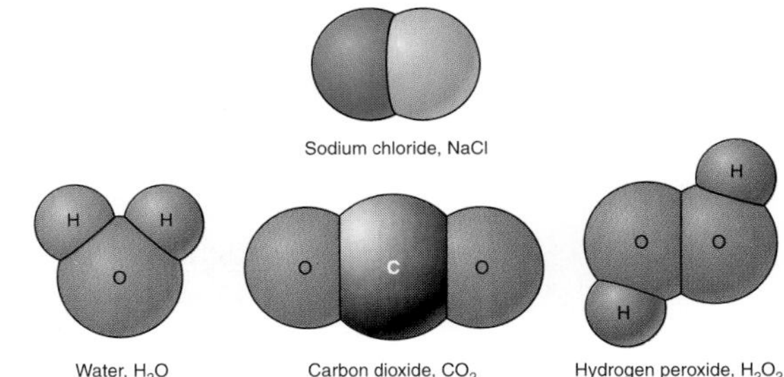

Figure 7-2 Compound molecules.

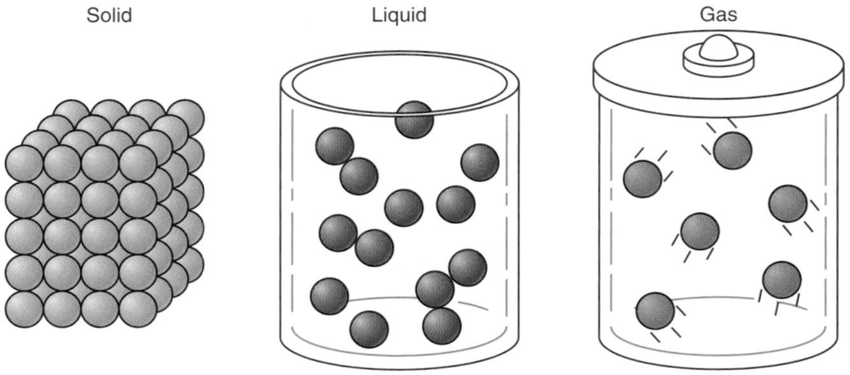

Solid Liquid Gas

Figure 7-3 Solids, liquids, and gases.

STATES OF MATTER

All matter exists in one of three different physical forms: solid, liquid, or gas. These three forms are called the "states of matter." Matter assumes one of these states depending on its temperature (Figure 7–3).

Like most other substances, water (H_2O) can exist in all three states of matter, depending on its temperature. For instance, when water freezes, it turns to ice. When ice melts, it turns to water. When water boils, it turns to steam. When steam cools, it turns to water. The form of the water changes according to changes in the temperature, but it is still water (H_2O). It does not become a different chemical. It stays the same chemical but in a different physical form.

The three different states of matter have the following distinct characteristics:

- Solids have a definite shape and volume. Ice is an example of a solid.
- Liquids have a definite volume but not a definite shape. Water is an example of a liquid.
- Gases do not have a definite volume or shape. Steam is an example of a gas.

PHYSICAL AND CHEMICAL PROPERTIES OF MATTER

Every substance has unique properties that allow us to identify it. The two different types of properties are physical and chemical.

Physical properties are those characteristics that can be determined without a chemical reaction and that do not cause a chemical change in the identity of the substance. Physical properties include color, odor, weight, density, specific gravity, melting point, boiling point, and hardness.

Chemical properties are those characteristics that can only be determined with a chemical reaction and that cause a chemical change in the identity of the substance. Rusting iron and burning wood are examples of a change in chemical properties. In both these examples, the chemical reaction known as "oxidation" creates a chemical change in the identity of the substance. The iron is chemically changed to rust, and the wood is chemically changed to ash.

Physical and Chemical Changes

Matter can be changed in two different ways: physically and chemically.

- A **physical change** is a change in the form or physical properties of a substance without the formation of a new substance. There is no chemical reaction involved, and no new chemicals are formed. A change in the state of matter is an example of a physical change. Solid ice undergoes a physical change when it melts into liquid water (Figure 7–4).

Another example of physical change is the change brought about by temporary haircolor. Temporary haircolor changes the appearance of the hair by physically adding color to the surface of the hair. There is no change in the chemical structure of the hair or its color. There is no chemical reaction and no new chemicals are formed.

- A **chemical change** is a change in the chemical composition of a substance, in which a new substance or substances are formed having properties different from the original. It is the result of a chemical reaction (Figure 7–5). As described above (iron into rust, wood into charcoal), oxidation is an example of a chemical reaction that causes a chemical change.

Permanent haircolor is an example of a chemical change. A chemical reaction (oxidation) develops the dye in the color and creates a chemical change in the hair. The hair is a different color because of changes in the chemical structure of both the dye and the hair. This is a chemical reaction and new chemicals are formed.

Pure Substances and Physical Mixtures

All matter can be classified as either a pure substance or a physical mixture. A **pure substance** is matter with a fixed chemical composition, definite proportions, and distinct properties. The two types of pure substances are elements and compounds.

Elemental molecules contain two or more atoms of the same element that are united chemically. Elements are pure substances. Aluminum foil is an

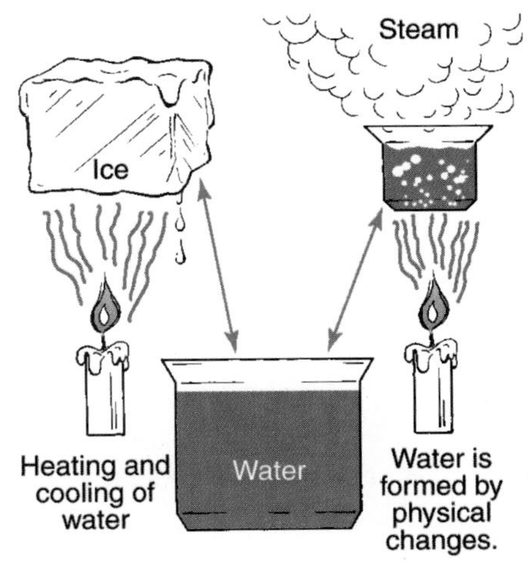

Figure 7–4 Physical changes.

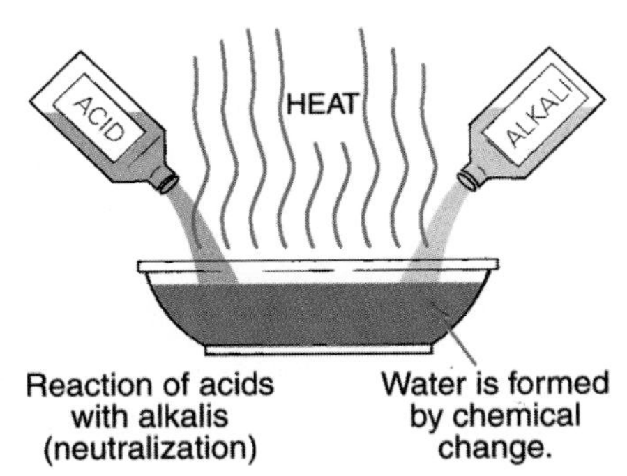

Figure 7–5 Chemical changes.

example of a pure substance; it is composed only of atoms of the element aluminum.

Chemical compounds are combinations of two or more atoms of different elements united chemically with a fixed chemical composition, definite proportions, and distinct properties. The properties of chemical compounds are different from the properties of the elements from which they were made. Water (H_2O) is a chemical compound. A water molecule is composed of two atoms of the element hydrogen (H) and one atom of the element oxygen (O).

A **physical mixture** is a combination of two or more substances united physically, not chemically, without a fixed composition and in any proportions. Physical mixtures are not the result of a chemical reaction. In a physical mixture, each substance holds on to its own identity and its own distinct properties. Pure air is a mixture of gases, mostly nitrogen and oxygen (Figure 7–6). (See Table 7–1 for a summary of the differences between chemical compounds and physical mixtures.)

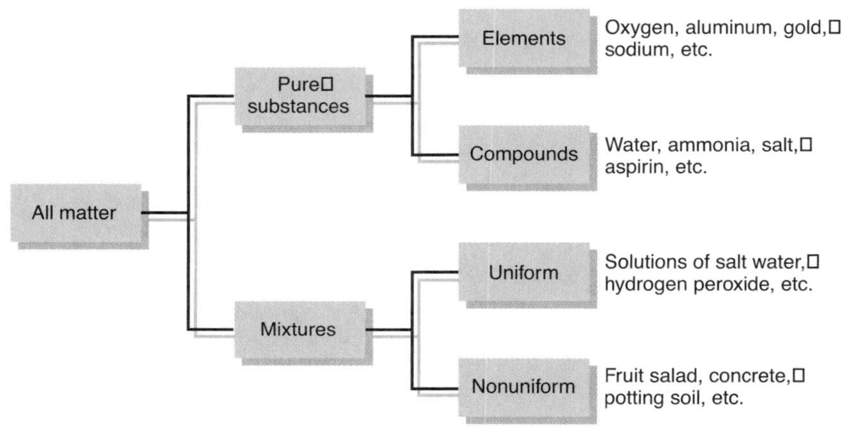

Figure 7–6 Pure substances and mixtures.

7

Chemical Compounds	Physical Mixtures
Involve a chemical reaction	Do not involve a chemical reaction
Change the chemical properties	Change only the physical properties
Mixed in definite proportions	Mixed in any proportions
Water or salt are examples	Salt water is an example
Pure hydrogen peroxide	Solution of hydrogen peroxide

Table 7–1 Chemical Compounds and Physical Mixtures

Solutions, Suspensions, and Emulsions

Solutions, suspensions, and emulsions are different types of physical mixtures, all of which contain two or more different substances.

A **solution** is a blended mixture of two or more solids, liquids, or gaseous substances. A **solute** is the dissolved substance in a solution. A **solvent** is a substance, usually liquid, which dissolves another substance to form a solution, with no change in chemical composition. If a gas or a solid is dissolved in a liquid, the gas or solid is the solute and the liquid is the solvent.

Miscible (MIS-uh-bul) liquids are mutually soluble, meaning that they can be mixed with each other in any proportion without separating. Water and alcohol are examples of miscible liquids. **Immiscible** liquids are not capable of being mixed. Water and oil are examples of immiscible liquids.

Solutions contain particles the size of a small molecule that are invisible to the naked eye. Solutions are usually transparent, although they may be colored. They do not separate on standing. Salt water is a solution of a solid dissolved in a liquid. Water is the solvent that dissolves the salt and holds it in solution. Air and hydrogen peroxide are other examples of solutions.

A **suspension** is a state in which solid particles are distributed throughout a liquid medium. Suspensions differ from solutions in that they contain larger particles, which are generally visible to the naked eye but not large enough to settle to the bottom. Suspensions are not usually transparent and may be colored. They have a tendency to separate over time.

A salad dressing made up of oil and vinegar is an example of a suspension, with the oil suspended in the vinegar. Salad dressing will separate on standing and must be shaken well before using. Many of the lotions used by hairstylists are suspensions and need to be shaken or mixed well before use.

An **emulsion** is a mixture of two or more immiscible substances united with the aid of a binder or emulsifier. The term "emulsify" means "to form an emulsion," a suspension of one liquid in another. Although emulsions have a tendency to separate over time, a properly formulated emulsion that is stored correctly should be stable for at least three years. (Table 7–2 offers a summary of the differences among solutions, suspensions, and emulsions.)

Surfactants are substances that act as a bridge to allow oil and water to mix, or emulsify. The term "surfactant" (sur-FAK-tant) is a contraction for "surface active agent" (surface active agent). A surfactant molecule has two distinct parts (Figure 7–7). The head of the surfactant molecule is **hydrophilic** (hy-drah-FIL-ik), meaning water-loving, and the tail is **lipophilic** (ly-puh-FIL-ik), meaning oil-loving. Since "like dissolves like," the hydrophilic head dissolves in water and the lipophilic tail dissolves in oil. So a surfactant molecule dissolves in both oil and water and joins them together to form an emulsion.

Did you know...

Soaps were the first surfactants. Soaps were made more than 5,000 years ago by boiling oil or animal fat with wood ashes. Modern soaps are made from animal, vegetable, or synthetic fats or oils by a process called sulfonation. Soaps are highly alkaline and combine with the minerals in hard water to form an insoluble film that coats and dulls the hair. Modern synthetic surfactants have overcome these disadvantages and are superior to soaps.

Solutions	Suspensions	Emulsions
Miscible	Slightly miscible	Immiscible
No surfactant	No surfactant	Surfactant
Small particles	Larger particles	Largest particles
Usually clear	Usually cloudy	Usually a solid color
Stable mixture	Unstable mixture	Limited stability
Solution of hydrogen peroxide	Calamine lotion	Shampoos and conditioners

Table 7–2 Solutions, Suspensions, and Emulsions

In an **oil-in-water emulsion (O/W)**, oil droplets are suspended in a water base. The droplets of oil are surrounded by surfactants with their lipophilic tails pointing in and their hydrophilic heads pointing out. Oil forms the internal portion of an O/W emulsion because the oil is completely surrounded by water (Figure 7–8). Oil-in-water emulsions usually contain a small amount of oil and a greater amount of water.

Mayonnaise is an example of an oil-in-water emulsion of two immiscible liquids. Although oil and water are immiscible, the egg yolk in mayonnaise emulsifies the oil droplets and distributes them uniformly in the water.

7

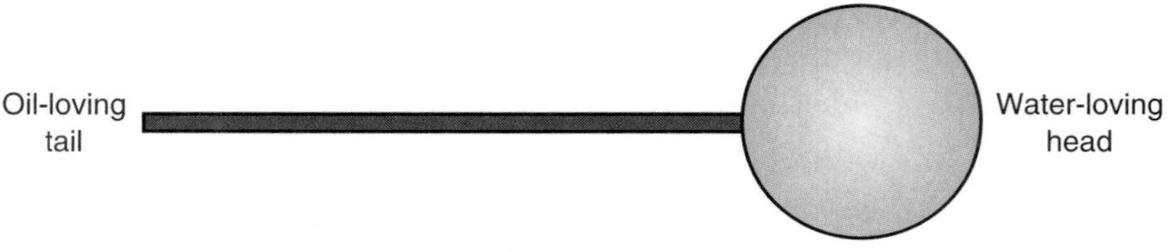

Figure 7–7 A surfactant molecule.

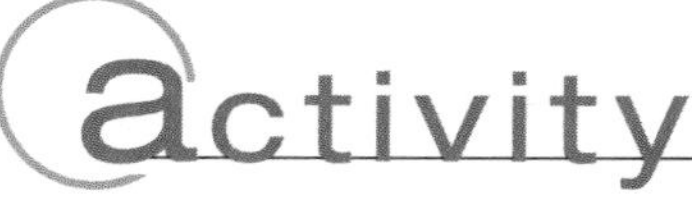

Have you ever heard the saying "Oil and water don't mix?" Pour some water into a glass, and then add a little cooking oil (or other oil). What happens? Stir the water briskly with a spoon, and then observe for a minute or two. What does the oil do?

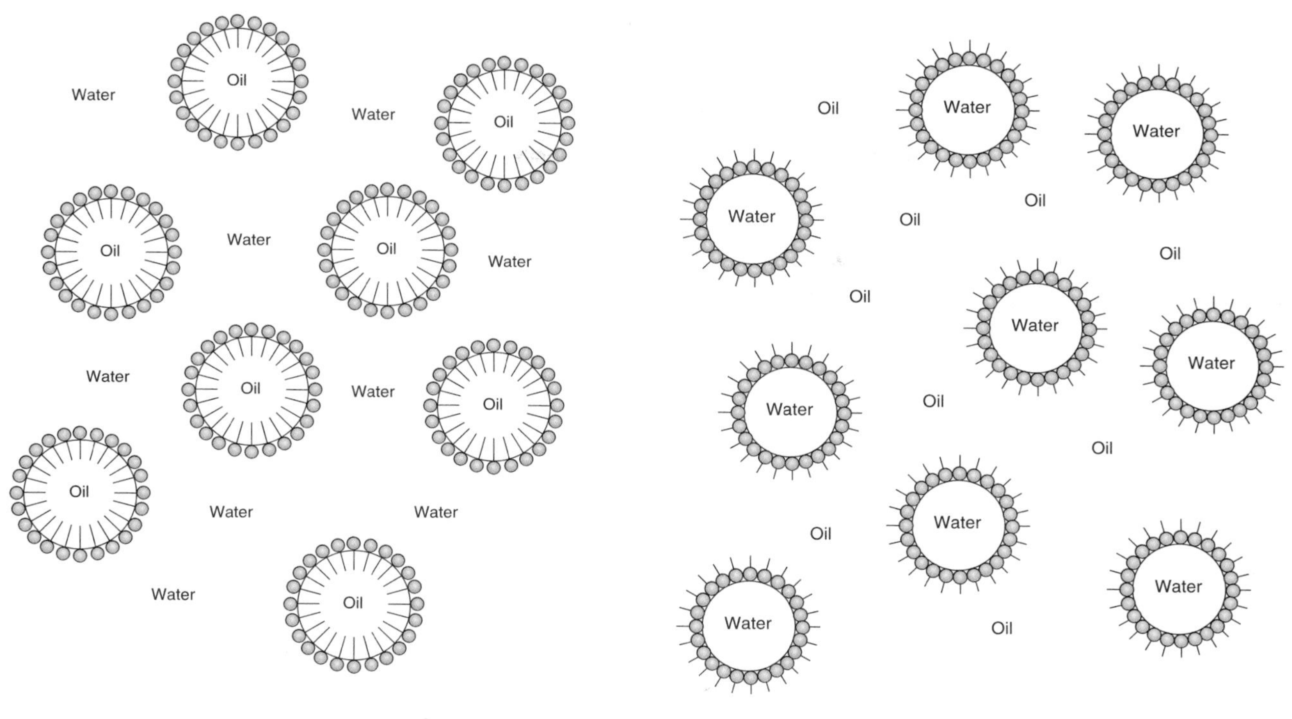

Figure 7–8 Oil-in-water emulsion.

Figure 7–9 Water-in-oil emulsion.

Without the egg yolk as an emulsifying agent, the oil and water would separate into two layers. Most of the emulsions used in a salon are oil-in-water. Haircoloring, shampoos, and conditioners are oil-in-water emulsions.

In a **water-in-oil emulsion (W/O)**, droplets of water are suspended in an oil base. The droplets of water are surrounded by surfactants with their hydrophilic heads pointing in and their lipophilic tails pointing out (Figure 7–9). Water forms the internal portion of a W/O emulsion because the water is completely surrounded by oil. Water-in-oil emulsions usually contain a smaller amount of water and a greater amount of oil. Cold cream is an example of a water-in-oil emulsion.

Other Physical Mixtures

Ointments, pastes, pomades, and styling waxes are semisolid mixtures made with any combination of petrolatum (petroleum jelly), oil, and wax. Medicated ointments are used to treat a variety of conditions. Hairstylists often use pomades and waxes to create today's latest styles.

Powders are a physical mixture of two solids. Free-flowing powders are rarely found in cosmetics. Powders that tend to stick together, such as talc, are far more common. Off-the-scalp powdered hair lighteners are physical mixtures that may separate during shipping and storage and should be thoroughly mixed before each use.

Common Product Ingredients

Some of the most common chemical ingredients used in salon products are described below.

Alcohol is a readily evaporating, colorless liquid obtained by the fermentation of starch, sugar, and other carbohydrates. Most people are familiar with **volatile** (VAHL-uh-tul) alcohols (those that evaporate easily) such as isopropyl alcohol (rubbing alcohol) and ethyl alcohol (alcoholic beverages). But you will encounter other kinds in your work. Fatty alcohols, such as cetyl alcohol and cetearyl alcohol, are nonvolatile oils that are used as conditioners.

Alkanolamines (al-kan-oh-LAH-mynz) are substances used to neutralize acids or raise the pH of many hair products. They are often used in place of ammonia because there is less odor associated with their use.

Ammonia (uh-MOH-nee-uh) is a colorless gas with a pungent odor, composed of hydrogen and nitrogen. In water solution, it is called ammonia water. It is used to raise the pH in permanent waving, haircoloring, and lightening substances (see discussion of pH below). Raising the pH allows the solution to penetrate the hair. Ammonium hydroxide and ammonium thioglycolate are examples of ammonia compounds that are used to raise the pH.

CAUTION

Formaldehyde, also known as formalin, is used in cosmetics as a preservative. It is toxic to inhale, a strong irritant, and carcinogenic (causing cancer). It may cause allergic reactions, even at low concentrations.

Glycerin (GLIS-ur-in) is a sweet, colorless, oily substance formed by the decomposition of oils, fats, or fatty acids. It is used as a solvent and as a moisturizer in skin and body creams.

Silicones are a special type of oil used in hair conditioners and as a water-resistant lubricant for the skin. Silicones are superior to plain oil because they are less greasy and form a "breathable" film that does not cause comedones (blackheads).

Volatile organic compounds (VOCs) are two or more elements combined chemically (compounds) that contain carbon (organic) and evaporate very quickly (volatile). The most common VOC used in hairsprays is SD alcohol. 2

7

Potential Hydrogen (pH)

Although pH is often discussed with regard to salon products, it is often one of the least understood properties. Understanding what pH is and how it affects the skin and hair is essential to understanding all chemical services.

Water and pH

We cannot begin to understand pH without first learning a bit about ions. An **ion** (EYE-ahn) is an atom or molecule that carries an electrical charge. **Ionization** (eye-ahn-ih-ZAY-shun) is the separating of a substance into ions. These ions have opposite electrical charges. An ion with a negative electrical charge is an **anion** (AN-eye-on). An ion with a positive electrical charge is a **cation** (KAT-eye-un).

In pure water, some of the water molecules naturally ionize into hydrogen ions and hydroxide ions. The pH scale measures those ions. The hydrogen ion (H+) is acidic. The hydroxide ion (OH) is alkaline. pH is only possible because of this ionization of water. Only aqueous (AY-kwee-us) (water) solutions have pH. Nonaqueous solutions (oil and alcohol) do not have pH. Without water, there is no pH.

In pure water, every water molecule that ionizes produces one hydrogen ion and one hydroxide ion (Figure 7–10). Pure water is neutral because it contains the same number of hydrogen ions as hydroxide ions, meaning it is neither acidic nor alkaline. Pure water is 50 percent acidic and 50 percent alkaline.

The pH Scale

You may have heard the terms "parts hydrogen" or "potential hydrogen" used to describe pH. In fact, the term **pH** originates from the French term *pouvoir hydrogene*, or "hydrogen power" and means the relative degree of acidity and alkalinity of a substance. Notice that pH is written with a small *p* (which represents a quantity) and a capital *H* (which represents the hydrogen ion, H^+). The symbol pH represents the quantity of hydrogen ions.

The pH values are arranged on a scale ranging from 0 to 14. A pH of 7 indicates a neutral solution, a pH below 7 indicates an acidic solution, and a pH above 7 indicates an alkaline solution (Figure 7–11).

The pH scale is a logarithmic scale. This means that in a pH scale, a change of one whole number represents a tenfold change in pH. A pH of 8 is 10 times more alkaline than a pH of 7. A change of two whole numbers indicates a change of 10 times 10, or a one hundredfold change. A pH of 9 is 100 times more alkaline than a pH of 7.

Pure water, with a pH of 7, is 100 times more alkaline than a pH of 5. Since the average pH of hair and skin is 5, pure water is 100 times more alkaline than your hair and skin, even though it has a neutral pH. Pure water can cause the hair to swell by as much as 20 percent.

Acids and Alkalis

All **acids** owe their chemical reactivity to the hydrogen ion (H^+). Acids have a pH below 7.0, taste sour, and turn litmus paper from blue to red. Acids contract and harden the hair. One such acid, thioglycolic acid, is used in permanent waving.

All **alkalis** (AL-kuh-lyz) owe their chemical reactivity to the hydroxide (OH^-) ion. The terms "alkali" and "base" are interchangeable. Alkalis have a

7

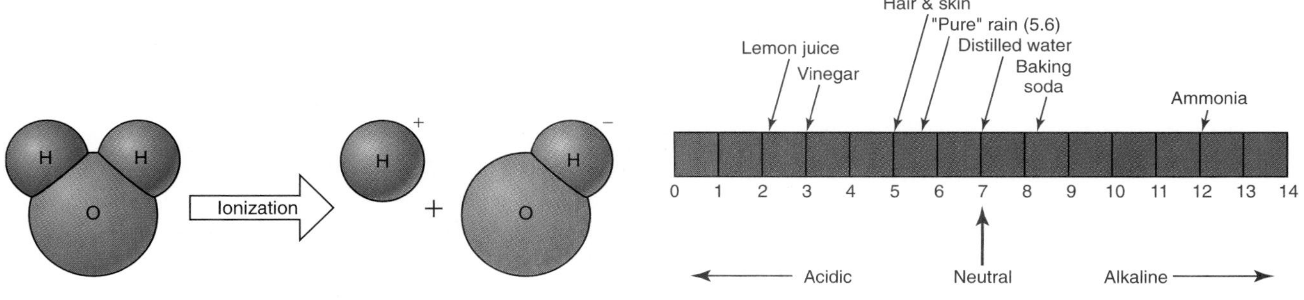

Figure 7-10 The ionization of water.

Figure 7-11 The pH scale.

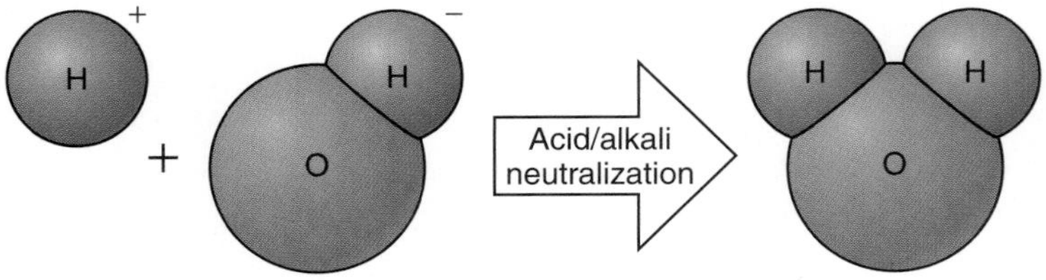

Figure 7-12 Acid/alkali neutralization reaction.

pH above 7.0, taste bitter, turn litmus paper from red to blue, and feel slippery and soapy on the skin. Alkalis soften and swell the hair. Sodium hydroxide, commonly known as lye, is a very strong alkali used in chemical drain cleaners and chemical hair relaxers.

ACID–ALKALI NEUTRALIZATION REACTIONS

Pure water (H_2O) naturally ionizes to create hydrogen (H^+) ions and hydroxide ions (OH^-). When acids (H^+) and alkalis (OH^-) are mixed together in equal proportions, they neutralize each other to form water (H_2O) (Figure 7–12). The neutralizing shampoos and normalizing lotions used to neutralize hydroxide hair relaxers work by creating an acid–alkali neutralization reaction (see Chapter 15). 3

Oxidation–Reduction (Redox) Reactions

Oxidation–reduction (redox) reactions are responsible for the chemical changes created by haircolors, hair lighteners, permanent wave solutions, and neutralizers. The chemical services that we take for granted would not be possible without oxidation–reduction (redox) reactions.

OXIDATION REACTIONS

Oxidation is a chemical reaction that combines an element or compound with oxygen to produce an oxide. When oxygen is added to a substance, some heat is almost always produced. Chemical reactions that are characterized by or formed with the giving off of heat are called **exothermic**

7

activity

Did you know that you can easily and safely test the pH of a solution? Litmus papers (pH test papers) can be used to indicate the pH of any aqueous solution. You can test haircolor, permanent waving solution, neutralizer, or your favorite shampoo and conditioner.

You will need litmus papers, several small open containers, bottled drinking water, stirring sticks, and some white towels. Place the product you want to test in a small, open cup or bowl. If the product is a powder or is extremely thick, add a small amount of bottled water and stir thoroughly. Dip the litmus paper into the product. Immediately place the paper on a white towel and compare the color obtained to the color on the package to determine the pH. Test anything you can think of. Be creative! What you discover may surprise you.

(ek-soh-THUR-mik). Exothermic permanent waves produce heat because of an oxidation reaction (see Chapter 15).

Slow oxidation takes place in oxidation haircolors and permanent wave neutralizers. If you pay close attention, you will notice an increase in the temperature of oxidation haircolors after the peroxide is added. **Combustion** (kum-BUS-chun) is the rapid oxidation of any substance, accompanied by the production of heat and light. Lighting a match is an example of rapid oxidation. You cannot have a fire without oxygen.

Reduction Reactions

When a substance is combined with oxygen, the substance is **oxidized**. When oxygen is subtracted from a substance, the substance is **reduced**, and the chemical reaction is called **reduction**. An **oxidizing agent** is a substance that releases oxygen. Hydrogen peroxide (H_2O_2) is an example of an oxidizing agent because it contains extra oxygen. Hydrogen peroxide can be thought of as water (H_2O) with an extra atom of oxygen. When hydrogen peroxide is mixed with an oxidation haircolor, oxygen is added to the

activity

This exercise demonstrates that oxidation reactions produce heat. You will need 2 ounces of haircolor, 2 ounces of peroxide, two 6-ounce cups or bowls, a stirring stick, towels, and a thermometer that measures room temperature.

1. Put 2 ounces of peroxide in one cup and 2 ounces of haircolor in another.
2. Dip the thermometer in the peroxide. Leave for two minutes and write down the starting temperature.
3. Wipe off the thermometer and do the same thing with the haircolor (Figure 7–13).
4. Add the peroxide to the haircolor and mix thoroughly. Dip the thermometer in the mixture and wait five minutes. Write down the temperature (Figure 7–14).

Is there a difference in the temperatures?

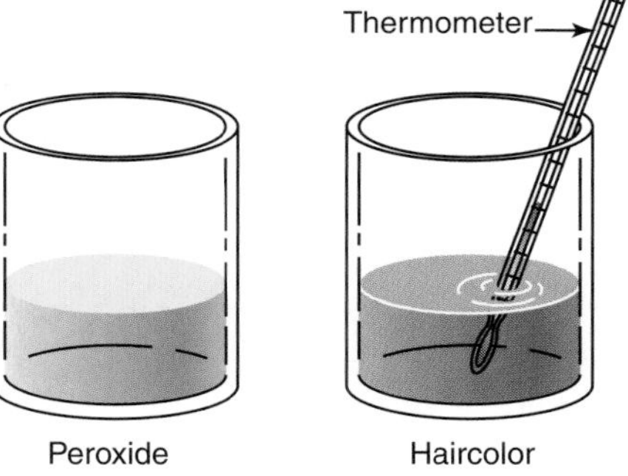

Figure 7–13 Take the temperature of the peroxide, then the haircolor.

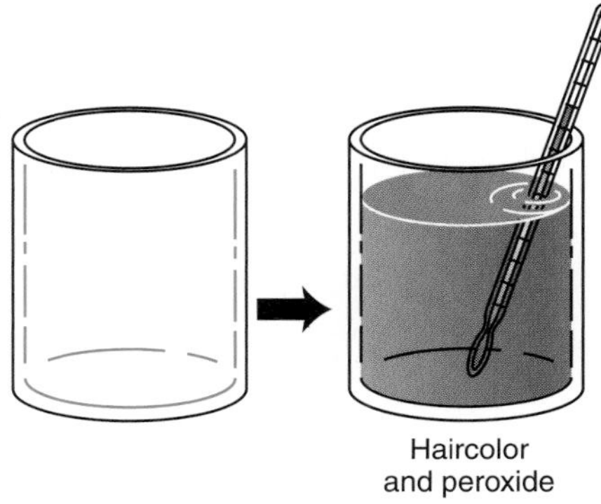

Figure 7–14 Take the temperature of peroxide and haircolor mixed together.

haircolor and the haircolor is oxidized. At the same time, oxygen is removed from the hydrogen peroxide and the hydrogen peroxide is reduced. In this example, haircolor is the reducing agent.

Redox Reactions

Oxidation and reduction always occur at the same time and are referred to as redox reactions. **Redox** is a contraction for reduction-oxidation. In redox reactions the oxidizing agent is reduced and the reducing agent is oxidized.

So far, we have considered oxidation only as the addition of oxygen, and reduction only as the removal of oxygen. Oxidation can also result from the removal of hydrogen, and reduction can also result from the addition of hydrogen.

Permanent waving is an example of this type of redox reaction. Permanent waving solution breaks certain bonds in the hair through a reduction reaction that adds hydrogen atoms to the hair. In this reaction, the hair is reduced and the perm solution is oxidized. Neutralizer then oxidizes the hair by removing the hydrogen atoms that were previously added by the perm solution. When the hair is oxidized, the neutralizer is reduced (see Chapter 15).

Oxidation is the result of either the addition of oxygen or the loss of hydrogen. Reduction is the result of either the loss of oxygen or the addition of hydrogen. 4

Electricity

Just as we have provided you with a very general overview of chemistry, we will do the same with electricity, since it, too, will play an important role in your work.

If you look out at lightning on a stormy night, what you are seeing is electricity. If you plug a poorly wired appliance into a socket and sparks fly out, what you are seeing is electricity. But even though you can see electricity, it is important to remember that electricity does not occupy space or have physical or chemical properties; therefore, it is not matter. If it is not matter, then what is it? **Electricity** is a form of energy that, when in motion, exhibits magnetic, chemical, or thermal effects. It is a flow of electrons, which are negatively charged subatomic particles.

An **electric current** is the flow of electricity along a conductor. All substances can be classified as conductors or insulators, depending on the ease with which an electric current can be transmitted through them.

A **conductor** is any substance, material, or medium that conducts electricity. Most metals are good conductors. Copper is a particularly good conductor and is used in electric wiring and electric motors. Although pure water does not conduct electricity, the ions in ordinary water make it a good

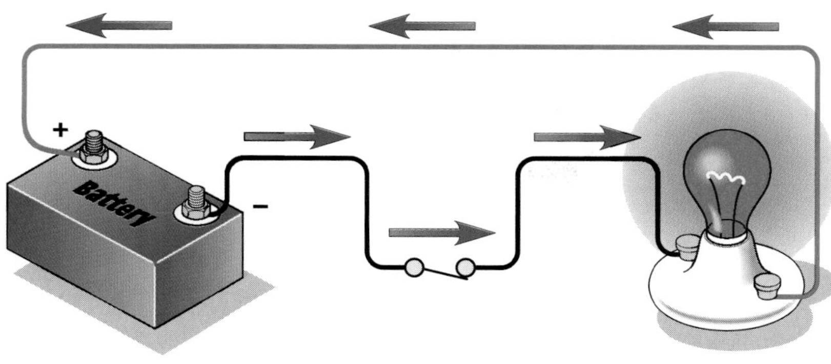

Figure 7–15 A complete electrical circuit.

conductor. This explains why you should not swim in a lake during a lightning storm.

An **insulator** (IN-suh-layt-ur) or **nonconductor** is a substance that does not easily transmit electricity. Rubber, silk, wood, glass, and cement are good insulators. Electric wires are composed of twisted metal threads (conductors) covered with rubber or silk (insulators). A **complete circuit** (SUR-kit) is the path of an electric current from the generating source through conductors and back to its original source (Figure 7–15).

Types of Electric Current

There are two kinds of electric current.

1. **Direct current (DC)** is a constant, even-flowing current that travels in one direction only and produces a chemical reaction. Flashlights, cellular telephones, and cordless electric clippers use the direct current produced by batteries. The battery in your car stores electrical energy. Without it, your car would not start in the morning. A **converter** is an apparatus that changes direct current to alternating current. Some cars have converters that allow you to use appliances that would normally be plugged into an electrical wall outlet with the car's battery instead.
2. **Alternating current (AC)** is a rapid and interrupted current, flowing first in one direction and then in the opposite direction. This current produces a mechanical action. Hair dryers and curling irons that plug into a wall outlet use alternating current. The generator in your car produces the electrical energy needed to recharge your car's battery. A **rectifier** is an apparatus that changes alternating current to direct current. Cordless electric clippers and battery chargers use a rectifier to convert the AC current from an electrical wall outlet to DC current needed to recharge the batteries. 5

Electrical Measurements

The flow of an electric current can be compared to water flowing through a garden hose. Individual electrons flow through a wire in the same way that individual water molecules flow through a hose.

7

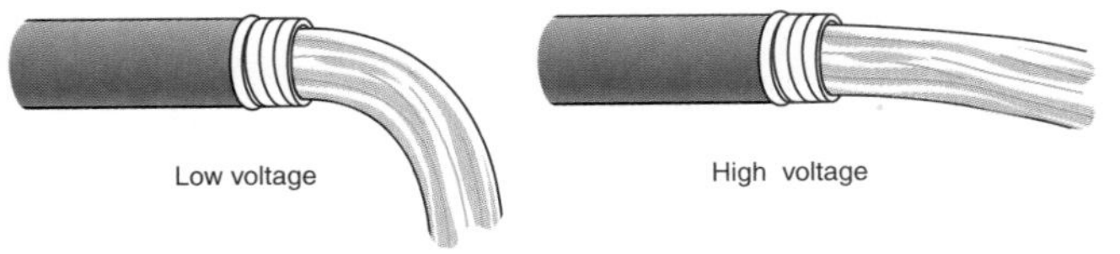

Low voltage

High voltage

Figure 7–16 Volts measure the pressure or force that pushes electrons forward.

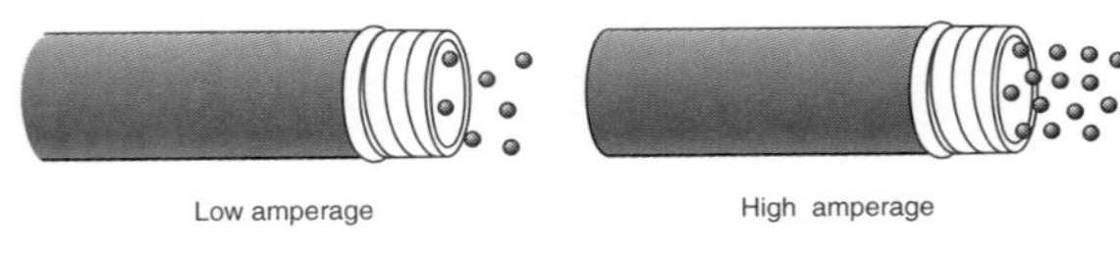

Figure 7–17 Amps measure the number of electrons flowing through the wire.

A **volt** (V), or voltage, is the unit that measures the pressure or force that pushes the flow of electrons forward through a conductor, much like the water pressure that pushes the water molecules through the hose. Without pressure, neither water nor electrons would flow. Car batteries are 12 volts, normal wall sockets that power your hair dryer and curling iron are 110 volts, and most air conditioners and clothes dryers run on 220 volts. A higher voltage indicates more pressure, more force, and more power (Figure 7–16).

An **amp** (A), or ampere (AM-peer), is the unit that measures the strength of an electric current (the number of electrons flowing through a wire). Just as a water hose must be able to expand as the amount of water flowing through it increases, so a wire must expand with an increase in the amount of electrons (amps). A hair dryer rated at 10 amps must have a cord that is twice as thick as one rated at 5 amps; otherwise the cord might overheat and start a fire. A higher amp rating indicates a greater number of electrons and a stronger current (Figure 7–17).

A **milliampere** (mil-ee-AM-peer) is one-thousandth of an ampere. The current for facial and scalp treatments is measured in milliamperes; an ampere current would be much too strong.

An **ohm** (O) is a unit that measures the resistance of an electric current. Current will not flow through a conductor unless the force (volts) is stronger than the resistance (ohms).

A **watt** (W) is a measurement of how much electric energy is being used in one second. A 40-watt light bulb uses 40 watts of energy per second. A **kilowatt** (K) is 1,000 watts. The electricity in your house is measured in kilowatt hours (kwh). A 1,000-watt (1-kilowatt) hair dryer uses 1,000 watts of energy per second.

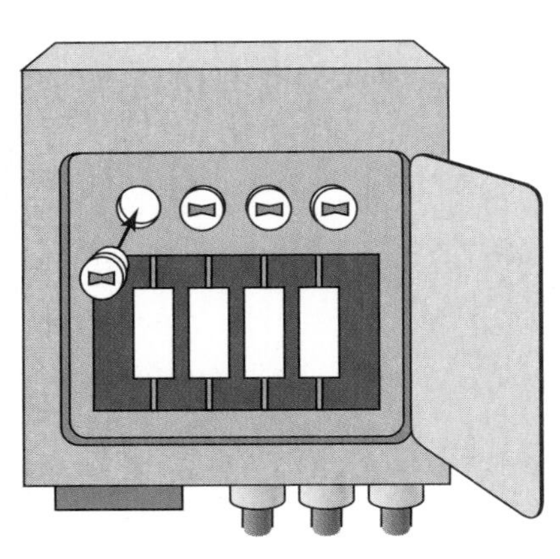

Figure 7–18 Fuse box.

Safety Devices

A **fuse** (FYOOZ) is a special device that prevents excessive current from passing through a circuit. It is designed to blow out or melt when the wire becomes too hot from overloading the circuit with too much current from too many appliances or from faulty equipment. To reestablish the circuit, disconnect the appliance, check all connections and insulation, and insert a new fuse (Figure 7–18).

A **circuit breaker** is a switch that automatically interrupts or shuts off an electric circuit at the first indication of overload. Circuit breakers have replaced fuses in modern electric circuits. They have all the safety features of fuses but do not require replacement and can simply be reset. Your hair dryer has a circuit breaker located in the electric plug designed to protect you and your client in case of an overload or short circuit. When a circuit breaker shuts off, you should disconnect the appliance and check all connections and insulation before resetting (Figure 7–19).

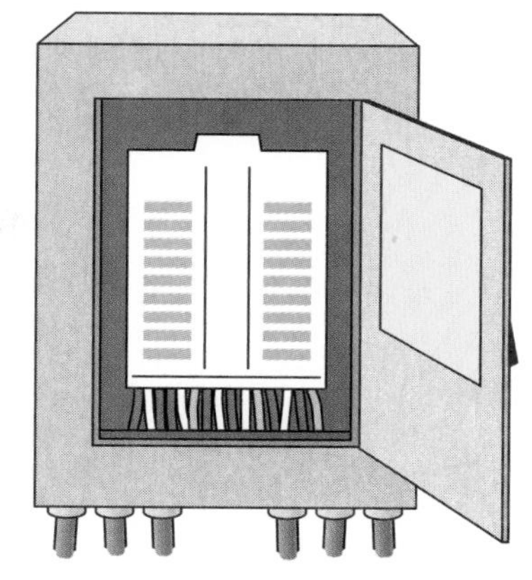

Figure 7–19 Circuit breakers.

Electrical Equipment Safety

When working with electricity, you must always be concerned with your own safety as well as the safety of your clients. All electrical equipment should be inspected regularly to determine whether or not it is in safe working order. Careless electrical connections and overloaded circuits can result in an electrical shock, a burn, or even a serious fire.

The principle of "grounding" is another important way of promoting electrical safety. All electrical appliances must have at least two electrical connections. The "live" connection supplies current to the circuit. The ground connection completes the circuit and carries the current safely away to the ground. If you look closely at electrical plugs with two rectangular prongs, you will see that one is slightly larger than the other. This guarantees that the plug can only be inserted one way, and protects you and your client from electrical shock in the event of a short circuit.

For added protection, some appliances have a third, circular, electrical connection that provides an additional ground. This extra ground is designed to guarantee a safe path of electricity if the first ground fails, or is improperly connected. Appliances with a third circular ground offer the most protection for you and your client (Figure 7–20).

Careful attention to electrical safety helps to eliminate accidents and to ensure greater client satisfaction. The following reminders will help ensure the safe use of electricity.

- all the electrical appliances you use should be UL certified (Figure 7–21)
- read all instructions carefully before using any piece of electrical equipment
- disconnect all appliances when not in use
- inspect all electrical equipment regularly

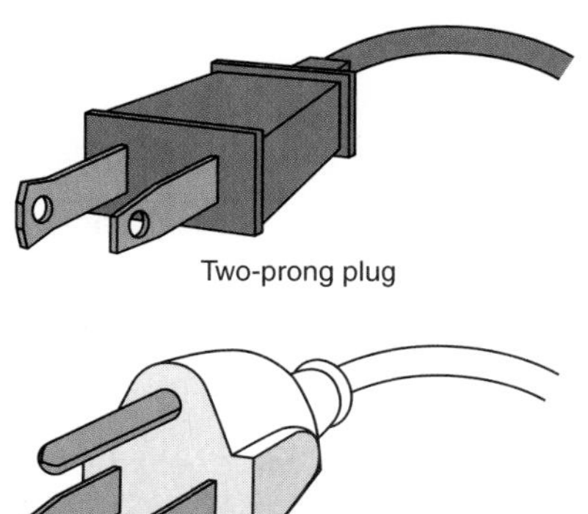

Figure 7–20 Two-prong and three-prong plugs.

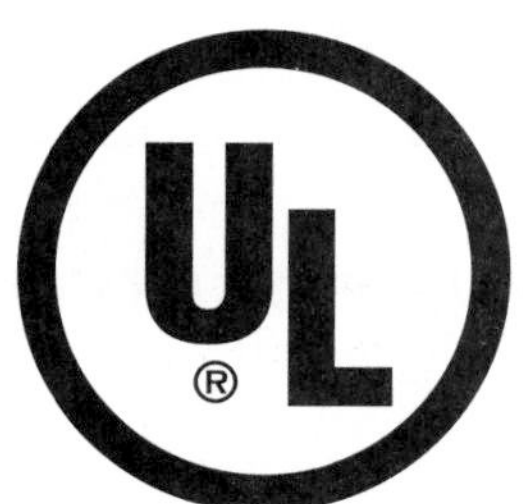

Figure 7–21 A UL symbol as it appears on electrical devices.

CAUTION

Underwriter's Laboratory (UL) certifies the safety of electrical appliances. Curling irons, hair dryers, and electric clippers that are UL approved are certified to be safe when used according to the manufacturers' directions. Always look for the UL symbol on electrical appliances and take the time to read and follow the manufacturers' directions.

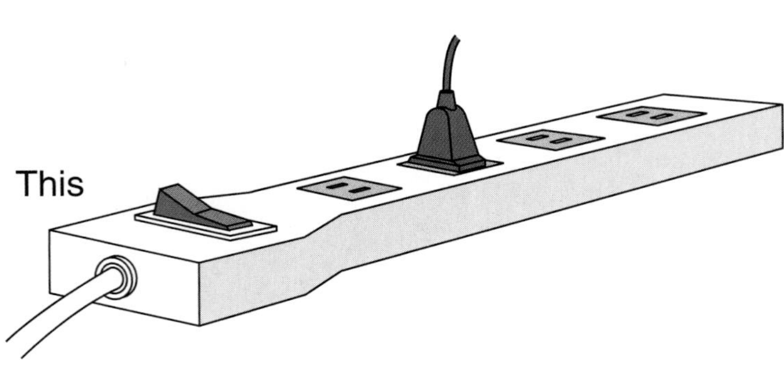

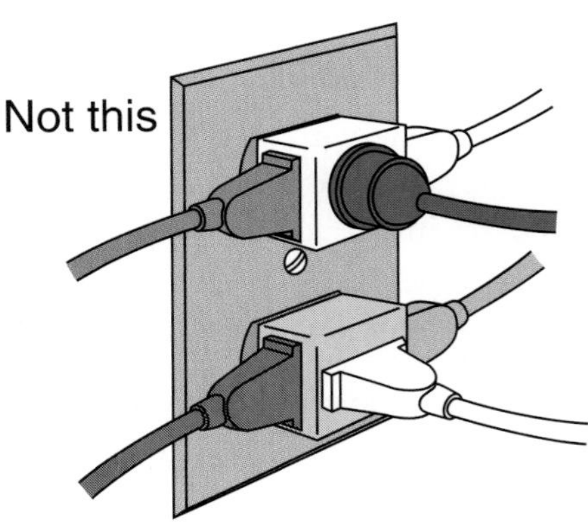

Figure 7-22 One plug per outlet.

CAUTION

Never tamper with wiring or electrical plugs to get them to fit into a receptacle they were not designed for.

7

- keep all wires, plugs, and electrical equipment in good repair
- use only one plug to each outlet; overloading may cause the fuse to blow out (Figure 7–22)
- you and your client should avoid contact with water and metal surfaces when using electricity, and do not handle electrical equipment with wet hands
- do not leave your client unattended while connected to an electrical device
- keep electrical cords off the floor and away from people's feet; getting tangled in a cord could cause you or your client to trip
- do not attempt to clean around electric outlets while equipment is plugged in
- do not touch two metal objects at the same time if either is connected to an electric current
- do not step on or place objects on electrical cords
- do not allow electrical cord to become twisted; it can cause a short circuit
- disconnect appliances by pulling on the plug, not the cord
- do not attempt to repair electrical appliances unless you are qualified

ELECTROTHERAPY

Electronic facial treatments are commonly referred to as **electrotherapy**. A **wall plate** (facial stimulator) is an instrument that plugs into an ordinary wall outlet and produces different types of electric currents that are used for facial and scalp treatments. These different currents are called **modalities**. Each modality produces a different effect on the skin.

An **electrode** is an applicator for directing the electric current from the machine to the client's skin. It is usually made of carbon, glass, or metal. Each modality requires two electrodes, one negative and one positive, to conduct the flow of electricity through the body (except the Tesla high-frequency).

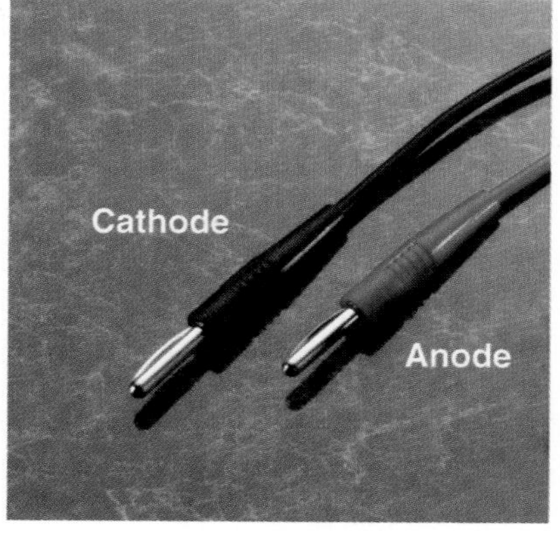

Figure 7-23 Anode and cathode.

Polarity

Polarity indicates the negative or positive pole of an electric current. Electrotherapy devices always have one negatively charged pole and one positively charged pole. The positive electrode is called an **anode** (AN-ohd). It is usually red and is marked with a "P" or a plus (+) sign. The negative electrode is called a **cathode** (KATH-ohd). It is usually black and is marked with an "N" or a minus (–) sign (Figure 7–23). If the electrodes are not marked, either of the following polarity tests will tell you which is which.

Separate the two tips of the conducting cords from each other and immerse them in a glass of salt water. Turn the selector switch of the appliance to galvanic current, and then turn up the intensity. More active bubbles will accumulate at the negative pole than at the positive pole.

Or, place the tips of the conducting cords on two separate pieces of moist blue litmus paper. The paper under the positive pole will turn red, while the paper under the negative pole will stay blue. If you use red litmus paper, the paper under the positive pole will remain red and the paper under the negative pole will turn blue.

Modalities

The four main modalities used in cosmetology are galvanic, faradic, sinusoidal, and Tesla high-frequency.

Galvanic Current

The most commonly used modality is **galvanic current**. It is a constant and direct current (DC), having a positive and negative pole, and producing chemical changes when it passes through the tissues and fluids of the body. Two different chemical reactions are possible, depending on the polarity (negative or positive) that is used (see Table 7–3). The **active electrode** is the electrode used on the area to be treated. The **inactive electrode** is the opposite pole from the active electrode.

CAUTION

Do not let the tips of the cords touch or you will cause a short circuit. The polarity tests can be dangerous and should only be performed with your instructor's supervision.

Iontophoresis

Iontophoresis (eye-ahn-toh-foh-REE-sus) is the process of introducing water-soluble products into the skin with the use of electric current, such as the use of the positive and negative poles of a galvanic machine. **Cataphoresis** (kat-uh-fuh-REE-sus) forces acidic substances into deeper tissues using galvanic current from the positive toward the negative pole. **Anaphoresis** (an-uh-for-EES-sus) is the process of forcing liquids into the tissues from the negative toward the positive pole. **Desincrustation** (des-in-krus-TAY-shun) is a process used to soften and emulsify grease deposits (oil) and blackheads in the hair follicles. This process is frequently used to treat acne, milia (whiteheads), and comedones.

Positive Pole (Anode)	Negative Pole (Cathode)
Produces acidic reactions	Produces alkaline reactions
Closes the pores	Opens the pores
Soothes nerves	Stimulates and irritates the nerves
Decreases blood supply	Increases blood supply
Contracts blood vessels	Expands blood vessels
Hardens and firms tissues	Softens tissues

Note that the effects produced by the positive pole are the exact opposite of those produced by the negative pole.

Table 7-3 Effects of Galvanic Current

CAUTION

Do not use the negative galvanic current on skin with broken capillaries, pustular acne conditions, or on a client with high blood pressure or metal implants.

FARADIC CURRENT

The **faradic current** is an alternating and interrupted current that produces a mechanical reaction without a chemical effect. It is used during scalp and facial manipulations to cause muscular contractions that tone the facial muscles. Benefits derived from faradic current include:

- improved muscle tone.
- removal of waste products.
- increased blood circulation.
- relief of blood congestion.
- increased glandular activity.
- stimulation of hair growth.
- increased metabolism.

SINUSOIDAL CURRENT

Sinusoidal current (sy-nuh-SOYD-ul) is similar to faradic current and is also used during scalp and facial manipulations. It is an alternating current that produces mechanical contractions that tone the muscles. Sinusoidal current has the following advantages.

- supplies greater stimulation, deeper penetration, and is less irritating than faradic current
- soothes the nerves and penetrates into deeper muscle tissue
- is best suited for the nervous client

TESLA HIGH-FREQUENCY CURRENT

The **Tesla high-frequency current** is a thermal or heat-producing current with a high rate of oscillation or vibration. It is commonly called the violet ray and is used for both scalp and facial treatments. Tesla current does not produce muscle contractions, and its effects can be either stimulating or soothing, depending on the method of application. The electrodes are made from either glass or metal, and only one electrode is used to perform a service (Figure 7–24). The benefits from the use of Tesla high-frequency current are:

- stimulated blood circulation.
- improved glandular activity.
- increased elimination and absorption.
- increased metabolism.
- improved germicidal action.
- relief of congestion.

CAUTION

Do not use faradic or sinusoidal currents if it causes pain or discomfort, if the face is very ruddy (red in color), or if your client has gold-filled teeth, high blood pressure, broken capillaries, or pustular skin conditions. Never use faradic or sinusoidal currents longer than 15 to 20 minutes.

Other Electrical Equipment

Conventional hood hair dryers or heat lamps are sources of dry heat that can be used to shorten chemical processing time. Since dry heat causes evaporation, the hair must be covered with a plastic cap to avoid drying the hair during a chemical process. Several small holes should be placed in the cap to allow for the escape of excess heat and any gases that might form.

Electric curling irons are available in many types and sizes. They have built-in heating elements and plug directly into a wall outlet.

Heating caps provide a uniform source of heat and can be used with hair and scalp conditioning treatments.

Several different types of haircolor processing machines or accelerating machines shorten the time it takes to process chemical hair services. These processors usually look similar to a hood dryer and dispense a hot water vapor inside the hood. A haircolor service processed with a machine at 90°F (32°C) will process twice as fast as it would at a normal room temperature of 72°F (22°C).

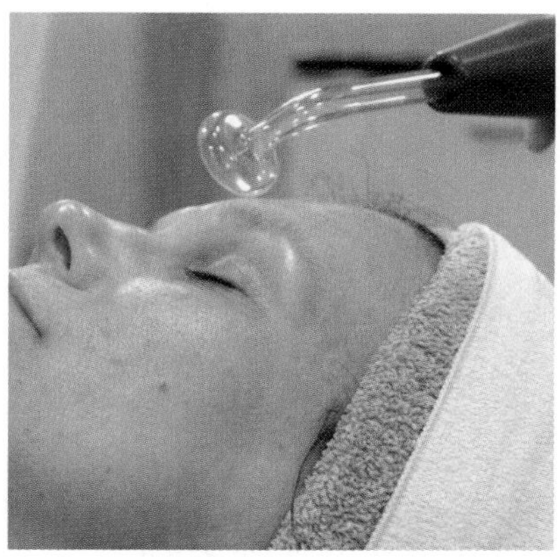

Figure 7–24 Applying high-frequency current with a facial electrode.

A steamer or vaporizer produces moist, uniform heat that can be applied to the head or face. Steamers warm and cleanse the skin by increasing the flow of both oil and sweat. Some steamers may also be used for hair and scalp conditioning treatments.

A vibrator is used in massage to produce a mechanical succession of manipulations. Use of a vibrator stimulates muscles, increases blood supply, soothes nerves, and increases glandular activity.

CAUTION

Tesla high-frequency current should not be used on clients who are pregnant, suffer from epilepsy (seizures) or asthma, or who have high blood pressure, a sinus blockage, a pacemaker, or metal implants.

LIGHT THERAPY

As a salon professional, you may use equipment to perform light therapy treatments. Before we explore the specific types of equipment involved, it is important to have some basic understanding of what light is and how it works.

insights

Dwight Miller

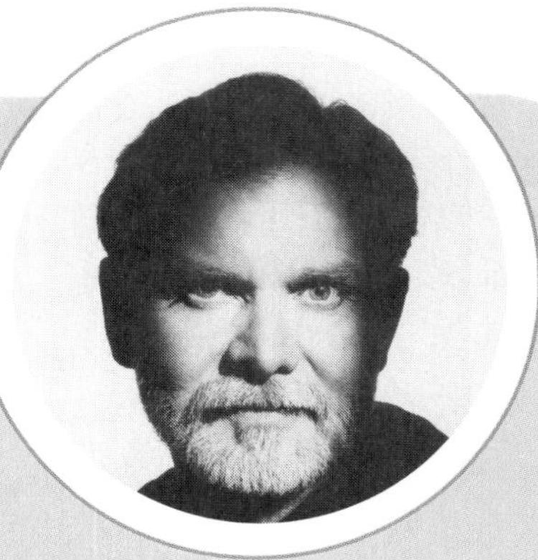

A hair artist with almost 40 years of experience in the industry, Dwight Miller is now involved with image and product development.

Right now, I'm working with a company in Korea and another in New York. I do everything from product creation to marketing the product and promoting it. I've been doing this since 1981—I just kind of fell into it. That's what I love: to do things I don't know anything about. I started in the industry that way.

I was in the Marine Corps when I first got into beauty school. I had never even thought about going to beauty school, but I was in L.A. with a friend who was going that route and I got interested in what he was doing. I didn't know anything about it, nothing at all. But I love the process of learning about something I don't know, erasing any preconceptions. I didn't have any natural talent, none at all, so I found two students who were the best, a guy and a girl, and I worked between them. I copied what they did, over and over again. I'd watch every movement and then I'd do it, practicing over and over until I got it right.

If you were to ask me what the three most important skills were for a cosmetologist to have, I'd say artistic talent would be third.
Technical skills, which you can acquire by the kind of practice I'm talking about, are second. But relationship-building comes first. You have to like people. When you're with a client, you have to keep in mind that you want the client to come back. Allude to what you'll do in the future. For instance, say, "Next time you come we'll do this" or "I'd like to try this next time." Plant the idea.

This is a great business, an amazing business. It's all about the caring relationships you build with people. You have a client with you for only 45 minutes, but during that time, you're totally with that person. Some people say you shouldn't talk about personal stuff, but I disagree. You should talk about your client's life, her kids, what she's doing. People talk to their hairdresser about things they don't tell anyone else. It's a very special relationship, more personal than with a doctor or a lawyer. Selling is important, but not just selling products. You're selling the client on yourself. You're selling the client on a kind of hairstyle. Products are just an add-on to the other kind of selling.

Visible light is electromagnetic radiation that we can see. **Electromagnetic radiation** is also called "radiant energy" because it carries, or radiates, energy through space on waves. These waves are similar to the waves caused when a stone is dropped on the surface of the water. The distance between two successive peaks is called the **wavelength**. Long wavelengths have low frequency, meaning the number of waves is less frequent (fewer waves) within a given length. Short wavelengths have higher frequency because the number of waves is more frequent (more waves) within a given length (Figure 7–25).

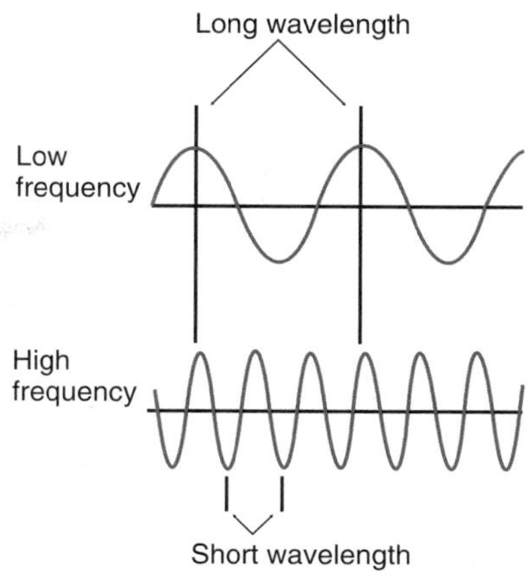

Figure 7–25 Long and short wavelengths.

The entire range of wavelengths of electromagnetic radiation (radiant energy) is called the "electromagnetic spectrum". Visible light is the part of the electromagnetic spectrum that we can see. Visible light makes up 35 percent of natural sunlight.

Ultraviolet rays and infrared rays are also forms of electromagnetic radiation, but they are invisible because their wavelengths are beyond the visible spectrum of light. Invisible rays make up 65 percent of natural sunlight (Figure 7–26).

Within the visible spectrum of light, violet has the shortest wavelength and red has the longest. The wavelength of infrared is just below red, and the wavelength of ultraviolet is just above violet. Infrared and ultraviolet rays are not really light at all. Again, they are the wavelengths of electromagnetic radiation that are just beyond the visible spectrum.

Therapeutic lamps are used to produce artificial light rays in the salon. These lamps are capable of producing the same rays that are produced by the sun. Three effects produced by therapeutic lamps are thermal (heat), mechanical, and chemical. 7✓

CAUTION

The vibrator should never be used when there is heart disease or when fever, abscesses, or inflammation are present.

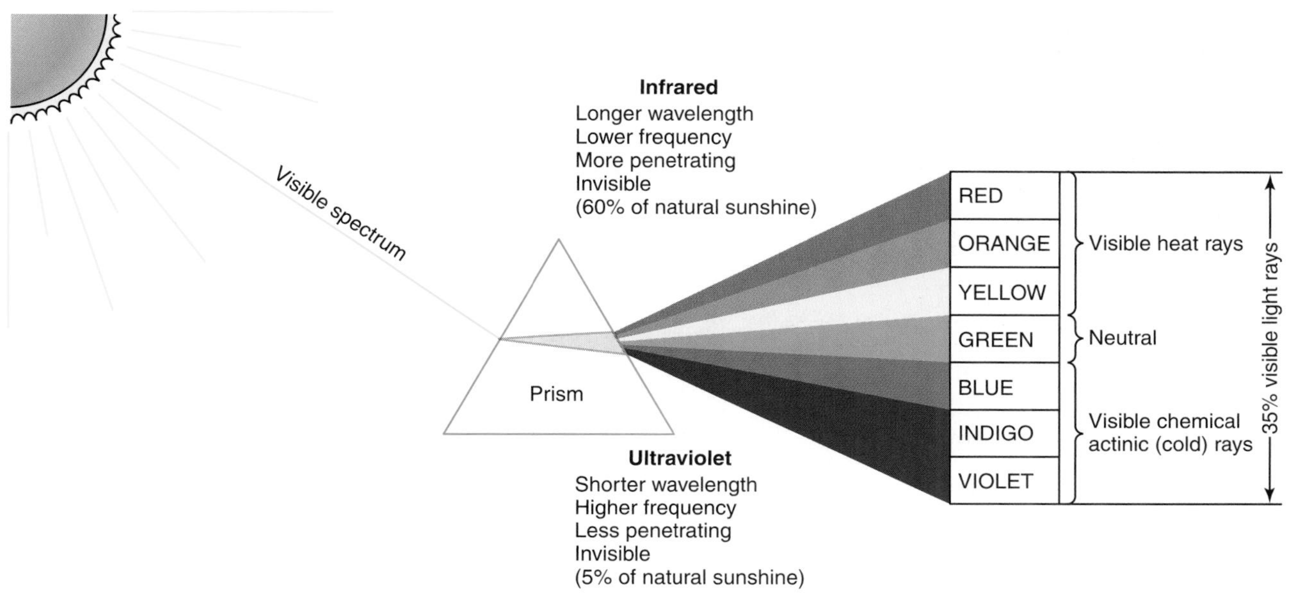

Figure 7–26 The visible spectrum.

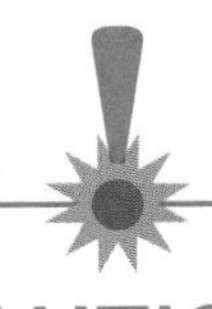

CAUTION

The client's eyes should always be protected during any light therapy treatment. Use cotton pads saturated with boric acid solution, witch hazel, or distilled water. To avoid damage to the eyes, both cosmetologist and client should always wear safety goggles when working with ultraviolet rays.

Ultraviolet Rays

Ultraviolet (UV) rays make up 5 percent of natural sunlight and are also referred to as cold rays or actinic rays. UV rays have short wavelengths, are the least penetrating rays, produce chemical effects, and kill germs.

Exposure to the sun can be beneficial if recommended guidelines are followed. Natural sunlight kills germs and produces vitamin D in the skin. UV radiation can be used to treat rickets (a disease characterized by soft and deformed bones), psoriasis, and acne. Exposure to UV rays also stimulates the skin's production of melanin, which causes a tan and helps protect the skin from further damage. But deep tanning is another matter: although a deep tan may look healthy, it is really a sign that the skin is under attack from UV radiation.

Over one million new cases of skin cancer are diagnosed each year. It is estimated that one in five Americans will develop skin cancer, and 90 percent of those cancers will be the result of exposure to UV radiation from the sun and from tanning beds.

Application of Ultraviolet Rays

Although the application of ultraviolet rays can be beneficial, it must be done with the utmost care. UV rays are applied with a lamp at a distance of 30 to 36 inches (76 to 91 cm). The therapy should begin with exposure times of two to three minutes with a gradual increase in exposure time to seven or eight minutes.

Infrared Rays

Infrared rays make up 60 percent of natural sunlight. Infrared rays have long wavelengths, penetrate the deepest, and produce the most heat.

Infrared lamps should be operated at a distance of at least 30 inches (76 cm), for an exposure time of about five minutes. Check the comfort of your client frequently during the service. Never leave the client unattended.

CAUTION

Overexposure to UV rays can produce painful burns and blistering, increase the risk of skin cancer, and cause premature aging of the skin. *Never* leave your client unattended during the exposure time.

Visible Light Rays

Visible light rays are the primary source of lights used for facial and scalp treatments. The bulbs used for therapeutic visible light therapy are white, red, and blue.

White light is referred to as "combination light" because it is a combination of all the visible rays of the spectrum. White light has the benefits of all the rays of the visible spectrum. **Blue light** should only be used on oily skin that is bare. It contains few heat rays, is the least penetrating, and has some germicidal and chemical benefits. **Red light** is used on dry skin in combination with oils and creams. Red light penetrates the deepest and produces the most heat. 8

YOU HAVE THE POWER

There are many benefits for the client who takes advantage of the various salon services that use chemicals and electricity. In the course of your career, developments in technology will undoubtedly introduce new, innovative salon services that were not available when this book was written. Your value as a salon professional depends on your ability to stay informed about these new developments.

While there is a great power connected to chemicals and electricity, always remember that there is a potential for injury as well. You need to learn as much as you can about the workings of chemistry and electricity in the salon, and to view your education as a lifelong learning experience.

Did you know...

Although salon lighting is not a form of light therapy, the quality of this light can have an effect on your work and your client's satisfaction. Fluorescent light is produced by fluorescent lamps and is much cooler (green–blue) than natural sunlight. Incandescent light is produced by standard (tungsten) light bulbs and is warmer (yellow–gold) than either natural sunlight or fluorescent light. Your client's hair and skin will appear more green–blue when viewed with fluorescent lighting and more golden when viewed with incandescent lighting.

Take caution when handling fluorescent light bulbs; they contain dangerous substances, including mercury. Be careful not to break fluorescent bulbs, and dispose of used bulbs properly.

7

chapter glossary

acid	solution that has a pH below 7.0, tastes sour, and turns litmus paper from blue to red
active electrode	electrode used on the area to be treated
alcohol	readily evaporating, colorless liquid obtained by the fermentation of starch, sugar, and other carbohydrates
alkali	solution that has a pH above 7.0, tastes bitter, and turns litmus paper from red to blue
alkanolamines	substances used to neutralize acids or raise the pH of many hair products; often used in place of ammonia
alternating current (AC)	rapid and interrupted current, flowing first in one direction and then in the opposite direction
ammonia	colorless gas with a pungent odor, composed of hydrogen and nitrogen; used as an alkalizing agent to raise the pH
amp	unit that measures the strength of an electric current (the number of electrons flowing through a wire)
anaphoresis	process of forcing liquids into the tissues from the negative toward the positive pole
anion	ion with a negative electrical charge
anode	positive electrode
atom	the smallest particle of an element that still retains the properties of that element
blue light	therapeutic light that should only be used on oily skin that is bare; contains few heat rays, is the least penetrating, and has some germicidal and chemical benefits
cataphoresis	process of forcing acidic substances into deeper tissues using galvanic current from the positive toward the negative pole
cathode	negative electrode
cation	ion with a positive electrical charge
chemical change	change in the chemical composition of a substance, in which a new substance or substances are formed having properties different from the original
chemical compounds	combinations of two or more atoms of different elements united chemically with a fixed chemical composition, definite proportions, and distinct properties
chemical properties	those characteristics that can only be determined with a chemical reaction and that cause a chemical change in the identity of the substance
chemistry	science that deals with the composition, structures, and properties of matter, and how matter changes under different chemical conditions
circuit breaker	switch that automatically interrupts or shuts off an electric circuit at the first indication of overload
combustion	rapid oxidation of any substance, accompanied by the production of heat and light
complete circuit	the path of an electric current from the generating source through conductors and back to its original source
compound molecules	chemical combinations of two or more atoms of different elements

conductor	any substance, material, or medium that conducts electricity
converter	apparatus that changes direct current to alternating current
direct current (DC)	constant, even-flowing current that travels in one direction only and produces a chemical reaction
desincrustation	process used to soften and emulsify grease deposits (oil) and blackheads in the hair follicles
electric current	flow of electricity along a conductor
electricity	form of energy that, when in motion, exhibits magnetic, chemical, or thermal effects; a flow of electrons
electrode	applicator for directing the electric current from the machine to the client's skin
electromagnetic radiation	also called radiant energy because it carries, or radiates, energy through space on waves
electrotherapy	electronic facial treatments
element	the simplest form of matter; cannot be broken down into a simpler substance without loss of identity
elemental molecules	molecules that contain two or more atoms of the same element that are united chemically
emulsion	mixture of two or more immiscible substances united with the aid of a binder or emulsifier
exothermic	characterized by or formed with the giving off of heat
faradic current	alternating and interrupted current that produces a mechanical reaction without a chemical effect
fuse	special device that prevents excessive current from passing through a circuit
galvanic current	constant and direct current (DC), having a positive and negative pole and producing chemical changes when it passes through the tissues and fluids of the body
glycerin	sweet, colorless, oily substance formed by the decomposition of oils, fats, or fatty acids
hydrophilic	capable of combining with or attracting water
immiscible	not capable of being mixed
inactive electrode	opposite pole from the active electrode
infrared rays	invisible rays that have long wavelengths, penetrate the deepest, and produce the most heat
inorganic chemistry	branch of chemistry dealing with compounds lacking carbon
insulator or nonconductor	substance that does not easily transmit electricity
ion	atom or molecule that carries an electrical charge
ionization	the separating of a substance into ions
iontophoresis	process of introducing water-soluble products into the skin with the use of electric current such as the use of the positive and negative poles of a galvanic machine

chapter glossary *(continued)*

kilowatt	1,000 watts
lipophilic	having an affinity or attraction to fat and oils
matter	any substance that occupies space, has physical and chemical properties, and exists in the form of a solid, liquid, or gas
milliampere	one-thousandth of an ampere
miscible	capable of being mixed with another liquid in any proportion without separating
modalities	currents used in electrical facial and scalp treatments
molecule	two or more atoms joined chemically
ohm	unit that measures the resistance of an electric current
oil-in-water (O/W) emulsion	oil droplets suspended in a water base
organic chemistry	study of substances that contain carbon
oxidation	chemical reaction that combines an element or compound with oxygen to produce an oxide
oxidize	to combine or cause an element to combine with oxygen
oxidizing agent	substance that releases oxygen
pH	relative degree of acidity and alkalinity of a substance
physical change	change in the form or physical properties of a substance without the formation of a new substance
physical mixture	combination of two or more substances united physically, not chemically, without a fixed composition and in any proportions
physical properties	those characteristics that can be determined without a chemical reaction and that do not cause a chemical change in the identity of the substance
polarity	negative or positive pole of an electric current
pure substance	matter with a fixed chemical composition, definite proportions, and distinct properties
rectifier	apparatus that changes alternating current to direct current
red light	therapeutic light used on dry skin in combination with oils and creams; penetrates the deepest and produces the most heat
redox	contraction for reduction-oxidation; chemical reaction in which the oxidizing agent is reduced and the reducing agent is oxidized
reduce	to subtract oxygen from or add hydrogen to a substance
reduction	the subtraction of oxygen from, or the addition of hydrogen to, a substance
silicones	special types of oil used in hair conditioners and as water-resistant lubricants for the skin

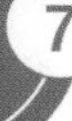

sinusoidal current	alternating current similar to faradic current; produces mechanical contractions and is used during scalp and facial manipulations
solute	the dissolved substance in a solution
solution	blended mixture of two or more solids, liquids, or gaseous substances
solvent	a substance, usually liquid, which dissolves another substance to form a solution, with no change in chemical composition
surfactants	surface active agents; substances that act as a bridge to allow oil and water to mix, or emulsify
suspension	state in which solid particles are distributed throughout a liquid medium
Tesla high-frequency current	thermal or heat-producing current with a high rate of oscillation or vibration; also called violet ray
therapeutic lamps	lamps used to produce artificial light rays in the salon
ultraviolet (UV) rays	invisible rays that have short wavelengths, are the least penetrating rays, produce chemical effects, and kill germs; also called cold rays or actinic rays
visible light	electromagnetic radiation that can be seen
volatile	easily evaporating
volatile organic compounds (VOCs)	two or more elements combined chemically (compounds) that contain carbon (organic) and evaporate very quickly (volatile)
volt	unit that measures the pressure or force that pushes the flow of electrons forward through a conductor
wall plate	instrument that plugs into an ordinary wall outlet and produces different types of electric currents that are used for facial and scalp treatments
water-in-oil (W/O) emulsion	droplets of water suspended in an oil base
watt	measurement of how much electric energy is being used in one second
wavelength	distance between two successive peaks of electromagnetic waves
white light	referred to as combination light because it is a combination of all the visible rays of the spectrum

review questions

1. What is chemistry?
2. Why is a basic understanding of chemistry important?
3. What is the difference between organic and inorganic chemistry?
4. What are atoms?
5. What are elements?
6. What are the physical and chemical properties of matter? Give examples.
7. What is the difference between physical and chemical changes? Give examples.
8. Describe the three states of matter.
9. Explain elements, compounds, and mixtures.
10. What is the difference between solutions, suspensions, and emulsions? Give examples.
11. Define pH and the pH scale.
12. Explain the difference between oxidation and reduction reactions.
13. Describe the two types of electric current and give examples of each.
14. List the four main types of electrical measurements. What do they measure?
15. List and describe the four main types of electrotherapy.
16. List and describe the five main types of light therapy.
17. What is electromagnetic radiation? What is visible light? What is white light?
18. Name two important precautions to observe when using light therapy.

HAIR CARE

part 3

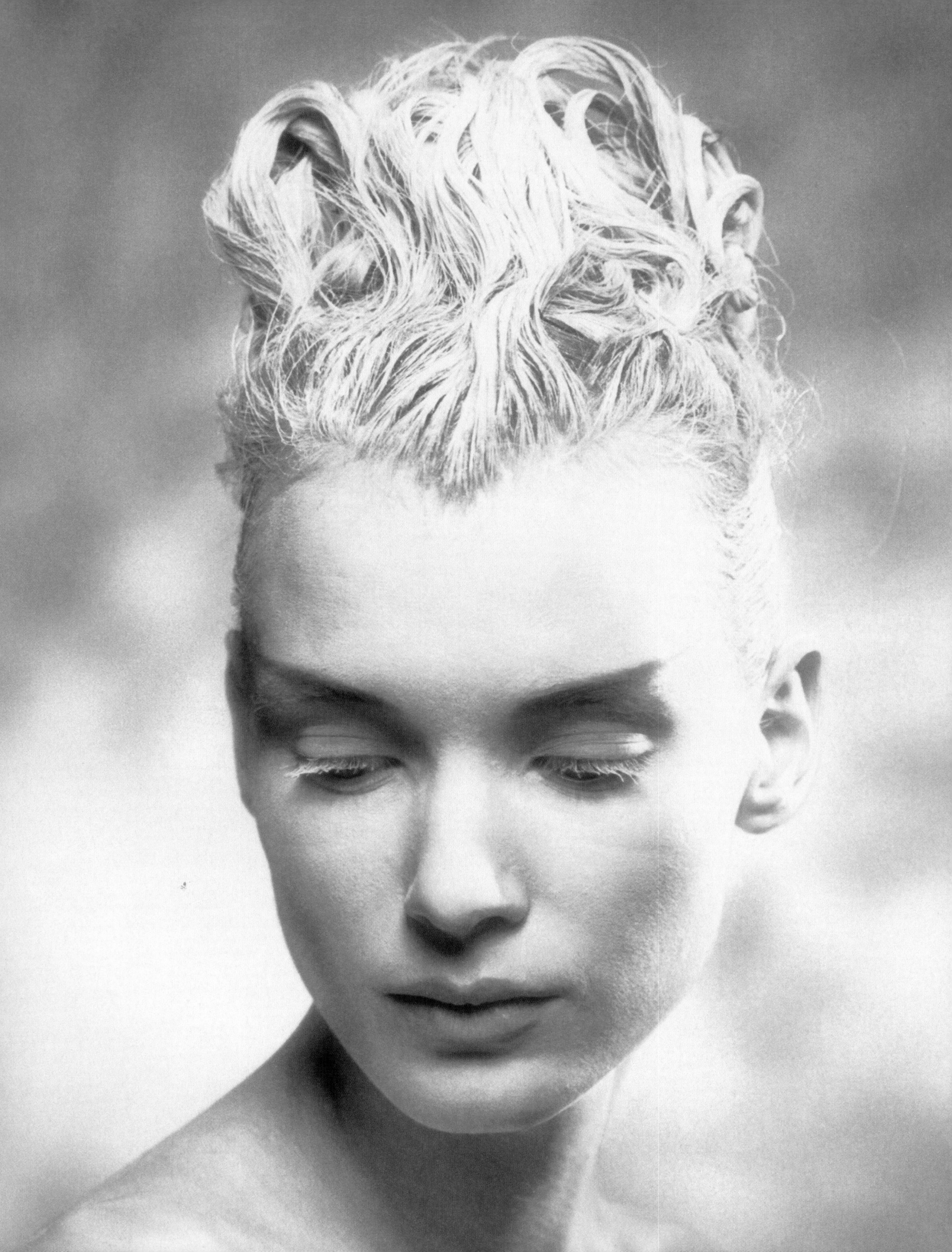

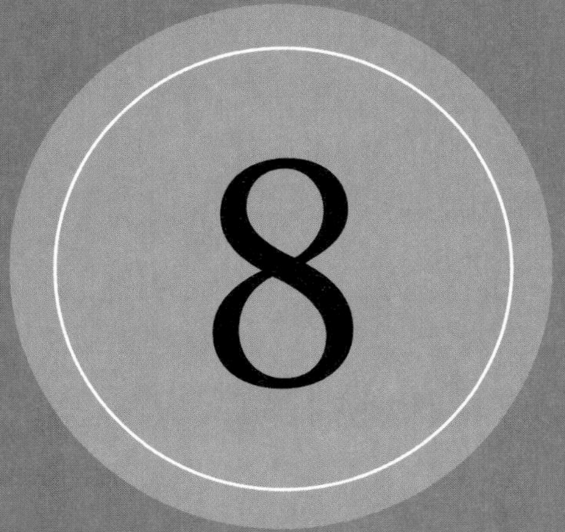

PROPERTIES OF THE HAIR AND SCALP

John Halal

PRESIDENT, HONORS BEAUTY COLLEGE, INDIANAPOLIS, IN

Chapter Outline

Structure of the Hair • The Chemical Composition of Hair
Hair Analysis • Hair Growth • Hair Loss
Disorders of the Hair • Disorders of the Scalp

Learning Objectives

After completing this chapter, you should be able to:

1. **Name and describe the structures of the hair root.**
2. **List and describe the three layers of the hair shaft.**
3. **Describe the three types of side bonds in the cortex.**
4. **List the factors that should be considered in a hair analysis.**
5. **Describe the process of hair growth.**
6. **Discuss the different types of hair loss and their causes.**
7. **Describe the various options for hair loss treatment.**
8. **Recognize hair and scalp disorders commonly seen in the salon and school, and know which can be treated there.**

National Skill Standards

This chapter provides you with the necessary information to master these National Industry Skill Standards for Entry-Level Cosmetologists.

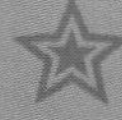
Consulting with clients to determine their needs and preferences.

Conducting services in a safe environment and taking measures to prevent the spread of infectious and contagious disease.

Key Terms

Page number indicates where in the chapter the term is used.

alopecia pg. 217
alopecia areata pg. 218
amino acids pg. 206
anagen pg. 215
androgenic alopecia pg. 217
arrector pili pg. 204
canities pg. 219
carbuncle pg. 222
catagen pg. 215
COHNS elements pg. 205
cortex pg. 205
cowlick pg. 212
cuticle pg. 204
dermal papilla (plural: papillae) pg. 204
disulfide bond pg. 207
eumelanin pg. 208
follicle pg. 204
fragilitas crinium pg. 220
furuncle pg. 222
hair bulb pg. 204
hair density pg. 210
hair elasticity pg. 211
hair porosity pg. 210
hair root pg. 205
hair shaft pg. 205
hair stream pg. 212
hair texture pg. 209
hydrogen bond pg. 207
hypertrichosis pg. 220
keratinization pg. 205
malassezia pg. 221
medulla pg. 205
melanin pg. 207
monilethrix pg. 220
pediculosis capitis pg. 222
peptide bond pg. 206
pheomelanin pg. 208
pityriasis pg. 220
pityriasis capitis simplex pg. 221
pityriasis steatoides pg. 221
polypeptide chain pg. 206
postpartum alopecia pg. 218
ringed hair pg. 220
salt bond pg. 207
scutula pg. 222
sebaceous glands pg. 204
sebum pg. 204
telogen pg. 215
terminal hair pg. 213
tinea pg. 221
tinea capitis pg. 221
tinea favosa pg. 222
trichology pg. 203
trichoptilosis pg. 220
trichorrhexis nodosa pg. 220
vellus or lanugo pg. 212
wave pattern pg. 208
whorl pg. 212

Although we no longer need hair for warmth and protection the way primitive man once did, hair still plays an enormous role in how we feel about ourselves. Our hair is one of the most dramatic and beautiful adornments we possess. In terms of color, texture, and style, hair makes a dramatic, personalized statement about who we are. The hairstyles we wear are an expression of the current mood of society and have always changed to reflect the changes in our attitude and culture.

All successful hairstyling services should be grounded in a thorough understanding of the growth, structure, and composition of hair. Hair, like people, comes in a variety of colors, shapes, and sizes. The scientific study of hair, its diseases, and care is called **trichology** (trih-KAHL-uh-jee), which comes from the Greek words *trichos* (hair) and *ology* (the study of). As a cosmetologist, you will need to know as much as you can about hair and how to keep it healthy. The more you learn and the more you understand how salon services affect different hair types, the more you will be able to achieve consistent results on your clients.

Did you know...

Although a healthy diet does not always guarantee healthy hair and scalp, you are what you eat. Your body cannot produce healthy hair without the proper nutrients. The body can produce 11 of the 20 amino acids that make up hair, but the remaining nine must come from your daily diet. Proteins like meat, fish, eggs, and dairy products are good sources of these amino acids, as are food combinations like peanut butter and bread, rice and beans, and beans and corn.

STRUCTURE OF THE HAIR

The integument (in-TEG-guh-ment) is the outer covering that encloses the entire body. It includes the hair, skin, and nails and is the largest and fastest-growing organ of the human body. Full-grown human hair is divided into two parts: the hair root and the hair shaft. The **hair root** is the part of the hair located below the surface of the scalp. The **hair shaft** is the portion of the hair that projects above the skin.

Structures of the Hair Root

The main structures of the hair root are the follicle, bulb, papilla, arrector pili muscle, and sebaceous glands (Figure 8–1).

The **follicle** (FAWL-ih-kul) is the tube-like depression or pocket in the skin or scalp that contains the hair root. Hair follicles are distributed all over the body, with the exception of the palms of the hands and the soles of the feet. The follicle extends downward from the epidermis (the outer layer of skin) into the dermis (the inner layer of skin), where it surrounds the dermal papilla. It is not uncommon for more than one hair to grow from a single follicle.

The **hair bulb** is the lowest area or part of a hair strand. It is the thickened, club-shaped structure that forms the lower part of the hair root. The lower part of the hair bulb fits over and covers the dermal papilla.

The **dermal papilla** (puh-PIL-uh) (plural: papillae) is a small, cone-shaped elevation located at the base of the hair follicle that fits into the hair bulb. The dermal papilla contains the blood and nerve supply that provides the nutrients needed for hair growth.

The **arrector pili** (ah-REK-tohr PY-ly) is a minute, involuntary muscle fiber in the skin inserted in the base of the hair follicle. Fear or cold causes it to contract, which makes the hair stand up straight, resulting in "goose bumps."

Sebaceous glands (sih-BAY-shus) are the oil glands of the skin, connected to the hair follicles. The sebaceous glands secrete an oily substance called **sebum** (SEE-bum), which lubricates the hair and skin.

Structures of the Hair Shaft

The three main layers of the hair shaft are the cuticle, cortex, and medulla (Figure 8–2).

The **cuticle** (KYOO-ti-kul) is the outermost layer of hair. It consists of a single, overlapping layer of transparent, scale-like cells that overlap like shingles on a roof. A healthy, compact cuticle layer is the hair's primary defense against damage.

A lengthwise section of hair shows that although the cuticle scales overlap, each individual cuticle scale is attached to the cortex (Figure 8–3). These overlapping scales makes up the cuticle layer. When viewed in cross-section,

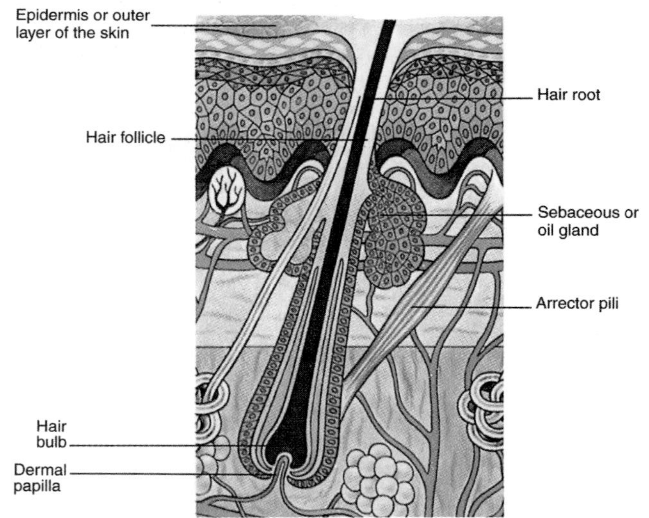

Figure 8–1 Structures of the hair.

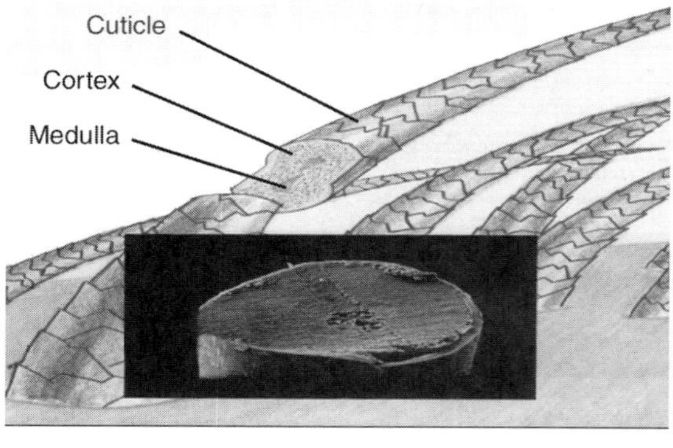

Figure 8–2 Cross-section of hair.

the scales can be seen to overlap, but it is important to note that hair has only one cuticle layer. Swelling the hair raises the cuticle layer and opens the space between the scales, which allows liquids to penetrate. If there were more than one cuticle layer and they were stacked on top of each other, nothing would be able to penetrate the hair.

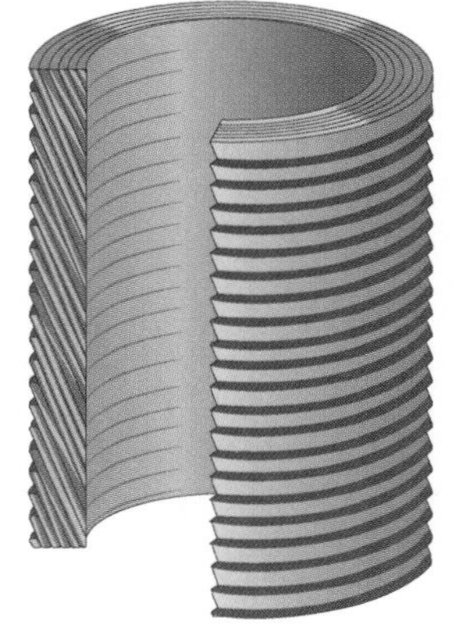

Figure 8–3 The cuticle layer.

A healthy cuticle layer protects the hair from penetration and prevents damage to hair fibers. Oxidation haircolors, permanent waving solutions, and chemical hair relaxers must have an alkaline pH in order to penetrate the cuticle layer and reach their target within the cortex.

The **cortex** is the middle layer of the hair. It is a fibrous protein core formed by elongated cells containing melanin pigment. About 90 percent of the total weight of hair comes from the cortex. The elasticity of the hair and its natural color are the result of the unique protein structures located within the cortex. The changes involved in oxidation haircoloring, wet setting, thermal styling, permanent waving, and chemical hair relaxing all take place within the cortex (Figure 8–4).

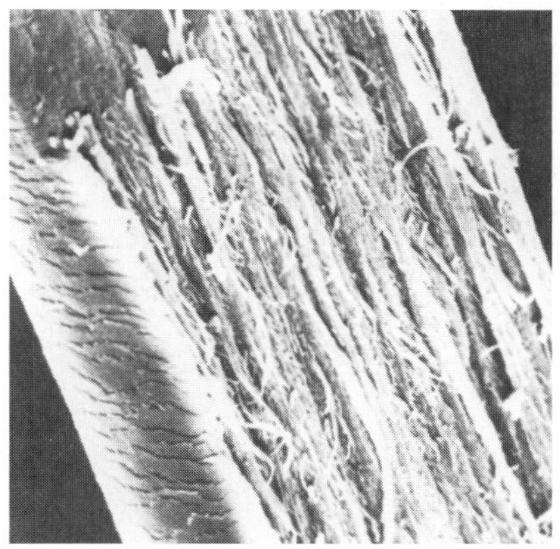

Figure 8–4 Hair shaft with part of cuticle stripped off, exposing the cortex.

The **medulla** (muh-DUL-uh) is the innermost layer, sometimes referred to as the pith of the hair. It is composed of round cells. It is quite common for very fine and naturally blonde hair to entirely lack a medulla. Generally, only thick, coarse hair contains a medulla. All male beard hair contains a medulla. Beard hair is generally much coarser and not as uniform as hair from the head of the same individual. As far as cosmetology is concerned, the medulla is an "empty" air space and is not involved in salon services. 2

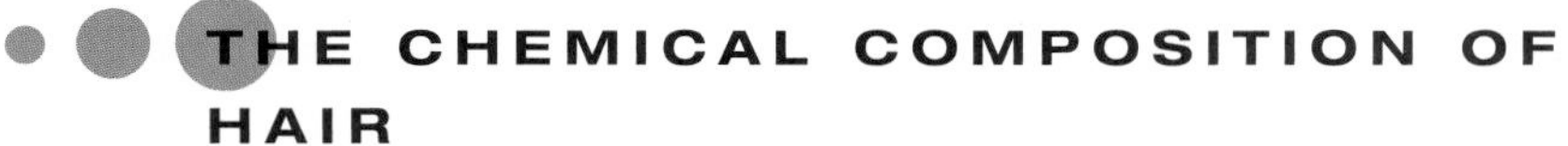

THE CHEMICAL COMPOSITION OF HAIR

Hair is composed of protein that grows from cells originating within the hair follicle. This is where the hair shaft begins. As soon as these living cells form, they begin their journey upward through the hair follicle. They mature in a process called **keratinization** (kair-uh-ti-ni-ZAY-shun). As these newly formed cells mature, they fill up with a fibrous protein called keratin, then move upward, lose their nucleus, and die. By the time the hair shaft emerges from the scalp, the cells of the hair are completely keratinized and are no longer living. The hair shaft that emerges from the scalp is a nonliving fiber composed of keratinized protein.

Hair is approximately 91 percent protein. The protein is made up of long chains of amino acids, which, in turn, are made up of elements. The elements that make up human hair are carbon, oxygen, hydrogen, nitrogen, and sulfur. These five elements are also the major elements found in skin and nails and are often referred to as the **COHNS elements**. Table 8–1 shows the percentages of each element in normal hair.

Element	Percentage in Normal Hair
Carbon	51%
Oxygen	21%
Hydrogen	6%
Nitrogen	17%
Sulfur	5%

Table 8–1 The COHNS Elements

The **amino acids** (uh-MEE-noh), the units of structure in protein, are linked together end to end like pop beads. The chemical bond that joins amino acids to each other is called a **peptide bond** or end bond. A long chain of amino acids linked by peptide bonds is called a **polypeptide chain** (pahl-ee-PEP-tyd). Polypeptide chains intertwine around each other in a spiral shape called a helix (HEE-liks) (Figure 8–5).

The Side Bonds of the Cortex

The cortex, middle layer of the hair, is made up of millions of polypeptide chains. These polypeptide chains are cross-linked together, like a ladder, by three different types of side bonds: hydrogen bonds, salt bonds, and disulfide bonds (Figure 8–6). These side bonds hold the hair fibers in place and account for the incredible strength and elasticity of human hair. These side bonds are essential to wet sets, thermal styling, permanent waving, and chemical hair relaxing (see Chapter 15).

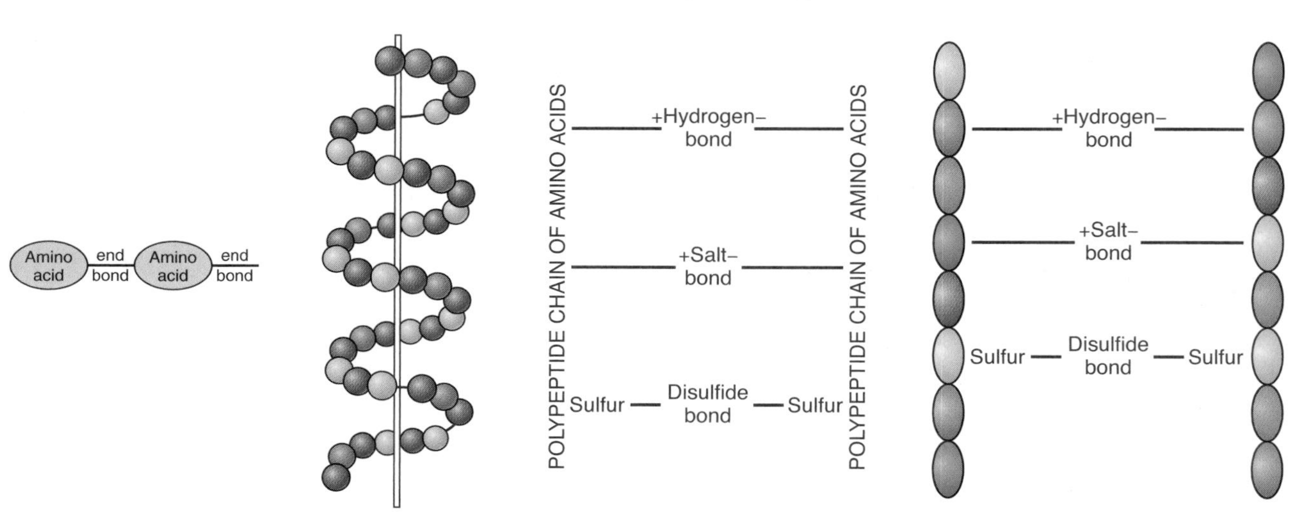

Figure 8–5 A polypeptide chain.

Figure 8–6 Side bonds.

A **hydrogen bond** is a physical side bond that is easily broken by water or heat. Although individual hydrogen bonds are very weak, there are so many of them that they account for about one-third of the hair's overall strength.

A **salt bond** is also a physical side bond, but it is broken by changes in pH. Salt bonds are easily broken by strong alkaline or acidic solutions and account for about one-third of the hair's overall strength.

A **disulfide bond** (dy-SUL-fyd) is a chemical side bond that differs greatly from the kind of physical bonding seen in a hydrogen or salt bond. A disulfide bond joins the sulfur atoms of two neighboring cysteine (SIS-ti-een) amino acids to create cystine (SIS-teen). Although there are far fewer disulfide bonds than hydrogen or salt bonds, disulfide bonds are much stronger and account for about one-third of the hair's overall strength. Disulfide bonds are not broken by heat or water. Permanent waves and chemical hair relaxers change the shape of hair by chemically changing the hair's disulfide bonds. 3 ✓

Thio permanent waves break disulfide bonds, which are re-formed by thio neutrilizers. Hydroxide chemical hair relaxers break disulfide bonds, which are converted to lanthionine bonds when the relaxer is rinsed from the hair. The disulfide bonds that are broken by hydroxide relaxers are broken permanently and can never be re-formed (see Chapter 15 and Table 8-2).

Hair Pigment

All natural hair color is the result of the pigment located within the cortex. **Melanin** (MEL-uh-nin) is the tiny grains of pigment in the cortex that give natural color to the hair. The two different types of melanin are eumelanin and pheomelanin.

Bond	Type	Strength	Broken By	Re-formed By
hydrogen	side bond	weak physical	water or heat	drying or cooling
salt	side bond	weak physical	changes in pH	normalizing pH
disulfide	side bond	strong chemical	1. thio perms and thio relaxers 2. hydroxide relaxers	1. oxidation with neutralizer 2. converted to lanthionine bonds
peptide	end bond	strong chemical	chemical depilatories	not re-formed; hair dissolves

Table 8-2 Bonds of the Hair

8

?

Did **you** know...

The term "hair color" refers to the color of hair created by nature. "Haircolor" (one word) is the term used in the beauty industry to refer to artificial haircoloring products. Gray hair is caused by the absence of melanin. Gray hair grows from the hair bulb in exactly the same way that pigmented hair grows and has exactly the same structure, but without the melanin pigment.

1. **Eumelanin** (yoo-MEL-uh-nin) provides brown and black color to hair.
2. **Pheomelanin** (fee-oh-MEL-uh-nin) provides natural hair colors from red and ginger to yellow/blonde tones.

All natural hair color is the result of the ratio of eumelanin to pheomelanin, along with the total number and size of pigment granules.

Wave Pattern

The **wave pattern** of the hair refers to the amount of movement in the hair strand and is described as straight, wavy, curly, or extremely curly (Figure 8–7). Wave pattern is the result of genetics and racial background. Although there are exceptions, as a general rule, Asians tend to have extremely straight hair, Caucasians tend to have straight to wavy hair, and African Americans tend to have extremely curly hair. But straight, curly, and extremely curly hair occurs in all races. This means that anyone of any race, or mixed race, can have hair with varying degrees of curliness from straight to extremely curly. It is also true that within races, individuals have hair with varying degrees of curliness.

The wave pattern may also vary from strand to strand on the same person's head. It is not uncommon for an individual to have different amounts of curl in different areas of the head. Individuals with curly hair often have straighter hair in the crown and curlier hair in other areas.

Several different theories seek to explain the cause of naturally curly hair, but there is no single, definite answer that explains why some hair grows straight and other hair grows curly. The most popular theory claims that the shape of the hair's cross-section determines the amount of curl. This theory states that hair with a round cross-section is straight, hair with an oval cross-section is wavy, and hair with a flat cross-section is curly. Although it is true that cross-sections of straight hair tend to be round and curlier hair tends to be more oval, modern microscopes have shown that a cross-section of hair can be almost any shape, including triangular, and that the shape of the cross-section does not always relate to the amount of curl.

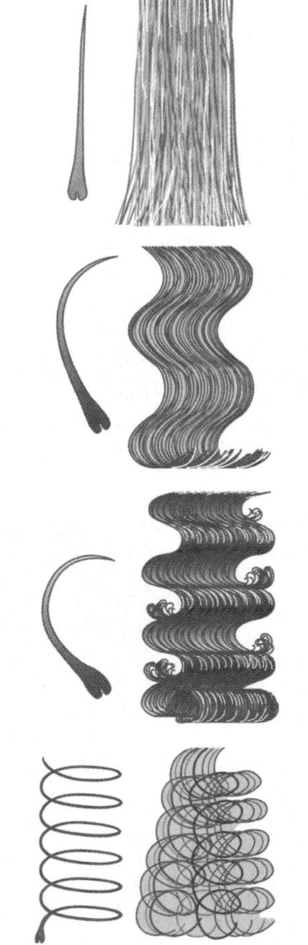

Figure 8–7 Straight, wavy, curly, and coiled hair strands.

Although it is still only a theory, it is now believed that natural curl is the result of one side of the hair strand growing faster than the other side. Since the side that grows faster is slightly longer than the slower growing side, tension within the strand causes the long side to curl around the short side. Hair that grows uniformly on both sides does not create tension and results in straight hair.

The hair's wave pattern is independent of its other properties. Hair has different diameters from fine to coarse, regardless of its wave pattern. All hair—extremely straight to extremely curly and everything in between—comes in different textures and densities.

Straight Hair

Straight hair can be any hair type without regard to texture or density. Like all other wave patterns, straight hair can be fine or coarse, dense or thin. Straight hair has a fairly regular and uniform diameter along a single strand. Cross-sections of straight hair are usually round.

Wavy Hair

Cross-sections of wavy hair are usually oval and have a fairly regular and uniform diameter along a single strand.

Extremely Curly Hair

Extremely curly hair grows in long twisted spirals. Cross-sections are highly oval and vary in shape and thickness along their length. Compared to straight or wavy hair, which tends to possess a fairly regular and uniform diameter along a single strand, extremely curly hair is quite irregular, showing varying diameters along a single strand.

Some extremely curly hair has a natural tendency to form a coil like a telephone cord or the spring in an ink pen. Coiled hair usually has a fine texture, with many individual strands winding together to form the coiled locks that characterize this type of hair. Coiled hair usually has low elasticity, breaks easily, and has a tendency to knot, especially on the ends. Gentle scalp manipulations, conditioning shampoo, and a detangling rinse help minimize tangles.

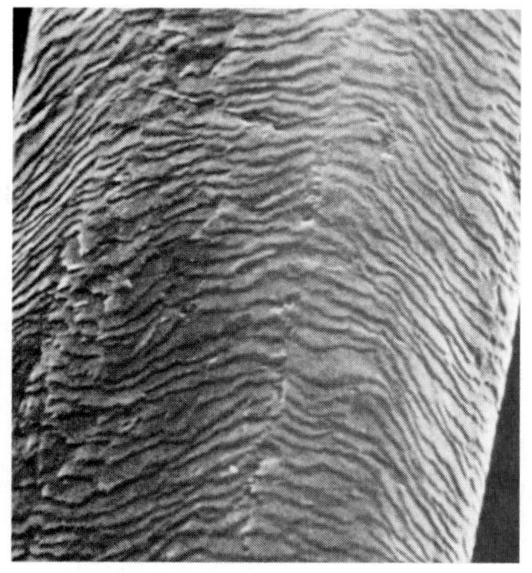

Figure 8-8 Coarse hair.

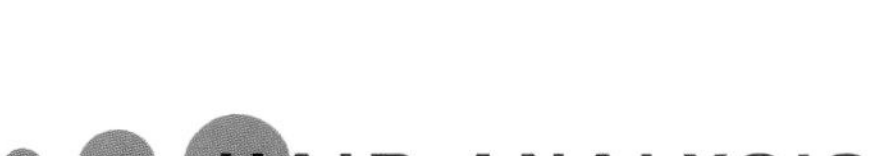

HAIR ANALYSIS

All successful salon services must begin with a thorough analysis of the client's hair type and its present condition in order to determine beforehand the results that can reasonably be expected from the service. Since different types of hair react differently to the same service, it is essential that a thorough analysis be performed prior to all salon services. Hair analysis is performed by observation using the senses of sight, touch, hearing, and smell. The four most important factors to consider in hair analysis are texture, porosity, elasticity, and density. Other factors that you should also be aware of are growth pattern as well as dryness and oiliness.

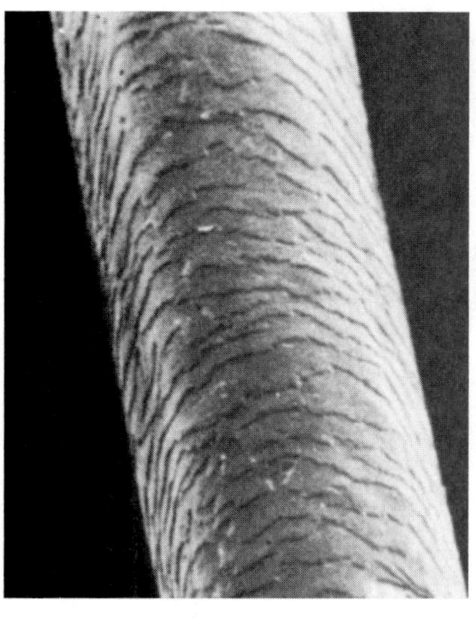

Figure 8-9 Medium hair.

Hair Texture

Hair texture is the thickness or diameter of the individual hair strand. Hair texture can be classified as coarse, medium, or fine and differs from individual to individual (Figure 8–8, Figure 8–9, and Figure 8–10). Hair texture can also vary from strand to strand on the same person's head. It is not uncommon for hair from different areas of the head to have different textures. Hair from the nape (back of the neck), crown, temples, and front hairline of the same person may all have different textures.

Coarse hair texture has the largest diameter. It is stronger than fine hair, for the same reason that a thick rope is stronger than a thin rope. Coarse hair also has a stronger structure. It usually requires more processing than medium or fine hair and may also be more resistant to that processing. It is usually more difficult for hair lighteners, haircolors, permanent waving solutions, and chemical hair relaxers to penetrate coarse hair.

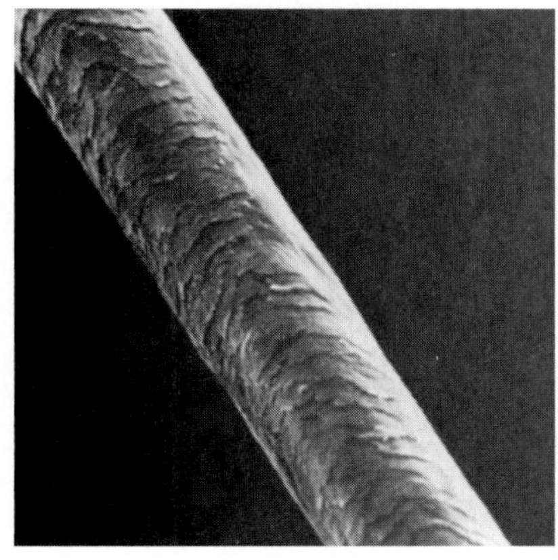

Figure 8-10 Fine hair.

8

Medium hair texture is the most common and is the standard to which other hair is compared. Medium hair is considered normal and does not pose any special problems or concerns.

Fine hair has the smallest diameter and is more fragile, easier to process, and more susceptible to damage from chemical services than coarse or medium hair.

Hair texture can be determined by feeling a single dry strand between the fingers. Take an individual strand from four different areas of the head—the front hairline, the temple, the crown, and the nape—and hold the strand securely with one hand while feeling it with the thumb and forefinger of the other hand. With a little practice, you will be able to feel the difference between coarse, medium, and fine hair diameters (Figure 8–11).

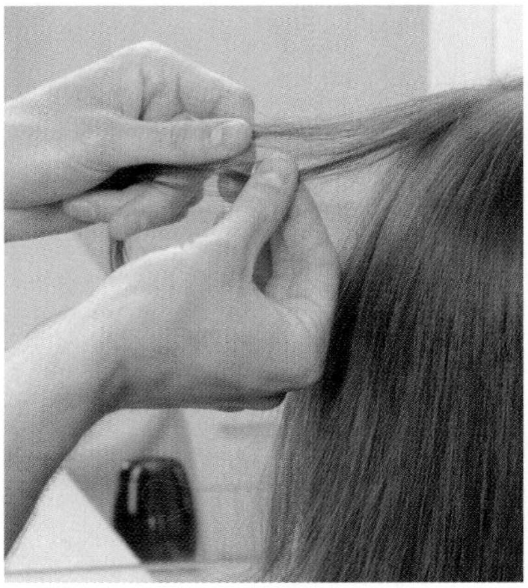

Figure 8-11 Testing for hair texture.

Hair Density

Hair density measures the number of individual hair strands on one square inch (2.5 cm) of scalp. It indicates how many hairs there are on a person's head. Hair density can be classified as low, medium, or high (or thin, medium, or thick-dense). Hair density is different from hair texture in that different individuals with the same hair texture can have different densities. Some individuals may have coarse hair texture (each hair has a large diameter), but low hair density (a low number of hairs on the head). Others may have fine hair texture (each hair has a small diameter), but high hair density (a high number of hairs on the head).

The average hair density is about 2,200 hairs per square inch. Hair with high density (thick or dense hair) has more hairs per square inch. Hair with low density (thin hair) has fewer hairs per square inch. The average head of hair contains about 100,000 individual hair strands. The number of hairs on the head generally varies with the color of the hair. Blondes usually have the highest density, and redheads tend to have the lowest (Table 8–3).

Hair Porosity

Hair porosity is the ability of the hair to absorb moisture. The degree of porosity is directly related to the condition of the cuticle layer. Healthy hair

Hair Color	Number of Hairs on Head
Blonde	140,000
Brown	110,000
Black	108,000
Red	80,000

Table 8-3 Number of Hairs on the Head by Hair Color

8

with a compact cuticle layer is naturally resistant to penetration. Porous hair has a raised cuticle layer that easily absorbs water.

Hair with low porosity is considered resistant hair (Figure 8–12). Chemical services performed on hair with low porosity require a more alkaline solution than those on hair with high porosity. Alkaline solutions raise the cuticle and permit uniform saturation and processing.

Hair with average porosity is considered normal hair (Figure 8–13). Chemical services performed on this type of hair will usually process as expected, according to the texture.

Hair with high porosity is considered overly porous hair and is the result of previous overprocessing (Figure 8–14). Overly porous hair is damaged, dry, fragile, and brittle. Chemical services performed on overly porous hair require less alkaline solutions with a lower pH. This will help prevent additional overprocessing.

The texture of the hair is not an indication of its porosity. Different degrees of porosity can be found in all hair textures. Although coarse hair normally has a low porosity and is resistant to chemical services, coarse hair can also have high porosity as the result of previous chemical services.

You can check porosity on dry hair by taking a strand of several hairs from four different areas of the head (the front hairline, the temple, the crown, and the nape). Hold the strand securely with one hand while sliding the thumb and forefinger of the other hand from the end to the scalp. If the hair feels smooth and the cuticle is compact, dense, and hard, it is considered resistant. If you can feel a slight roughness, it is considered porous. If the hair feels very rough, dry, or breaks, it is considered overly porous (Figure 8–15).

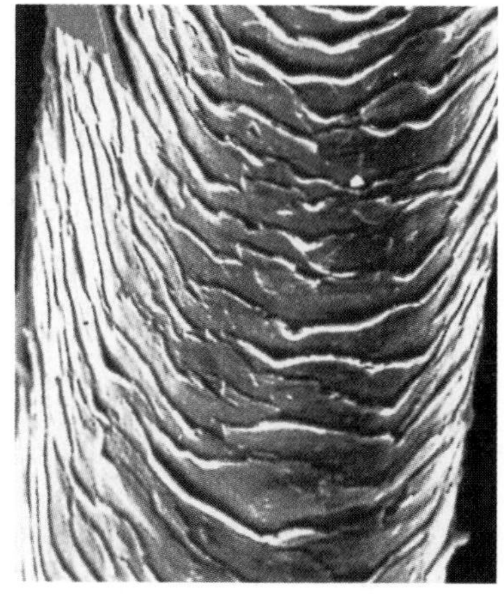

Figure 8–12 Low porosity (resistant hair).

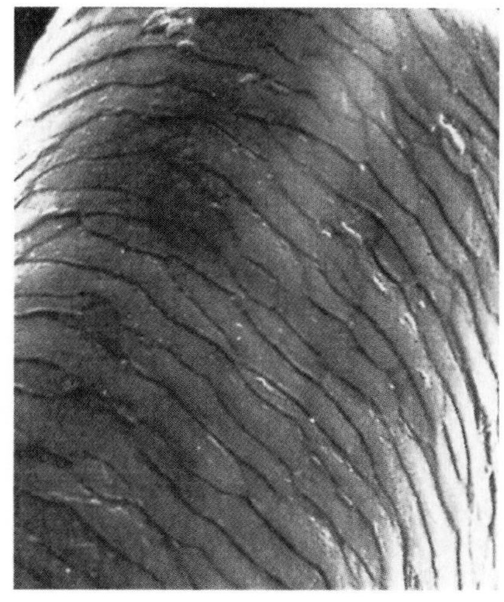

Figure 8–13 Average porosity (normal hair).

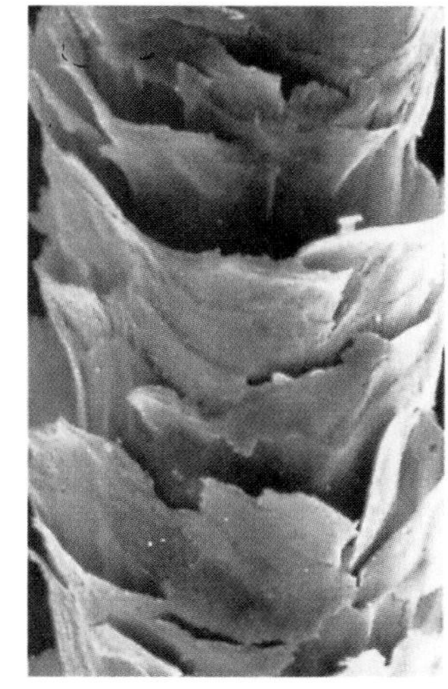

Figure 8–14 High porosity (overly porous).

Hair Elasticity

Hair elasticity is the ability of the hair to stretch and return to its original length without breaking. Hair elasticity is an indication of the strength of the side bonds that hold the hair's individual fibers in place. Wet hair with normal elasticity will stretch up to 50 percent of its original length and return to that same length without breaking. Dry hair stretches about 1/5 of its length. Hair with normal elasticity holds the curl from wet sets and permanent waves without excessive relaxing.

Hair with low elasticity is brittle and breaks easily. Hair with low elasticity may not be able to hold the curl from wet setting, thermal styling, or permanent waving. Hair with low elasticity is the result of weak side bonds that usually result from previous overprocessing. Chemical services performed on hair with low elasticity require a milder solution with a lower pH. Such a solution minimizes damage and helps prevent additional overprocessing.

Check elasticity on wet hair by taking an individual strand from four different areas of the head (the front hairline, the temple, the crown, and the nape). Hold a single strand of wet hair securely and try to pull it apart (Figure 8–16). If the hair stretches and returns to its original length without breaking, it has normal elasticity. If the hair breaks easily or fails to return to its original length, it has low elasticity. 4 ✓

8

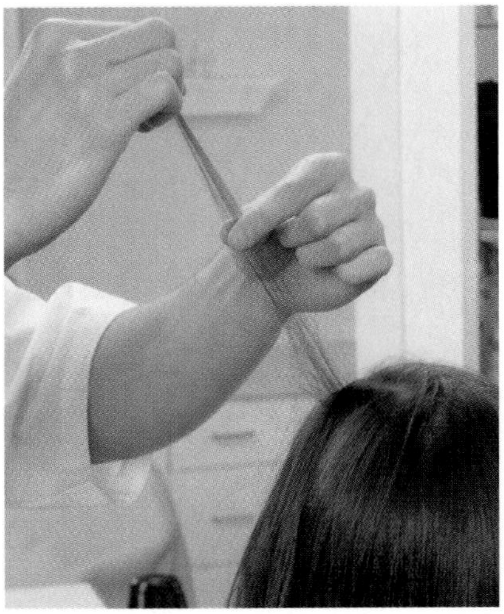

Figure 8–15 Testing for hair porosity.

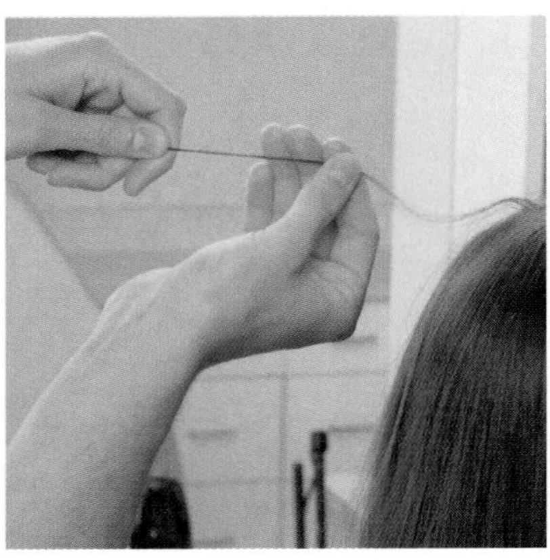

Figure 8–16 Testing for hair elasticity.

Growth Patterns

It is important when shaping and styling hair to consider the hair's growth patterns. Hair follicles do not usually grow perpendicular to the scalp. Most hair follicles grow at an angle other than 90 degrees, and most hair grows in a direction other than straight out from the head. The growth patterns result in hair streams, whorls, and cowlicks.

- A **hair stream** is hair flowing in the same direction. It is the result of follicles sloping in the same direction. Two streams flowing in opposite directions form a natural part in the hair.
- A **whorl** is hair that forms in a circular pattern, as on the crown. A whorl normally forms in the crown with all the hair from that point growing down.
- A **cowlick** is a tuft of hair that stands straight up. Cowlicks are usually more noticeable at the front hairline, but they may be located anywhere.

Dry Hair and Scalp

Dry hair and scalp is caused by inactive sebaceous glands and is aggravated by a dry winter or desert climate. The lack of natural oils (sebum) leads to a flaky scalp and hair that appears dull, dry, and lifeless. Dry hair and scalp should be treated with products that contain moisturizers and emollients. Frequent shampooing should be avoided, along with the use of strong soaps, detergents, or products with a high alcohol content because they may aggravate the condition. Dry hair should not be confused with overly porous hair that has been damaged by thermal styling, environmental forces, or chemical services.

Oily Hair and Scalp

Oily hair and scalp is caused by overactive sebaceous glands and is characterized by a greasy buildup on the scalp and an oily coating on the hair. Oily hair and scalp can be treated with clarifying or normalizing shampoos. A well-balanced diet, exercise, regular shampooing, and good personal hygiene are essential to control oily hair and scalp.

HAIR GROWTH

The two main types of hair found on the body are vellus (or lanugo) and terminal hair (Figure 8–17).

Vellus or **lanugo** (luh-NOO-goh) hair is short, fine, and downy. Vellus hair is not pigmented and almost never has a medulla. It is commonly found on infants and can be present on children until puberty. On adults, vellus hair is usually found in places that are normally considered hairless (forehead, eyelids, and bald scalp), as well as nearly all other areas of the body, except the palms of the hands and the soles of the feet. Women normally retain 55 percent more vellus hair than men. Vellus hair helps in the efficient evaporation of perspiration.

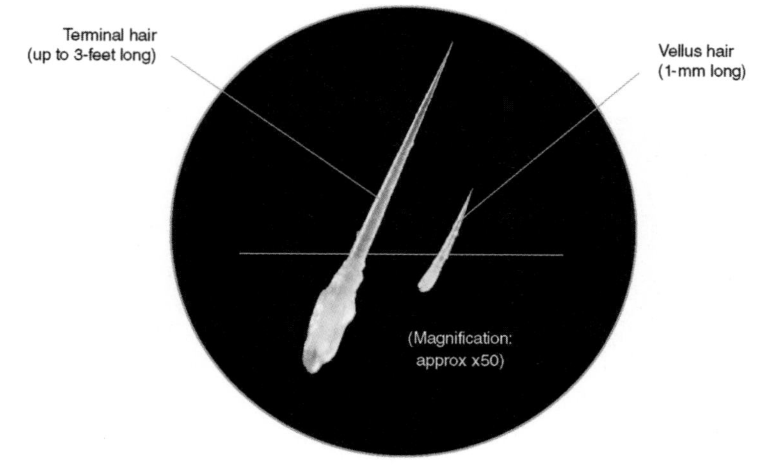

Figure 8–17 Terminal and vellus hair.

Terminal hair is the long, soft hair found on the scalp, legs, arms, and bodies of males and females. Terminal hair is coarser than vellus hair and, with the exception of gray hair, it is pigmented. It usually has a medulla and is easily distinguished from vellus hair by its dark color and coarse texture. Hormonal changes during puberty cause some areas of fine vellus hair to be replaced with thicker terminal hair. All hair follicles are capable of producing either vellus or terminal hair, depending on genetics, age, and hormonal changes.

The Growth Cycles of Hair

Hair growth occurs in cycles. Each complete cycle has three phases that are repeated over and over again throughout life. The three phases are anagen, catagen, and telogen (Figure 8–18).

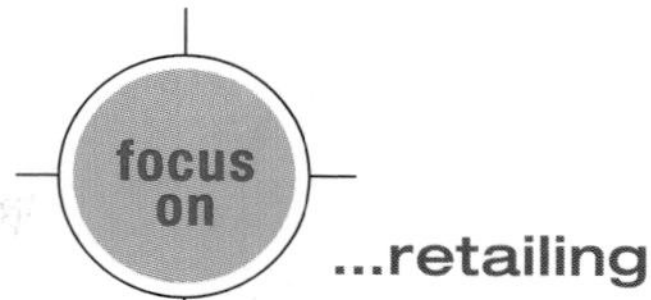

...retailing

Did you know that selling retail products increases client retention? A client who takes home a retail product is more than twice as likely to return for services.

Recommending products for home use is an important part of a successful career as a hairstylist. Your client needs to know which products to use and how to use them.

A complete hair analysis will enable you to recommend the right products for your client with confidence. It is your job to know more about your client's specific needs than anyone else and recommend the right products to satisfy those needs. Your clients do not want to make these decisions by themselves. They want your advice. Do not disappoint them.

8

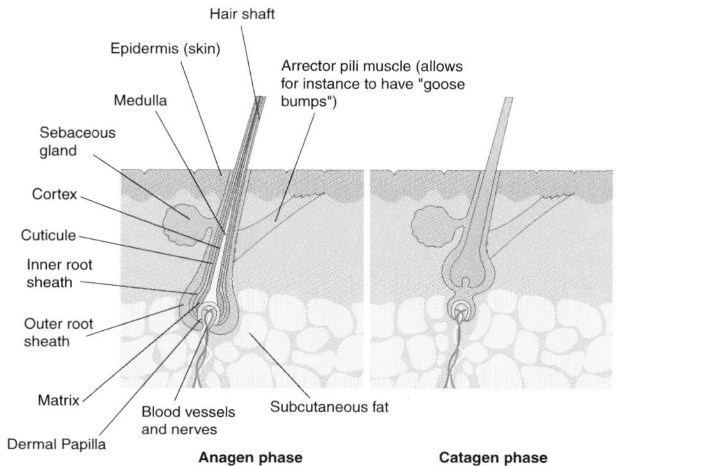

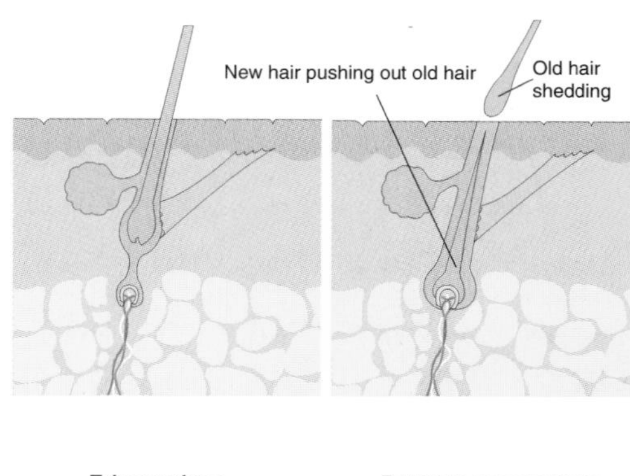

Figure 8–18 Cycles of hair growth.

insights

Jeffrey Paul

The path taken by Jeffrey Paul, owner of Jeffrey Paul's for Restoring Beautiful Hair in Rocky River, Ohio, has taken him places he never could have anticipated.

I was a very high-profile salon stylist. I studied in Europe; I was on stage with Sassoon and Paul Mitchell; I did the Saudi Arabian royal family, *Vogue* models, even the President of the United States. I had the kind of career that anybody who sets out to be a hairdresser would want. Then my nine-year-old niece got cancer. "Uncle Jeff," she cried, "don't let me lose my hair." She was trying out for gymnastics, and I promised her she would be able to perform without a problem.

I had made wigs in Europe as part of my training, but of course that was more for fashion. With the help of various specialists and a manufacturer, we made a child's wig that would stay on through anything, even gymnastics. Well, when I went to see my niece compete, she flew off the apparatus, looked up at me in the audience, and pointed to her head. My wife and I just looked at each other because we knew that God was changing my life somehow.

Six months later, I opened a small cosmetic therapy center. The very day we opened, both my mother and my sister were diagnosed with cancer. Believe me, I learned a lot about cancer, about survival, and about the compassion necessary to help someone deal with hair loss. Research has shown that for women the prospect of losing their hair is more devastating than the prospect of losing their life. Nobody believes that until you've been there with someone going through hair loss. When you help people repair their image, they have better survival rates because their immune systems are less compromised by stress and distress.

Once the media got wind of what we were doing with our hair loss treatments, everything exploded. I began hearing about kids who needed wigs but couldn't afford them, so we set up a nonprofit organization, Wigs for Kids, that over the years has helped thousands of children. We've never turned one away. But the problem of hair loss goes way beyond medical issues and treatment. Women from the ages of 29 to 79 have hair loss and thinning at very serious rates. Between 25 and 30 million women in the U.S. alone experience hair loss, often as a result of menopause and other genetic causes.

When we train cosmetologists in hair replacement, we always begin by focusing on the consultation. When a woman admits she has hair loss, it is like an alcoholic or drug addict admitting they have a problem. It requires great trust and compassion. We always say that trust in the hair replacement process is the greatest tool you have, greater than your shears, greater than the hairpiece. Once we have trained a person, we also help them make financial headway. We teach them how to set up the proper room and we develop a business plan for them. But this work is not for everyone. You have to want to help people. That's a given.

Anagen: The Growth Phase

During the **anagen** (AN-uh-jen) or growth phase, new hair is produced. The hair actively manufactures new keratinized cells in the hair follicle. During this phase, hair cells are produced faster than any other normal cell in the human body.

The average growth of healthy scalp hair is about 1/2 inch (1.25 centimeters) per month. The rate of growth varies on different parts of the body, between sexes, and with age. Scalp hair grows faster on women than on men. Scalp hair grows rapidly between the ages of 15 and 30, but slows down sharply after the age of 50.

About 90 percent of scalp hair is growing in the anagen phase at any one time. For each specific hair, the anagen phase generally lasts from three to five years, but in some cases, it can last as long as ten years.

Catagen: The Transition Phase

The **catagen** (KAT-uh-jen) phase is the brief transition period between the growth and resting phases of a hair follicle. It signals the end of the growth phase. During the catagen phase, the follicle canal shrinks and detaches from the dermal papilla. The hair bulb disappears and the shrunken root end forms a rounded club.

Less than 1 percent of scalp hair is in the catagen phase at any one time. The catagen phase is very short and lasts from one to two weeks.

Telogen: The Resting Phase

The **telogen** (TEL-uh-jen) or resting phase is the final phase in the hair cycle and lasts until the fully grown hair is shed. The hair is either shed during the telogen phase or remains in place until the next anagen phase, when the new hair growing in pushes it out.

About 10 percent of scalp hair is in the telogen phase at any one time. The telogen phase lasts for approximately three to six months. As soon as the telogen phase ends, the hair returns to the anagen phase and begins the entire cycle again. On average, the entire growth cycle repeats itself once every four to five years. 5✓

The Truth About Hair Growth

As a stylist, you may hear myths and opinions about hair growth from your clients or from other stylists. Here are some myths and facts about hair growth.

activity

Break up into groups of two or more in the classroom and analyze each other's hair. Hair analysis includes evaluating texture, density, porosity, and elasticity. Wave patterns, growth patterns, and the oiliness or dryness of the hair and scalp should also be noted. Follow the procedures in this textbook and use the same terminology. Write down results and present an oral report to the class. What is the most common texture among your classmates? The most common density?

MYTH: Shaving, clipping, and cutting the hair makes it grow back faster, darker, and coarser.

FACT: Shaving or cutting the hair has no effect on hair growth. When hair is blunt cut to the same length, it grows back more evenly. Although that may make it seem to grow back faster, darker, and coarser, shaving or cutting hair has no effect on hair growth.

MYTH: Scalp massage increases hair growth.

FACT: There is no evidence that any type of stimulation or scalp massage increases hair growth. Minoxidil and finasteride are the only treatments that have been proven to increase hair growth and are approved for that purpose by the Food and Drug Administration (FDA).

MYTH: Gray hair is coarser and more resistant than pigmented hair.

FACT: Other than the lack of pigment, gray hair is exactly the same as pigmented hair. Although gray hair may be resistant, it is not resistant simply because it is gray, and it is not more resistant than the pigmented hair on the same person's head. The pigmented hair on the same person's head is just as resistant as the gray hair. Gray hair is simply more noticeable than pigmented hair.

MYTH: The amount of natural curl is determined by racial background.

FACT: Anyone of any race, or mixed race, can have hair from straight to extremely curly. It is also true that within races, individuals have hair with different degrees of curliness.

MYTH: Hair with a round cross-section is straight, hair with an oval cross-section is wavy, and hair with a flat cross-section is curly.

FACT: Cross-sections of straight hair tend to be round and curlier hair tends to be more oval, but cross-sections of hair can be almost any shape, including triangular, and the shape of the cross-section does not always relate to the amount of curl or the shape of the follicle.

HAIR LOSS

Under normal circumstances, we all lose some hair every day. Normal daily hair loss is the natural result of the three phases of the hair's growth cycle. The growth cycle provides for the continuous growth, fall, and replacement of individual hair strands. Hair that is shed in the telogen phase is replaced by a new hair, in that same follicle, in the next anagen phase. This natural shedding of hair accounts for normal daily hair loss. Although estimates of the rate of hair loss have long been quoted at 100 to 150 hairs per day, recent measurements indicate that the average rate of hair loss is closer to 35 to 40 hairs per day.

Over 63 million people in the United States suffer from abnormal hair loss (alopecia). As a professional hairstylist, it is likely that you will be the first person that many of these people come to with questions about their hair loss. It is important that you have a basic understanding of the different types of hair loss and the products and services that are available.

The Emotional Impact of Hair Loss

Although the medical community does not recognize hair loss as a medical condition, the anguish felt by many of those who suffer from abnormal hair loss is very real, and all too often overlooked. Results from a study that investigated perceptions of bald and balding men showed that compared to men who had hair, bald men were perceived as:

- less physically attractive (by both sexes).
- less assertive.
- less successful.
- less personally likable.
- older (by about five years).

Results of a study investigating how bald men perceive themselves showed that greater hair loss had a more significant impact than moderate hair loss. Men with more severe hair loss:

- experience significantly more negative social and emotional effects.
- are more preoccupied with their baldness.
- make some effort to conceal or compensate for their hair loss.

For women, abnormal hair loss is particularly devastating. Women who experience hair loss try to disguise it from everyone, even their doctor. Women also tend to worry that their hair loss is a symptom of a serious illness. Studies indicate that women have a greater emotional investment in their appearance, and, although abnormal hair loss is not as common in women as it is in men, it can be very traumatic. The vast majority of women with abnormal hair loss feel anxious, helpless, and less attractive. Many think they are the only ones who have the problem.

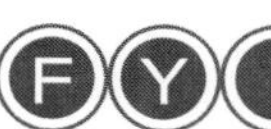

The mission of the National Alopecia Areata Foundation (NAAF) is to support research to find a cure or acceptable treatment for alopecia areata, to support those with the disease, and to educate the public.

The National Alopecia Areata Foundation
P.O. Box 150760
San Rafael, CA 94915-0760
(415) 456-4644
www.alopeciaareata.com
info@NAAF.org

Types of Abnormal Hair Loss

Abnormal hair loss is called **alopecia** (al-oh-PEE-shah). The most common types of abnormal hair loss are androgenic alopecia, alopecia areata, and postpartum alopecia.

Androgenic Alopecia

Androgenic alopecia (an-druh-JEN-ik) or androgenetic (an-druh-je-NET-ik) alopecia is the result of genetics, age, and hormonal changes that cause miniaturization of terminal hair, converting it to vellus hair (Figure 8–19). Androgenic alopecia can begin as early as the teens and is frequently seen by the age of 40. By age 35, almost 40 percent of both men and women show some degree of hair loss.

In men, androgenic alopecia is known as male pattern baldness and usually progresses to the familiar horseshoe-shaped fringe of hair. In

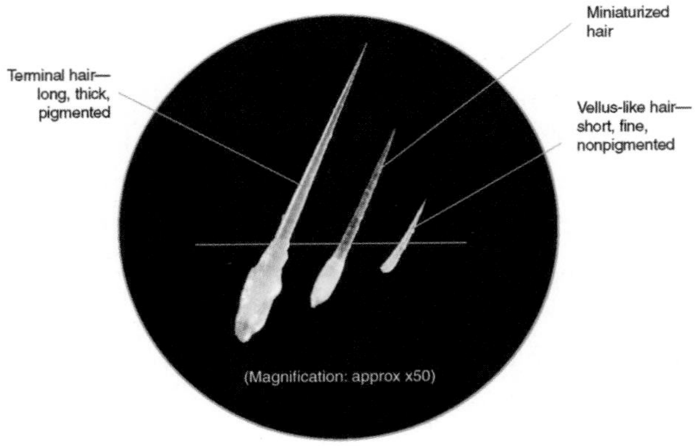

Terminal hair—long, thick, pigmented

Miniaturized hair

Vellus-like hair—short, fine, nonpigmented

(Magnification: approx x50)

Figure 8–19 Miniaturization of the hair follicle.

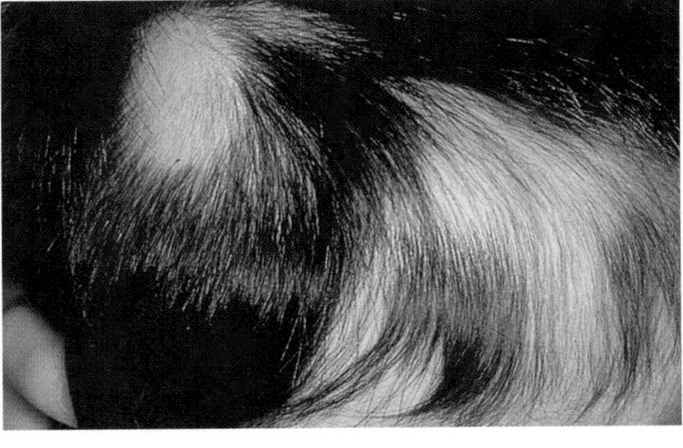

Figure 8–20 Alopecia areata.

women, it shows up as a generalized thinning over the entire crown area. Androgenic alopecia affects about 40 million men and 20 million women in the United States.

Alopecia Areata

Alopecia areata (air-ee-AH-tah) is characterized by the sudden falling out of hair in round patches or baldness in spots, and may occur on the scalp and elsewhere on the body. It is a highly unpredictable skin disease that affects almost five million people in the United States alone.

Alopecia areata is an autoimmune disease that causes the affected hair follicles to be mistakenly attacked by a person's own immune system, with white blood cells stopping the hair growth (anagen) phase. Alopecia areata usually begins with one or more small, round, smooth bald patches on the scalp and can progress to total scalp hair loss (alopecia totalis), or complete body hair loss (alopecia universalis).

Alopecia areata occurs in males and females of all ages and races and most often begins in childhood. The scalp usually shows no signs of inflammation. Alopecia areata occurs in individuals who have no obvious skin disorder or disease (Figure 8–20).

Postpartum Alopecia

Postpartum alopecia is temporary hair loss experienced at the conclusion of a pregnancy. For some women, pregnancy seems to disrupt the normal growth cycle of hair, with very little normal hair loss during pregnancy, but sudden and excessive shedding from three to nine months after delivery. Although this is usually very traumatic to the new mother, the growth cycle generally returns to normal within one year after the baby is delivered.

Hair Loss Treatments

Of all the treatments that are said to counter hair loss, there are only two products—minoxidil and finasteride—which have been proven to stimulate hair growth and are approved by the FDA for that purpose.

Minoxidil is a topical (applied to the surface of the body) medication that is applied to the scalp twice a day, and has been proven to stimulate hair growth. It is sold over-the-counter (OTC) as a nonprescription drug. Minoxidil is available for both men and women and comes in two different strengths: 2% regular and 5% extra strength. It is not known to have any negative side effects.

Finasteride is an oral prescription medication for men only. Although finasteride is more effective and convenient than minoxidil, possible side effects include weight gain and loss of sexual function. Women may not use this treatment, and pregnant women or those who might become pregnant are cautioned not to even touch the drug because of the strong potential for birth defects.

In addition to the treatments described above, there are also several surgical options available. Transplants, or hair plugs, are probably the most common permanent hair replacement technique. The process consists of removing small sections of hair, including the follicle, papilla, and bulb, from an area where there is a lot of hair (usually in the back) and transplanting them into the bald area. These sections, or bulbs, grow normally in the new location. Only licensed surgeons may perform this procedure, and several surgeries are usually necessary to achieve the desired results. The cost of each surgery ranges from $8,000 to over $20,000.

Hairstylists can offer a number of nonmedical options to counter hair loss. Some salons specialize in nonsurgical hair replacement systems such as wigs, toupees, hair weaving, and hair extensions. With proper training, you can learn to fit, color, cut, and style wigs and toupees. Hair weaving and hair extensions allow you to enhance a client's natural hair and create a look that boosts self-esteem (see Chapter 14). 7

Abnormal hair loss is an unwanted side effect of chemotherapy or radiation cancer treatments. Look Good . . . Feel Better (LGFB) is a free, national public service program that teaches beauty techniques to women with cancer, helping them boost their self-image and camouflage their hair loss. The program is open to all women cancer patients actively undergoing treatment for cancer. Each year, approximately 30,000 women participate in LGFB group sessions, and more than 200,000 women have been served by the organization since it was founded.

Look Good … Feel Better
800-395-LOOK, 800-395-5665
www.lookgoodfeelbetter.org

DISORDERS OF THE HAIR

The following disorders of the hair range from those that are commonplace and not particularly troublesome to those that are far more unusual or distressing.

Canities

Canities (kah-NISH-ee-eez) is the technical term for gray hair. Canities results from the loss of the hair's natural melanin pigment. Other than the absence of pigment, gray hair is exactly the same as pigmented hair. The two types of canities are congenital and acquired.

1. Congenital canities exists at or before birth. It occurs in albinos, who are born without pigment in the skin, hair and eyes, occasionally in individuals with normal hair. A patchy type of congenital canities may develop either slowly or rapidly, depending on the cause of the condition.
2. Acquired canities develops with age and is the result of genetics. Although genetics is also responsible for premature canities,

acquired canities may develop due to worry, anxiety, or prolonged illness.

Ringed Hair

Ringed hair is a variety of canities, characterized by alternating bands of gray and pigmented hair throughout the length of the hair strand.

Hypertrichosis

Hypertrichosis (hi-pur-trih-KOH-sis), or hirsuties (hur-SOO-shee-eez) is a condition of abnormal growth of hair. It is characterized by the growth of terminal hair in areas of the body that normally grow only vellus hair. A mustache or light beard on women are examples of hypertrichosis. Treatments include wax hair removal, tweezing, chemical depilatories, shaving, mechanical epilators, and electrolysis (see Chapter 18).

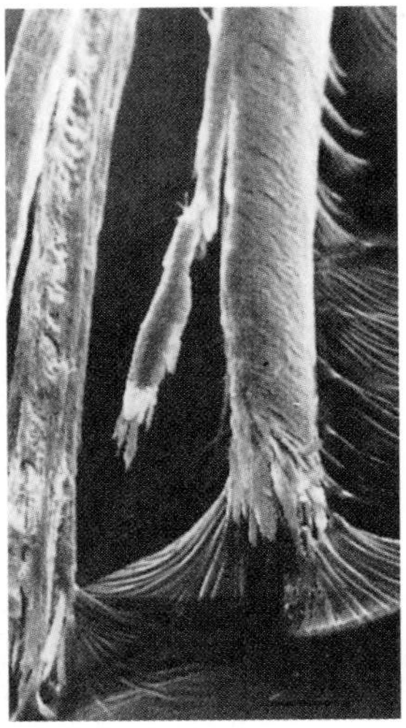

Trichoptilosis

Trichoptilosis (trih-kahp-tih-LOH-sus) is the technical term for split ends (Figure 8–21). Treatments include hair conditioning to soften and lubricate dry ends. The split ends may also be removed by cutting.

Figure 8–21 Trichoptilosis.

Trichorrhexis Nodosa

Trichorrhexis nodosa (trik-uh-REK-sis nuh-DOH-suh), or knotted hair, is characterized by brittleness and the formation of nodular swellings along the hair shaft (Figure 8–22). The hair breaks easily, and the broken fibers spread out like a brush along the hair shaft. Treatments include softening the hair with conditioners and moisturizers.

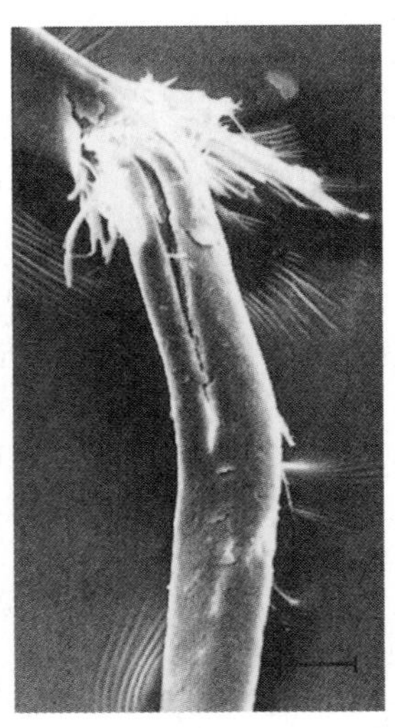

Figure 8–22 Trichorrhexis nodosa.

Monilethrix

Monilethrix (mah-NIL-ee-thriks) is the technical term for beaded hair (Figure 8–23). The hair breaks easily between the beads or nodes. Treatments include hair and scalp conditioning.

Fragilitas Crinium

Fragilitas crinium (fruh-JIL-ih-tus KRI-nee-um) is the technical term for brittle hair. The hairs may split at any part of their length. Treatments include hair and scalp conditioning.

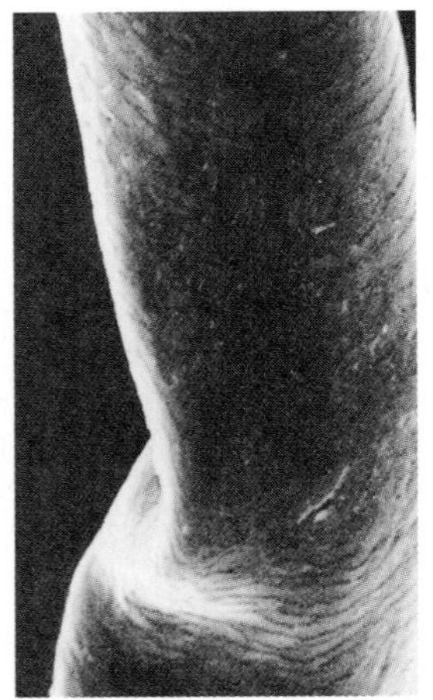

Figure 8–23 Monilethrix.

DISORDERS OF THE SCALP

The skin is in a constant state of renewal. The outer layer of skin that covers your body is constantly being shed and replaced by new cells from below. The average person sheds about nine pounds of "dead" skin each year. The skin cells of a normal, healthy scalp fall off naturally as small, dry flakes, without being noticed.

Dandruff can easily be mistaken for dry scalp because the symptoms of both conditions are a flaky, itchy, irritated scalp, but a dry scalp is dry, unlike the oily scalp that is common to dandruff. And the flakes from a dry scalp are much smaller and less noticeable than the larger flakes associated with dandruff. Dry scalp can result from contact dermatitis, sunburn, or extreme age and is usually worse in cold, dry climates.

Dandruff

Pityriasis (pit-ih-RY-uh-sus) is the medical term for dandruff, which is characterized by the excessive production and accumulation of skin cells. Instead of the normal shedding of individual skin cells, one at a time, dandruff results from the accumulation of clumps of cells large enough to be visible on the scalp, hair, or shoulders.

Although the cause of dandruff has been debated for over 150 years, current research confirms that dandruff is the result of a fungus originally named pityrosporum (spores of the scalp) and recently reclassified as **malassezia** (mal-uh-SEEZ-ee-uh).

Malassezia is a naturally occurring fungus that is present on all human skin but only develops the symptoms of dandruff when it grows out of control. Some individuals are also more susceptible to malassezia's irritating effects, and other factors like stress, age, hormones, and poor hygiene can cause the fungus to multiply and dandruff symptoms to worsen.

Older antidandruff treatments that relied on sulfur and coal tar were harsh to the skin and left the hair unmanageable. Modern antidandruff shampoos contain the antifungal agents pyrithione zinc, selenium sulfide, or ketoconazole that control dandruff by suppressing the growth of malassezia. Antidandruff shampoos that contain pyrithione zinc are available in a variety of formulas for all hair types and are gentle enough to be used everyday, even on color-treated hair. Frequent use of an antidandruff shampoo is essential for controlling dandruff. And although good personal hygiene and proper sanitation techniques are important, dandruff is not contagious.

The two principle types of dandruff are pityriasis capitis simplex and pitryiasis steatoides:

Pityriasis capitis simplex (pit-ih-RY-uh-sus KAP-ih-tis SIM-pleks) is the technical term for classic dandruff that is characterized by scalp irritation, large flakes, and an itchy scalp. The scales may attach to the scalp in masses, scatter loosely in the hair, or fall to the shoulders. Regular use of antidandruff shampoos, conditioners, and topical lotions are the best treatment.

Pityriasis steatoides (pit-ih-RY-uh-sus stee-uh-TOY-deez) is a more severe case of dandruff characterized by an accumulation of greasy or waxy scalp scales, mixed with sebum, that stick to the scalp in crusts. When accompanied by redness and inflammation the medical term is **seborrheic dermatitis** (seb-oh-REE-ik dur-muh-TY-tis). Occasionally, seborrheic dermatitis can also be found in the eyebrows or beard. A client with this condition should be referred to a physician.

Vegetable Parasitic Infections (Tinea)

Tinea (TIN-ee-uh) is the medical term for ringworm. It is characterized by itching, scales, and, sometimes, painful circular lesions. Several such patches may be present at one time. Ringworm is caused by vegetable parasites (fungi).

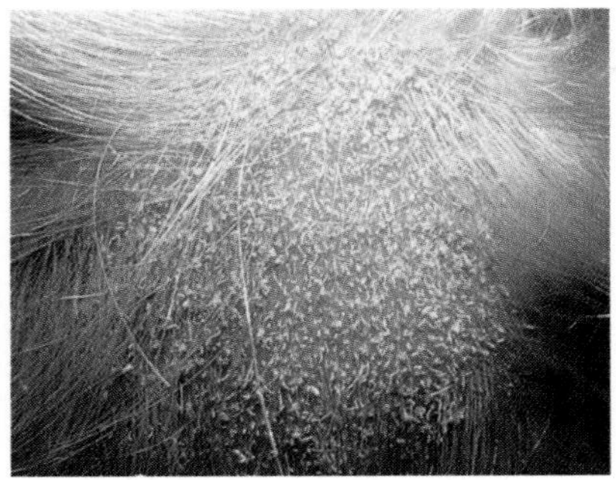

Figure 8-24 Tinea capitis.

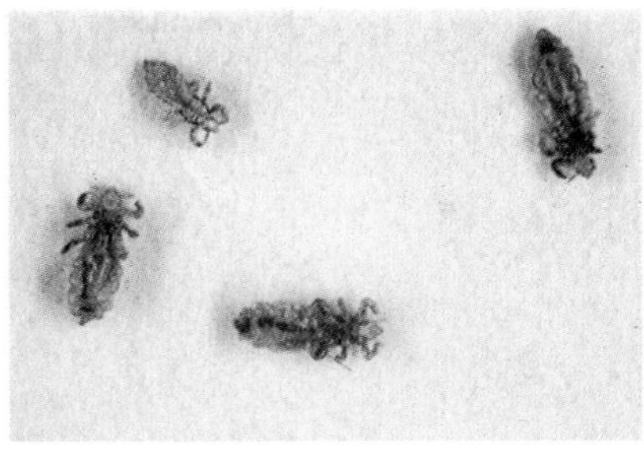

Figure 8-25 Head lice.

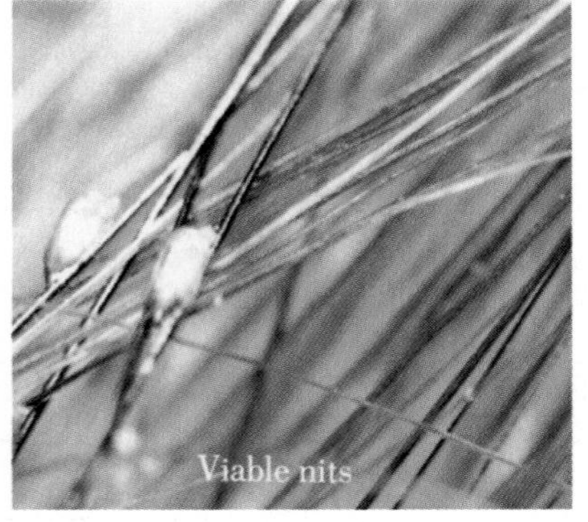

Figure 8-26 Nits (lice eggs).

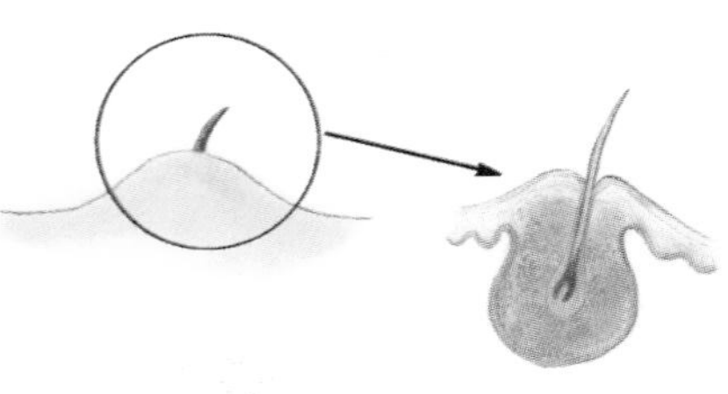

Figure 8-27 Furuncle (boil).

All forms of tinea are contagious and can be easily transmitted from one person to another. Infected skin scales or hairs that contain the fungi are known to spread the disease. Bathtubs, swimming pools, and unsanitary personal articles are also sources of transmission. Practicing approved sanitization and disinfection procedures will help prevent the spread of this disease. A client with this condition should be referred to a physician for medical treatment.

Tinea capitis (KAP-ih-tis) is commonly known as ringworm of the scalp. It is characterized by red papules, or spots, at the opening of the hair follicles (Figure 8–24). The patches spread and the hair becomes brittle and lifeless. Hair often breaks off, leaving only a stump, or may be shed from the enlarged open follicle.

Tinea favosa (fah-VOH-suh), also known as tinea favus (FAY-vus) or honycomb ringworm, is characterized by dry, sulfur-yellow, cup-like crusts on the scalp called **scutula** (SKUCH-ul-uh), which have a distinctive odor. Scars from favus are bald patches that may be pink or white and shiny.

Animal Parasitic Infections

Scabies "itch" is a highly contagious skin disease caused by the itch mite burrowing under the skin (see Figure 5–7 in Chapter 5). Vesicles (blisters) and pustules (inflamed pimples with pus) usually form on the scalp from the irritation caused by this animal parasite. Excessive itching results in scratching the infected areas and makes the condition worse. Practicing approved sanitization and disinfection procedures will help prevent the spread of this disease. A client with this condition should be referred to a physician for medical treatment.

Pediculosis capitis (puh-dik-yuh-LOH-sis KAP-ih-tis) is the infestation of the hair and scalp with head lice (Figure 8–25 and Figure 8–26). As these animal parasites feed on the scalp, itching occurs and the scratching that usually results can cause an infection. Head lice are transmitted from one person to another by contact with infested hats, combs, brushes, and other personal articles. You can distinguish them from dandruff flakes by looking closely at the scalp with a magnifying glass.

Practicing approved sanitization and disinfection procedures will help prevent the spread of this disease. Several nonprescription medications are available. A client with this condition should be referred to a physician or pharmacist.

Staphylococci Infections

The two most common types of staphylococci infections are furuncles and carbuncles.

A **furuncle** (FYOO-rung-kul) or boil is an acute, localized bacterial infection of the hair follicle that produces constant pain (Figure 8–27). It is limited to a specific area and produces a pustule perforated by a hair.

A **carbuncle** (KAHR-bung-kul) is an inflammation of the subcutaneous tissue caused by staphylococci. It is similar to a furuncle but is larger.

Practicing approved sanitization and disinfection procedures will help prevent the spread of these diseases. A client with either condition should be referred to a physician for medical treatment. 8

chapter glossary

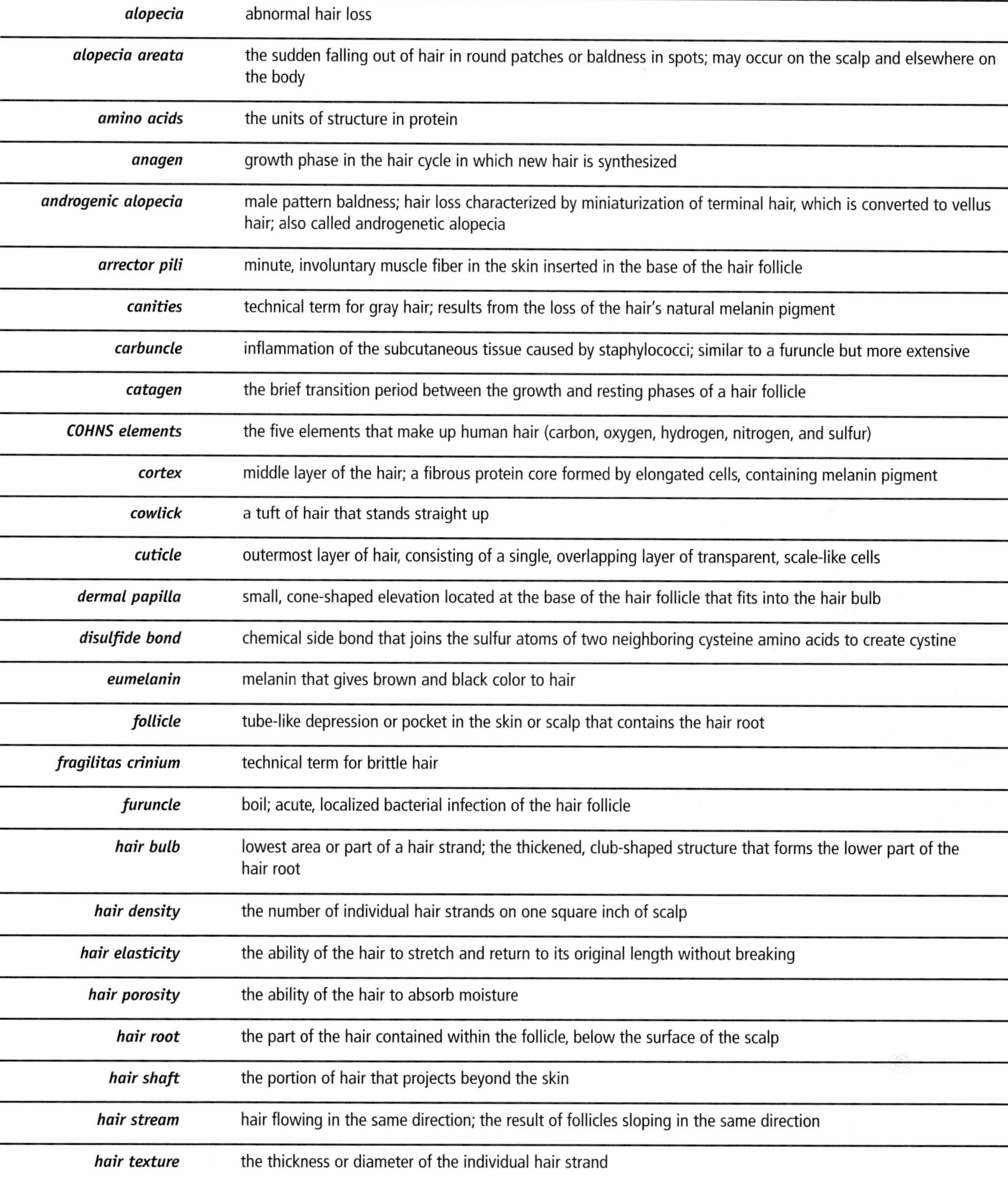

alopecia	abnormal hair loss
alopecia areata	the sudden falling out of hair in round patches or baldness in spots; may occur on the scalp and elsewhere on the body
amino acids	the units of structure in protein
anagen	growth phase in the hair cycle in which new hair is synthesized
androgenic alopecia	male pattern baldness; hair loss characterized by miniaturization of terminal hair, which is converted to vellus hair; also called androgenetic alopecia
arrector pili	minute, involuntary muscle fiber in the skin inserted in the base of the hair follicle
canities	technical term for gray hair; results from the loss of the hair's natural melanin pigment
carbuncle	inflammation of the subcutaneous tissue caused by staphylococci; similar to a furuncle but more extensive
catagen	the brief transition period between the growth and resting phases of a hair follicle
COHNS elements	the five elements that make up human hair (carbon, oxygen, hydrogen, nitrogen, and sulfur)
cortex	middle layer of the hair; a fibrous protein core formed by elongated cells, containing melanin pigment
cowlick	a tuft of hair that stands straight up
cuticle	outermost layer of hair, consisting of a single, overlapping layer of transparent, scale-like cells
dermal papilla	small, cone-shaped elevation located at the base of the hair follicle that fits into the hair bulb
disulfide bond	chemical side bond that joins the sulfur atoms of two neighboring cysteine amino acids to create cystine
eumelanin	melanin that gives brown and black color to hair
follicle	tube-like depression or pocket in the skin or scalp that contains the hair root
fragilitas crinium	technical term for brittle hair
furuncle	boil; acute, localized bacterial infection of the hair follicle
hair bulb	lowest area or part of a hair strand; the thickened, club-shaped structure that forms the lower part of the hair root
hair density	the number of individual hair strands on one square inch of scalp
hair elasticity	the ability of the hair to stretch and return to its original length without breaking
hair porosity	the ability of the hair to absorb moisture
hair root	the part of the hair contained within the follicle, below the surface of the scalp
hair shaft	the portion of hair that projects beyond the skin
hair stream	hair flowing in the same direction; the result of follicles sloping in the same direction
hair texture	the thickness or diameter of the individual hair strand

chapter glossary *(continued)*

hair texture	the thickness or diameter of the individual hair strand
hydrogen bond	physical side bond that is easily broken by water or heat
hypertrichosis	condition of abnormal growth of hair, characterized by the growth of terminal hair in areas of the body that normally grow only vellus hair; also called hirsuties
keratinization	the process of being keratinized; as newly formed cells in the hair mature, they fill up with keratin, move upward, lose their nucleus, and die; the hair shaft is a nonliving fiber composed of keratinized protein
malassezia	reclassified term for the fungus originally named pityrosporum
medulla	innermost layer of the hair, sometimes referred to as the pith; composed of round cells; often absent in fine hair
melanin	tiny grains of pigment in the cortex that give natural color to the hair
monilethrix	technical term for beaded hair
pediculosis capitis	infestation of the hair and scalp with head lice
peptide bond	chemical bond that joins amino acids to each other; also called end bond
pheomelanin	melanin that provides natural hair colors from red and ginger to yellow/blonde tones
pityriasis	dandruff; an inflammation of the skin characterized by the formation and flaking of fine, thin scales
pityriasis capitis simplex	technical term for scalp inflammation marked by dry dandruff, thin scales, and an itchy scalp
pityriasis steatoides	scalp inflammation marked by fatty (greasy or waxy) types of dandruff
polypeptide chain	long chain of amino acids linked by peptide bonds
postpartum alopecia	temporary hair loss experienced at the conclusion of a pregnancy
ringed hair	variety of canities, characterized by alternating bands of gray and pigmented hair throughout the length of the hair strand
salt bond	physical side bond that is broken by changes in pH
scutula	dry, sulfur-yellow, cup-like crusts on the scalp in tinea favosa or favus
sebaceous glands	oil glands of the skin, connected to the hair follicles
sebum	fatty or oily secretion of the sebaceous glands, which lubricates the hair and skin
telogen	resting phase; the final phase in the hair cycle that lasts until the fully grown hair is shed
terminal hair	the long, soft hair found on the scalp, also on legs, arms, and body of both males and females
tinea	medical term for ringworm; contagious condition caused by vegetable parasites
tinea capitis	ringworm of the scalp
tinea favosa	ringworm characterized by dry, sulfur-yellow, cup-like crusts on the scalp, called scutula; also known as tinea favus or honeycomb ringworm
trichology	the science dealing with the hair, its diseases, and care

trichoptilosis	technical term for split ends
trichorrhexis nodosa	knotted hair, characterized by brittleness and the formation of nodular swellings along the hair shaft
vellus or lanugo	short, fine, downy hair that appears on the body, with the exception of the palms of the hands and the soles of the feet
wave pattern	amount of movement in the hair strand; described as straight, wavy, curly, and extremely curly
whorl	hair that forms in a circular pattern, as on the crown

review questions

1. Name and describe the five main structures of the hair root.
2. Name and describe the three layers of the hair.
3. Explain the process of keratinization.
4. List and describe the three types of side bonds.
5. What are the differences between end bonds and side bonds?
6. Name and describe the two types of melanin responsible for natural hair color.
7. What four factors about the hair should be considered in a hair analysis?
8. Name and describe the different types of hair and their locations on the body.
9. What are the three phases of the hair growth cycle? What occurs during each one?
10. What is the reason for normal daily hair loss?
11. What are the most common types of abnormal hair loss?
12. What are the only two approved hair loss treatments?
13. Name the two main types of dandruff. Can either one be treated in the salon?
14. Which of these scalp and hair disorders cannot be treated in the salon: tinea capitis, trichoptilosis, trichorrhexis nodosa, ringed hair, tinea favosa, carbuncles, hypertrichosis, pediculosis capitis, scabies, monilethrix, fragilitas crinium, canities, and furuncles.

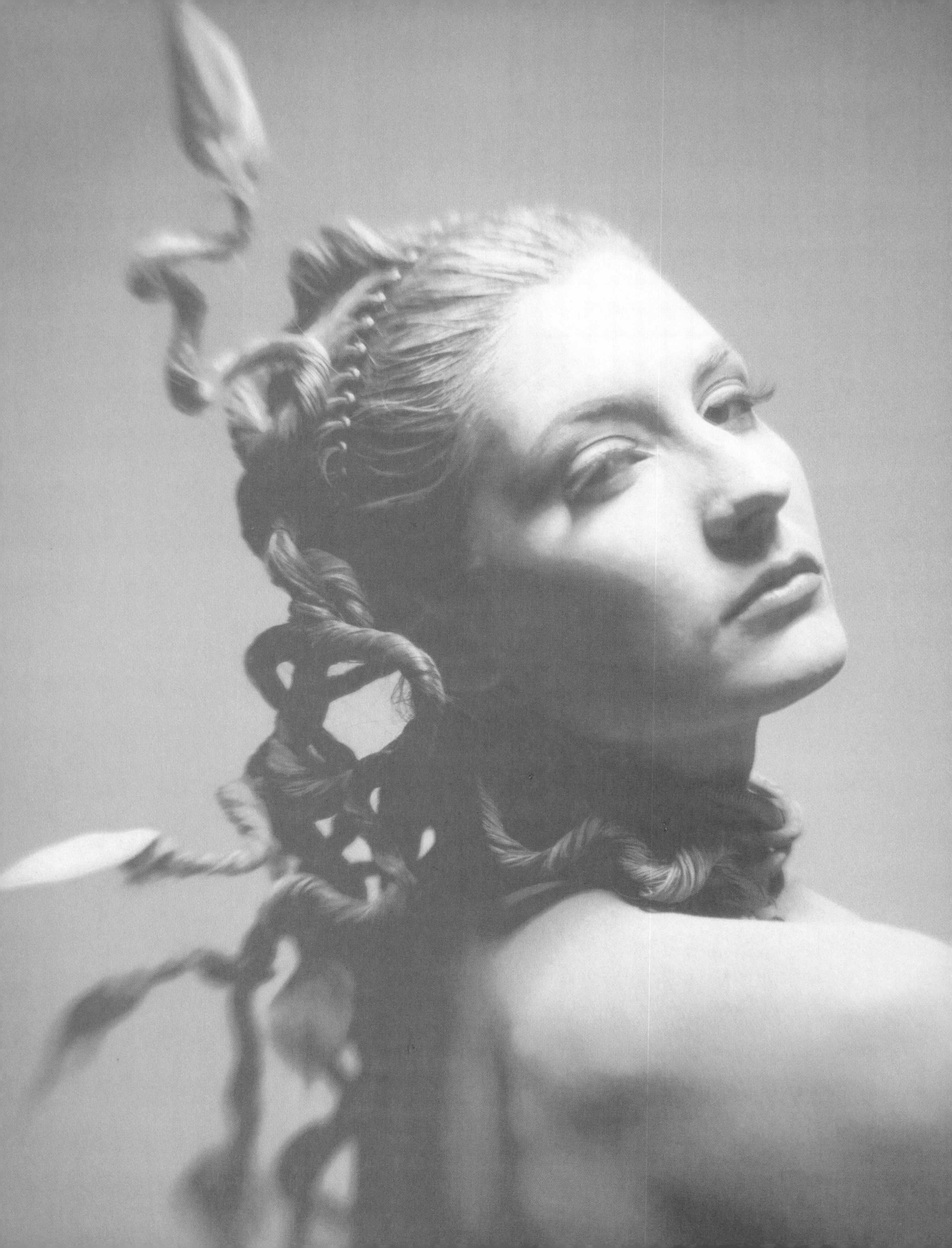

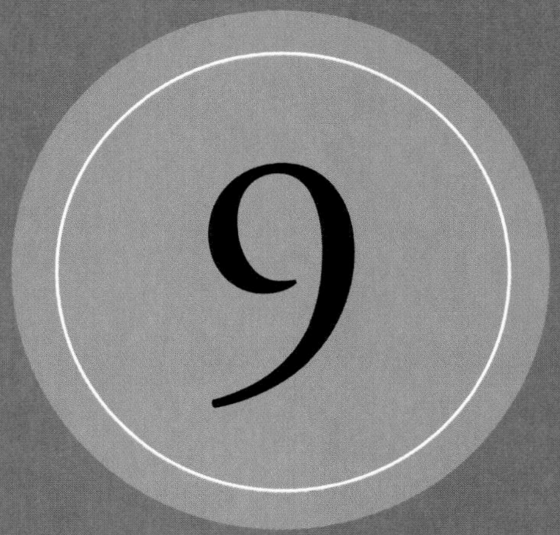

PRINCIPLES OF HAIR DESIGN

Mary Brunetti

FREELANCE AND CELEBRITY HAIRSTYLIST,
1991 NORTH AMERICAN HAIRSTYLIST OF THE YEAR

Chapter Outline

Learning Objectives

After completing this chapter, you should be able to:

1. **List the five elements of hair design.**
2. **List the five principles of hair design.**
3. **Identify different facial shapes.**
4. **Demonstrate how to design hairstyles to enhance or camouflage facial features.**
5. **Explain design considerations for men.**

National Skill Standards

This chapter provides you with the necessary information to master these National Industry Skill Standards for Entry-Level Cosmetologists.

Consulting with clients to determine their needs and preferences.

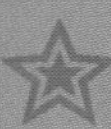
Providing styling and finishing techniques to complete a hairstyle to the satisfaction of the client.

Key Terms

Page number indicates where in the chapter the term is used.

asymmetrical balance
pg. 238

balance
pg. 237

concave
pg. 245

contrasting lines
pg. 233

convex
pg. 245

diagonal lines
pg. 231

emphasis
pg. 238

form
pg. 230

fringe
pg. 248

harmony
pg. 238

horizontal lines
pg. 231

parallel
pg. 231

proportion
pg. 236

profile
pg. 245

rhythm
pg. 238

space
pg. 231

symmetrical balance
pg. 237

transitional lines
pg. 233

vertical lines
pg. 231

Design is the foundation of any artistic application. All designers—architects, clothing designers, interior designers, and others—have a strong visual orientation. So do you, if you have chosen to pursue a career in hairstyling and beauty.

As a stylist, your goal is to learn how to design the appropriate hairstyle for your client. That process begins with analyzing the entire person, using the elements and principles of design with an understanding of how they can enhance your client's positive features and minimize negative features. This is only possible if you have a firm grounding in the philosophy of design. A good grasp of the philosophy of design will help you develop real artistic skill and judgment. Over time, you will become more and more competent with your design skills.

It takes practice and experience to recognize facial types and to make the appropriate design decisions. Choosing the best possible design for your client will determine whether you are known as a good stylist or a great one.

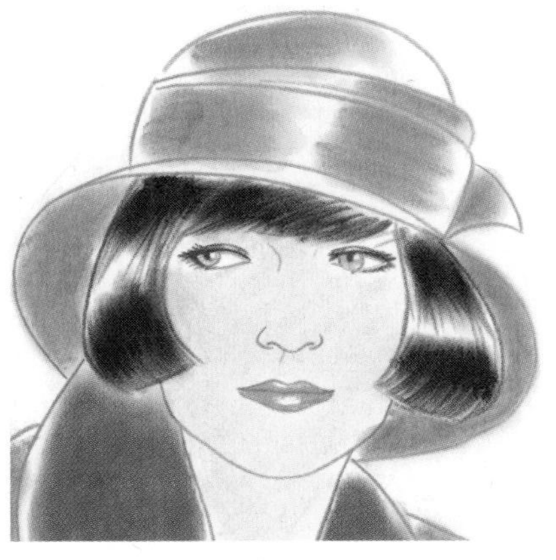

Figure 9–1 A bob haircut from the 1920s.

PHILOSOPHY OF DESIGN

A good designer always visualizes the finished product before beginning a project. For instance, when an architect designs a building, he first visualizes it completed, then takes the necessary steps backward to create the design. The first step in this creative process has to do with inspiration.

Inspiration can come to you from almost anywhere during the course of a day. A newspaper, the TV, the radio, faces on the bus, food, furniture, toys, and so on often spark the creative process. One of the most common sources of inspiration is nature itself. Ocean waves have inspired painters, poets, composers, and hairstylists, as have the shapes and colors of a flower, a leaf, or a star. Sometimes, you may find yourself looking to the past for inspiration. Hairstyles from earlier times might inspire you, as you seek to reinvent them in a way that makes sense for contemporary life (Figure 9–1 and Figure 9–2). Looking at the fashion pages of magazines is always inspiring, because hair typically follows fashion.

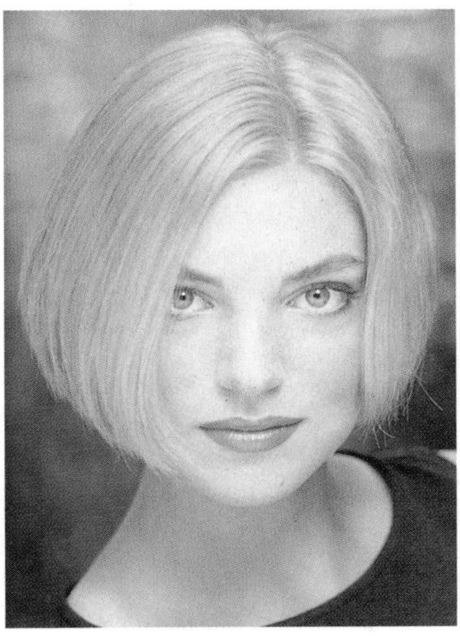

Figure 9–2 A contemporary bob.

Once you are inspired, you will then decide which applications and tools are needed to achieve your design, such as cutting shears, Velcro rollers, permanent wave, haircolor, and so forth. It is always a good idea when working out a design to practice first on a mannequin head. There is always the chance, as you develop or practice a technique, that your concept might turn into something entirely different from what you set out to do. This kind of spontaneity is what makes the creative process exciting and satisfying.

As a designer, you will need to develop a strong visual understanding of which hairstyles work best on which face shapes and body types. As noted, it takes time to train your eye to recognize the correct design decision. Even with all the instruction you will be getting in this chapter, you cannot achieve a trained eye simply through book-learning. It will benefit you to review these pages over and over, but do not get frustrated if it takes a while for this strong visual understanding to sink in. Sometimes, the best teacher is time and the trial and error that comes with experience. All experienced stylists have a significant number of "design mistakes" in their histories.

Learning the rules—the foundation of your craft—is imperative. This foundation will make you a truly talented stylist. Once you have your skills down to a science, your creative juices can kick in and you can move beyond the basics.

Having a strong foundation in technique and skills will allow you to take calculated risks. It is important in this field to take those risks. Too many stylists confine themselves to the basics where they feel safe. But "safe" can translate into "dull." If you are looking for a satisfying career over the long run, do not allow yourself to become what is typically known in the industry as a "cookie cutter" hairdresser who learns a new haircut and then gives it to everyone who sits in her chair for the next month. Always explore new possibilities, catering to each client's individual needs and lifestyle. Otherwise, you may find yourself in a styling rut, typically known as "the box." Great hairstylists find inspiration everywhere, keep an eye out for what is new in the industry, and dedicate themselves to their continuing education. Remember that, as a stylist, you are a designer, and designers are always growing and learning.

ELEMENTS OF HAIR DESIGN

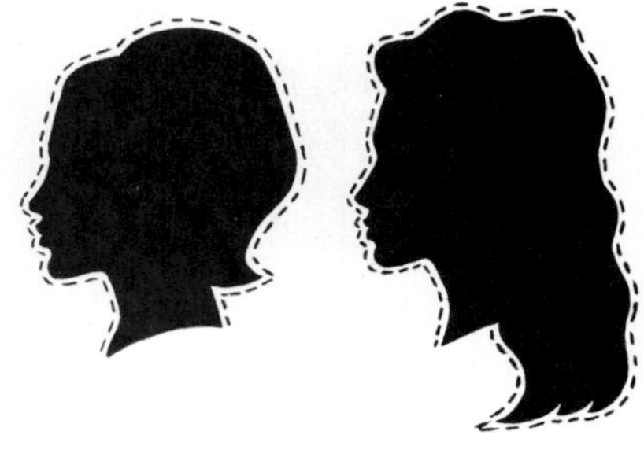

Figure 9-3 The outline of the hairstyle is the form.

To begin to understand the creative process involved in hairstyling, it is critical to learn the five basic elements of hair design. These elements are form, space, line, color, and wave pattern.

Form

Form is the outline of the overall hairstyle as seen from all angles. It is three-dimensional and changes as it is viewed from different angles. The silhouette is typically the aspect of the overall design that a client will react to first. Generally, it is best to use forms that are simple and pleasing to the eye. The hair form should be in proportion to the shape of the head and face, the length and width of the neck, and the shoulder line (Figure 9–3).

Space

Space is the area that the hairstyle occupies, also thought of as the area inside the form. Space may also be called volume. It is three-dimensional, and has length, width, and depth (Figure 9–4). The space may contain curls, curves, waves, straight hair, or a combination of these.

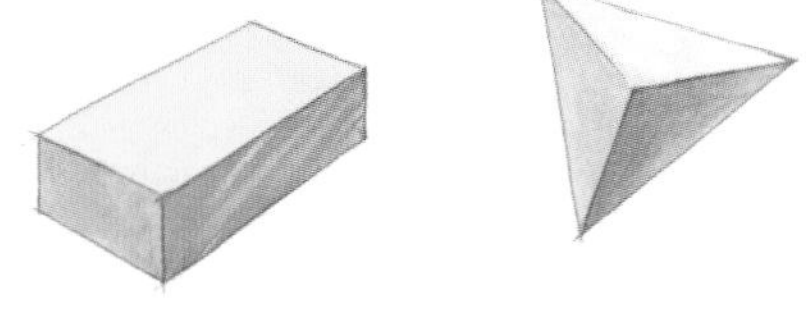

Figure 9–4 Space is three-dimensional.

Line

The eye follows the lines in a design. Lines create the form, design, and movement of a hairstyle. They can be straight or curved. There are four basic types of lines.

1. **Horizontal lines** are **parallel**—extending in the same direction and maintaining a constant distance apart—to the floor or horizon. A horizontal line creates width in hair design because the eye follows the line from the center out to the ends (Figure 9–5).
2. **Vertical lines** are straight up and down. They make a hairstyle appear longer and narrower as the eye follows the lines up and down (Figure 9–6).
3. **Diagonal lines** are positioned between horizontal and vertical lines. They are often used to emphasize or minimize facial features. Diagonal lines are also used to create interest in hair design (Figure 9–7).

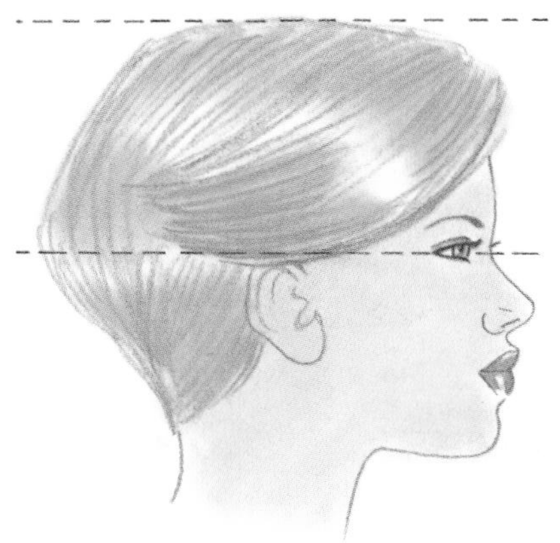

Figure 9–5 Horizontal lines in a hairstyle.

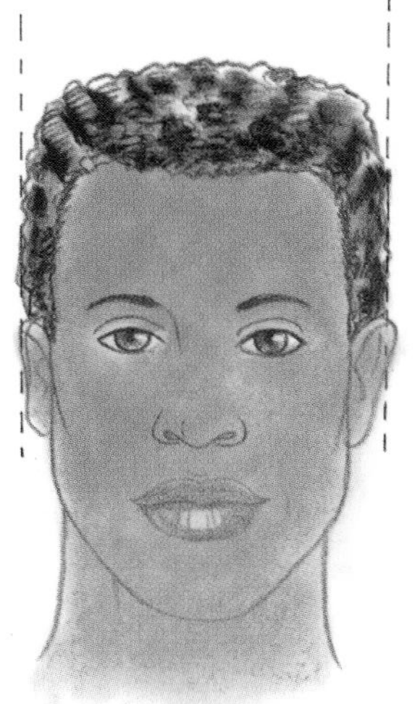

Figure 9–6 Vertical lines in a hairstyle.

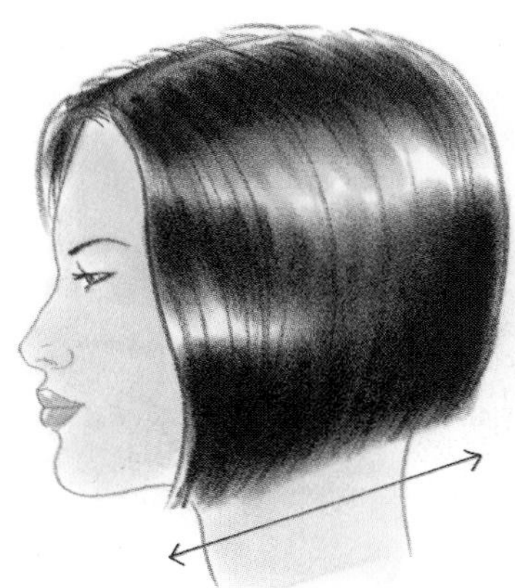

Figure 9–7 Diagonal lines in a hairstyle.

9

insights

Sonny Betts

The owner of a successful salon in St. Paul, Minnesota, Sonny Betts has spent 22 years in the industry but keeps looking ahead.

For me, the greatest challenge in becoming a cosmetologist was getting the big picture. I had a hard time understanding how shape is perceived and how it's executed. Sure, I studied it all in beauty school, but I didn't have that "Aha!" moment until I had been in the industry for about three years. I was going at it pretty randomly and then one day, miraculously, it clicked for me. Taking a lot of classes was crucial. I'm one of those goal-oriented people, and I just always took extra training in anything I could get ahold of.

I'm very passionate about what I do. I love making people feel really good about themselves. I think the key to success as a stylist, to building that loyal client base, is making yourself available. In the world we live in today, people are so stretched. Both parents are working long hours. So putting in your time at night and working on Saturdays shows that you're accommodating those clients.

This business is all about service, when you come down to it. It's about giving a good cut, talking to the client about the products that will work well at home so that they can duplicate what you've done in the salon, doing a makeup touch-up before they leave your chair, and closing the deal. A lot of people in the field go blank when you say, "closing the deal." It means getting the client to buy the products you're promoting, scheduling their next service, upselling their next service—that kind of thing.

It's funny: you have to be good at selling, but you have to not think of it as selling. You have to think of it as helping people look their best. Most hairdressers don't go into this business to be salespersons. If that were the case, they would have gone into another line of work. I think one reason a lot of hairdressers are not successful is because they feel they have to sell. If only they took a different approach and looked at it from the angle of helping their clients, it would be so much easier. The selling gets easier when you've got the passion.

People who are really passionate about their craft will succeed, even if they're working in a salon that's not in a great location. Word of mouth will get out. This holds true for any field you go into: if you're not passionate about something, you'll just be average; but if you're passionate about it, then you'll be extremely successful.

4. **Curved lines** soften a design. They can be large or small, a full circle, or just part of a circle (Figure 9–8). They can be placed horizontally, vertically, or diagonally. Curved lines repeating in opposite directions create a wave (Figure 9–9).

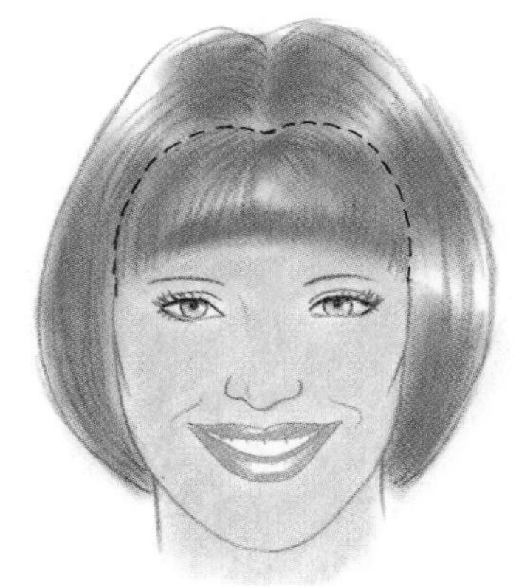

Figure 9-8 Curved lines in a hairstyle.

Designing with Lines

Four kinds of hairstyles can be developed based on the type of lines you choose.

1. Single-line hairstyles are best worn on clients who require the minimum of care when styling their hair. An example of this is the one-length hairstyle (Figure 9–10).
2. Repeating lines are parallel lines in a hairstyle. They can be straight or curved. The repetition of lines creates more interest in the design. A finger wave is an example of a style using curved, repeating lines (Figure 9–11).
3. **Contrasting lines** are horizontal and vertical lines that meet at a 90-degree angle. These lines create a hard edge. Contrasting lines in a design are usually reserved for clients with the personality to carry off a strong look (Figure 9–12).
4. **Transitional lines** are usually curved lines that are used to blend and soften horizontal or vertical lines (Figure 9–13).

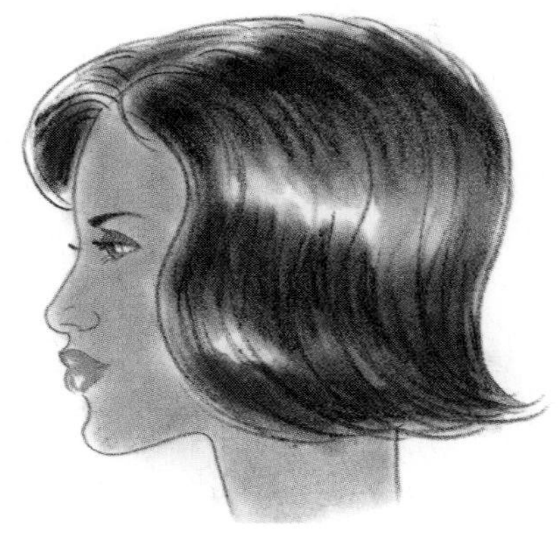

Figure 9-9 Wave.

Color

Color plays an important role in hair design, both visually and psychologically. It can also be used to make all or part of the design appear larger or smaller. Color can help create textures and lines and can tie the design elements together. In Chapter 16, you will learn more about creating hair designs that include haircolor as an important element.

The power of color is something that most people are not consciously aware of. Certain colors tend to evoke certain reactions. Lighter colors seem

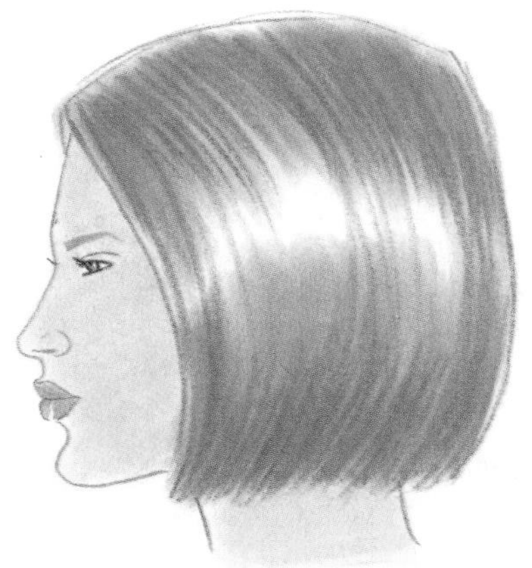

Figure 9-10 Single-line hairstyle.

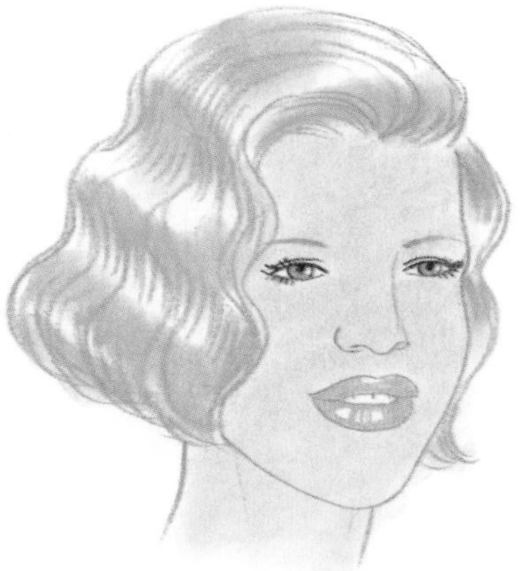

Figure 9-11 Repeating lines in a hairstyle.

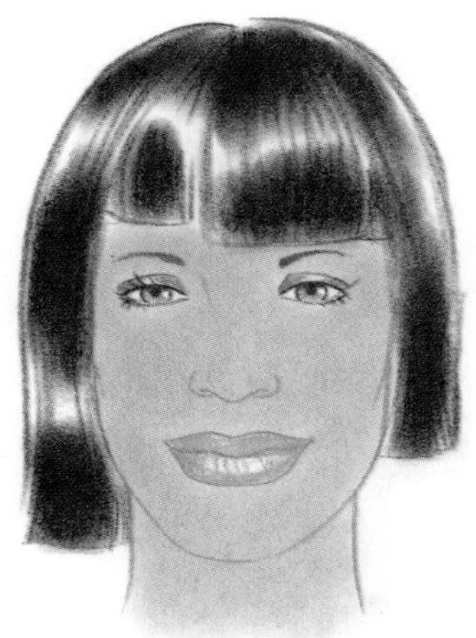

Figure 9-12 Contrasting lines.

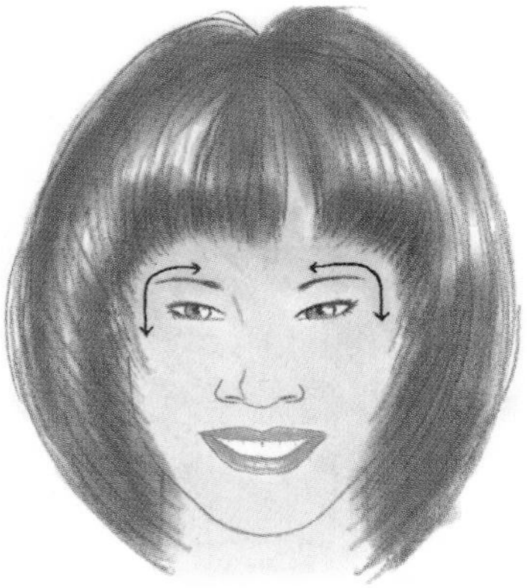

Figure 9-13 Transitional lines.

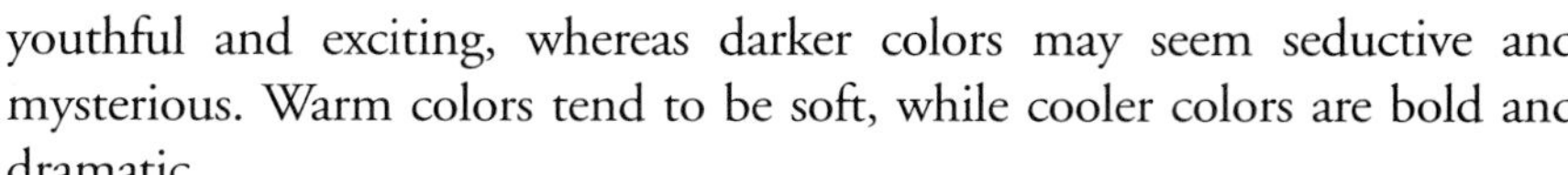

youthful and exciting, whereas darker colors may seem seductive and mysterious. Warm colors tend to be soft, while cooler colors are bold and dramatic.

Creating Dimension with Color

Light colors and warm colors create the illusion of volume. Dark and cool colors recede or move in toward the head, creating the illusion of less volume. The illusion of dimension, or depth, is created when colors that are warm and cool alternate with those that are light and dark (Figure 9–14 and Figure 9–15).

Creating Lines with Color

Using a lighter color, you can draw a line in the hairstyle in the direction you want the eye to travel. A single line of color or a series of repeated lines can create a bold, dramatic accent (Figure 9–16).

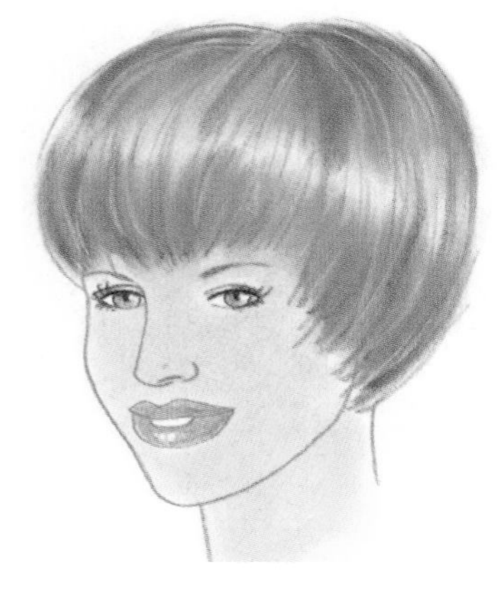

Figure 9-14 Light colors appear closer to the surface.

Color Selection

Before choosing a color, be sure that the tone is compatible with the skin tones of the client. In other words, if a client has gold tones in her skin, select warm hair colors, not transparent cool tones. When using two or more colors, choose colors with similar tones within two levels of each other. When using high-contrast colors, use one color sparingly. Too much contrast will create an attention-grabbing look and should only be used on clients who are very trendy and can carry off a bold look (Figure 9–17).

Wave Pattern

All hair has a natural wave pattern, which is described as straight, wavy, curly, or extremely curly (see Chapter 8). This wave pattern must be taken into consideration when designing a style for your client. For example, straight hair reflects light better than other wave patterns, so it reflects the most light

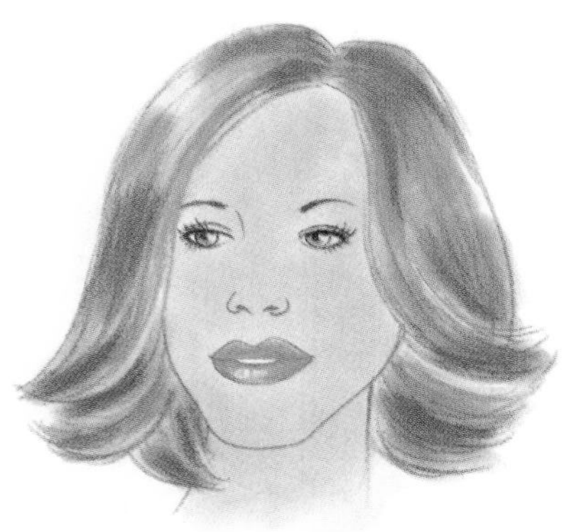

Figure 9-15 Creating dimension with color.

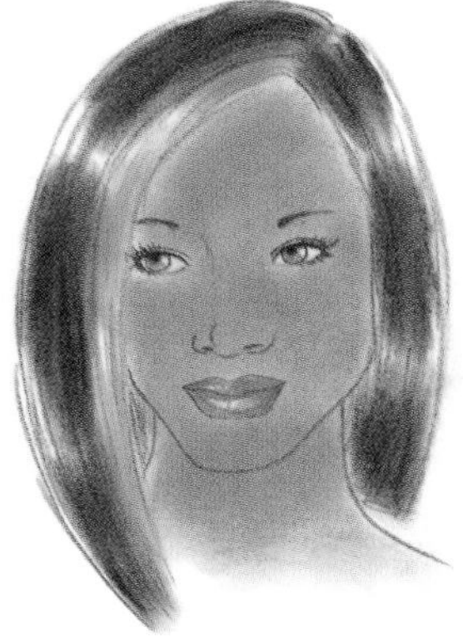

Figure 9-16 Contrasting color accents the line.

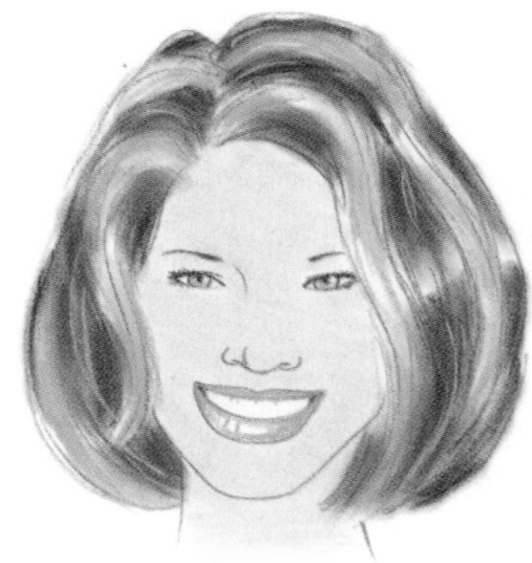

Figure 9-17 Vivid color contrast.

when it is cut to one length (Figure 9–18). Wavy hair can be combed into waves that create horizontal lines (Figure 9–19). Curly and extremely curly hair does not reflect much light and could be coarse to the touch. It creates a larger form than straight or wavy hair (Figure 9–20 and Figure 9–21).

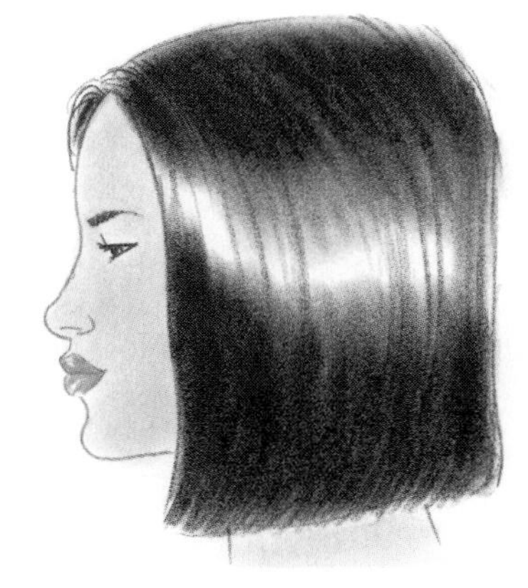

Figure 9-18 Straight hair.

Creating Wave Patterns with Styling Tools

Wave patterns can be created temporarily with the use of heat or wet styling techniques. Curling irons or hot rollers can be used to create a wave or curl. Curly hair can be straightened with a blow-dryer or flat iron (Figure 9–22). Crimping irons are used to create interesting and unusual wave patterns like zigzags. Hair can also be wet-set with rollers or pin curls to create curls and waves. Finger waves are another way of creating temporary wave pattern changes (Figure 9–23, Figure 9–24, and Figure 9–25). You will learn more about styling techniques in the chapters that follow.

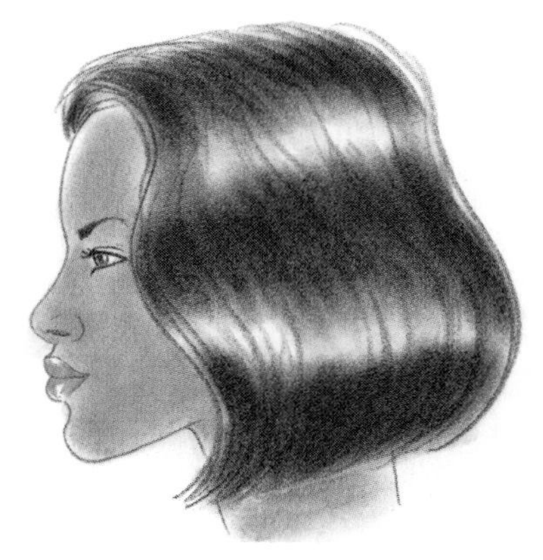

Figure 9-19 Wavy hair.

Changing Wave Patterns with Chemicals

Chemical wave pattern changes are considered permanent (Figure 9–26). They last until the new growth is long enough to alter the design. Curly hair can be straightened with relaxers, while straight hair can be curled with permanent waves. These techniques are covered in detail in Chapter 15.

Tips for Designing with Wave Patterns

Using too many wave pattern combinations together could create a look that is overly busy. This is fine for a young client who wants to achieve a multitextured look, but this would be less appropriate for a conservative professional client. Smooth wave patterns accent the face and are particularly useful when you wish to narrow a round head shape (Figure 9–27). Curly wave patterns take attention away from the face and can be used to soften square or rectangular features (Figure 9–28). 1

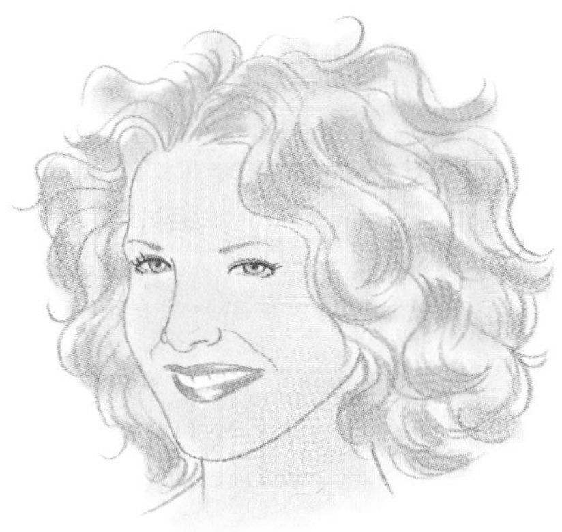

Figure 9-20 Curly hair.

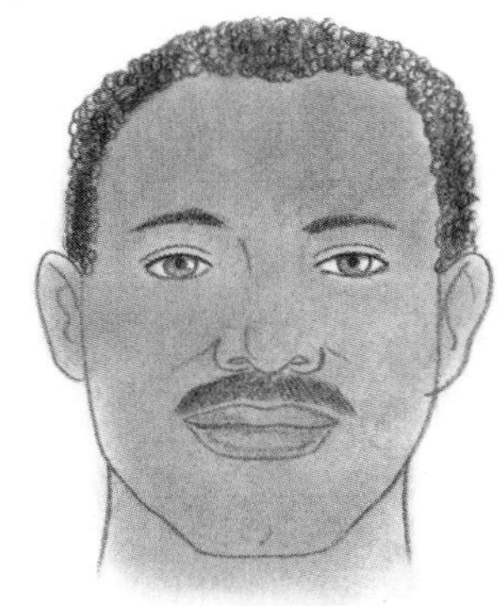

Figure 9-21 Very curly hair.

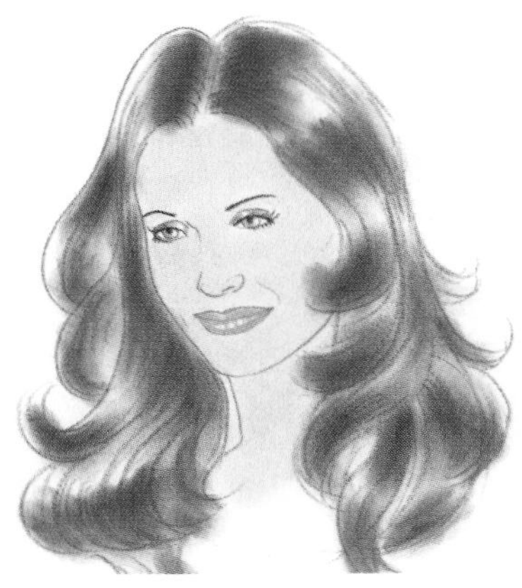

Figure 9-22 Wave patterns can be altered temporarily.

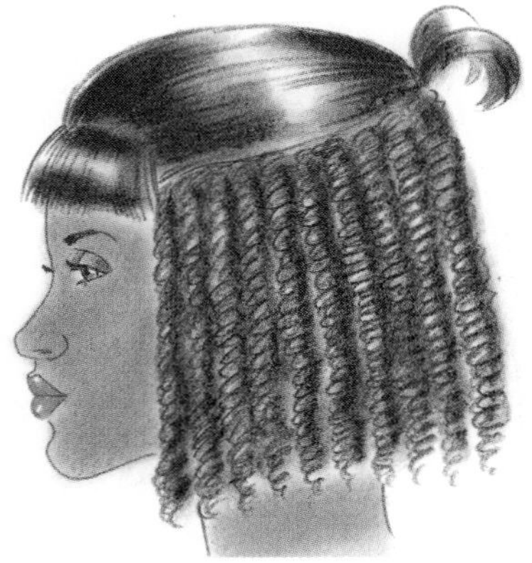

Figure 9-23 Combining wave patterns.

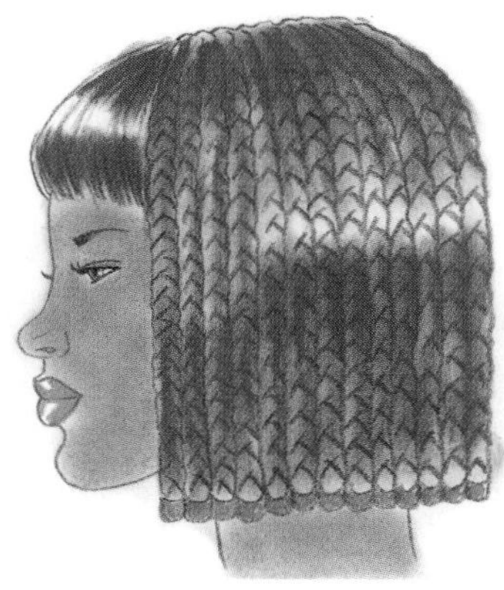

Figure 9-24 Fine braids create temporary waves.

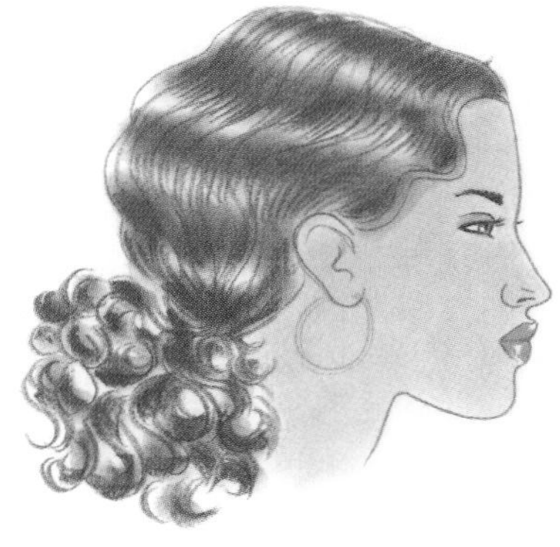

Figure 9-25 Finger waves and curls.

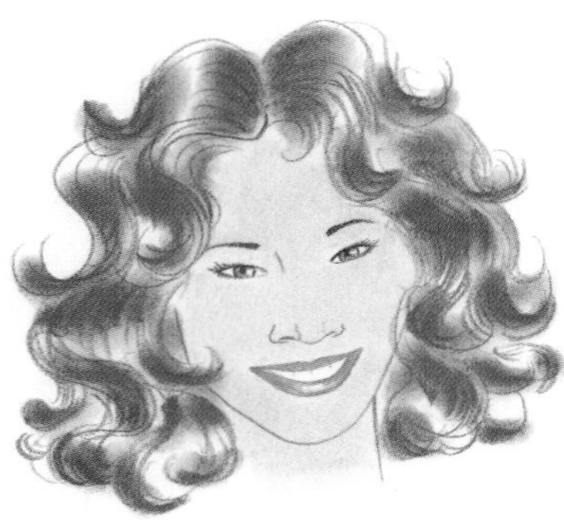

Figure 9-26 Chemically altered hairstyle.

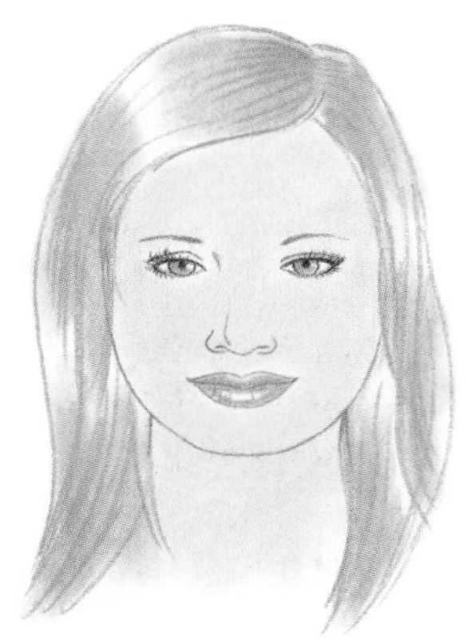

Figure 9-27 Straight wave patterns are flattering on round faces.

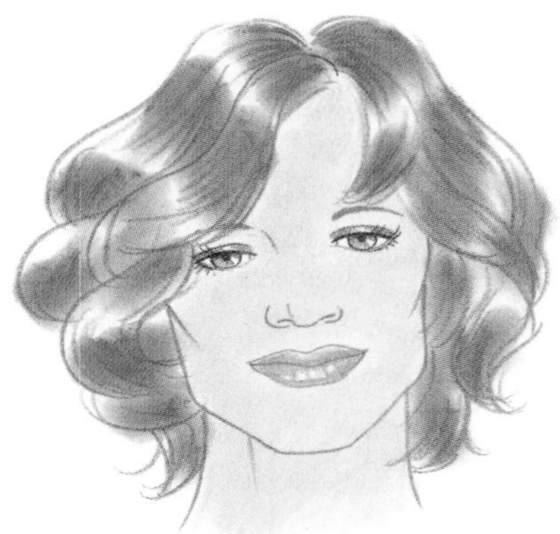

Figure 9-28 Curly wave patterns soften angular faces.

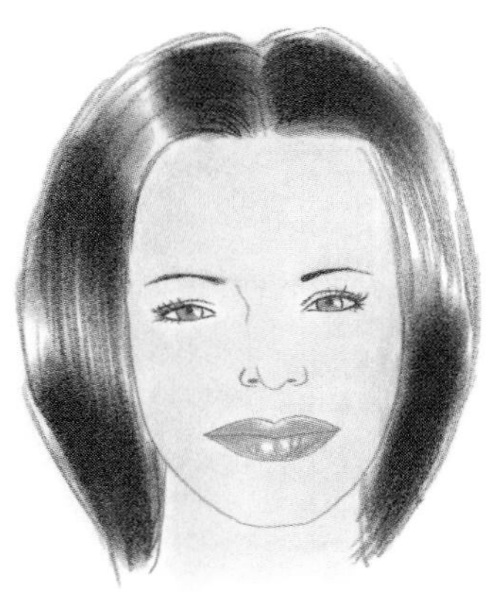

Figure 9-29 Facial features out of proportion.

PRINCIPLES OF HAIR DESIGN

There are certain principles by which we judge the quality of a hairstyling design. The better you understand these principles, the more confident you can feel about creating styles that are pleasing to the eye. The five principles important for art design are also the basis of hair design. They are proportion, balance, rhythm, emphasis, and harmony.

Proportion

Proportion is the harmonious relationship between parts or things, or the comparative relation of one thing to another. For example, a 60-inch TV set might be considered out of proportion in a very small bedroom. A 20-inch TV would be more proportionate to the room. A person with a very small chin and a very wide forehead might be said to have a head shape that is out of proportion. The right hairstyle would go a long way toward correcting the problem, giving the illusion of proper proportion (Figure 9–29 and Figure 9–30).

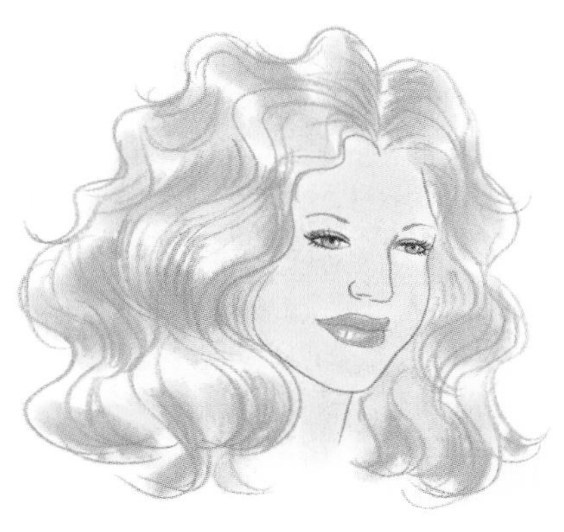

Figure 9-30 Hair out of proportion to face.

Body Proportion

It is essential when designing hairstyles that you take into account the client's body proportions. Problems in body proportion become more obvious if the hair form is too small or too large. When choosing a style for a woman with large hips or broad shoulders, for instance, you would normally create a style with more volume (Figure 9–31). But the same large hair form would appear out of proportion on a petite woman (Figure 9–32). When designing a hairstyle, keep in mind that the hair should not be wider than the center of the shoulders, regardless of the body structure.

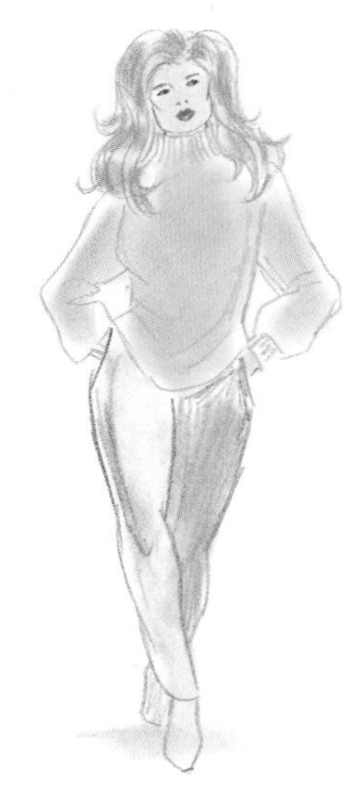

Figure 9-31 A large hairstyle balances a large body structure.

Balance

Balance means harmony or proportion; in hairstyling, it signifies the proper degree of height and width. Balance can be symmetrical or asymmetrical. If you are dissatisfied with a finished hair design, it is often because the style is out of balance. To measure symmetry, divide the face into four equal parts. Where the lines cross is the central axis, the reference point for judging the balance of the hair design. You can then decide if the hairstyle looks pleasing to the eye and is in correct balance (Figure 9–33).

In **symmetrical balance**, the design is similar on both sides of the face. Both sides of the hairstyle are the same distance from the center, the same length, and have the same volume when viewed from the front. The sides may have the same shape or a different shape but will still have the same volume. These shapes are generally less trendy than asymmetrical styles (Figure 9–34, Figure 9–35, and Figure 9–36).

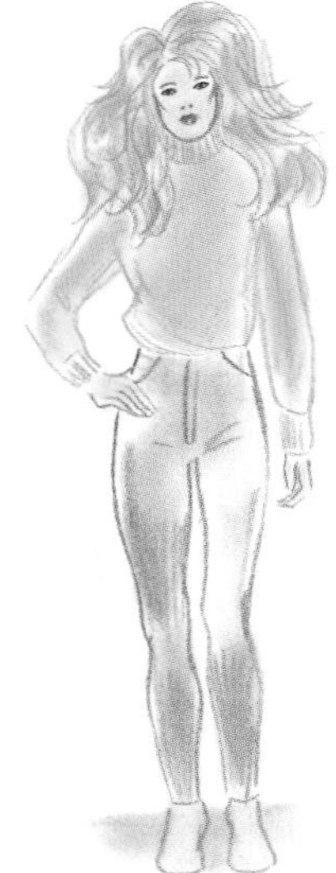

Figure 9-32 A large hairstyle makes a petite woman look smaller.

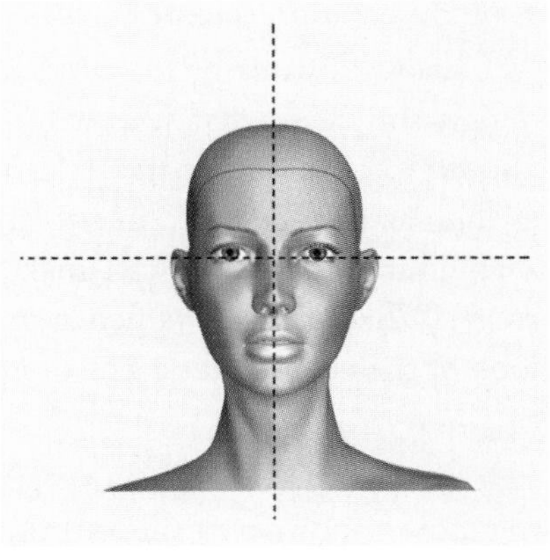

Figure 9-33 Measuring symmetry of the head.

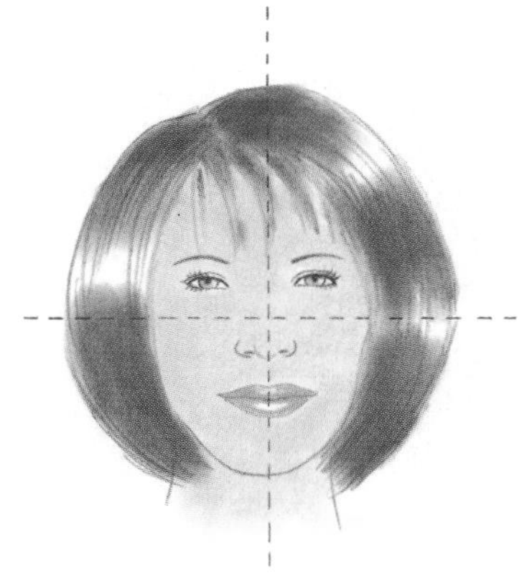

Figure 9-34 Both sides equidistant from center.

9

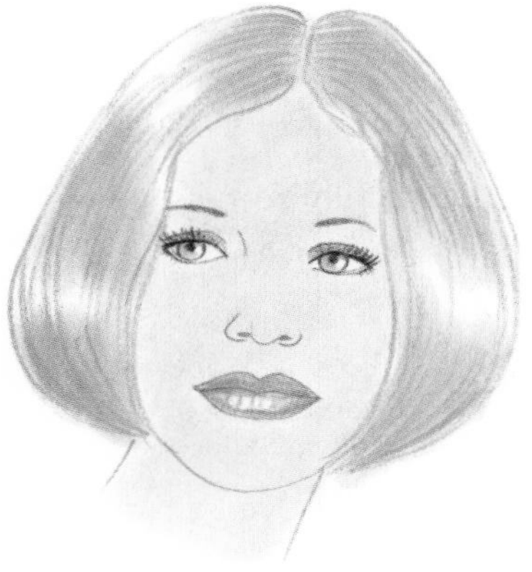

Figure 9-35 Perfect symmetry.

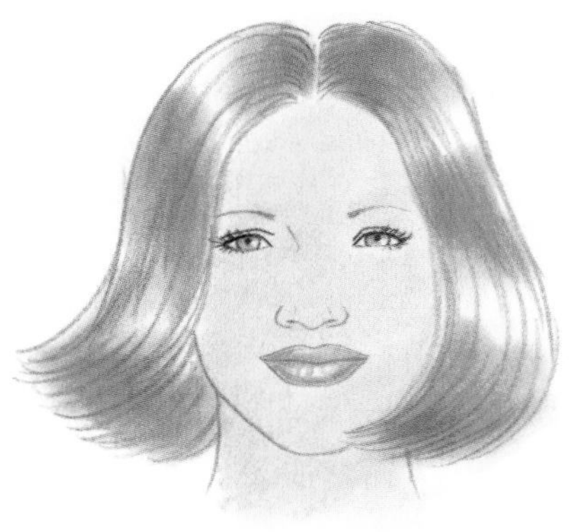

Figure 9-36 Symmetry with different shapes, same volume.

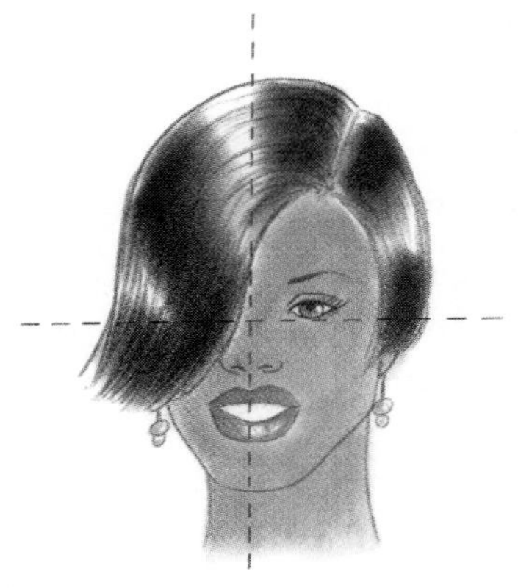

Figure 9-37 Horizontal asymmetry.

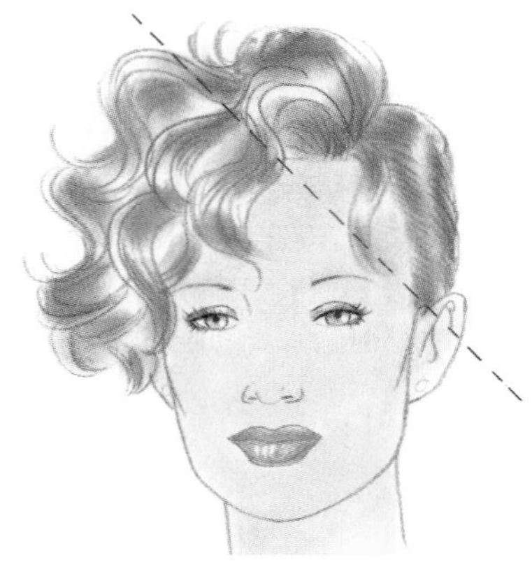

Figure 9-38 Diagonal asymmetry.

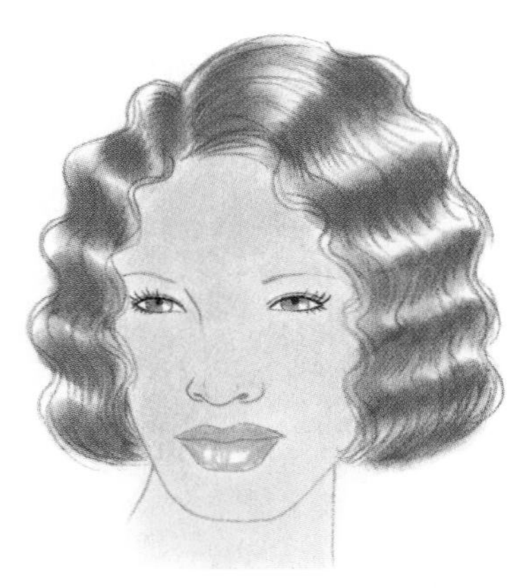

Figure 9-39 Fast rhythm.

Asymmetrical balance features unequal proportions designed to balance facial features. Opposite sides of the hairstyle are different lengths or have a different volume. Asymmetry can be horizontal or diagonal (Figure 9–37 and Figure 9–38).

Rhythm

Rhythm is the regular, recurrent pattern of movement in a hairstyle. It can be fast or slow. A fast rhythm moves quickly; tight curls are an example. A slow rhythm can be seen in larger shapings or long waves (Figure 9–39 and Figure 9–40).

Emphasis

The **emphasis** in a hairstyle is where the eye turns first before traveling to the rest of the design. A hairstyle may be well balanced, with good rhythm and harmony, and still lack flair. An interesting hairstyle should have an area of focus or emphasis. You can create emphasis by using:

- wave patterns (Figure 9–41).
- color (Figure 9–42).
- change in form (Figure 9–43).
- ornamentation (Figure 9–44).

Choose the area of the head or face you want to emphasize. Keep the design simple so that it is easy for the eye to follow from the point of emphasis to the rest of the style. You can have multiple points of emphasis as long as they decrease in size and importance. Be careful not to use too many, however, as this can make the design too busy. Remember, less is more. When using ornaments, make sure they are appropriate to the total look of the client and do not overpower the hairstyle.

Harmony

Harmony—the orderly and pleasing arrangement of shapes and lines—is the most important of the art principles. Harmony holds all the elements of the design together. When a style is harmonious, it has a pleasing form with interesting lines, a pleasing color or combination of colors, and the right

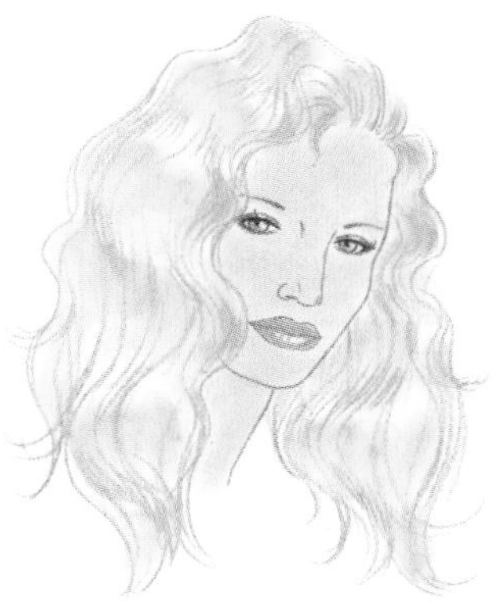
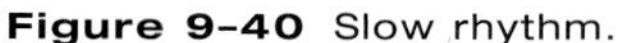

Figure 9-40 Slow rhythm.

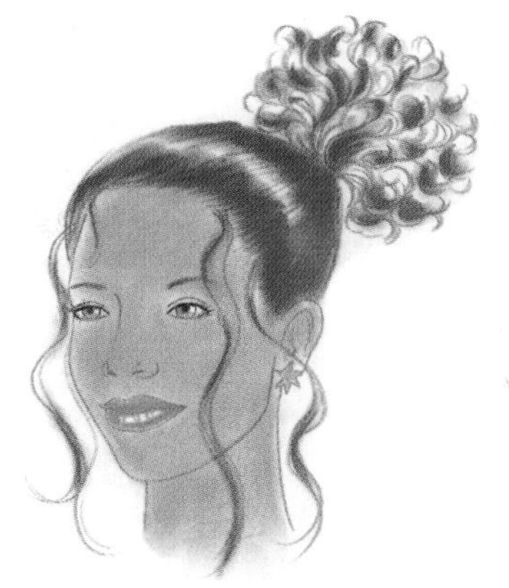

Figure 9-41 Creating emphasis with different wave patterns.

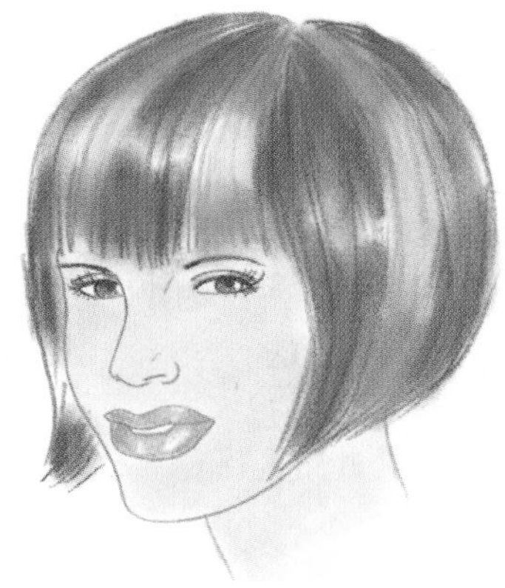

Figure 9-42 Creating emphasis with color.

balance and rhythm for the design. A harmonious style is in proportion to the client's facial and body structure and includes an area of emphasis from which the eyes move to the rest of the style.

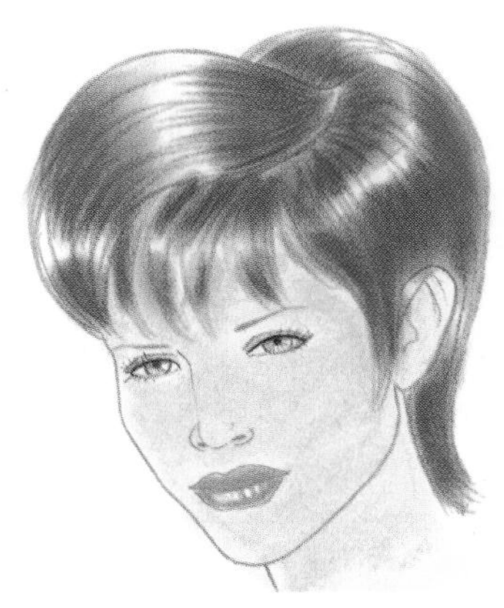

Figure 9-43 Creating emphasis with form changes.

CREATING HARMONY BETWEEN HAIRSTYLE AND FACIAL STRUCTURE

The principles of modern hairstyling and makeup are there to guide you as you decide how best to achieve a beautiful appearance for your client. The most favorable results are obtained when each of your client's facial features is properly analyzed for strengths and shortcomings. Your job is to accentuate a client's best features and to downplay those features that do not add to the person's attractiveness. Every hairstyle you create for every client should be properly proportioned to body type and correctly balanced to the head and facial features, and it should attractively frame the face. An artistic and suitable hairstyle takes into account characteristics of the client such as:

- shape of the head; front view (face shape), profile, and back view.
- features (perfect as well as imperfect features).
- body posture.

How Hair Types Influence Hair Design Decisions

The characteristics of your client's hair type are of prime importance to the selection of a hairstyle. Hair type is based on two major characteristics: wave patterns and hair texture.

All hair has natural wave patterns that must be taken into consideration when designing a style for your client. These wave patterns are straight, wavy, curly, and extremely curly.

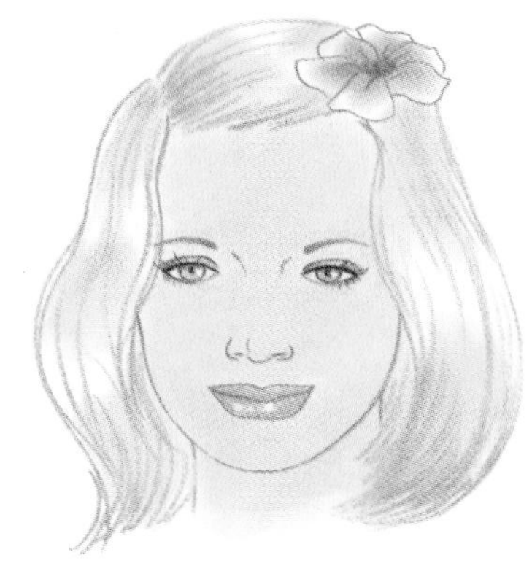

Figure 9-44 Ornament as focal point.

Similarly, hair texture is an important factor in the choice of style, in terms of both appearance and maintenance. The basic hair textures are fine, medium, and coarse. Keep in mind the following guidelines for each type of hair:

- *Fine, straight hair.* This combination usually hugs the head shape due to the fact that there is no body or volume. The silhouette is small and narrow. If this is not appropriate for the client, based on the characteristics of her features or her body structure, think about what styling aids or chemical services can be recommended to achieve the most flattering style. Left in its natural state, the hair does not offer enough support for versatility in styling.
- *Straight, medium hair.* This type of hair offers more versatility in styling. The hair responds well to blow-drying with various sized brushes and has a good amount of movement. It also responds well to rollers and thermal styling.
- *Straight, coarse hair.* This hair is hard to curl and carries more volume than the previous two types. It casts a slightly wider silhouette and responds well to thermal styling. Blow-drying with round brushes can make this hair look too "poofy" because the hair shaft itself is very wide in diameter. Flat brushes are fine for blow-dry styling. Chemical services may take a little longer to process.
- *Wavy, fine hair.* This type of hair can appear fuller with the appropriate haircut and style. With layering, it will look fuller, and it responds well to blow-drying and chemical services. Do not overdo any of these services, however, as this hair can be fragile. If the desired result is straight hair, it will straighten easily by blow-drying, but you may sacrifice volume. If diffused, the hair will have a fuller appearance.
- *Wavy, medium hair.* There are many, many options available in styling. If this hair is diffused dry, it could look curly. If it is blow-dried, you can easily get it straight. This type of hair offers the most versatility in styling.
- *Wavy, coarse hair.* The silhouette could get very wide here, and the hair could appear unruly if it is not shaped properly. Blow-drying tends to be much easier for the stylist than for the client. If the client is not good at working with her own hair, try to work out a flattering shape that is easily maintained. Chemical services like mild relaxers work very well. Sometimes, the client feels that her hair leaves her trapped between being too wavy to be left in a straight style, but not curly enough for a curly style. A soft perm could easily bring her to a wash-and-wear curly style. It is up to you to educate the client toward the right decision and to teach her how to maintain her style at home.
- *Curly, fine hair.* If this hair is left too long, it could separate and reveal too much of the client's scalp unless the hair is abundant. It will respond well to a mild relaxer, and to color. Blow-drying could be difficult unless the hair is cut into short layers, but if the client is going to be in humidity, the hair will just end up curly again.
- *Curly, medium hair.* This creates a wide silhouette, and looks romantic if left natural. Shape the hair appropriately, keeping in mind where the

weight line of the haircut will fall, and make sure that where it falls will be flattering to the client. The wide silhouette should be in proportion to the client's body shape and not overwhelm it. This hair responds well to relaxers and color.

- *Curly, coarse hair.* This hair needs lots of heavy styling product to weight it down. It is easy for this hair to look as though it overwhelms any client. Keep in mind while cutting this combination that the hair will shrink considerably when dry, making it appear much shorter to the client.
- *Very curly, fine hair.* The most flattering shape for the client must be determined, and then—for ease of styling—the hair is generally best left short. If the hair is left long, the silhouette will be wide and extremely voluminous. Chemical services take well, but be careful with relaxing, as the hair could be fragile. Hair pressing (temporary straightening) is an option, but do not overdo it.
- *Extremely curly, medium hair.* This silhouette can get very wide, as the hair can look wider, rather than longer, as it grows. Chemical relaxers work very well to make the shape narrower, and hair pressing is a good option, too. Thermal styling could follow the pressing. If the hair is left in its natural state, cropping close to the head in a flattering shape is great for ease of styling and low maintenance.
- *Extremely curly, coarse hair.* This silhouette will be extremely wide without proper maintenance. Chemical relaxing is recommended, if not to straighten the hair, then to relax it enough to make it easier to style. Once this is accomplished, other thermal services will be easier to perform. This hair is often too thick to tie back in a ponytail, so if the client does not want any chemical services, try short, cropped layers to make the silhouette narrower.

Facial Types

A client's facial shape is determined by the position and prominence of the facial bones. A good way to determine facial shape is to pull all the client's hair completely off the face, using a towel or ponytail, so that you can observe the client's face in the mirror. There are seven basic facial shapes: oval, round, square, oblong, triangle (pear-shaped), inverted triangle (heart-shaped), and diamond. To recognize each facial shape and to be able to style the hair in the most flattering design with that facial shape in mind, you should be acquainted with the characteristics of each. Remember, when designing a style for your client's facial type, you generally try to create the illusion of an oval-shaped face.

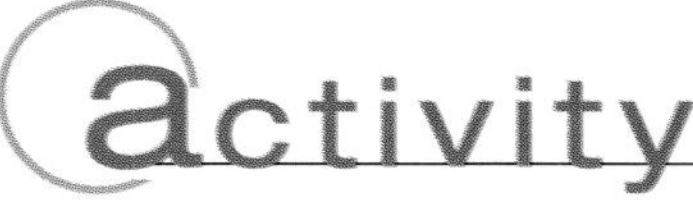

Bring to class some pictures of models and celebrities from magazines, and review them with your classmates to analyze facial shapes and what styles work or do not work with each. If any of these celebrities was your client, what hairstyle would you suggest?

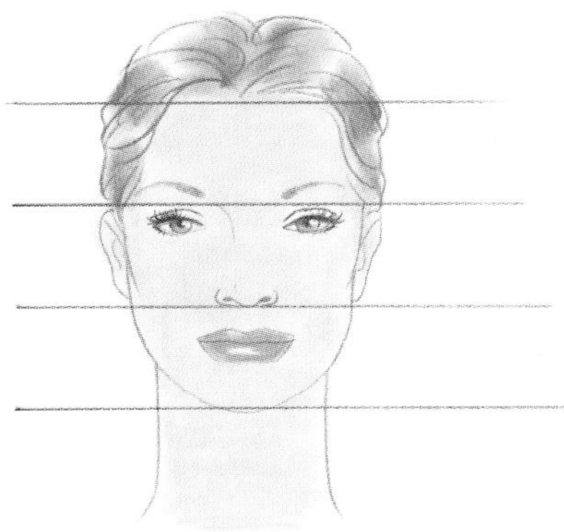

Figure 9-45 Ideal facial proportions.

The face can be divided into three zones: forehead to eyebrow, eyebrows to end of nose, and end of nose to bottom of chin. Keep in mind that when you design hairstyles, you will be trying to create the illusion that each client has the ideal face shape, which is generally recognized as an oval (Figure 9–45).

Oval Facial Type

The contour and proportions of this ideal face shape form the basis for modifying all other facial types.

Facial contour: The oval face is about one and a half times longer than its width across the brow. The forehead is slightly wider than the chin (Figure 9–46). A person with an oval face can wear any hairstyle unless there are other considerations, such as eyeglasses, length and shape of nose, or profile (see sections on special considerations).

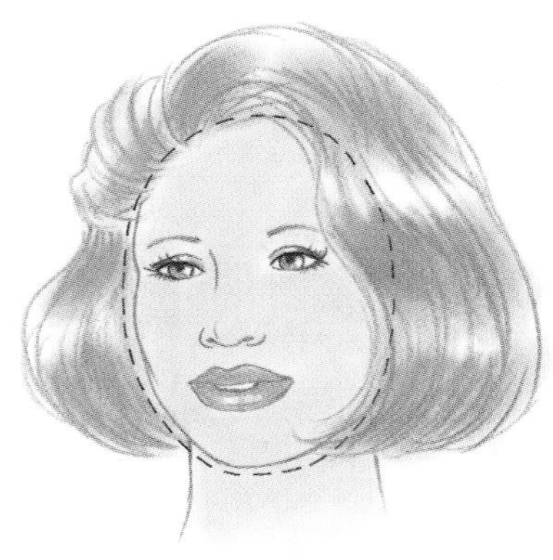

Figure 9-46 Oval face.

Round Facial Type

Facial contour: Round hairline and round chin line; wide face.

Aim: To create the illusion of length to the face, which makes the face appear slimmer.

Styling choice: Create a hairstyle that has height or volume on top and closeness or no volume at the sides (Figure 9–47).

Square Facial Type

Facial contour: Wide at the temples, narrow at the middle third of the face, and squared off at the jaw.

Aim: To offset or round out the square features.

Styling choice: Soften the hair around the temples and jaw, bringing the shape or silhouette close to the head form. Create volume around the areas between the temples and jaw, by adding width around the ear area, for example (Figure 9–48).

Triangular (Pear-Shaped) Facial Type

Facial contour: Narrow forehead, wide jaw and chin line.

Aim: To create the illusion of width in the forehead.

9

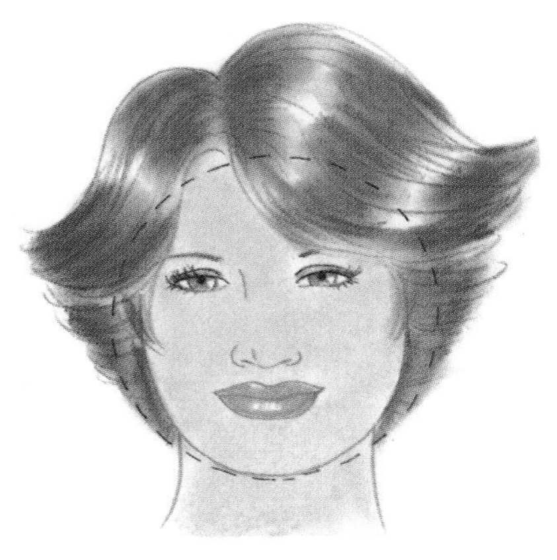

Figure 9-47 Round face.

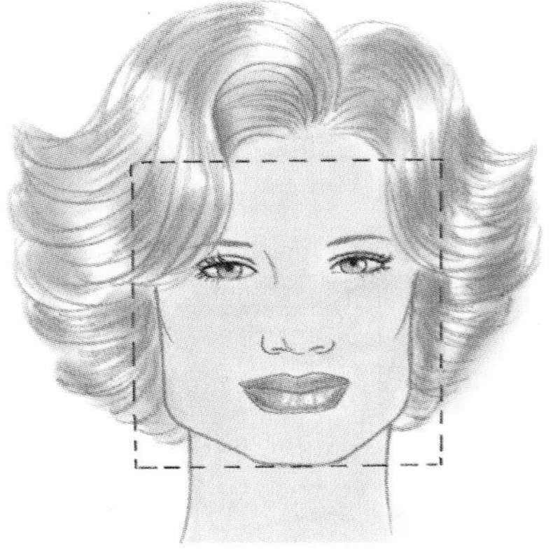

Figure 9-48 Square face.

Styling choice: Build a hairstyle that has volume at the temples and some height at the top. You can disguise the narrowness of the forehead with a soft fringe (Figure 9–49).

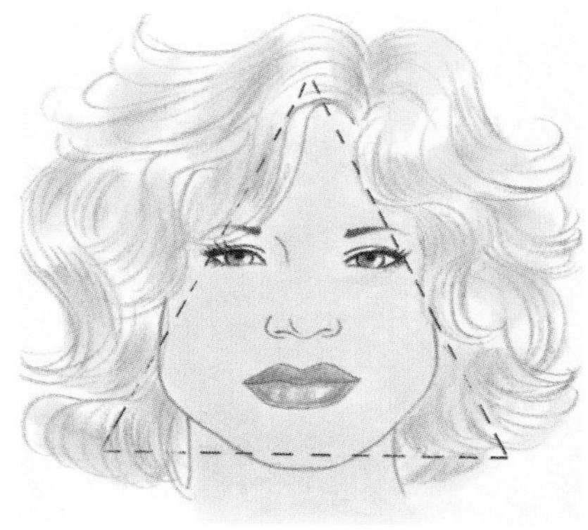

Figure 9-49 Triangular (pear-shaped) face.

Oblong Facial Type

Facial contour: Long, narrow face with hollow cheeks.

Aim: To make the face appear shorter and wider.

Styling choice: Keep the hair fairly close to the top of the head. Add volume on the sides to create the illusion of width. The hair should not be too long, as this would elongate the oblong shape of the face. Chin length is the most effective (Figure 9–50).

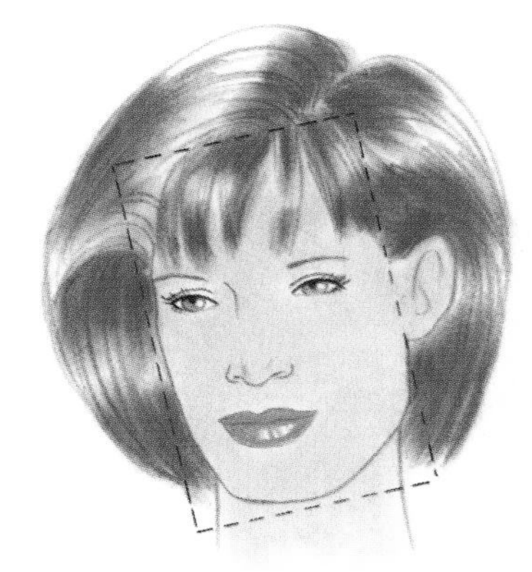

Figure 9-50 Oblong face.

Diamond Facial Type

Facial contour: Narrow forehead, extreme width through the cheekbones, and narrow chin.

Aim: To reduce the width across the cheekbone line.

Styling choice: Increasing the fullness across the jawline and forehead while keeping the hair close to the head at the cheekbone line helps create an oval appearance. Avoid hairstyles that lift away from the cheeks or move back from the hairline on the sides near the ear area (Figure 9–51).

Inverted Triangle Facial Type

Facial contour: Wide forehead and narrow chin line.

Aim: To decrease the width of the forehead and increase the width in the lower part of the face.

Styling choice: To reduce the width of the forehead, by styling the hair close to the head with no volume. A fringe is recommended. Gradually increase the width of the silhouette as you style the middle third of the shape in the cheekbone area and near the ears, and keep the silhouette to its widest at the jaw and neck area (Figure 9–52). 3

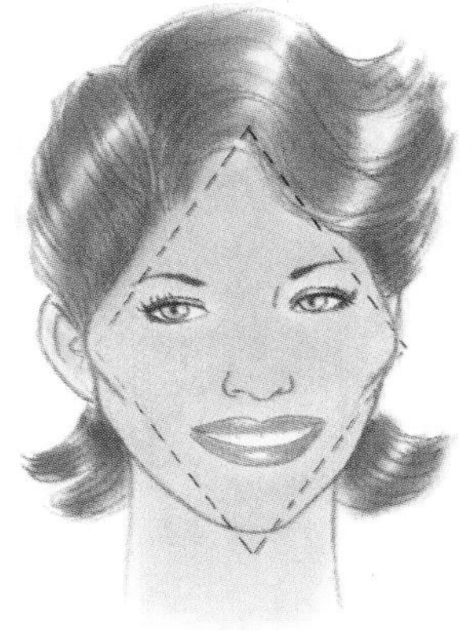

Figure 9-51 Diamond face.

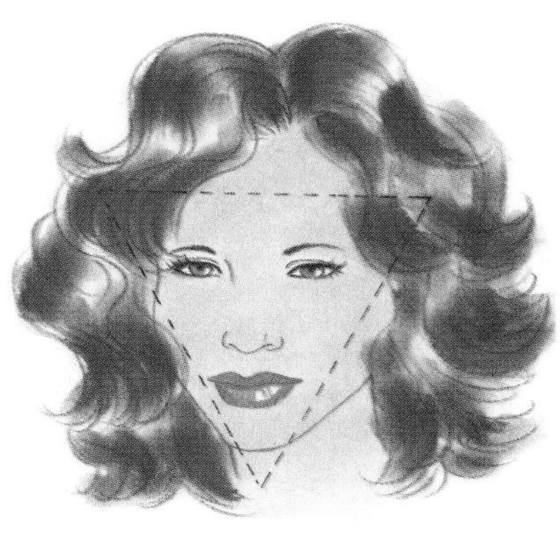

Figure 9-52 Inverted triangle-shaped face.

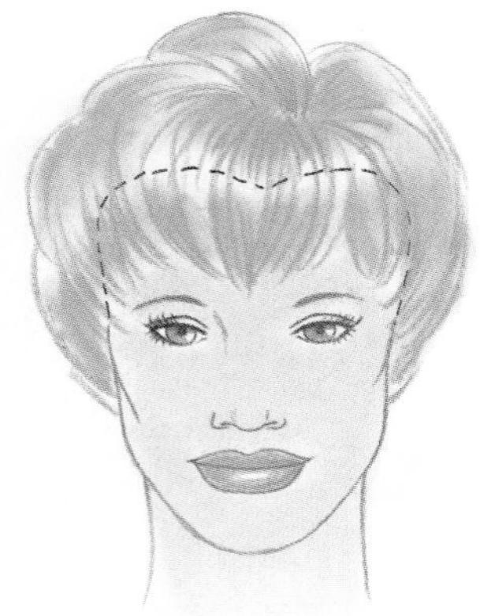

Figure 9-53 Wide forehead.

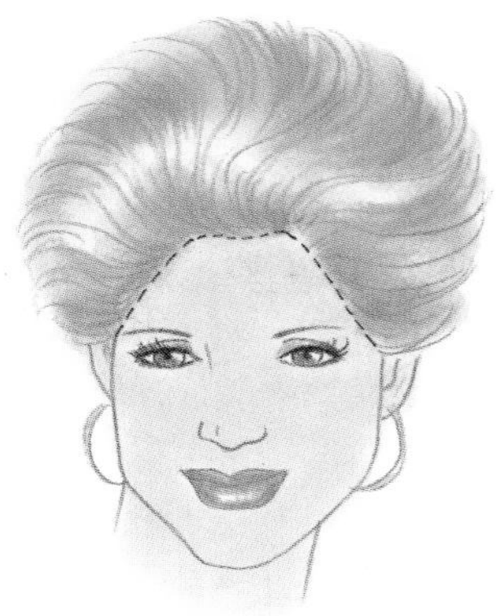

Figure 9-54 Narrow forehead.

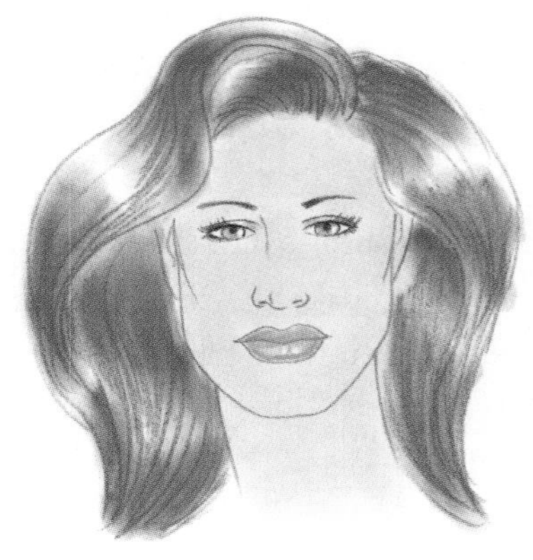

Figure 9-55 Close-set eyes.

Special Considerations

An understanding of facial features and proportions will make it easier for you to analyze each client's face. With this understanding, you can then apply the design principles you have learned to help correct for structural problems. Dividing the face into three sections is one way to do this analysis (See Figure 9–33).

The Top Third of the Face

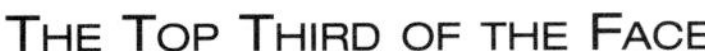

Wide forehead: Direct hair forward over the sides of the forehead (Figure 9–53).

Narrow forehead: Direct hair away from the face at the forehead. Lighter highlights can be used at the temples to create the illusion of width (Figure 9–54).

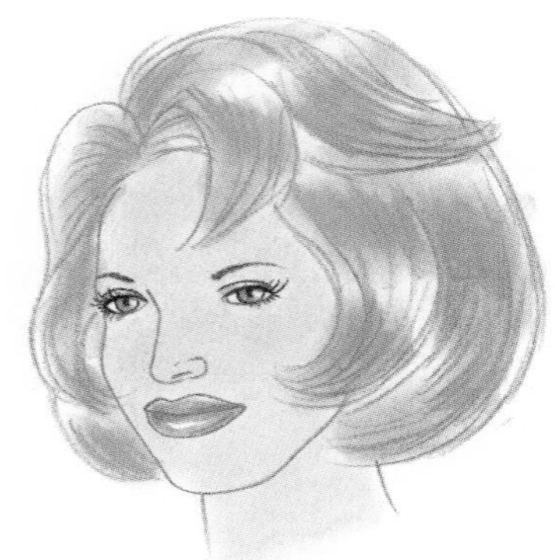

Figure 9-56 Wide-set eyes.

The Middle Third of the Face

Close-set eyes: Usually found on long, narrow faces. Direct hair back and away from the face at the temples. A side movement from a diagonal back part with some height is advisable. A slight lightening of the hair at the corner of the eyes will give the illusion of width (Figure 9–55).

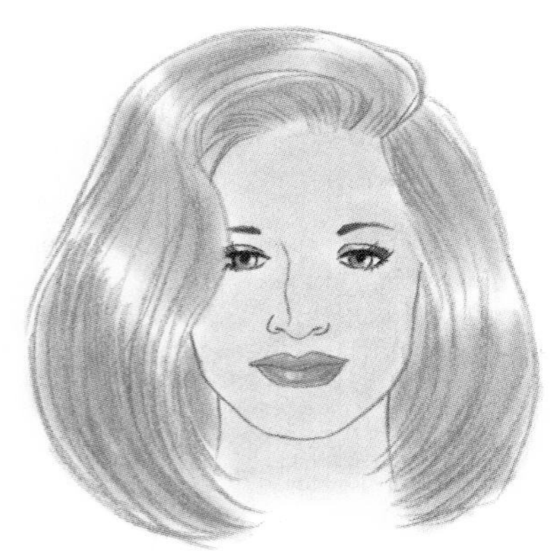

Figure 9-57 Crooked nose.

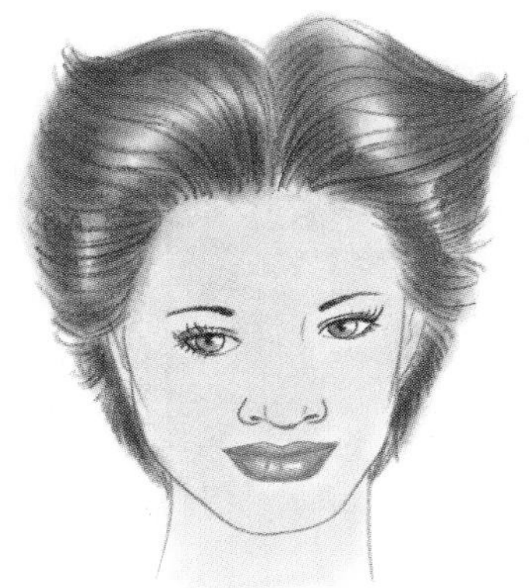

Figure 9-58 Wide nose.

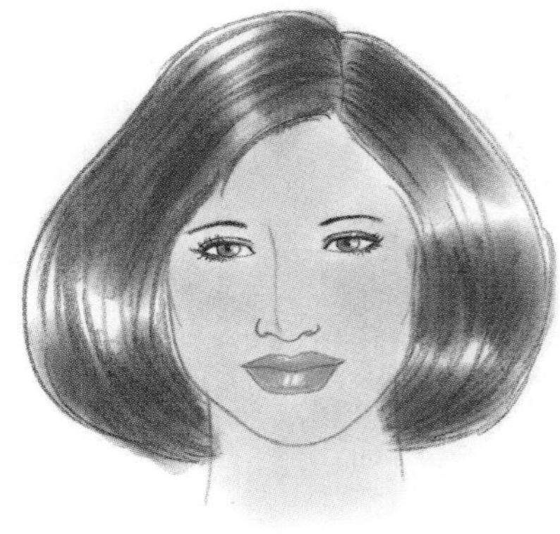

Figure 9-59 Long, narrow nose.

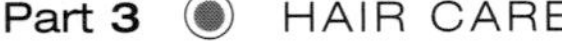

Wide-set eyes: Usually found on round or square faces. Use a higher half bang to create length in the face. This will give the face the illusion of being larger and will make the eyes appear more proportional. The hair should be slightly darker at the sides than the top (Figure 9–56).

Crooked nose: Asymmetrical, off-center styles are best, as they attract the eye away from the nose. Any well-balanced style will accentuate the fact that the face is not even (Figure 9–57).

Wide, flat nose: Draw the hair away from the face and use a center part to help elongate and narrow the nose (Figure 9–58).

Long, narrow nose: Stay away from styles that are tapered close to the head on the sides, and have height on top. Middle parts or too much hair directed toward the face are also poor choices. This will only accentuate any long, narrow features on the face. Instead, select a style where the hair moves away from the face, creating the illusion of wider facial features (Figure 9–59).

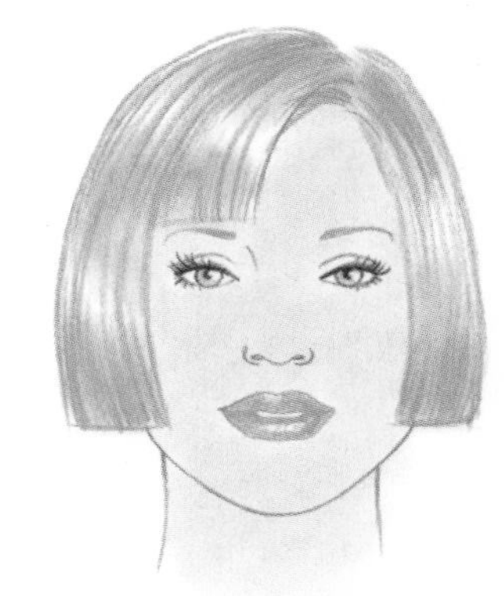

Figure 9-60 Round jaw.

The Lower Third of the Face

Round jaw: Use straight lines at the jawline (Figure 9–60).

Square jaw: Use curved lines at the jawline (Figure 9–61).

Long jaw: Hair should be full and fall below the jaw to direct attention away from it (Figure 9–62).

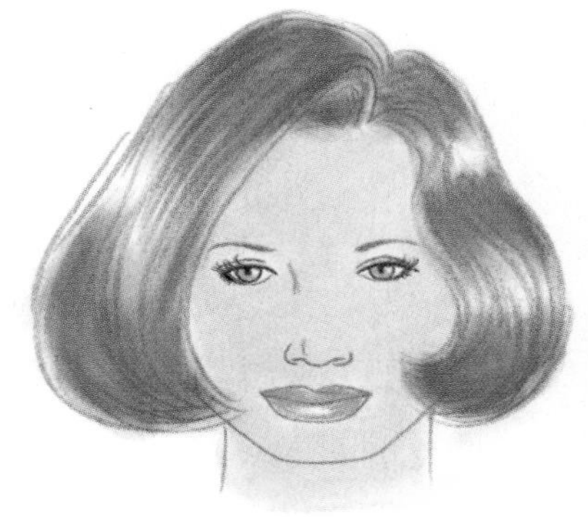

Figure 9-61 Square jaw.

Profiles

The **profile** is the outline of the face, head, or figure seen in a side view. There are three basic profiles.

1. The straight profile is considered the ideal. It is neither **convex** (curving outward) nor **concave** (curving inward), although even a straight profile has a very slight curvature. Generally, all hairstyles are flattering to the straight or normal profile (Figure 9–63).
2. The convex profile has a receding forehead and chin. It calls for an arrangement of curls or bangs over the forehead. Keep the style close to the head at the nape and move hair forward in the chin area (Figure 9–64 and Figure 9–65).

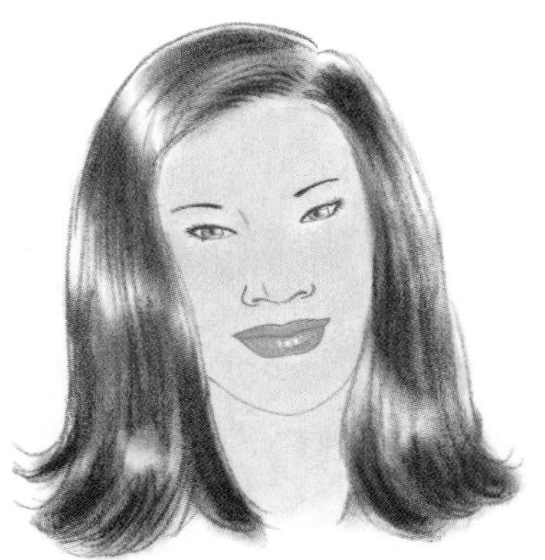

Figure 9-62 Long jaw.

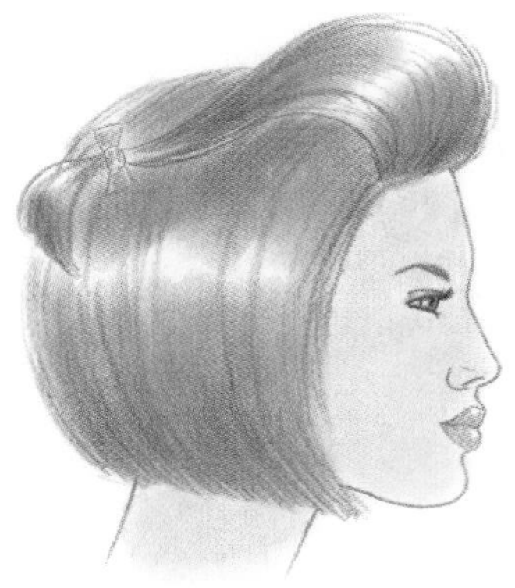

Figure 9-63 Straight profile.

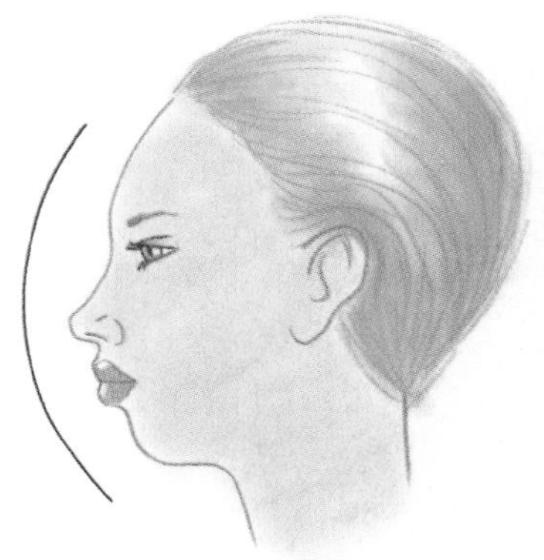

Figure 9-64 Convex profile.

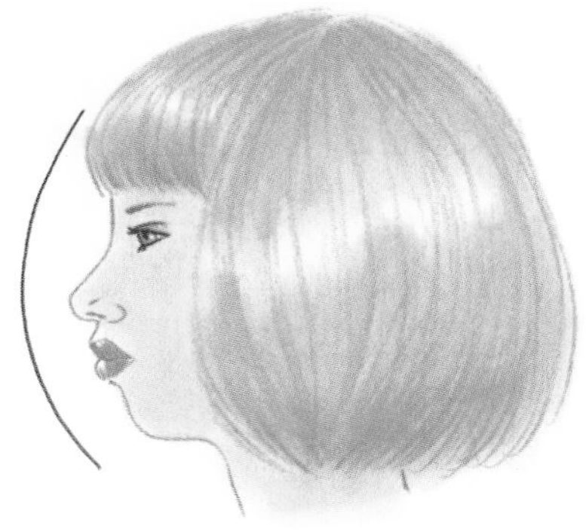

Figure 9-65 Styling for convex profile.

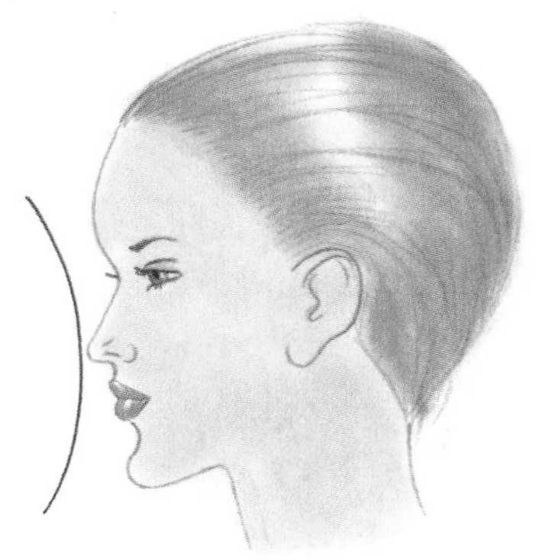

Figure 9-66 Concave profile.

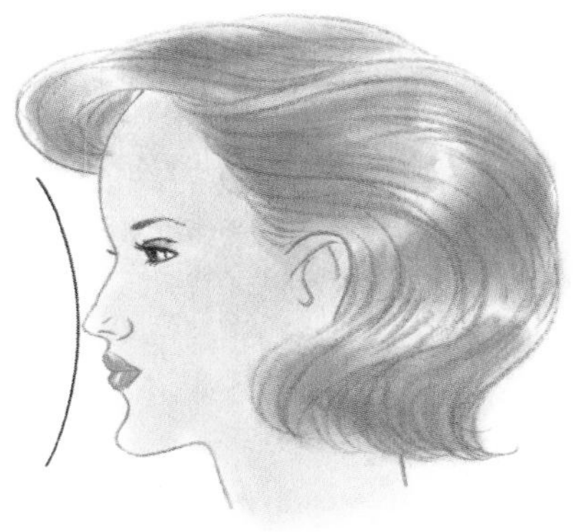

Figure 9-67 Styling for concave profile.

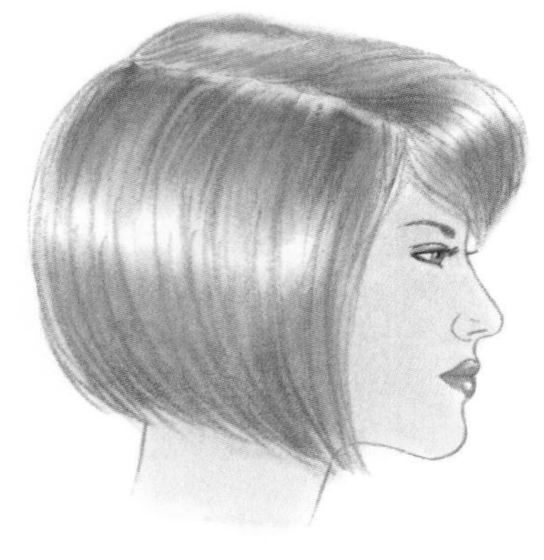

Figure 9-68 Receding forehead.

3. The concave profile has a prominent forehead and chin, with other features receded inward. It should be accommodated by softly styling the hair at the nape with an upward movement. Do not build hair onto the forehead (Figure 9–66 and Figure 9–67).

Various hair designs can help balance other disproportionate areas of the profile.

Receding forehead: Direct the bangs over the forehead with an outwardly directed volume (Figure 9–68).

Large forehead: Use bangs with little or no volume to cover the forehead (Figure 9–69).

Small nose: A small nose is considered a child-like quality; therefore it is best to design a hairstyle that is not associated with children. Hair should be swept off the face, creating a line from nose to ear. The top hair should be moved off the forehead to give the illusion of length to the nose (Figure 9–70).

Prominent nose: To draw attention away from the nose, bring hair forward at the forehead with softness around the face (Figure 9–71).

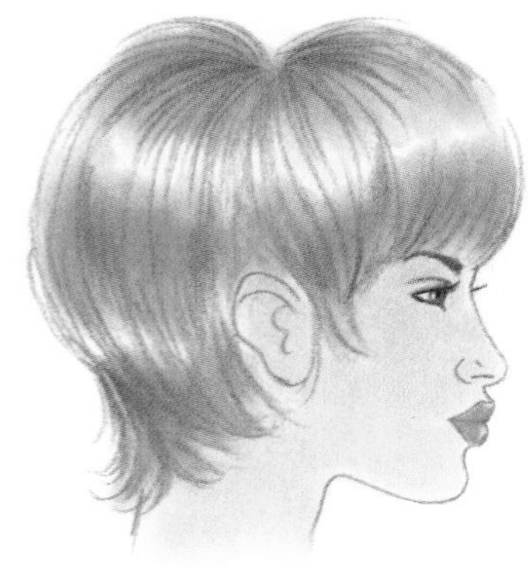

Figure 9-69 Large forehead.

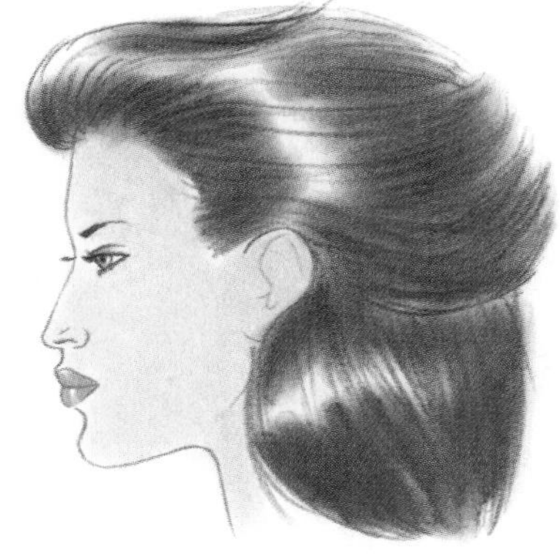

Figure 9-70 Small nose.

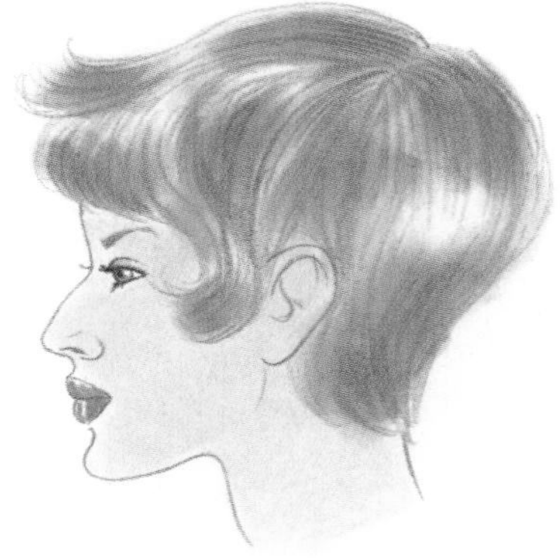

Figure 9-71 Prominent nose.

Receding chin: Hair should be directed forward in the chin area (Figure 9–72).

Small chin: Move the hair up and away from the face along the chin line (Figure 9–73).

Large chin: The hair should be either longer or shorter than the chin line so as to not draw attention to the chin (Figure 9–74).

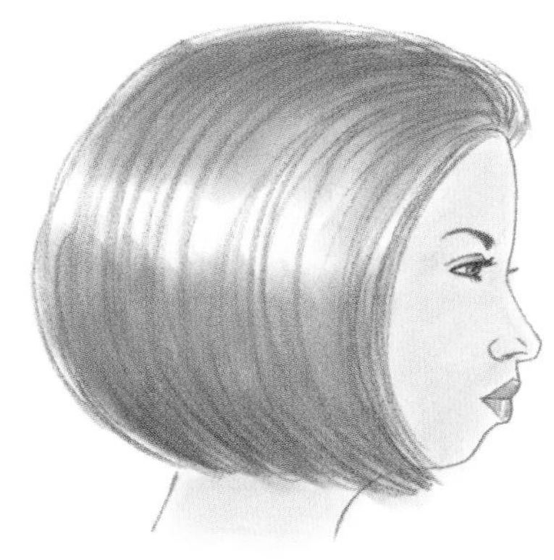

Figure 9–72 Receding chin.

Head Shape

Not all head shapes are round. It is important to feel the head shape before deciding on a hairstyle. Design the style with volume in areas that are flat or small while reducing volume in areas that are large or prominent (Figure 9–75).

Styling for People Who Wear Glasses

Eyeglasses have become a fashion accessory, and many people change their glasses with their clothes. It is important for you to know whether your clients ever wear glasses so you can take that into account when designing the appropriate hairstyle. Keep in mind that when a client puts on her glasses, the arm of the glasses (the part that rests on the ear) can push the hair at the ear and cause it to stick out.

If you are choosing a short haircut, you may want to reconsider the length of the hair around the ear, opting to either leave it a little longer or cut the hair above and around the ear. For styling purposes, choose a style in which there is enough hair covering the ear (fine hair may "pop" out at the ear), or direct the hair away from the face, so that the arms of the glasses are not an issue. 4

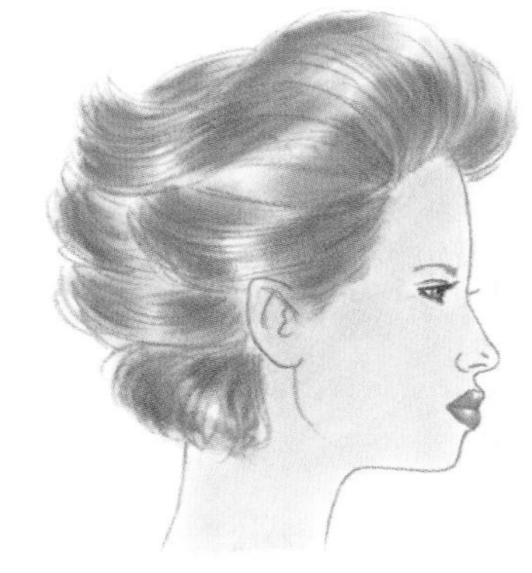

Figure 9–73 Small chin.

Hair Parts

Hair parts can be the focal point of a hairstyle. Because the eye is drawn to a part, you must be careful how you use it. First of all, the part must always be neat, without hairs straggling from one side to another, and it must be straight and directed positively. It is usually best to use a natural part if at all possible. You may, however, want to create a part according to your client's

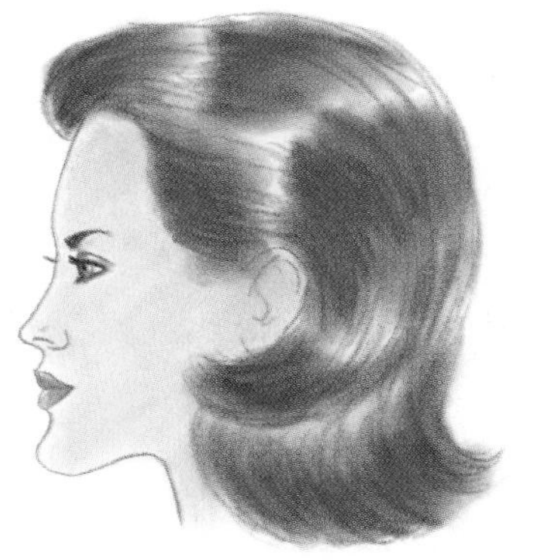

Figure 9–74 Large chin.

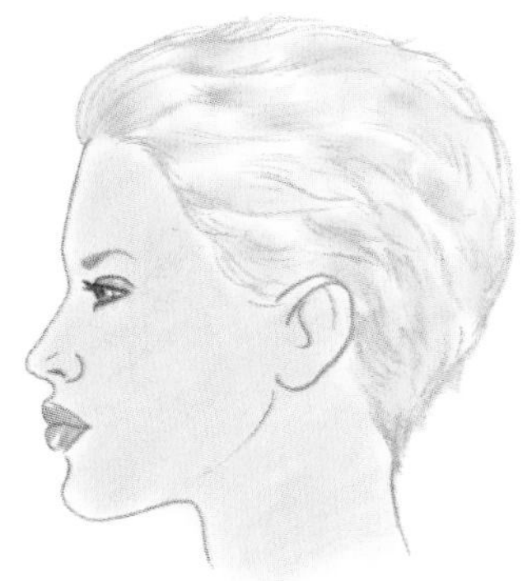

Figure 9–75 Perfect oval.

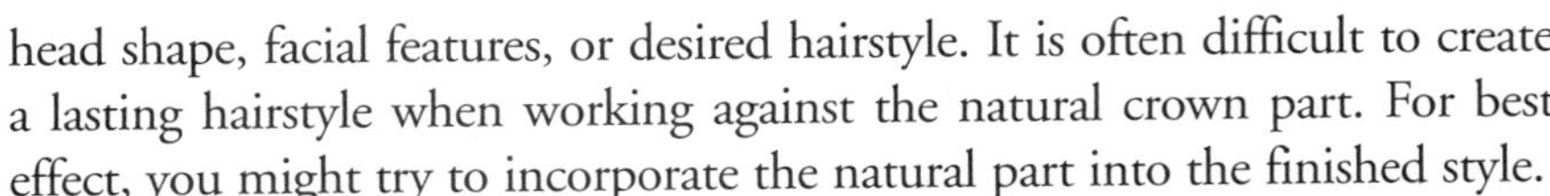

head shape, facial features, or desired hairstyle. It is often difficult to create a lasting hairstyle when working against the natural crown part. For best effect, you might try to incorporate the natural part into the finished style.

The following are suggestions for hair parts that suit the various facial types.

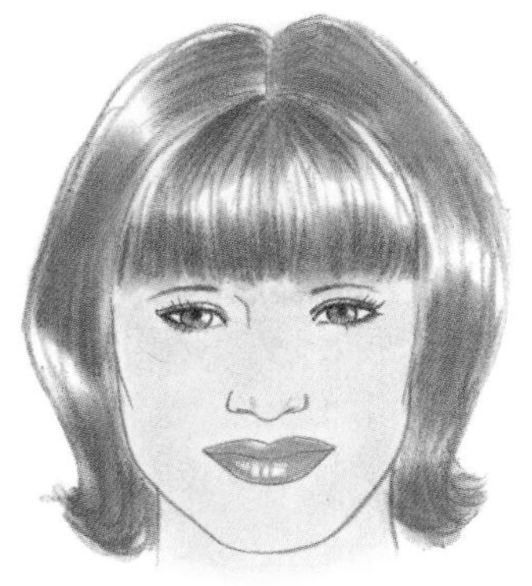

Figure 9-76 Triangular part.

Parts for the Fringe (Bangs)

The **fringe**, or bangs area, is the triangular section that begins at the apex, or high point of the head, and ends at the front corners. The fringe is parted in three basic ways.

1. The triangular part is the basic parting for fringe sections (Figure 9–76).
2. The diagonal part gives height to a round or square face and width to a long, thin face (Figure 9–77).
3. The curved part is used for a receding hairline or high forehead (Figure 9–78).

Style Parts

There are four other parts that can be used to highlight facial features.

1. Side parts are used to direct hair across the top of the head. They help develop height on top and make thin hair appear fuller (Figure 9–79).
2. Center parts are classic. They are used for an oval face, but also give an oval illusion to wide and round faces. Do not use center parts on people with prominent noses (Figure 9–80).
3. Diagonal back parts are used to create the illusion of width or height in a hairstyle (Figure 9–81).
4. Zigzag parts create a dramatic effect (Figure 9–82).

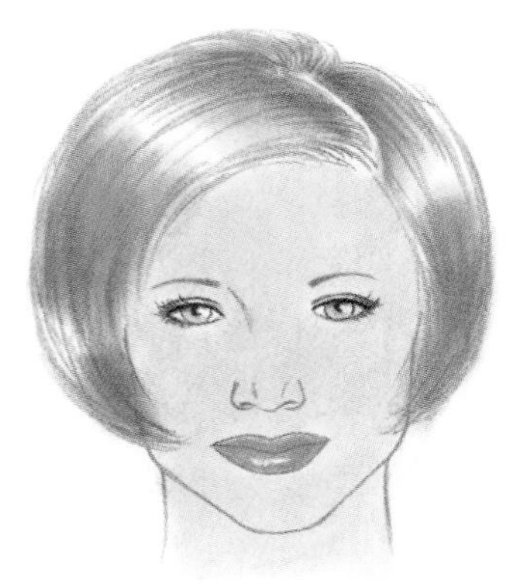

Figure 9-77 Diagonal part in fringe.

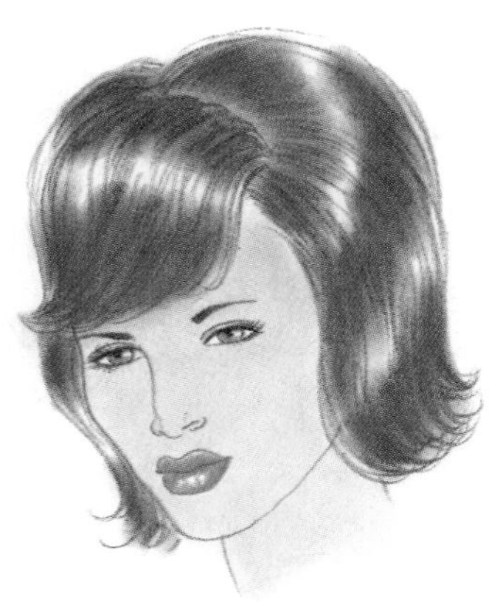

Figure 9-78 Curved part.

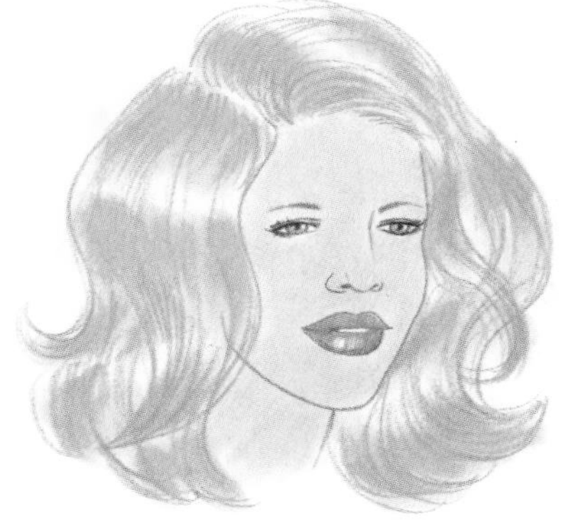

Figure 9-79 Side part.

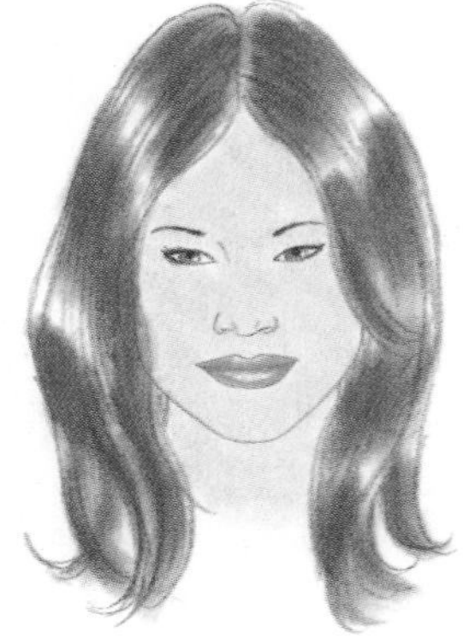

Figure 9-80 Center part.

Client Consultation: A Sample Dialogue

The design process does not spring forth from the stylist alone. It is a collaboration, beginning with the client consultation. Ellen, a new client at the salon, has just met Mark, who is going to style her hair (Figure 9–83). Let us have a look at how Mark handles the consultation.

Mark: Hello, Ellen. My name is Mark and I'll be styling your hair today. Is there anything particular you had in mind?

Ellen: Well, I don't want it cut too short, and I like to keep my ears covered. I have a picture I tore out from a magazine.

Mark notices that the picture Ellen has is of a model with a different kind of hair texture and a cut about three inches shorter than what Ellen currently has.

Mark: This is lovely. I could achieve this look for you with a permanent wave and a haircut. I would have to cut about three inches off the length and add some layers. But I don't know how much time you have in the morning to spend on your hair. I also need to know if you're currently taking any medications, because they could have a negative effect on your perm.

Ellen: Well, let's keep it about an inch longer than this picture. I'm not sure about the layering. My mornings are very busy, getting my son off to school and getting myself ready to go to work. And no, I'm not taking any medications.

Mark realizes that Ellen is looking for a wash-and-wear style consistent with her lifestyle needs. He believes as well that the layering would help soften the lines of Ellen's square face.

Mark: Well, I can show you how to style your hair with gel. That would cut your styling time in half by diffusing your curls. I think it would be fine to leave it an inch longer, but I really do feel that the layering would be most flattering to your features and would soften the whole look.

Ellen: Okay, that sounds great. Let's do it!

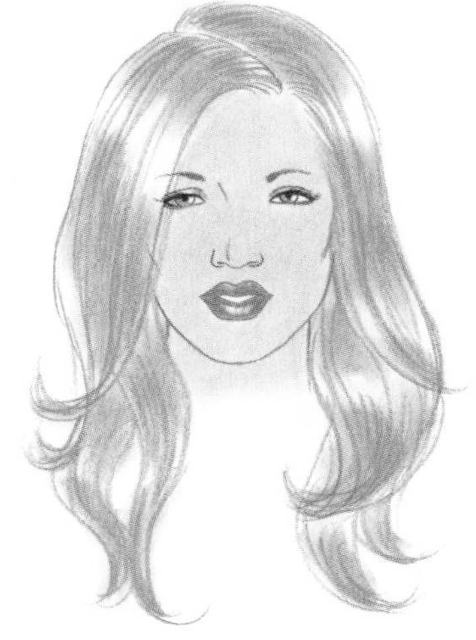

Figure 9–81 Diagonal part.

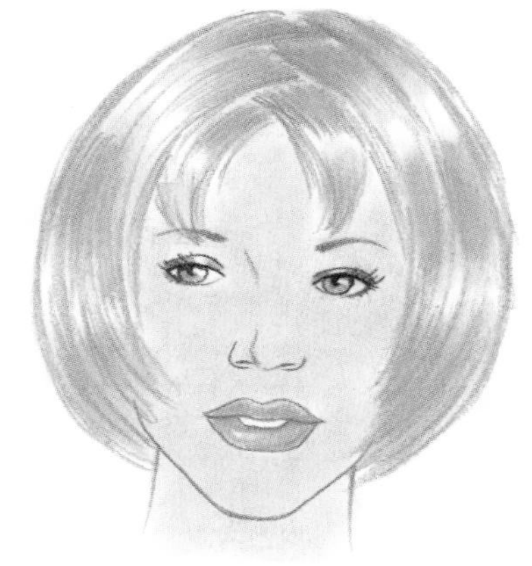

Figure 9–82 Zigzag part.

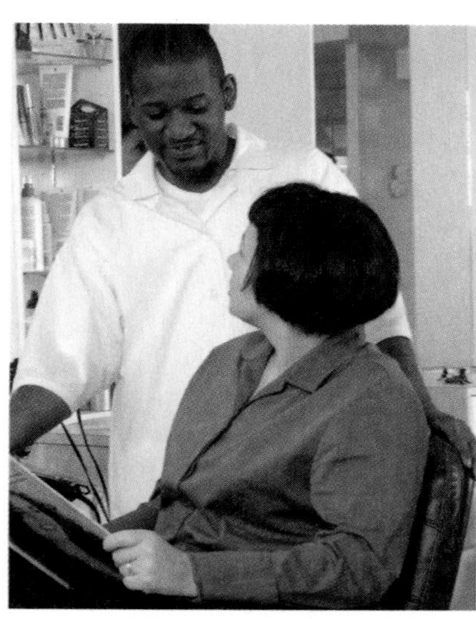

Figure 9–83 A client consultation.

DESIGNING FOR MEN

All the design principles and elements you have just read about pertain to men's hairstyles as well as to women's. Men's styles have run the gamut since the early 1960s, when the Beatles hit the music and fashion scene and greatly revolutionized men's style. Now all hair lengths are acceptable for men, giving them more choices than ever. As a professional, you should recommend styles that are flattering, and that are appropriate for the client's career, hair type, and lifestyle.

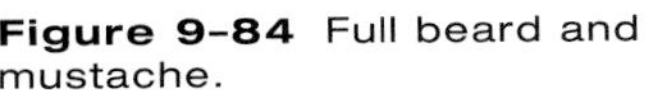

Figure 9–84 Full beard and mustache.

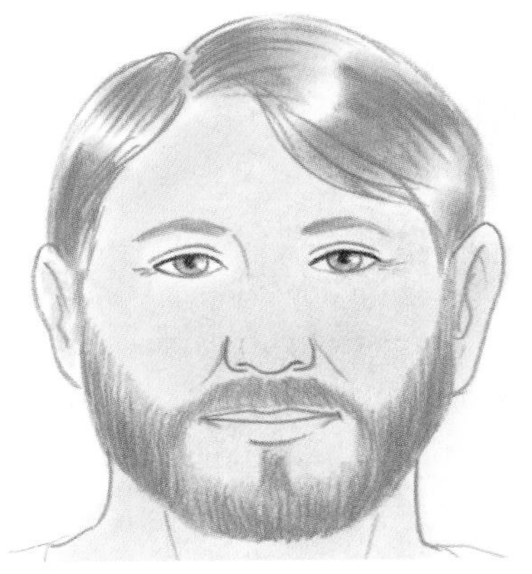

Figure 9–85 Closely trimmed beard and mustache.

Choosing Mustache and Beard Shapes

Mustaches and beards can be a great way to discreetly disguise a facial flaw on a male client. For example, if a man does not have a prominent chin when you look at his profile, a neatly trimmed full beard and mustache could camouflage that feature (Figure 9–84). If a man has a wide face and full cheeks, a fairly close-trimmed beard and mustache would be very flattering (Figure 9–85).

A man who is balding with closely trimmed hair also could look very good in a closely groomed beard and mustache. Sideburns, mustaches without beards, and beard shapes are, to some extent, dictated by current trends. No matter what the trend calls for, it is important that the shapes appear well groomed and are flattering to the client.

chapter glossary

asymmetrical balance	hairstyle design that features unequal proportions designed to balance facial features
balance	harmony or proportion; in hairstyling, it signifies the proper degree of height and width
concave	curving inward
contrasting lines	horizontal and vertical lines that meet at a 90-degree angle
convex	curving outward
diagonal lines	lines positioned between horizontal and vertical lines
emphasis	in a hairstyle, the place where the eye turns first before traveling to the rest of the design
form	the outline of the overall hairstyle as seen from all angles
fringe	triangular section that begins at the apex, or high point of the head, and ends at the front corners; bangs
harmony	orderly and pleasing arrangement of shapes and lines
horizontal lines	lines parallel to the floor or horizon
parallel	extending in the same direction and maintaining a constant distance apart
proportion	the harmonious relationship between parts or things, or the comparative relation of one thing to another
profile	outline of the face, head, or figure seen in a side view
rhythm	regular, recurrent pattern of movement in a hairstyle
space	the area that the hairstyle occupies; also thought of as the area inside the form
symmetrical balance	hairstyle design that is similar on both sides of the face
transitional lines	usually curved lines that are used to blend and soften horizontal or vertical lines
vertical lines	lines that are straight up and down

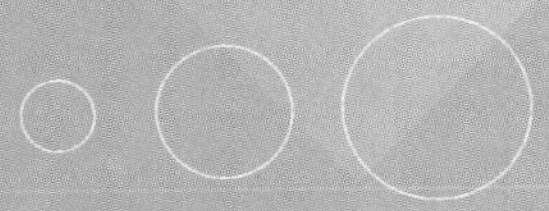

review questions

1. Name the five elements of design.
2. Name the five principles of hair design.
3. Why must the stylist consider the client's entire body when designing a hairstyle?
4. What are symmetrical and asymmetrical balance?
5. What is considered the most important art principle and why?
6. Explain the general principles of highlighting or camouflaging facial features.
7. List and describe the seven facial shapes.
8. Name at least five facial features that must be considered when designing a hairstyle.
9. What is the difference between a convex and concave profile?
10. How do the elements and principles of hair design apply to men?

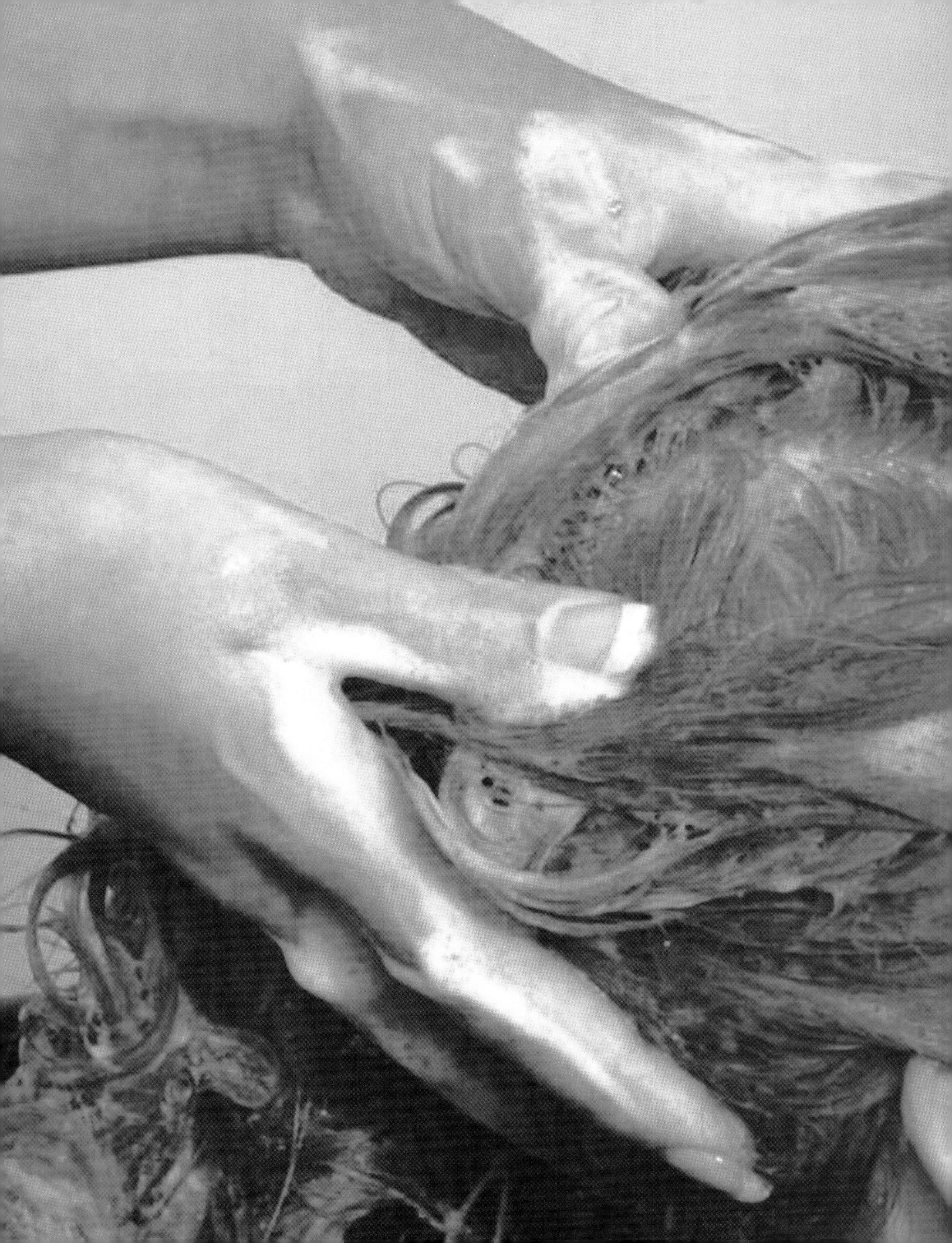

SHAMPOOING, RINSING, AND CONDITIONING

Mary Brunetti

FREELANCE AND CELEBRITY HAIRSTYLIST,
1991 NORTH AMERICAN HAIRSTYLIST OF THE YEAR

Chapter Outline

Learning Objectives

After completing this chapter, you should be able to:

1. Explain pH and its importance in shampoo selection.
2. Explain the role of surfactants in shampoo.
3. Discuss the uses and benefits of various types of shampoos and conditioners.
4. Perform proper scalp manipulations as part of a shampoo service.
5. Demonstrate proper shampooing and conditioning procedures.
6. Describe general hair and scalp treatments.

National Skill Standards

This chapter provides you with the necessary information to master these National Industry Skill Standards for Entry-Level Cosmetologists.

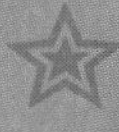
Consulting with clients to determine their needs and preferences.

Conducting services in a safe environment and taking measures to prevent the spread of infectious and contagious disease.

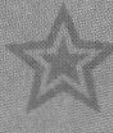
Using a variety of salon products while providing client services.

Effectively marketing professional salon products.

Key Terms

Page number indicates where in the chapter the term is used.

acid-balanced shampoo pg. 262

balancing shampoos pg. 262

clarifying shampoos pg. 262

color-enhancing shampoos pg. 263

conditioners pg. 263

conditioning or moisturizing shampoos pg. 262

deep conditioning treatments pg. 265

dry or powder shampoo pg. 262

hard water pg. 259

humectants pg. 264

hydrophilic pg. 260

instant conditioners pg. 264

lipophilic pg. 260

medicated shampoos pg. 262

medicated scalp lotions pg. 265

moisturizers pg. 264

nonstripping pg. 262

protein conditioners pg. 264

scalp astringent lotions pg. 265

scalp conditioners pg. 265

soft water pg. 259

spray-on thermal protectors pg. 265

When a client visits a salon for the first time, she starts to make judgments almost immediately. The judgments begin with the kind of reception she finds at the desk. Is she greeted by name? Does the receptionist tell her where she can hang her coat? These things are important. Even more important is the kind of attention she gets when she moves into the salon itself. The first part of a client's hair service will most likely be the shampoo. The shampoo can be a source of either pleasure or unpleasantness. The way it goes may determine whether or not the client will make a return visit.

In some salons, the stylist is the one who gives the client the shampoo. In other salons, there may be a separate shampoo person. Either way, the client will often draw conclusions about the professionalism of the salon on the basis of how the shampoo is performed. While shampooing is an important preliminary step for a variety of hair services, it also has a psychological impact. The shampoo is an opportunity to provide the client with quality relaxing time in the salon, free from the stresses of the day. And if the experience is pleasurable, the client is more likely to enjoy the rest of the service as well (Figure 10–1).

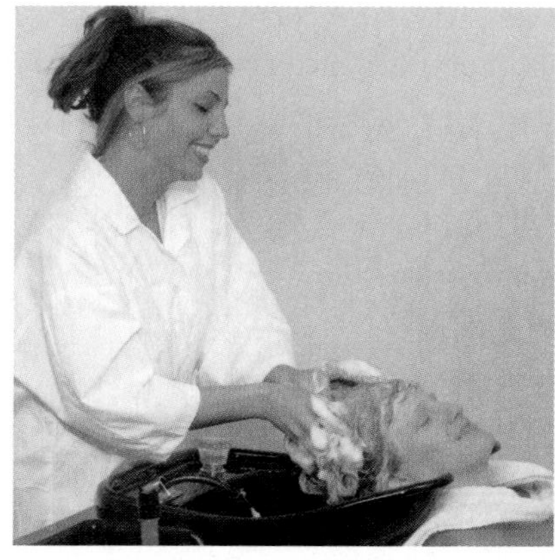

Figure 10–1 The shampoo is an enjoyable salon experience.

One concern for a client might be the new hairstyle she is about to try out. If she is nervous about that or any other service she is scheduled to receive, you can relieve some of that stress right there at the shampoo bowl. This is also where you will begin your analysis of the client's hair and scalp. In salons where shampoos are performed by separate shampoo persons, it is important for the stylist to see what the client's hair looks like before it is wet. The shampoo person should also alert the stylist to any existing hair or scalp conditions, diseases, or disorders. A client with an infectious disease should not be treated in the salon and should be referred to a physician.

The primary purpose of a shampoo is, obviously, to cleanse the hair and scalp prior to receiving a service. To be effective, a shampoo must remove all dirt, oils, cosmetics, and skin debris without adversely affecting either the scalp or hair. The scalp and hair need to be cleansed regularly to combat the accumulation of oils and perspiration, which mix with the natural scales and dirt to create a breeding ground for disease-producing bacteria that can cause scalp disorders. Hair should be shampooed as often as necessary, depending on how quickly the scalp and hair become soiled. As a general rule, oily hair should be shampooed more often than normal or dry hair. It should not be shampooed too often, however, for excessive shampooing strips the hair of its protective oil, or sebum, which, in small amounts, seals and protects the hair's cuticle.

focus on ...retailing

The proper home hair care products can make all the difference when a client uses them correctly. It is your job to educate clients as to what products to use and why. Otherwise, they are likely to make their own uninformed decisions, buying inferior products at the drugstore or supermarket. The wrong products can make even a good haircut look bad and can affect the success of a chemical service. Professional products are also guaranteed when purchased in the salon. Remember, you want your clients to look their best so they can act as good advertising for your skills and talents. In the words of Vidal Sassoon: "If you don't look good, we don't look good!"

UNDERSTANDING SHAMPOO

There are many types of shampoos on the market. As a professional cosmetologist, you should make it your goal to become skilled at selecting shampoos the composition and action of which best match the services you will be performing. Always read labels and accompanying literature carefully so that you can make informed decisions about the use of various shampoos. The careful attention you give your products will also serve you well as you recommend these retail items for purchase by your clients.

Select a shampoo according to the condition of the client's hair. Hair can usually be characterized as oily, dry, normal, or chemically treated. Your client might even have an oily scalp with dry hair, due to overprocessing. Hair is not considered normal or virgin if it has been lightened, colored, permed, chemically relaxed, abused by the use of harsh shampoos, or damaged by improper care and exposure to the elements, such as wind, sun, cold, or heat.

The pH Scale

Chapter 7 of this book provides you with an overview of important chemistry basics like pH and surfactants. You can refer back to that chapter as necessary, but let us review pH here as it applies to shampoo.

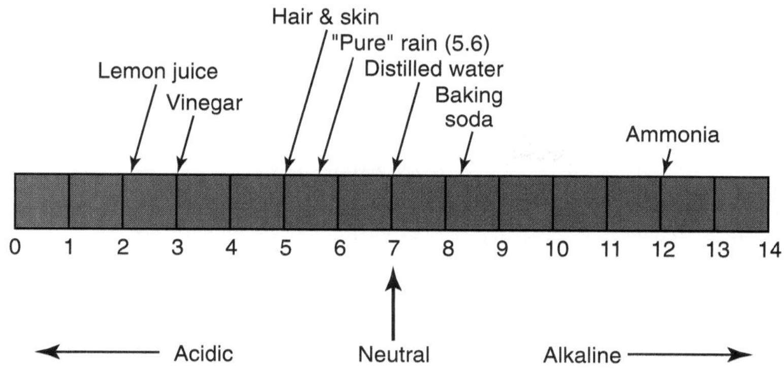

Figure 10-2 The pH scale.

Understanding pH levels will help you select the proper shampoo for your client. The amount of hydrogen in a solution, which determines whether it is more alkaline or acid, is measured on a pH scale that has a range from 0 to 14. A shampoo that is more acid can have a pH rating from 0 to 6.9; a shampoo that is more alkaline can have a pH rating from 7.1 to 14. The higher the pH rating (more alkaline), the stronger and harsher the shampoo. A high-pH shampoo can leave the hair dry, brittle, and more porous, and it can cause fading in color-treated hair. 1

The Chemistry of Water

Water is the most abundant and important chemical on the earth. It is essential to the life process. It is the "universal solvent," meaning that it is capable of dissolving more substances than any other solvent.

Fresh water from lakes and streams is purified by sedimentation (a treatment that causes matter to sink to the bottom) and filtration (passing of water through a porous substance, such as a filter paper or charcoal) to remove suspended clay, sand, and organic material. Small amounts of chlorine are then added to kill bacteria. Boiling water at a temperature of 212° Fahrenheit (100° Celsius) will also destroy most microbes. Water can be further treated by distillation, a process of heating water so it becomes a vapor, then condensing the vapor so that it collects as a liquid. This process is often used in the manufacturing of cosmetics.

Water is of crucial importance in the cosmetology industry because it is used for shampooing, mixing solutions, and other functions. Depending on the kinds and amounts of minerals present in water, water can be classified as either hard or soft. You will be able to make a more professional shampoo selection if you know whether the water in your salon is hard or soft.

Soft water is rain water or chemically softened water. It contains small amounts of minerals and, therefore, allows soap and shampoo to lather freely. For this reason, it is preferred for shampooing. **Hard water** contains certain minerals that lessen the ability of soap or shampoo to lather readily. However, a chemical process can soften hard water.

The Chemistry of Shampoos

To determine which shampoo will leave your client's hair in the best condition for the intended service, you must understand the chemical ingredients regularly found in shampoos. Most shampoos share many ingredients in common. It is often the small differences in formulation that make one shampoo better than another for a particular hair texture or condition.

Water is the main ingredient in all shampoos. Generally it is not just plain water, but purified or deionized (ions removed) water. Water is usually the first ingredient listed, which indicates that the shampoo contains more water than anything else. From there on, ingredients are listed in descending order, according to the percentage of each ingredient in the shampoo.

Surfactants

The second ingredient that most shampoos have in common is the primary surfactant or base detergent. These two terms, surfactant and detergent, mean the same thing: cleansing or "surface active agent."

A surfactant molecule has two ends: a **hydrophilic** (hy-drah-FIL-ik) or water-attracting "head," and a **lipophilic** (ly-puh-FIL-ik) or oil-attracting "tail." During the shampooing process, the hydrophilic head attracts water, and the lipophilic tail attracts oil. This creates a push-pull process that causes the oils, dirt, and deposits to roll up into little balls that can be lifted off in the water and rinsed from the hair (Figure 10–3, Figure 10–4, Figure 10–5, and Figure 10–6).

Other ingredients are added to the base surfactants to create a wide variety of shampoo formulas. Moisturizers, oils, proteins, preservatives, foam enhancers, and perfumes are all standard components of shampoo. 2

Types of Shampoo

Shampoo products account for the highest dollar expenditure in hair care products. Consumer studies show that the most vigorous growth in the shampoo market is found in those products that are retailed through professional salons. This is good news for salon professionals, but never allow yourself to be overconfident if you want to succeed at sales. You will

10

activity

Here's a good exercise for getting a sense of what retailing is all about. List all the hair products used in your school, along with what types of hair these products are best used on. Analyze the hair of one or two classmates and recommend a particular shampoo and conditioner. List the benefits of each product for that particular "client." With your instructor's guidance, you might even try using your recommended choices on your classmates. Keep a record of what products you use, how the hair feels and behaves afterward, and your classmates' own opinions about the products.

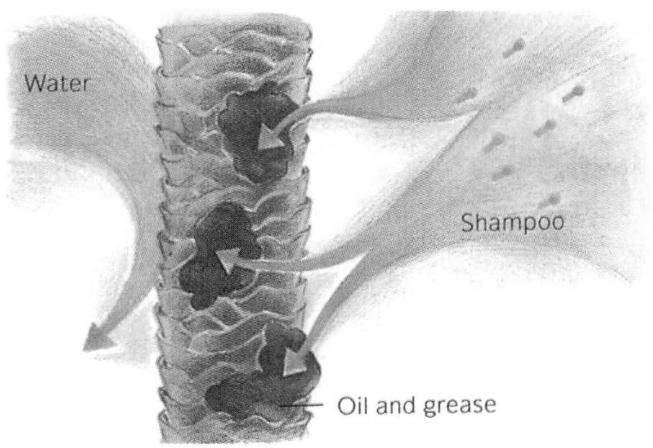

Figure 10-3 The tail of the shampoo molecule is attracted to oil and dirt.

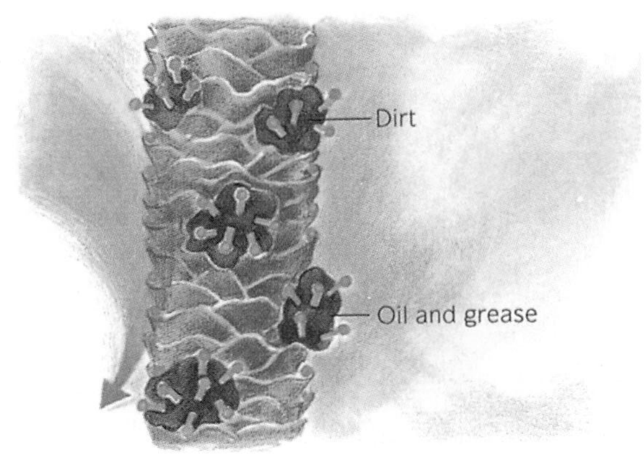

Figure 10-4 Shampoo causes oils to roll up into small globules.

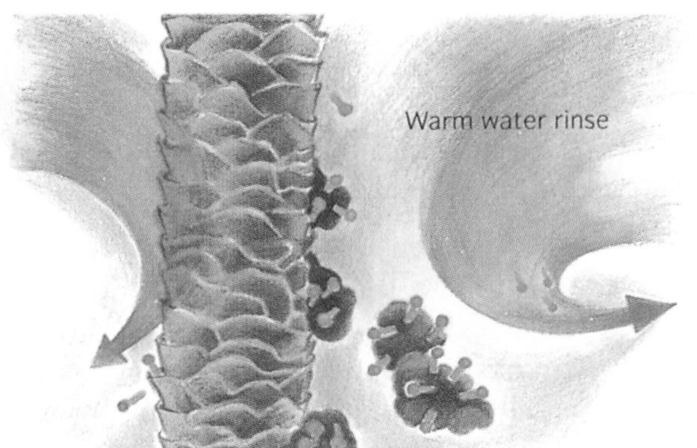

Figure 10-5 During rinsing, the heads of the shampoo molecules attach to water molecules and cause debris to roll off.

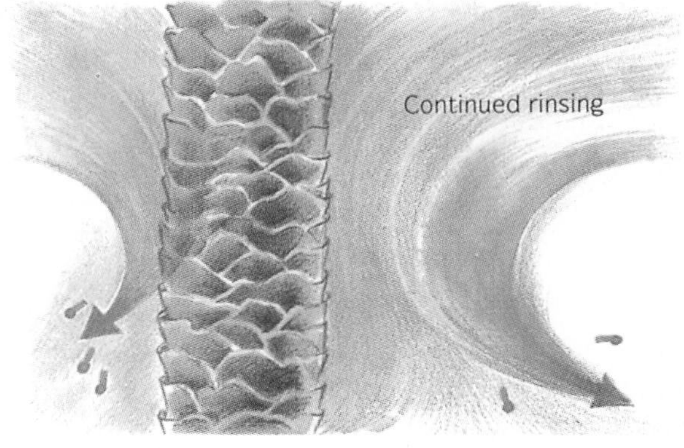

Figure 10-6 Thorough rinsing washes away debris and excess shampoo.

have to be as knowledgeable and sophisticated as possible about the products you are selling and as proficient as you can be in demonstrating their use. Clients are becoming increasingly informed about beauty products from reading about them in beauty magazines and other consumer reports. Your credibility as a professional will be in question if your client is better informed than you are.

Thousands of good shampoos exist, one for every type of hair or scalp condition. There are shampoos for dry, oily, fine, coarse, limp, lightened, permed, relaxed, or chemically untreated hair. There are shampoos that add a slight amount of color to highlighted hair, and those that cleanse hair of styling buildup, mineral deposits, and so forth. There are shampoos that deposit a coating on the hair, and shampoos that strip coating off the hair. The list of ingredients is your key to determining which shampoo will leave a client's hair lustrous and manageable, which will treat a scalp or hair condition, or which will prepare hair for chemical treatment. Most shampoos share many common ingredients, and it is your responsibility as a professional cosmetologist to understand the chemical composition in order to select the best shampoo for each particular service and client.

Now that you are familiar with pH and the chemistry of water and shampoo, let us look at some of the different types of shampoos.

Acid-balanced or Everyday Shampoo

An **acid-balanced shampoo** is one that is balanced to the pH of skin and hair (4.5 to 5.5). Any shampoo can become acid-balanced by the addition of citric, lactic, or phosphoric acid. Some experts believe that an acid pH of 4.5 to 5.5 is essential to prevent excessive dryness and hair damage during the cleansing process. Acid-balanced shampoo helps to close the hair cuticle and is recommended for hair that has been color-treated or lightened.

?

Did you know...

In the 1960s, when Jheri Redding founded four hair care companies—Redken, Jhirmack, Nexxus, and Jheri Redding Products—he revolutionized the salon industry by being the first to market pH-balanced shampoos. He went around the country, staging demonstrations that showed how more acidic shampoos (pH below 7) outperformed those that were more alkaline. When Redding dipped a piece of litmus paper into his shampoo, it would come up a glowing orange, pink, or gold. The litmus test on his competitors' products would come up a murky purple or black. Most cosmetic chemists agree that a low pH is good for any hair, especially treated hair. Redding was right!

Conditioning or Moisturizing Shampoos

Conditioning or **moisturizing shampoos** are designed to make the hair smooth and shiny, to avoid damage to chemically treated hair, and to improve the manageability of the hair. Protein and biotin are just two examples of conditioning agents that boost shampoos so they can meet current grooming needs. These conditioning agents restore moisture and elasticity, strengthen the hair shaft, and add volume. They also are **nonstripping**, meaning they do not remove artificial color from the hair.

Medicated Shampoos

Medicated shampoos contain special chemicals or drugs that are very effective in reducing excessive dandruff or relieving other scalp conditions. Some of these medicated shampoos have to be prescribed by a physician. They are generally quite strong and could affect the color of tinted or lightened hair. In some cases, the shampoo must sit on the scalp for a longer period of time than other shampoos in order for the active ingredient to work. Always read the manufacturers' instructions carefully.

Clarifying Shampoos

Clarifying shampoos contain an acidic ingredient such as cider vinegar to cut through product buildup that can flatten hair. They also increase shine. These shampoos should not be used on a regular basis. They should be used only when a buildup is evident, perhaps once a week to once every two weeks, depending on how much styling product a client tends to use.

Balancing Shampoos

For oily hair and scalp, **balancing shampoos** wash away excess oiliness, while keeping the hair from drying out.

Dry or Powder Shampoos

Sometimes, the state of a client's health makes a wet shampoo uncomfortable or hard to manage. For instance, an elderly client may experience some discomfort at the shampoo bowl due to pressure on the back of the neck. In such a case, it is advisable to use a **dry** or **powder shampoo**, which cleanses the hair without the use of soap and water. The powder picks up dirt and oils as you brush or comb it through the hair. It also adds volume to the hair. Follow the manufacturers' recommended directions. Never give a dry shampoo before performing a chemical service.

Color-Enhancing Shampoos

Color-enhancing shampoos are created by combining the surfactant base with basic colors. They are similar to temporary color rinses in that they are attracted to porous hair and give only slight color changes that are removed with plain shampooing. Color shampoos are used to brighten, to add some slight color, and to eliminate unwanted color tones.

Shampoos for Hairpieces and Wigs

Prepared wig cleaning solutions are available for these hair enhancements (see Chapter 14).

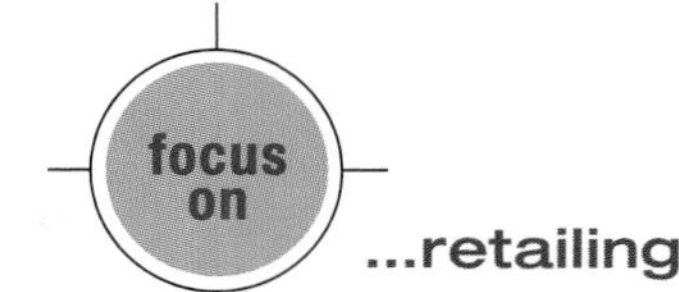

...retailing

Some stylists view the shampoo as "down time" and use it to chatter about what they did the evening before. Your time, and your client's time, can be better used. You can begin to establish your professional relationship during the shampoo by giving the client information as to what you are doing and why. Let the client know what shampoo you are using and why you have selected it. Mention that these products are available for purchase, and emphasize their benefits. There is no need to be pushy or to see this as being pushy. Chances are the client will be eager to make a purchase based on your advice and will thank you for your recommendation.

CONDITIONERS

Conditioners are special chemical agents applied to the hair to deposit protein or moisturizer, to help restore its strength and give it body, or to protect it against possible breakage. Conditioners are a temporary remedy for hair that feels dry, appears damaged, or is damaged. They can only repair to a certain extent; they cannot "heal" damaged hair, and cannot improve the quality of new hair growth.

Heredity, health, and diet control the texture and structure of the hair. However, conditioners are valuable because they can minimize the damage to hair during a cosmetology service, and can restore luster, shine, manageability, and strength while the damaged hair grows long enough to be cut off and replaced by new hair.

Conditioners can sometimes give the false impression that the hair has been restored to its original healthy condition. But habitual use can lead to a buildup on the hair, making it heavy and oily. The stylist should know when to choose between a cream rinse, which simply removes tangles, and a conditioning treatment, which truly repairs damaged hair. Conditioners, also known as "reconstructors" or even "hair masks," are available in three basic types.

1. *Rinse-through.* Finishing rinses or cream rinses that are rinsed out after they are worked through the hair for detangling.
2. *Treatment or repair.* Deep, penetrating conditioners that are left on the hair for 10 to 20 minutes, restoring protein and moisture. Sometimes, it is necessary for the client to sit under a hooded dryer for deeper penetration.
3. *Leave-in.* Applied to the hair and not rinsed out.

CAUTION

Even though a product may be formulated to improve the quality of the hair, it can become damaging over time if used incorrectly. Conditioners can build up on the hair shaft and make your hair heavy and oily, leading you to think it is time to shampoo again. This constant shampooing strips the hair shaft of its protective oils, which prompts you to condition your hair more, creating a vicious cycle. If you use a gentle shampoo that is appropriate for your hair type with a little conditioner only when you need it, you can avoid this problem. Pass this insight on to your clients.

Most conditioners contain silicone along with moisture-binding **humectants** (hew-MECK-tents), substancess that absorb moisture or promote the retention of moisture. This reflects light and makes the hair appear shiny. Other ingredients reduce frizz and bulk up the hair. Most treatments and leave-ins contain proteins, which penetrate the cortex and reinforce the hair shaft from within.

Conditioners affect the hair in different ways:

The cuticle, or outermost layer, is made up of overlapping scales. A healthy cuticle lies down smoothly and reflects light, giving the appearance of shiny hair. Conditioners smooth the cuticle and coat the hair shaft to achieve the same effect. So do detangling rinses or cream rinses, although they are not as heavy.

The cortex makes up 90 percent of the hair strand. It can be penetrated with protein conditioners to reconstruct the hair. Moisturizing conditioners also contain humectants that attract moisture from the air and are absorbed into the cortex (Figure 10–7).

Instant Conditioners

Within the classification of **instant conditioners** fall those products that either remain on the hair for a very short period (one to five minutes) or are left in the hair during styling ("leave-in" conditioners). Instant conditioners contain humectants to improve the appearance of dry, brittle hair.

Most conditioners fall in the pH range of 3.5 to 6.0 and restore the pH balance after an alkaline chemical treatment. Those conditioners designed primarily to balance pH are considered instant because of their short application time. They generally contain an acid that balances the alkalinity of a prior chemical service.

Moisturizers

Heavier and creamier than instant conditioners, **moisturizers** also have a longer application time (10 to 20 minutes). They contain many of the same ingredients as instant conditioners but are formulated to be more penetrating and to have longer staying power. Some moisturizers involve the application of heat.

Quaternary ammonium compounds (quats) are included in the chemical formulation of moisturizers for their ability to attach themselves steadfastly to hair fibers and to provide longer lasting protection than the instant conditioners.

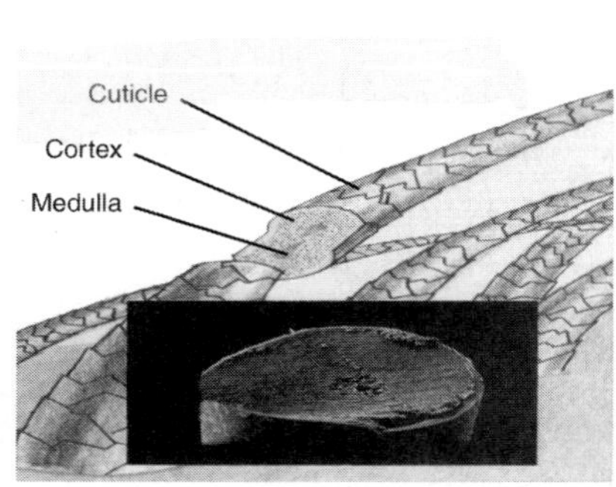

Figure 10-7 The cuticle, cortex, and medulla of the hair shaft.

Protein Conditioners

Protein conditioners are designed to slightly increase hair diameter with a coating action, thereby adding body to the hair. They are often referred to as protein treatments and facilitate the hair setting process. Protein conditioners are available in several strengths. Choose the strength appropriate to the condition, texture, and quality of the hair you are treating.

Concentrated protein conditioners characteristically have a brown liquid appearance. They are used to improve the strength of the hair and to temporarily close split ends. These conditioners are designed to pass through the cuticle, penetrate into the cortex, and replace the keratin that has been lost from the hair. They improve appearance, equalize porosity, and increase elasticity. The excess conditioner must be rinsed from the hair before setting. Concentrated protein treatments are generally not given immediately after a chemical treatment, as they can alter the desirable rearrangement of protein bonds formed by a permanent wave, relaxer, or haircoloring.

Deep Conditioning Treatments

Deep conditioning treatments, also known as hair masks or conditioning packs, are chemical mixtures of concentrated protein in the heavy cream base of a moisturizer. They penetrate several cuticle layers and are the chosen therapy when an equal degree of moisturizing and protein treatment is required.

Other Conditioning Agents

Among the other conditioning agents with which you should be familiar are:

- **spray-on thermal protectors**, which are applied to hair prior to any thermal service to protect the hair from the harmful effects of blow-drying, thermal irons, or electric rollers.
- **scalp conditioners**, which are products, usually in a cream base, used to soften and improve the health of the scalp. They contain moisturizing and emollient ingredients.
- **medicated scalp lotions**, which are conditioners that promote healing of the scalp.
- **scalp astringent lotions**, which remove oil accumulation from the scalp and are used after a scalp treatment and before styling. (Table 10-1 on the following page lists products suitable for different hair types.)

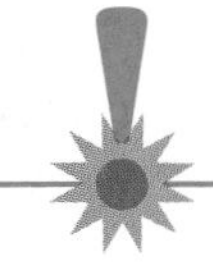

BRUSHING THE HAIR

Correct hair-brushing stimulates the blood circulation to the scalp; helps remove dust, dirt, and hair spray buildup from the hair; and gives hair added shine. You should include a thorough hair-brushing as part of every shampoo and scalp treatment, regardless of whether your client's hair and scalp are dry or oily. But keep these exceptions in mind:

- do not brush before giving a chemical service
- do not brush if the scalp is irritated
- never brush the scalp

CAUTION

Hair services that should not be preceded by brushing, shampooing, or massage include:

- **single-process and double-process haircolor.**
- **highlighting.**
- **most chemical relaxers (follow manufacturers' directions).**
- **some temporary and semi-permanent haircolor (follow manufacturers' directions).**

If shampooing is recommended, shampoo gently to avoid scalp irritation.

Hair Type	Fine	Medium	Coarse
Straight	Volumizing shampoo Detangler, if necessary Protein treatments	Acid-balanced shampoo Finishing rinse Protein treatments	Moisturizing shampoo Leave-in conditioner Moisturizing treatments
Wavy, Curly, Extremely Curly	Fine hair shampoo Light leave-in conditioner Protein treatments Spray-on thermal protectors	Acid-balanced shampoo Leave-in conditioner Moisturizing treatment	Moisturizing shampoo Leave-in conditioner Protein and moisturizing treatments
Dry & Damaged (Perms, Color, Relaxers, Blow-drying, Sun, Hot Irons)	Gentle cleansing shampoo Light leave-in conditioner Protein and moisturizing repair treatments Spray-on thermal protection	Shampoo for chemically treated hair Moisturizing conditioner Protein and moisturizing repair treatments	Deep-moisturizing shampoo for damaged hair Leave-in conditioner Deep conditioning treatments and hair masks

Table 10-1 Matching Products to Hair Types

Also, never use a comb to loosen scales from the scalp. The most highly recommended hairbrushes are those made from natural bristles. Natural bristles have many tiny overlapping layers or scales, which clean and add luster to the hair. Hairbrushes with nylon bristles are shiny and smooth and are fine for hairstyling.

To brush the hair, first part it through the center from front to nape. Then part a section about ½ inch (1.25 cm) off the center parting to the crown of the head. Hold this section of hair in your left hand (Figure 10–8). Rotate the brush by turning the wrist slightly and sweep the bristles the full length of the hair shaft (Figure 10–9). Repeat three times. Then part the hair again ½ inch from the first parting and continue until the entire head has been brushed.

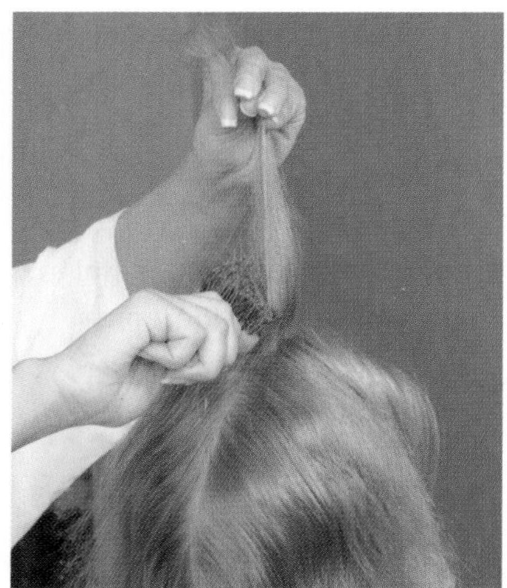

Figure 10-8 Begin the brushing stroke.

SCALP MASSAGE

The two basic requisites for a healthy scalp are cleanliness and stimulation. Since the same manipulations are given with all scalp treatments, you should learn to give them with a continuous, even motion, which will stimulate the scalp and help to relax the client. Scalp massage is most effective when given

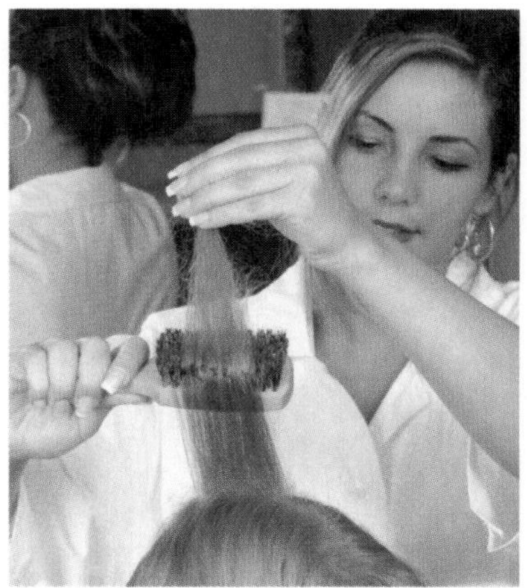

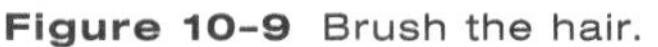

Figure 10–9 Brush the hair.

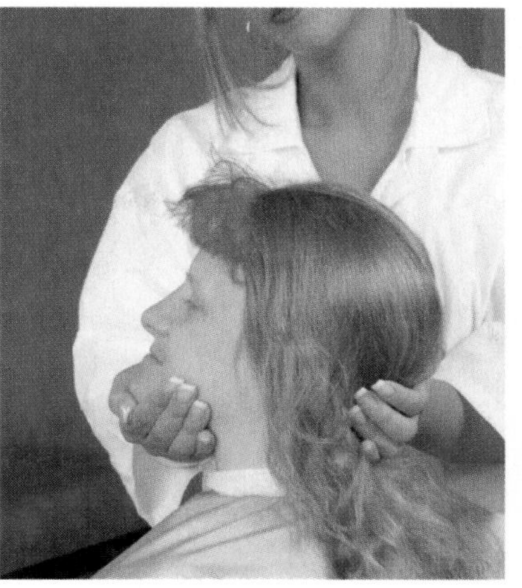

Figure 10–10 Relaxing movement.

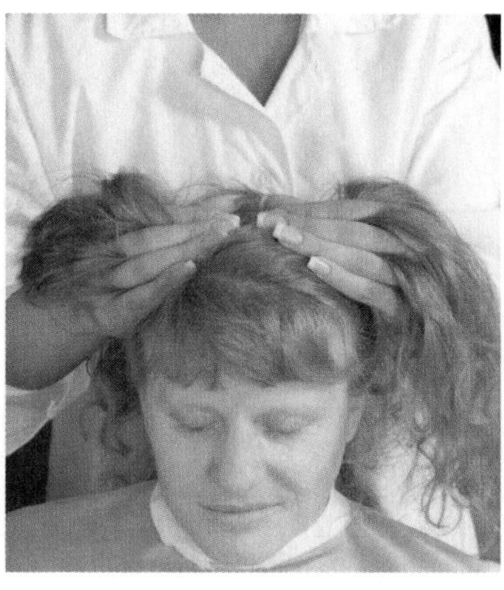

Figure 10–11 Sliding movement.

as a series of treatments once a week for a normal scalp and more frequently when scalp disorders are present, in conjunction with treatment by a dermatologist. Do not massage or manipulate a client's scalp if abrasions are present.

Scalp massage is performed prior to the shampoo. It is a luxurious "extra" service that will keep your clients coming back to you. Knowing the muscles, the location of blood vessels, and the nerve points of the scalp and neck will help guide you to those areas most likely to benefit from massage movements. For this information, refer to Chapter 6.

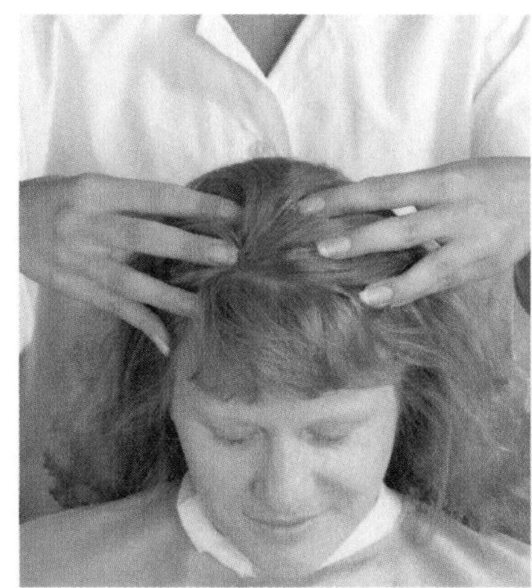

Figure 10–12 Sliding and rotating movement.

Scalp Manipulation Technique

There are several ways to effectively manipulate the scalp. The following routines may be adjusted following your instructor's recommendations.

With each massage movement, place the hands under the hair so the length of the fingers, balls of the fingertips, and cushions of the palms can stimulate the muscles, nerves, and blood vessels of the scalp area.

1. *Relaxing movement:* Cup the client's chin in your left hand; place your right hand at the base of her skull, and rotate the head gently. Reverse positions of your hands and repeat (Figure 10–10).
2. *Sliding movement:* Place your fingertips on each side of the client's head; slide your hands firmly upward, spreading the fingertips until they meet at the top of the head. Repeat four times (Figure 10–11).
3. *Sliding and rotating movement:* Same as (2), except that after sliding the fingertips 1 inch (2.5 cm), rotate and move the client's scalp. Repeat four times (Figure 10–12).
4. *Forehead movement:* Hold the back of the client's head with your left hand. Place your stretched thumb and the fingers of your right hand on the client's forehead. Move your hand slowly and firmly upward to 1 inch past the hairline. Repeat four times (Figure 10–13).

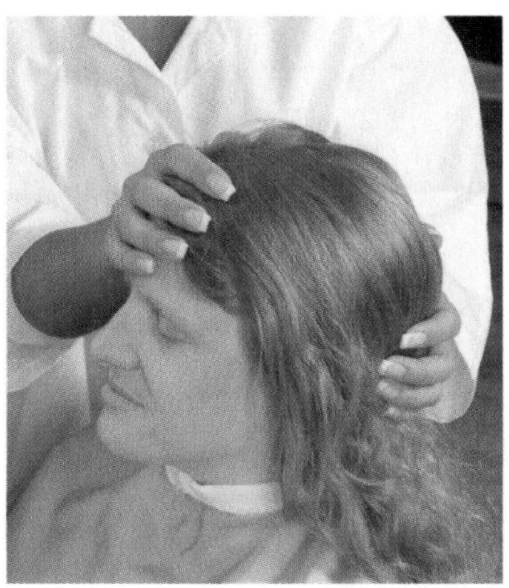

Figure 10–13 Forehead movement.

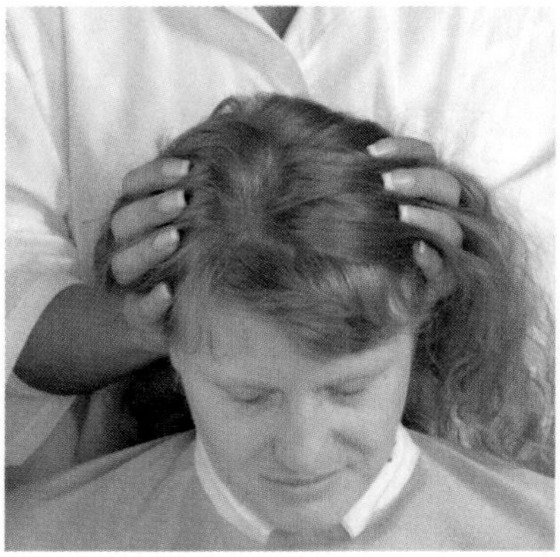

Figure 10–14 Scalp movement.

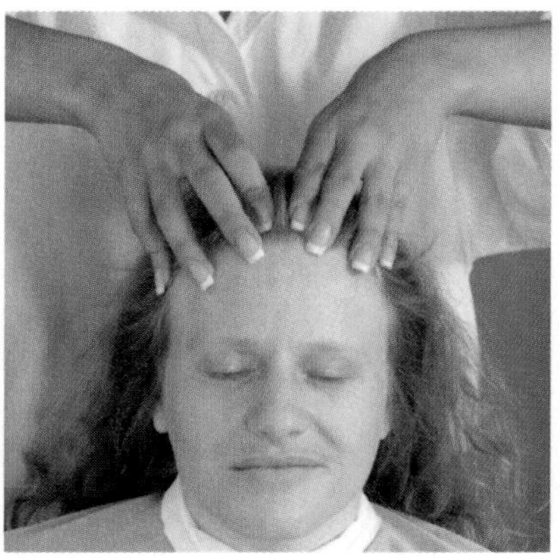

Figure 10–15 Hairline movement.

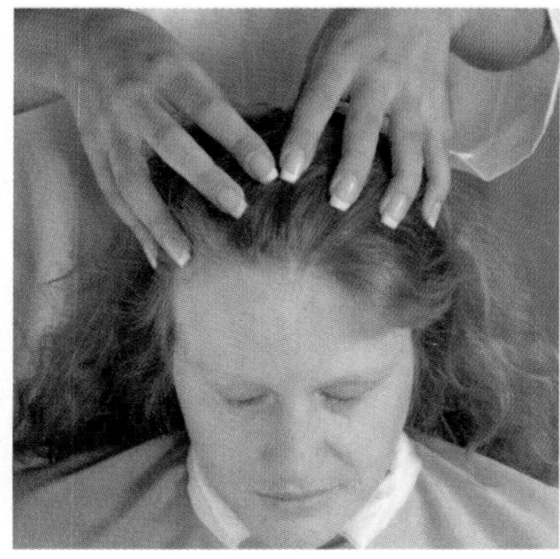

Figure 10–16 Front scalp movement.

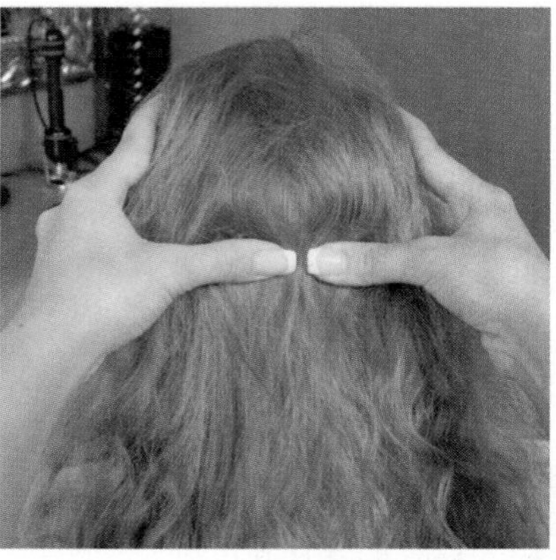

Figure 10–17 Back scalp movement.

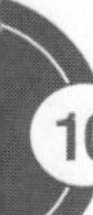

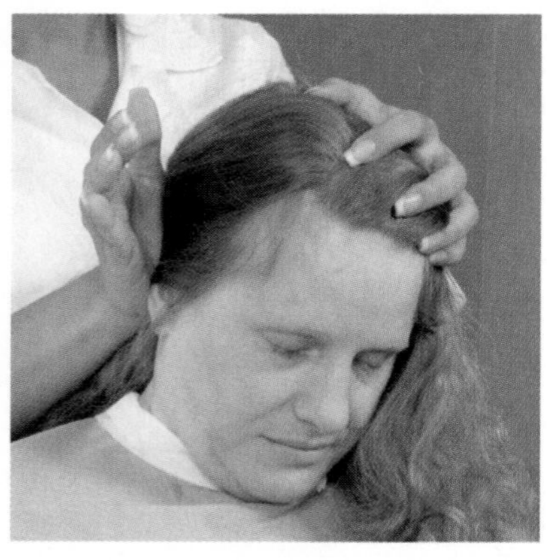

Figure 10–18 Ear-to-ear movement.

5. *Scalp movement:* Place the palms of your hands firmly against the client's scalp. Lift the scalp in a rotary movement, first with your hands placed above her ears, and second with your hands placed at the front and back of her head (Figure 10–14).
6. *Hairline movement:* Place the fingers of both hands at the client's forehead. Massage around her hairline by lifting and rotating (Figure 10–15).
7. *Front scalp movement:* Dropping back 1 inch, repeat the preceding movement over entire front and top of the scalp (Figure 10–16).
8. *Back scalp movement:* Place the fingers of each hand on the sides of the client's head. Starting below her ears, manipulate the scalp with your thumbs, working upward to the crown. Repeat four times. Repeat thumb manipulations, working toward the center back of the head (Figure 10–17).
9. *Ear-to-ear movement:* Place your left hand on the client's forehead. Massage from the right ear to the left ear along the base of the skull with the heel of your hand, using a rotary movement (Figure 10–18).
10. *Back movement:* Place your left hand on the client's forehead and stand to her left. Using your right hand, rotate from the base of the client's neck, along the shoulder, and back across the shoulder blade to the spine. Slide your hand up the client's spine to the base of her neck. Repeat on the opposite side (Figure 10–19).
11. *Shoulder movement:* Place both your palms together at the base of the client's neck. Using a rotary movement, catch the muscles in your palms and massage along the shoulder blades to the point of her shoulders, then back again. Then massage from the shoulders to the spine and back again (Figure 10–20).

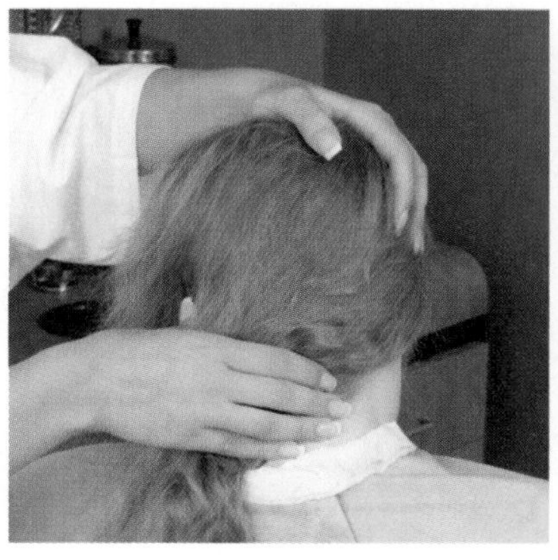

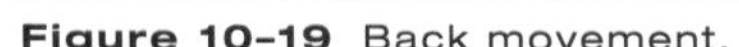

Figure 10–19 Back movement.

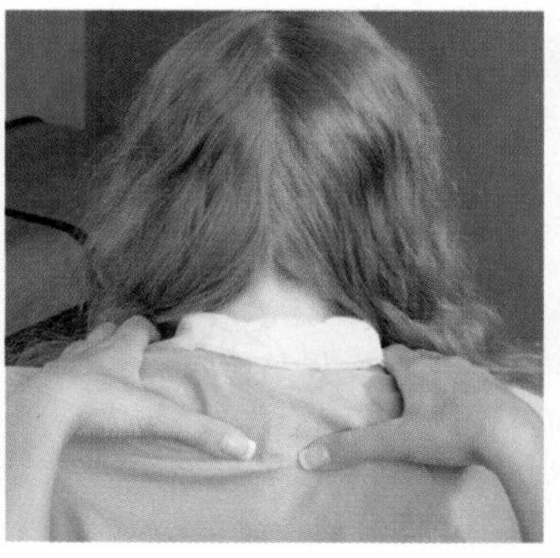

Figure 10–20 Shoulder movement.

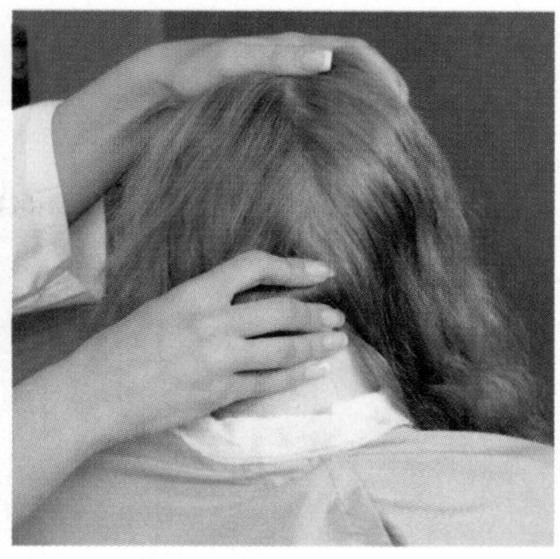

Figure 10–21 Spine movement.

12. *Spine movement:* Massage from the base of the client's skull down the spine with a rotary movement. Using a firm finger pressure, bring your hand slowly to the base of the client's skull (Figure 10–21). 4 ✓

THE SHAMPOO PROCEDURE

Before getting into the actual specifics of the shampoo procedure, it is important to say a few words about posture. Maintaining good posture will protect you against the muscle aches, back strain, discomfort, fatigue, and other physical problems that can result when performing shampoos. Correct posture will also help you maintain an attractive image, always an important consideration given your role as a model to your clients. The most important rule regarding posture is to always keep your shoulders back while performing the shampoo. This way, you will avoid slumping over the client. Remember, too, to hold your abdomen in, thereby lifting your upper body. Free-standing shampoo bowls allow for healthier body alignment and help reduce strain on the back and shoulders (Figure 10–22).

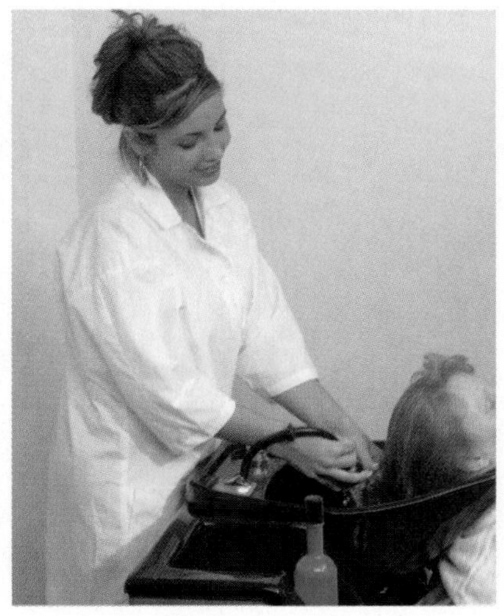

Figure 10–22 Correct posture at the shampoo bowl.

Shampooing Chemically Treated Hair

Chemically treated hair tends to be drier and more fragile than nonchemically treated hair. Therefore, a mild shampoo formulated especially for chemically treated hair is recommended. Chemically treated hair also tends to tangle. To remove tangles, comb gently from the nape and work to the frontal area. Do not force the comb through the hair. Use a conditioner, if necessary. Hair that has been relaxed or straightened tends to be less tangled, but it may mat if not moisturized properly before drying.

PROCEDURE

BASIC SHAMPOO

Implements and Materials

The following are routinely used when performing the shampoo service.

- towels
- shampoo cape
- shampoo
- conditioner (optional)
- comb and hairbrush

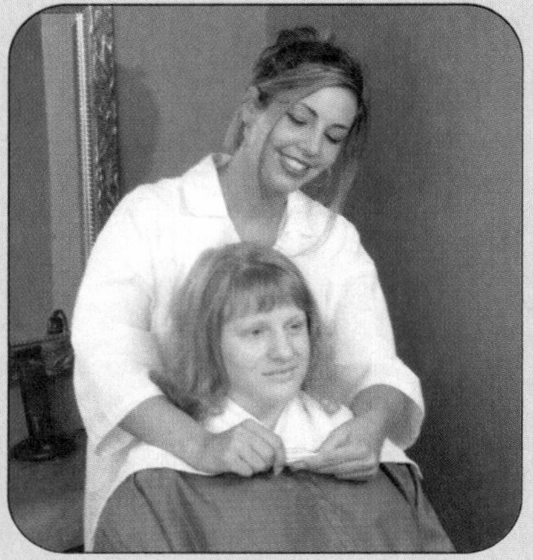

Figure 10-23 Cross ends of the towel under the chin.

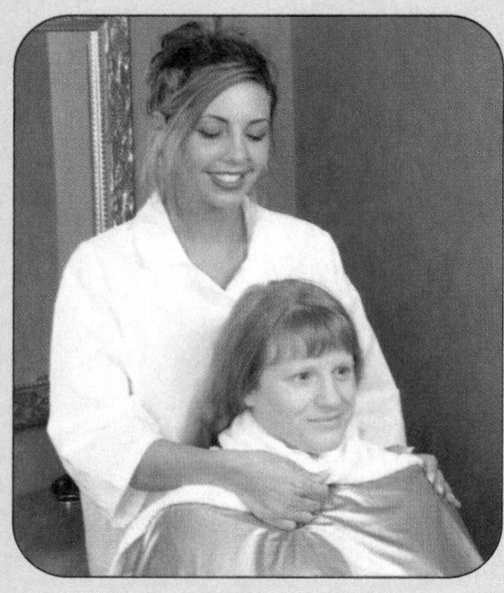

Figure 10-24 Place another towel over cape.

Preparation

1. Seat your client at your workstation, making sure she is comfortable.
2. Consult on which hair services your client will be receiving on this visit.
3. Wash your hands with soap and warm water.
4. Drape the client for the shampoo. Turn the client's collar to the inside, if necessary. Place a towel lengthwise across the client's shoulders, crossing the ends beneath the chin (Figure 10–23).
5. Place the cape over the towel and fasten in the back so that the cape does not touch the client's skin.
6. Place another towel over the cape and secure in the front (Figure 10–24).
7. Remove all hairpins and combs from the hair.
8. Ask the client to remove earrings and glasses and keep them in a safe place.
9. Examine the condition of the client's hair and scalp, and determine the appropriate shampoo and conditioner to be used.
10. Brush the hair thoroughly.
11. Massage the scalp.

Procedure

1. Seat the client comfortably at the shampoo sink.
2. Supporting the client's head with one hand, draw the back of the cape over the outside of the shampoo chair to keep water from running down the client's back (Figure 10–25).
3. Adjust the volume and temperature of the water spray. Consider the client's preference when adjusting the water temperature. Turn on the cold water first and gradually add warm water until you obtain a comfortably warm temperature. Test the temperature of the water by spraying it on the inner side of your wrist. Monitor the temperature of the water throughout the shampoo by keeping one finger over the edge of the spray nozzle and in contact with the water.
4. Wet the hair thoroughly with warm water spray. Lift the hair and work it with your free hand to saturate the scalp. When working around the hairline, shift your hand to protect the client's face, ears, and neck from the spray. If you wish, you can place your little finger behind the client's ear and cup your hand to make a shield, thus preventing water from running into the client's ear. You can also bend the ear inward to keep water out (Figure 10–26, Figure 10–27, and Figure 10–28).
5. Apply small quantities of shampoo to the hair, beginning at the hairline and working back. Work into a lather using the pads or cushions of the fingers. Do not use your fingernails.
6. Manipulate the scalp.
   a. Begin at the front hairline and work in a back-and-forth movement until the top of the head is reached (Figure 10–29).
   b. Continue in this manner to the back of the head, shifting your fingers back 1 inch (2.5cm) at a time.

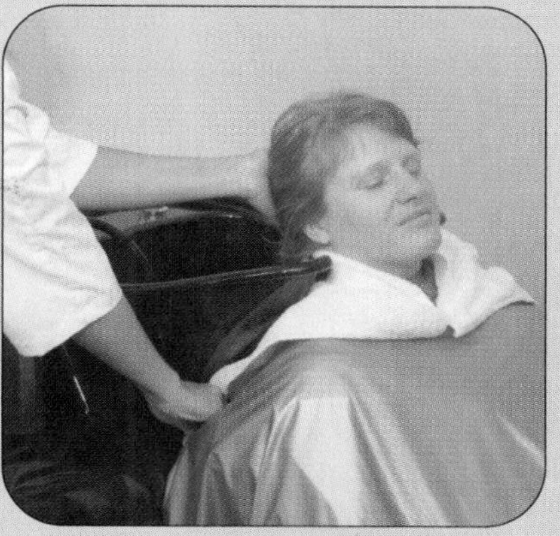

Figure 10–25 Adjust cape over back of shampoo chair.

CAUTION

In massaging or manipulating the scalp while shampooing, do not use firm pressure if:

- **you will be giving the client a chemical service after the shampoo.**
- **the client's scalp is tender or sensitive.**
- **the client asks for less pressure.**

10

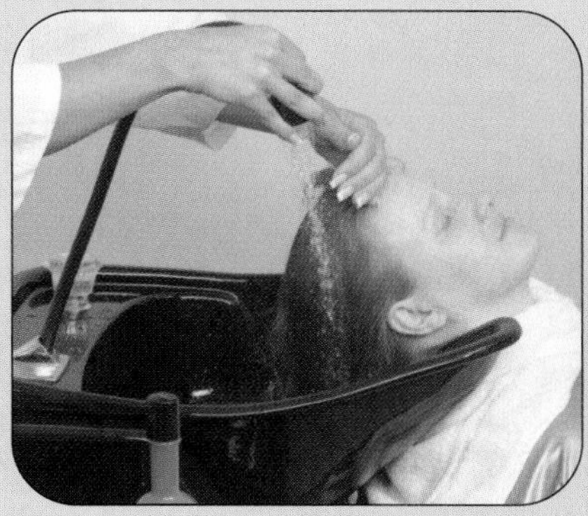

Figure 10–26 Protect the face.

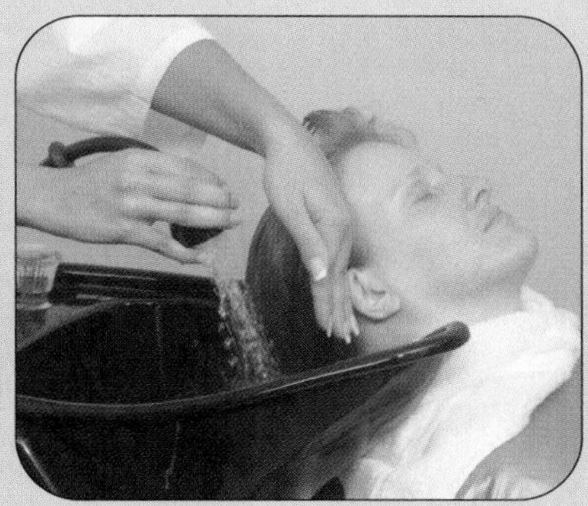

Figure 10–27 Protect the ears.

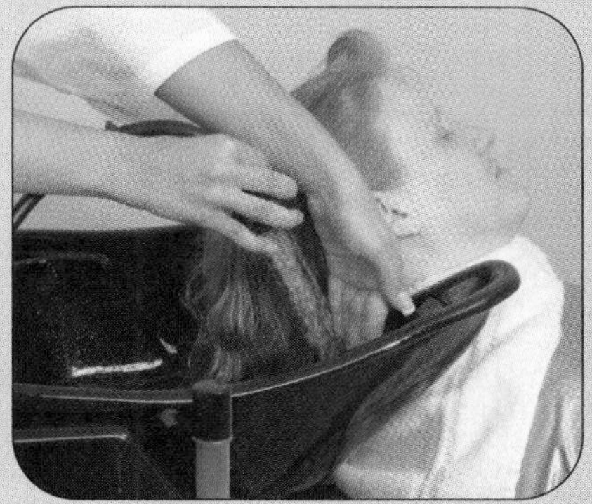

Figure 10–28 Protect the neck.

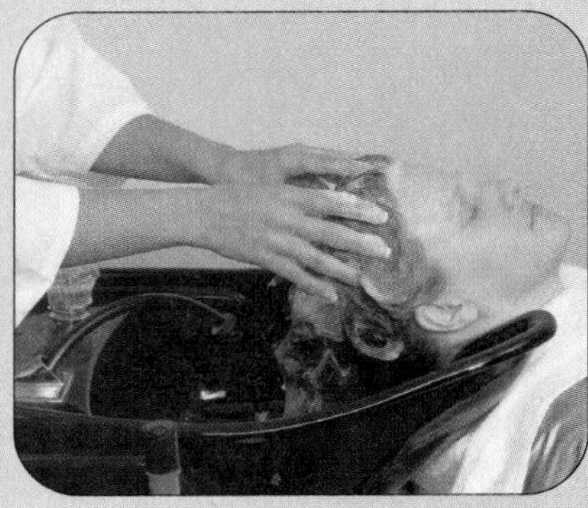

Figure 10-29 Manipulate the scalp.

c. Lift the client's head with one hand. With the other hand, manipulate the scalp above the ear, and using the same movement, work to the back of the head (Figure 10–30).

d. Drop your fingers down 1 inch and repeat the process until that side of the head is covered.

e. Beginning at the other ear, repeat steps c and d.

f. Allow the client's head to relax and work around the hairline with your thumbs in a rotary movement.

g. Repeat these movements until the scalp has been thoroughly massaged.

h. Remove excess shampoo and lather by squeezing the hair.

7. Rinse hair thoroughly with a strong spray of lukewarm water. Lift the hair at the crown and back with the fingers of your left hand to permit the spray to rinse the hair thoroughly (Figure 10–31). Cup your left hand along the nape and pat the hair, forcing the spray of water against the base scalp area.
8. If required, apply shampoo again. Repeat the procedure using steps 5, 6, and 7 as outlined. You will need less shampoo because partially clean hair lathers more easily.
9. Gently squeeze excess water from the hair. Apply conditioner, avoiding the base of the hair near the scalp. Gently comb the conditioner through, distributing it with a wide-tooth comb, while the client remains in a reclining position, with her head in the shampoo bowl (Figure 10–32).
10. Leave the conditioner on for the recommended time. Some conditioners are left on less than 1 minute, and some for 10 to 20 minutes. If you are rinsing out in less than 1 minute, it is fine to keep the client in a reclining position, as long as she is comfortable. Rinse the conditioner out thoroughly and finish with a cool water rinse to seal the cuticle.

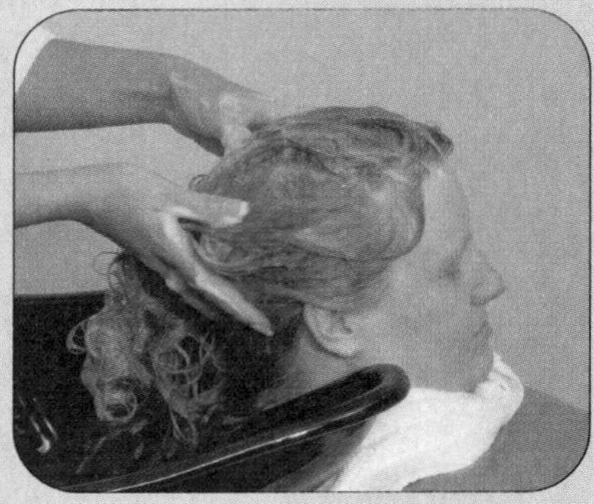

Figure 10-30 Lift the client's head.

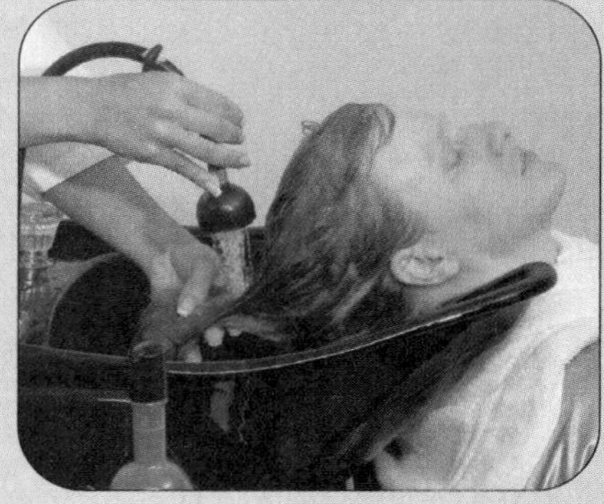

Figure 10-31 Rinse the client's hair.

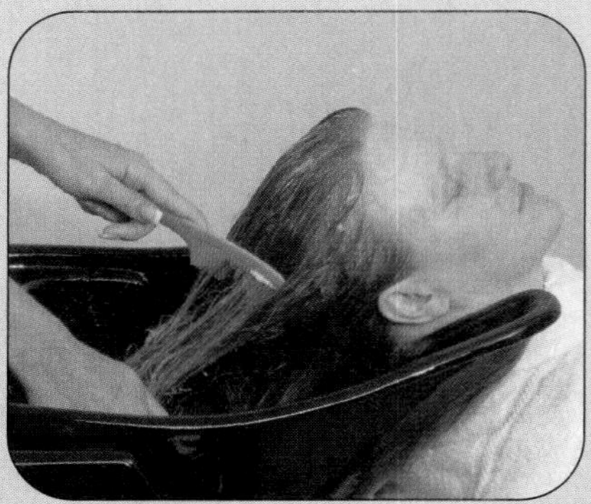

Figure 10-32 Comb conditioner through client's hair.

11. If the conditioner is to remain on the head for more than 1 minute, place a plastic cap on the client's head and have her sit upright for the recommended time (Figure 10–33). If you have applied a deep conditioning treatment, you may have to place the client under a heated dryer for the recommended time. Always follow the manufacturer's directions carefully.
12. Partially towel dry.
    a. While still at the shampoo bowl, remove excess moisture from the hair.
    b. Wipe excess moisture from around the client's face and ears with the ends of the towel.
    c. Lift the towel over the back of the client's head and drape the head with the towel.
    d. Place your hands on top of the towel and blot out excess water. Do not rub, as rubbing will tangle the hair (Figure 10–34).
13. Clean out the shampoo bowl, removing any loose hair.
14. Comb the client's hair, beginning with the ends at the nape of the neck.
15. Change the drape, if necessary.
16. Style the hair as desired.

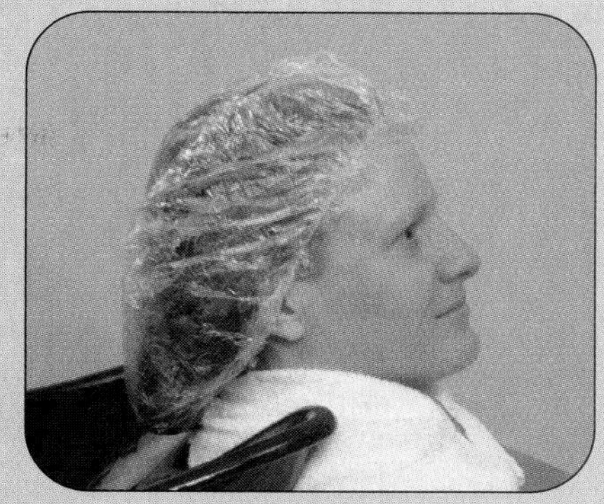

Figure 10–33 Some conditioners require a plastic cap.

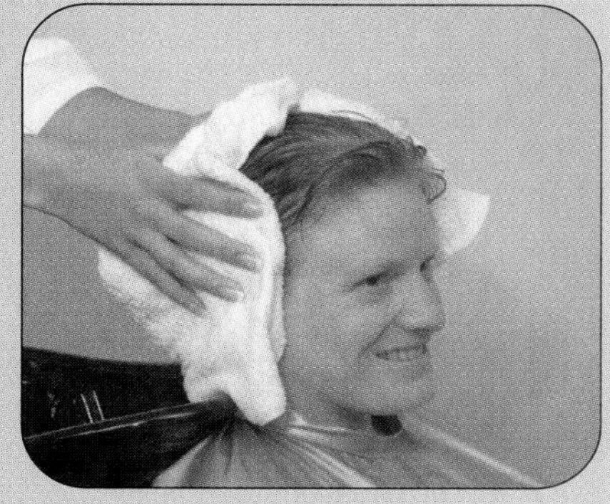

Figure 10–34 Towel-blot the client's hair.

Cleanup and Sanitation

1. Discard used materials, and place unused supplies in their proper place.
2. Place used towels in the towel hamper.
3. Disinfect combs and brushes for the required time.
4. Sanitize the shampoo bowl. The neck of the bowl should be disinfected after each client.
5. Wash your hands with soap and warm water. 5 ✓

completed!

insights

Pat Grant-Williams

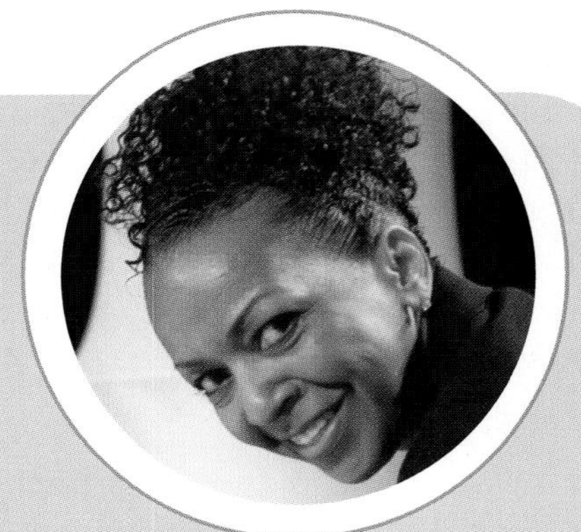

Teaching and education are central to the cosmetology profession. Pat Grant-Williams, artistic director of Colomer USA and owner and president of Hair & Beyond, Inc., has spent 20 years in the field, both behind the chair and training others.

I have a degree in journalism, but I didn't like what I was doing, so I became a freelance makeup artist for Lancôme Cosmetics, where I met Floyd Kenyatta. He asked me to do makeup for one of his shows, and then I started shampooing in his salon. One day he wasn't there, so I curled one of his clients, and from that day on, I was styling hair (much to my mother's dismay—she expected that I was going to become a journalist).

I love what I do—and that's so important. You have to love what you do. I love every aspect of this business. I get to make a difference in people's lives every day just by touching them, and there is no greater pleasure than that. I still work behind the chair three days a week. I don't think I could be an artistic director without being behind the chair. I need to keep my hand in it. What I love most is creating a style for a customer, maintaining healthy hair, and seeing the smile on her face when I turn her around to look in the mirror.

The most challenging thing for me is when a client has had a bad experience elsewhere and consequently has a negative opinion of hairdressers and salons. A client having lost her hair for whatever reason is very troubling for me as a stylist, especially if she had it done by a "professional."

Our industry is not looked on as a major player, even though we are the second most licensed entity in the United States after motor vehicles operators. There is a lot of education still needed, and that is what my struggle is every day: to change the way the laws are written for people who work in this business.

As artistic director, I train all of the hairdressers who work for us. I recruit and train them, and teach onstage for us globally. I also get to use my journalistic skills, helping to write the packaging instructions and writing the scripts for our videos. This year, I'm being named Global Ambassador in the beauty industry. It's like the Academy Awards of hair. Last year, Floyd Kenyatta won. Following in his footsteps is a major honor, and it's very humbling for me.

Applying Dry Shampoos

Sometimes, as stated earlier, the state of a client's health makes a wet shampoo uncomfortable or hard to manage. For instance, an elderly client may experience some discomfort at the shampoo bowl due to pressure on the back of the neck. In such cases, it is advisable to use a dry or powder shampoo. A dry shampoo can be applied at the stylist's station, with the client draped as for a chemical service. Follow the manufacturers' recommended directions, as they will vary. For the most part, you will be applying the powder directly onto the hair from scalp to the ends, then brushing through with a natural bristle brush to remove oil and dirt (Figure 10–35).

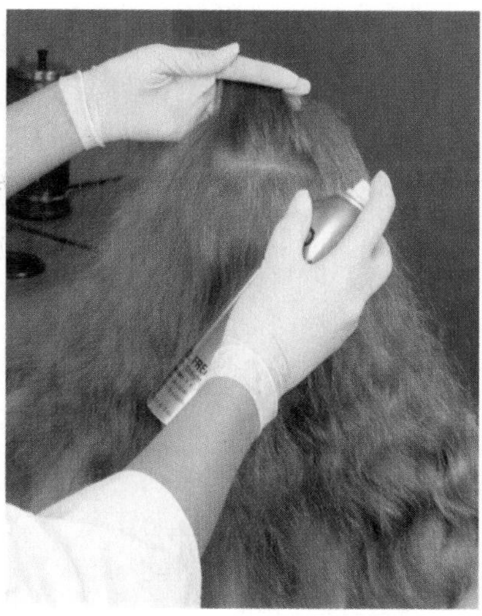

Figure 10-35 Applying powder dry shampoo.

Shampooing Clients with Special Needs

Clients with disabilities or those who are wheelchair-bound will usually tell you how they prefer to be shampooed. Some clients in wheelchairs will allow you to shampoo their hair while they remain seated in their wheelchairs, facing the shampoo bowl and bending forward, with a towel to protect their face. If the wheelchair is the correct height in relation to the shampoo bowl, shampoo as normal while the client remains in the wheelchair. Sometimes, a client will arrive in the salon with her hair freshly shampooed from home, and sometimes a dry shampoo is appropriate. The same goes for clients with other special needs. Always ask their preferences and keep their comfort and safety a priority.

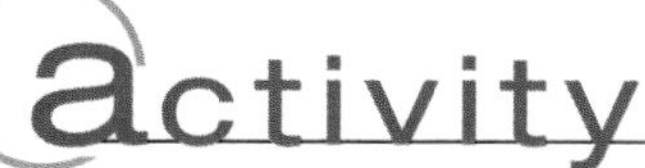

Role-playing is a good way to practice recommending retail products to clients. Pair off with a classmate. One takes the role of the stylist and the other plays a client. Your "scene" might go like this.

Stylist: Have you encountered any problems with your scalp or hair since your last salon visit, Mrs. Benson? Any itchiness or flaking?

Mrs. Benson: No. I don't usually have scalp problems this time of year. But in the winter I do.

Stylist: Any dryness?

Mrs. Benson: Well, ever since I started having my hair highlighted, it does feel a little drier.

Stylist: Chemical services often dry the hair. I'm going to use a shampoo for color-treated hair and finish with a moisturizing conditioner.

Mrs. Benson: That sounds good. But won't the conditioner make my hair feel limp?

Stylist: I'll use a light-weight conditioner. It'll leave your hair silky and shiny. If you like it you can purchase some before you leave. You know, using the right shampoo and conditioner will help keep your hair healthy in between visits to the salon.

Mrs. Benson: Great! Let's do it!

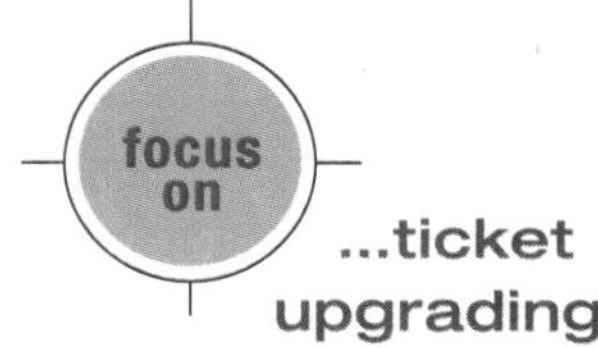

...ticket upgrading

The shampoo procedure offers an excellent opportunity to acquaint clients with products and services particularly suited for their hair, and also to make a sale. Imagine the following exchange:

Stylist: I notice that your hair ends feel very dry and brittle today. I can apply a moisturizing conditioner for you right here at the sink that I'm sure will make your hair feel silkier and look shinier. I just want you to know that there will be a slight charge.

Client: You're right, the ends have felt dry lately. Go ahead, and add it to my bill.

10

GENERAL HAIR AND SCALP TREATMENTS

CAUTION

Do not use high-frequency current on hair treated with tonics or lotions that contain alcohol.

The purpose of a general scalp treatment is to keep the scalp and hair in a clean and healthy condition. A stylist should recommend a hair or scalp treatment only after having performed a hair and scalp examination. If the client does not have the time to sit for a treatment, recommend scheduling the treatment at a later, more convenient time. If the client does request a treatment at that time, it should be given either before or after the shampoo, depending on which treatment is given.

For a discussion of the uses and benefits of light therapy and electrotherapy, refer back to Chapter 7.

Normal Hair and Scalp Treatments

1. Drape the client.
2. Brush the hair for about five minutes.
3. Apply scalp conditioner.
4. Apply infrared lamp for about five minutes.
5. Manipulate the scalp for 10 to 20 minutes.
6. Shampoo the hair.
7. Towel dry the hair to remove excess moisture.
8. Apply suitable scalp lotion and/or styling aids.
9. Style the hair.

Dry Hair and Scalp Treatments

This treatment should be used when there is a deficiency of natural oil on the scalp and hair. Select scalp preparations containing moisturizing and emollient ingredients. Avoid the use of strong soaps, preparations containing a mineral oil or sulfonated oil base, greasy preparations, and lotions with a high alcohol content. In this treatment, a scalp steamer, which resembles a hooded dryer, will be used.

1. Drape the client.
2. Brush the client's hair for about five minutes.
3. Apply the scalp preparation for this condition.
4. Apply the scalp steamer for seven to ten minutes, or wrap the head in warm steam towels for seven to ten minutes.
5. Give a mild shampoo.
6. Towel dry the hair and scalp thoroughly.
7. Apply moisturizing scalp cream sparingly with a rotary, frictional motion.
8. Stimulate the scalp with direct high-frequency current, using the glass rake electrode, for about five minutes.
9. Rinse the hair thoroughly.
10. Style the hair.

Oily Hair and Scalp Treatments

Excessive oiliness is caused by overactive sebaceous (oil) glands. Manipulate the scalp and knead it to increase blood circulation to the surface. Any hardened sebum in the pores of the scalp will be removed with gentle pressing or squeezing. To normalize the function of these glands, excess sebum should be flushed out with each treatment.

1. Drape the client.
2. Brush the client's hair for about five minutes.
3. Using a cotton pledget, apply a medicated scalp lotion to the scalp only (Figure 10–36).
4. Apply infrared lamp for about five minutes.
5. Manipulate the scalp. (*Optional:* Faradic or sinusoidal current may be used) (Figure 10–37).
6. Shampoo with a corrective shampoo for oily hair.
7. Towel dry the hair.
8. Apply direct high-frequency current for three to five minutes (Figure 10–38).
9. Apply a scalp astringent and/or suitable styling aids.
10. Style the hair.

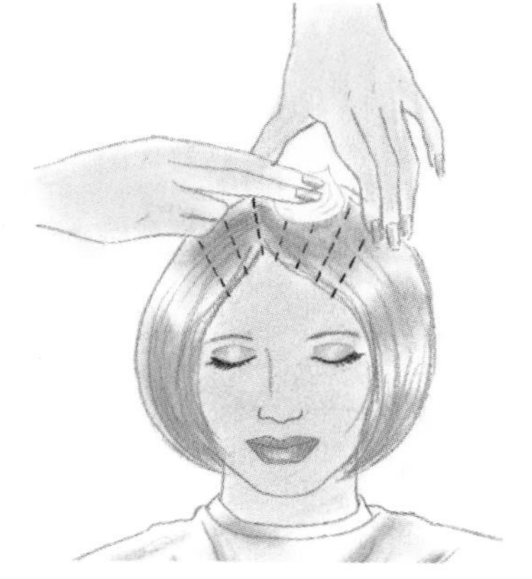

Figure 10-36 Apply scalp lotion with cotton pledget.

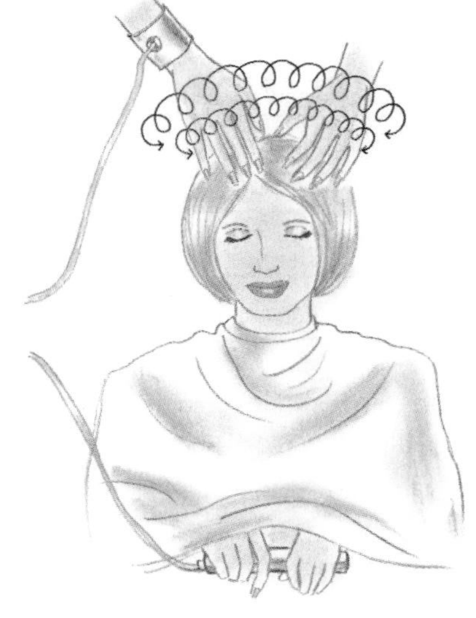

Figure 10-37 Manipulate the scalp with faradic current while the client holds the electrode.

Antidandruff Treatments

Dandruff is the result of a fungus called malassezia. Antidandruff shampoos, conditioners, and topical lotions contain antifungal agents that control dandruff by suppressing the growth of malassezia. Moisturizing salon treatments also soften and loosen scalp scales that stick to the scalp in crusts.

1. Drape the client.
2. Shampoo with an antidandruff shampoo.
3. Towel dry the hair.
4. Apply an antidandruff conditioner or lotion.
5. Apply heat with an infrared lamp or scalp steamer for about five minutes (optional).
6. Shampoo with an antidandruff shampoo.
7. Style the hair.
8. Because of the ability of the fungus to resist treatment, additional salon treatments and the frequent use of antidandruff products at home should be recommended. 6 ✓

Caution: Some antidandruff lotions are alcohol based and should not be used in conjunction with infrared lamps.

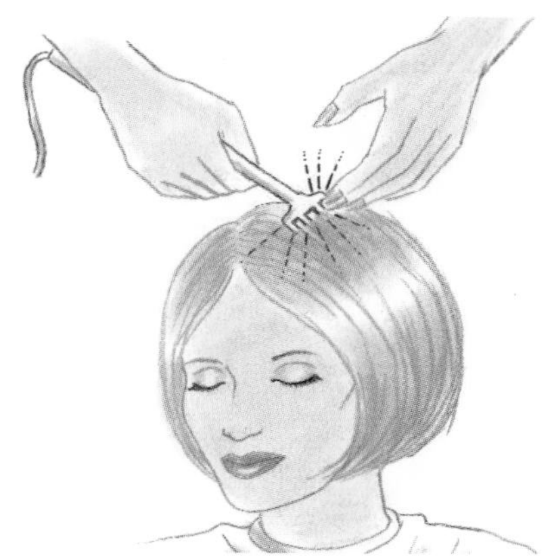

Figure 10-38 Apply high-frequency current.

chapter glossary

acid-balanced shampoo	shampoo that is balanced to the pH of skin and hair (4.5 to 5.5)
balancing shampoos	shampoos that wash away excess oiliness from oily hair and scalp, while keeping the hair from drying out
clarifying shampoos	shampoos containing an acidic ingredient such as cider vinegar to cut through product buildup that can flatten hair; also increase shine
color-enhancing shampoos	shampoos created by combining the surfactant base with basic dyes
conditioners	special chemical agents applied to the hair to deposit protein or moisturizer, to help restore its strength and give it body, or to protect it against possible breakage
conditioning or moisturizing shampoos	shampoos designed to make the hair smooth and shiny, avoid damage to chemically treated hair, and improve manageability
deep conditioning treatments	chemical mixtures of concentrated protein and the heavy cream base of a moisturizer; used to provide an equal degree of moisturizing and protein treatment
dry or powder shampoo	shampoo that cleanses the hair without the use of soap and water
hard water	water containing certain minerals that lessen the ability of soap or shampoo to lather readily
humectants	substances that absorb moisture or promote the retention of moisture
hydrophilic	capable of combining with or attracting water
instant conditioners	conditioners that either remain on the hair for a very short period (1 to 5 minutes) or are left in the hair during styling ("leave in" conditioners)
lipophilic	having an affinity for attracting fat and oils
medicated shampoos	shampoos containing special chemicals or drugs for reducing excessive dandruff or relieving other scalp conditions
medicated scalp lotions	conditioners that promote healing of the scalp
moisturizers	products formulated to add moisture to dry hair, with a heavier formulation than instant conditioners and a longer application time
nonstripping	descriptive of products that do not remove artificial color from the hair
protein conditioners	products designed to slightly increase hair diameter with a coating action, thereby adding body to the hair
scalp astringent lotions	products used to remove oil accumulation from the scalp; used after a scalp treatment and before styling
scalp conditioners	products, usually in a cream base, used to soften and improve the health of the scalp
soft water	rain water or chemically softened water that lathers easily with soap or shampoo
spray-on thermal protectors	products applied to hair prior to any thermal service to protect it from the harmful effects of blow-drying, thermal irons, or electric rollers

review questions

1. Why is pH an important factor in shampoo selection?
2. Name four ways in which water can be purified.
3. What is the chemical action of surfactants in shampoo?
4. What shampoo and/or conditioner is appropriate for use on dandruff? On product buildup? On damaged hair?
5. What is the action of conditioner on the hair?
6. What is the purpose of brushing the hair prior to shampooing?
7. Describe the draping procedure for a shampoing service.
8. What hair services should not be preceded by shampooing, brushing, or massage?
9. Describe the hair and scalp treatment for oily hair, dry hair, and dandruff.

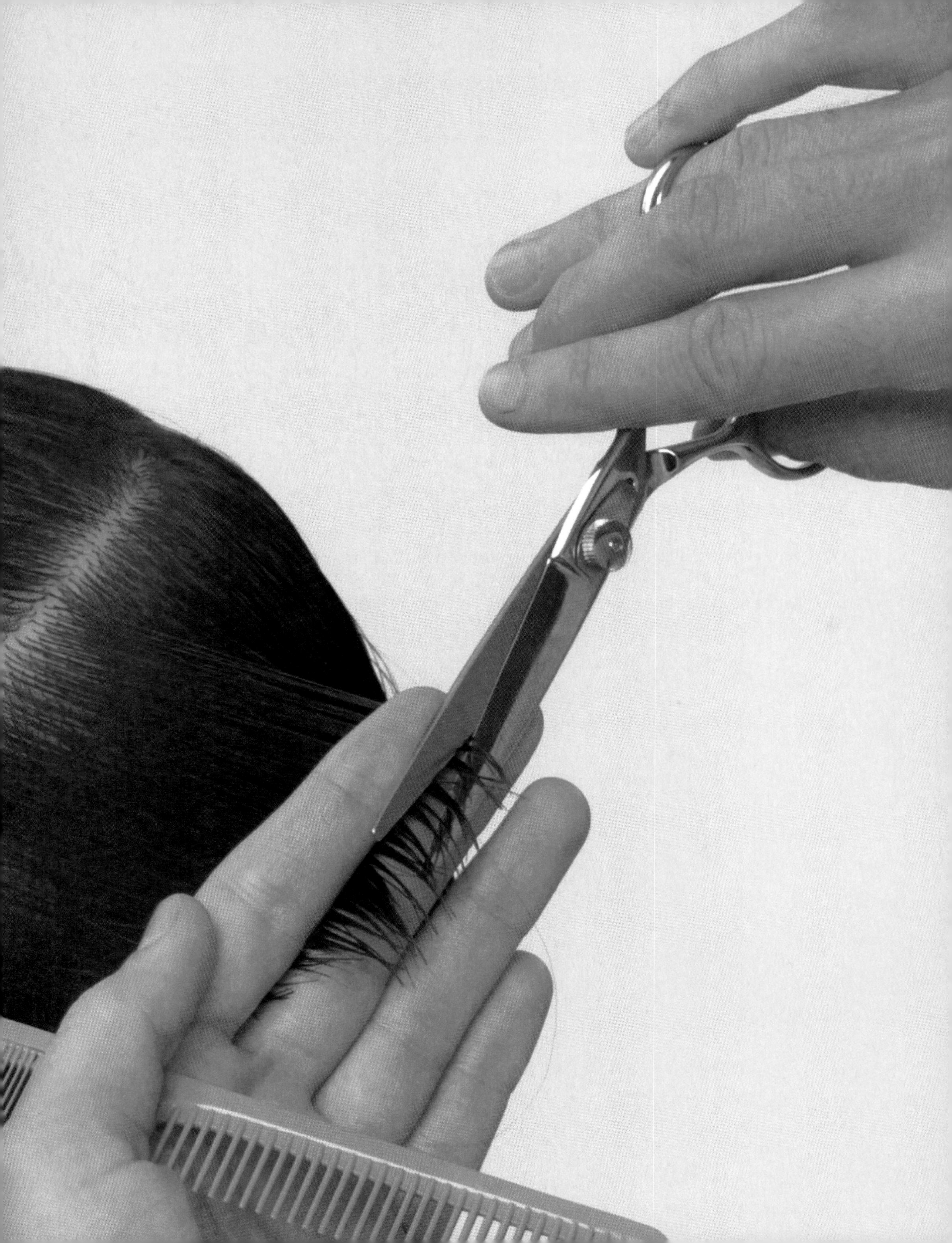

HAIRCUTTING

Ruth Roche

FOUNDER/EDUCATION DIRECTOR, RARE NYC, AN ACADEMY FOR LICENSED COSMETOLOGISTS

Chapter Outline

Learning Objectives

After completing this chapter, you should be able to:

1. Identify reference points on the head form and understand their role in haircutting.
2. Define angles, elevations, and guidelines.
3. List the factors involved in a successful client consultation.
4. Demonstrate the safe and proper use of the various tools of haircutting.
5. Demonstrate mastery of the four basic haircuts.
6. Demonstrate mastery of other haircutting techniques.

National Skill Standards

This chapter provides you with the necessary information to master these National Industry Skill Standards for Entry-Level Cosmetologists.

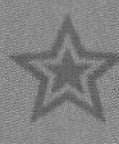
Providing a haircut in accordance with a client's needs or expectations.

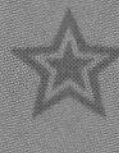
Consulting with clients to determine their needs and preferences.

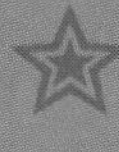
Conducting services in a safe environment and taking measures to prevent the spread of infectious and contagious diseases.

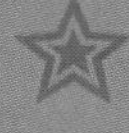
Using a variety of salon products while providing client services.

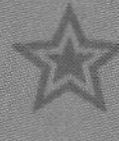
Effectively marketing professional salon products.

Key Terms

Page number indicates where in the chapter the term is used.

angle pg. 286
apex pg. 284
beveling pg. 286
blunt haircut pg. 300
carving pg. 332
clipper-over-comb pg. 337
cross-checking pg. 302
crown pg. 285
cutting line pg. 287
distribution pg. 326
elevation pg. 287
four corners pg. 285
free-hand notching pg. 332
fringe pg. 285
graduated haircut/graduation pg. 301
growth pattern pg. 293
guideline pg. 287
hairline pg. 293
head form pg. 283
interior guideline pg. 320
layered haircut/layers pg. 301
line pg. 286
long layered haircut pg. 301
nape pg. 285
notching pg. 331
occipital bone pg. 284
overdirection pg. 289
palm-to-palm pg. 299
parietal ridge pg. 284
part/parting pg. 287
perimeter pg. 287
point cutting pg. 331
razor-over-comb pg. 335
razor rotation pg. 335
reference points pg. 284
section pg. 287
shears-over-comb pg. 329
slicing pg. 332
slide cutting pg. 329
slithering pg. 332
stationary guideline pg. 288
subsections pg. 287
tapers pg. 336
tension pg. 298
texturizing pg. 331
traveling guideline pg. 288
uniform layers pg. 317
weight line pg. 300

As a student of cosmetology, it is important to develop a strong foundation in haircutting on which you will build for the rest of your career. Without this foundation of basic skills and techniques, the services and creativity you will be able to provide to your clients may be limited. The best way to build this foundation is by paying close attention to the instruction you are receiving. The more familiar you become with basic haircutting and shaping techniques and the more comfortable you are with shears, razors, and clippers, the more solid that foundation will be. Practice will not necessarily make perfect, but practice—lots and lots of practice—will help you to achieve excellence. And excellence is the goal that you, your instructors, and your school all strive for.

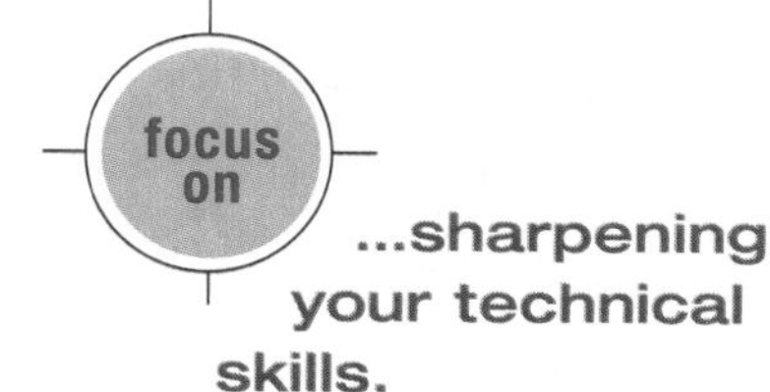

...sharpening your technical skills.

While you're in school, there may be many things you will be asked to learn and master that will have you wondering, "Why do I need to know this?" Here is some good advice: learn and master everything you can. Trends come and go, and believe it or not, what is out of style today may be hot again tomorrow. With your imagination and skill, you may become a trend-setter yourself. You may even bring back finger waves to a world bored out of its mind with straight hair!

BASIC PRINCIPLES OF HAIRCUTTING

Great haircuts, or shapes, come about when you have a solid understanding of the important steps of the haircutting process. The process begins with combing the hair. Next, the hair needs to be parted, in order to create the uniform work areas on which you will be working. It may also be necessary to elevate, or raise, the hair while cutting to create a graduated effect or layers. The core of the process, however, has to do with understanding the physics of hair. This basically means that for every action or technique you use on the hair, there will be an expected and predictable result. When you understand the physics of hair, you can create whatever shape you choose.

Every time you comb, lift, and cut the ends of the hair, you create a haircut. When the hair falls back to its natural position, it falls into a shape, or formation, based on the execution of the essential steps described above.

Head Form: Anatomy of the Skull

It is necessary to understand the shape of the skull in order to create consistent and successful results in haircutting. The shape of the head or skull, also referred to as the **head form** or head shape, plays a major role in guiding you to the desired end result. Hair responds differently on different areas of the head, depending on the end-result length and the cutting technique used. An awareness of where the head form curves, turns, and

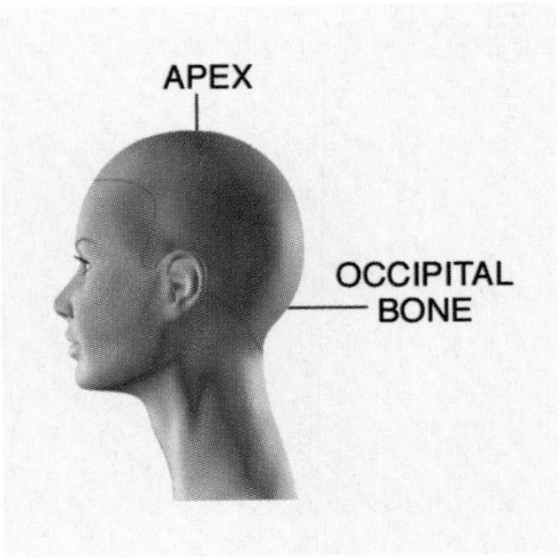

Figure 11-1 Reference points.

changes will produce the best haircutting results and will help you achieve the look that you and your clients are seeking.

Reference points are points on the head that mark where the surface of the head changes or the behavior of the hair changes, such as the ears, jawline, occipital bone, or apex. These points are used to establish design lines that are proportionate (Figure 11–1).

Reference Points

A thorough understanding of head form and reference points will guide you in the following ways:

- it will help ensure balance within the design, so that both sides of the haircut turn out the same
- it will allow you to recreate the same haircut again and again
- it will tell you where and when it is necessary to change technique in order to make up for irregularities in the head form (for example, if a client has a flat crown, you may choose to adapt your technique in that area to achieve more volume)

These are the specific reference points with which you will need to become thoroughly familiar.

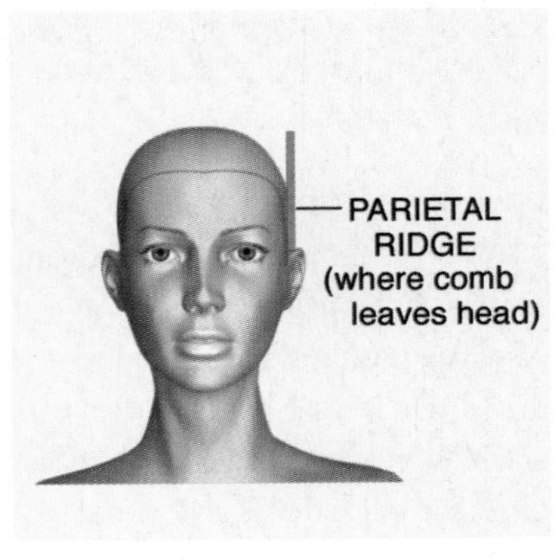

Figure 11-2 The parietal ridge.

- *Parietal ridge.* The **parietal ridge** is the widest area of the head, starting at the temples and ending at the bottom of the crown. This area is easily found by placing a comb flat on the head at the sides. Where the head starts to curve away from the comb is the parietal ridge. This is also referred to as the crest area (Figure 11–2).
- *Occipital bone.* The bone that protrudes at the base of the skull is the **occipital bone**. To find the occipital bone, simply feel the skull, or place a comb flat against the nape area and observe where the comb leaves the head (Figure 11–3).
- *Apex.* The **apex** is the highest point on the top of the head. This area is easily located by placing a comb flat on the top of the head. The comb will rest on that highest point (Figure 11–4).

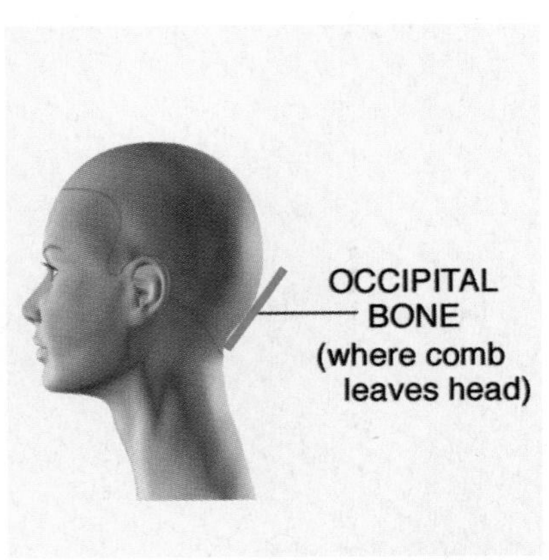

Figure 11-3 The occipital bone.

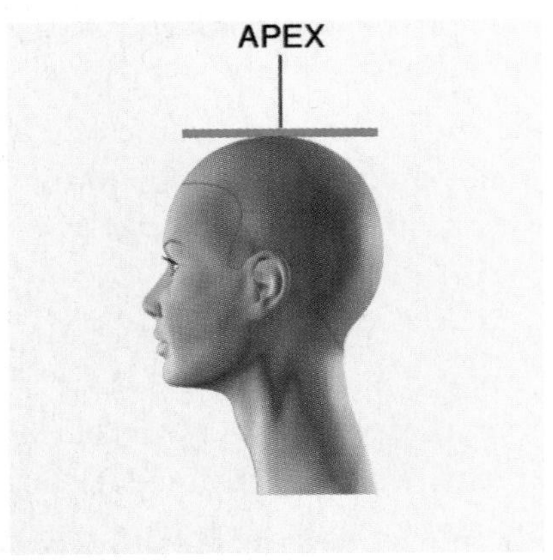

Figure 11-4 The apex.

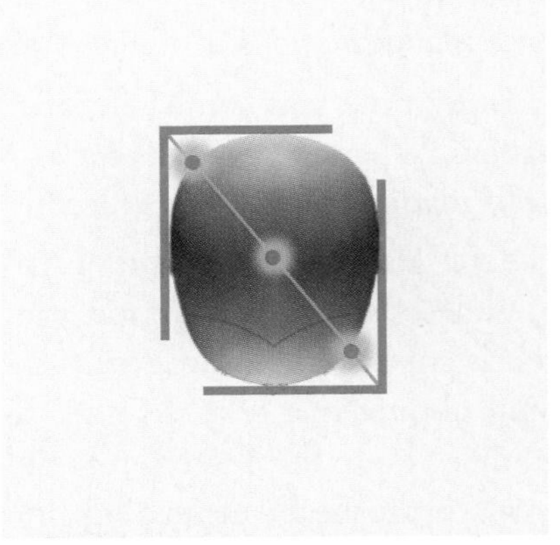

Figure 11-5 Locating the four corners.

- *Four corners.* The **four corners** may be located in two different ways: (1) place two combs flat against the side and back, locating the back corner at the point where the two combs meet (Figure 11–5); and (2) make two diagonal lines crossing the apex of the head, pointing directly to the front and back corners (Figure 11–6).

You will not necessarily use every reference point for every haircut, but it is important to know where they are. The location of the four corners, for example, signals a change in the shape of the head, from flat to round and vice versa. This change in the surface can have a significant effect on the outcome of the haircut. For example, the two front corners represent the widest points in the fringe (bangs) area. Cutting past these points can cause the fringe to end up on the sides of the haircut once it is dry, creating an undesirable result.

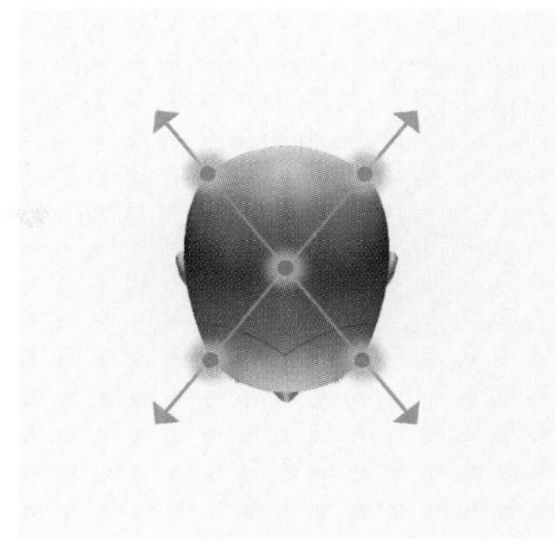

Figure 11-6 Another way to locate the four corners.

Areas of the Head

Knowing the reference points gives you a clear understanding of the areas of the head, which is crucial to successful haircutting skills (Figure 11–7). The areas of the head are as follows.

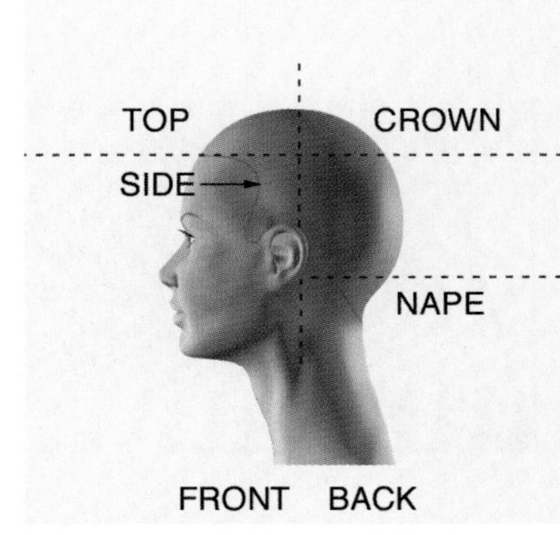

Figure 11-7 The areas of the head.

- *Top.* By locating the parietal ridge, you can identify which hair grows on the top of the head. The hair here "lies" on the head form. Hair that falls below the parietal, or crest, "hangs" due to gravity. In other words, hair on the top of the head behaves differently than hair on the sides and back. You can locate the top by parting the hair at the parietal ridge, continuing all the way around the head.
- *Front.* By making a parting or drawing a line from the apex to the back of the ear, you can separate the hair that falls naturally in front of the ear from the hair that falls naturally behind the ear. Everything that falls in front of the ear is considered the front.
- *Sides.* The sides can be located easily. They include all hair from the back of the ear forward, and below the parietal ridge.
- *Crown.* The **crown** is the area between the apex and the back of the parietal ridge. On many people, the crown is flat and is often the site of cowlicks or whorls. It is extremely important to pay extra attention to this area when performing any haircutting service.
- *Nape.* The **nape** area is the back part of the neck and consists of the hair below the occipital bone. The nape can be located by taking a horizontal parting or making a horizontal line across the back of the head at the occipital bone.
- *Back.* By making a parting or drawing a line from the apex to the back of the ear, you can locate the back of the head, which consists of all the hair that falls naturally behind the ear. In essence, once you have identified the front, you have identified the back.
- *Fringe (bangs) area.* The **fringe** area is a triangular section that begins at the apex and ends at the front corners (Figure 11–8). This area can be located by placing a comb on top of the head so that the middle of the comb is balanced on the apex. The spot at which the comb leaves the head

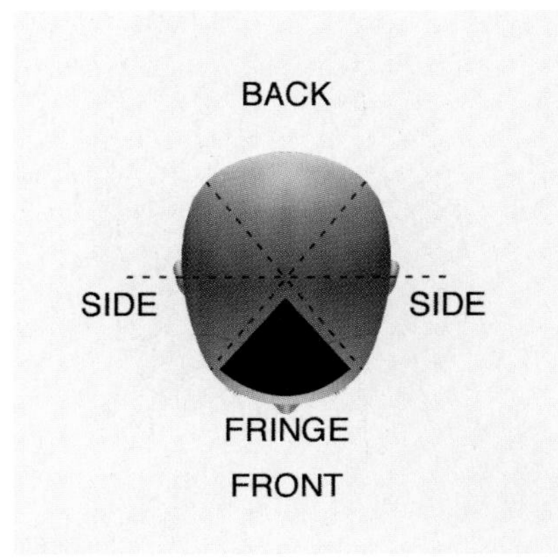

Figure 11-8 The fringe area.

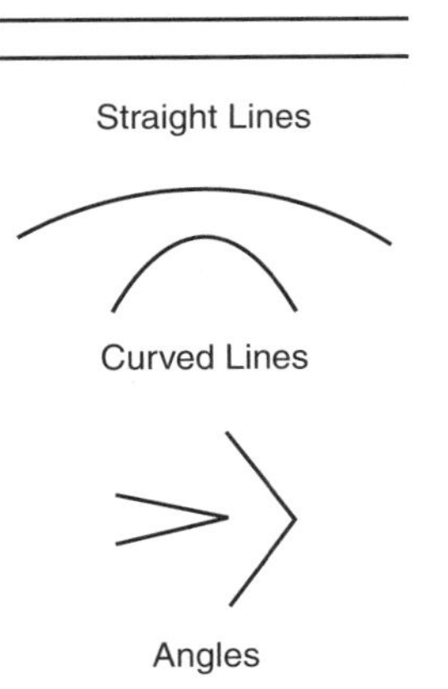

Figure 11-9 Lines and angles.

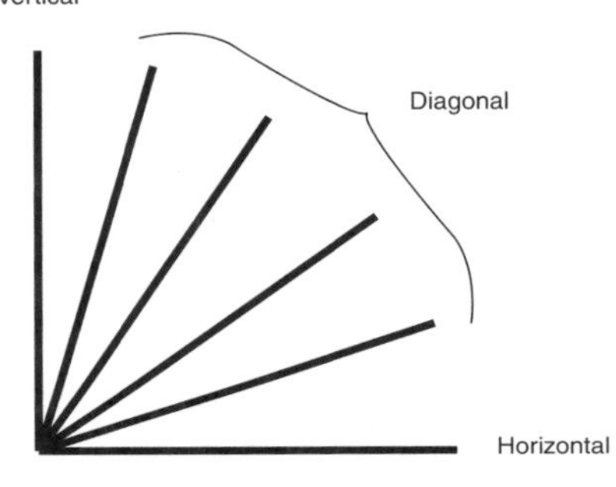

Figure 11-10 Horizontal, vertical, and diagonal lines.

in front of the apex is where the fringe area begins. Notice how the fringe area, when combed into natural falling position, falls no farther than the outer corners of the eyes.

Lines and Angles

Every haircut is made up of lines and angles. A **line** is a thin continuous mark used as a guide. An **angle** is the space between two lines or surfaces that intersect at a given point.

Two basic lines are used in haircutting: straight and curved. The head itself is made up of curved and straight lines, or surfaces. When you cut lines into the hair, the hair falls into a shape based on the lines you have cut (Figure 11–9).

There are three types of straight lines in haircutting: horizontal, vertical, and diagonal (Figure 11–10).

1. *Horizontal lines* are parallel to the horizon, or the floor; they are level, the opposite of vertical. They direct the eye from one side to the other. Usually, horizontal lines are used to create one-length and low-elevation haircuts. Horizontal lines build weight (Figure 11–11).
2. *Vertical lines* are usually described in terms of up and down as opposed to left and right. They are perpendicular to the floor. Vertical lines help to create graduated or layered haircuts and are used with higher elevations. Vertical lines remove weight (Figure 11–12).
3. *Diagonal lines* are between horizontal and vertical. They have a slanting or sloping direction. Diagonal lines are used to create **beveling**, a technique for creating fullness in a haircut by cutting the ends of the hair at a slight taper. Diagonal lines can be used to create stacking and to blend long layers to short layers (Figure 11–13).

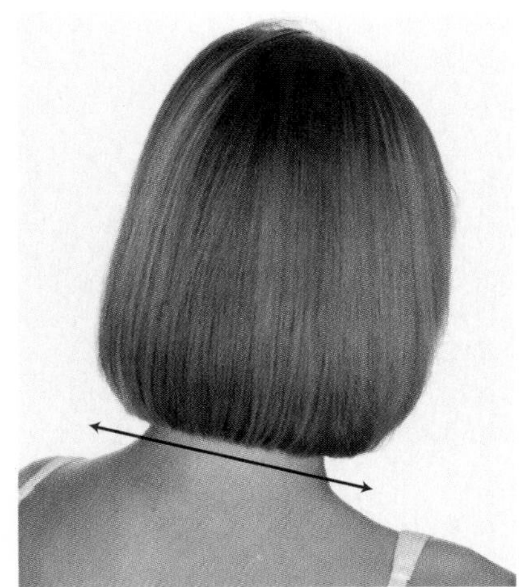

Figure 11-11 Horizontal line on a haircut.

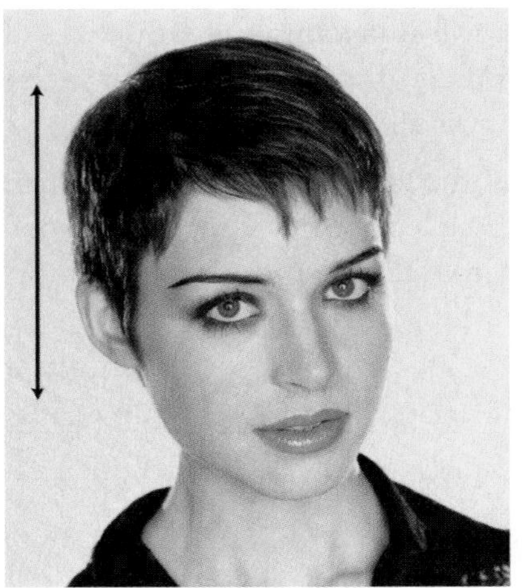

Figure 11-12 Vertical lines on a haircut.

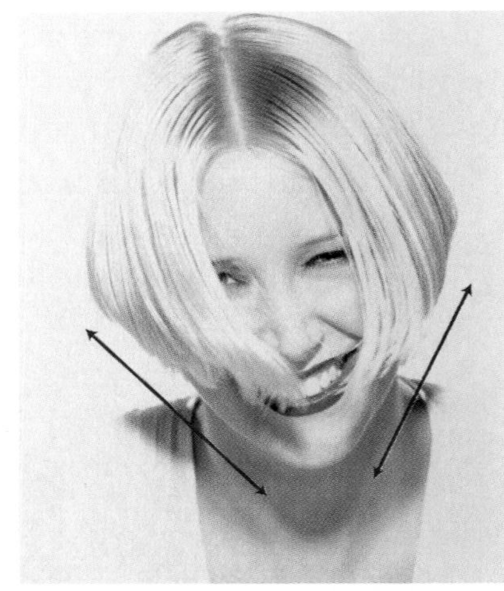

Figure 11-13 Diagonal lines on a haircut.

Angles are extremely important elements in creating a strong foundation and consistency in haircutting (Figure 11–14). Although this is basic geometry, it is important to haircutting because this is how shapes are created. Angles are particularly important in two instances: elevation and cutting line.

Elevation

The hair is parted into uniform working areas, called **sections**, for control during haircutting. Each section is further divided into smaller parts called **subsections**. A **part** or **parting** is the line dividing the hair to the scalp that separates one section of hair from another or creates subsections.

The angle or degree at which a subsection of hair is held, or elevated, from the head when cutting is called **elevation**. Elevation is an action that occurs when you lift a subsection of hair above 0 degrees. It is sometimes referred to as "projection" or simply "lifting" the hair. Elevation creates graduation and layers and is usually described in degrees (Figure 11–15). In a blunt or one-length haircut, there is no elevation (0 degrees). If a haircut is not one length, you can be sure that elevation was used.

Once you understand the effects of elevation, you can create any shape you desire. When a client brings in a picture of a haircut she would like, you should be able to examine the picture and determine which elevation was used, as well as the cutting line. A firm grasp of the principle of elevation will eliminate guesswork and will point you toward complete artistic freedom in coming up with new and innovative haircuts.

The most commonly used elevations are 45 and 90 degrees. A general rule of thumb is, the more you elevate the hair, the more graduation you create. When you elevate the hair below 90 degrees, you are building weight. When you elevate the hair at 90 degrees or higher, you begin to remove weight, or layer the hair. The length to which you cut the hair also affects the end result. The weight of hair when it is longer often makes it appear heavier or less layered, due to gravity. On the other hand, curly hair shrinks when it dries, so you usually use less elevation than on straighter textures, or leave the hair a bit longer.

Cutting Line

The **cutting line** is the angle at which the fingers are held when cutting, and ultimately the line that is cut. It is also known as finger angle, finger position, cutting position, cutting angle, and shears angle. This angle creates the end-result shape. The angle can be described in a few different ways: horizontal, vertical, or diagonal, or by using degrees (Figure 11–16, Figure 11–17, and Figure 11–18).

Guidelines

A **guideline** (sometimes called a guide) is a section of hair that determines the length the hair will be cut, located either at the **perimeter** (outer line) or the interior (inner or internal part) of the cut. It is usually the first section you cut when creating a shape. Two basic guidelines in haircutting are stationary and traveling.

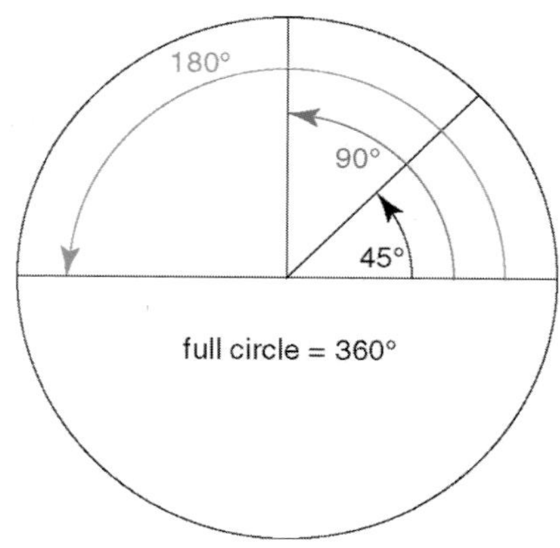

Figure 11–14 Angles.

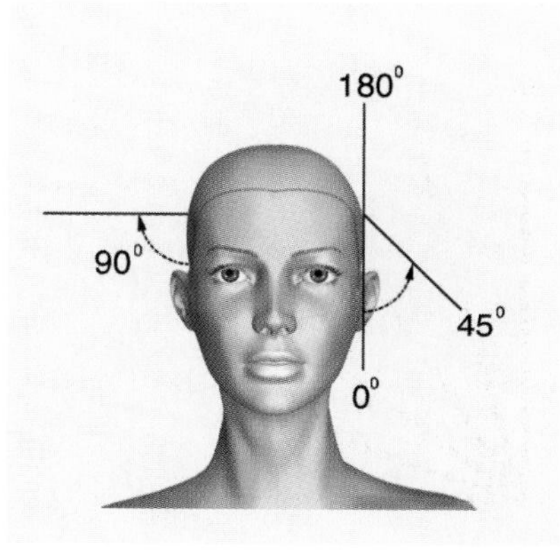

Figure 11–15 Angles relative to the head form.

11

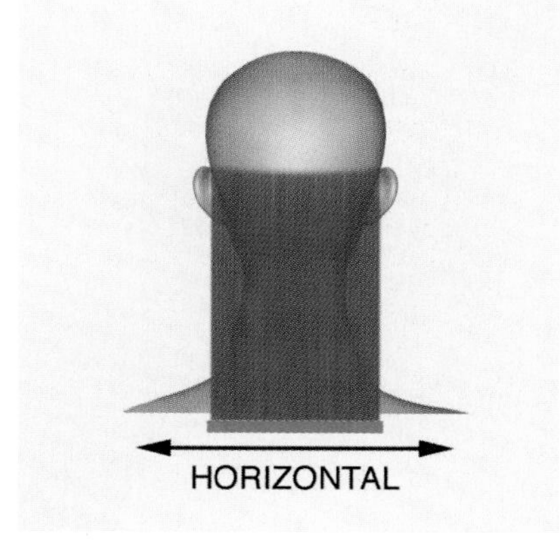

Figure 11–16 Horizontal cutting line.

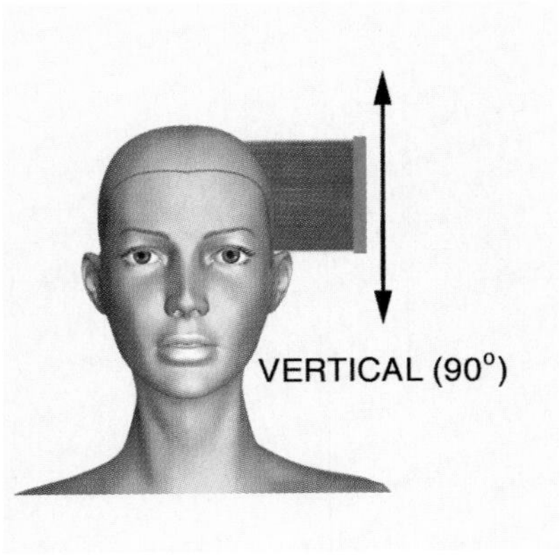

Figure 11-17 Vertical cutting line.

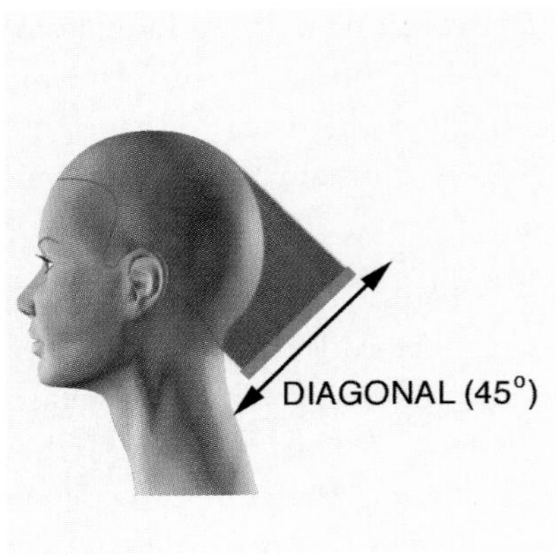

Figure 11-18 Diagonal cutting line.

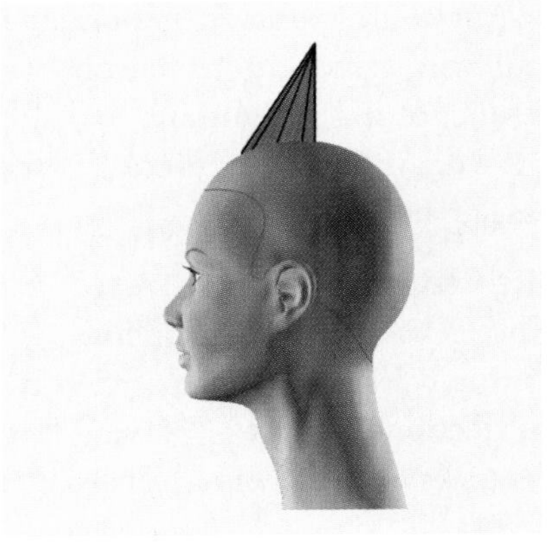

Figure 11-19 Stationary guideline.

- A **stationary guideline** is one that does not move (Figure 11–19). All other sections are combed to the stationary guideline and cut at the same angle and length. Stationary guidelines are used mostly in blunt (one-length) haircuts (Figure 11–20), or when using overdirection to create a length or weight increase in a haircut (Figure 11–21).
- A **traveling guideline**, or movable guideline, moves as the haircut progresses. It travels with you as you work through the haircut (Figure 11–22). When you use a traveling guide, you take a small slice of the previous subsection and move it to the next position, or subsection, where it becomes your new guideline. Traveling guidelines are most often used when creating layered or graduated haircuts (Figure 11–23 and Figure 11–24). When you are creating uniform layers, you use a traveling guide, with no overdirection, to create the same length throughout the entire haircut.

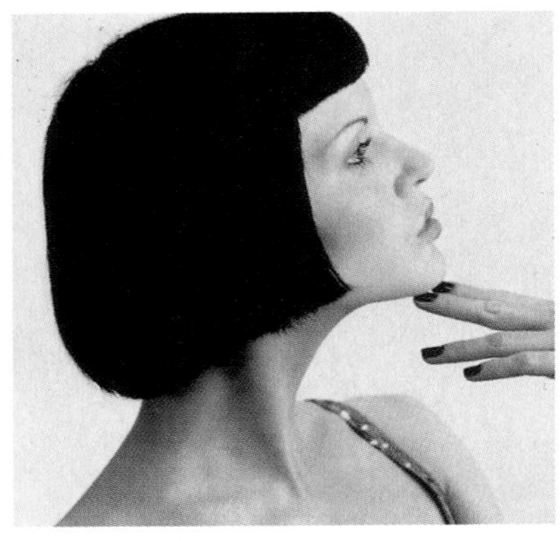

Figure 11-20 Blunt (one-length) haircut.

EXAMPLES

Let us look at some of the different shapes that can be created by using different elevations, cutting lines, and stationary and traveling guidelines.

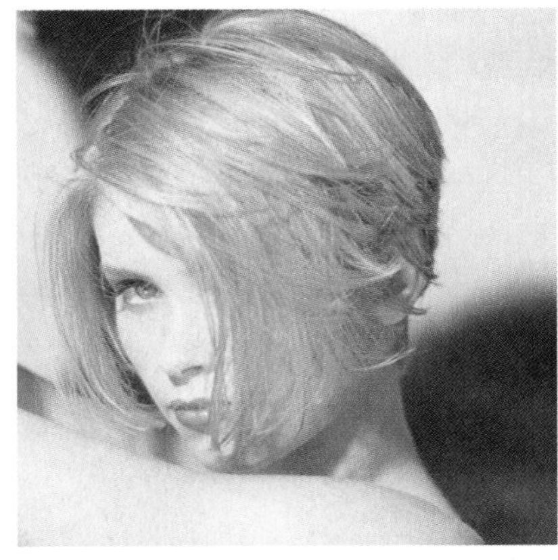

Figure 11-21 Layered haircut.

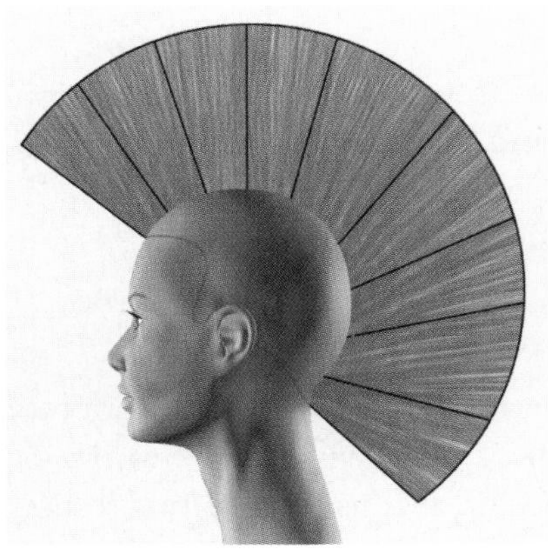

Figure 11-22 Traveling guideline.

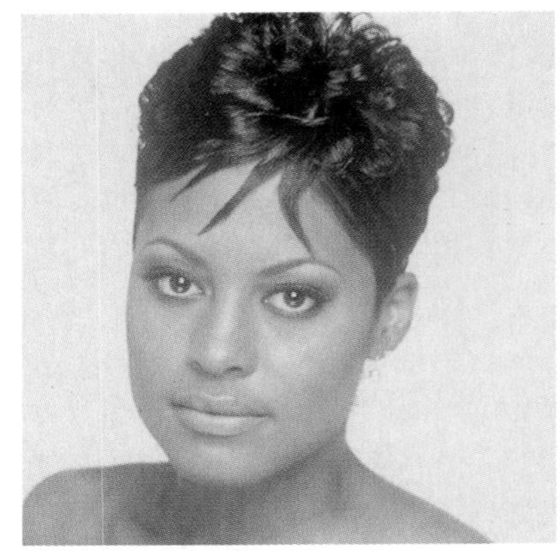

Figure 11-23 Uniform layered haircut.

Keep in mind the varying amount of weight that results from these different combinations.

Figure 11–25 and Figure 11–26 show a blunt (one-length haircut) cut with no elevation, a diagonal cutting line, and a stationary guideline. To achieve the layered shape in Figure 11–27 and Figure 11–28, a 90-degree elevation was used, with a vertical cutting line and a traveling guideline. The next shape (Figure 11–29 and Figure 11–30) was cut using a 45-degree elevation throughout the sides and back, creating a stacked effect with a diagonal (45-degree) cutting line. The top was cut using a 90-degree elevation (layered) and the entire shape was created using a traveling guideline.

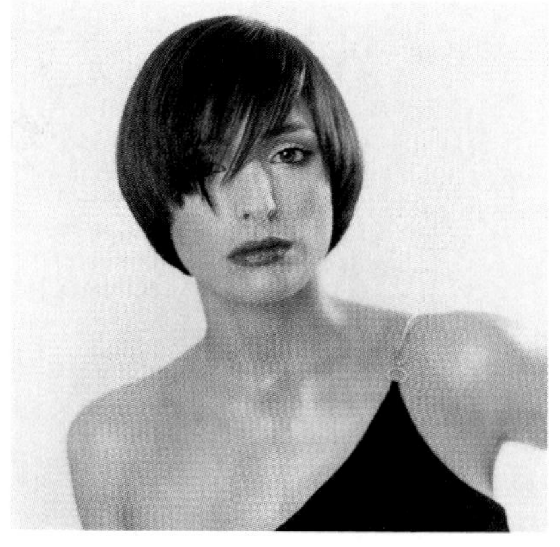

Figure 11-24 Graduated haircut.

Overdirection

Overdirection is a unique action that can best be understood by comparing it to elevation. Whereas elevation is simply the degree to which you lift a subsection away from the head, overdirection occurs when you comb the hair away from its natural falling position, rather than straight out from the

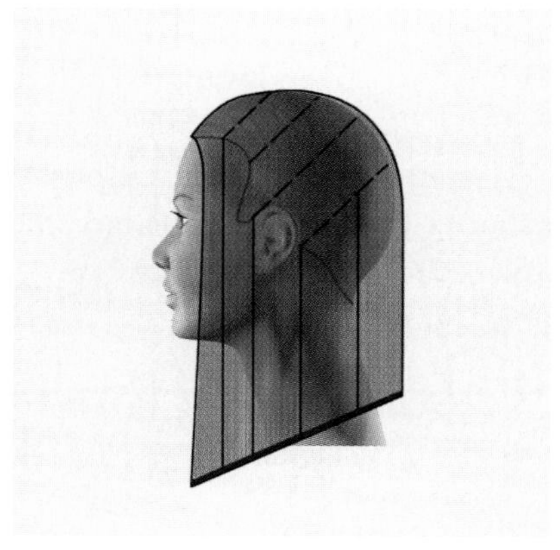

Figure 11-25 Blunt cut variation: design.

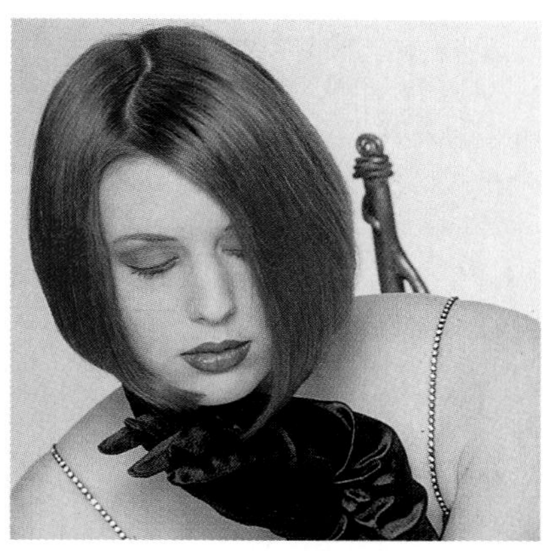

Figure 11-26 Finished blunt cut variation.

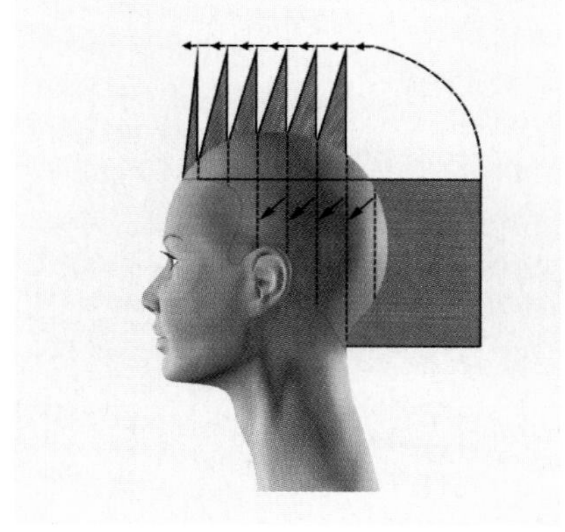

Figure 11-27 Layered cut variation: design.

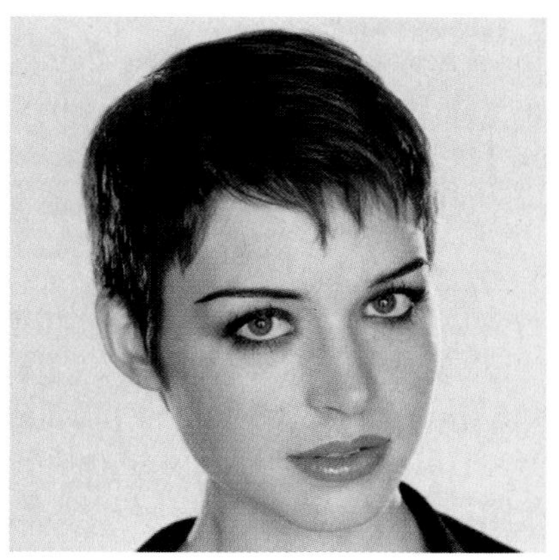

Figure 11-28 Finish layered cut variation.

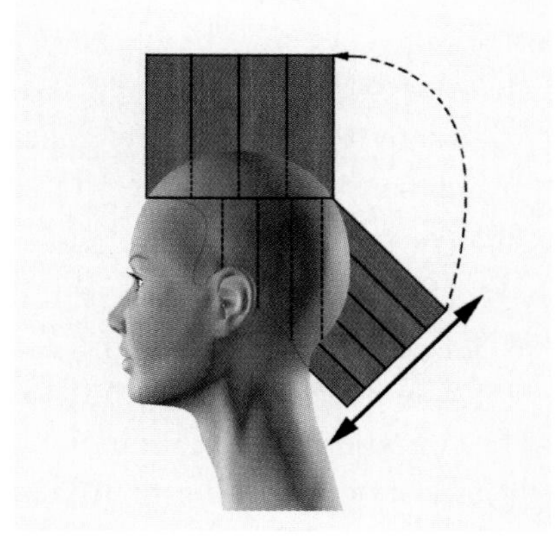

Figure 11-29 Graduated cut variation: design.

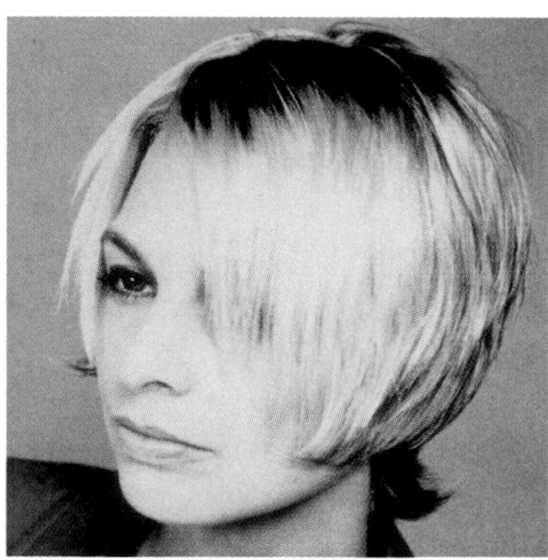

Figure 11-30 Finished graduated cut variation.

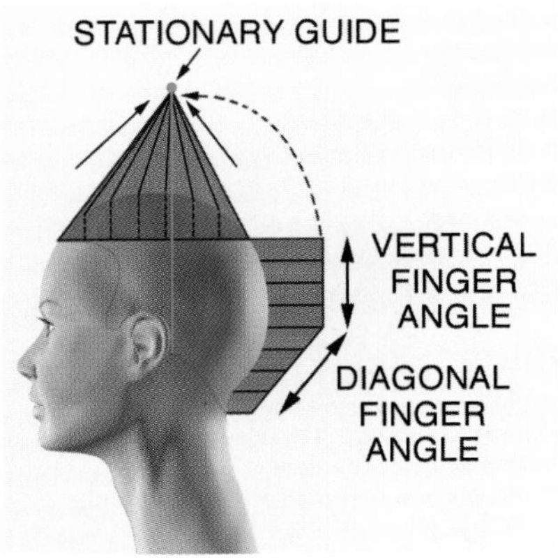

Figure 11-31 Overdirection in layered cut: design.

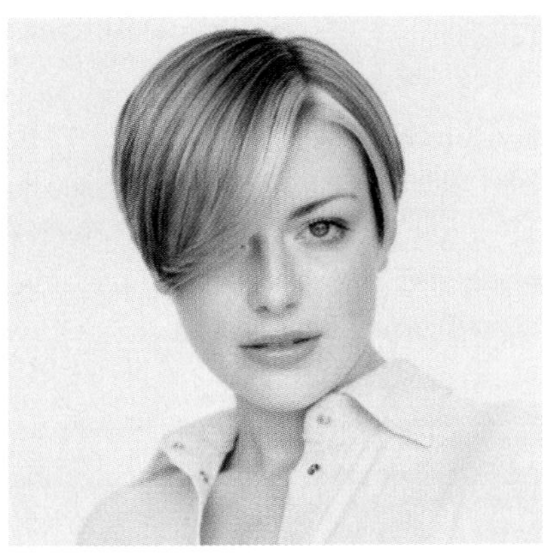

Figure 11-32 Finish layered cut.

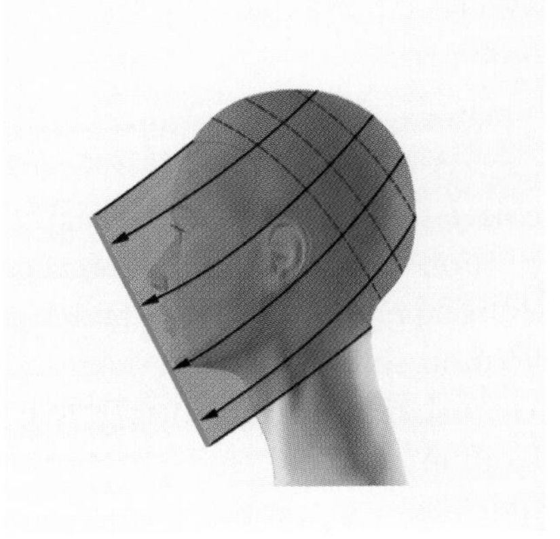

Figure 11-33 Overdirection in long layered cut: design.

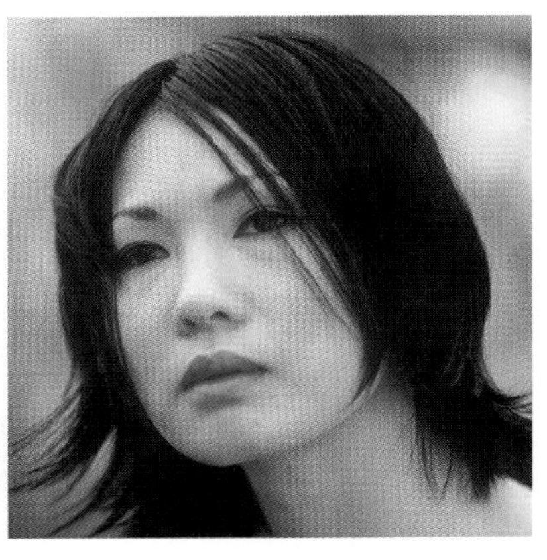

Figure 11-34 Finished long layered cut.

head, toward a guideline. Overdirection is used mostly in graduated and layered haircuts, and in those situations where you want to create a length increase in the design.

For example, if you are working on a layered haircut and want the hair to be longer toward the front, you can overdirect the sections to a stationary guide at the back of the ear. (Figure 11–31 and Figure 11–32). Or, if you are creating a long layered haircut, with shorter layers around the face and longer layers in the back, you can overdirect sections to a stationary guide at the front (Figure 11–33 and Figure 11–34).

CLIENT CONSULTATION

A great haircut always begins with a great consultation. Often, when clients come to you, they are feeling that there is a lot at stake. They may be preparing for an important event, such as a party, a business event, or a wedding. They may be in the market for a new look, wanting to change their appearance and, by extension, the way they feel about themselves. Always perform a complete consultation before beginning the haircut to ensure that both of you are on the same wavelength and that the haircut is suitable.

A consultation is a conversation between you and your client during which you find out what the client is looking for, offer suggestions and professional advice, and come to a decision about the most suitable haircut. The purpose of the consultation is to open the lines of communication, have an understanding of what the client wants, ensure that the client understands what you would like to do, and together determine the end result. Together you may share thoughts about the best haircut for the client's face shape and can discuss the nature of the client's hair whether it is thick or thin, fine or coarse, or straight or curly. If the client has a particular look in mind, the two of you can discuss whether that look will be appropriate.

It can be difficult when a client asks for something that you know will not be the best look for that person. This is when you will want to draw on skills such as gentle persuasion and positive reinforcement. A true professional can offer alternative suggestions that will work with the client's hair texture, face shape, and lifestyle. It is within the framework of the consultation that you will hone those skills that led you into this people-oriented profession in the first place.

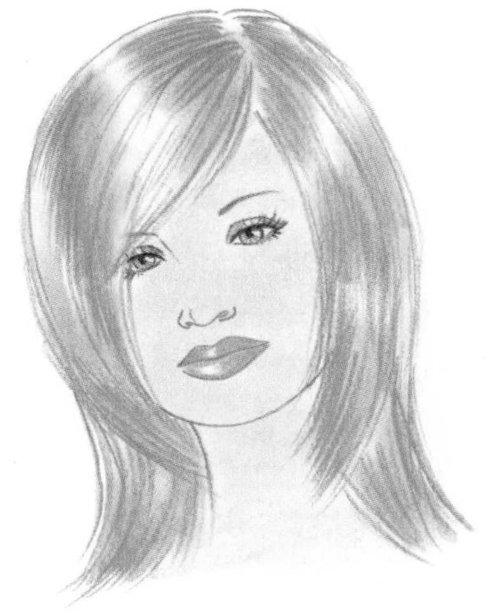

Figure 11-35 Wide face with suitable hairstyle.

The Desired Look

A great place to start with the consultation is to ask the client what she wants. Sometimes, she may not be able to answer that question and may ask you for some suggestions. Either way, this is the first step in the consultation. There are several points to focus on here. How much time is the client willing to spend on her hair every day? What is her lifestyle? Does she want something that is classic or something trendy? For example, if a client with naturally curly thick hair is asking for a haircut that is primarily designed for straight hair, will she be willing to take the time to blow-dry it straight every day? This is also the time when you will want to analyze hair density and texture, growth patterns, and hairline. If the client has hair that grows straight up in the nape and is requesting a short haircut that is soft and wispy at the hairline, you know the hairline will not lie down, so you may need to suggest other alternatives that will work with that kind of hairline.

Face Shape

Another part of consultation is analyzing the face shape. A great haircut is not only technically sound, but it suits the client's face shape. To analyze the shape of a client's face, pull all the hair away with a clip, or wrap the hair in a towel. Look for the widest areas, the narrowest areas, and the balance of the features. A quick way to analyze a face shape is to determine if it is predominantly wide or long. Look for the features that you want to bring out, and those you might want to deemphasize. See Chapter 9 for examples of face shapes.

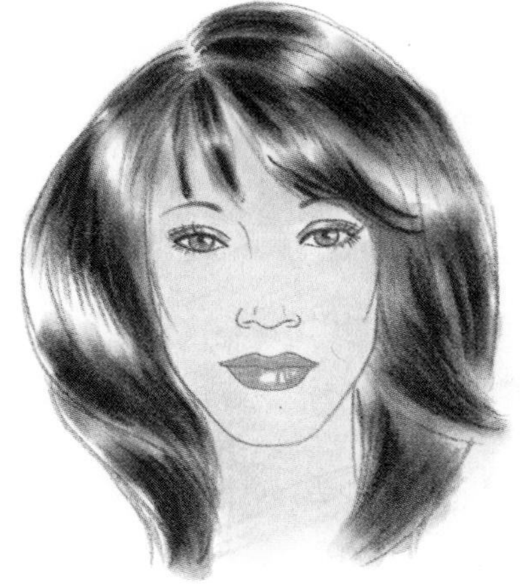

Figure 11-36 Narrow face with suitable hairstyle.

By analyzing face shape, you can begin to make decisions about the most suitable haircut, or shape, for the client. An important thing to remember is that weight and volume draw attention to an area. For example, if a client has a wide face, a hairstyle with fuller sides makes the face appear wider, whereas a narrower shape will give length to the face. On the other hand, if the client has a long face, a hairstyle with fullness on the sides will add width. Or if a client has a narrow forehead, you can add visual width by increasing volume or weight in that area. In order to balance out face shapes or draw the eye away from certain areas, you need to add or remove weight or volume in other areas. Figure 11–35 and Figure 11–36 illustrate two face shapes and haircuts that help create balance.

Another important point to consider is the client's profile, or how she looks from the side. Turn the chair so you can see your client from the side

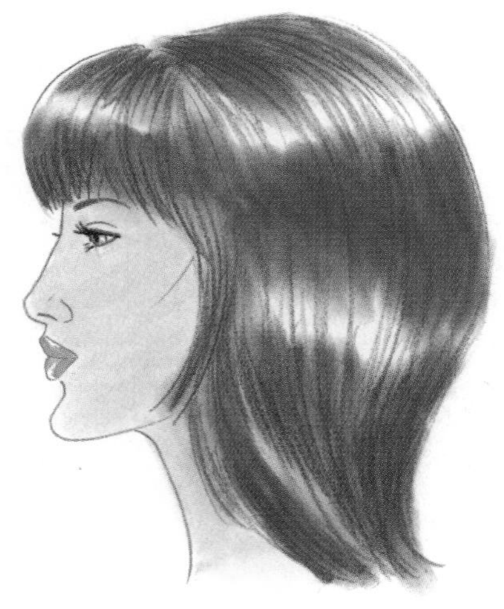

Figure 11–37 Flattering style for client with prominent chin.

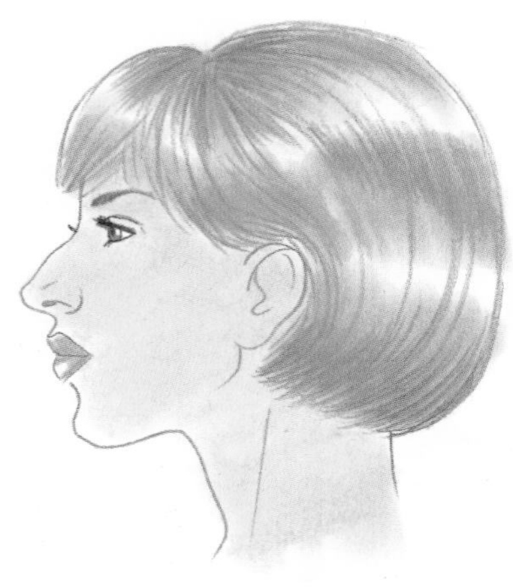

Figure 11–38 Flattering style for client with prominent nose.

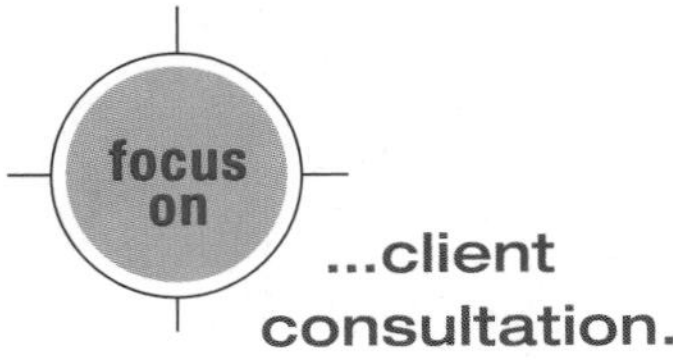

...client consultation.

During the consultation, it is helpful to use parts of the body as points of reference when describing the length of the haircut. For example, you could say, "Would you like your hair to be chin-length or shoulder-length?"

in the mirror. Pull the hair away from the face and up and away from the neck. What do you see? Look for features to emphasize, such as a nice jaw line or lovely neck; or features to draw attention away from, such as a prominent or receding chin, a double chin, or a prominent nose. The haircut you choose should flatter the client by emphasizing good features and taking attention away from features that are not as flattering. For example, if a client has a prominent chin, you will want to balance the shape by adding volume or weight somewhere else (Figure 11–37). If the client has a prominent nose, you can balance the shape from the profile by adding weight in an appropriate place (Figure 11–38).

The consultation is also the time to decide on which what kind of part the client will wear. Will you be working with her natural part, a center part, or a side part?

Hair Analysis

There are five characteristics that determine the behavior of the hair (see Chapter 8 for a more thorough discussion):

- density
- texture
- wave pattern
- hairlines
- growth pattern

Hair Density

Hair density is the number of individual hair strands on one square inch of scalp. It is usually described as thin, medium, or thick.

Hair Texture

Hair texture is the general quality and feel of the hair. It is based on the thickness or diameter of each hair strand, usually classified as coarse, medium, and fine. A fine hair strand is much "skinnier" than a coarse hair strand. A client may, in fact, have a fine texture of hair with a thick density, meaning the individual hairs are fine, but there are a lot of them. Or a client may have a coarse texture but a thin density, meaning the individual hairs are "fatter" but they are spaced farther apart. Or the client may have a coarse texture and a thick density, which translates into a substantial amount of hair.

Why are density and texture important? Because different hair types respond differently to the kind of cutting they receive. Some hair types need more layers; some need more weight. For example, coarse hair tends to stick out more, especially if it is cut too short, whereas fine hair can be cut to very short lengths and still lie flat. However, if a client has fine (texture) and thin (density) hair, cutting too short can result in an unflattering look, with the scalp showing through (Table 11–1).

Wave Pattern

The wave pattern, or the amount of movement in the hair strand, varies from client to client, as well as within the same head of hair. A client may

Texture	Density: Thin	Density: Medium	Density: Thick
Fine	Limp, needs weight	Great for many cuts, especially blunt and low elevation. Razor cuts are good.	Usually needs more texturizing. Suitable for many haircuts.
Medium	Needs weight. Graduated shapes work well.	Great for most cuts. Hair can handle texturizing.	Many shapes are suitable. Texturizing usually necessary.
Coarse	Maintain some weight. Razor cuts not recommended.	Great for many shapes. Razor cuts appropriate if hair is in good condition.	Very short cuts do not work. Razors may frizz and "expand" hair. Maintain some length to weigh hair down.

Table 11-1 Density and Texture

have stick-straight hair (no wave), wavy hair, curly hair, extremely curly hair, or anything in between.

Imagine the same haircut cut at the same length on different types of hair: fine thin hair (Figure 11–39), thick coarse hair (Figure 11–40), and medium curly hair (Figure 11–41).

Hairlines and Growth Patterns

Both the hairline and the growth patterns are important to examine. The hairline is the hair that grows at the outermost perimeter along the face, around the ears, and on the neck. The growth pattern is the direction in which the hair grows from the scalp, also referred to as natural fall or natural

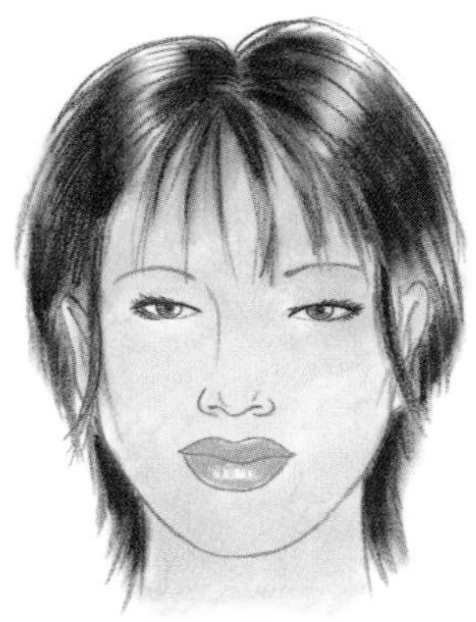

Figure 11-39 Uniform layered cut on fine, thin hair.

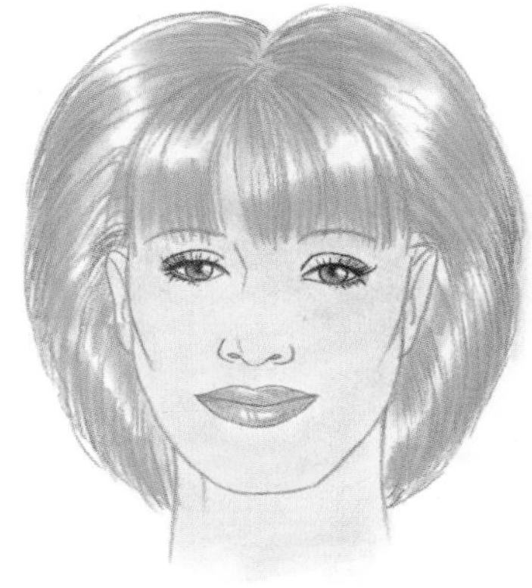

Figure 11-40 Uniform layered cut on thick, coarse hair.

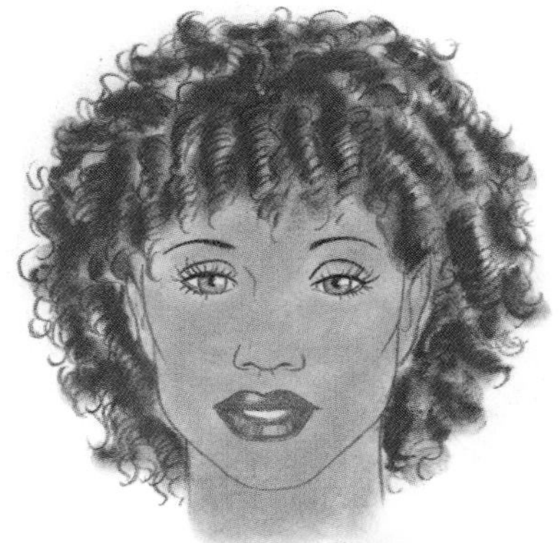

Figure 11-41 Uniform layered cut on medium curly hair.

Did you know...

Hair shrinks when it dries. Once you and the client have decided on the length, keep in mind that the hair will shrink ¼ inch (.6 cm) to ½ inch (1.25 cm) after it is dry. In other words, you need to cut the hair ¼ to ½ inch longer than the desired length. If the hair is curly, it will shrink even more, ½ to 2 inches (5 cm). Be sure to check with your instructor when deciding on the length for curly-haired clients.

falling position. Cowlicks, whorls, and other growth patterns affect where the hair ends up once it is dry (see Chapter 8). You may need to use less tension when cutting these areas to compensate for hair being pushed up when it dries, especially in the nape, or to avoid getting a "hole" around the ear in a one-length haircut. Another crucial area is the crown (on many people, there are some wild things going on up there!). 3

TOOLS, BODY POSITION, AND SAFETY

Anyone cutting hair is only as good as his tools. You need to understand the function and characteristics of your tools, how to use them in way that is safe for both yourself and your client, and how to position your body so that your energy and effectiveness are maximized and protected.

Haircutting Tools

There are several tools that are indispensable for haircutting. Understanding these different implements, or tools, and the different results you can get from them is vital to creating a great haircut. To do your best work, buy and use only superior implements from a reliable manufacturer, use them properly, and take good care of them.

- *Haircutting shears.* Mainly used to cut blunt or straight lines in hair. May also be used to "slide cut," "point cut," and for other texturizing techniques (discussed later in this chapter). The words *shears* and *scissors* are sometimes used interchangeably (Figure 11–42a and Figure 11–42b).
- *Thinning shears.* Mainly used to remove bulk from the hair. Sometimes referred to as texturizing shears, tapering shears, or notching shears. Many different types of thinning shears are used today, with varying amounts of teeth in the blades. A general rule of thumb is that the more teeth there are, the less hair is removed. Notching shears are usually designed to remove more hair, with larger teeth set farther apart.

11

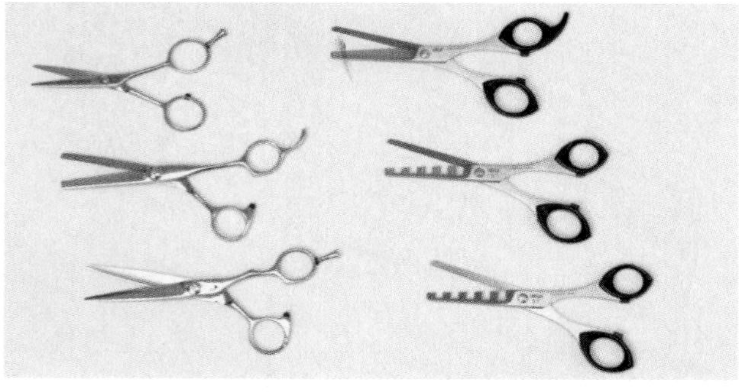

Figure 11-42a Haircutting shears and thinning shears.

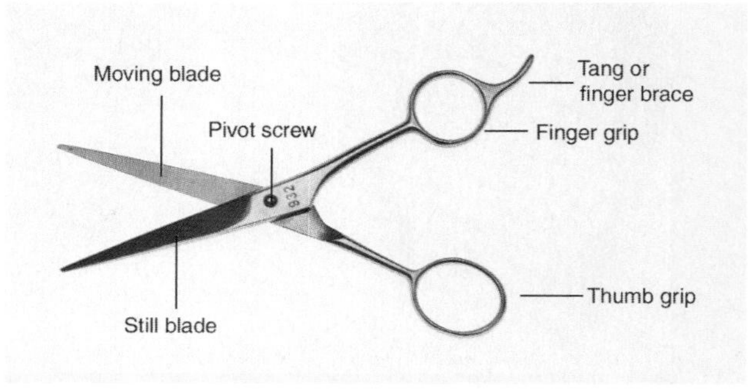

Figure 11-42b Parts of haircutting shears.

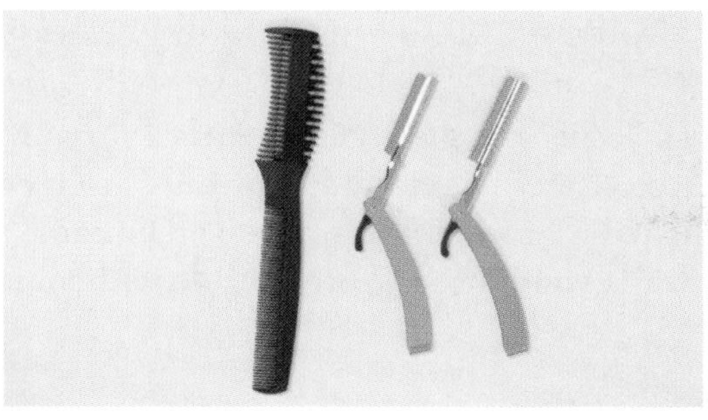

Figure 11-43a Razors.

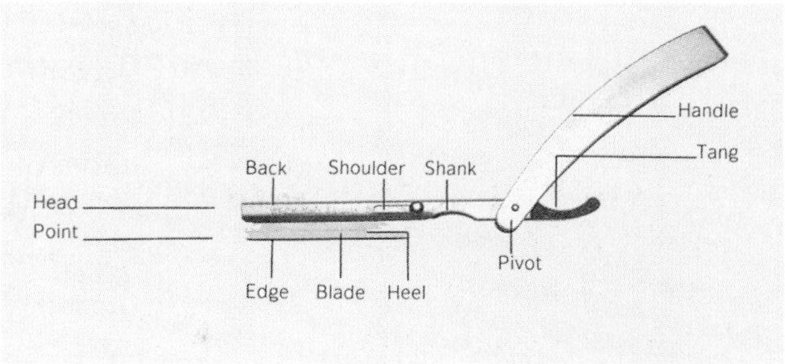

Figure 11-43b Parts of a razor.

- *Straight razor or razor shaper.* Mainly used when a softer effect is desired on the ends of the hair. Razors can be used to create an entire haircut, to thin hair out, or to texturize in certain areas. Razors come in different shapes and sizes, with or without guards (Figure 11–43a and Figure 11–43b).
- *Clippers.* Mainly used when creating short tapers, short haircuts, fades, and flat tops. Clippers can be used without a guard to "shave" hair right to the scalp, with cutting guards at various lengths, or in the "clipper-over-comb" technique (Figure 11–44).
- *Edgers.* A smaller version of clippers, mainly used to remove excess or unwanted hair at the neckline and around the ears, mostly on haircuts for men and very short haircuts for women.
- *Wide-tooth comb.* Mainly used to detangle hair. Rarely used when performing a haircut.
- *Sectioning clips.* These come in a variety of shapes, styles, and sizes and can be made of plastic or metal. In general, two types are used: jaw clips and duckbill clips. Both come in large and small sizes.
- *Barber comb.* Mainly used for close tapers in the nape and sides when using the shears-over-comb technique. The narrow end of the comb allows the shears to get very close to the head.
- *Styling or cutting comb.* Also referred to as all-purpose comb, used for most haircutting procedures. It can be 6 to 8 inches (15 to 20 cm) in length and has fine teeth at one end, wider teeth at the other (Figure 11–45).

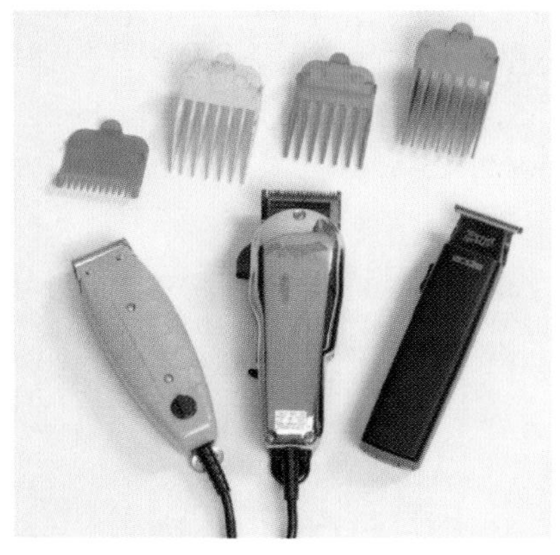

Figure 11-44 Clippers and edgers.

Holding Your Tools

The way you hold your tools is important for two reasons.

1. Proper holding gives you the most control and the best results when cutting hair.
2. Proper holding can help you avoid muscle strain in your hands, arms, neck, and back.

Holding the Shears

1. Open your right hand (left hand if you are left-handed), and place the ring finger in the finger grip of the still blade and the little finger in the finger brace (tang) (Figure 11–46).

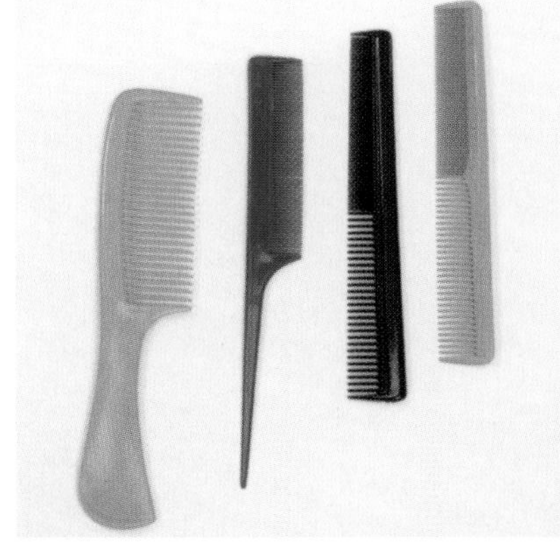

Figure 11-45 From left to right: wide-tooth comb, tail comb, barber comb, and styling comb.

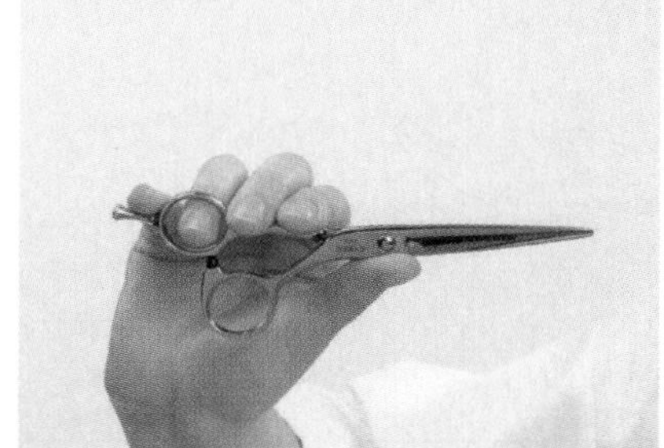

Figure 11-46 Proper placement of ring finger and little finger.

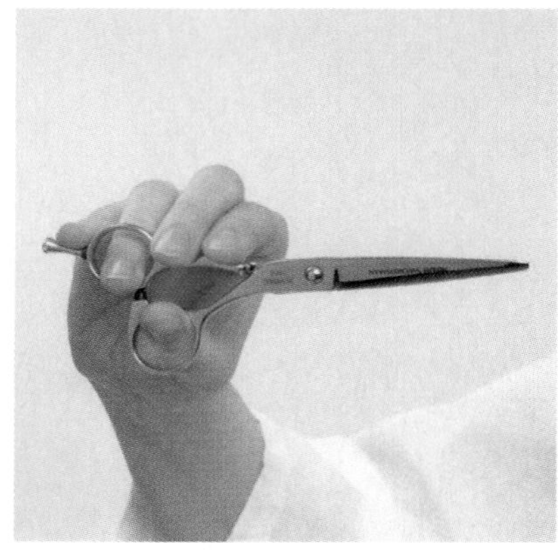

Figure 11-47 Proper placement of thumb.

2. Place the thumb in the finger grip (thumb grip) of the moving blade (Figure 11–47).
3. Practice opening and closing the shears. Concentrate on moving only your thumb. A great way to get the feel of this is to lay the still blade against the palm or forefinger of your other hand, which holds it still while you move the other blade with your thumb (Figure 11–48).

Holding the Shears and Comb

During the haircutting process, you will be holding both the comb and the shears at the same time. You may be tempted to put the comb down while cutting, but in the long run this wastes a lot of time. It is best to learn early how to hold both tools during the entire haircutting process. In general, your cutting hand (your dominant hand) does most of the work. It holds the shears, parts the hair, combs the hair, and cuts the hair. Your holding hand does just that: it holds the sections of hair and the comb while cutting. The holding hand is the means by which you maintain control while cutting.

- *Palming the shears.* Remove your thumb from the thumb grip, leaving your ring and little fingers in the grip and finger rest. Curl your fingers in to "palm" the shears, which keeps them closed while you comb or part the hair (Figure 11–49). This allows you to hold the comb and the shears at the same time. While palming the shears, hold the comb between thumb, index, and middle fingers (Figure 11–50).
- *Transferring the comb.* After you have combed a subsection into position, you will need to free up your cutting hand. Once your fingers are in place at the correct cutting position, transfer the comb by placing it between the thumb and index finger of your holding hand (the hand holding the subsection) (Figure 11–51). You are now ready to cut the subsection.

Holding the Razor

The straight razor or shaping razor is a versatile tool that can be used for an entire haircut, or for detailing and texturizing. Holding and working

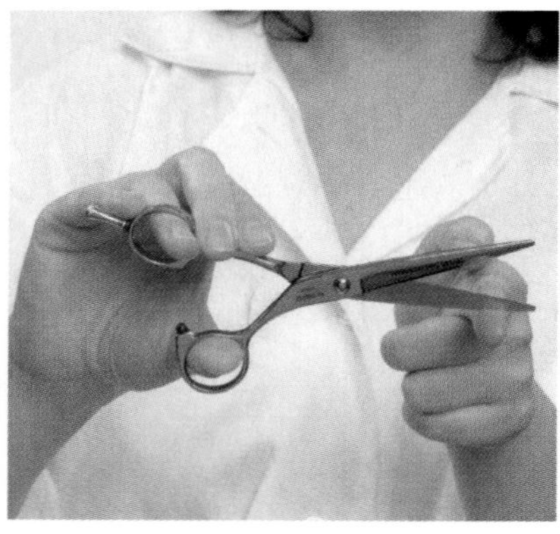

Figure 11-48 Still and moving blades.

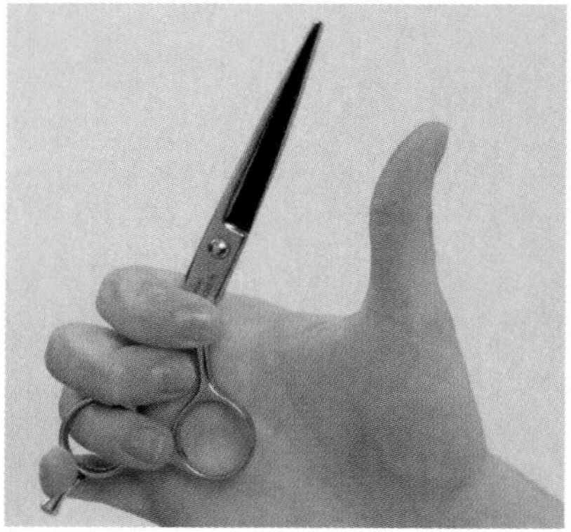

Figure 11-49 Palming the shears.

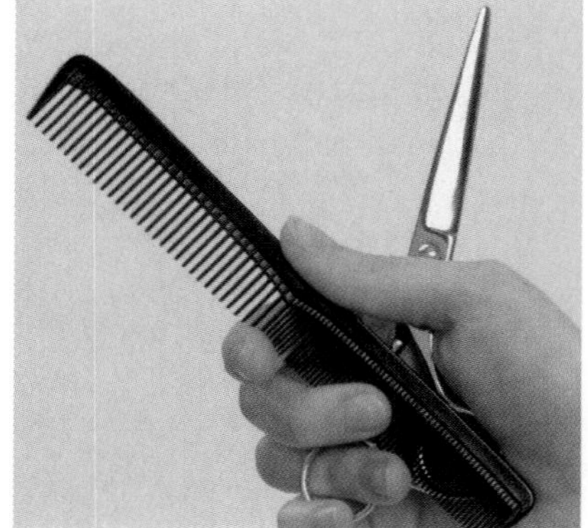

Figure 11-50 Holding comb and shears.

with a razor feels very different from holding and working with shears. The more you practice holding and palming the razor, the more comfortable you will become with this tool. There are two methods for holding the razor for cutting.

1. Method A
   a. Open the razor so that the handle is higher than the shank. Place the thumb on the thumb grip and the index, middle, and ring fingers on the shank.
   b. Place the little finger in the tang, underneath the handle (Figure 11–52).
   c. When cutting a subsection, position the razor on top of the subsection, the part facing you, for maximum control (Figure 11–53).
2. Method B
   a. Open the razor until the handle and shank form a straight line.
   b. Place the thumb on the grip and wrap the fingers around the handle (Figure 11–54).

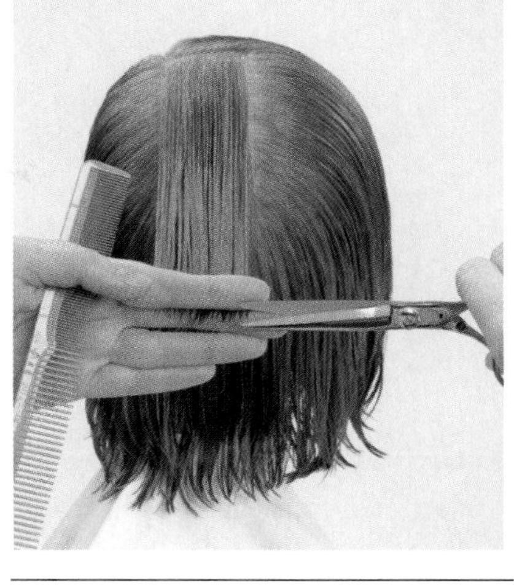

Figure 11-51 Transferring the comb.

Just as you need to be able to hold the comb and the shears in your cutting hand while working, you also need to palm the razor so that you can comb and section hair during a haircut. Curl in your ring finger and little finger to palm the razor. Hold the comb between your thumb and index and middle fingers (Figure 11–55). Most accidents with razors happen while combing the hair, not when cutting the hair, because of a loose grip when palming. Be sure to practice keeping a firm grip on the razor with the ring and little fingers, which keeps the open blade from sliding and cutting your hand while you comb the hair.

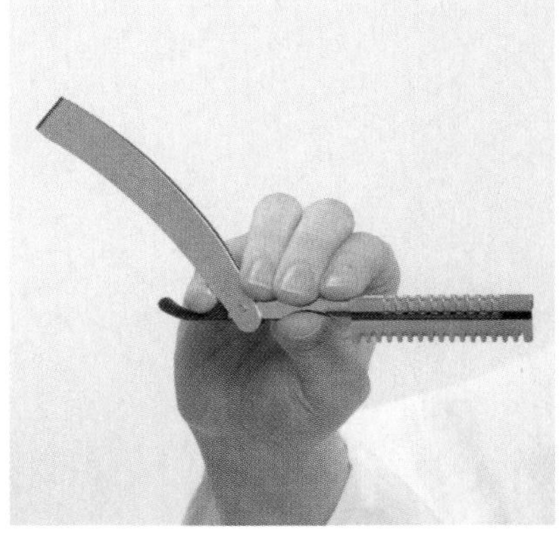

Figure 11-52 Holding razor properly.

Handling the Comb

Both the wide and fine teeth of the comb are regularly used when cutting hair. The wide teeth are used for combing and parting hair, while the finer

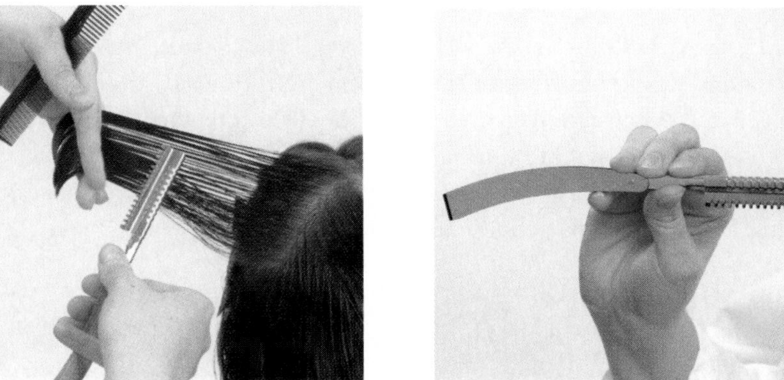

Figure 11-53 Holding razor for cutting.

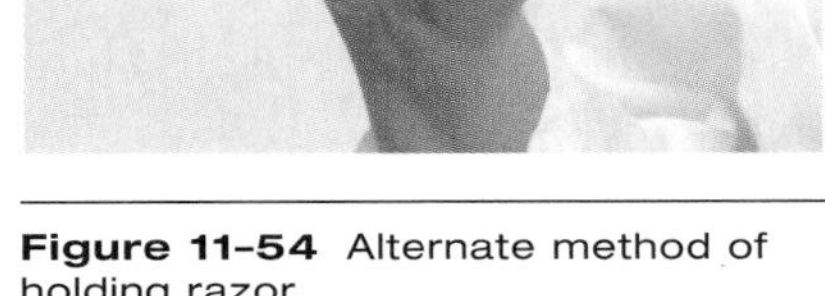

Figure 11-54 Alternate method of holding razor.

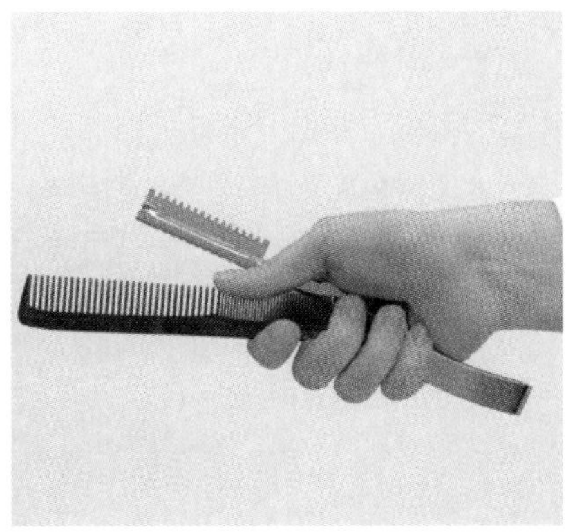

Figure 11-55 Palming the razor.

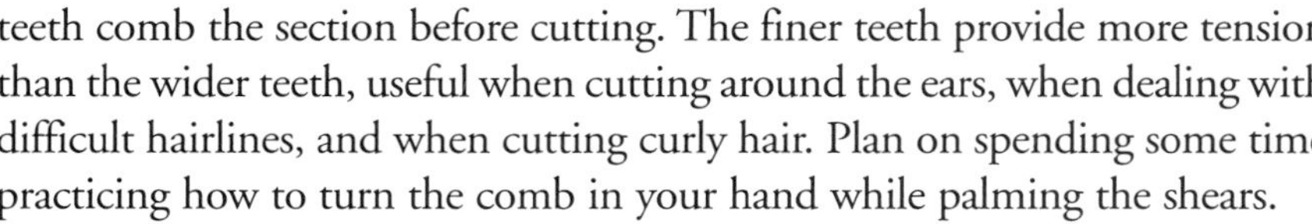

teeth comb the section before cutting. The finer teeth provide more tension than the wider teeth, useful when cutting around the ears, when dealing with difficult hairlines, and when cutting curly hair. Plan on spending some time practicing how to turn the comb in your hand while palming the shears.

focus on ...sharpening your technical skills.

Learning how to control your shears is so important because there are many techniques that can be difficult to learn if you are not holding the shears properly (for example, shears-over-comb and point cutting).

Tension

Tension in haircutting is the amount of pressure applied when combing and holding a subsection, created by stretching or pulling the subsection. Tension ranges from minimum to maximum. You control tension with your fingers when you hold the subsection of hair between them. The teeth of the comb also affect tension; greater tension can be achieved with closer and finer teeth.

Consistent tension is important for consistent, even results in a haircut. Use maximum tension on straight hair where you want precise lines. With curly or wavy hair, however, a lot of tension will result in the hair shrinking even more than usual when it is dry. Minimum tension should be used around the ears or on hairlines with strong growth patterns.

Posture and Body Position

Posture, which is how you stand, and body position, which is how you hold your body when cutting hair, are important habits to be aware of. As a working cosmetologist, you will be spending many hours on your feet. Good posture and body position will help you avoid back problems in the future and ensure better haircutting results. The correct body position will help you move more efficiently through the haircut and thereby maintain more control over the process.

- *Position the client.* Not only is your body position important, but your client's is also. Make sure your client is sitting up straight and that her legs are not crossed. Gentle reminders as the haircutting session progresses may be necessary. Remember, you can move the client by turning the chair, which gives you the option to either keep your body in the same place or angle the client's chair so you can see what you are doing in the mirror.
- *Center your weight.* When working, keep your body weight centered and firm. Stand with your knees slightly bent, rather than locked. Instead of bending at the waist, bend one knee if you need to lean slightly one way or the other.
- *Stand in front of your section.* When cutting hair, a general rule of thumb is to stand directly in front of the area you are cutting. By doing this, you keep your body weight centered, and you will automatically find yourself moving around the head during a haircutting service. If you wish to stay standing in the same place, or want to be able to view what you are doing in the mirror, you may choose to move the chair.

CAUTION

Make a habit of always maintaining correct body posture and hand position while cutting. Back and wrist strain may result if you neglect this important point.

Hand Positions for Different Cutting Angles

As a general rule, always stand in front of the area you are working on, and position your hands according to the cutting line.

- *Cutting over your fingers.* There are some situations in which you will be cutting over your fingers or on top of your knuckles. This hand position is used most often when cutting uniform or increasing layers. In this case, you will usually stand to the side of the section on which you are working (Figure 11–56).

- *Cutting below the fingers.* When cutting a one-length bob or a heavier graduated haircut, it is customary to use a horizontal cutting line. In this case, you will be cutting below your fingers, or on the inside of your knuckles (Figure 11–57).
- *Cutting palm-to-palm.* When cutting with a vertical or diagonal cutting line, cutting palm-to-palm is the best way to maintain control of the subsection, especially with regard to elevation and overdirection. Cutting **palm-to-palm** means that the palms of both hands are facing each other while cutting. This is different from cutting on the top of your fingers or knuckles. Cutting palm-to-palm also helps to prevent strain on your back as you work (Figure 11–58 and Figure 11–59).

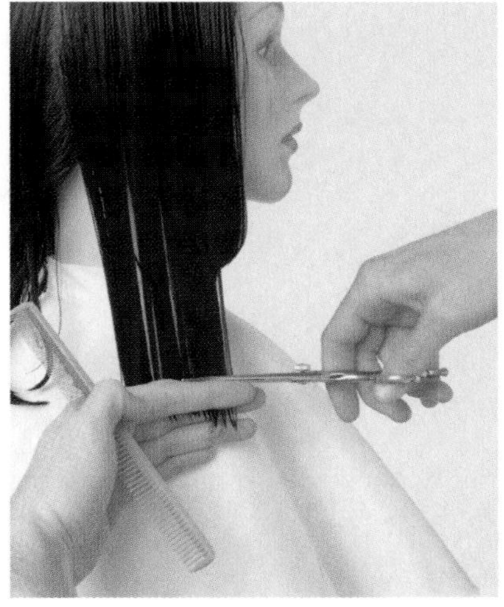

Figure 11-56 Cutting over the fingers.

Safety in Haircutting

It is absolutely essential for you to keep in mind that when you are cutting hair, accidents can happen. You will be handling sharp tools and instruments, and you must always safeguard yourself and your client by following the proper precautions.

- Always palm the shears and the razor when combing or parting the hair. This keeps the points of the shears closed and pointed away from the client while combing, which prevents you from cutting yourself or the client. Palming the shears also reduces strain on the index finger and thumb while combing the hair.
- Do not cut past the second knuckle when cutting underneath your fingers or the inside of your hand. The skin is soft and fleshy past the second knuckle and is easy to cut.
- When cutting around the ears or in the case of shorter haircuts, take extra care not to accidentally cut the ear.
- When cutting bangs or any area close to the skin, balance the shears by placing the tip of the index finger of your left hand (right hand if you cut

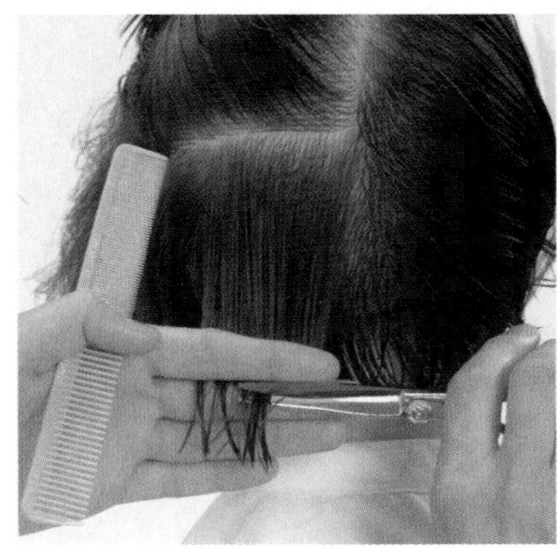

Figure 11-57 Cutting below the fingers.

11

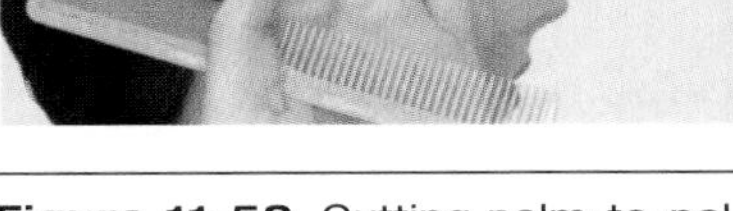

Figure 11-58 Cutting palm-to-palm, vertical cutting line.

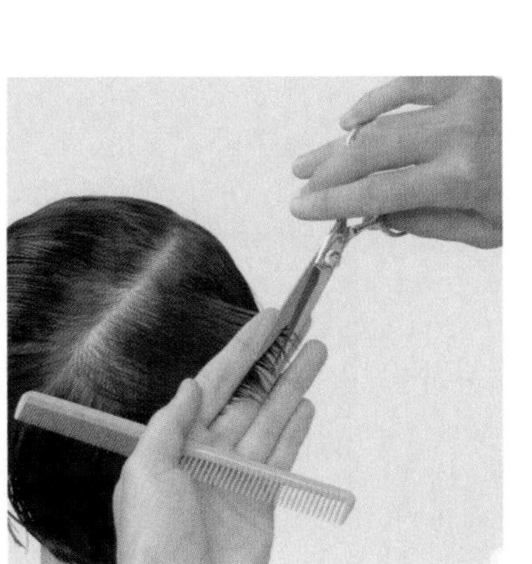

Figure 11-59 Cutting palm-to-palm, diagonal cutting line.

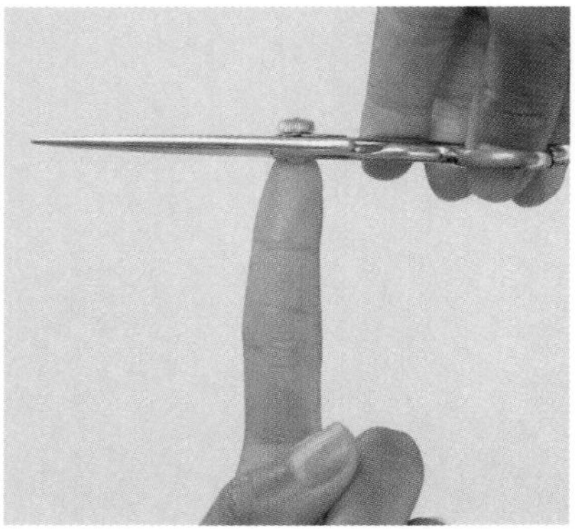

Figure 11–60 Balancing shears.

left-handed) on the pivot screw and the knuckles of your left hand against the skin (Figure 11–60). This prevents the client from being accidentally poked with the shears if she moves suddenly. This also helps to balance your shears and cut a cleaner line.

- When working with a razor, always use a guard. Once you are comfortable with holding, palming, and cutting with the razor, you may practice without a guard, but *always let your instructor be your guide.*
- Take extra care when removing and disposing of the razor blade. Place the blade in its original sleeve or wrap it in a paper towel to protect anyone from getting cut.

Sanitation and Disinfection Guidelines

1. Wash your hands with soap and warm water before and after each service.
2. Before blow-drying your client, sweep up cut hair and dispose of properly.
3. Drape the client properly for the shampoo and the haircutting procedures.
4. Always sanitize combs, brushes, shears, clips, and other implements after each haircut by washing thoroughly and placing in a disinfectant solution or by another method approved by your regulatory agency. See Chapter 5 for disinfection and storage procedures.
5. Replace the blade in your razor prior to each new client. Discard used blades in a puncture-proof container.
6. Keep your shears in good working order by lubricating with a few drops of oil and wiping with a chamois (or dry cloth).
7. Sanitize your workstation after each haircutting service.

Check with the regulatory agency of your state or province for the approved method of disinfecting shears, razors, combs, and brushes.

BASIC HAIRCUTS

The art of haircutting is made up of variations on four basic haircuts: blunt, graduated, layers, and long layers. A thorough grounding in these basic haircuts is essential before you can begin experimenting with other cuts and effects.

In a **blunt haircut**, also known as a one-length haircut, all the hair comes to one hanging level, forming a weight line or area. The **weight line** is a visual "line" in the haircut, where the ends of the hair hang together. The blunt cut is also referred to as a zero-elevation cut or no-elevation cut because it is cut with no elevation or overdirection. It is cut with a stationary guide. The cutting line can be horizontal, diagonal, or rounded. Blunt haircuts are excellent for finer and thinner hair types, because all the hair is cut to one length, therefore making it appear thicker (Figure 11–61).

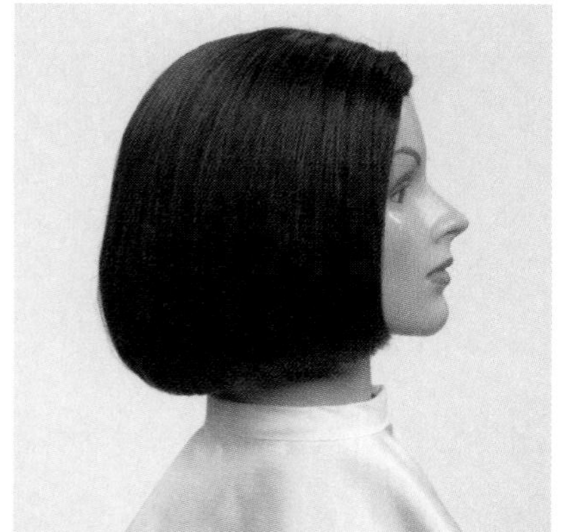

Figure 11–61 Blunt haircut.

A **graduated haircut** is a graduated shape or wedge, an effect or haircut that results from cutting the hair with tension, low to medium elevation, or overdirection. The most common elevation is 45 degrees. In a graduated haircut, there is a visual buildup of weight in a given area. The ends of the hair appear to be "stacked." There are many variations and effects you can create with graduation simply by adjusting the degree of elevation, the amount of overdirection, or your cutting line (Figure 11–62).

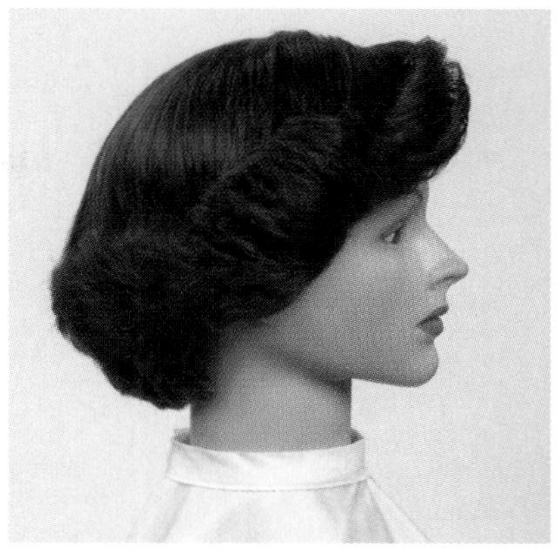

Figure 11-62 Graduated haircut.

A **layered haircut** is a graduated effect achieved by cutting the hair with elevation or overdirection. The hair is cut at higher elevations, usually 90 degrees and above. Layered haircuts generally have less weight than graduated haircuts. In a graduated haircut, the ends of the hair appear closer together. In a layered haircut, the ends appear farther apart. Layers create movement and volume in the hair by releasing weight. A layered haircut can be created with a traveling guide, a stationary guide, or both (Figure 11–63).

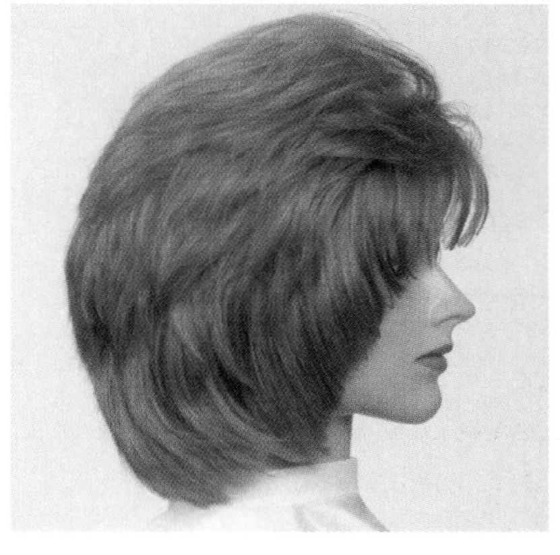

Figure 11-63 Layered haircut.

Another basic haircut is the **long layered haircut**. The hair is cut at a 180-degree angle. This technique gives more volume to hairstyles and can be combined with other basic haircuts. The resulting shape will have shorter layers at the top and increasingly longer layers toward the perimeter (Figure 11–64).

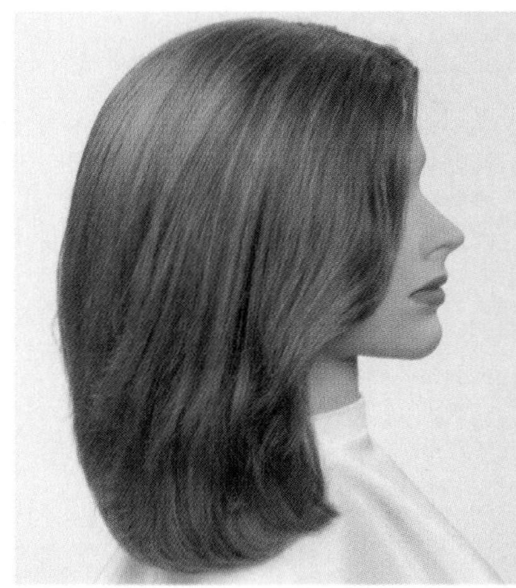

Figure 11-64 Long layered haircut.

By mastering these four basic concepts, you will be able to create any haircut you want. Every haircut is made up of one, two, or all three of these basic techniques. Add a little texturizing, slide cutting, or shears-over-comb, and you've got advanced haircutting. Advanced haircutting is simply learning the basics and then applying them in any combination to create unlimited shapes and effects. Take the time now to practice discipline and precision in your work.

General Haircutting Tips

- *Always take consistent and clean partings*, which ensure an even amount of hair in each subsection and produce more precise results.
- *Take extra care* when working in the crown and neckline, which sometimes have very strong growth patterns.
- *Another danger zone* is the hair that grows around the ear or hangs over the ear in a finished haircut. Allow for the protrusion of the ear by either keeping more weight in this area or cutting with minimal tension.
- *Always use consistent tension.* Tension may range from maximum to minimum. You can maintain light tension by using the wide teeth of the comb and by not "pulling" the subsection too tightly. Whatever tension you are using, it should be consistent within the area on which you are working.
- *Pay attention to head position.* If the head is not upright, it can be hard to judge elevation and overdirection.
- *Maintain an even amount of moisture in the hair.* Dry hair responds to cutting differently than wet hair, and may give you uneven results in the finished haircut.
- *Always work with your guideline.* If you cannot see the guide, your subsection is too thick. Go back and take a smaller subsection before

cutting. Taking too large a subsection can result in a large mistake. By using smaller sections, if a mistake is made, it is small and therefore easier to correct.

- *Always cross-check the haircut.* **Cross-checking** is parting the haircut in the opposite way from which you cut it, to check for precision of line and shape. For example, if you use vertical partings in a haircut, cross-check the lengths with horizontal partings (Figure 11–65).
- *Use the mirror to see your elevation.* You can also turn the client sideways so that you can see one side in the mirror while working on the opposite side. This helps create even lines and maintains visual balance while working.
- Always check that both sides are even by standing in front of your client as well.
- Remember that curly hair shrinks more than straight hair, anywhere from ½ to 2 inches (1.25 to 5 cm). Always leave the length longer than the desired end result.

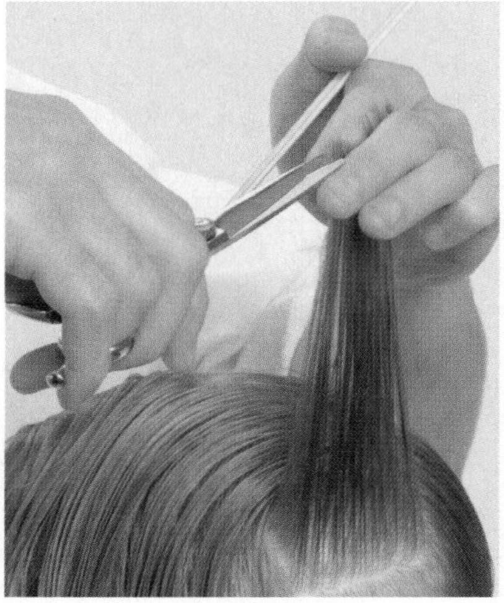

Figure 11-65 Cross-checking.

The Blunt Haircut

The client's head should be upright and straight for this cut. If you tilt the head forward, the hair will not fall in its natural falling position. If you attempt to cut a blunt haircut with the head forward, you will make two unfortunate discoveries: the line will not fall as you cut it, and you will have created some graduation where you did not intend to.

Blunt haircuts may be performed by either holding the sections between the fingers or using the comb to hold the hair, and always with little to no tension. If the hair length is past the shoulders, sections need to be held between the fingers, with minimal tension.

In the following haircut procedure, you will be working with a horizontal cutting line and a center part.

PROCEDURE

BLUNT HAIRCUT

Implements and Materials

- towels
- shampoo cape
- shampoo and conditioner
- cutting cape
- wide-tooth comb
- cutting or styling comb
- four sectioning clips
- haircutting shears
- water spray bottle
- neck strip

Preparation

1. Perform the client consultation and hair analysis.
2. Drape the client for shampooing, using two towels.
3. Shampoo and condition the hair as necessary.
4. Towel-dry the hair. Remove the towel around the neck and dispose of properly, leaving the second towel in place to prevent excess water from dripping on the client.
5. Escort the client back to the styling chair. Secure a neck strip around the client's neck (Figure 11–66). Place a cape over the neck strip and fasten in the back. Fold the neck strip down over the cape so that no part of the cape touches the client's skin (Figure 11–67).

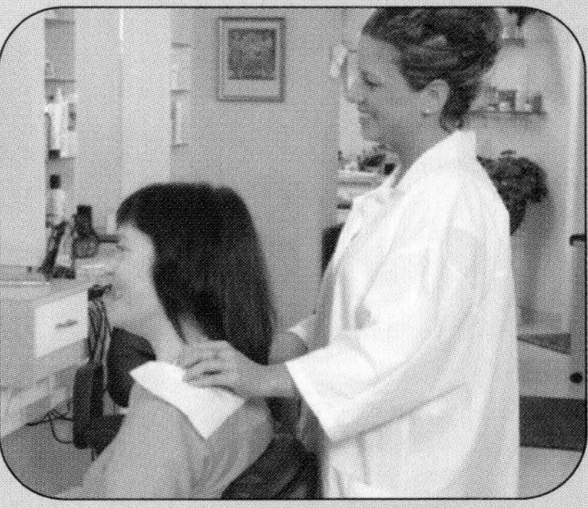

Figure 11–66 Place a neck strip around the client's neck.

Procedure

1. Detangle the hair with the wide-tooth comb. Then comb the hair back and away from the face to find the natural part, or part the hair the way the client will be wearing it.

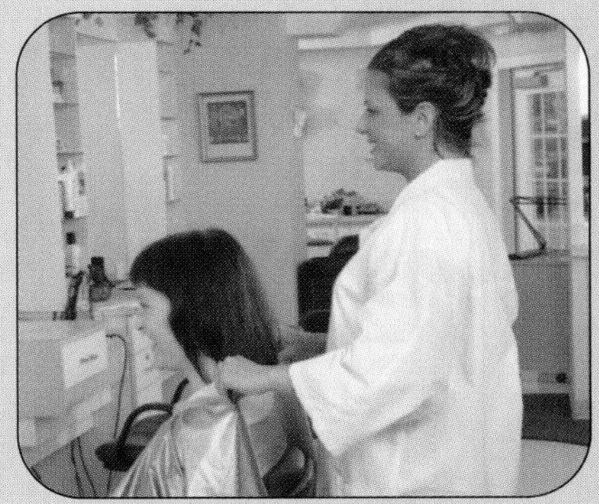

Figure 11–67 Fold the neck strip down.

11

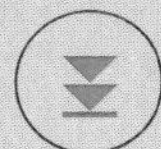

Here's a tip:

The density (thickness) of the hair will determine the size of the subsection. The thicker the hair, the narrower the subsection; the thinner the hair, the wider the subsection. In other words, to create narrower subsections, your partings need to be closer together. To create wider subsections, your partings should be farther apart. If there is too much hair in one subsection, it becomes difficult to control the hair, because the hair is "pushed" away as you close the shears, producing an uneven line.

2. Take a center part that runs from the front hairline to the nape, dividing the head in two (Figure 11–68).
3. Find the apex of the head. Take a parting that runs from the apex to the back of the ear on both sides, and clip. You have now divided the head into four sections (Figure 11–69).
4. Beginning in the nape, on the left side, take a horizontal parting $^{1}/_{4}$ to $^{1}/_{2}$ inch (.6 to 1.25 cm) from the hairline, depending on the density of the hair. This creates the first subsection (Figure 11–70 and Figure 11–71).
5. With the client's head upright, comb the subsection in a natural fall from scalp to ends. With your dominant hand, comb the subsection again, stopping just above the cutting line. Make sure the comb is horizontal and just above the cutting line (desired length). Cut the subsection straight across against the skin, remembering to keep your shears horizontal and parallel to the floor (Figure 11–72). Repeat on the right-hand side, using the length of your first subsection as a guide (Figure 11–73). Check to make sure your cutting line is straight before moving on. You have now created your guideline for the entire haircut.

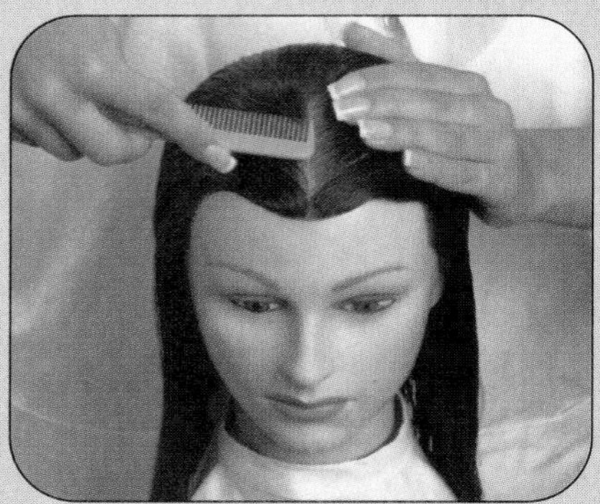

Figure 11–68 Center part.

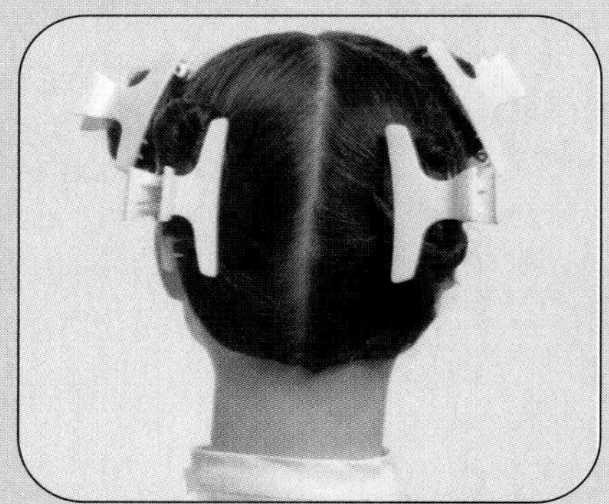

Figure 11–69 Hair parted into four sections.

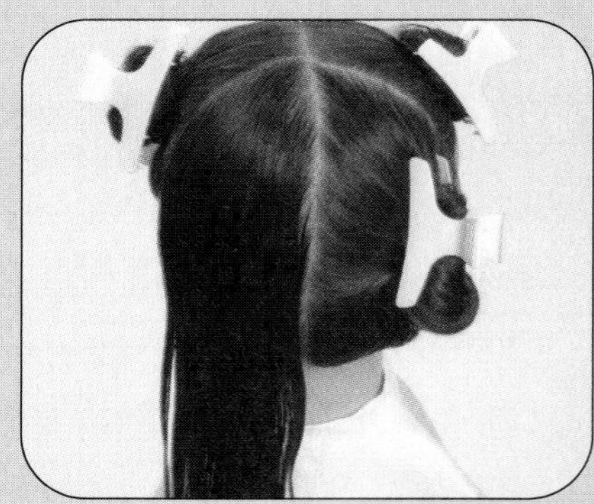

Figure 11–70 One section prepared for parting.

11

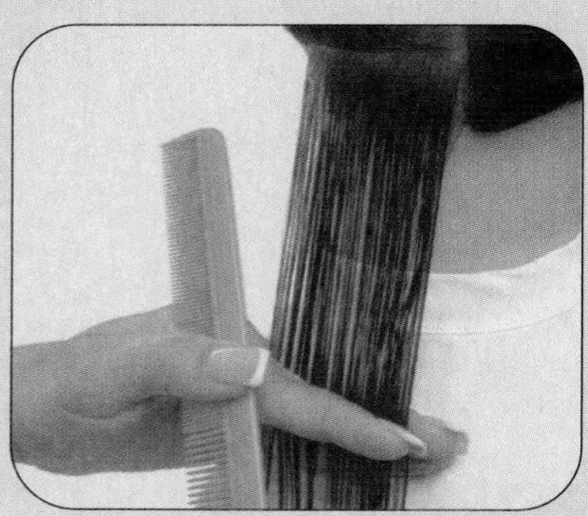

Figure 11–71 First subsection.

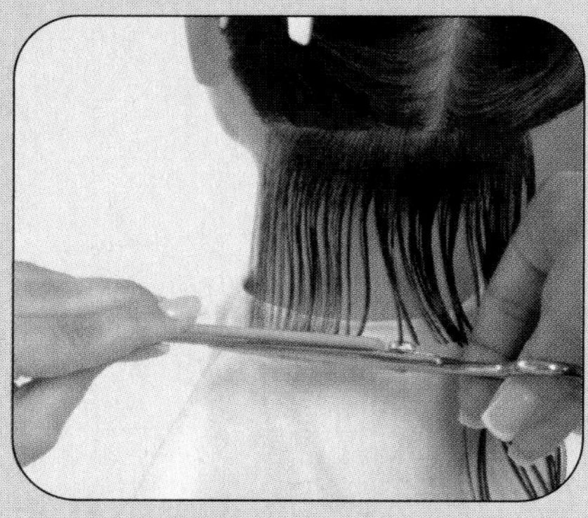

Figure 11–72 Cut first subsection on left.

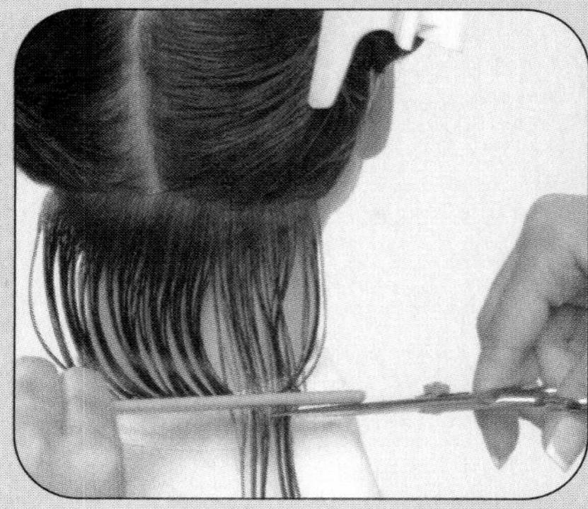

Figure 11–73 Cut first subsection on right.

6. If the hairline lies down nicely, an alternate way of cutting a blunt line in the nape is to comb down the subsection and hold the hair against the skin with the edge of your nondominant hand. Cut the guideline below your hand, making sure your shears are horizontal and parallel to the floor (Figure 11–74).
7. Returning to the left side, take another horizontal parting, creating a subsection the same size as your previous subsection. A general rule of thumb is you should be able to see the guideline through the new subsection. If you cannot see the guide, take a smaller subsection. Comb the hair down in a natural fall, and cut the length to match the guide (Figure 11–75). Repeat on the right side (Figure 11–76).
8. Continue working up the back of the head, alternating from the left section to the right section, using $^1/_2$ inch subsections.
9. When you reach the crown area (danger zone), pay close attention to the natural fall of the hair. Comb the hair into its natural falling position, and cut with little or no tension to match the guide (Figure 11–77). You have now completed the back of the haircut.

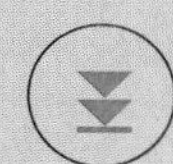

Here's a tip:

Using the comb to control the hair allows you to cut with very little tension. This allows the hair to do what it wants to naturally and still maintain a clean line.

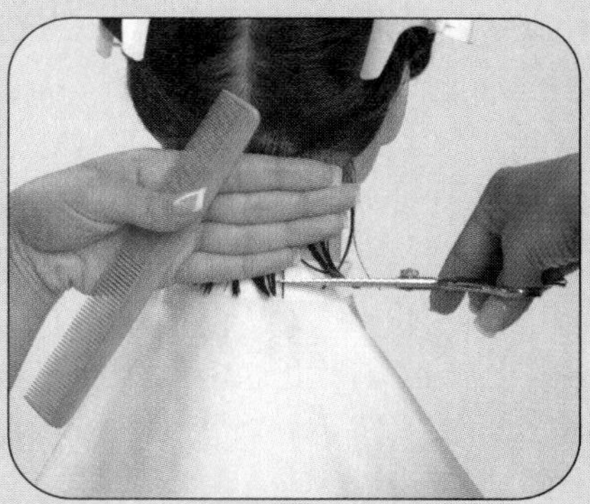

Figure 11–74 Hold the hair against the skin.

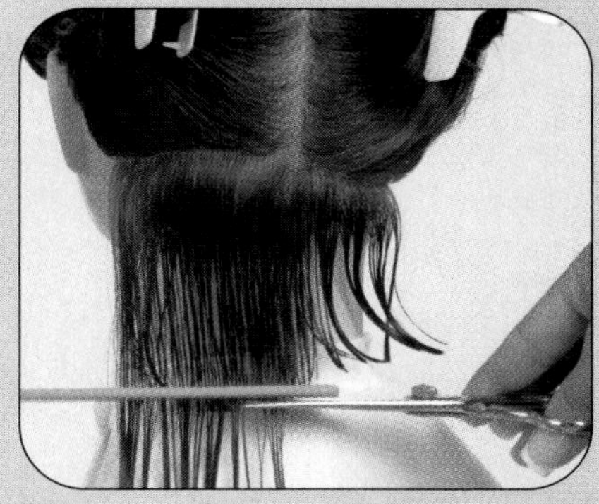

Figure 11–75 Second subsection on left.

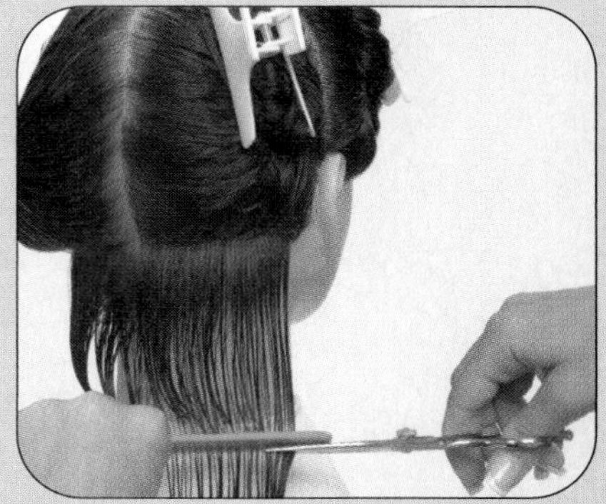

Figure 11–76 Second subsection on right.

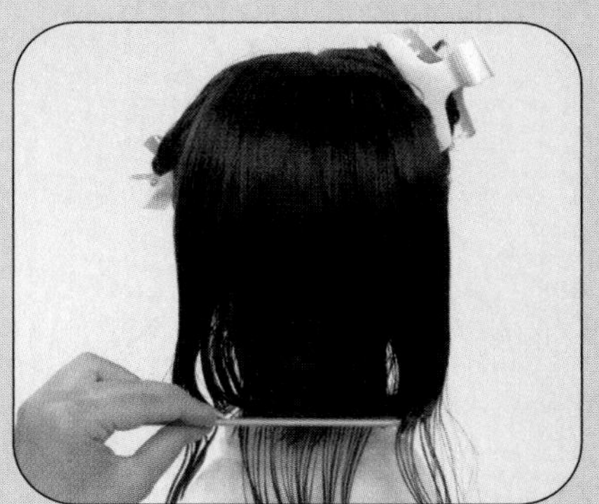

Figure 11–77 Comb the crown into natural fall.

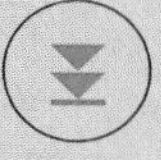

Here's a tip:

The crown area is called the "danger zone" because it is where irregular growth patterns are most apparent. The crown is particularly problematic when you are dealing with blunt haircuts. Look at the scalp to see the natural growth pattern. You may even want to leave this area out until the very end of the haircut, or cut it slightly longer than the guideline. Once the hair is dry, you can see where it falls, then match the length to the guideline. Another danger zone is around the ears. Because ears do not lie flat against the head, you need to take special steps to keep a clean cutting line. Always work with very little tension, or no tension, around the ears, unless you are working with shorter layers.

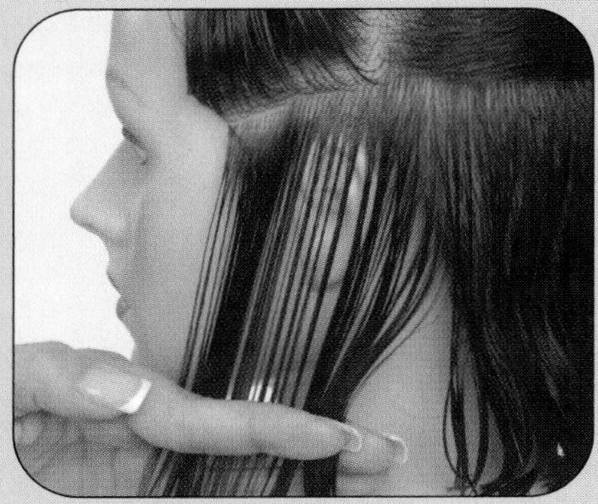

Figure 11-78 Take a horizontal parting on the left side.

10. Now move to the sides of the haircut. Beginning on the left side, take a horizontal parting and part off a portion from the back area to match (Figure 11–78). This will ensure that you maintain consistency with the blunt line when connecting the back to the sides. Be sure to take a subsection that is large enough to give you an even amount of hair at the cutting line, allowing for the protrusion of the ear. Comb the hair from scalp to ends, release the subsection, and allow the hair to hang in a natural fall. Using the wide teeth, place the comb back into the subsection just below the ear. Slide the comb down to just above the cutting line. Holding the comb parallel to the floor, cut the hair straight across just below the comb, connecting the line to the back (Figure 11–79). Repeat on the right-hand side (Figure 11–80).
11. When working on the right side (left side if you are left-handed), your shears will be pointing toward the back. To maintain consistency in your line, take smaller subsections, connecting at the ear first, and gradually move forward with the line until you reach the face.
12. An alternative way to approach the right side (left side if you are left-handed) is to turn your wrist so that your palm is facing upward and your shears are pointed toward the face. This requires that you position your body slightly behind the section you are working on, with your elbow dropped down. Either method gives you a consistent result in your line (Figure 11–81).
13. Before moving on, check that both sides of the haircut are even. Stand behind the client and check the lengths on both sides while looking in the mirror. Make any adjustments needed (Figure 11–82).
14. Continue working up the left side with horizontal partings, until all the hair has been cut to match the guide. When cutting the hair that falls along the face, make sure to comb the hair so it lies on the side, not the front, of the face. Repeat on the right side.

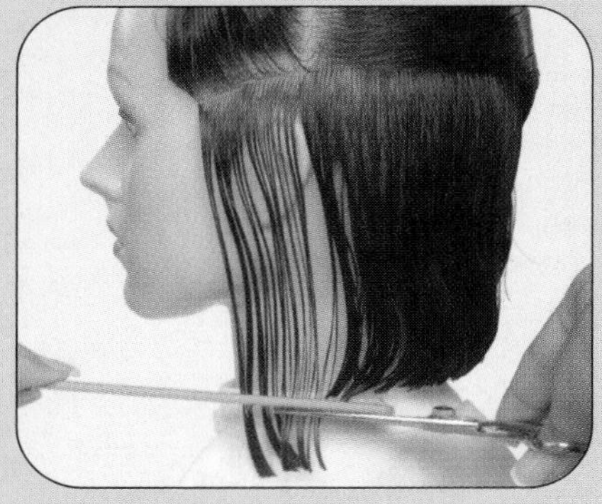

Figure 11-79 Cut the first subsection.

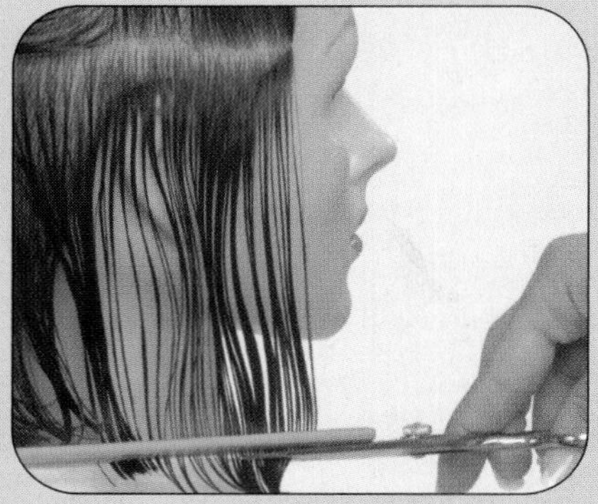

Figure 11-80 Repeat on the right.

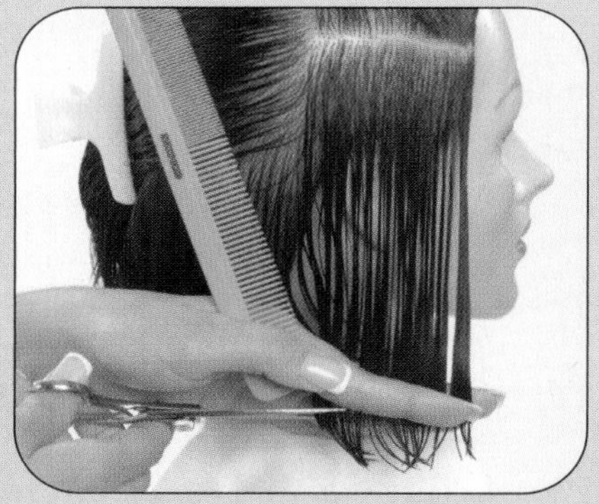

Figure 11-81 Cutting on the right side.

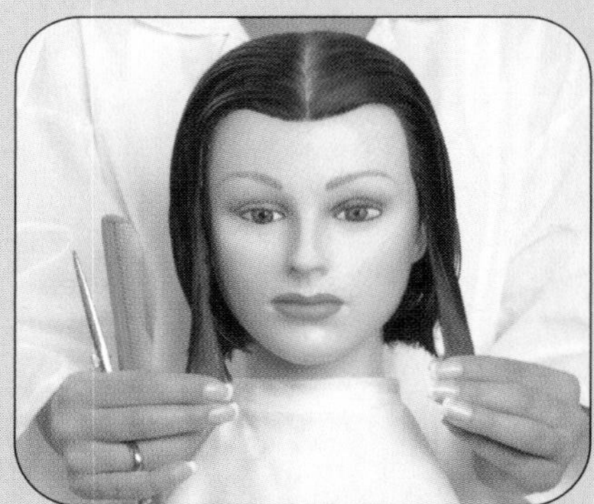

Figure 11-82 Check both sides.

15. Cross-check the haircut using vertical sections, making sure you do not overdirect the hair. Elevate the hair slightly and cut off any excess hair, removing only minimal amounts (Figure 11–83).
16. Sweep up cut hair from the floor and dispose of properly.
17. Blow-dry the haircut. In order to get a true reading of the haircut, it is best to perform a smooth blow-dry, with very little lift at the scalp.
18. Once the haircut is dry, have the client stand. Check the line in the mirror. You should see an even, horizontal line all the way around the head. This is the time to clean up any hair at the neckline and to check where the hair falls when dry (Figure 11–84). Use the wide teeth of the comb to connect the crown area. If this section was left longer during the haircut, now is the time to connect it into the line (Figures 11–85a, b, and c).
19. Remove the drape and neck strip from the client and dispose of properly.
20. Brush loose hair from the client's neck and face. Escort the client to the reception area.

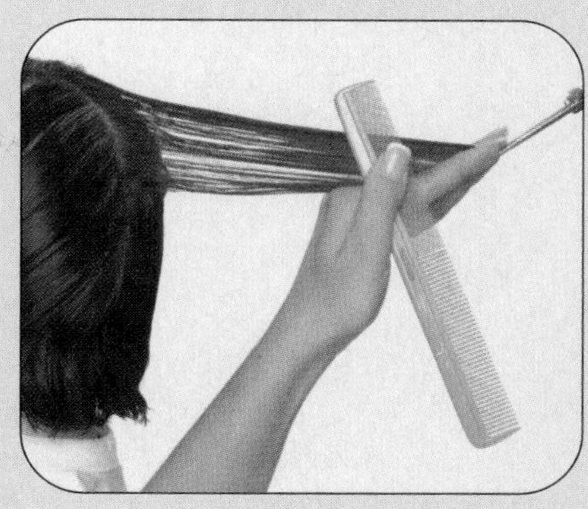

Figure 11–83 Cross-check with vertical subsections.

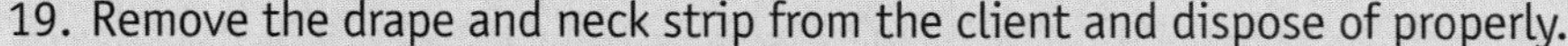

Cleanup and Sanitation

1. Disinfect all shears, combs, and brushes used during the haircut by immersing in a hospital-level disinfectant.
2. Sanitize your workstation, making sure it is clean and neat for your next client.
3. Wash your hands with soap and warm water.

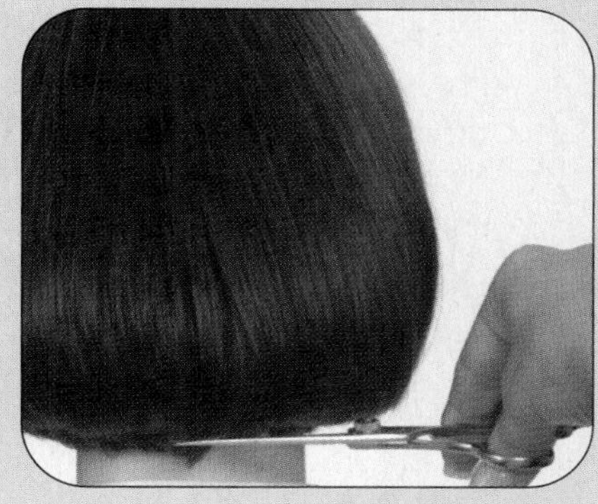

Figure 11–84 Clean up the neckline.

11

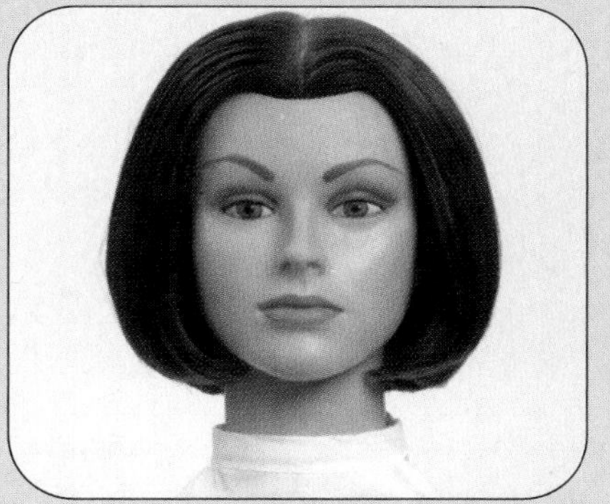

Figure 11–85a Finished blunt haircut.

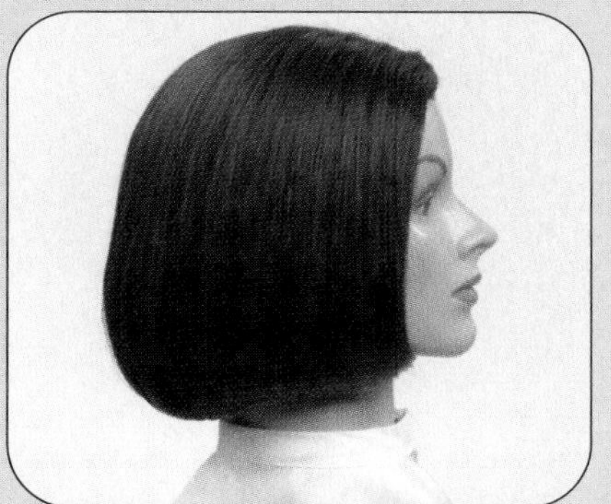

Figure 11–85b

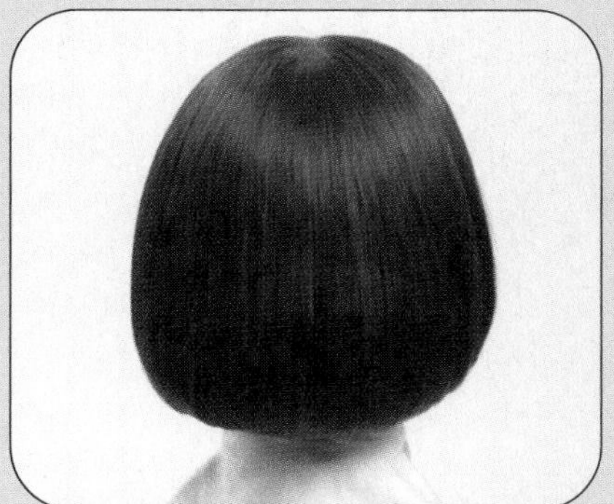

Figure 11–85c

completed!

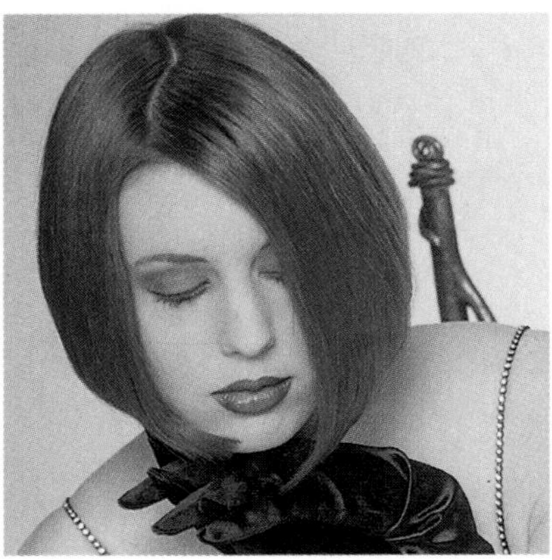

Figure 11-86 A-line bob.

Other Blunt Haircuts

The blunt haircut described above is the basis for a variety of other classic cuts.

- In a classic A-line bob, a diagonal cutting line (finger angle) is used (Figure 11–86).
- In this longer blunt haircut (Figure 11–87) the fringe has been left long and was cut with a horizontal finger angle. When blunt-cutting longer hair, hold the hair between the fingers with very little tension.
- Figure 11–88 illustrates a blunt haircut on curly hair. Notice how the hair naturally "graduates" itself when it dries.
- In a classic pageboy, or "bowl" shape, the perimeter is curved, using a combination of horizontal and curved lines (Figure 11–89).

Tips for Blunt Haircuts

- Always cut with minimal or no tension.
- Work with the natural growth patterns of the hair, keeping the client's head upright.
- Always comb the section twice before cutting, to ensure that you have combed the hair clean from the parting to the ends. If using the wide teeth of the comb while cutting, always comb the section first with the fine teeth, then turn the comb around, and recomb with the wide teeth.
- Always maintain an even amount of moisture in the hair.
- Pay close attention to growth patterns in the crown and hairline.
- Take precautions to allow for the protrusion of the ear, to avoid getting a "hole."

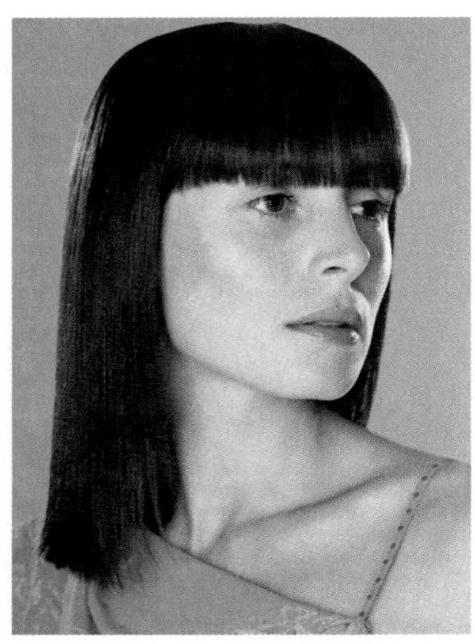

Figure 11-87 Longer blunt cut with one-length bangs.

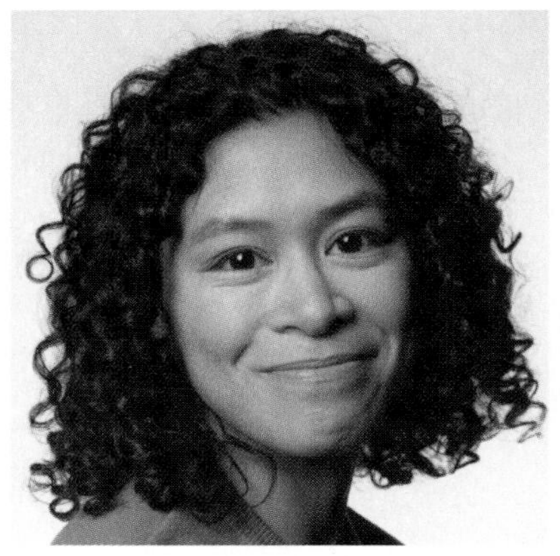

Figure 11-88 Blunt cut on curly hair.

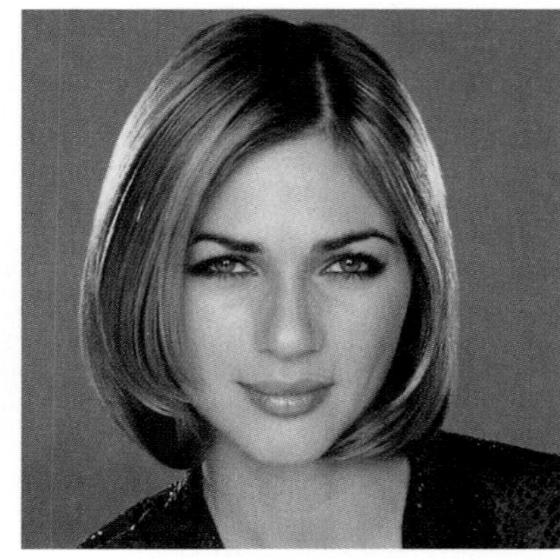

Figure 11-89 Classic blunt pageboy.

insights

Mary Brunetti

A thirty-year veteran of the industry, Mary had no trouble getting her first job, but, without sufficient training, she almost had trouble keeping it. Continuing education came to the rescue.

There is no substitute for a good education and well-practiced skills. Investing in our careers takes time and money. I'll never forget what the legendary Vidal Sassoon once said: "If you think education is expensive, try ignorance!" I learned this the hard way.

I became a hairdresser in 1973, when the licensing laws were first changed to allow cosmetologists to service both men and women in the same salon. "Unisex" hair salons were popping up everywhere, and the need for stylists with strong skills was overwhelming. I recognized the opportunity, went to cosmetology school, and got my first job at a very busy salon in New York City. They had a training program in place to strengthen the skills of new stylists. At that time, my skills were substandard at best, but I was more interested in just earning a living and enjoying all my free time and socializing, so I ignored the training classes. Why bother, if I was already making money?

One busy day in the salon, however, the head of the training program actually took the brush out of my hand while I was working on a client. What an embarrassment! But he was right. I wasn't taking my craft seriously. He told me to go home and seriously consider if this was what I wanted to do as a career. If I came back, I could start training seriously. (I wound up marrying him, but that's another story.)

From that point on, my perspective changed. I trained hard to be the best I could. I took pride in my work and realized that hairdressers actually have the power to make their clients feel better about themselves. And that's a great feeling. Pretty soon, doors started to open for me. Now I was prepared. Soon I was styling the hair of models for fashion magazines. Then I was asked to educate stylists at major hair shows. I won national awards. I have to say, it's wonderful to be recognized in such a way by your peers and the people you greatly respect. Now I style the hair of a celebrity for a popular TV talk show and make appearances on the show doing makeovers. What a career! And all because I began to take what I do seriously, and I put in the time to learn from those who had something to teach me.

Don't miss this vital step. Take school seriously. There's no replacement for a strong foundation in the basic skills of your trade. When opportunities present themselves, you'll be ready!

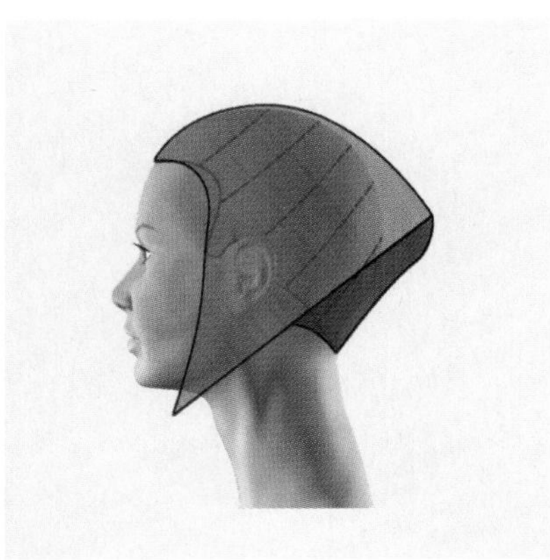

Figure 11-90 Graduated bob: design.

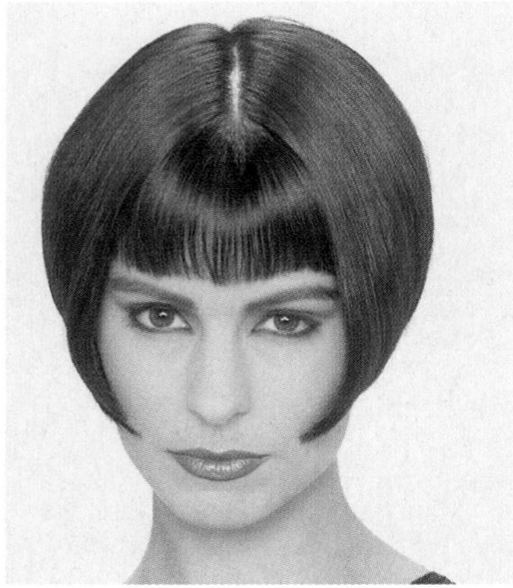

Figure 11-91 Finished graduated bob.

The Graduated (45-Degree) Haircut

In this basic haircut, you will be working with a vertical cutting line and a 45-degree elevation as well as a 90-degree elevation. Although you will use a center part, keep in mind that this haircut can also work with a side part or a fringe. You will be using a stationary guideline and a traveling guideline. Remember, a stationary guideline is a guideline that does not move. All other sections are combed toward the guideline and are cut to match it. A traveling guideline moves with you as you work through the haircut.

Other Graduated Haircuts

Let us take a look at some other types of graduated haircuts, created with different cutting angles.

- In the classic graduated bob made popular by Vidal Sassoon, diagonal sections and finger angles are used to create a rounded or beveled effect. This haircut begins in the back, using a 45-degree elevation throughout, and gradually incorporates the sides and top. If you find that the hairline grows up or toward the center, you can use the shears-over-comb technique to blend it (Figure 11–90 and Figure 11–91).

activity

Here's a great way to understand what a graduated haircut looks like. Hold a telephone book by the spine with the pages hanging down. The edges of the pages make a straight line, just like a blunt haircut (Figure 11–92).

Now turn the book the other way, open it in the middle, and let the pages flop down on either side. The edges of the pages make a beveled line, just like a graduated haircut (Figure 11–93).

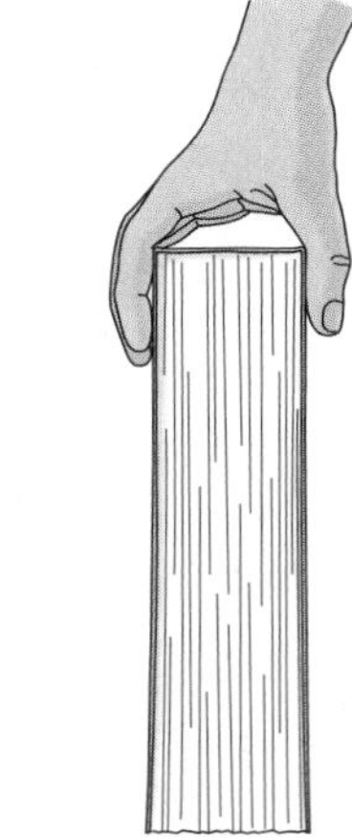

Figure 11-92 Straight or "blunt" hanging line.

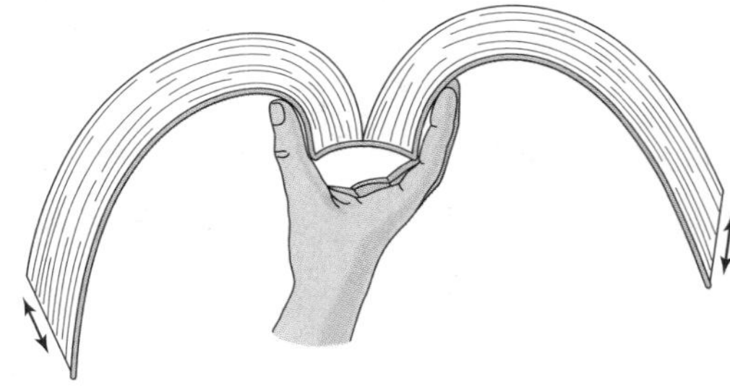

Figure 11-93 Beveled or "graduated" hanging line.

11

PROCEDURE

GRADUATED HAIRCUT

Implements and Materials

See list of implements and materials for Procedure 3—blunt haircut.

Preparation

Follow preparation steps for Procedure 3—blunt haircut.

Procedure

1. Part the hair into six sections. Begin with a part from the front hairline just above the middle of each eyebrow back to the crown area and clip the hair in place (Figure 11-94). Establish another part from the crown area where section one ends to the back of each ear, forming side sections two and three (Figure 11-95). Clip these sections in place. Part the hair down the center of the back to form sections four and five (Figure 11-96). Take a horizontal part from one ear to the other across the nape area, about 1 inch (2.5 cm) above the hairline. This section (six) is your horizontal guide section (Figure 11-97).

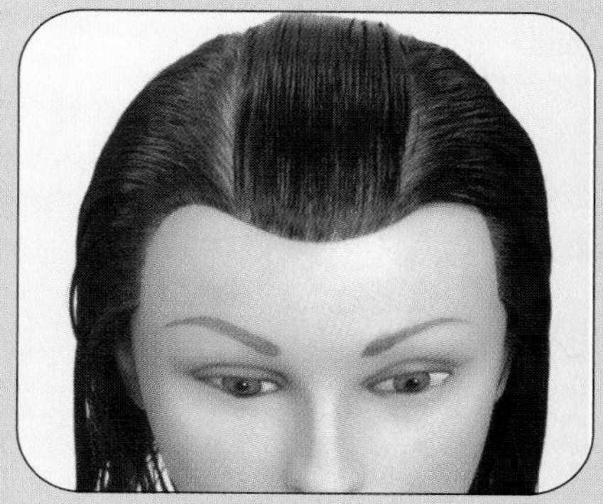

Figure 11-94 Part off section 1.

11

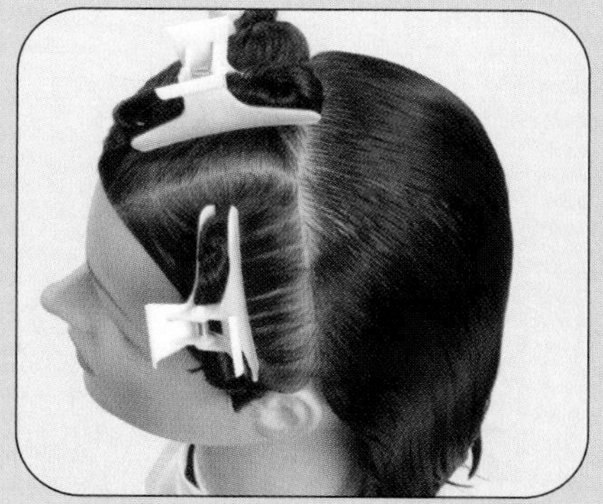

Figure 11-95 Form sections 2 and 3.

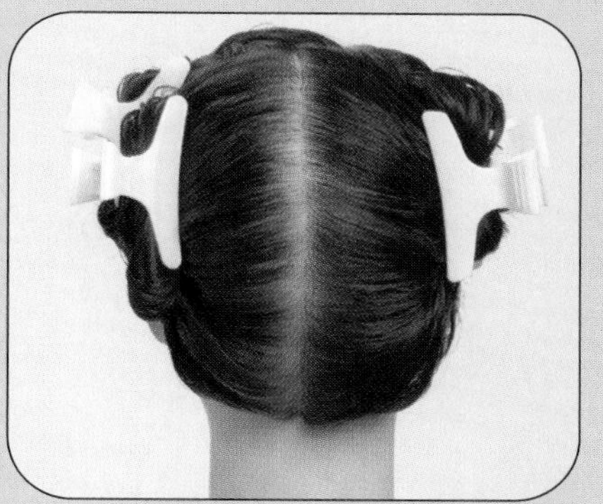

Figure 11-96 Form sections 4 and 5.

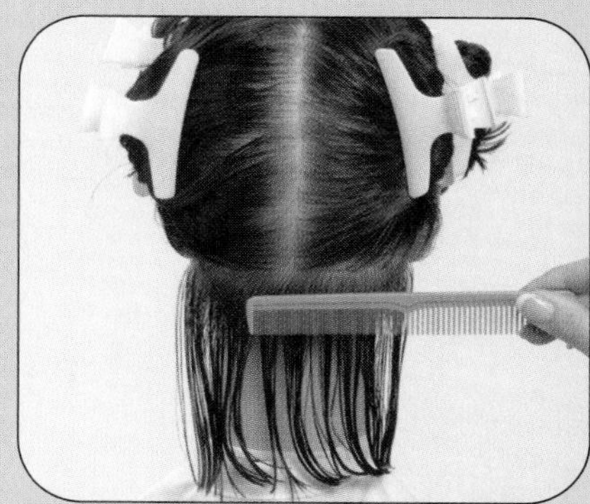

Figure 11-97 Finished sectioning.

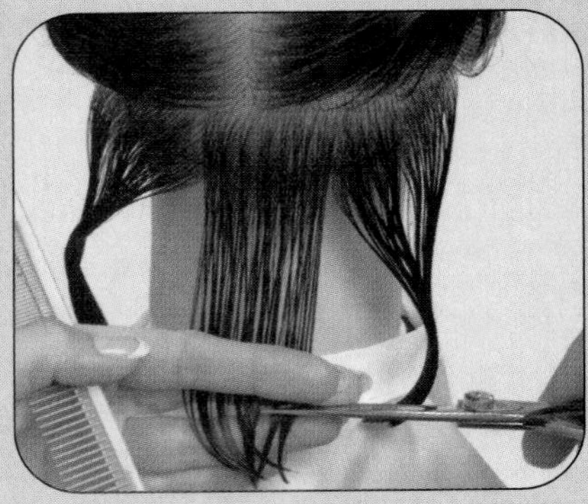

Figure 11-98 Cut the first nape section (guideline).

2. Establish your guideline by first cutting the center of the nape section to the desired length. Use a horizontal cutting line parallel to the fingers (Figure 11–98). Cut the right and left sides of the nape section the same length as the center guideline (Figure 11–99).
3. Working upward in the left back section, measure and part off the first horizontal section approximately 1 inch wide (Figure 11–100).
4. Beginning at the center part, establish a vertical subsection approximately ½ inch (1.25 cm) wide. Extend the subsection down to include the nape guideline. Comb the subsection smooth at a 45-degree angle to the scalp (Figure 11–101). Hold your fingers at a 90-degree angle to the strand and cut (Figure 11–102).
5. Proceed to cut the entire horizontal section by parting off vertical subsections and cutting in the same manner as Step 4. Check each section vertically and horizontally throughout the haircut. Each completed section will serve as a guideline for the next section.
6. Part off another horizontal section approximately 1 inch wide. Beginning at the center, create another vertical subsection that extends down and includes the previously cut strands (Figure 11–103). Comb the hair smoothly at a 45-degree elevation to the head. Hold the fingers

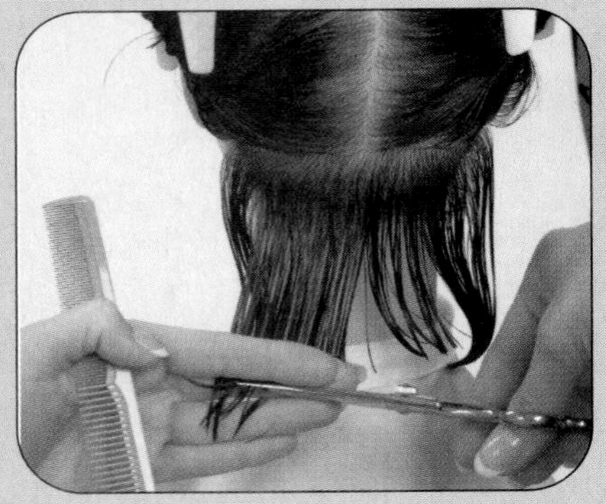

Figure 11-99 Finish cutting nape section.

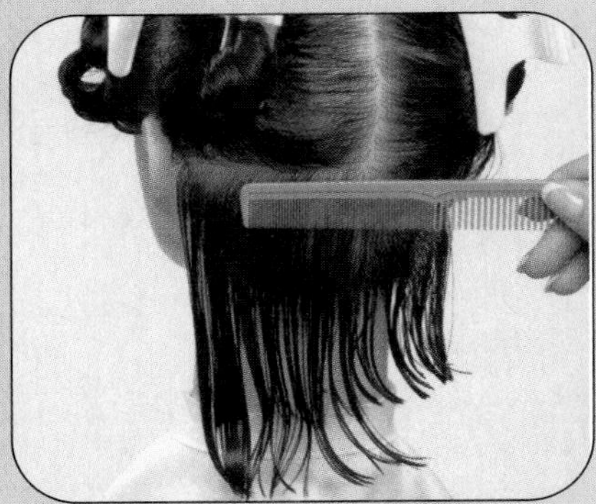

Figure 11–100 Measure off first horizontal section with comb.

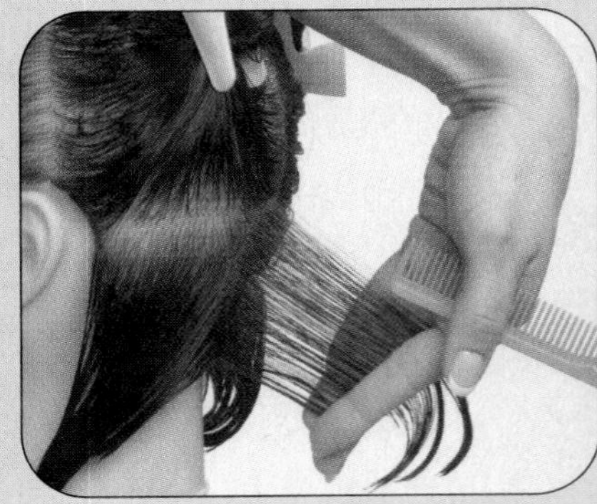

Figure 11–101 Comb first vertical subsection.

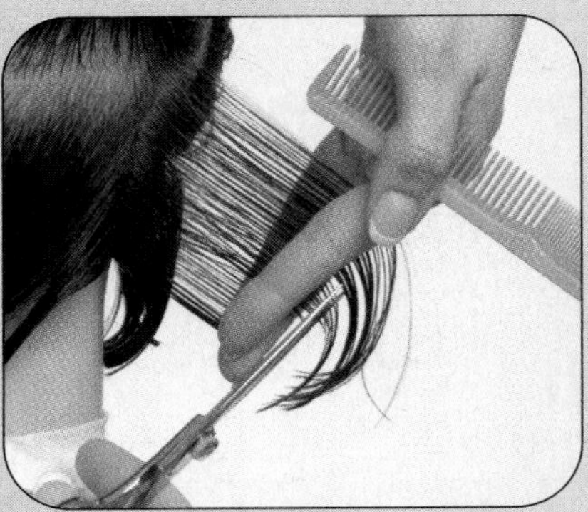

Figure 11–102 Cut first vertical subsection.

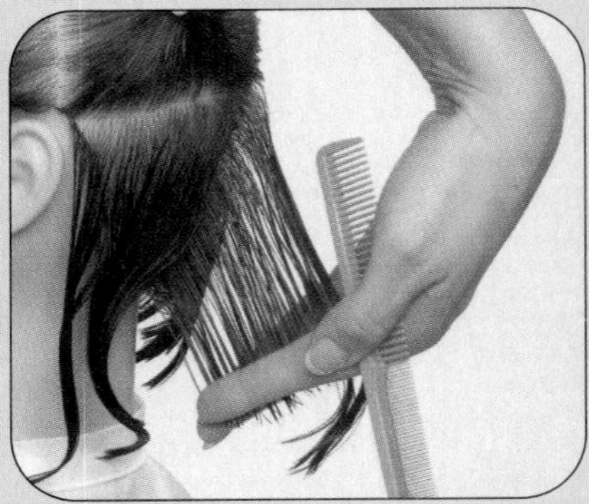

Figure 11–103 Create first vertical subsection in new section.

and shears at a 90-degree angle to the subsection and cut (Figure 11–104). Cut the entire horizontal section in this manner. Make sure the second section blends evenly with the previously cut section.

7. Continue taking horizontal sections throughout the left and right back sections and follow the same cutting procedure. The hair will gradually become longer as it reaches the apex. For example, if your nape guide was 2.5 (6.25 cm) inches long, your upper crown section will be approximately 6 inches (15 cm) long (Figure 11–105).
8. Maintain the length in the upper crown by holding each vertical subsection throughout the crown area at a 90-degree angle while cutting (Figure 11–106). After checking the back and crown for even blending, proceed to the left side section.
9. Establish a narrow guide section on the left side at the hairline approximately ½ inch wide. The side guideline should be the same length as the nape (Figure 11–107). Move to the right side of the head and establish a matching guideline there. This will help ensure that both side sections will be the same length when the right side section is cut later (Figure 11–108).
10. Establish a ½ inch side section that curves and follows the hairline above the ear back to the nape section. Smoothly comb the section, including the side guideline and part of the nape section (Figure 11–109).

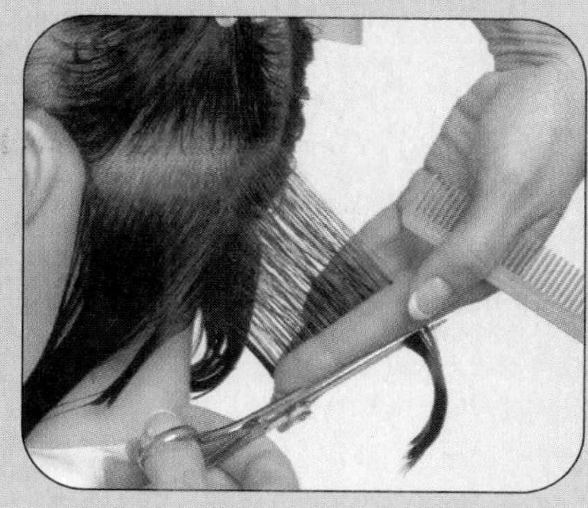

Figure 11–104 Cut subsection.

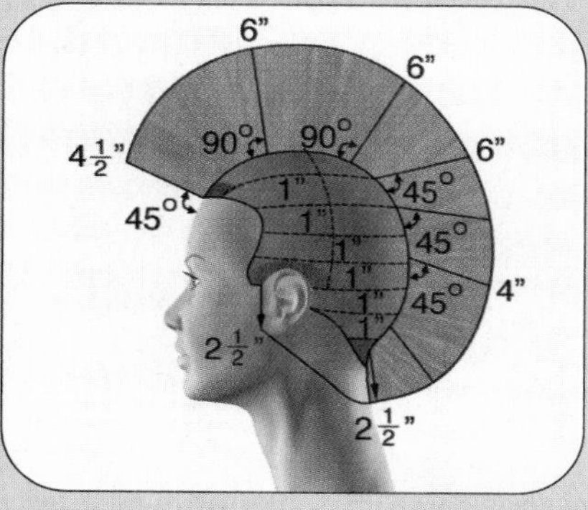

Figure 11–105 Graduated cutting design.

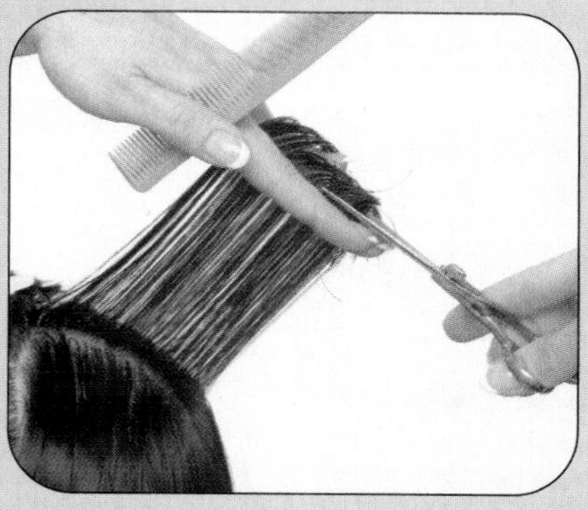

Figure 11–106 Cut hair in crown at 90 degrees.

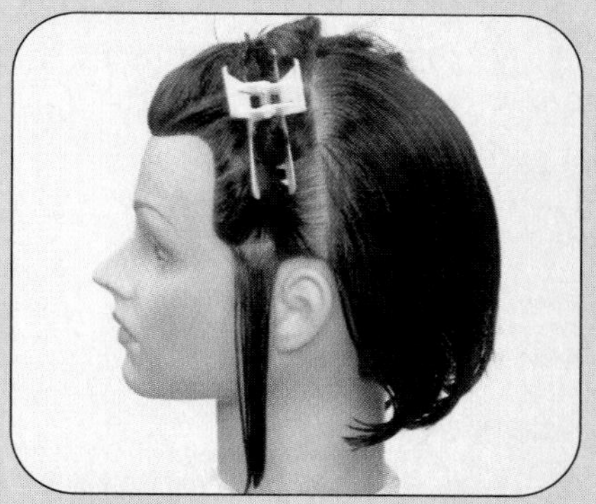

Figure 11–107 Establish guide section on the left.

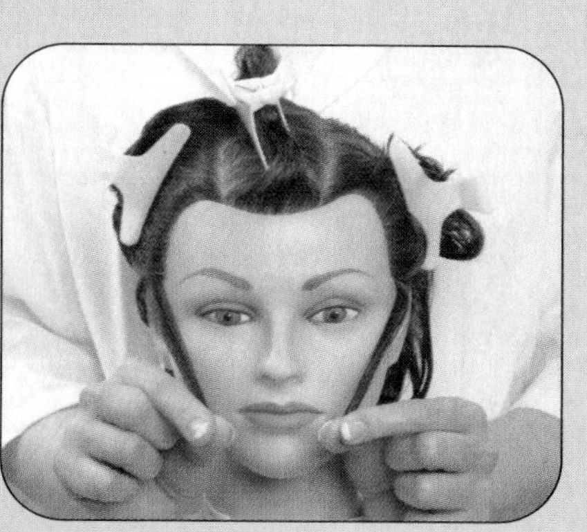

Figure 11–108 Check that both sections are the same length.

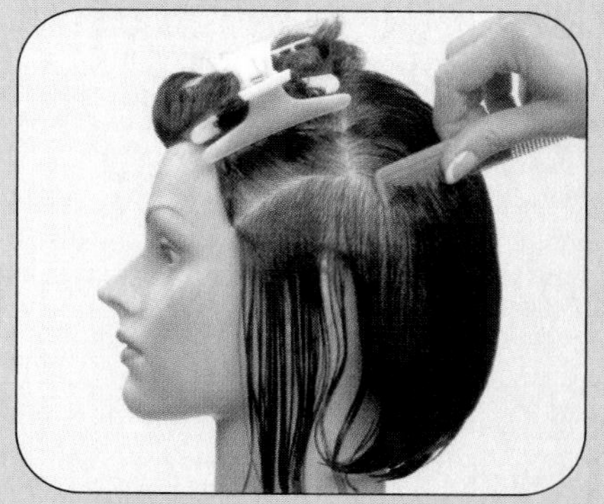

Figure 11–109 Establish side section.

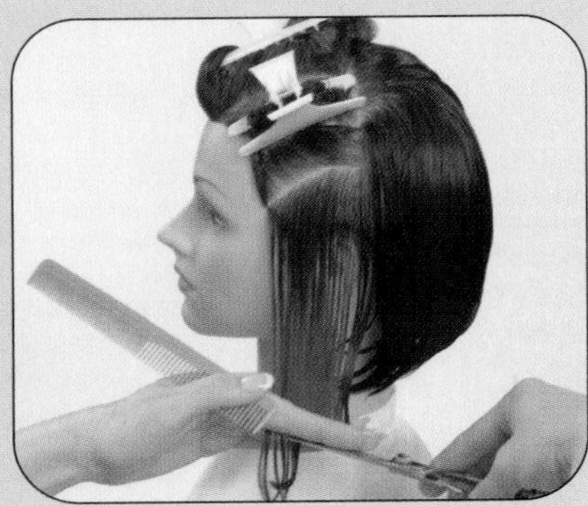

Figure 11–110 Cut hair from nape guide to side guide.

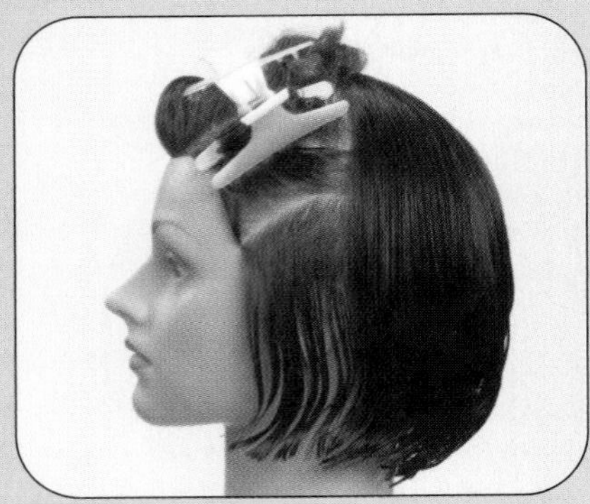

Figure 11–111 Finished side section.

11. Holding the hair with little or no tension, cut the hair from the nape guide to the side guide. Note that the fingers are held at a slight angle to connect the two guides (Figure 11–110 and Figure 11–111).
12. Establish a horizontal section on the left side. The width of this section will vary because of the irregular hairline around the ear (Figure 11–112).
13. Starting at the ear, part a ½ inch vertical subsection. Include the underlying guideline and a small portion of the nape section (Figure 11–113).
14. Continue the same cutting procedure followed thus far. Take vertical subsections, comb smoothly, elevate at a 45-degree angle from the head, holding the fingers at a 90-degree angle to the strand. Cut the section even with the side guideline and nape section. Be sure to hold the vertical subsections straight out from the head at 45 degrees, not pulled to the right or left (Figure 11–114).
15. Continue establishing horizontal sections on the left side of the head and following the same cutting procedure. Check each section horizontally to ensure the ends are evenly blended. Add strands from the back section when checking to ensure that the two sections are uniform in length.
16. When the left side section is complete, the strands in the uppermost part of the section should be the same length as those in the upper crown area. In the final 1-inch section, comb the vertical subsections

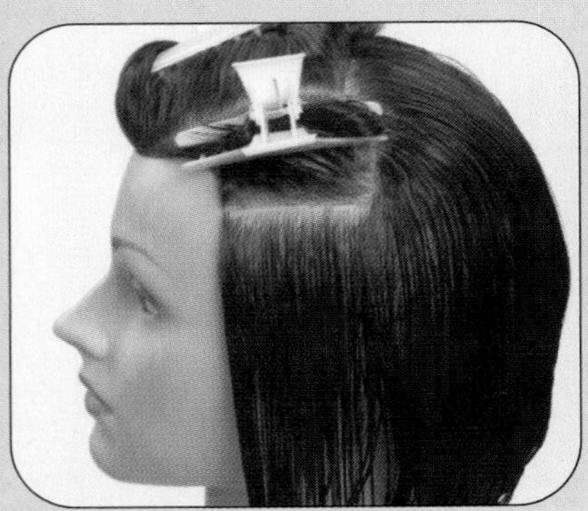

Figure 11–112 Establish horizontal section on left side.

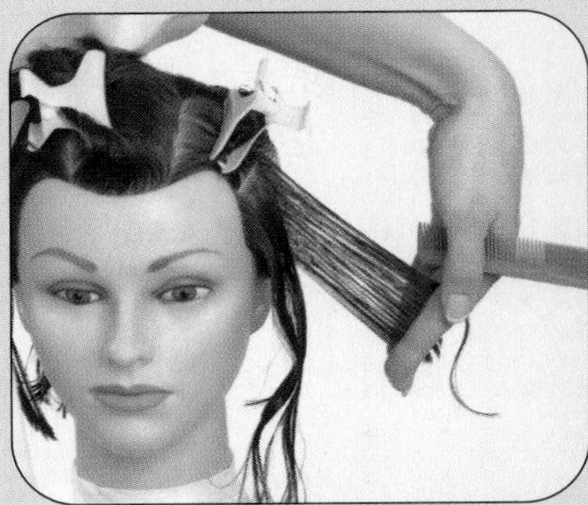

Figure 11–113 Part first vertical subsection.

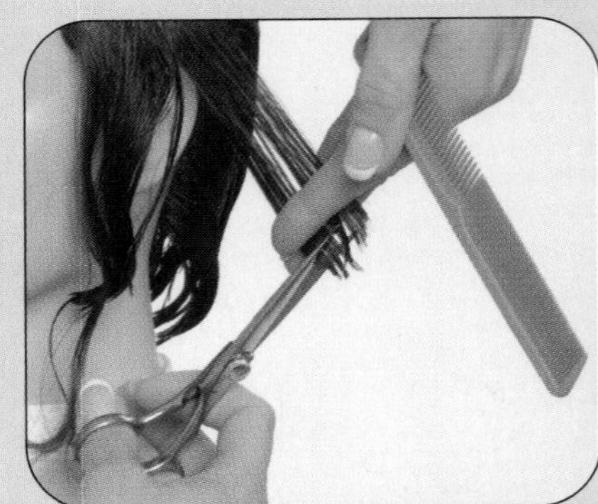

Figure 11–114 Hold vertical subsection straight out from the head at 45 degrees.

and hold them at a 90-degree angle to the head. Position your fingers at 90 degrees to the strand and cut parallel to your fingers (Figure 11–115). Check the completed section horizontally to make sure the ends are even (Figure 11–116).

17. Move to the right side of the head and cut the hair in the same manner as you did on the left side, using the previously established guide. Once the back and both sides are complete, move to the fringe and top areas.
18. You can create a variety of fringe designs by cutting the fringe length close to that of the side guideline. Create a fringe guide section along the hairline about ½ inch wide. Starting at the center part and working on the left side of the forehead, cut to the desired length (Figure 11–117).
19. Comb the fringe section, including the center guide strand and a small portion of the side area. Connecting the two guidelines will determine the angle of the cut (Figure 11–118).
20. Cut this fringe section at a low elevation. Check the cut for evenness and accuracy (Figure 11–119).
21. Establish a 1-inch section parallel to the fringe guideline. Beginning in the center, take narrow vertical subsections about ½ inch wide that include the underlying guideline. Comb the strand smoothly and elevate from the head at 45 degrees. Continue this cutting procedure throughout the fringe area (Figure 11–120). The fringe section should blend evenly with the side section.

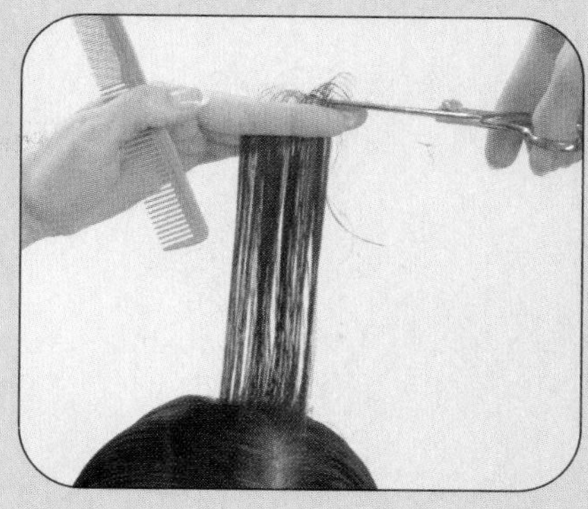

Figure 11–115 Blend subsections.

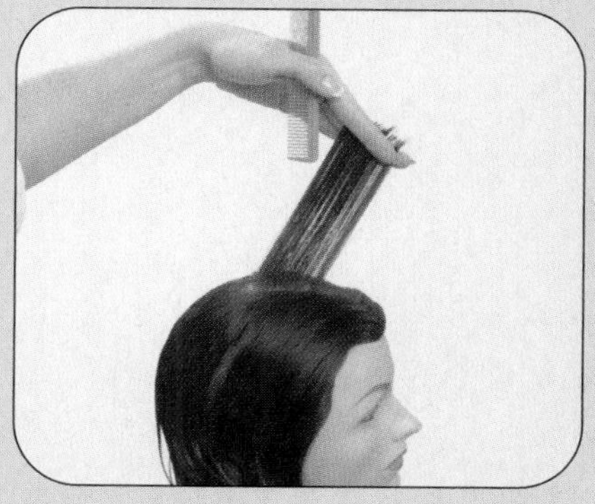

Figure 11–116 Cross-check section horizontally.

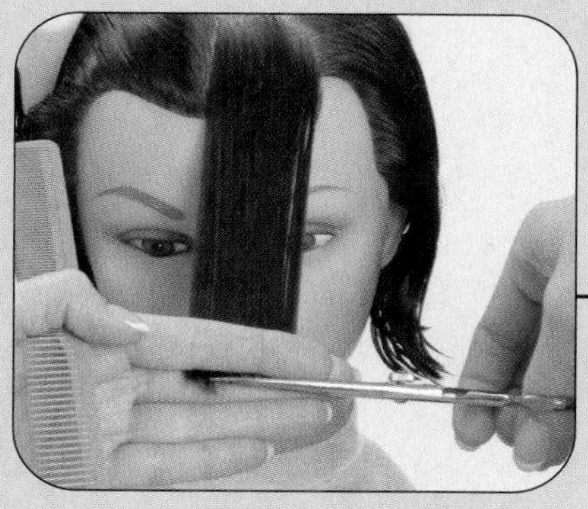

Figure 11–117 Cut fringe guide section.

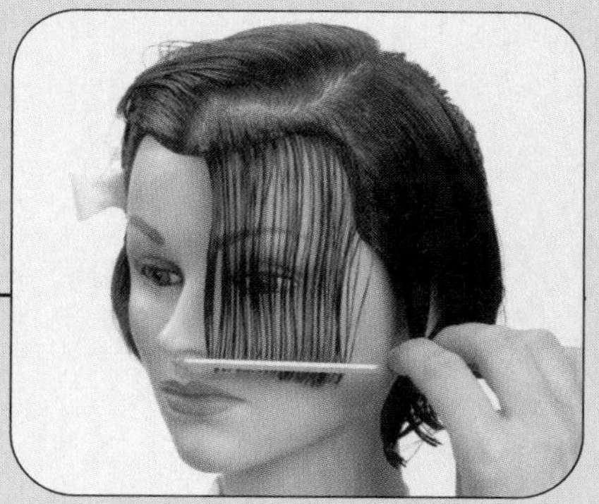

Figure 11–118 Comb fringe section.

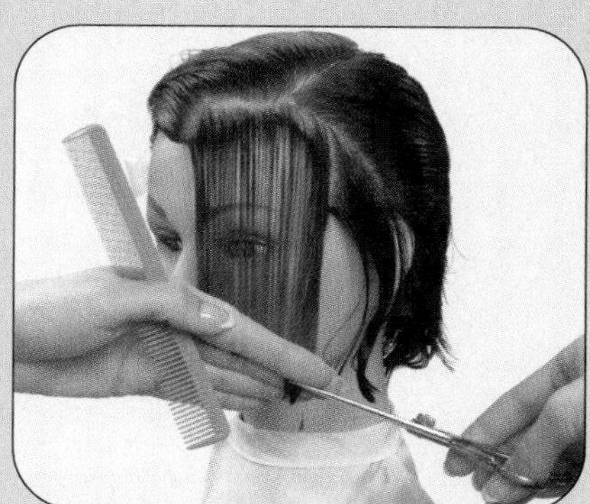

Figure 11–119 Cut fringe section at low elevation.

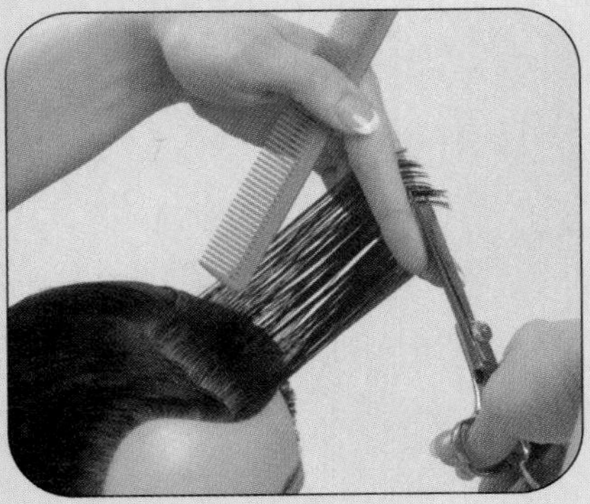

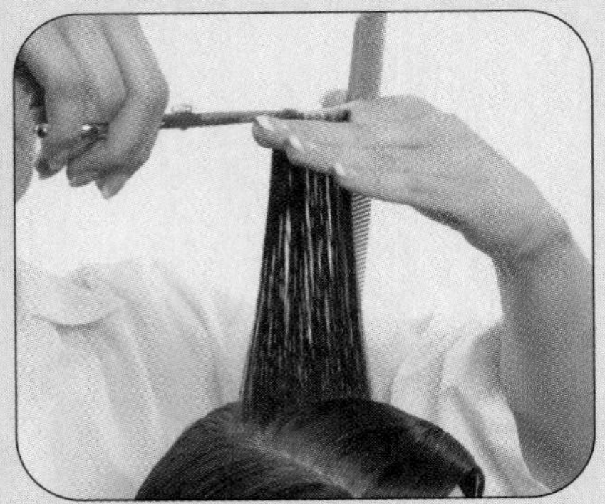

Figure 11–120 Cut vertical subsections in fringe area.

22. Cut the remainder of the fringe area on the right side of the head in the same manner as you did on the left side.
23. Finish the top section by taking 1/2-inch vertical subsections parallel to the center part. Hold the hair up from the head at a 90-degree angle. Include hair from the crown and fringe areas and cut to blend the section with the two precut sections. Continue cutting in this manner until the remainder of the top section is cut. Hold the hair up from the head at a 90-degree angle and check the completed cut. Trim any uneven ends. The fringe guide gradually increases in length to the preestablished length in the top and crown areas (Figure 11–121).
24. Blow-dry the haircut and view the design, movement, and evenly blended ends (Figures 11–122a, b, and c).
25. Follow cleanup and sanitation steps in Procedure 3—blunt haircut.

Figure 11–121 Cut top section.

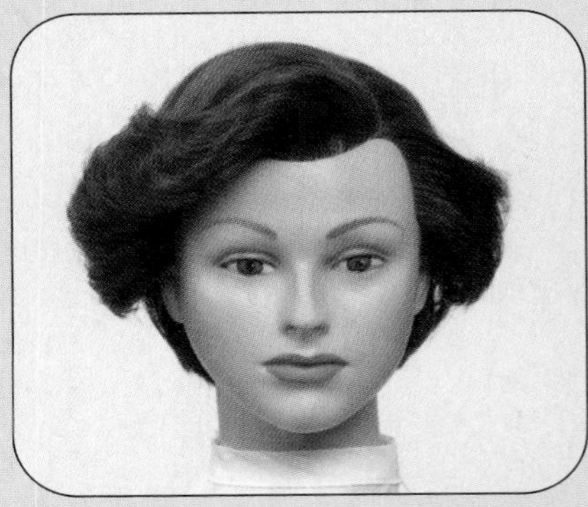

Figure 11–122a Finished graduated cut.

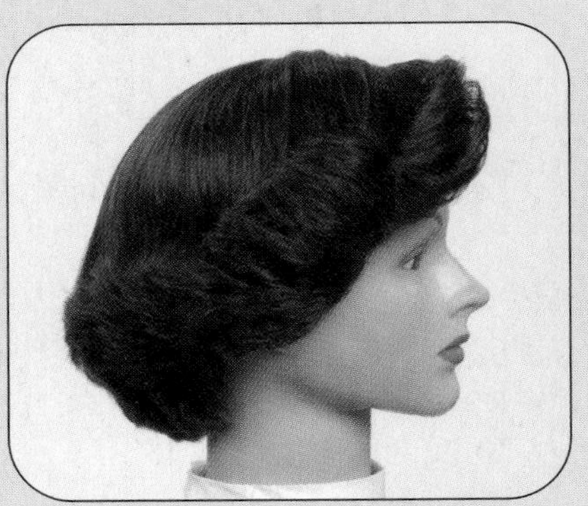

Figure 11–122b

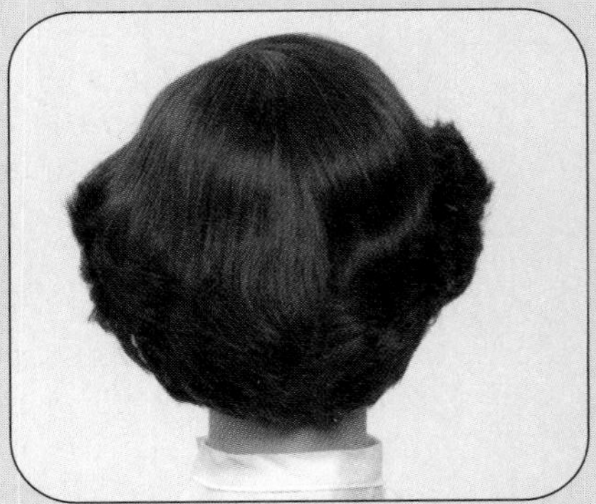

Figure 11–122c

completed!

- In the example in Figure 11–123 and Figure 11–124, you can see a shorter shape that has "rounded" weight. This haircut is created using diagonal partings that connect at the back of the ear. In front of the ear, the diagonal partings point down toward the face. Behind the ear, the diagonal partings point down toward the back. The sides are elevated and overdirected to the back of the ear, producing more length toward the face. The back is cut using a traveling guideline, with each section overdirected to the previous section.

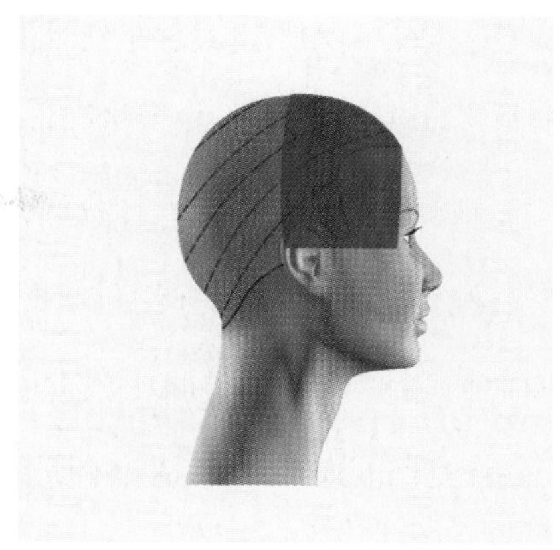

Figure 11–123 Classic (round) graduated cut: design.

Tips for Graduated Haircuts

- Heavier graduated haircuts (those cut with lower elevations) work well on hair that tends to "expand" when dry. Coarse textures and curly hair will appear to graduate more than straight hair. Keep your elevation below 45 degrees when working on these hair types.
- Fine hair responds well to graduation. Because graduation builds weight, you can make thin or fine hair appear thicker and fuller. However, if hair is both fine and thin, avoid creating heavy weight lines. Softer graduation, using diagonal partings, will create a softer weight line. If hair has medium density but is fine in texture, it is safe to elevate more, because there is enough density to support it.
- Check the neckline carefully before cutting the nape short. If the hairline grows straight up, you may want to leave the length longer and the graduation lower, so that it falls below the hairline. You can also blend in a tricky hairline by using the shears-over comb technique, which is explained later in this chapter.
- Always use the fine teeth of the comb and maintain even tension to ensure a precise line.

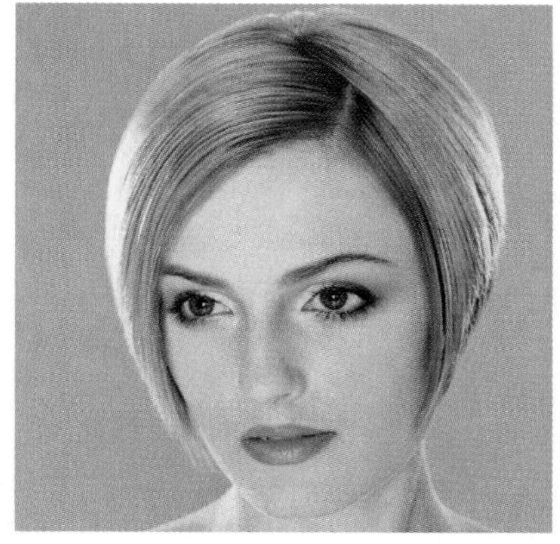

Figure 11–124 Finished classic (round) graduated cut.

The Uniform Layered (90-Degree) Haircut

The third basic haircut is the layered haircut created with **uniform layers**. All the hair is elevated to 90 degrees and cut at the same length. Your guide for this haircut is an interior traveling guideline. An **interior guideline** is inside the haircut rather than on the perimeter. The resulting shape will appear soft and rounded, with no built-up weight or corners. The perimeter of the hair will fall softly, because of the vertical sections on the interior that reduce weight.

Long Layered (180-Degree) Haircut

In this haircut you will use increased layering, which features progressively longer layers. Your guide is an interior guide, beginning at the top of the head. All remaining hair will be elevated up (180 degrees) to match the guide.

Other Examples of Layered Haircuts

There are many variations on the basic layered haircut.

- If you follow the uniform layering technique but cut the hair much shorter, to 1 inch (2.5 cm) or so, you will create a "pixie," "crop," or

PROCEDURE

UNIFORM LAYERED HAIRCUT

Implements and Materials

See list of implements and materials for Procedure 3—blunt haircut.

Preparation

Follow preparation steps for Procedure 3 —blunt haircut.

Procedure

1. To create the guideline, take two partings ½ inch (1.25 cm) apart, creating a section that runs from the front hairline to the bottom of the nape. Comb all other hair out of the way (Figure 11–126).
2. Beginning at the crown, comb the section straight out from the head, keeping your fingers parallel to the head form, and cut to the desired length. Continue working forward to the front hairline, making sure to stand to the side of the client (Figure 11–127 and Figure 11–128).
3. Continue cutting the guideline from the crown to the nape, rounding off any corners as you go along and making sure that your fingers are parallel to the head form (Figure 11–129 and Figure 11–130).

11

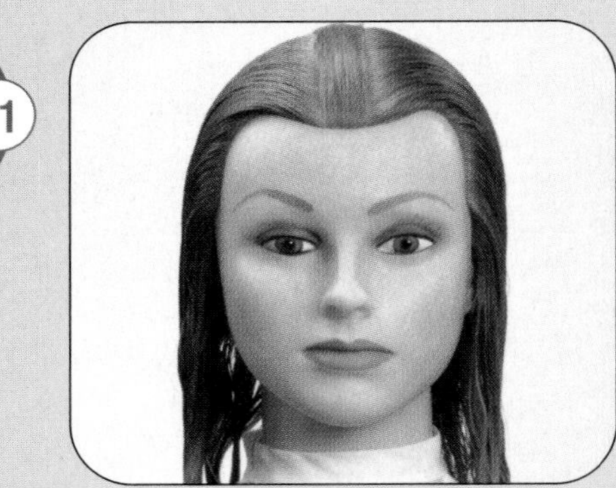

Figure 11-126 Part off guideline section.

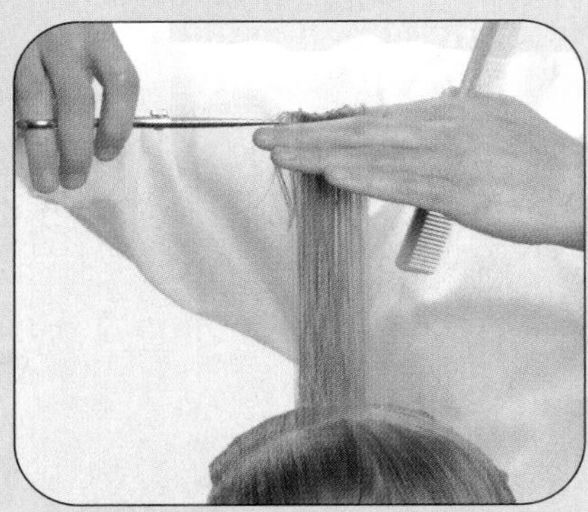

Figure 11-127 Part out first section in the crown and cut.

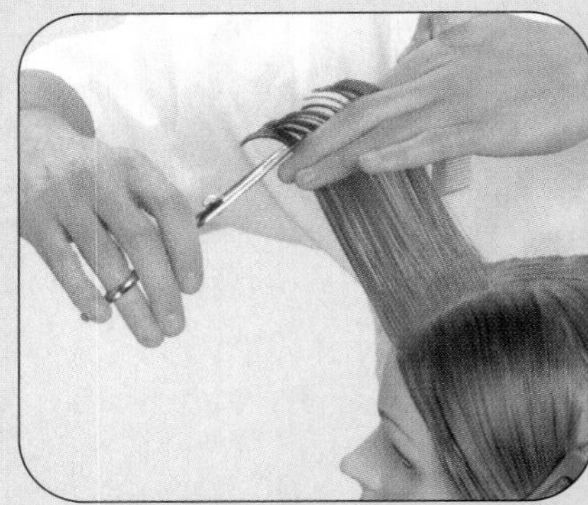

Figure 11-128 Cut front section.

4. To maintain control and consistency while working through the haircut, separate the sides from the back by parting the hair from the apex to the back of the ear. Work through the back areas first. The parting pattern will be wedge-shaped, where each section begins at the same point in the crown and is slightly wider at the bottom of the nape (Figure 11–131a and Figure 11–131b).
5. Work through the right side first. Take a vertical parting that begins at the crown and connects with the guideline, creating a vertical section that ends at the hairline. Keep the sections small to maintain control. Beginning at the crown and using the previously cut guideline, comb the new section to the guide, and elevate the hair straight out from the head, with no overdirection. Cut the line by keeping your fingers parallel to the head and matching the guideline (Figure 11–132).
6. Continue working with a traveling guideline to the back of the ear (Figure 11–133). Repeat on the left side. When working on the left side of the back, shift your body position so that the tips of your shears are pointing down and the fingers holding the section are pointing up. By shifting your hand position, you will be able to control the section. In essence, you are reversing the hand position you used when you cut the right side of the back (Figure 11–134).

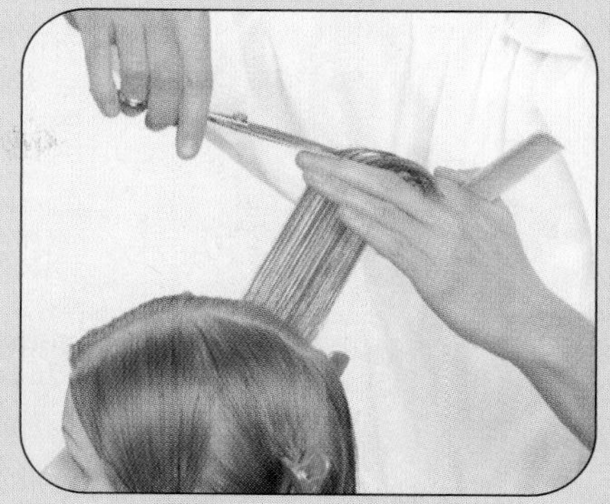

Figure 11–129 Connect crown to back.

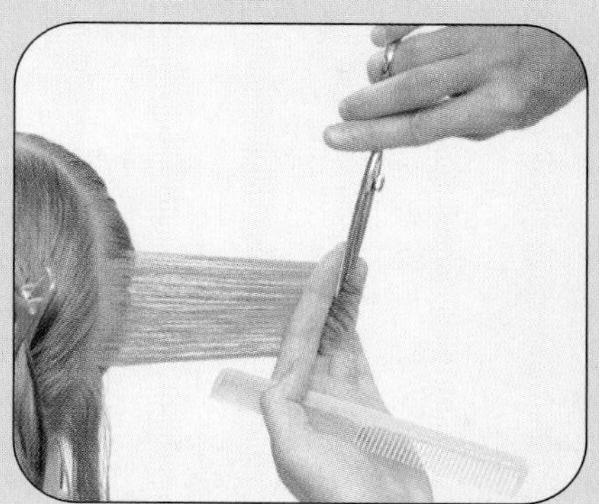

Figure 11–130 Connect back to nape.

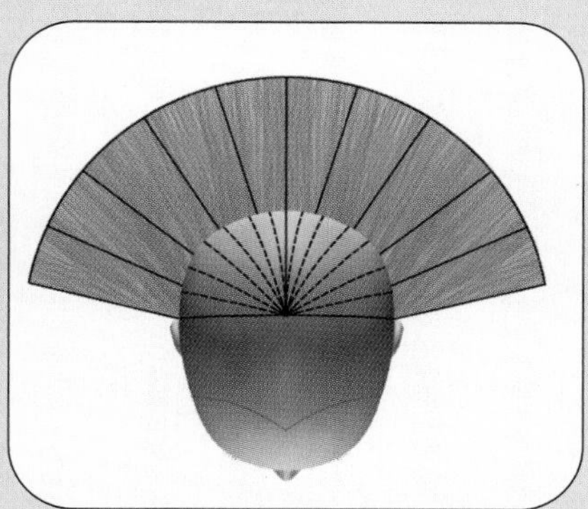

Figure 11–131a Wedge-shaped partings.

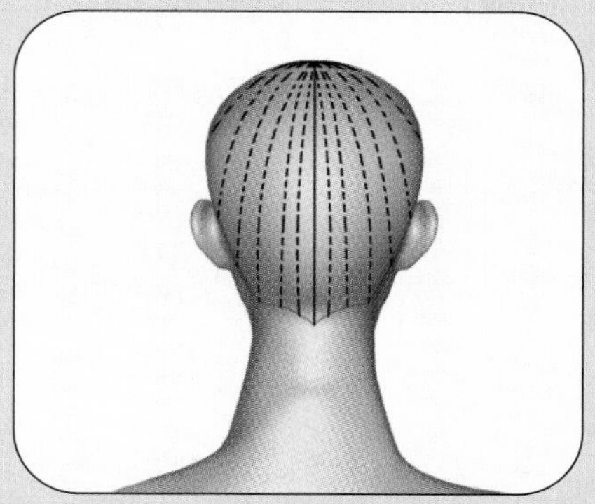

Figure 11–131b Wedge-shaped partings.

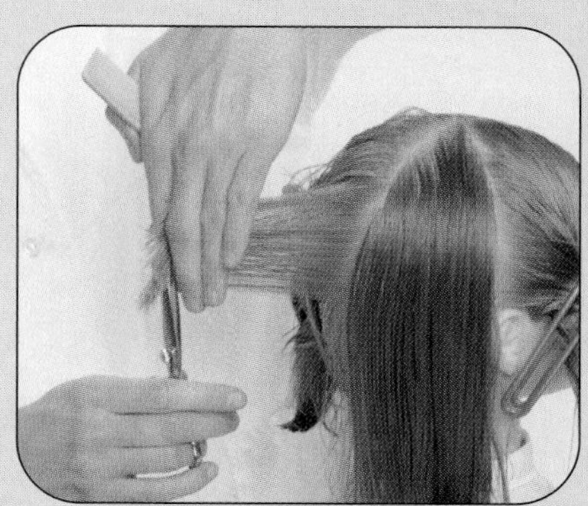

Figure 11–132 Cut second section on right back side.

11

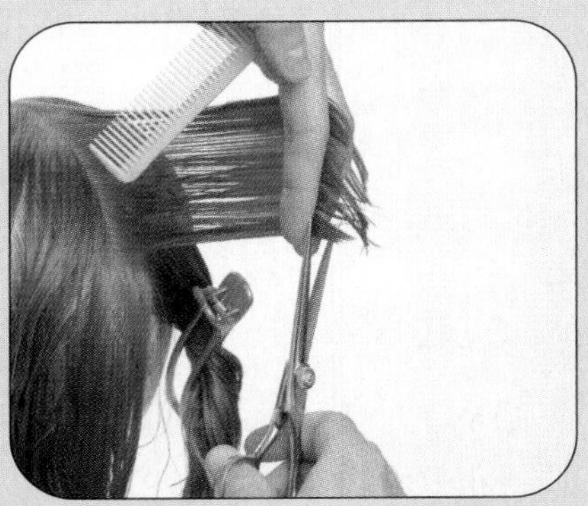

Figure 11–133 Cut section at back of the ear.

7. Cross-check the entire back area. Take horizontal sections and elevate the hair at 90 degrees from the head. As you are checking, you should see a line that runs parallel to the shape of the head (Figure 11–135).
8. Section off the top area by taking a parting that begins at the recession area and ends at the crown, just above the parietal ridge on both sides. Clip the sides out of the way (Figure 11–136).
9. Cut the top area using vertical partings. Using the previously cut center section as a guideline, connect to the crown, holding each section straight up at 90 degrees from the head form. Make sure you do not overdirect the hair (Figure 11–137 and Figure 11–138).
10. Cross-check the top, using horizontal partings and elevating the hair 90 degrees from the head form (Figure 11–139).

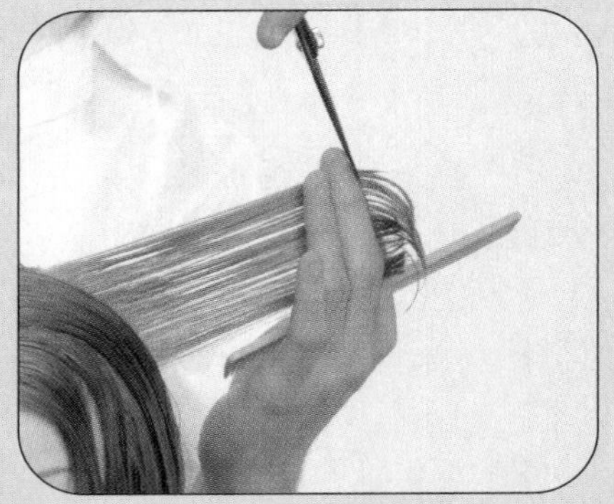

Figure 11–134 Shift hand position.

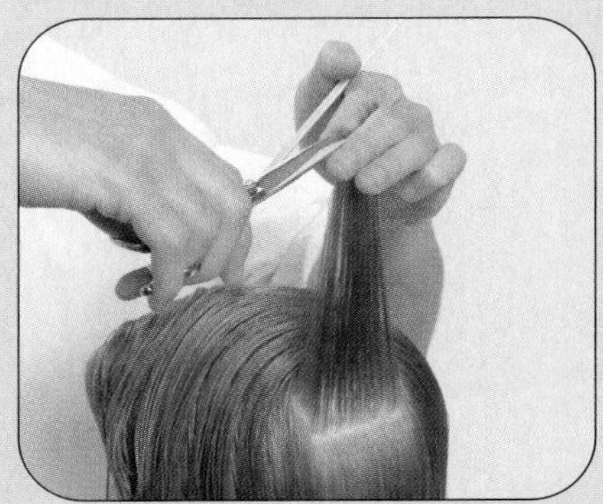

Figure 11–135 Cross-check back area.

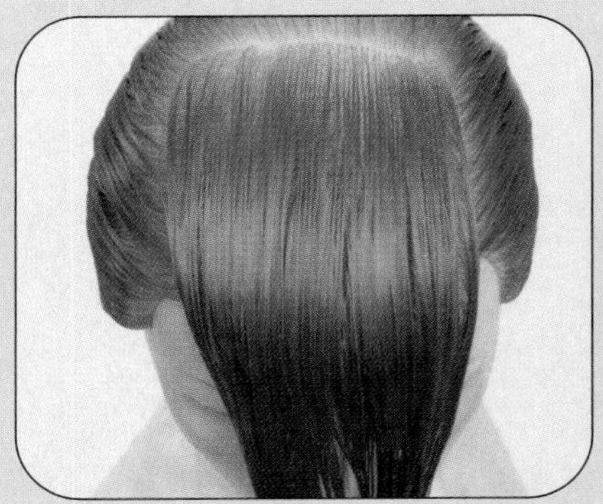

Figure 11–136 Section off the top area.

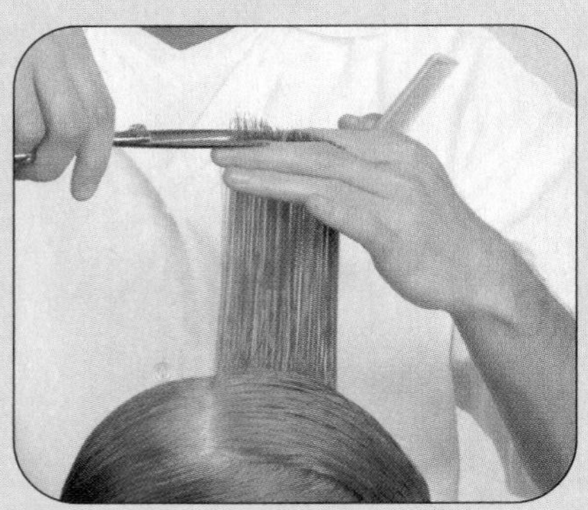

Figure 11–137 Match the first section to the guideline.

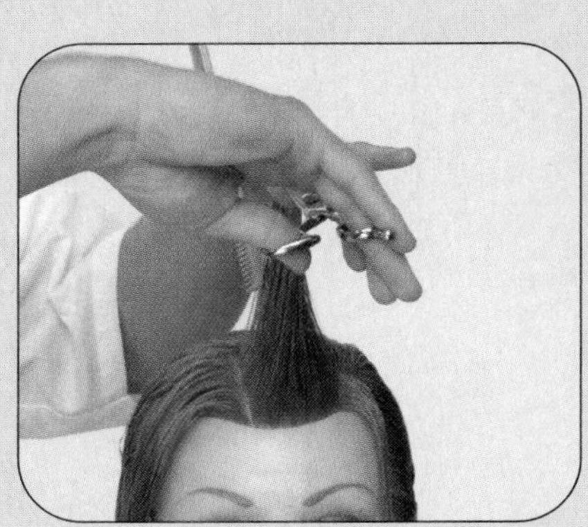

Figure 11–138 Complete last section of top area.

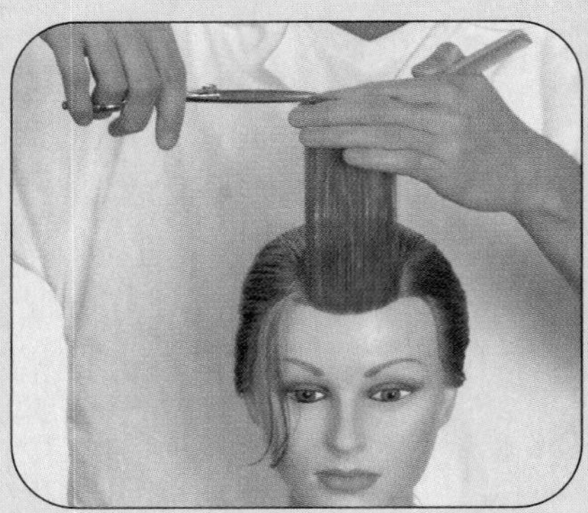

Figure 11–139 Cross-check the top.

11. Now move to the right side. Work from the back of the ear toward the face, using vertical sections, and connect to the previous section at the back of the ear and the top. Comb the hair straight out from the head form at 90 degrees, removing any corners as you go (Figure 11–140 and Figure 11–141). Repeat on the left side, shifting body position so that the tips of your shears are pointing down and the fingers holding the section are pointing up.
12. Cross-check the side sections, using horizontal partings and combing the hair straight out at 90 degrees.
13. Comb the hair down. Notice the soft perimeter and rounded head shape (Figure 11–142).
14. Blow-dry the haircut, using a vent brush to encourage movement, and complete (Figures 11–143a, b, and c).
15. Follow cleanup and sanitation steps in Procedure 3— blunt haircut.

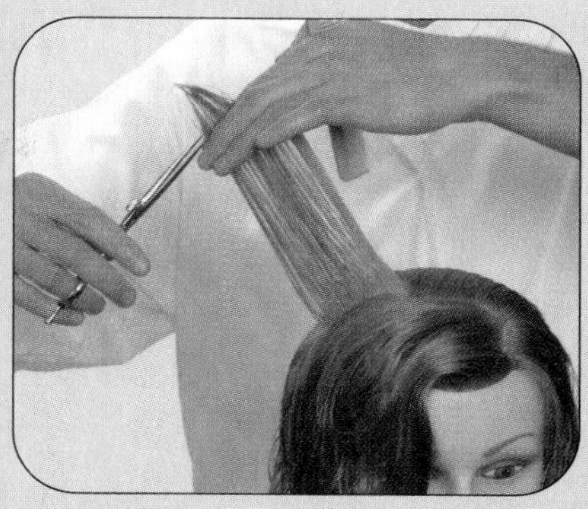

Figure 11–140 Connect at back of ear and top.

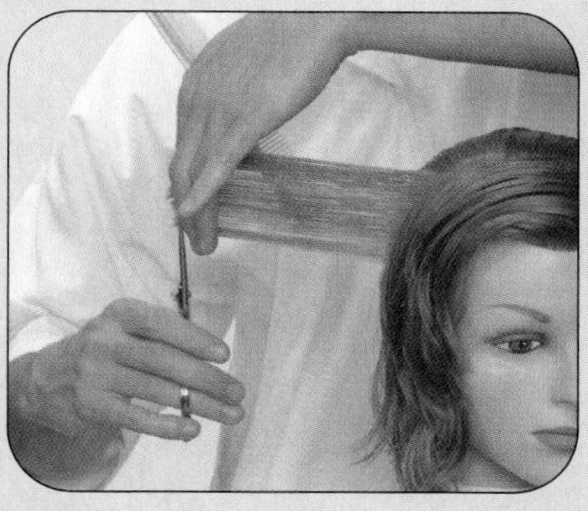

Figure 11–141 Connect lower portion of vertical section.

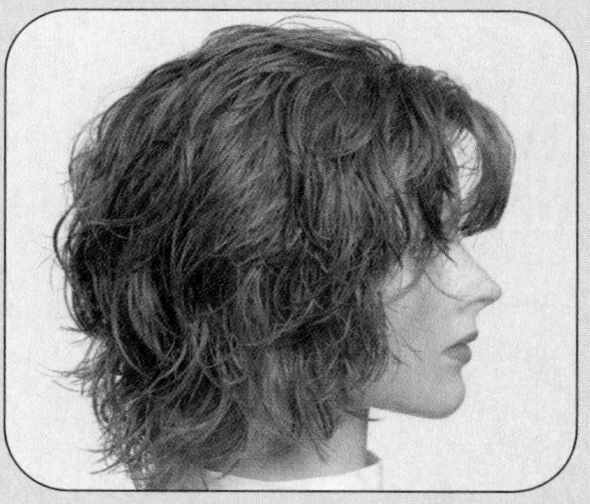

Figure 11–142 Finished haircut, wet profile.

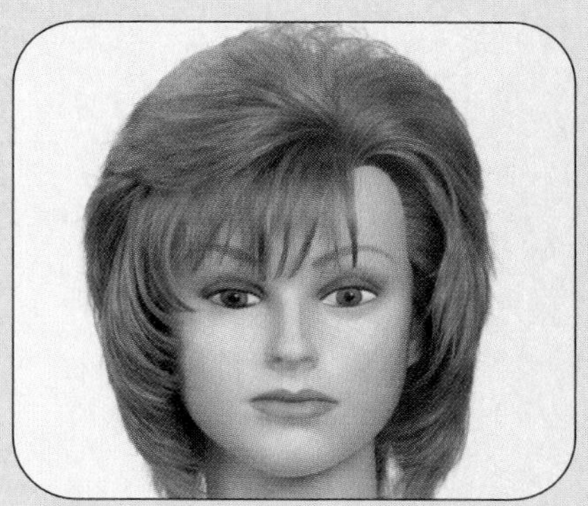

Figure 11–143a Finished uniform-layer haircut.

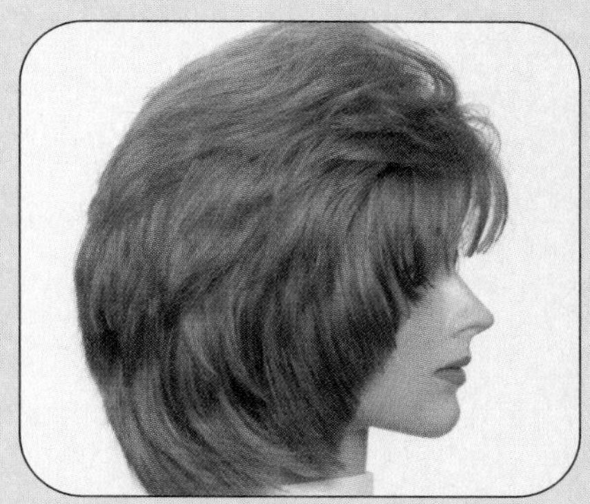

Figure 11–143b

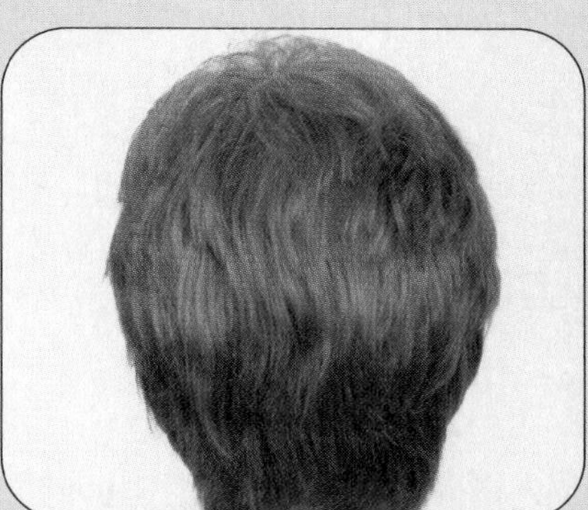

Figure 11–143c

completed!

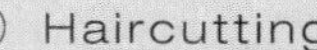

PROCEDURE

LONG LAYERED (180-DEGREE) HAIRCUT

Implements and Materials

See list of implements and materials for Procedure 3—blunt haircut.

Preparation

Follow preparation steps for Procedure 3—blunt haircut.

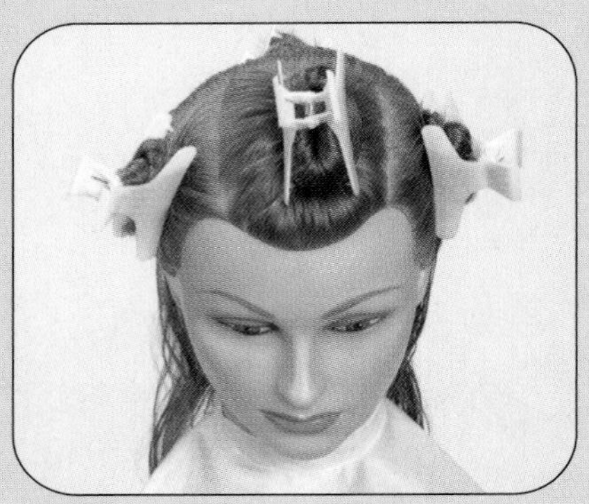

Figure 11-144 Five sections.

Procedure

1. Part the hair into five cutting sections (Figure 11–144).
2. Begin at the top of the crown by taking a ½ inch (1.25 cm) subsection across the head. Comb straight up from the head form and cut straight across (Figure 11–145).
3. Work to the front of the top section by taking a second ½ inch subsection. Direct the first subsection (guideline) to the second one and cut to the same length (Figure 11–146).
4. Continue, using the previously cut subsection as your guideline to cut a new ½-inch subsection throughout the top section (Figure 11–147).

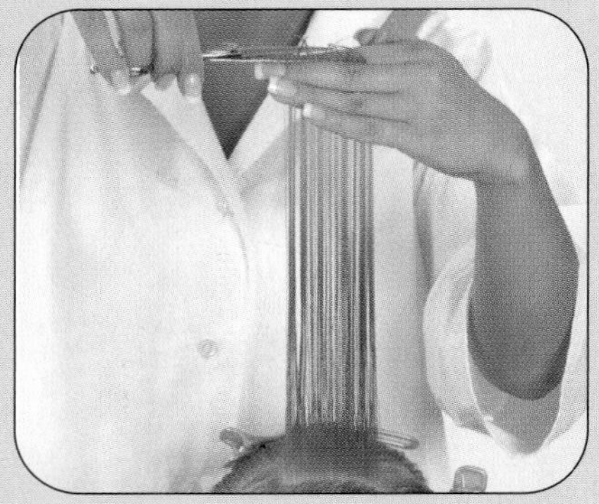

Figure 11-145 Cut the first subsection.

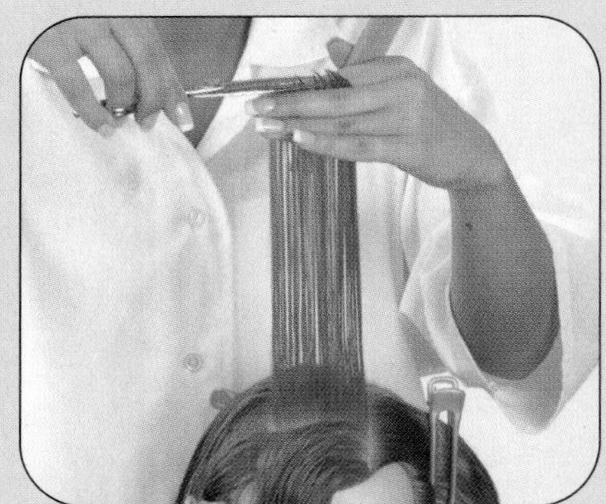

Figure 11-146 Cut the second subsection.

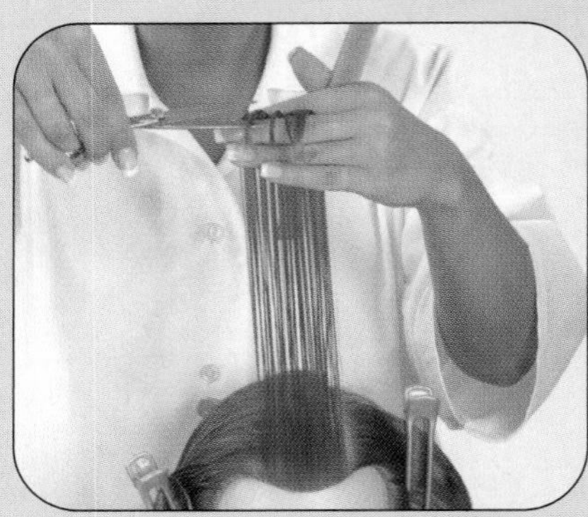

Figure 11-147 Continue cutting through top section.

5. On the left front section, using ½-inch horizontal subsections, comb the hair straight up and match to the previously cut hair (guideline) in the top section (Figure 11–148). Continue working down the side, using ½-inch subsections until the hair no longer reaches the guide.
6. Repeat on the right side (Figure 11–149).
7. At the top of the left rear section, using ½-inch horizontal subsections, comb the hair straight up from the head form, matching the length to the top section (guideline) and cut straight across (Figure 11–150).
8. Continue, using ½-inch horizontal subsections and working from top to bottom until the hair no longer reaches the guideline.
9. Repeat on the right side until the hair no longer reaches the guideline (Figure 11–151).
10. Blow-dry the hair (Figures 11–152a, b, and c).

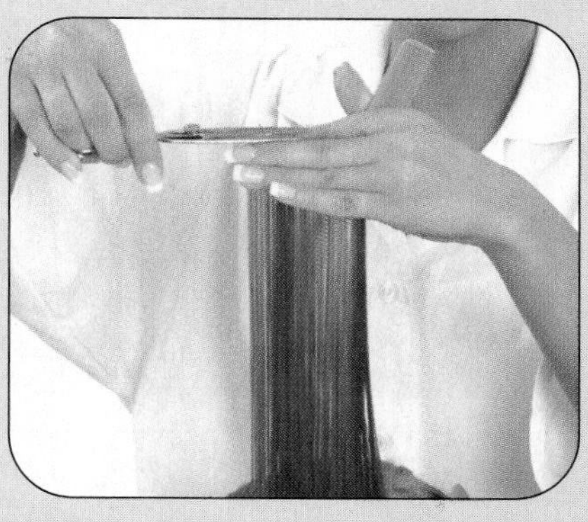

Figure 11-148 Match hair to guideline and cut.

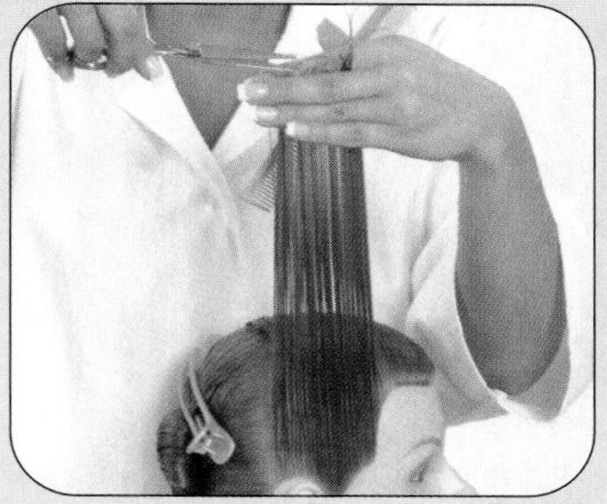

Figure 11-149 Repeat on the right side.

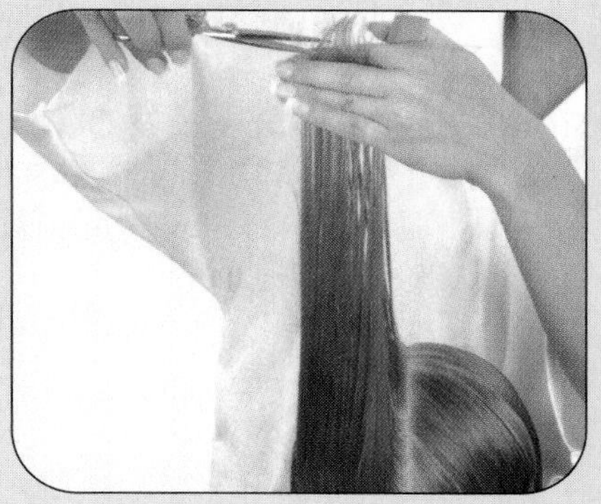

Figure 11-150 Cut left rear section.

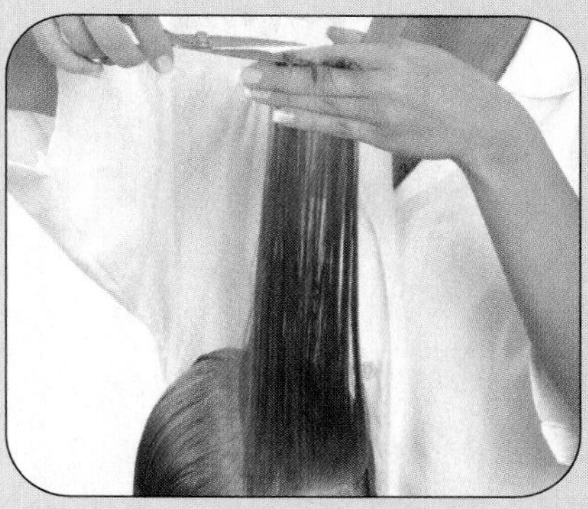

Figure 11-151 Work down the rear section.

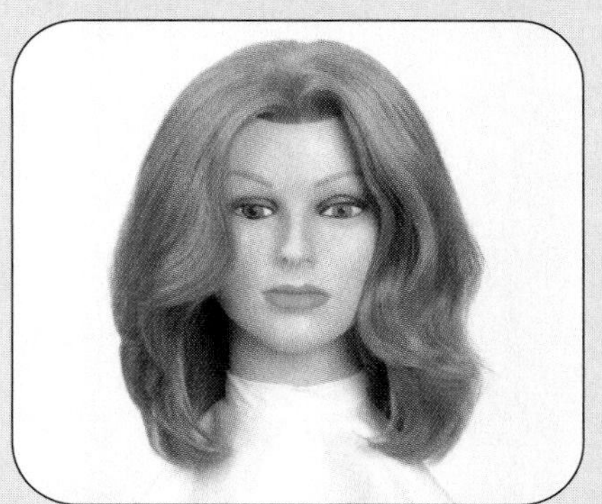

Figure 11-152a Finished long-layered haircut.

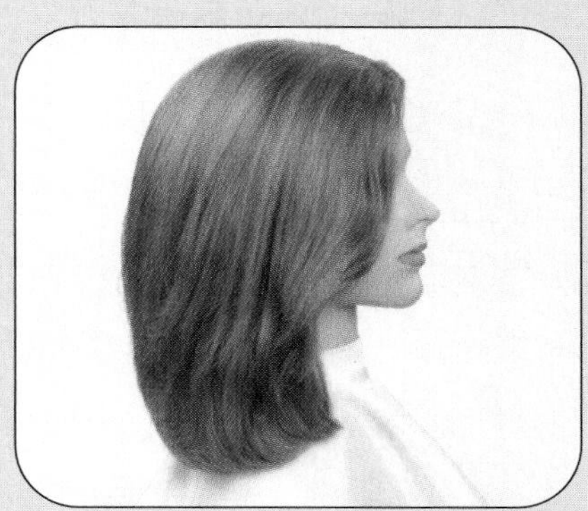

Figure 11-152b

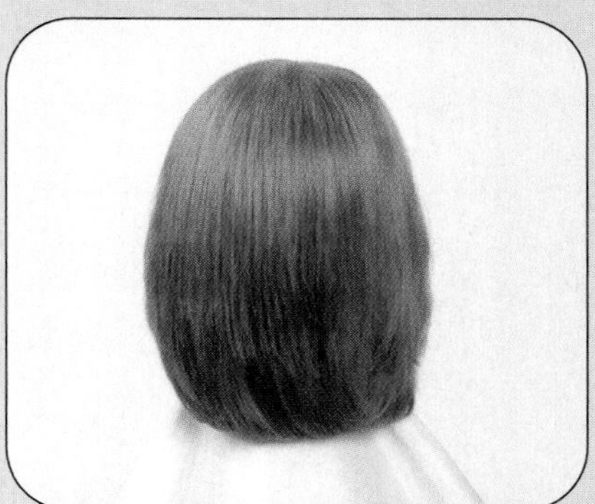

Figure 11-152c

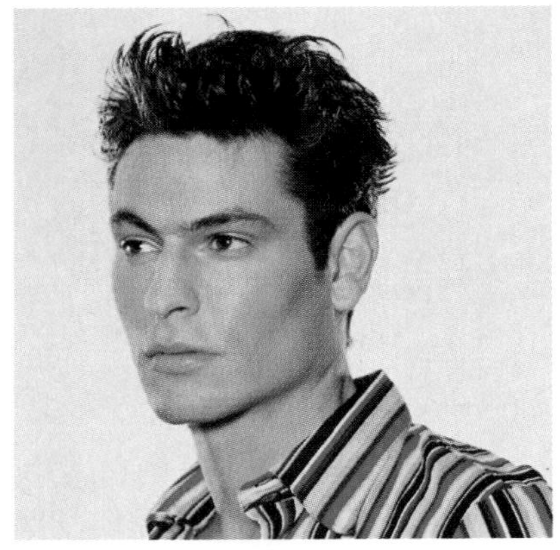

Figure 11-153 Short crop, men's cut.

"Caesar" haircut. This hairstyle is flattering on both men and women (Figure 11–153).

- If you follow the same method but keep the "corners" by keeping your fingers vertical and not following the head form, you can create a square shape, which is common in a man's basic haircut (Figure 11–154 and Figure 11–155).
- You can create a layered haircut with longer perimeter lengths, otherwise known as a "shag," by cutting the top area the same as for uniform layers and then elevating the side and back sections straight up (180 degrees), blending them into the top lengths (Figure 11–156 and Figure 11–157).

Tips for Layered Haircuts

- Cut the interior first. Then you can then go back to the perimeter edges and cut stronger lines, cut out around the ears, or texturize where needed.
- When layering hair short, you will achieve the best results on medium to thicker densities. Cutting thin hair too short can expose the scalp.
- Coarse hair tends to stick out if cut shorter than 3 inches. This hair texture needs the extra length to hold it down.
- When working on longer layered shapes in which you want to maintain thickness at the bottom, remember to keep the top sections longer. Cutting the top layers too short will take too much hair away from the rest of the haircut, and may leave you with a collapsed shape that is stringy at the bottom.
- If the client has long hair, past the shoulder blades, use slide cutting (explained later in this chapter) to connect the top sections to the lengths. This will maintain maximum length and weight at the perimeter of the haircut. 5

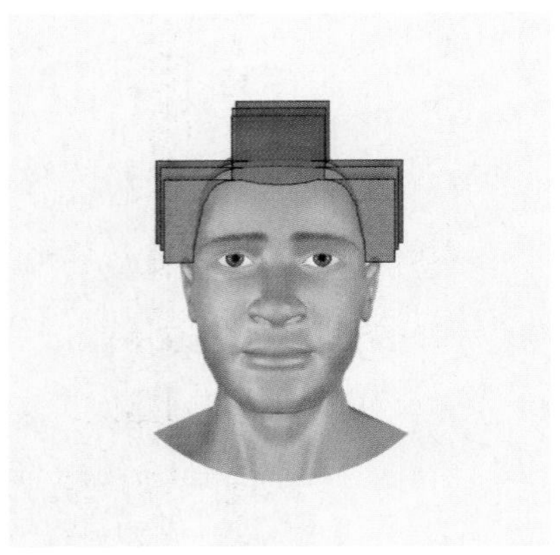

Figure 11-154 Basic men's haircut design.

11

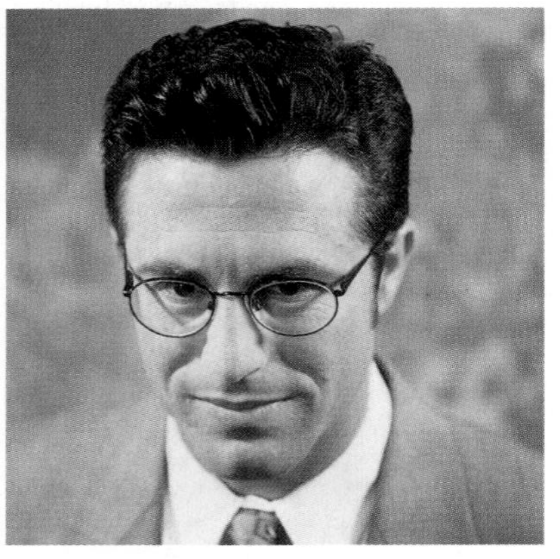

Figure 11-155 Basic men's haircut.

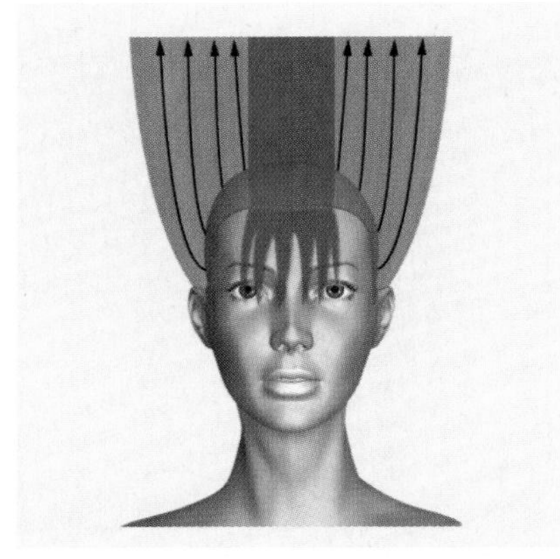

Figure 11-156 Long shag design.

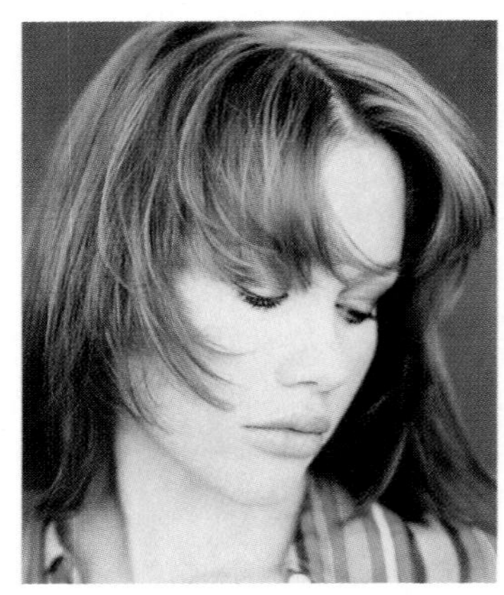

Figure 11-157 Long shag haircut.

CUTTING CURLY HAIR

Curly hair can be a challenge to cut. Once you gain enough confidence, it can be a lot of fun to work with. However, it is essential to understand how curly hair behaves after it has been cut and dried. Although you can apply any cutting technique to curly hair, you will get very different results with each one than you get when cutting straight hair. Curl patterns can range from slightly wavy to extremely curly, and curly-haired clients may have fine, medium, or coarse textures, with density ranging from thin to thick.

Tips for Cutting Curly Hair

- Curly hair shrinks much more after it dries than straight hair. The curlier the hair, the more it will shrink. For every 1/4 inch (.6 cm) you cut when the hair is wet, it will shrink up to 1 inch (2.5 cm) when dry. Always keep this in mind when consulting with your client.
- Use minimal tension and/or the wide teeth of your comb. If you use a lot of tension when cutting curly hair, you will be stretching the wet hair even more, and the hair will shrink that much more when it dries.
- Curly hair naturally "graduates" itself. If the shape you want to create has strong angles, you need to elevate less than when working with straight hair.
- Curly hair expands more than straight hair. This means that you will generally need to leave lengths longer, which ultimately helps weigh the hair down and keeps the shape from shrinking or ending up too short.
- In general, a razor should not be used on curly hair. Doing so can weaken the cuticle and cause the hair to frizz.
- Choose your texturizing techniques carefully. Avoid using the razor, and work mostly with point cutting and freehand notching to remove bulk and weight. (These techniques are discussed later in this chapter.)

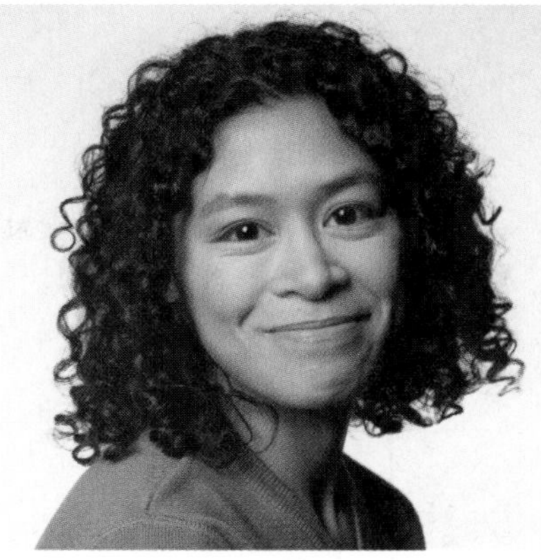

Figure 11-158 Blunt cut on curly hair.

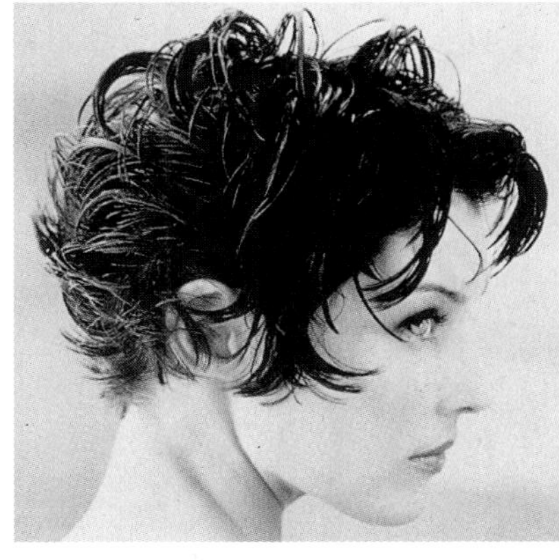

Figure 11-159 Graduated cut on curly hair.

Examples of Basic Haircuts on Curly Hair

Let us take a look at some of the basic haircuts and how they work on curly hair. In Figure 11–158, notice how the hair appears stacked, even though it was cut with a blunt technique. Although the hair was not elevated, it appears graduated. Notice how the volume in the graduated haircut (Figure 11–159) is above the ears. The hair shrinks as it dries, resulting in a weight line that has graduated itself even higher. In the next example (Figure 11–160), notice the round shape. This is a uniform-layered cut on curly hair and was cut the same way as it was in Figure 11–143.

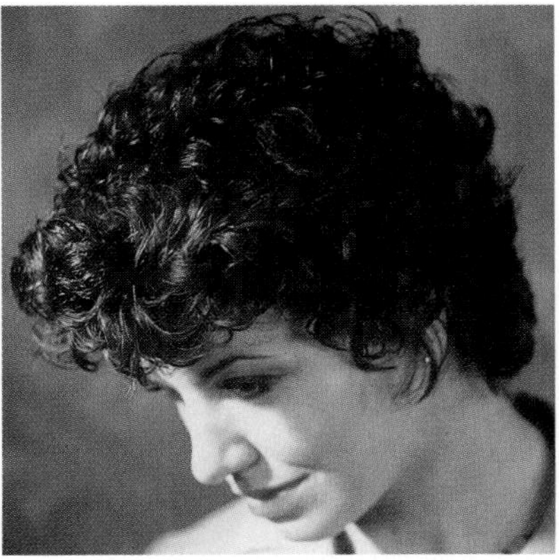

Figure 11-160 Uniform layered cut on curly hair.

OTHER CUTTING TECHNIQUES

Besides the basic haircuts, there are many techniques you can use to create different effects in the behavior and appearance of the hair. You can make

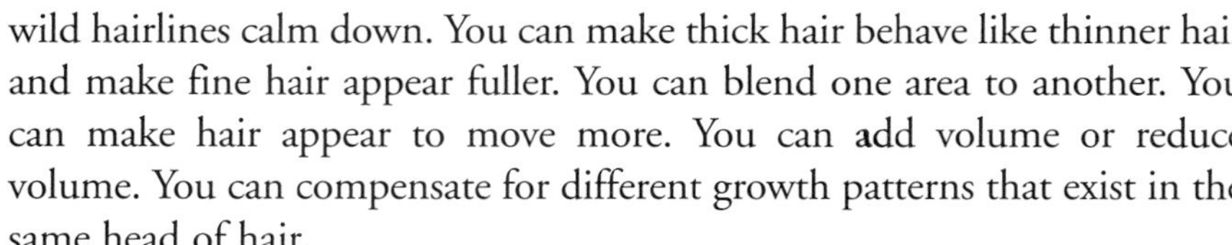

wild hairlines calm down. You can make thick hair behave like thinner hair and make fine hair appear fuller. You can blend one area to another. You can make hair appear to move more. You can add volume or reduce volume. You can compensate for different growth patterns that exist in the same head of hair.

Figure 11-161 Fringe area.

Cutting the Fringe (Bangs)

Because much of our haircutting history comes from England, you will often hear the word "fringe" used instead of "bangs." The two words mean essentially the same thing. The fringe area is the hair that lies between the two front corners, or approximately between the outer corners of the eyes (Figure 11–161). See Figure 11-8.

It is important to work with the natural **distribution** (where and how hair is moved over the head) when locating the fringe area. Every head is different, and you need to make sure that you cut only the hair that falls in that area. Otherwise, you can end up with short pieces falling where they don't belong, which will ruin the haircut. When creating bangs, you do not always cut all the hair in this area, but you never cut more unless you are blending to the sides or the top.

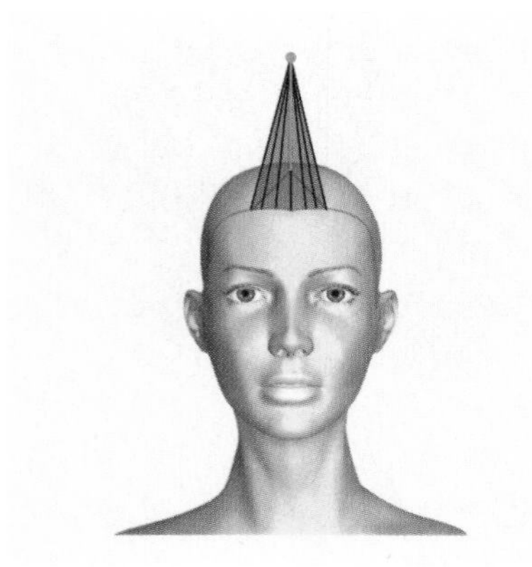

Figure 11-162 Layered fringe design.

Let us have a look at some different types of fringes.

- In Figure 11–162 and Figure 11–163, the fringe is cut using a stationary guide, elevating at 90 degrees straight up from the head form.
- Short bangs make a strong statement. In Figure 11–164 and Figure 11–165, they are combined with a shorter layered haircut. Notice that the line is curved. It has been cut with low elevation, so that it remains more solid-looking and not too heavy.
- In Figure 11–166 and Figure 11–167, the fringe is very long and was cut with the slide cutting technique to create a wispy effect.
- Sometimes, only a few pieces are cut in the fringe area. This keeps the hair out of the face. In this case, you will not be cutting all the hair in the fringe

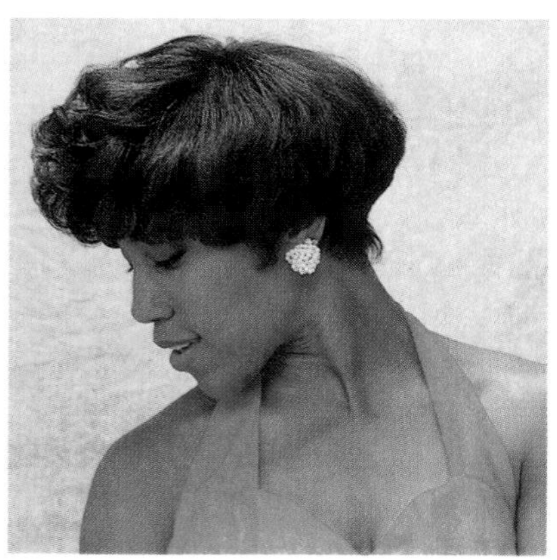

Figure 11-163 Layered fringe cut.

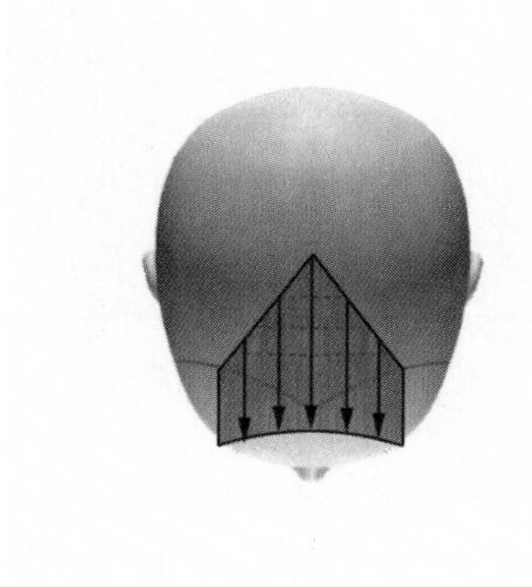

Figure 11-164 Short, curved fringe design.

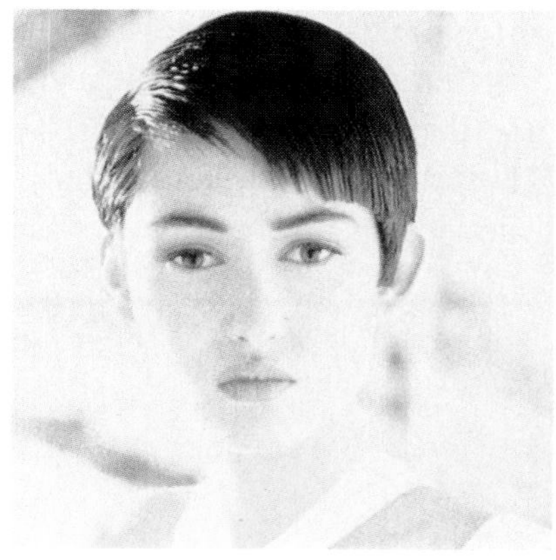

Figure 11-165 Short, curved fringe cut.

area. You will cut only a small portion of this area and might even use a razor for that purpose (Figure 11–168 and Figure 11–169).

Depending on the haircut, a fringe can be blended or not. If you are working with a blunt haircut and the fringe is one length, you usually will not need to blend it in. If you are working with layered or graduated shapes, you may want to blend the length of the fringe into the sides and/or the top (Figure 11–170 and Figure 11–171).

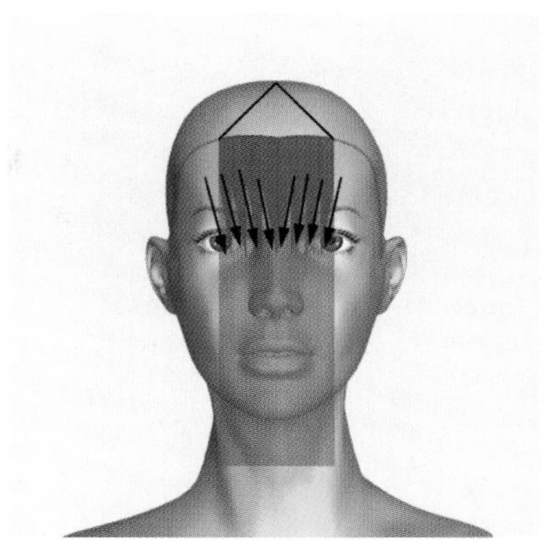

Figure 11-166 Long fringe design.

Razor Cutting

Razor cutting provides an entirely different kind of result from other haircutting procedures. In general, razor cuts lend a softer appearance than shear cuts. The razor is an excellent choice when working with medium to fine hair textures. The entire haircut moves and blends more. When you work with shears, you usually cut the ends of the hair blunt. When you work with the razor, however, the ends are cut at an angle and the line is not blunt, which produces softer shapes with more visible separation, or a "feathered"

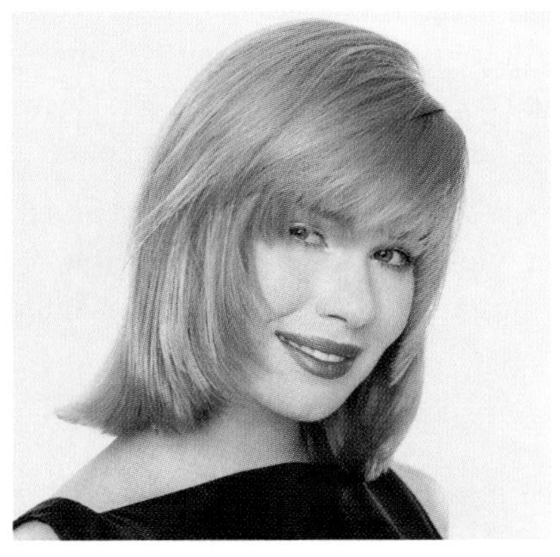

Figure 11-167 Long fringe cut.

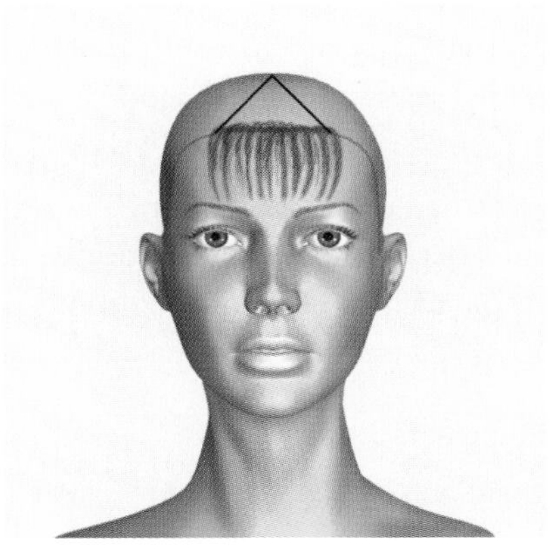

Figure 11-168 Wispy fringe design.

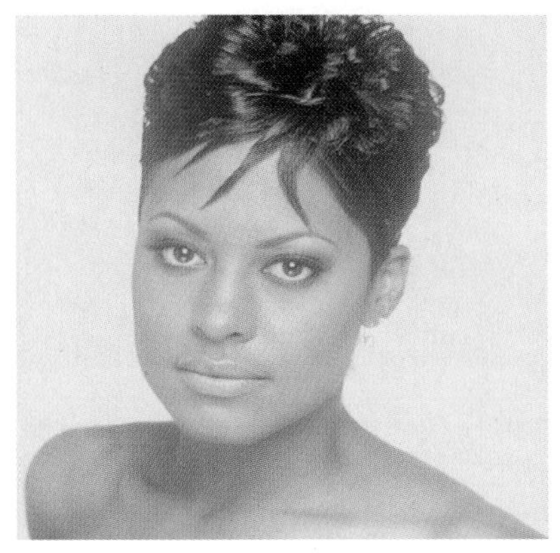

Figure 11-169 Wispy fringe cut.

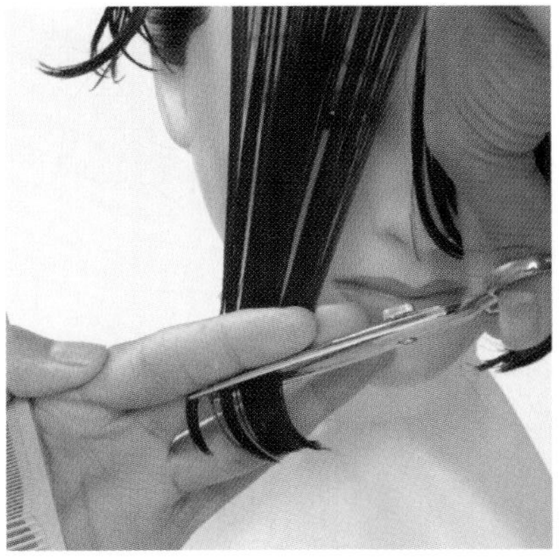

Figure 11-170 Blend fringe to sides.

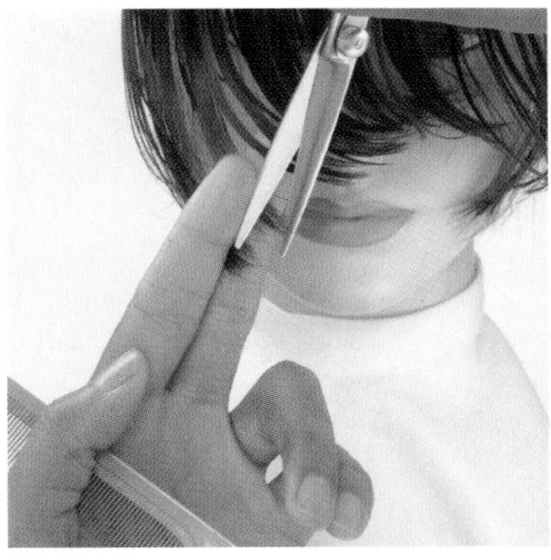

Figure 11-171 Blend fringe to layered top.

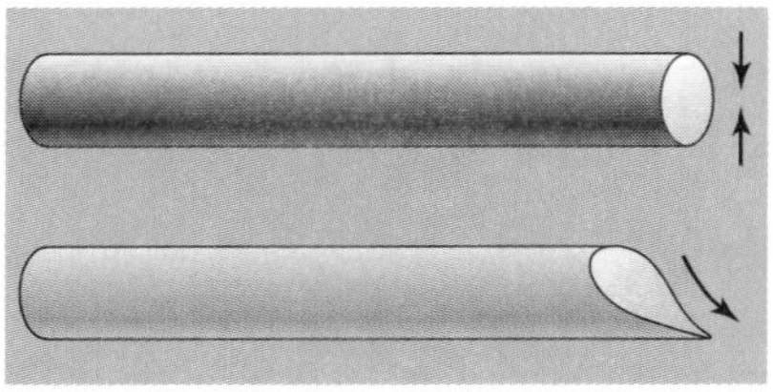

Figure 11-172 Razor-cut and shears-cut strands.

effect, on the ends. With the razor, there is only one blade cutting the hair, and it is a much finer blade than the shears. With the shears, there are two blades that close on the hair, creating blunt ends (Figure 11–172).

Any haircut you can create with shears can also be done with the razor. You will be able to cut horizontal, vertical, and diagonal lines. The main difference is that the guide is above your fingers, whereas with shears the guide is usually below your fingers. Razor cutting is an entirely different experience from cutting with shears. The best way to get comfortable with the razor is to practice, practice, practice. Before cutting with a razor, review how to properly hold the razor in the "Tools, Safety, and Body Position" section of this chapter.

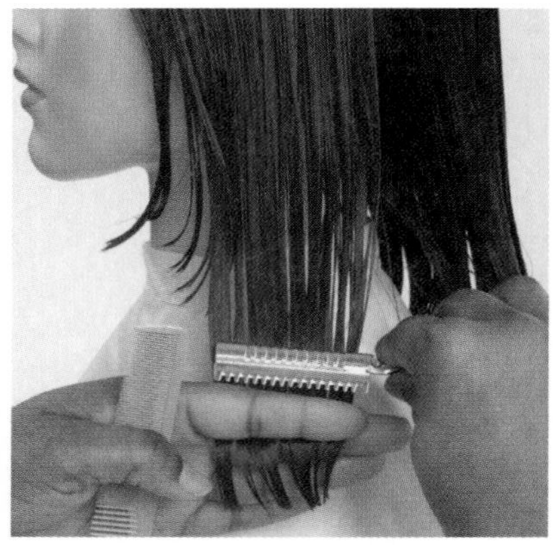

Figure 11-173 Razor cutting parallel to subsection.

There are two commonly used methods for cutting with a razor. In the first method, the razor is kept more parallel to the subsection (Figure 11–173). This technique is mainly used to thin the ends of the hair, and the entire length of the blade is used. The other approach is to come into the subsection with the blade at an angle (about 45 degrees). Here you are using about one-third of the blade to make small strokes as you work through the subsection (Figure 11–174). If the blade is not entering the hair at an angle and you attempt to "push" the razor through the hair, you will be putting added stress on the hair, and you risk losing control (Figure 11–175). Always remember that the blade needs to be at an angle when entering the hair.

When cutting a section, you usually move from top to bottom or side to side, depending on the section and finger angle. Here are some examples of razor techniques and hand positions on a vertical subsection (Figure 11–176) and a horizontal subsection (Figure 11–177).

Razor Cutting Tips

- Always check with your instructor before performing a razor cut. Make sure that the hair is in good condition. Never use a razor on curly hair, coarse wiry hair, or overprocessed, damaged hair.

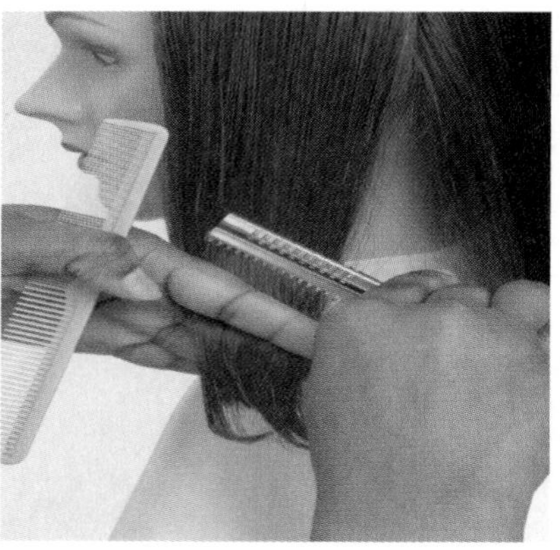

Figure 11-174 Razor cutting at a 45-degree angle.

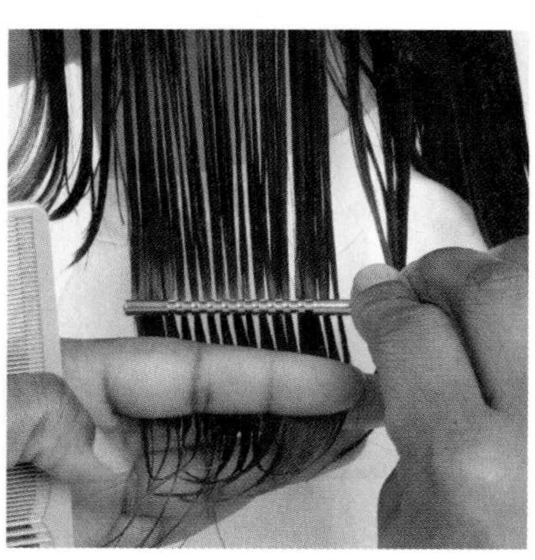

Figure 11-175 Incorrect razor angle.

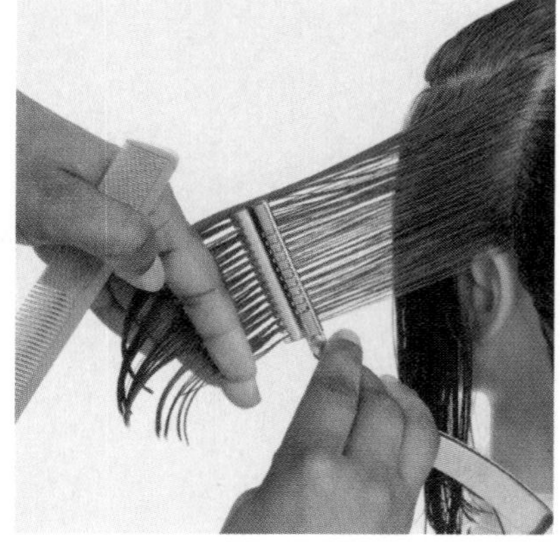

Figure 11-176 Hand position on vertical section.

- Always use a guard.
- Always use a new blade. Working with a dull blade is painful for the client and puts added stress on the hair. Discard used blades in a puncture-proof container.
- Keep the hair wet. Cutting dry hair with a razor can make the hair frizz and can be painful for the client.
- Always work with the razor at an angle. Never force the razor through the hair.

Slide Cutting

Slide cutting is a method of cutting or thinning the hair in which the fingers and shears glide along the edge of the hair to remove length. It is useful for removing length, blending shorter lengths to longer lengths, and texturizing. Slide cutting is a perfect way to layer very long hair and keep weight at the perimeter. Rather than opening and closing the shears, you keep them partially open as you "slide" along the edge of the section. This technique should only be performed on wet hair with razor-sharp shears.

There are two methods of holding the subsection when slide cutting. It is important to visualize the line you wish to cut before you begin (Figure 11–178). In one method, you hold the subsection with tension beyond the cutting line (Figure 11–179). In the other method, you place your shears on top of your knuckles, then use both hands to move simultaneously out to the length.

Shears-over-Comb

Shears-over-comb (also called scissors-over-comb) is a barbering technique that has crossed over into cosmetology. In this technique, you hold the hair in place with the comb while you use the tips of the shears to remove the lengths. Shears-over-comb is used to create very short tapers and allows you to cut from an extremely short length to longer lengths. In most cases, you start at the hairline and work your way up to the longer lengths.

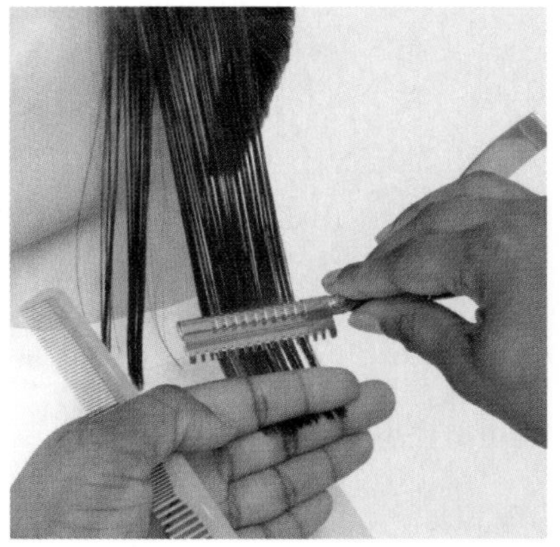

Figure 11–177 Hand position on horizontal section.

CAUTION

Always check with your instructor to see if the hair type you are working on is suitable for the razor. Coarse, wiry hair, curly hair, or damaged hair is not suitable for razor cuts. The razor may tend to make these hair types frizzier. Fine and medium hair textures in good condition are suitable for razor cuts.

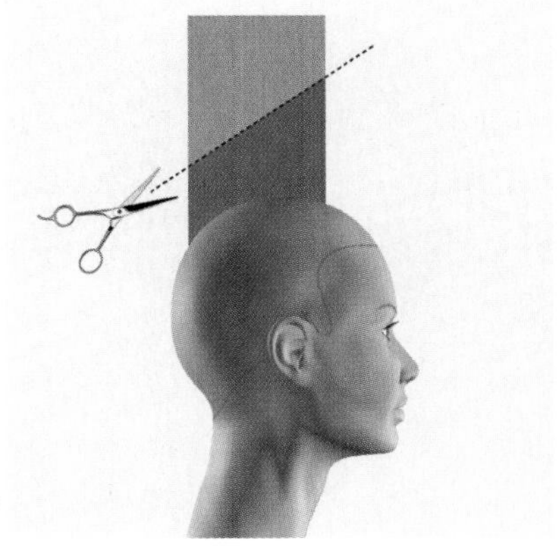

Figure 11–178 Visualize your cutting line first.

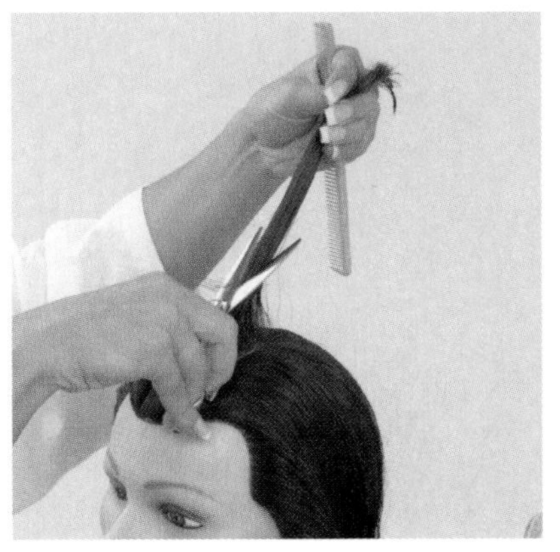

Figure 11–179 Slide cutting.

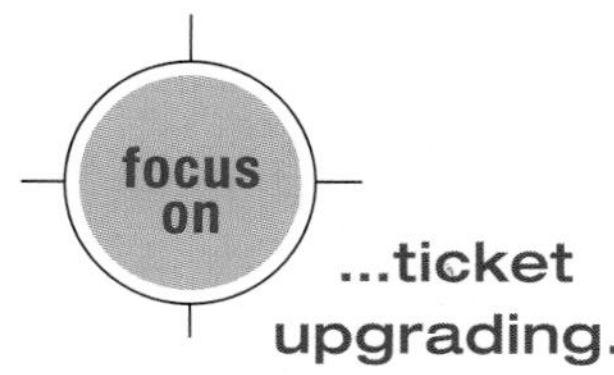

Figure 11-180 Shears-over-comb technique.

It is best to use this technique on dry hair, because that way you can see exactly how much hair you are cutting and will therefore maintain control. Lift (elevate) the hair away from the head using the comb, and allow the comb to act as your guide. Do not hold the hair between your fingers. Let the shears and comb move simultaneously up the head. It is crucial that one blade stays still and remains parallel to the spine of the comb as you move the thumb blade to close the shears. Strive for continual motion. Stopping the motion may cause "steps" or visible weight lines in the hair. Practice moving the comb and shears simultaneously, keeping the bottom blade still and opening and closing the shears with your thumb (Figure 11–180).

These are the basic steps when working with the shears-over-comb technique.

1. Stand directly in front of the section on which you are working. The area you are cutting should be at eye level.
2. Place the comb, teeth first, into the hairline, and turn the comb so that the teeth are angled away from the head (Figure 11–181).
3. With the still blade parallel to the spine of the comb, begin moving the comb up the head, continually opening and closing the thumb blade smoothly and quickly.
4. Angle the comb farther away from the head as you reach the area you are blending to avoid cutting into the length (weight) (Figure 11–182).

focus on ...ticket upgrading.

What is ticket upgrading? Suppose that, in addition to her haircut, your client wants highlights, but color is not your specialty. If you refer the client to the color specialist in the salon, you have increased her total ticket. This is called ticket upgrading, or upselling, and means greater profits for the salon as well as increased income for you when other stylists return the favor.

Shears-over-Comb Tips

- Work with small areas at a time (no wider than the blade).
- Always start at the hairline and work up toward the length. You may even run the comb again through a previously cut section, on your way up to the new area.
- Cross-check by working across the area diagonally.
- Use a barber comb to cut areas very close (usually on sideburns and hairlines where the hair is cut close to the scalp). Switch to a regular cutting comb as you work up into the longer lengths.

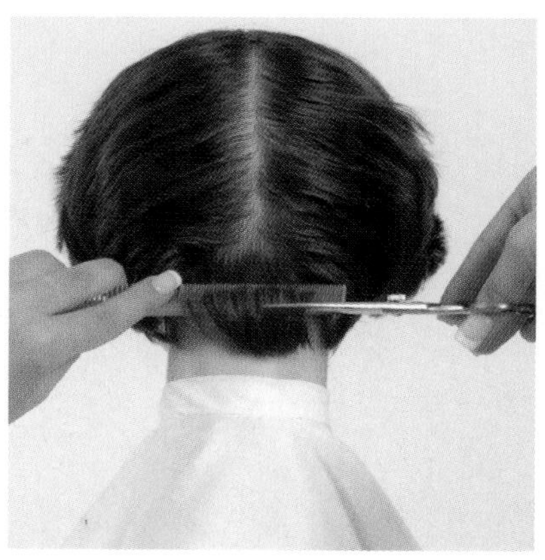

Figure 11-181 Comb position.

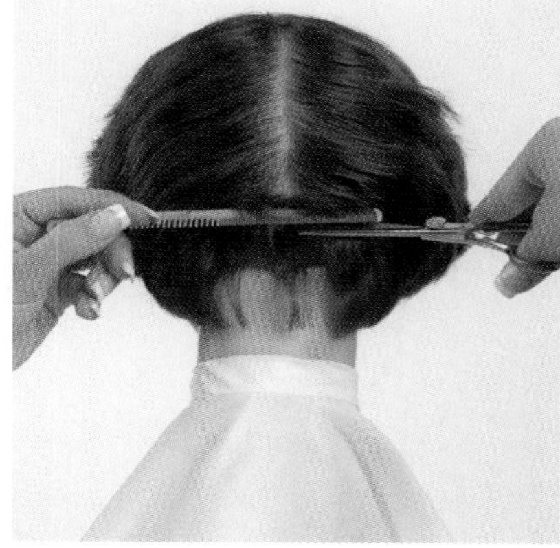

Figure 11-182 Reaching the weight line.

Texturizing

Texturizing is a commonly used technique within the professional hair industry. Today's haircuts generally require some form of texturizing. **Texturizing** is the process of removing excess bulk without shortening the length. It also means to cut for effect within the hair length, causing wispy or spiky effects. The term "texturize" should not be confused with hair texture, which is simply the diameter of the hair strand itself.

Texturizing techniques can be used to add volume, remove volume, make hair "move," and blend one area into another. It can also be used to compensate for different densities that exist within the same head of hair. Texturizing can be done with cutting shears, thinning shears, or a razor. There are many texturizing techniques, and a number of them will be explained in this section. Be sure to practice all the techniques, so that you learn the different effects they create and draw on them as the need arises with your clients.

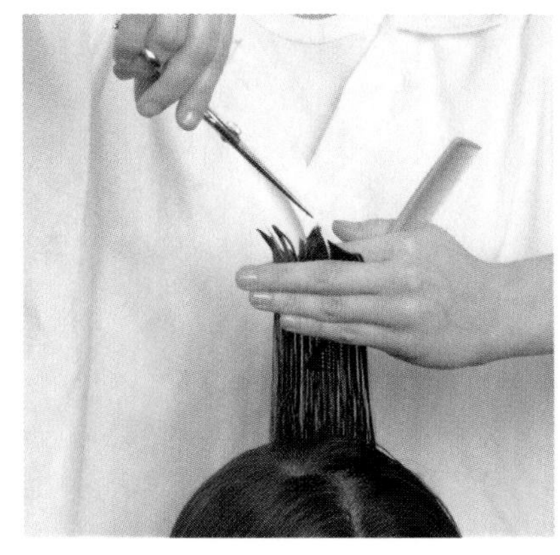

Figure 11–183 Point cutting.

Texturizing with Shears

- **Point cutting** is a technique performed on the ends of the hair using the tips, or points, of the shears. This can be done on wet or dry hair. It is very easy to do on dry hair because the hair stands up and away from your fingers. Hold the hair 1 to 2 inches (2.5 to 5 cm) from the ends. Turn your wrist so that the tips of the shears are pointing into the ends, with your palm facing away from you. Open and close the shears by moving your thumb as you work across the section. As you close the shears, move them away from your fingers to avoid cutting yourself. Move them back in toward your fingers as you open them (Figure 11–183). In essence, you are cutting "points" in the hair. A more vertical shears angle removes less hair (Figure 11–184). The more diagonal the shears angle, the more hair is taken away, and the chunkier the effect (Figure 11–185).
- **Notching** is another version of point cutting. Notching is more aggressive and creates a chunkier effect. Notching is done toward the ends. Hold the section about 3 inches (7.5 cm) from the ends. Place the tips of your shears about 2 inches (5 cm) from the ends. Close your shears as you quickly move them out toward the ends. If you are working on very thick hair, you can repeat the motion every 1/8 inch (.3 cm). On medium to fine

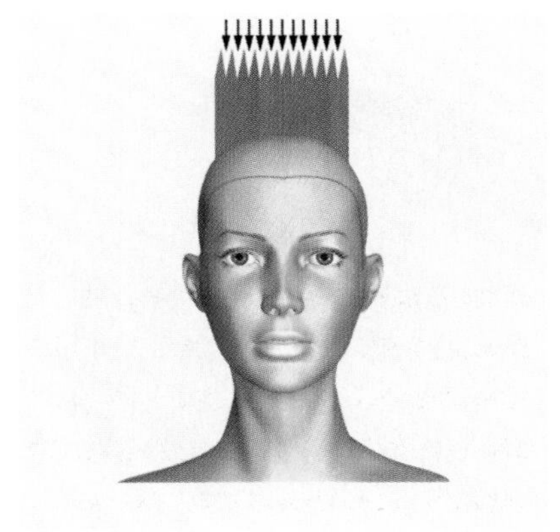

Figure 11–184 Point cutting with steeper shears angle.

11

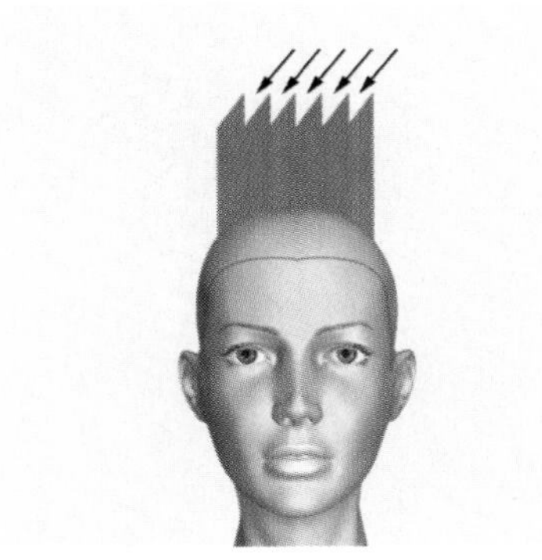

Figure 11–185 Point cutting with flatter shears angle.

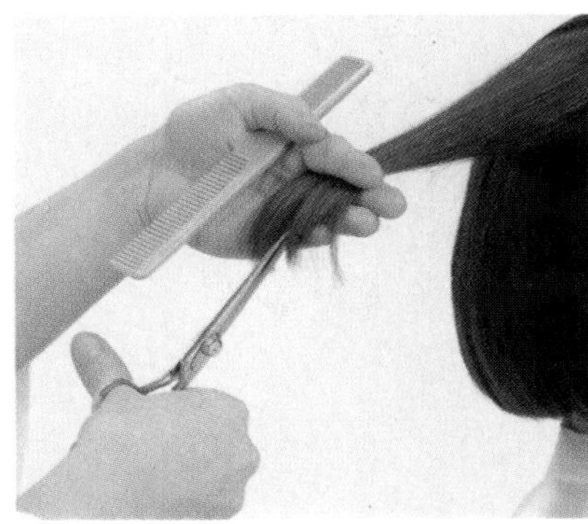

Figure 11–186 Notching.

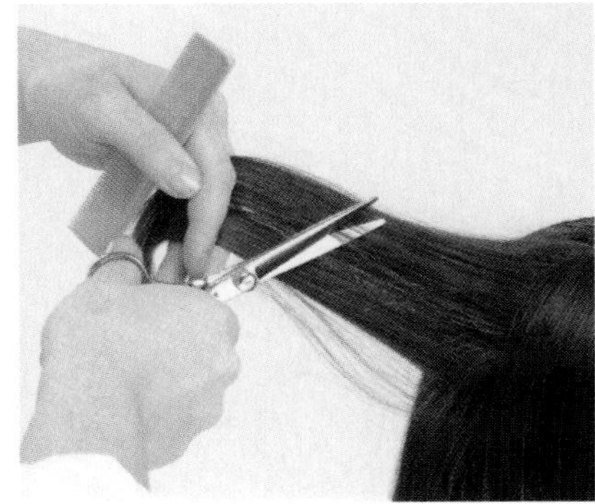

Figure 11–187 Free-hand notching.

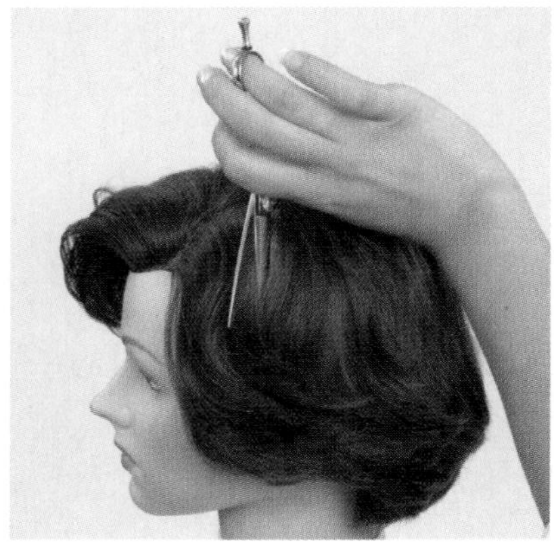

Figure 11-188 Slithering.

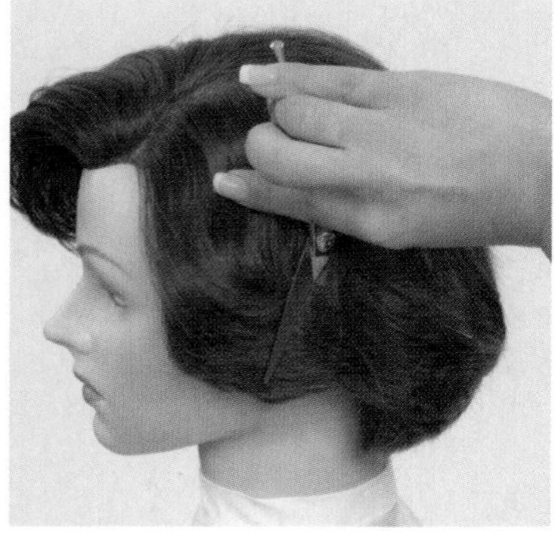

Figure 11-189 Ideal open position.

hair, place your "notches" further apart. This technique can be done on wet or dry hair (Figure 11–186).

- **Free-hand notching** also uses the tips of the shears. Do not slide the shears, but simply snip out pieces of hair at random intervals. This technique is generally used throughout the interior of the section, rather than at the ends. It works particularly well on curly hair, where it is not desirable to add too many layers but, rather, where you would choose to release the curl and remove some density (Figure 11–187).
- **Slithering** or effilating is the process of thinning the hair to graduated lengths with shears. In this technique, the hair strand is cut by a sliding movement of the shears, with the blades kept partially opened (Figure 11–188). Slithering reduces volume and creates movement.
- **Slicing** is a technique that removes bulk and adds movement through the lengths of the hair. When slicing, never completely close the shears. Use only the portion of the blades near the pivot. This prevents removing large pieces of hair (Figure 11–189 and Figure 11–190). This technique can be performed within a subsection or just on the surface of the hair, with haircutting or texturizing shears (Figure 11–191 and Figure 11–192). To slice an elevated subsection, work with either wet or dry hair. When slicing on the surface of the haircut, it is best to work on dry hair, because you can see exactly how much hair you are taking away.
- **Carving** is a version of slicing that creates a visual separation in the hair. It works best on short hair (1-½ to 3 inches, or 3.75 to 7.5 cm, in length). This technique is done by placing the still blade into the hair and resting it on the scalp. Move the shears through the hair, gently opening and partially closing the shears as you move, thus "carving" out areas (Figure 11–193). The more horizontal your shears, the more hair you remove. The more vertical, the less hair you remove.
- By carving the ends, you can add texture and separation to the perimeter of a haircut by holding the ends of a small strand of hair between your thumb and index fingers, and carving on the surface of that strand. Begin carving about 3 inches from the ends toward your fingers.

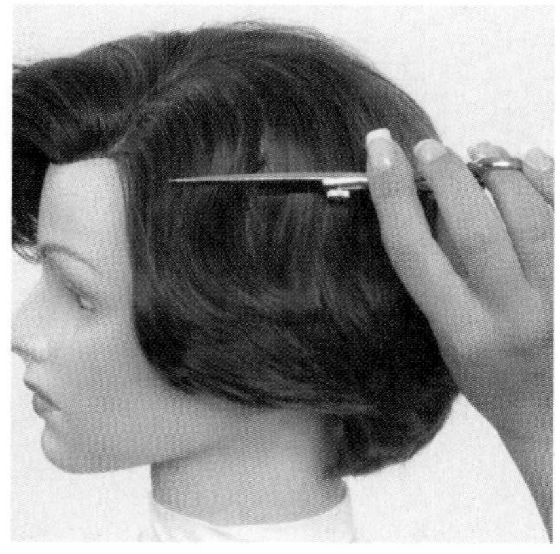

Figure 11-190 Slicing with shears.

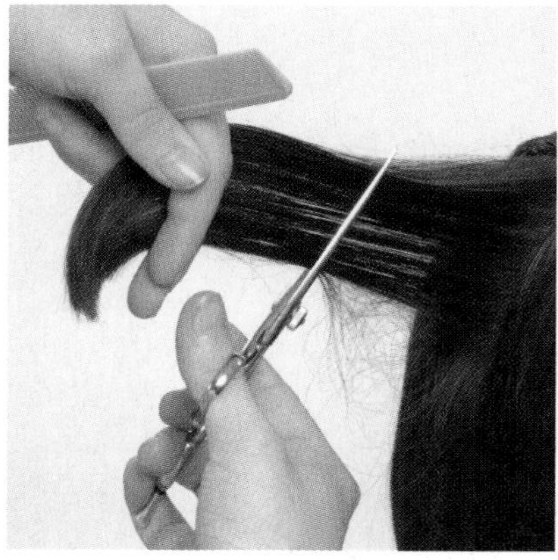

Figure 11-191 Slicing through a subsection with texturizing shears.

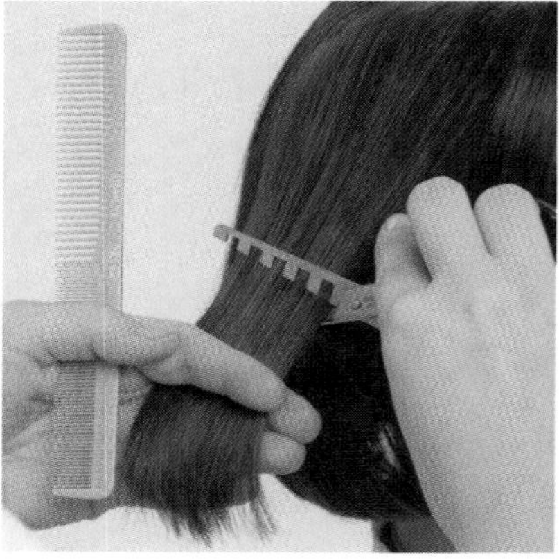

Figure 11-192 Slicing through the surface with texturizing shears.

Texturizing with Thinning Shears

- *Removing bulk (thinning).* Thinning shears were originally created for the purpose of thinning out hair and blending. Many clients are afraid of the word "thinning." A more modern choice of words would be "removing bulk" or "removing weight." When using the thinning shears for this purpose, it is best to follow the same sectioning as in the original haircut. Comb the subsection out from the head and cut it with the thinning shears, at least 4 to 5 inches (10 to 12.5 cm) from the scalp (Figure 11–194). On longer lengths, you may need to repeat the process again as you move out toward the ends. On coarse hair textures, stay farther away from the scalp, as sometimes the shorter hairs will poke through the haircut. On blunt haircuts, avoid thinning the top surfaces, as you may see visible lines where the hair is cut with the thinning shears. When working on curly hair, it is best to use the free-hand notching technique rather than thinning shears.
- *Removing weight from the ends.* You can also use thinning shears to remove bulk from the ends. This process works well on many hair textures. It can be used on both thin and thick hair, and it helps taper the perimeter of both graduated and blunt haircuts. Elevating each subsection out from the head, place the thinning shears into the hair at and angle and close the shears a few times as you work out toward the ends (Figure 11–195).
- *Thinning shears-over-comb.* Practicing the shears-over-comb technique with the thinning shears is a particularly effective way of mastering this technique. This technique, which is useful for blending weight lines on finer textures of hair, can be used as well on thick and coarse haircuts that are cut very short, especially in the sides and the nape. It helps the hair to lie closer to the head.
- *Other thinning shears techniques.* Any texturizing technique that can be performed with regular haircutting shears may also be performed with the thinning shears. When working on very fine or thin hair, try using the thinning shears for carving, point cutting, and slicing. This keeps you from overtexturizing and removing too much weight.

Texturizing with the Razor

- *Removing weight.* You can use the razor to thin out the ends of the hair. On damp hair, hold the section out from the head, with your fingers at the ends. Place the razor flat to the hair, 2 to 3 inches (5 to 7.5 cm) away from your fingers. Gently stroke the razor, removing a thin "sheet" of hair from the area (Figure 11–196). This tapers the ends of the section, and can be used on any area of the haircut where this effect is desired.
- *Free-hand slicing.* This technique can be used throughout the section or at the ends, and should be done on wet hair. When working in the midshaft of the subsection, comb the hair out from the head, and hold it with your fingers close to the ends. With the tip of the razor, slice out pieces of hair. The more vertical the movement, the less hair you remove. The more horizontal the movement, the more hair you remove. This technique releases weight from the subsection, allowing it to move more

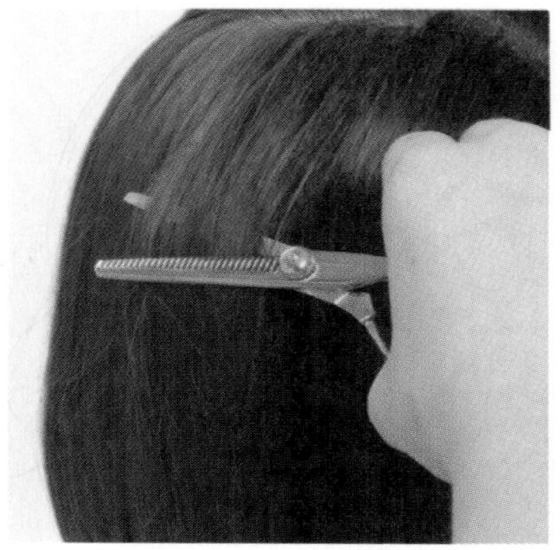

Figure 11–193 Carving through a short haircut.

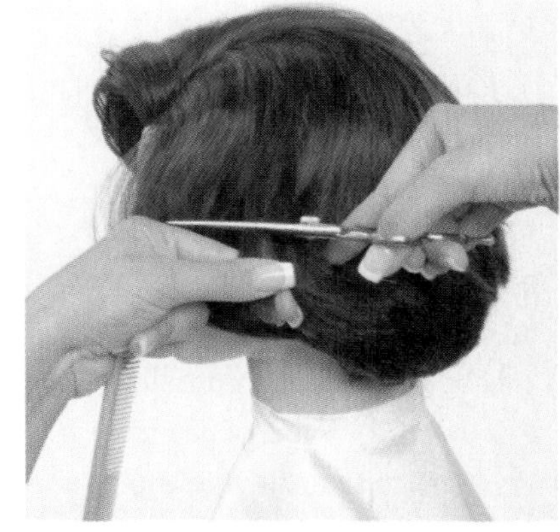

Figure 11–194 Thinning out the midsection.

11

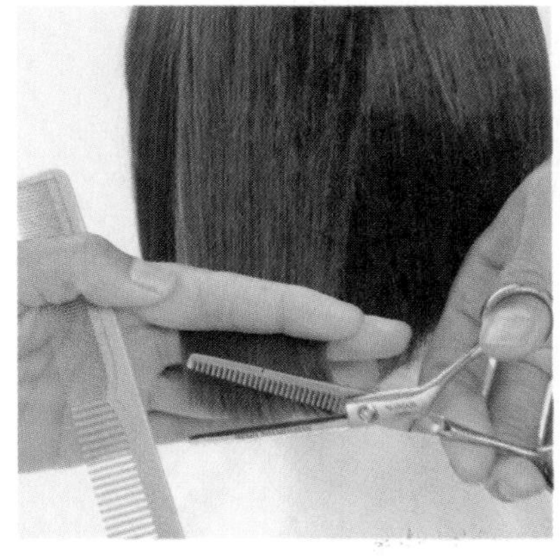

Figure 11–195 Thinning out the ends.

Figure 11-196 Tapering the ends with the razor.

(Figure 11–197). You can also use free-hand slicing on the ends of the hair to produce a softer perimeter or to create separation throughout the shape. In this case, hold the ends of a small piece of hair in your fingertips. Beginning about 3 inches from your fingers, slice down one side of the piece toward your fingers (Figure 11–198).

- *Razor-over-comb.* In this technique, the comb and the razor are used on the surface of the hair. Using the razor on the surface softens weight lines and causes the area to lie closer to the head. This technique is used mainly on shorter haircuts. There are two approaches. The first is to place the comb into the hair, with the teeth pointing down, a few inches above the area on which you will be working. Make small, gentle strokes on the surface of the hair with the razor. Move the comb down as you move the razor down (Figure 11–199). This is a great technique for tapering in the nape area or softening weight lines.

  The second way, referred to as **razor rotation**, is very similar to razor-over-comb. The difference is that you make small circular motions. Begin by combing the hair in the direction you will be moving in. Place the razor on the surface of the hair. Then allow the comb to follow the razor, combing through the area just cut, and then comb back into the section or onto a new section. This helps soften the texture of the area and gives direction to the haircut (Figure 11–200).

CAUTION

During the thinning process, remember that you can always go back and remove more hair if necessary. However, once the hair has been cut, it is impossible to replace, and you might have difficulty achieving the desired hairstyle.

11

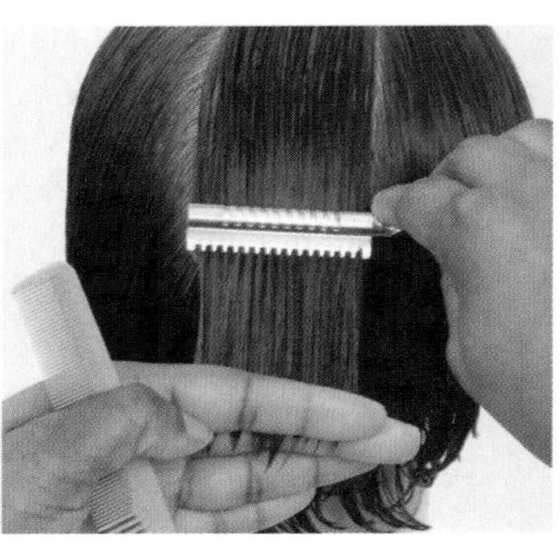

Figure 11-197 Slicing the midshaft.

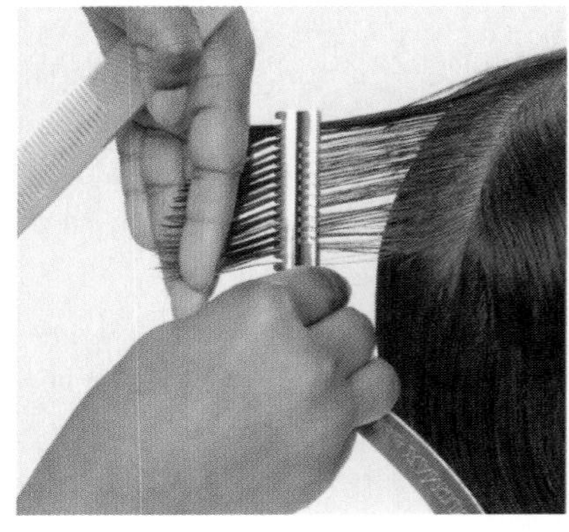

Figure 11-198 Slicing the perimeter.

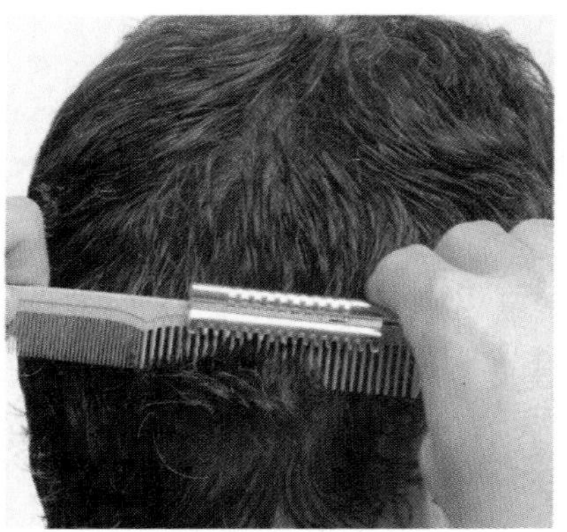

Figure 11-199 Razor-over-comb technique.

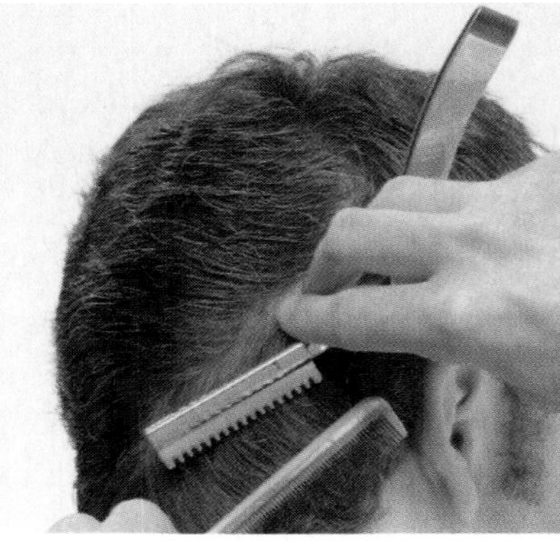

Figure 11-200 Razor rotation.

Basic Haircuts Enhanced with Texturizing Techniques

Consider these three basic haircuts and see how texturizing techniques can change the appearance of each haircut.

1. Figure 11–201 shows a blunt haircut before freehand razor slicing, and Figure 11–202 shows the same haircut after the technique has been used.
2. Figure 11–203 shows a graduated haircut before freehand shears slicing, and Figure Figure 11–204 shows the haircut after.
3. Figure 11–205 shows a uniform layered haircut, and Figure 11–206 shows the same haircut after notching on the ends and free-hand notching on the interior.

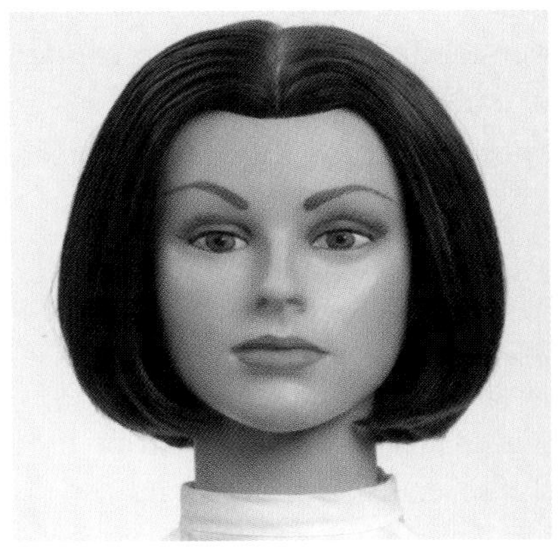

Figure 11-201 Blunt hair cut before texturizing.

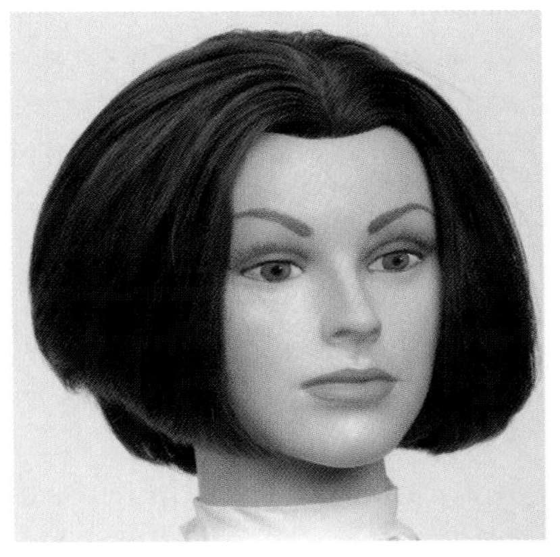

Figure 11-202 Texturized blunt haircut.

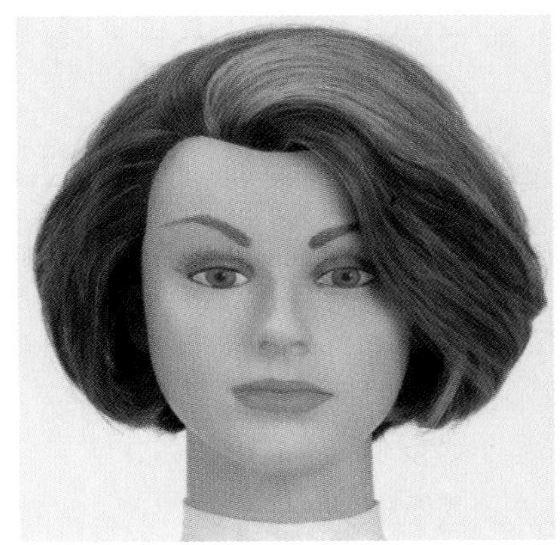

Figure 11-203 Graduated haircut before texturizing.

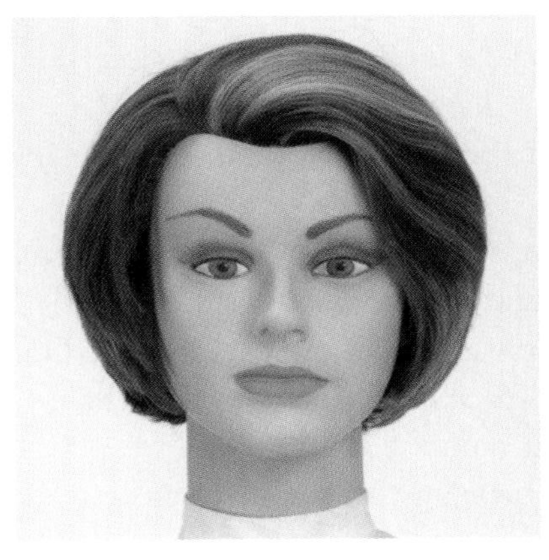

Figure 11-204 Texturized graduated haircut.

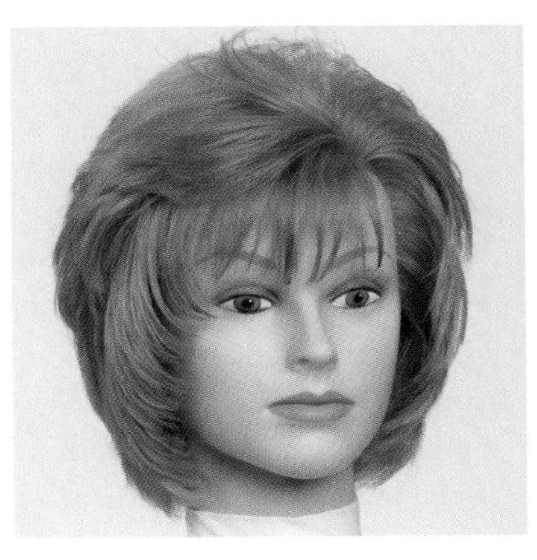

Figure 11-205 Uniform layered haircut before texturizing.

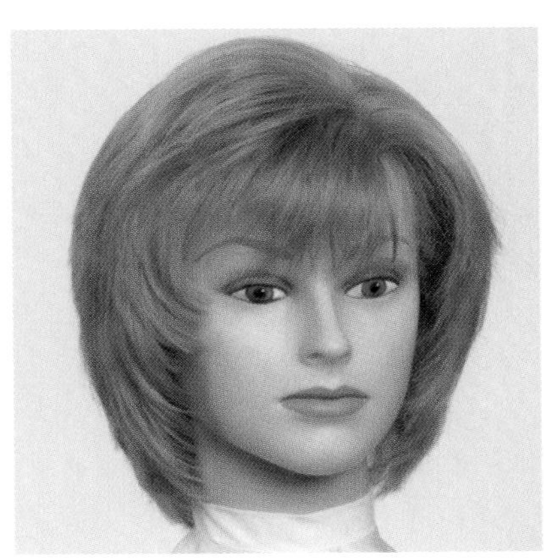

Figure 11-206 Texturized uniform layered haircut.

CLIPPERS, EDGERS, AND TRIMMERS

One last category of tools with which all stylists should be familiar is clippers, edgers, and trimmers, which offer versatile solutions for many haircutting challenges.

Clippers are electric devices that cut the hair by using two moving blades held in place by a metal plate with teeth. The action of the blades is faster than the eye can see. Clippers are mainly used for cutting shorter haircuts, and can be used to create **tapers**, which sit very close to the hairline and gradually get longer as you move up the head. While men have been getting clipper cuts for years, clippers are increasingly being used for haircuts on women today. Clippers can be used:

- without length guards, to remove hair completely (especially useful for cleaning up necklines and around the ears).
- without length guards, to taper hairlines from extremely short lengths into longer lengths, using the **clipper-over-comb** technique (this technique is very similar to shears-over-comb, except that the clippers move sideways across the comb rather than bottom to top).
- with length guards, which are attachments that fit over the blade plate and vary in size from 1/8 inch to 1 inch.

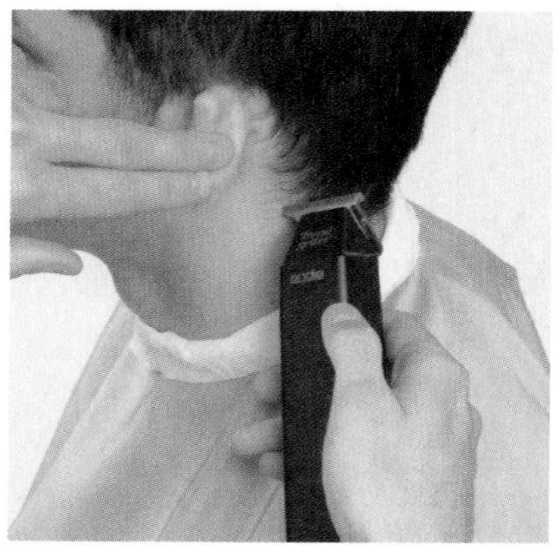

Figure 11-207 Edger cutting around the ear.

Tools for Clipper Cutting

There are several tools to have on hand when clipper cutting. Although you will not necessarily use each tool for every haircut, it is important to understand in which situations these tools are used (refer to Figure 11–44.)

- *Clippers.* Clippers come in different shapes and sizes. They can be used with or without attachments. Edgers, also called trimmers, are usually cordless, smaller-sized clippers. They are mainly used to clean the necklines and around the ears (Figure 11–207). Clean clippers and edgers after each use with a clipper brush. Disinfect the detachable blade and heel after each use as well. Follow the manufacturers' instructions for care and cleaning.
- *Length guard attachments.* When attached to the clippers, length guards allow you to cut all the hair evenly to that exact length. They range from 1/8 to 1 inch (.3 to 2.5 cm) wide, and can be used in different combinations to create different lengths.
- *Haircutting shears.* Used mainly for removing length and detailing the haircut.
- *Thinning shears.* Also called blending or tapering shears, these are great for removing excess bulk and for blending one area with another.
- *Combs.* In a regular cutting comb, the wider-spaced teeth are geared for combing and cutting, while the finer-spaced teeth are used for detailing, shears-over-comb, and clipper-over-comb techniques. The classic barbering comb is often used in the nape, at the sides, and around the ears, and allows you to cut the hair very short and close to the head. The wide-toothed comb is used when cutting thicker and longer lengths, where detailing is not required.

Basic Clipper Techniques

Basic techniques with clippers include clipper-over-comb and clipper cutting with length guard attachments.

Clipper-Over-Comb

The clipper-over-comb technique allows you to cut the hair very close to the scalp and create a flat-top or square shape. The way you use the comb is the same as when you are working with shears-over-comb. The main difference is that the clippers move across the comb, which requires that you keep the comb in position as you cut. The angle at which you hold the comb determines the amount of hair that is cut.

Clippers are most accurate when used on dry hair. Use the lever switch on the clipper or a numbered attachment to vary the distance that the clipper is held from the head.

Here are some tips for working with the clipper-over-comb technique, which will be illustrated in the procedure for the men's basic clipper cut later in this chapter.

1. Stand directly in front of the section on which you are working. The area you are cutting should be at eye level.
2. Place the comb, teeth first, into the hairline, and turn the comb so that the teeth are angled slightly away from the head. Always work against the growth patterns of the hair to ensure that you are lifting the hair away from the head and cutting evenly.
3. Hold the comb stationary and cut the length against the comb, moving the clippers from right to left. (If you are left-handed, you will move the clippers left to right.)
4. Although your movements should be fluid, remember to stop momentarily to cut the section. Remove the comb from the hair and begin the motion again, using the previously cut section underneath as your guideline. Continue working up the head toward the weight or length.

Clipper Cutting with Attachments

Using the length guard attachments is a quick and easy way to create short haircuts. With practice, clipper-cutting with attachments allows you to create many different shapes. For example, you can use the 1/4-inch guide in the nape and sides. Switch to the 1/2-inch guide as you reach the parietal area, which would maintain more length at the parietal and produce a square shape.

Using Edgers and Trimmers

- Using edgers around the ears. When cutting a clean line around the ears, use both hands to hold the edger sideways. Using just the outer edge on the skin, arc the edger up and around the ear (Figure 11–208). As you reach the area behind the ear, use the comb to hold the hair in place, and continue with the arcing motion (Figure 11–209).
- Using edgers at the neckline. Clean up hair on the neck that grows below the design line (Figure 11–210). Edgers also help create more defined lines at the perimeter (Figure 11–211).

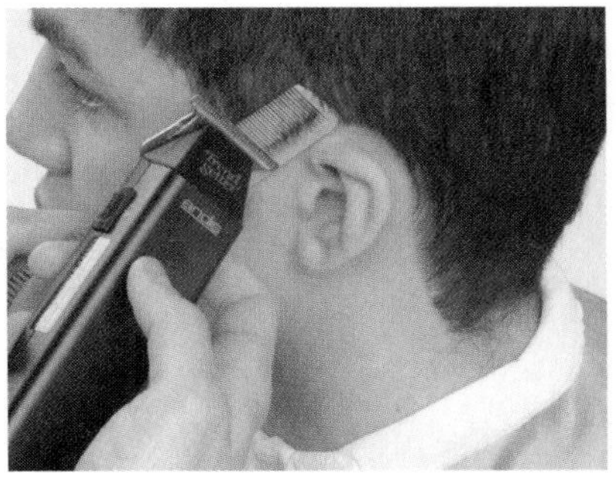

Figure 11-208 Arcing edger at front of the ear.

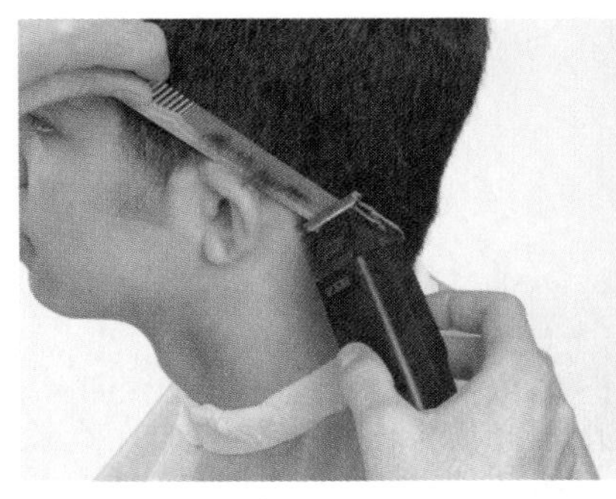

Figure 11-209 Arcing edger at back of ear with comb.

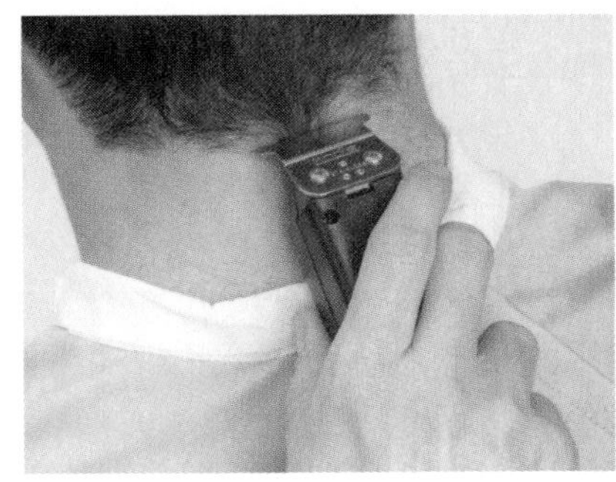

Figure 11-210 Cleaning up neck hair.

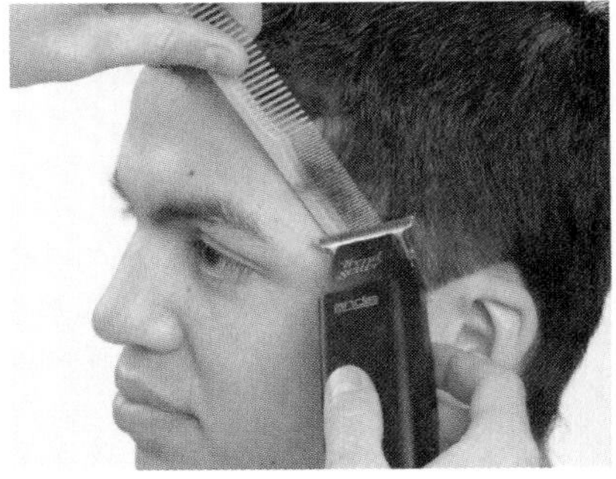

Figure 11-211 Edging line at side perimeter.

Men's Basic Clipper Cut

In this cut, the hair is close-cropped along the bottom and sides and becomes longer as you travel up the head. The distance between the comb and the scalp determines the amount of hair to be cut. The clipper can be positioned horizontally, vertically, or diagonally.

Tips for Clipper Cutting

- Always work against the natural growth patterns, especially in the nape. This ensures that you are elevating the hair away from the head and cutting the hair evenly.
- Always work with small sections. When using the clipper-over-comb technique, do not try to cut all the way across the entire length of the comb. The area you are cutting should be no wider than 3 inches.

activity

Part of your job as a salon professional will be to determine your client's overall needs and make suggestions that will enhance the service you've performed. In the following "scene," a stylist suggests an additional service to a haircut client. This is known as ticket upgrading or upselling. Read this dialogue over, then choose a partner with whom to role-play a similar scene. Focus on a different type of problem, such as oily hair. Or try suggesting a service from another stylist, such as a color or texture service, always keeping in mind what would benefit this particular client.

Stylist: Ms. Sanchez, I'm really glad you came in today for a trim. Your hair feels quite dry.

Ms. Sanchez: I know. I've been spending a lot of time at the pool. It really has dried out something awful.

Stylist: Are you finding that your hair is harder to style in this condition? Are you having trouble getting the volume you're used to?

Ms. Sanchez: Absolutely. And it's so dull! It just lies there on top of my head. Do you think it's just too long?

Stylist: Well, that may be part of it. To tell you the truth, a haircut would help. I'd also suggest a deep conditioning treatment. I can apply the treatment after the shampoo. If you have the time, I'd like to leave it on for 15 or 20 minutes to get the reconstruction process started. You may want to pick up a tube of the reconstructor to use at home, once or twice a week (Figure 11–125).

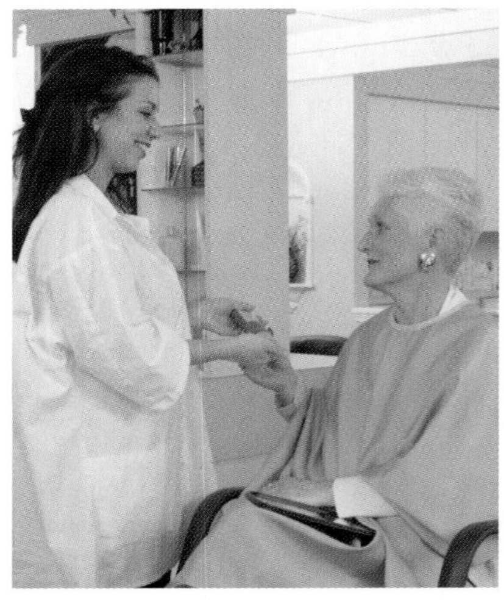

Figure 11–125 Ticket upgrading.

Ms. Sanchez: What's that going to cost?

Stylist: It will be an additional $5. A tube of the conditioner is $15 for eight ounces, or about eight treatments at home. I'm suggesting this because I think your hair really needs it—and I want you to be happy with the feel of your hair again. What do you say? Should I go ahead and apply the treatment?

Ms. Sanchez: Okay. Let's try it and see if it makes a difference!

PROCEDURE

MEN'S BASIC CLIPPER CUT

Implements and Materials

- cutting cape
- neck strip
- haircutting comb
- barber comb
- haircutting shears
- clipper
- trimmer
- small-number guard attachment (optional)

Procedure

1. The hair should be clean and dry for this haircut (Figure 11–212).
2. Make a horseshoe parting about 2 inches (5 cm) below the apex of the head, beginning and ending at the front hairline (Figure 11–213). Comb the hair above the part forward.
3. Starting in the nape area, place the haircutting comb against the scalp, teeth up. Angle the comb against the scalp from 0 to 45 degrees, allowing for the natural contour of the head. Cut the hair that extends through the teeth of the comb (Figure 11–214).
4. Repeat Step 3 as you move up the back of the head. Blend the lengths over the curve of the head by cross-cutting horizontally, from side to side (Figure 11–215). Shape the back center area first, from the nape to the parietal ridge. Then, still using the clipper-over-comb technique, cut both sides of the back, from ear to ear.

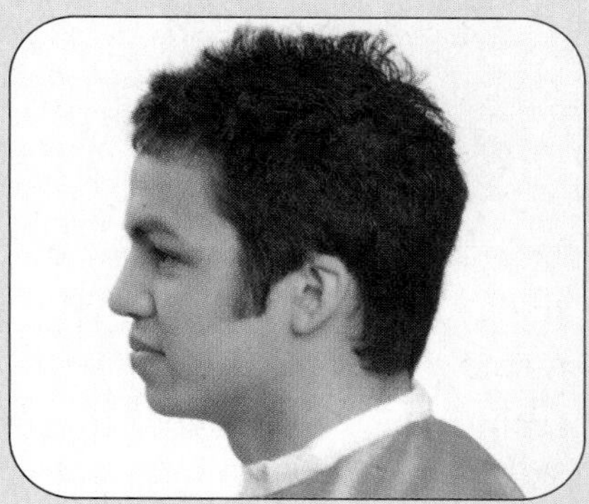

Figure 11-212 Client before clipper cut.

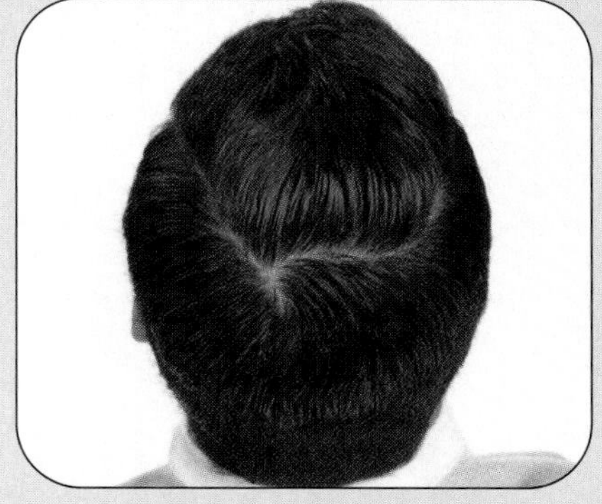

Figure 11-213 Make a horseshoe part.

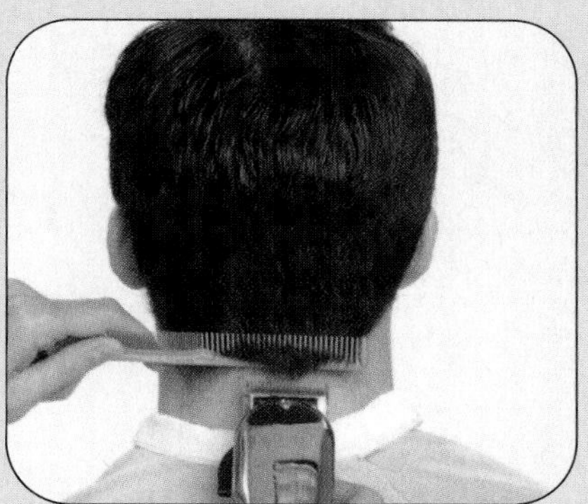

Figure 11-214 Cut at the nape.

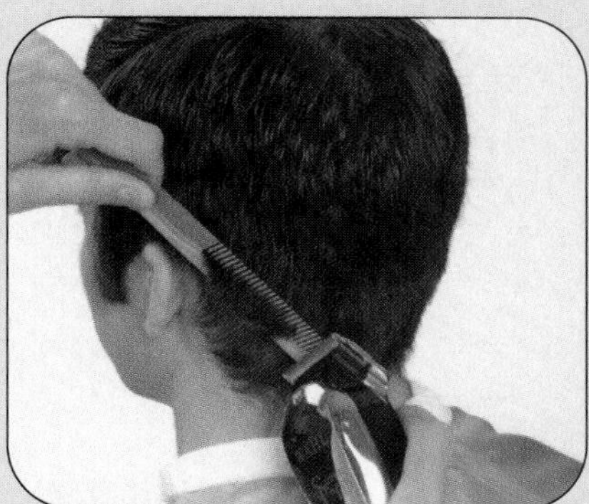

Figure 11-215 Cross-cut the back of the head.

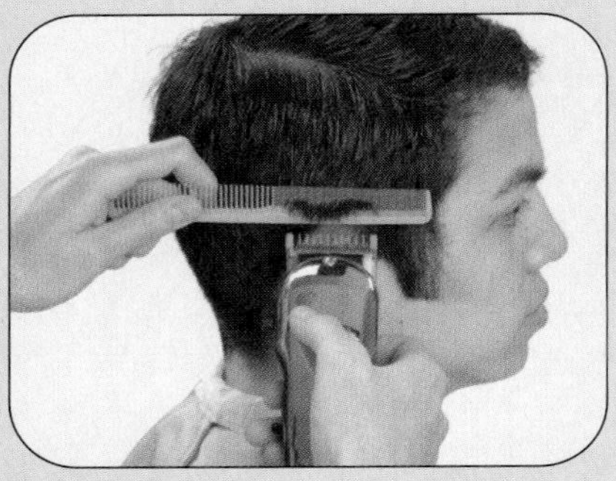

Figure 11-216 Cut from sideburn to parietal ridge.

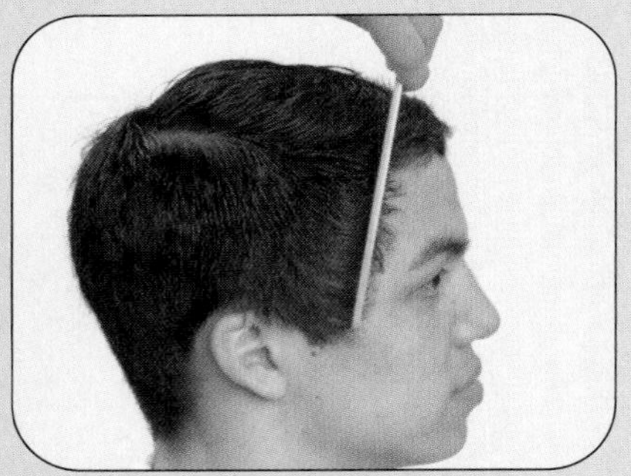

Figure 11-217 Measure from eyebrow to natural hairline.

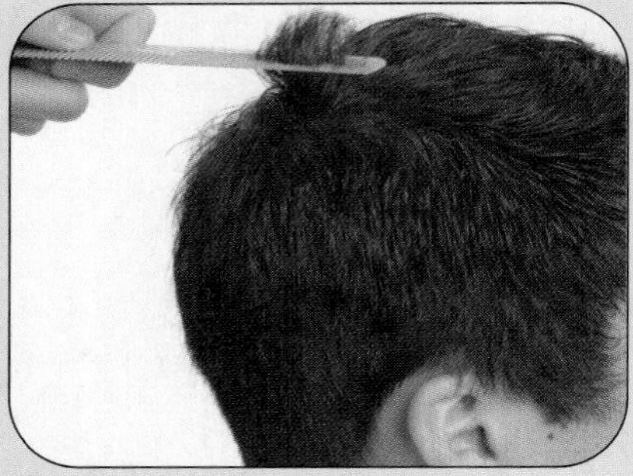

Figure 11-218 Cut guideline at crown.

5. Carefully blend the lengths over the curve of the head by cross-cutting.
6. Using a small number attachment on the clipper, cut up each side from the sideburn to the parietal ridge (Figure 11–216). The hair lengths will be very close to the scalp. If the client wants longer sides, the weight on the top should not overpower the sides; it should blend. If the sides are very short, the top should be cut shorter to blend.
7. Measure the distance between the eyebrows and the natural hairline to establish an appropriate guideline for the length in the crown area (Figure 11–217).
8. Cut a narrow guideline at the crown end of the horseshoe parting. Determine the length by the forehead measurement (Figure 11–218). Beginning at the crown end, cut the top area with the clipper to the exact length of the initial crown guideline. As you move toward the forehead, pull the hair back toward the guideline in order to increase the length at the forehead (Figure 11–219).
9. Using the clipper and attachment, shorten and shape the hair around the ears and sideburns (Figure 11–220). Continue to cut the hair until the shape of the head and the length of the hair are in harmony. To blend or outline the perimeter of the haircut, you may use a clipper or trimmer (Figure 11–221). The shears-over-comb or clipper-over-comb technique, using the front teeth of a barber comb, may also be employed here.
10. Follow cleanup and sanitation steps in Procedure 3—blunt haircut.

11

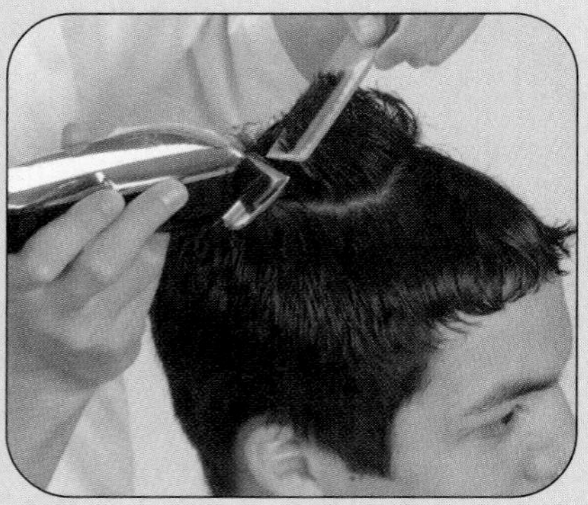

Figure 11-219 Bring hair toward guideline.

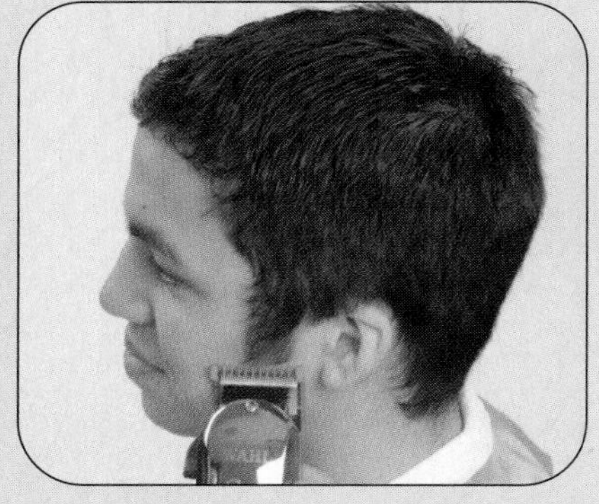

Figure 11-220 Shape hair around ears and sideburns.

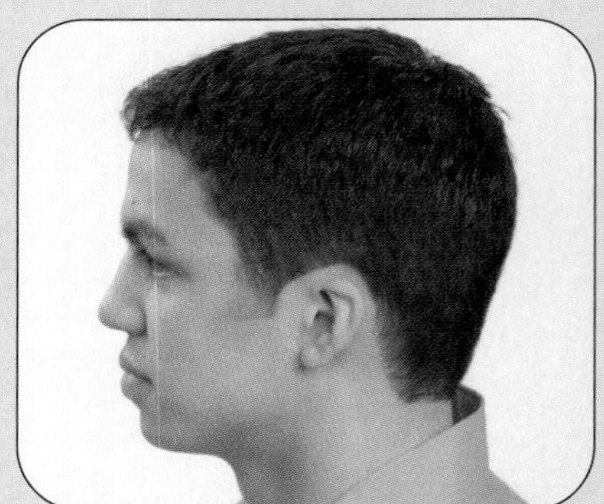

Figure 11-221 Finished clipper cut.

completed!

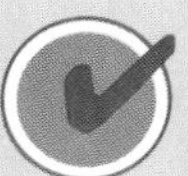

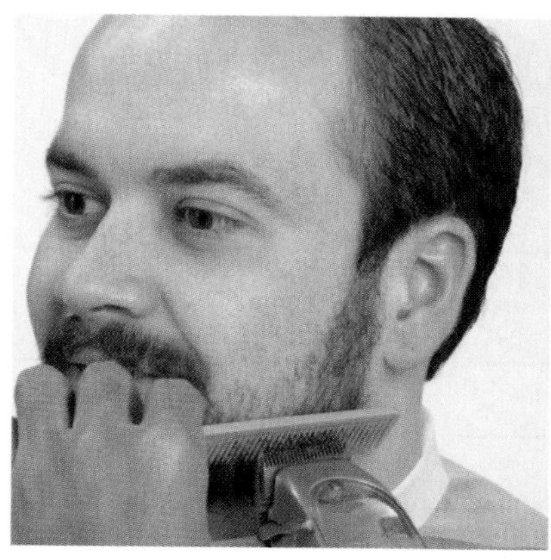

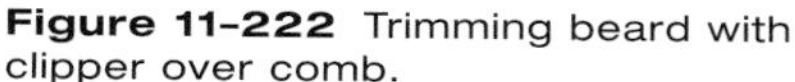

Figure 11-222 Trimming beard with clipper over comb.

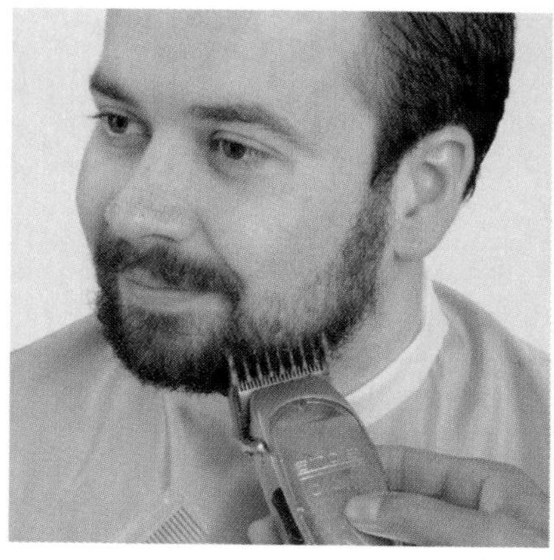

Figure 11-223 Trimming beard with clipper and guard.

- When using the clipper-over-comb technique, the angle of the comb determines the cutting angle. If the comb is parallel to the head, you will cut the hair the same length as you move up the head. If the comb is angled away from the head as you move, you begin to build length.

Trimming Facial Hair

Clippers and edgers can be used to trim beards and mustaches as well. The technique is very similar to shears-over-comb and clipper-over-comb. When removing length, use the comb to control the hair, and always cut against the comb (Figure 11–222). You can also use the length guard attachments to trim a beard to the desired length (Figure 11–223). If you choose to use haircutting shears to trim facial hair, you may want to keep a less expensive pair for this purpose. Facial hair is very coarse and may dull your haircutting shears.

Some male clients have excess hair in their ears. When performing a haircut or trimming facial hair, always check the ears and ask the client if he'd like you to remove any excess hair you may find. Carefully snip away the hair with your shears, using extreme caution.

chapter glossary

angle	the space between two lines or surfaces that intersect at a given point; in haircutting, the hair is held away from the head to create an angle of elevation
apex	highest point on the top of the head
beveling	tapering the ends of the hair
blunt haircut	haircut in which all the hair comes to one hanging level, forming a weight line or area; it is cut with no elevation or overdirection; also referred to as a one-length, zero-elevation, or no-elevation cut
carving	haircutting technique done by placing the still blade into the hair and resting it on the scalp, then moving the shears through the hair while opening and partially closing the shears
clipper-over-comb	haircutting technique similar to shears-over-comb, except that the clippers move sideways across the comb rather than bottom to top
cross-checking	parting the haircut in the opposite way from which you cut it, to check for precision of line and shape
crown	area of the head between the apex and the back of the parietal ridge
cutting line	the angle at which the fingers are held when cutting, and ultimately the line that is cut; also known as finger angle, finger position, cutting position, cutting angle, and shears angle
distribution	where and how hair is moved over the head; the direction hair is combed in relation to its base parting
elevation	angle or degree at which a subsection of hair is held, or elevated, from the head when cutting; also referred to as projection
four corners	points on the head that signal a change in the shape of the head, from flat to round or vice versa
free-hand notching	notching technique in which pieces of hair are snipped out at random intervals
fringe	triangular section that begins at the apex and ends at the front corners
graduated haircut/ graduation	graduated shape or wedge; an effect or haircut that results from cutting the hair with tension, low to medium elevation, or overdirection; has a stacked area around the exterior
growth pattern	the direction in which the hair grows from the scalp; also referred to as natural fall or natural falling position
guideline	section of hair, located either at the perimeter or the interior of the cut, that determines the length the hair will be cut; also referred to as a guide; usually the first section that is cut to create a shape
hairline	the hair that grows at the outermost perimeter along the face, around the ears, and on the neck
head form	the shape of the head or skull; greatly affects the way the hair falls and behaves; also called head shape
interior guideline	guideline that is inside the haircut rather than on the perimeter
layered haircut/layers	graduated effect achieved by cutting the hair with elevation or overdirection; the hair is cut at higher elevations, usually 90 degrees or above, which removes weight

line	thin continuous mark; in haircutting, may be the guideline, cutting line, or perimeter; can be straight or curved, horizontal, vertical, or diagonal.
long layered haircut	haircut in which the hair is cut at a 180-degree angle; the resulting shape has shorter layers at the top and increasingly longer layers toward the perimeter
nape	back part of the neck; the hair below the occipital bone
notching	version of point cutting in which the tips of the shears are moved toward the hair ends rather than into them; creates a chunkier effect
occipital bone	hindmost bone of the skull below the parietal bones; protrudes at the base of the skull
overdirection	combing a section away from its natural falling position, rather than straight out from the head, toward a guideline; used to create increasing lengths in the interior or perimeter
palm-to-palm	cutting position in which the palms of both hands are facing each other
parietal ridge	the widest area of the head, usually starting at the temples and ending at the bottom of the crown
part/parting	a line dividing the hair to the scalp that separates one section of hair from another or creates subsections; generally created with a comb
perimeter	the outer line of a hairstyle, the silhouette line; sometimes referred to as the exterior
point cutting	haircutting technique in which the tips of the shears are used to cut "points" into the ends of the hair
razor-over-comb	texturizing technique in which the comb and the razor are used on the surface of the hair
razor rotation	texturizing technique similar to razor-over-comb, done with small circular motions
reference points	points on the head that mark where the surface of the head changes or the behavior of the hair changes, such as ears, jawline, occipital bone, apex, etc.; used to establish design lines that are proportionate
section	to divide the hair by parting into uniform working areas for control; sections are created when two partings are made parallel to one another
shears-over-comb	haircutting technique in which the hair is held in place with the comb while the tips of the shears are used to remove the lengths
slicing	technique that removes bulk and adds movement through the lengths of the hair; the shears are not completely closed, and only the portion of the blades near the pivot is used
slide cutting	method of cutting or thinning the hair in which the fingers and shears glide along the edge of the hair to remove length
slithering	process of thinning the hair to graduated lengths with shears; cutting the hair strand by a sliding movement of the shears while keeping the blades partially opened; also called effilating
stationary guideline	guideline that does not move
subsections	smaller sections within a larger section of hair, used to maintain control of the hair while cutting

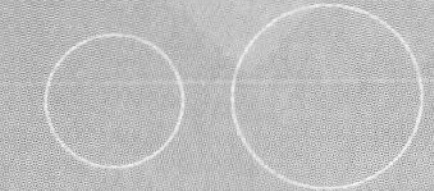

chapter glossary *(continued)*

tapers	haircuts in which there is an even blend from very short at the hairline to longer lengths as you move up the head; "to taper" is to narrow progressively at one end
tension	amount of pressure applied when combing and holding a section, created by stretching or pulling the section
texturizing	removing excess bulk without shortening the length; changing the appearance or behavior of hair, through specific haircutting techniques, using shears, thinning shears, or a razor
traveling guideline	guideline that moves as the haircutting progresses, used often when creating layers or graduation; also referred to as moving or movable guidelines
uniform layers	effect produced by cutting the hair at the same length consistently, using a 90-degree elevation
weight line	A visual "line" in the haircut, where the ends of the hair hang together; the line of maximum length within the weight area: heaviest perimeter area of a 0-degree (one-length) or 45-degree (graduated) cut

review questions

1. What are reference points and what is their function?
2. What are the main areas of the head and how do you find them?
3. Define elevation and describe the different effects it creates.
4. What is the difference between traveling and stationary guidelines, and when do you use each?
5. Define overdirection.
6. What are the important points to cover with a client during a haircutting consultation?
7. Explain the difference between hair density and hair texture.
8. Where are the danger zones in a haircut, and why do you need to be aware of them?
9. What is palm-to-palm cutting?
10. Explain the importance of proper posture and body position.
11. List disinfection and sanitation procedures that must be followed after performing a haircut.
12. Name and describe the four basic types of haircuts.
13. Define cross-checking.
14. Describe the shears-over-comb technique.
15. Name and describe three different texturizing techniques performed with shears.

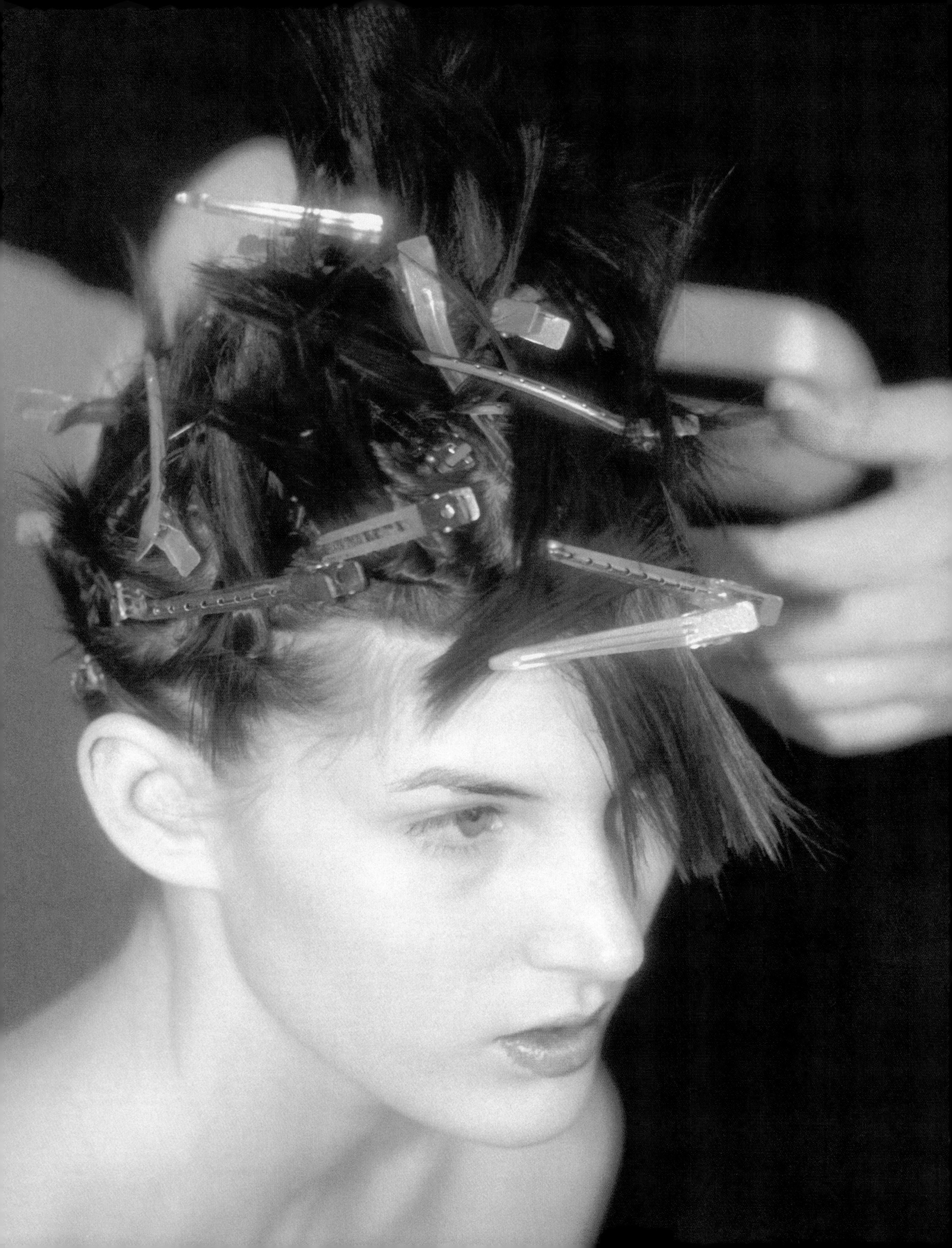

HAIRSTYLING

Mary Brunetti

FREELANCE AND CELEBRITY HAIRSTYLIST,
1991 NORTH AMERICAN HAIRSTYLIST OF THE YEAR

Chapter Outline

**Client Consultation • Wet Hairstyling Basics • Finger Waving
Pin Curls • Roller Curls • Comb-out Techniques • Hair Wrapping
Blow-dry Styling • Styling Long Hair • Thermal Hairstyling
Thermal Hair Straightening (Hair Pressing)**

Learning Objectives

After completing this chapter, you should be able to:

1. Demonstrate the techniques of a) finger waving, b) pin curls, c) roller setting, and d) hair wrapping.
2. Demonstrate mastery of various blow-dry styling techniques.
3. Demonstrate three basic techniques of styling long hair.
4. Demonstrate the proper use of thermal irons.
5. Demonstrate various thermal iron manipulations and explain how they are used.
6. Describe the three types of hair pressing.
7. Demonstrate the procedures involved in soft pressing and hard pressing.

National Skill Standards

This chapter provides you with the necessary information to master these National Industry Skill Standards for Entry-Level Cosmetologists.

Consulting with clients to determine their needs and preferences.

Conducting services in a safe environment and taking measures to prevent the spread of infectious and contagious diseases.

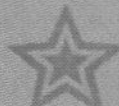
Marketing professional salon products.

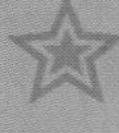
Using a variety of salon products while providing client services.

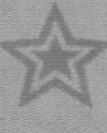
Providing styling and finishing techniques to complete a hairstyle to the satisfaction of the client.

Key Terms

Page number indicates where in the chapter the term is used.

back-brushing pg. 369

back-combing pg. 369

barrel curls pg. 364

base pg. 358

blow-dry styling pg. 373

carved curls pg. 361

cascade or stand-up curls pg. 364

circle pg. 358

closed center curls pg. 359

curl pg. 365

concentrator pg. 376

diffuser pg. 376

double press pg. 409

finger waving pg. 351

foam or mousse pg. 378

full-base curl pg. 406

full-stem curl pg. 359

gel pg. 378

hair pressing pg. 409

hair spray or finishing spray pg. 379

half base pg. 366

half-base curl pg. 406

half-stem curl pg. 359

hard press pg. 409

liquid gel or texturizer pg. 378

medium press pg. 409

no-stem curl pg. 359

off base pg. 366

off-base curl pg. 406

on base pg. 366

open center curls pg. 359

pomade or wax pg. 379

ribboning pg. 361

ridge curls pg. 361

rod pg. 387

shaping pg. 359

shell pg. 387

silicone shiner pg. 379

skip waves pg. 361

soft press pg. 409

spiral curl pg. 404

stem pg. 358

straightening gel pg. 378

thermal waving and curling pg. 387

updo pg. 379

volume-base curl pg. 405

volumizer pg. 379

waving lotion pg. 358

Now that you know how to properly cleanse, condition, and shape your client's hair, you are ready to style. In fact, you are more than ready, because the styling of hair is no doubt what attracted you to this profession in the first place. You see yourself as an artist, a kind of sculptor, and hair is your "clay." Sometimes, the hair is full and luxurious; sometimes, it is thin or coarse or fine. But whatever the case, you are there to meet the challenge and come up with the solution. Your understanding of basic facial anatomy and facial shapes will be crucial as you determine styles that work well for your clients.

There is a wide range of styling options from which you can choose. One fact about fashion is that no style ever really goes away. While pin curls and finger waves may remind you of the old days, these techniques are very much a part of the hairstyling scene today. If you are skilled in a full range of styling techniques, you will be a very busy person indeed. You might wind up working in film or television, where period styles often need to be recreated. And you will be the one to whom clients flock when they are bored with the hairstyles they have been wearing (Figure 12–1).

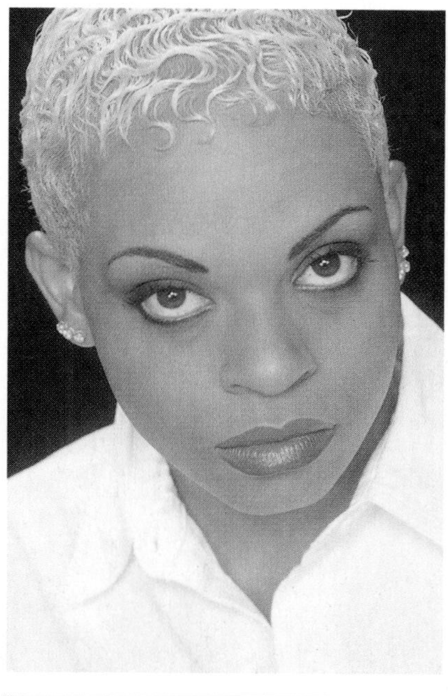

Figure 12–1 An updated finger wave style.

Consider the following fable. A stylist is asked to create a soft and romantic hairstyle on a beautiful model for the cover of a popular trade magazine. The model's hair is straight and long, so the stylist first gives her a basic pattern roller set, using electric rollers, a technique she learned 25 years earlier in beauty school. After combing out the model's hair, she creates a style using pinning and teasing techniques also learned in school. Then she adds soft finger-waved sides for a more romantic look. The result is a stunningly stylish look, achieved by using three different techniques the stylist learned a quarter of a century earlier.

The moral of the story? Never forget, or stop practicing, what you have learned. The reason this particular stylist is called on for exciting jobs is that she is well practiced in the skills of her craft. Many stylists choose to forget these skills once they leave cosmetology school, thinking they will never have any use for them. They typically complain about getting stuck in the "box," but many times, the box is of their own making.

An expert stylist is the one clients turn to when they have a big event coming up and need a more dramatic evening look. If you are not familiar with different styling techniques and your client's particular requests force you to refer her to another stylist in the salon, you might risk losing that client altogether. As a true professional, you will want to know all you can about your trade. This means being able to perform a variety of techniques on all hair textures, from extremely curly to bone-straight.

CLIENT CONSULTATION

The client consultation is the first step in the hairstyling process and cannot be skipped. Encourage your client to look through magazines to find a style she likes or, better yet, offer her the portfolio you keep on hand that is filled with pictures of current hairstyling trends. When guiding your client toward the appropriate design decision, take into consideration all that you have learned in Chapter 9 regarding face shapes, hair types, and lifestyle needs. And always remember that the consultation is a two-way street. You and the client need to listen to each other.

Often, your role in the consultation will be as a problem-solver. For example, on your client's last visit to a salon, she asked for a hairstyle that was not right for her type of hair. Because the stylist did not suggest something more appropriate, the outcome was disappointing. Now you are being asked to "fix" it. If you can come up with an entirely different style, one that is both flattering and easy to manage, the client who has come to you in an emergency may turn into a regular customer. Just remember that no matter what the client says, what she really wants is a style that is flattering and easy to maintain. Your job is to find these solutions for all kinds of clients on all kinds of occasions. It is a challenge, but the challenge is half the fun of being in this profession.

WET HAIRSTYLING BASICS

Wet hairstyling tools include:

- rollers (plastic)
- clips (duckbill, sectioning, finger waving, double prong, and single prong)
- pins (bobby pins and hairpins)
- clamps (sectioning clamps) (Figure 12–2)
- combs
- brushes

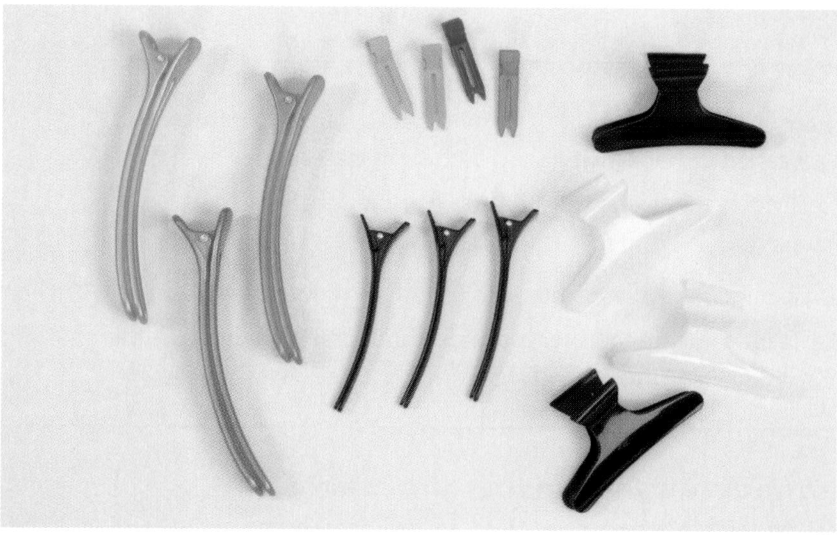

Figure 12-2 Clips (duckbill, sectioning, and double prong) and sectioning clamps.

FINGER WAVING

Finger waving is the process of shaping and directing the hair into a pattern of "S" shaped waves through the use of the fingers, combs, and waving lotion. Finger waving was all the rage back in the 1920s—1930s, which may have you wondering why you are being asked to learn it today. In addition to its use as a current style, finger waving teaches you the technique of moving and directing hair. It also helps you develop the coordination and finger strength required for professional hairstyling. In addition, it provides valuable training in molding hair to the curved surface of the head. In short, finger waving is an excellent introduction to hairstyling.

PROCEDURE

PREPARING THE HAIR FOR WET STYLING

Implements and Materials

- towels
- plastic cape
- shampoo
- conditioner
- neck strip

Preparation

1. Wash your hands with soap and warm water.
2. Perform the client consultation and hair analysis.
3. Drape the client for a shampoo service.
4. Shampoo the client's hair and condition if necessary. Towel-dry the hair.
5. Remove any tangles with a wide-tooth comb, starting at the ends and working up to the scalp.

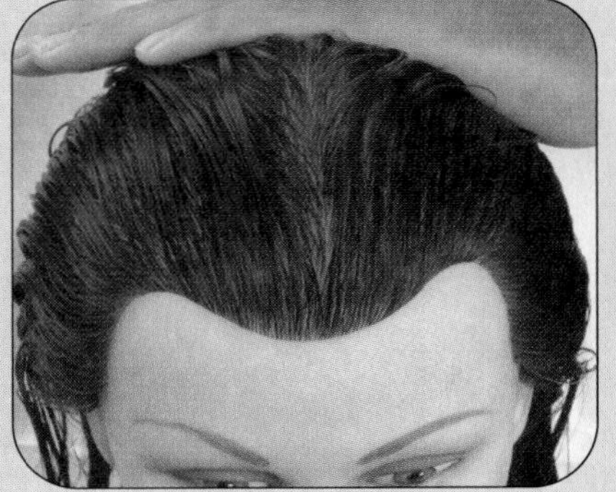

Figure 12-3 Push the hair forward.

Procedures for Parting the Hair

You can create a part elsewhere on the head if the client is more comfortable wearing it someplace else or if your design works better with the part placed elsewhere.

1. Comb wet hair straight back from the hairline.
2. Push the hair gently forward with the palm of the hand (Figure 12–3).
3. Use your comb and other hand to separate the hair where it parts (Figure 12–4).

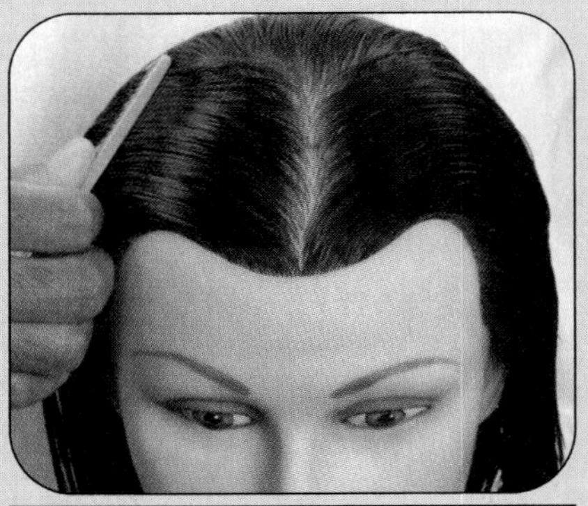

Figure 12-4 Find the natural part.

If the client's natural part works well with your hair design, use it.

1. Lay the wide-tooth end of a styling comb flat at the hairline.
2. Draw the comb back to the end of the desired part (Figure 12–5).
3. Hold the hair with the index finger on one side of the part. Pull the rest of the hair down with the comb (Figure 12–6).

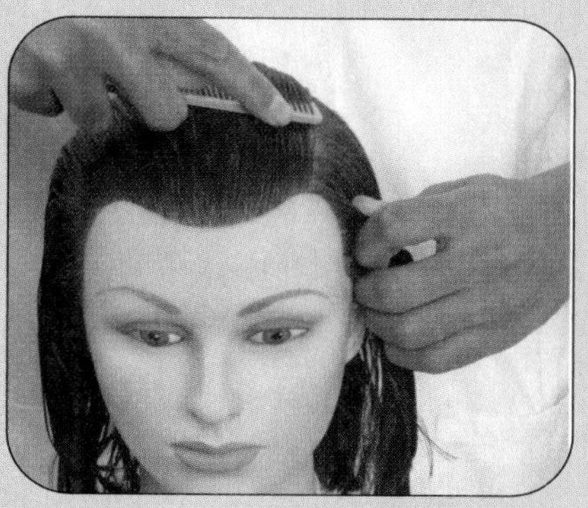

Figure 12-5 Part the wet hair.

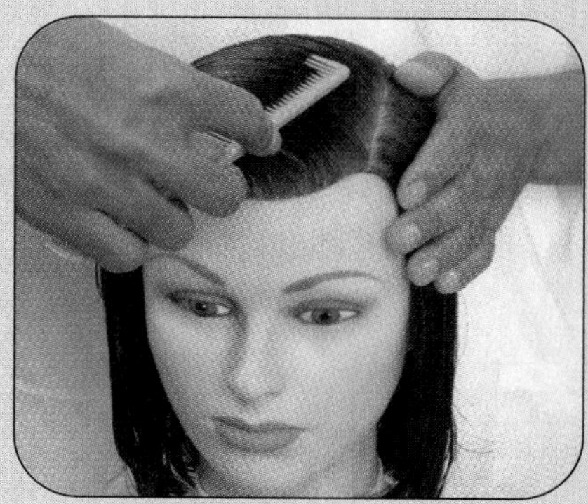

Figure 12-6 Comb the hair from the part.

completed!

PROCEDURE

HORIZONTAL FINGER WAVING

Finger waves may be started on either side of the head. In this procedure, the hair is parted on the left side of the head and the wave is started on the right (heavy) side. Apply lotion to one side of the head at a time; this prevents it from drying and requiring additional applications.

Implements and Materials

Use the list of implements and materials under. Procedure No. 8—preparing the hair for wet styling, and add the following:

- styling comb
- waving lotion or styling gel
- hairnet
- hairpins
- cotton or gauze

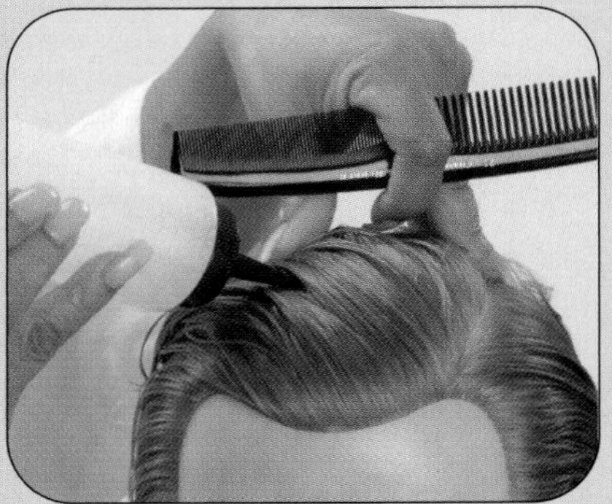

Figure 12-7 Comb waving lotion through the section.

Figure 12-8 Shape the top area.

Preparation

Follow the steps for Procedure 8—preparing the hair for wet styling.

Procedure

1. Part the hair, comb it smooth, and arrange it according to the planned style. Using the wide teeth of the comb will allow the hair to move more easily. Always follow the natural growth pattern when combing and parting the hair.
2. Apply waving lotion with an applicator bottle to the side of the hair you are working on first while the hair is damp. Then comb the lotion through the section (Figure 12–7).
3. Begin the first wave on the right side of the head. Using the index finger of your left hand as a guide, shape the top hair with a comb into the beginning of the "S" shaping, using a circular movement. Starting at the hairline, work toward the crown in $1\frac{1}{2}$ to 2-inch (3.7 to 5 cm) sections at a time (Figure 12–8).

4. To form the first ridge, place the index finger of your left hand directly above the position for the first ridge. With the teeth of the comb pointing slightly upward, insert the comb directly under the index finger. Draw the comb forward about 1 inch (2.5 cm) along the fingertip (Figure 12–9).
5. With the teeth still inserted in the ridge, flatten the comb against the head in order to hold the ridge in place (Figure 12–10).
6. Remove your left hand from the client's head and place your middle finger above the ridge with your index finger on the teeth of the comb. Draw out the ridge by closing the two fingers and applying pressure to the head (Figure 12–11). Do not try to increase the height or depth of a ridge by pinching or pushing with your fingers; such movements will create overdirection of the ridge and uneven hair placement.
7. Without removing the comb, turn the teeth downward, and comb the hair in a semicircular direction to form a dip in the hollow part of the wave (Figure 12–12).
8. Follow this procedure, section by section, until the crown has been reached, where the ridge phases out (Figure 12–13). The ridge and wave of each section should match evenly, without showing separations in the ridge and the hollow part of the wave.
9. To form the second ridge, begin at the crown area (Figure 12–14). The movements are the reverse of those followed in forming the first ridge. Draw the comb from the tip of the index finger toward the base. All movements are followed in a reverse pattern until the hairline is reached, completing the second ridge (Figure 12–15).

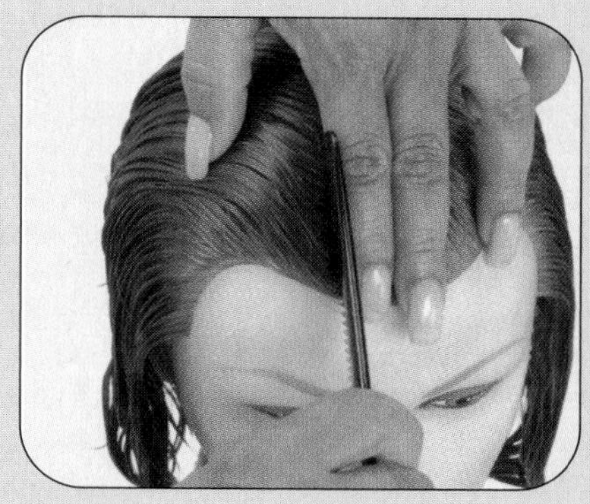

Figure 12-9 Draw hair toward the fingertip.

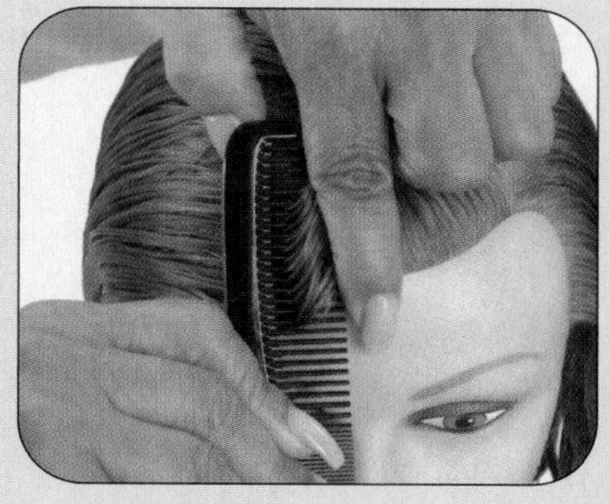

Figure 12-10 Flatten the comb against the head.

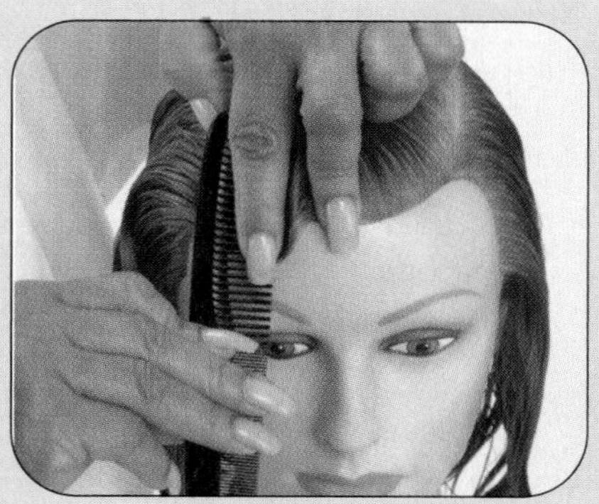

Figure 12-11 Emphasize the ridge.

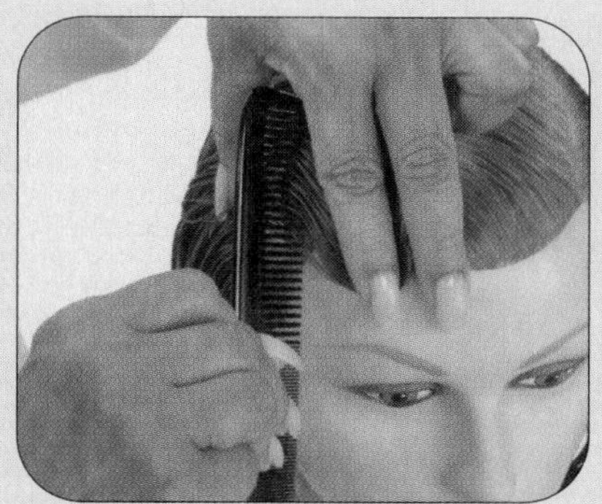

Figure 12-12 Comb hair in semicircular direction.

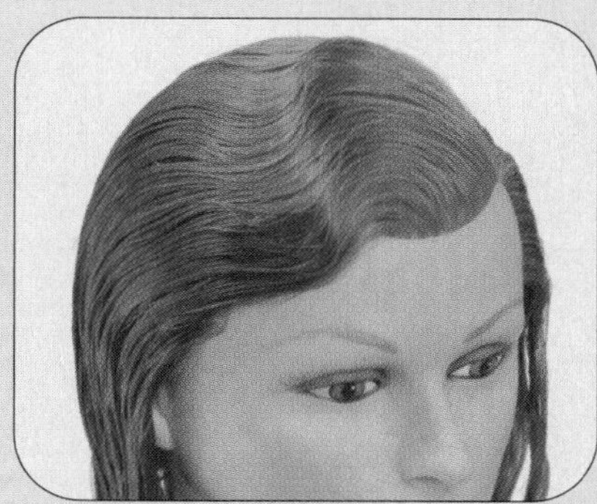

Figure 12-13 Completed first ridge.

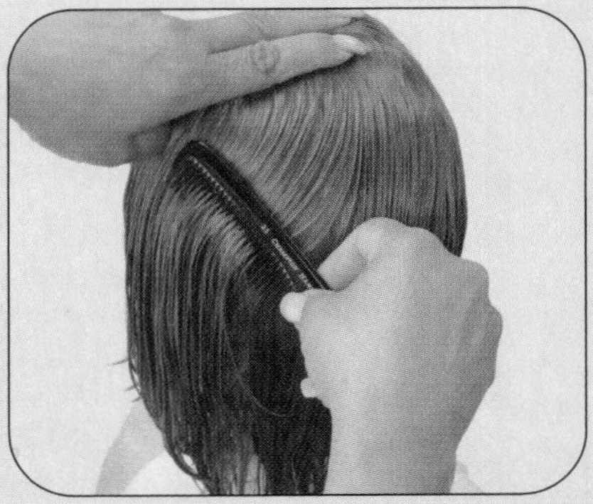

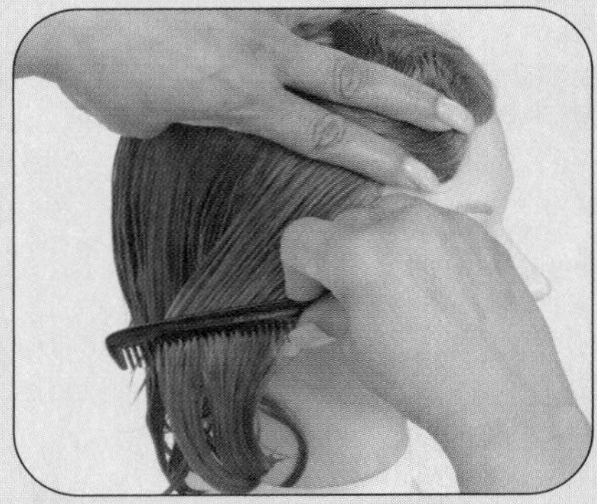

Figure 12–14 Start the second ridge.

10. Movements for the third ridge closely follow those used to create the first ridge. However, the third ridge is started at the hairline and is extended back toward the back of the head (Figure 12–16).
11. Continue alternating directions until the side of the head has been completed.
12. Use the same procedure for the left (light) side of the head as you used for finger waving the right (heavy) side of the head. First, shape the hair by combing it in the direction of the first wave (Figure 12–17).
13. Starting at the hairline, form the first ridge, section by section, until the second ridge of the opposite side is reached (Figure 12–18).
14. Both the ridge and the wave must blend without splits or breaks, with the ridge and wave on the right side of the head (Figure 12–19).
15. Start with the ridge and wave in the back of the head and proceed, section by section, toward the left side of the face.

Figure 12–15 Complete second ridge.

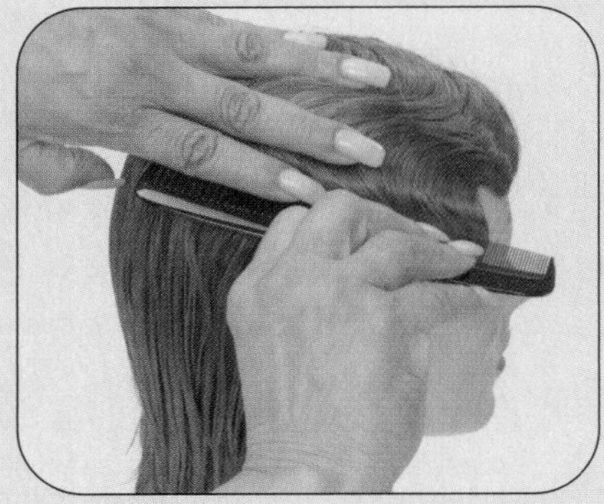

Figure 12–16 Start the third ridge.

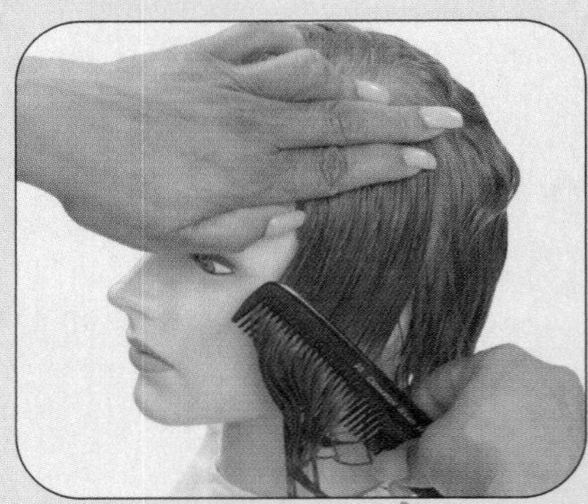

Figure 12–17 Shape the left side.

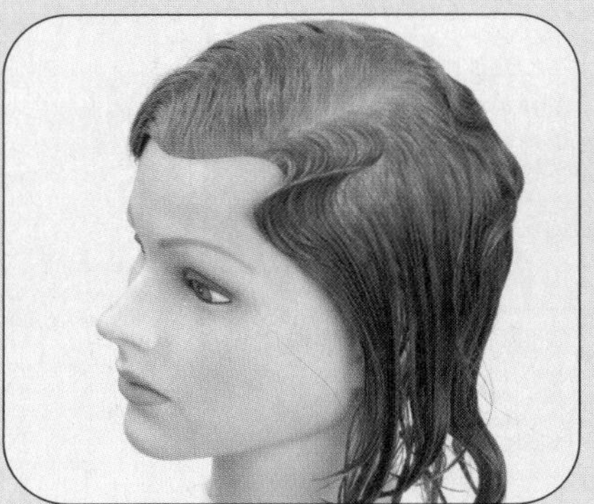

Figure 12–18 Start first ridge at hairline.

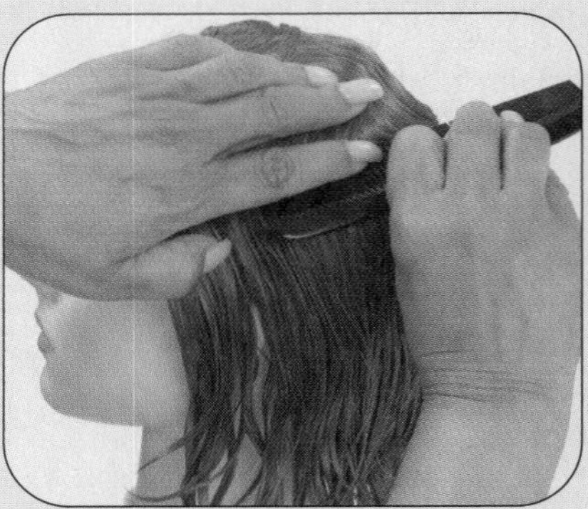

Figure 12–19 Ridge and wave matched in crown area.

16. Continue working back and forth until the entire side is completed (Figure 12–20).
17. Place a net over the hair, secure it with hairpins or clips if necessary, and protect the client's forehead and ears with cotton, gauze, or paper protectors while under the hood dryer. Adjust the dryer to medium heat and allow the hair to dry thoroughly.
18. Remove the client from under the dryer and let the hair cool down. Remove all clips or pins and the hairnet from the hair.
19. Comb out or brush the hair into a soft, waved hairstyle. Add a finishing spray for hold and shine (Figure 12–21 and Figure 12–22). For a retro, avant garde, or dramatic look, do not comb or brush, but perhaps add a hair ornament such as a rhinestone clip in the hollow portion of a wave.

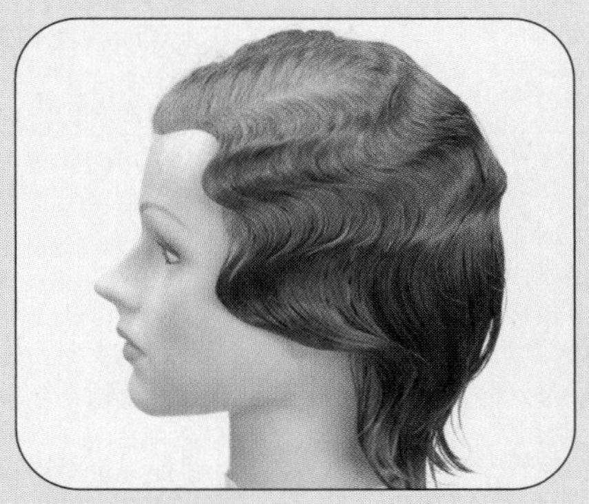

Figure 12-20 Left side completed.

Cleanup and Sanitation

1. Disinfect brushes, combs, hairpins, clips, cape, and hairnet after each use.
2. Sanitize your workstation.
3. Wash your hands with soap and warm water.

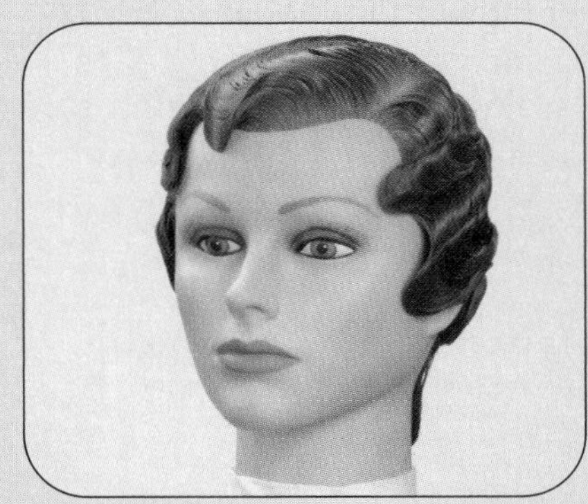

Figure 12-21 Finished hairstyle.

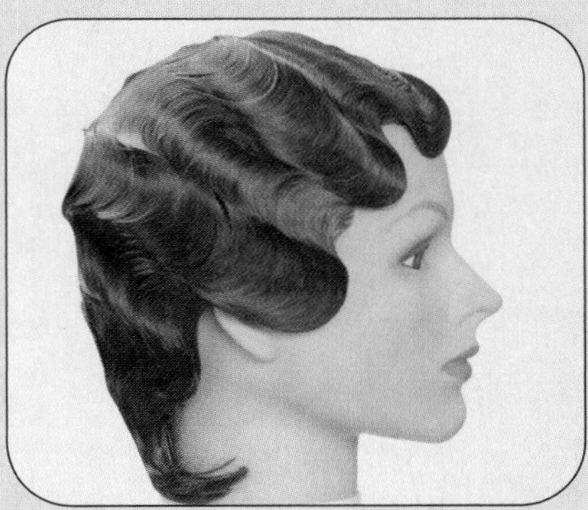

Figure 12-22 Side view.

completed!

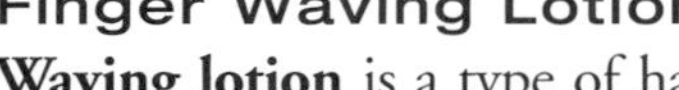

Finger Waving Lotion

Waving lotion is a type of hair gel that makes the hair pliable enough to keep it in place during the finger waving procedure. It is made from karaya gum, taken from trees found in Africa and India. Karaya gum is diluted for use on fine hair, or it can be used in a more concentrated consistency on regular or coarse hair. A good waving lotion is harmless to the hair and does not flake when it dries. Be sure not use too much of it at any one time. You will know if you have used too much as the hair will be too wet and the waving lotion will drip. Liquid styling gels are also commonly used in conjunction with finger waving, and in some cases, have phased out traditional karaya gum products.

Other Methods of Finger Waving

Instead of completing one side before beginning the other, you may want to complete the first ridge on one side of the head and then move to the other side to form the first ridge on that side. After joining the two, you can then repeat in this manner until you are finished with the entire head.

In vertical finger waving, the ridges and waves run up and down the head. Horizontal finger waves are sideways and parallel around the head. The procedure is the same for both.

PIN CURLS

Pin curls serve as the basis for patterns, lines, waves, curls, and rolls that are used in a wide range of hairstyles. You can use them on straight, permanent waved, or naturally curly hair. Pin curls work best when the hair is properly layered and is smoothly wound. This makes springy and long-lasting curls with good direction and definition.

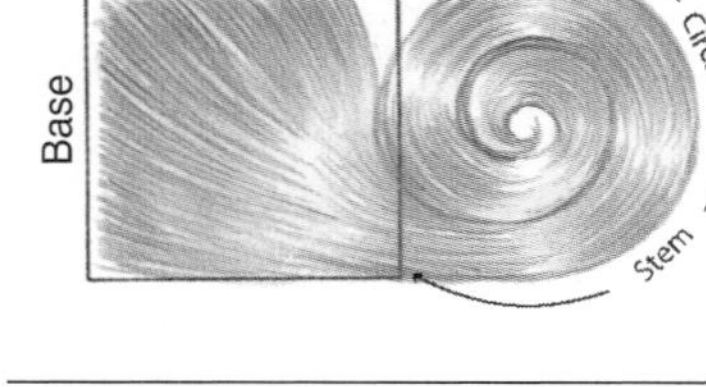

Figure 12-23 Parts of a curl.

Parts of a Curl

Pin curls are made up of three principal parts: base, stem, and circle (Figure 12–23).

1. The **base** is the stationary, or nonmoving, foundation of the curl, which is the area closest to the scalp.
2. The **stem** is the section of the pin curl, between the base and first arc (turn) of the circle, that gives the circle its direction and movement.
3. The **circle** is the part of the pin curl that forms a complete circle. The size of the circle determines the width of the wave and its strength.

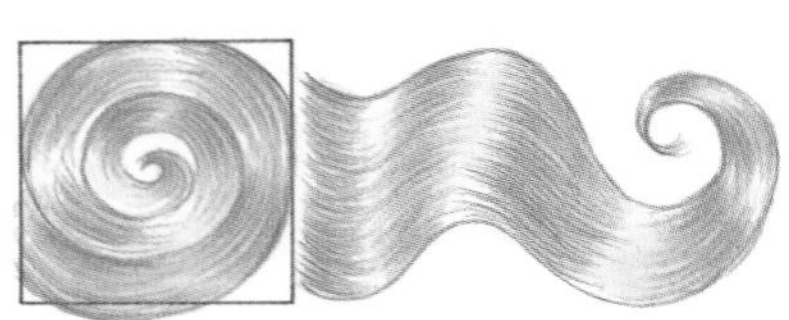

Figure 12-24 No-stem curl opened out.

Mobility of a Curl

The stem determines the amount of mobility, or movement, of a section of hair. Curl mobility is classified as no stem, half stem, and full stem.

- The **no-stem curl** is placed directly on the base of the curl. It produces a tight, firm, long-lasting curl and allows minimum mobility (Figure 12–24).
- The **half-stem curl** permits medium movement; the curl (circle) is placed half off the base. It gives good control to the hair (Figure 12–25).
- The **full-stem curl** allows for the greatest mobility. The curl is placed completely off the base. The base may be a square, triangular, half-moon, or rectangular section, depending on the area of the head in which the full-stem curls are used. It gives as much freedom as the length of the stem will permit. If it is exaggerated, the hair near the scalp will be flat and almost straight. It is used to give the hair a strong, definite direction (Figure 12–26).

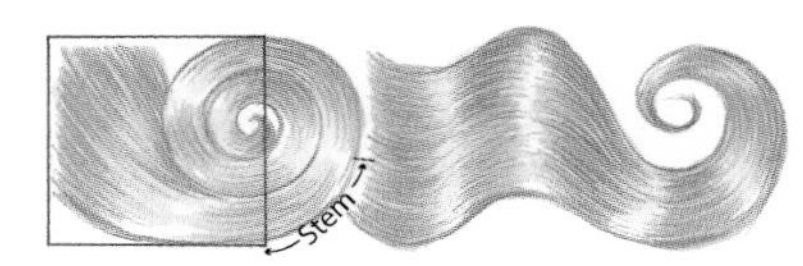

Figure 12-25 Half-stem curl opened out.

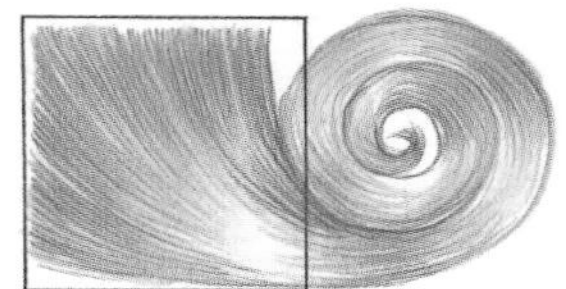

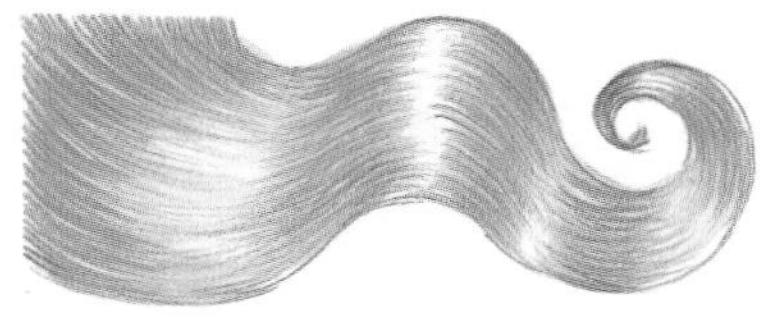

Figure 12-26 Full-stem curl opened out.

Shaping for Pin Curl Placements

A **shaping** is a section of hair that is molded in a circular movement in preparation for the formation of curls. Shapings are either open end or closed end. Always begin a pin curl at the open end, or convex side, of a shaping (Figure 12–27 and Figure 12–28).

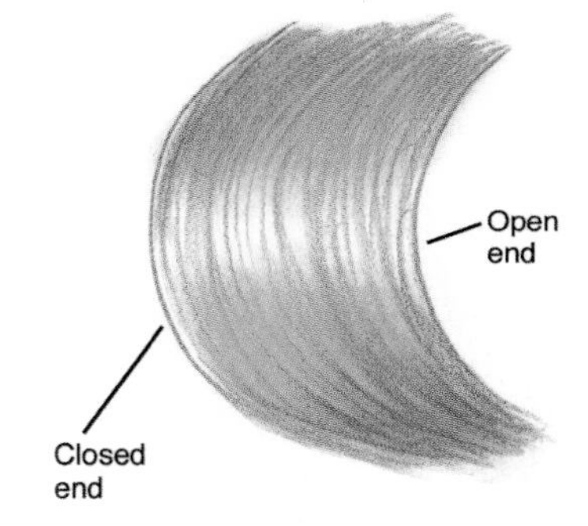

Figure 12-27 Closed and open ends of a curl.

Open and Closed Center Curls

Open center curls produce even, smooth waves and uniform curls. **Closed center curls** produce waves that get smaller in size toward the end. They are good for fine hair or if a fluffy curl is desired. Notice the difference in the waves produced by pin curls with open centers and those with closed centers. The width of the curl determines the size of the wave. If you make pin curls with the ends outside the curl, the resulting wave will be narrower near the scalp and wider toward the ends (Figure 12–29 and Figure 12–30).

Curl and Stem Direction

Curls may be turned toward the face, away from the face, upward, downward, or diagonally. The finished result will be determined by the direction in which the stem of the curl is placed.

The terms clockwise curls and counterclockwise curls are used to describe the direction of pin curls. Curls formed in the same direction as the

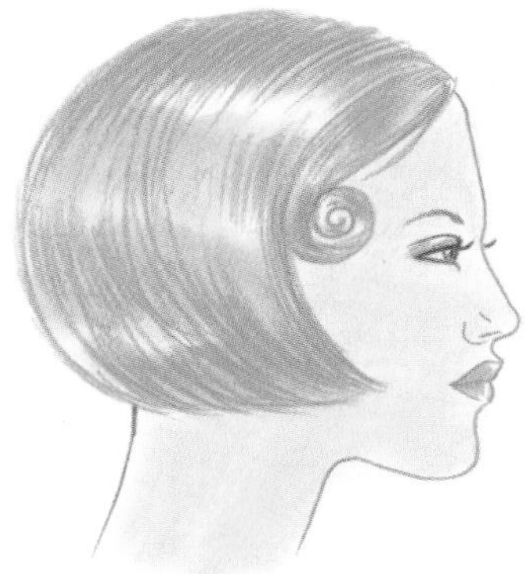

Figure 12-28 Curl in the shaping.

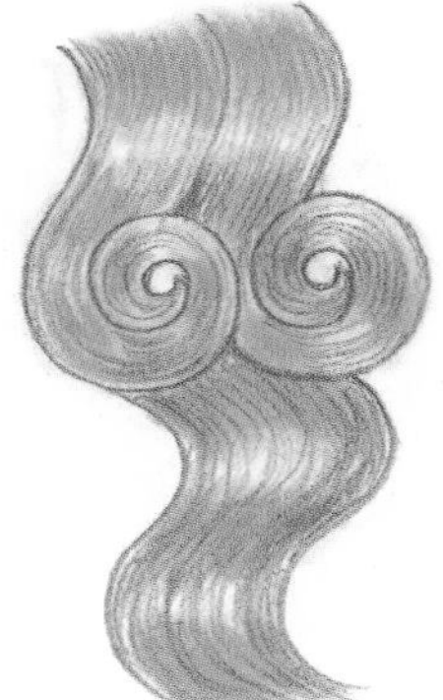

Figure 12-29 Curl with open center.

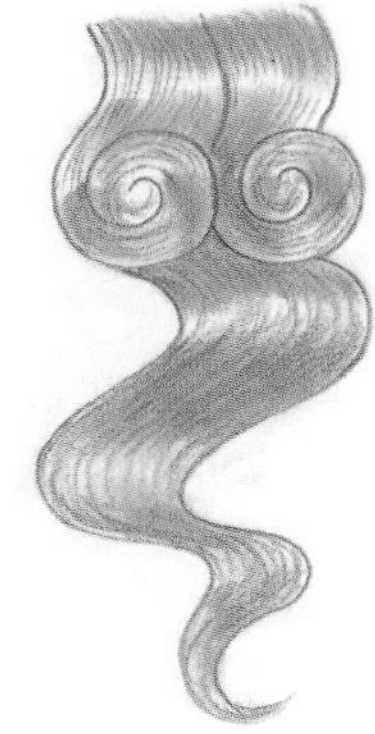

Figure 12-30 Curl with closed center.

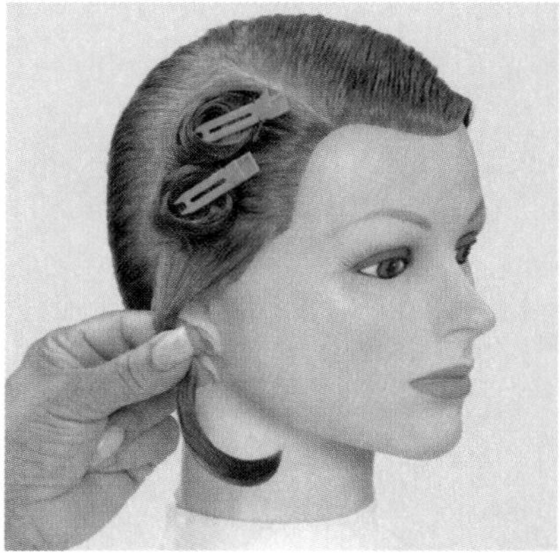

Figure 12-31 Rectangular base pin curls.

movement of the hands of a clock are known as clockwise curls. Curls formed in the opposite direction are known as counterclockwise curls.

Pin Curl Foundations or Bases

Before you begin to make pin curls, divide the wet hair into sections or panels. Then subdivide each section into the type of base required for the various curls. The most commonly shaped base you will use is the arc base (half-moon or "C" shape). Others are rectangular, triangular, or square.

To avoid splits in the finished hairstyle, you must use care when selecting and forming the curl base. When the sections of hair are as equal as possible, you will get curls that are similar to one another. Each curl must lie flat and smooth on its base. If too far off the base, the curl will lie loose away from the scalp. The shape of the base, however, does not affect the finished curl.

- *Rectangular base pin curls* are usually recommended at the side front hairline for a smooth, upsweep effect (Figure 12–31). To avoid splits in the comb-out, the pin curls must overlap.
- *Triangular base pin curls* are recommended along the front or facial hairline to prevent breaks or splits in the finished hairstyle. The triangular base allows a portion of the hair from each curl to overlap the next and can be combed into a wave without splits (Figure 12–32).
- *Arc base pin curls*, also known as half-moon or "C" shape base curls, are carved out of a shaping. Arc base pin curls give good direction and may be used at the hairline or in the nape (Figure 12–33).
- *Square base pin curls* are suitable for curly hairstyles without much volume or lift. They can be used on any part of the head and will comb out with lasting results. To avoid splits in the comb-out, stagger the sectioning as shown in the illustration (square base, bricklay fashion) (Figure 12–34).

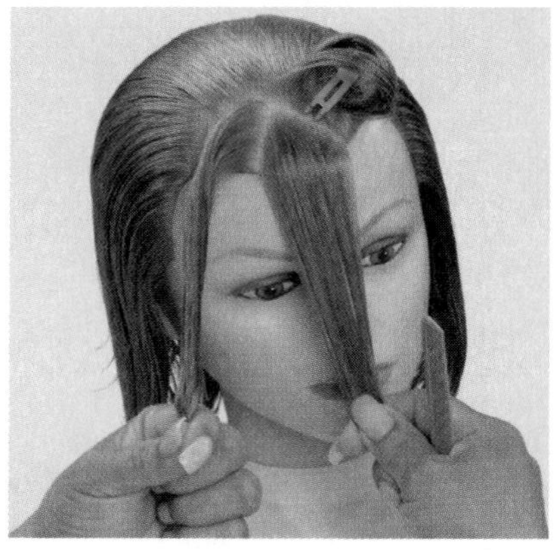

Figure 12-32 Triangular base pin curls.

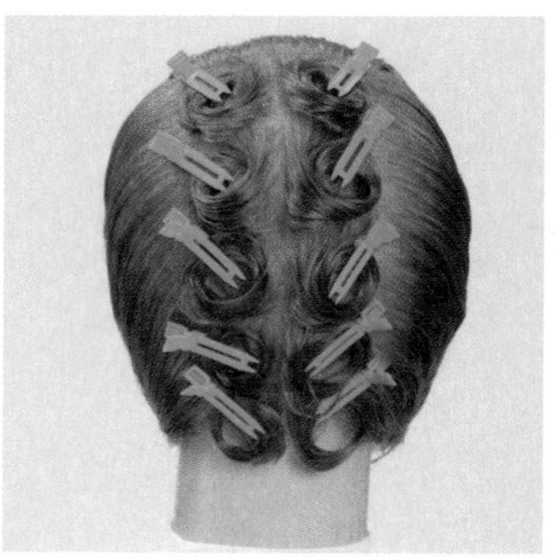

Figure 12-33 Arc base pin curls.

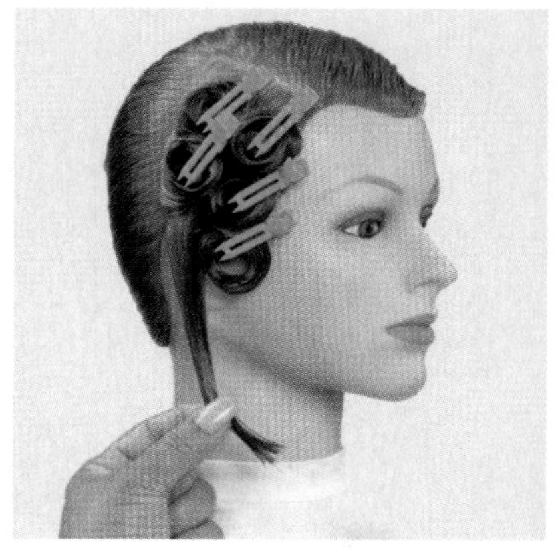

Figure 12-34 Square base pin curls.

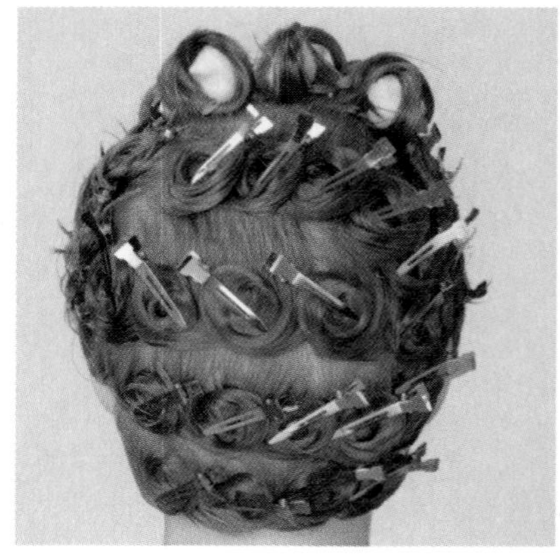

Figure 12-35 Setting pattern for wave.

Pin Curl Techniques

There are a number of different methods used to make pin curls. We will illustrate several methods below, but your instructor might demonstrate other methods that are equally correct.

One important technique to learn is called **ribboning**, which involves forcing the hair between the thumb and the back of the comb to create tension. You can also ribbon hair by pulling the strands while applying pressure between your thumb and index finger out toward the ends of the strands.

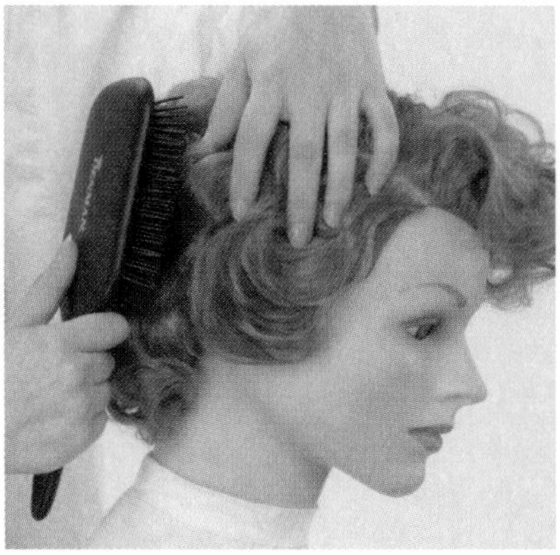

Carved Curls or Sculptured Curls

Pin curls sliced from a shaping and formed without lifting the hair from the head are referred to as **carved curls**. The technique of **ribboning**, described above, also features in this method.

Figure 12-36 Comb-out of wave setting.

Designing With Pin Curls

- To create a wave, use two rows of pin curls. Set one row clockwise and the second row counterclockwise (Figure 12–35 and Figure 12–36).
- **Ridge curls** are pin curls placed immediately behind or below a ridge to form a wave (Figure 12–37 and Figure 12–38).
- **Skip waves** are two rows of ridge curls, usually on the side of the head. They create a strong wave pattern with well-defined lines between the waves. This technique represents a combination of finger waving and pin curls (Figure 12–39 and Figure 12–40).

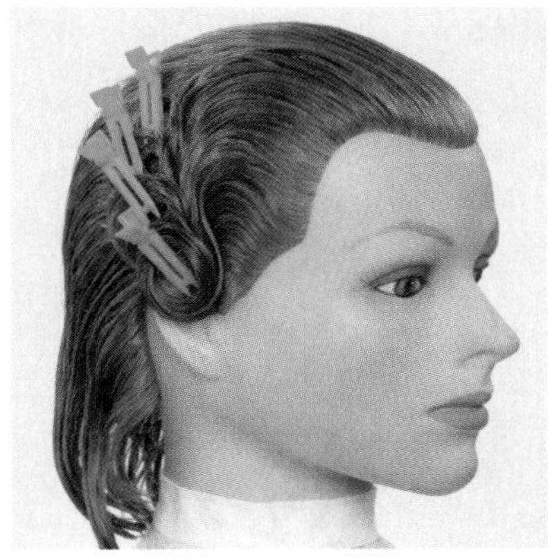

Figure 12-37 Setting pattern for ridge curl.

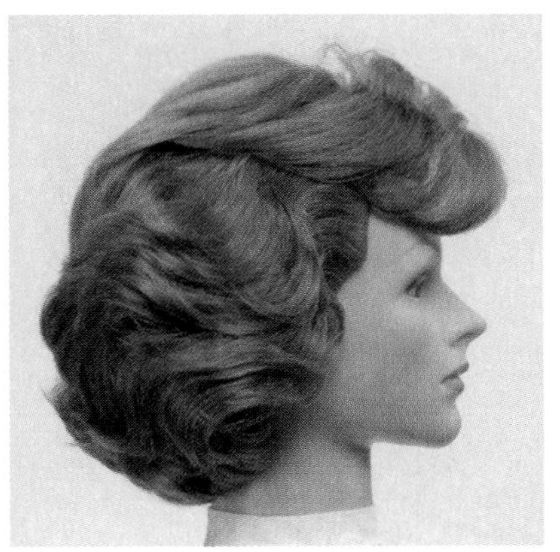

Figure 12-38 Comb-out for ridge curl.

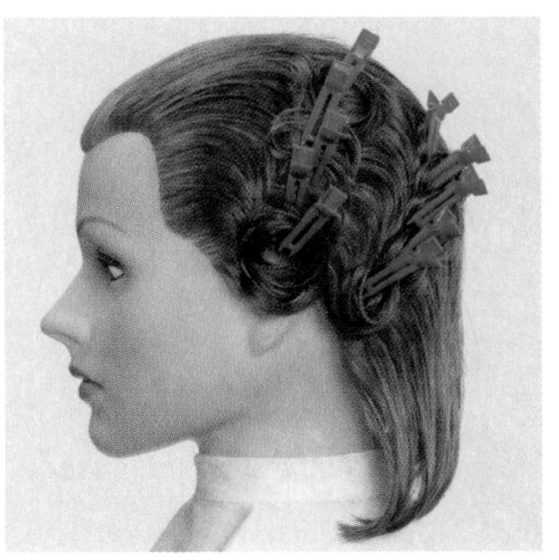

Figure 12-39 Setting pattern for skip wave.

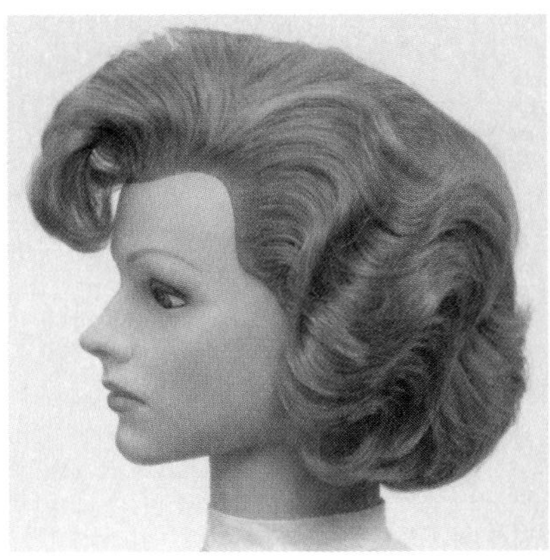

Figure 12-40 Comb-out of skip wave setting.

PROCEDURE

CARVED OR SCULPTURED CURLS

Implements and Materials

Use the list of implements and materials under Procedure 8—preparing the hair for wet styling and add the following:

- styling comb
- setting lotion
- double prong clips

Preparation

1. Follow the steps in Procedure 8—preparing the hair for wet styling
2. Apply a gel or setting lotion and comb the hair smoothly.

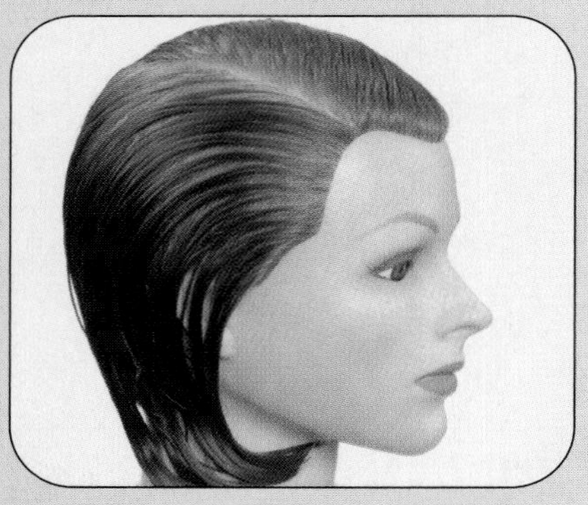

Figure 12-41 Form the first shaping.

12

Procedure

1. Form the first shaping (Figure 12-41).
2. Start making curls at the open end of the shaping. Slice a strand to create the first curl (Figure 12-42). Point your left index finger down and hold the strand in place.
3. Ribbon the strand (Figure 12-43).
4. Wind the curl forward, keeping the hair ends inside the center of the curl (Figure 12-44).
5. Hold the curl in the shaping and anchor it with a clip (Figure 12-45).

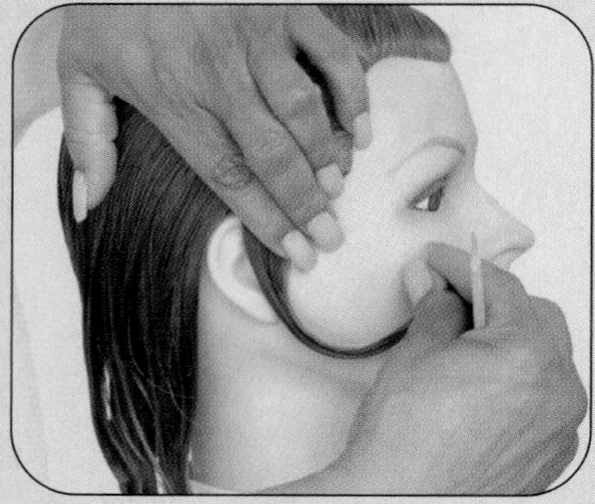

Figure 12-42 Slicing.

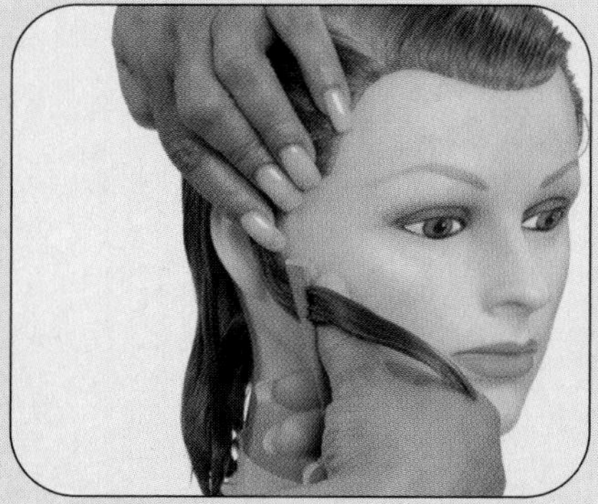

Figure 12-43 Ribbon the strand.

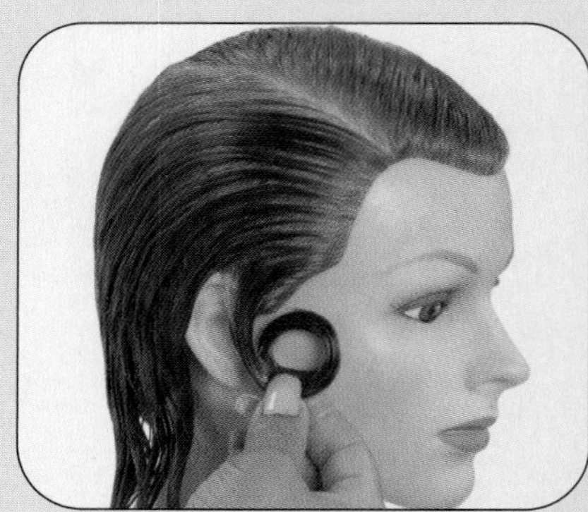

Figure 12-44 Wind the curl.

Follow the steps below to anchor pin curls correctly so that the curls hold firmly where you have placed them. This will allow you to comb the hair into the style you have planned.

1. To anchor pin curls, start at the open end of the curl. This is the side opposite the stem (Figure 12–46).
2. The clip should enter the circle parallel to the stem. Open the clip and place one prong above and one prong below one side of the circle. The upper prong should enter the hair in the center of the circle. The curl should be in the gap between the prongs. To avoid an indentation ("dent") in the curl, do not pin across the circle (Figure 12–47 and Figure 12–48).
3. If any clips touch the skin, place cotton between the skin and the clip to keep the skin from burning when the client is placed under the hood dryer.

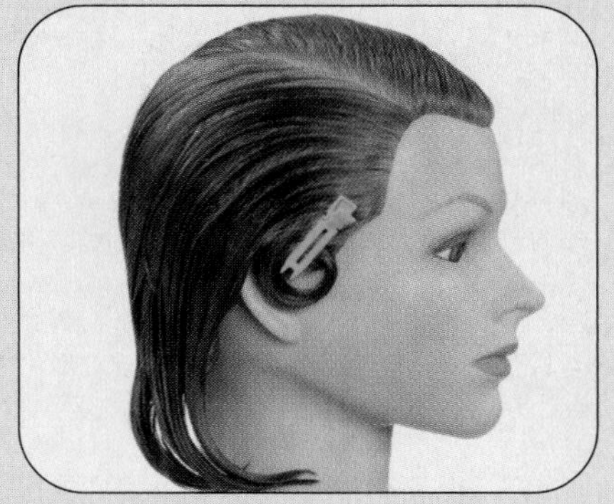

Figure 12–45 Anchor the curl.

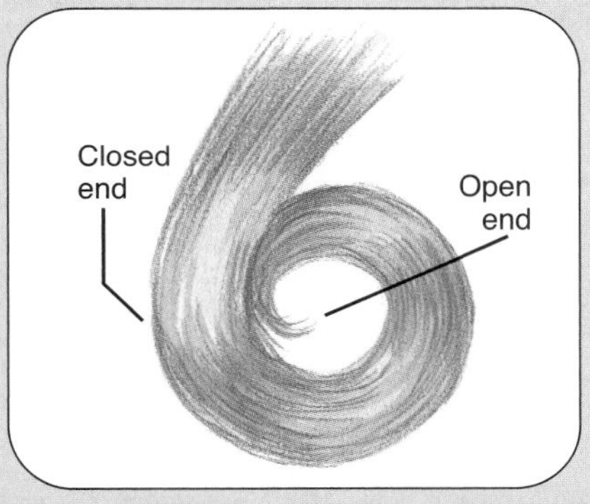

Figure 12–46 Closed and open ends of curl.

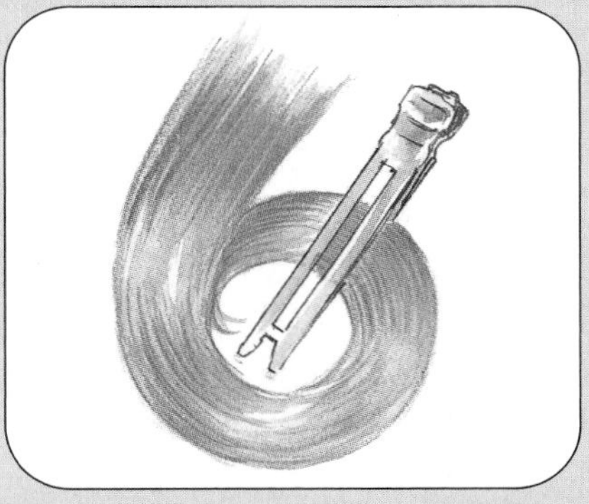

Figure 12–47 Correct placement of clip.

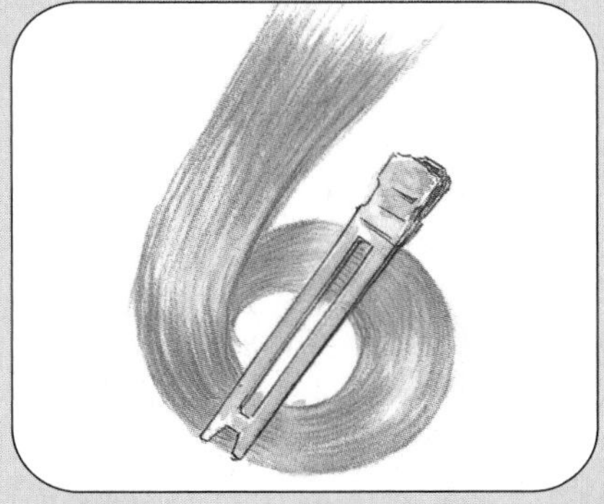

Figure 12–48 Incorrect placement of clip.

12

completed!

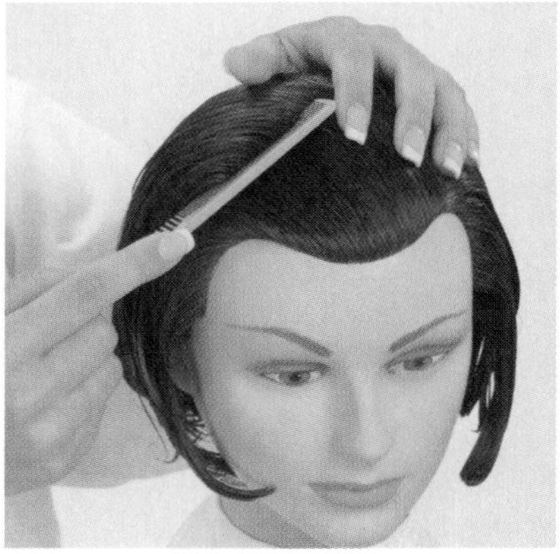

Figure 12–49 Comb, divide, and smooth section.

CREATING VOLUME WITH PIN CURLS

One of the best things about pin curls is that they contribute to the volume of the hair. Two types of pin curls that are particularly effective in this respect are:

- **cascade or stand-up curls**, which are used to create height in the hair design. They are fastened to the head in a standing position to allow the hair to flow upward and then downward. The size of the curl determines the amount of height in the comb-out (Figure 12–49, Figure 12–50, Figure 12–51, Figure 12–52, Figure 12–53, Figure 12–54, and Figure 12–55).
- **barrel curls**, which have large center openings and are fastened to the head in a standing position on a rectangular base. They have the same effect as stand-up pin curls. A barrel curl is similar to a roller but does not have the same tension as a roller when it is set.

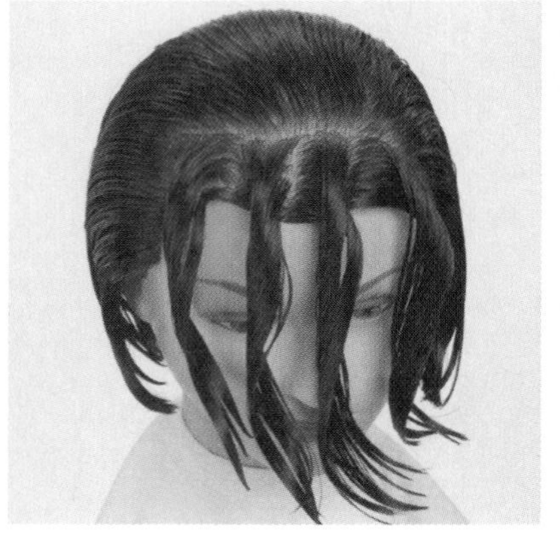

Figure 12–50 Divide section into strands.

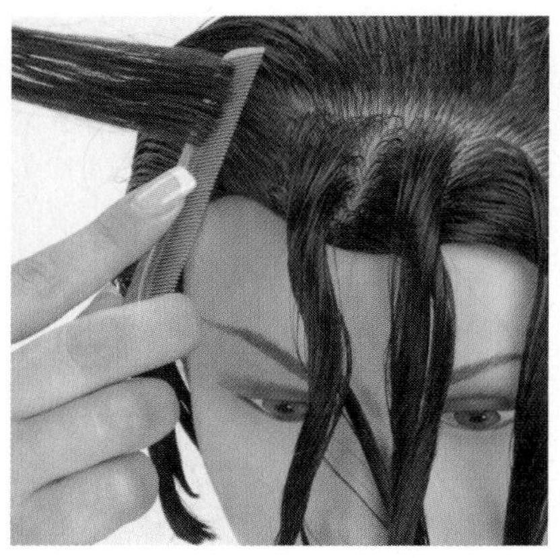

Figure 12–51 Ribbon the strand.

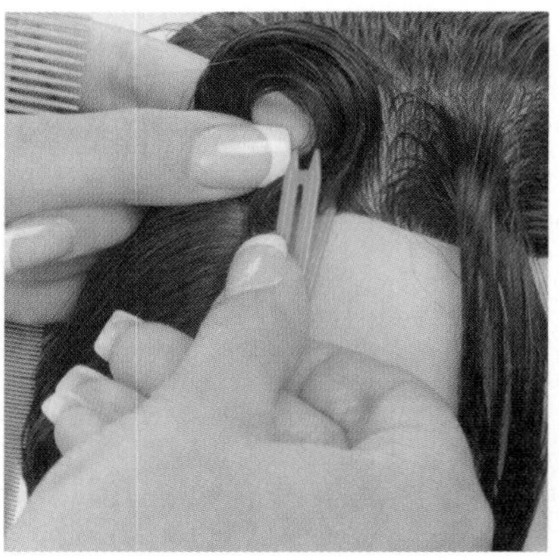

Figure 12–52 Direct the strand.

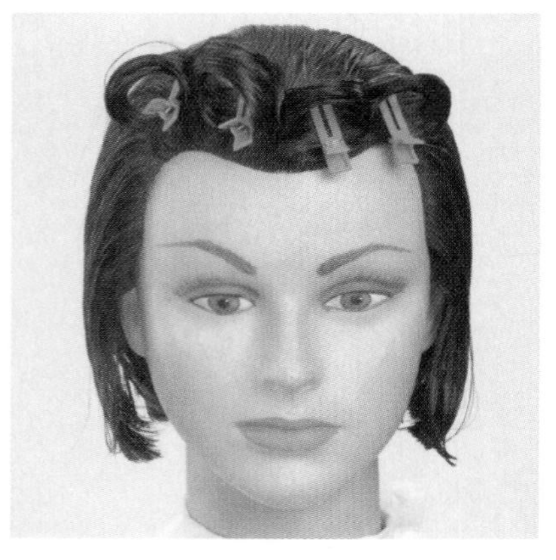

Figure 12–53 Anchor curl at base.

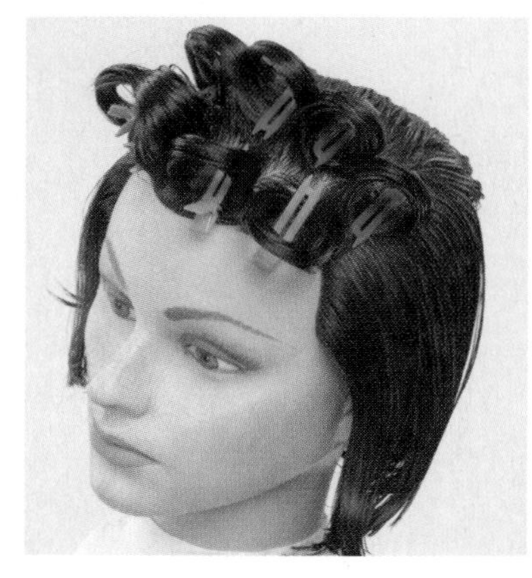

Figure 12–54 Top setting.

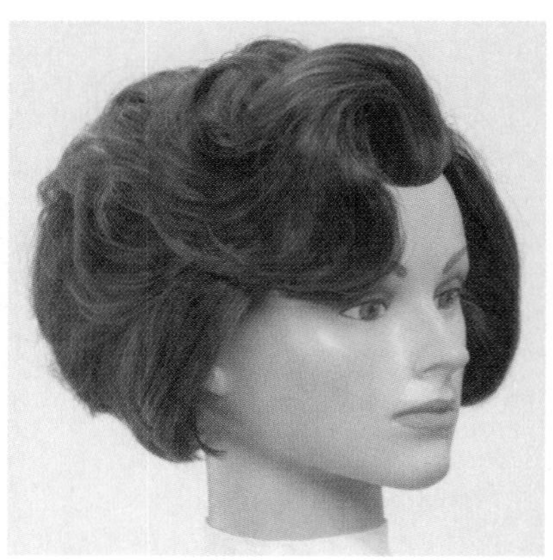

Figure 12–55 Comb out as you would a roller set.

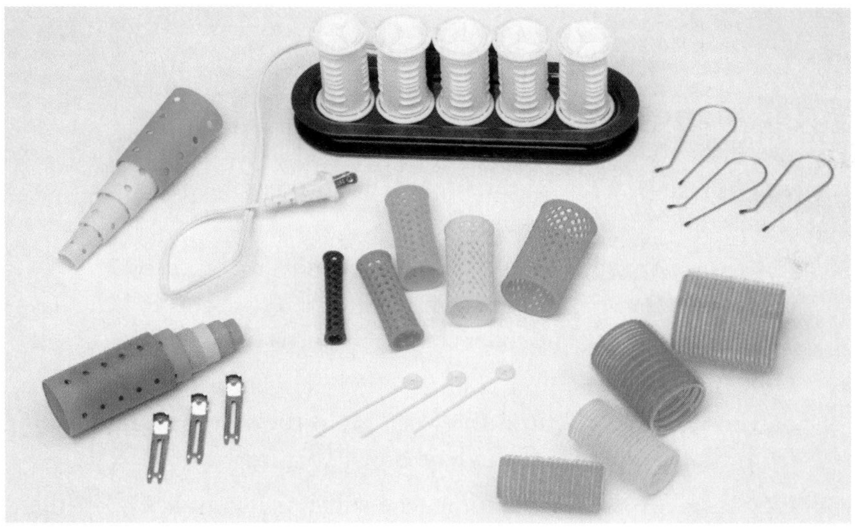

Figure 12–56 Rollers: plastic, mesh, hot, and Velcro.

ROLLER CURLS

Rollers are used to create many of the same effects as stand-up pin curls. Rollers have the following advantages over pin curls.

- Because a roller holds the equivalent of two to four stand-up curls, the roller is a much faster way to set the hair.
- The hair is wrapped around the roller with tension, which gives a stronger and longer-lasting set.
- Rollers come in a variety of shapes, widths, and sizes, which broadens the creative possibilities for any style (Figure 12–56).

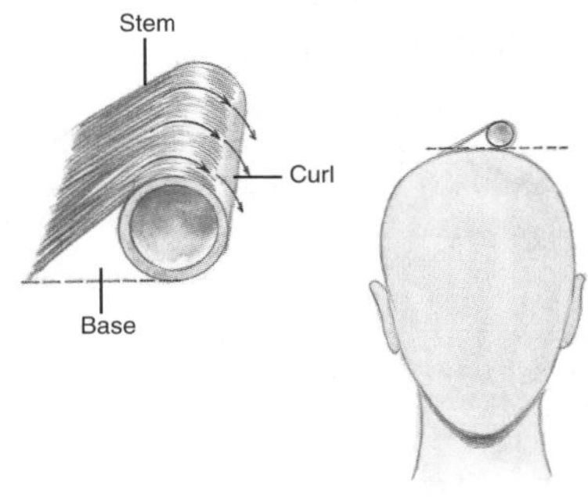

Figure 12–57 Parts of a roller curl.

Parts of a Roller Curl

It is important for you to be able to identify the three parts of a roller curl (Figure 12–57).

- **Base**. The panel of hair on which the roller is placed. The base should be the same length and width as the roller. The type of base affects the volume.
- **Stem**. The hair between the scalp and the first turn of the roller. The stem gives the hair direction and mobility.
- **Curl** or circle. The hair that is wrapped around the roller. It determines the size of the wave or curl.

Choosing Your Roller Size

The relationship between the length of the hair and the size of the roller will determine whether the result will be a C shape, a wave, or a curl. These three shapes are created as follows.

1. One complete turn around the roller will create a C-shaped curl (Figure 12–58).

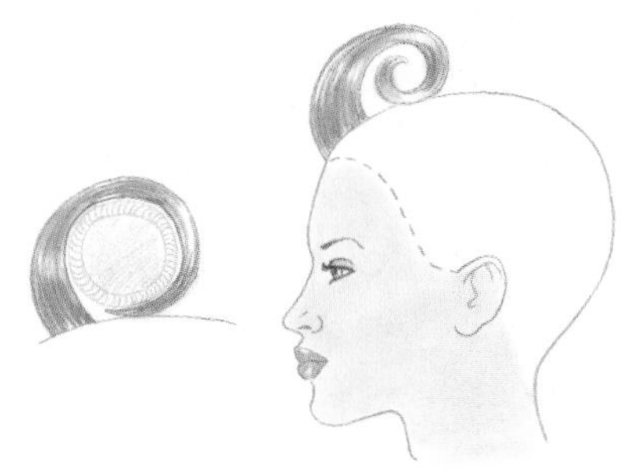

Figure 12–58 C-shaped curl.

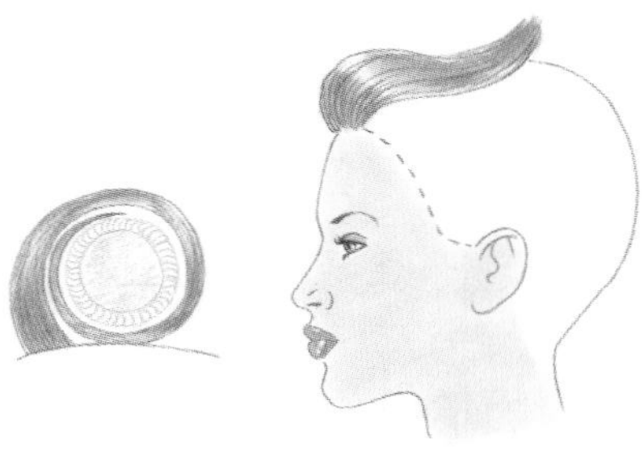

Figure 12-59 Wave.

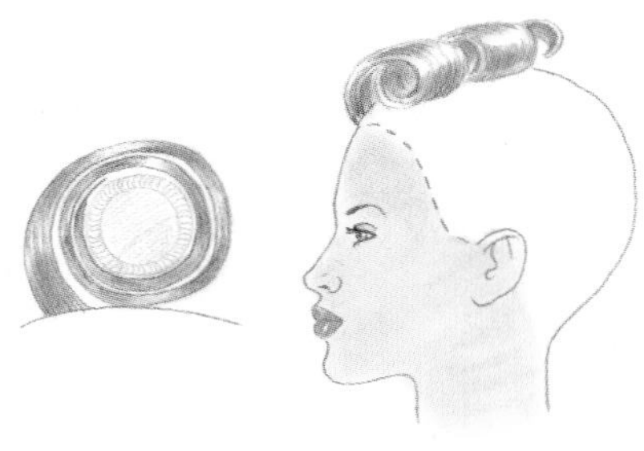

Figure 12-60 Curl.

2. One-and-a-half turns will create a wave (Figure 12–59).
3. Two-and-a-half turns will create curls (Figure 12–60).

Roller Placement

The size of the roller and how it sits on its base will determine the volume achieved. The general rule of thumb is that the larger the roller, the greater the volume. There are three kinds of bases.

1. **On base**. For full volume, the roller sits directly on its base. Overdirect the strand slightly in front of the base and roll the hair down to the base. The roller should fit on the base (Figure 12–61).
2. **Half base**. For medium volume, the roller sits halfway on its base and halfway behind the base. Hold the strand straight up from the head and roll the hair down (Figure 12–62).
3. **Off base** For the least volume, the roller sits completely off the base. Hold the strand 45 degrees back from the base and roll the hair down (Figure 12–63).

Hot Rollers

Hot rollers are used on dry hair only. They are heated either electrically or by steam, and are a great time-saver in the salon. Follow the same setting patterns as with wet setting, but allow the hot roller to stay on the hair for only about 10 minutes. Hot rollers usually come with their own clips to secure them. A thermal protector can be sprayed on the hair prior to the set. Some manufacturers have spray-on products to apply to each section of hair that help it take a stronger set.

Velcro Rollers

As with hot rollers, Velcro rollers are used on dry hair only. Using them on wet hair will snag and pull the hair. If you have a client who needs more body than can be achieved with a round brush and less volume than a hot roller or wet set will produce, try Velcro rollers. When they are used after

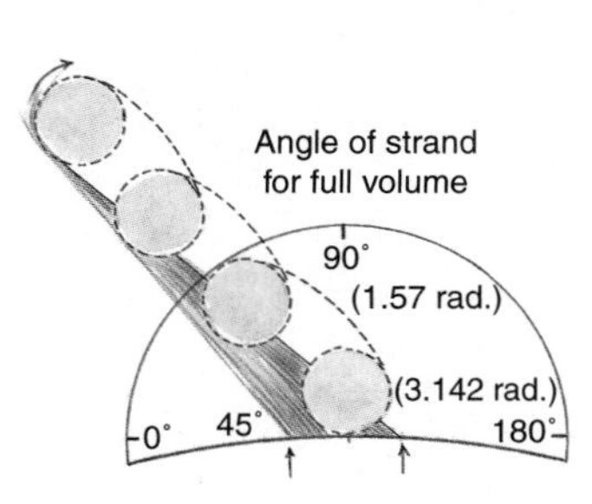

Figure 12-61 On base roller: full volume.

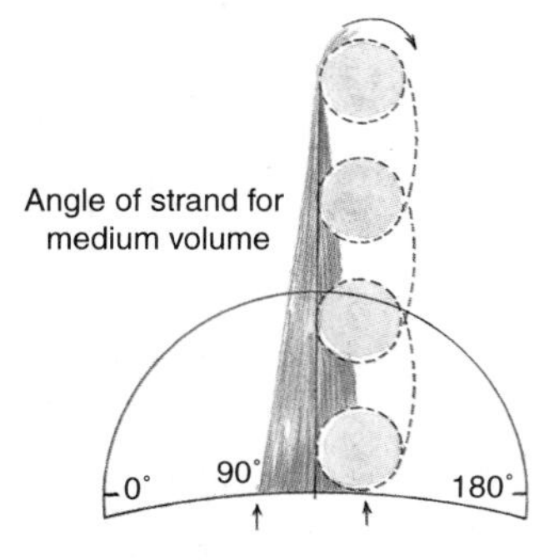

Figure 12-62 One-half base roller: medium volume.

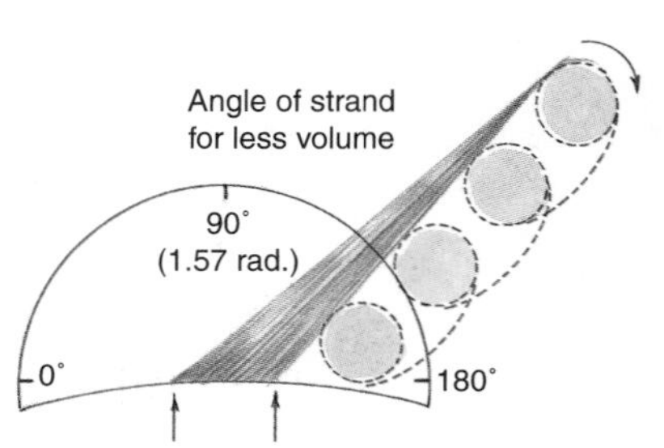

Figure 12-63 Off base roller: less volume.

PROCEDURE

WET SET WITH ROLLERS

Implements and Materials

Use the list of implements and materials under Procedure 8—preparing the hair for wet styling and add the following:

- rollers of various sizes made from plastic, wire with mesh covering, or sponge
- setting or styling lotion
- Clips (double or single prong)
- tail comb

Preparation

1. Follow the steps under Procedure 8—preparing the hair for wet styling
2. Apply a setting or styling lotion.

Procedure

1. Comb the hair in the direction of the setting pattern. Shapings may be used to accent the design.
2. Starting at the front hairline, part off a section the same length and width as the roller. Choose the type of base according to the desired volume. Comb the hair out from the scalp to the ends using the fine teeth of the comb. Repeat several times to make sure that the hair is smooth (Figure 12–64).

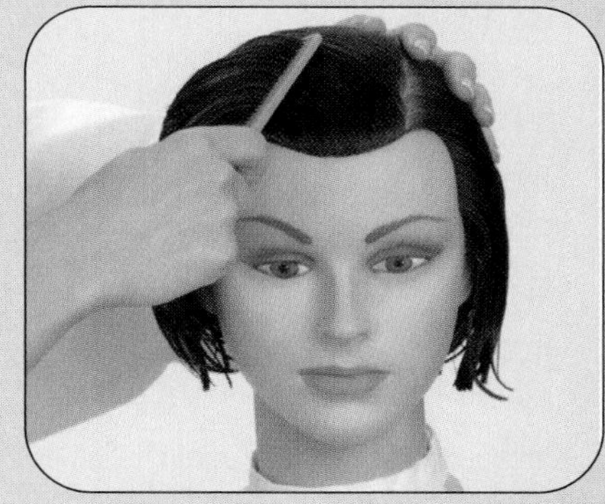

Figure 12–64 Comb section from scalp to ends.

3. Hold the hair with tension between the thumb and middle finger of the left hand. Place the roller below the thumb of the left hand. Do not bring together the ends of the hair(Figure 12–65).Wrap the ends of the hair smoothly around the roller until the hair catches and does not release.

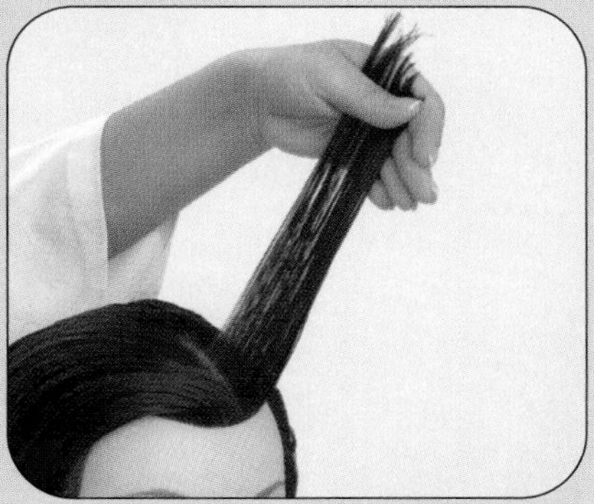

Figure 12–65 Right way to hold hair.

12

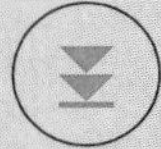

Here's a tip:

For added volume, back-comb the hair at the base a little before placing the roller in.

4. Place the thumbs over the ends of the roller and roll the hair firmly to the scalp (Figure 12–66a and Figure 12–66b).
5. Clip the roller securely to the scalp hair (Figure 12–67). Roll the remainder of the hair according to the desired style.
6. Place the client under a hood dryer. Set the dryer at a temperature that is comfortable for the client.
7. When the hair is dry, allow it to cool, then remove the rollers (Figure 12–68).
8. Comb out and style the hair as desired (see Procedure 12—combing out a wet set).

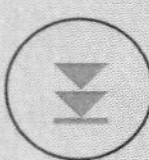

Here's a tip:

When clipping the roller, it is important to secure the roller properly to the head. A loose roller will lose its tension, resulting in a weak set. If the clip is placed at an angle against the hair, the sharp metal edge can cause the hair to break. Hold the roller against the scalp, maintaining the tension. Open the clip and slide it into the center of the roller. Place one end under the roller and one end inside the roller.

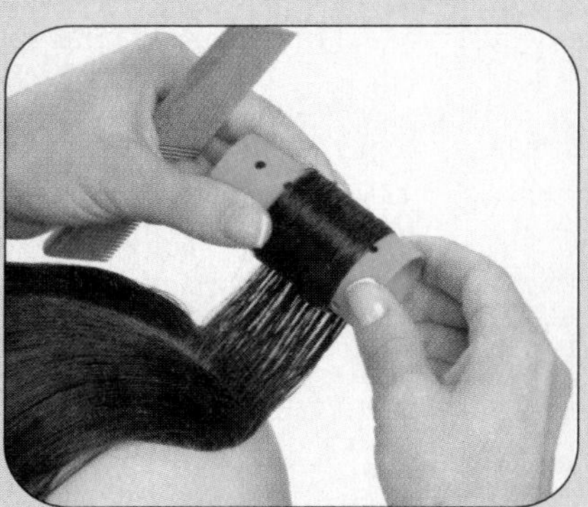

Figure 12-66a Wind the roller.

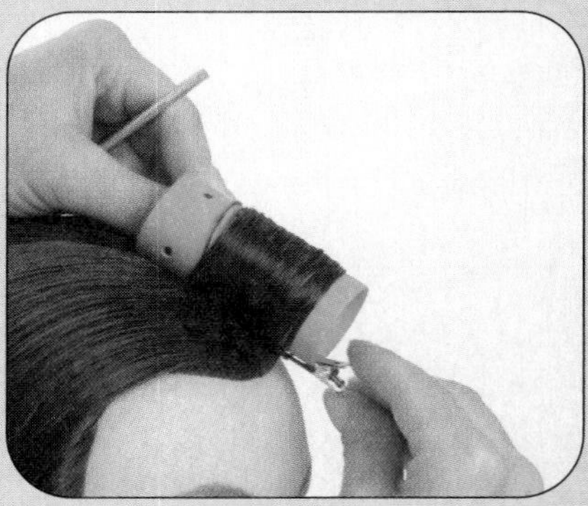

Figure 12-66b Clip the roller.

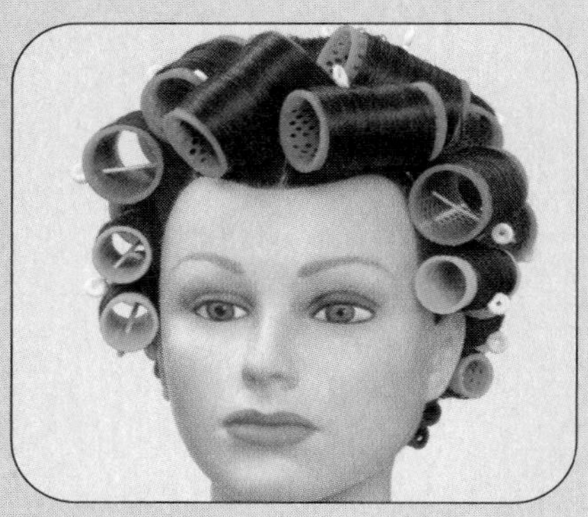

Figure 12-67 A finished roller set.

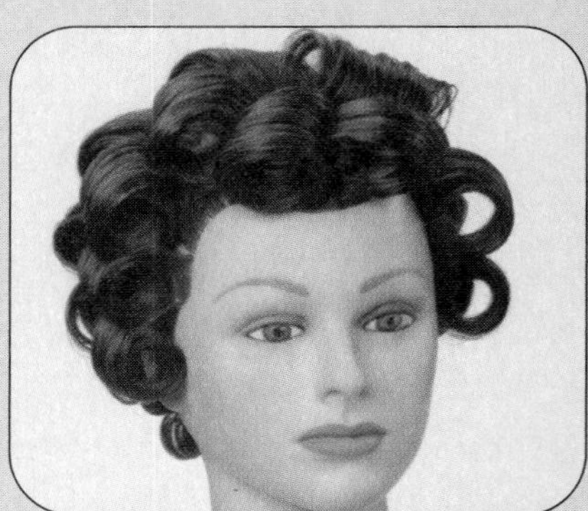

Figure 12-68 Remove the rollers.

12

completed!

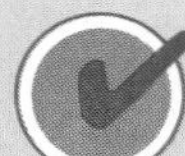

the hair is blow-dried, they may provide just the amount of volume you are looking for.

Velcro rollers need to stay in the hair for only 5 to 10 minutes, depending on how much set you want in the hair. Follow the same setting patterns as with wet setting, but keep in mind that no clipping is necessary to secure the roller. The Velcro fabric grips the hair well and stays in place on its own. Mist the entire head with hairspray, then either place the client under a hooded dryer for 5 to 10 minutes or use the diffuser attachment on your blow-dryer for the recommended time to give a soft set to the hair. For an even softer look, do not apply heat after the rollers are put in; just have your client sit for a few minutes. This would be a good time to instruct the client on how she can repeat the process at home in order to maintain the style.

Velcro rollers are not allowed by state boards in some states and provinces because of the difficulty of sanitizing them properly. Check with your regulatory agency to determine if you can use them.

Always remove any hair from Velcro and electric rollers after use. See Chapter 5, page 113, for instructions on disinfecting rollers.

COMB-OUT TECHNIQUES

Good sets lead to good comb-outs. To achieve success as a hairstylist, first master the skills of shaping and molding hair and then practice fast, simple, and effective methods for comb-outs. If you follow a well-structured system of combing out hairstyles, you will save time, get more consistent results, and build an appreciative and loyal clientele. One procedure for combing out is outlined below.

Back-Combing and Back-Brushing Techniques

Back-combing and back-brushing are the best ways to lift and increase volume, as well as to remove indentations caused by roller setting. **Back-combing**, also called teasing, ratting, matting, or French lacing, involves combing small sections of hair from the ends toward the scalp, causing shorter hair to mat at the scalp and form a cushion or base. **Back-brushing**, also called ruffing, is used to build a soft cushion or mesh two or more curl patterns together for a uniform and smooth comb-out.

During the 1950s and 1960s, women typically had their hair wet-set and combed out, and the set would last an entire week with back-combing and back-brushing. Now these techniques are used for styling updos or to add a little height to a hairstyle, after hot roller setting or blow drying. They are still useful techniques.

PROCEDURE

COMBING OUT A WET SET

Implements and Materials

- cloth cape
- neck strip
- cushioned paddle brush
- pick (optional)

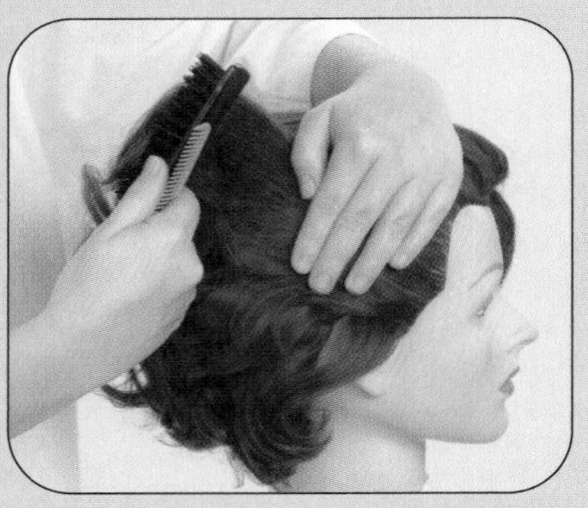

Figure 12-69 Brush out the hair.

Figure 12-70 Direct hair into desired pattern.

Procedure

1. Drape the client for the comb-out by securing a neck strip around the client's neck and placing a cloth cape over the neck strip so that the cape does not come into contact with the client's skin.
2. After removing the rollers and clips, brush the hair through and relax the set. Smooth the hair and brush it into a semi-flat condition that permits you to position the lines for the planned hairstyle (Figure 12–69). It is essential that you perform this procedure correctly in order to achieve a smooth, flowing, and finished coiffure. When combing out a curly style, use a pick or pick comb to lift and separate the curls before brushing out the hair.
3. After you have thoroughly brushed the hair, direct it into the general pattern desired. You may accomplish this by placing your hand on the client's head and gently pushing the hair forward so that the waves fall into the planned design. Lines of direction should be slightly overemphasized to allow for some relaxation during the comb-out process (Figure 12–70).
4. Back-comb areas that require volume and back-brush sections that need to be brought into the set (see section following). Accentuate and develop lines and style. Take one section at a time, placing the proper lines, ridges, volumes, and indentations into the hairstyle. You can create softness and evenness of flow by blending, smoothing, and combing (Figure 12–71). Avoid exaggerations and overemphasis. Finished patterns should reflect rhythm, balance, and smoothness of line.

5. Final touches make hairstyles look professional, so take your time. After completing the comb-out, you can use the tail of a comb to lift areas where the shape and form are not as full as you want them to be. Every touch during the final stage must be very lightly done. When you have completed your finishing touches, check the entire set for structural balance and then lightly spray the hair with a finishing spray (Figure 12–72).

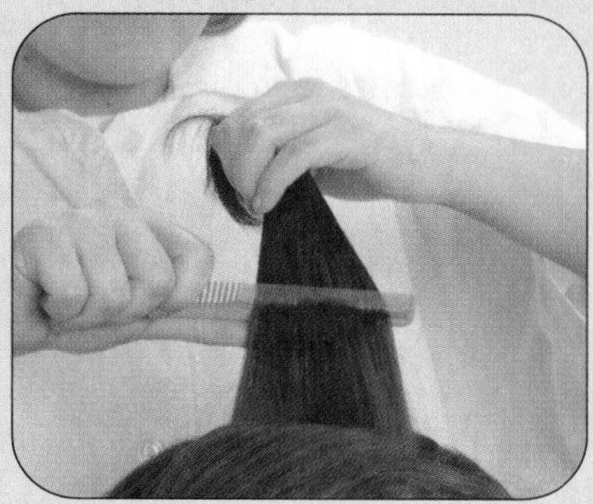

Figure 12–71 Blend sections with back-combing.

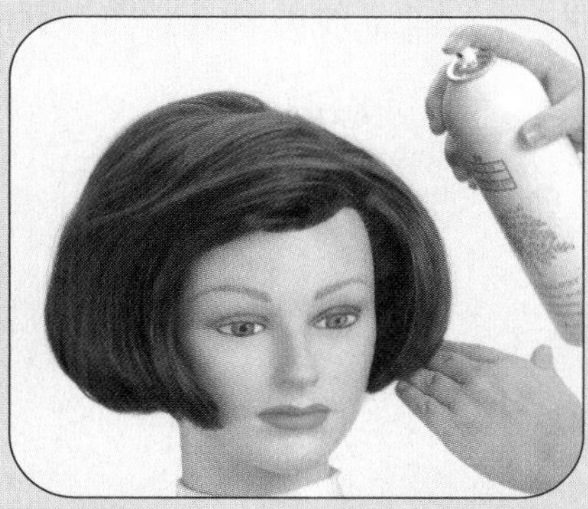

Figure 12–72 Apply finishing spray to complete style.

Cleanup and Sanitation

1. Discard the neck strip and place the cape in the appropriate hamper for laundering.
2. Thoroughly remove all hair from brushes and combs and disinfect.
3. Disinfect rollers, clips, and picks.
4. Sanitize your workstation.
5. Wash your hands with soap and warm water.

completed!

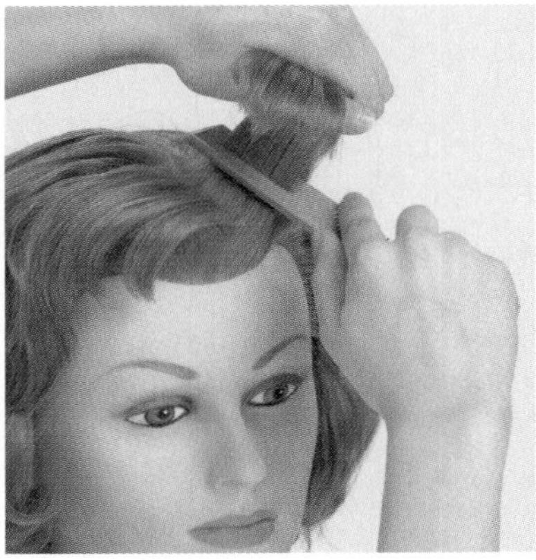

Figure 12–73 Insert comb.

Back-combing Technique

1. Starting in the front, pick up a section of hair no more than an inch in thickness and no more than 2 inches to 3 inches (5 to 7.5 cm) wide.
2. Insert the fine teeth of your comb into the hair at a depth of about 1 ½ inches (3.75 cm) from the scalp (Figure 12–73).
3. Press the comb gently down to the scalp, rotating it down and out of the hair. Repeat this process, working up the section until the desired volume is achieved (Figure 12–74).
4. If you wish to create a cushion (base), the third time you insert the comb use the same rotating motion, but firmly push the hair down to the scalp. Slide the comb out of the hair (Figure 12–75).
5. Repeat this process, working up the strand until the desired volume is achieved.
6. To smooth the hair that is back-combed, hold the teeth of the comb or the bristles of a brush at a 45-degree angle, pointed away from you, and lightly move the comb over the surface of the hair (Figure 12–76).

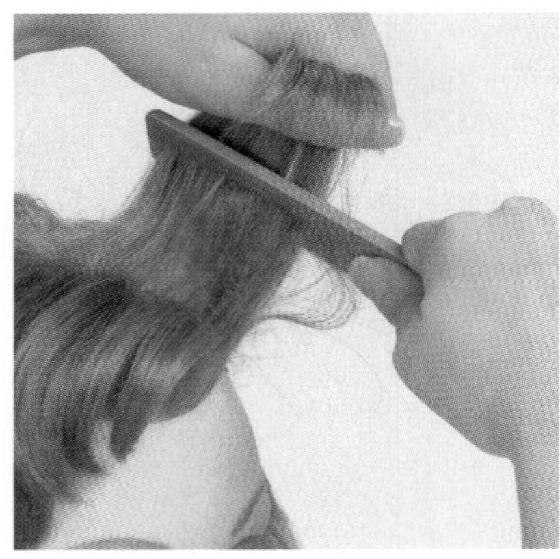

Figure 12–74 Press comb down.

Back-brushing Technique

1. Pick up and hold a strand straight out from the scalp.
2. Maintaining a slight amount of slack in the strand, place a teasing brush or a grooming brush near the base of the strand. Push and roll the inner edge of the brush with the wrist until it touches the scalp (Figure 12–77). For interlocking to occur, the brush must be rolled. Then remove the brush from the hair with a turn of the wrist, peeling back a layer of hair. The hair will be interlocked to form a soft cushion at the scalp (Figure 12–78a and Figure 12–78b).

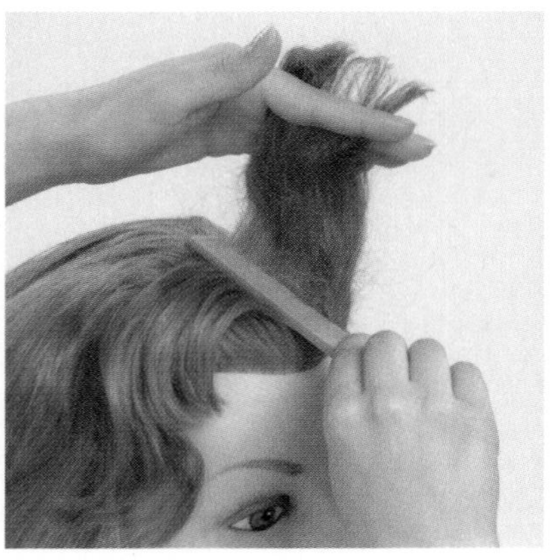

Figure 12–75 Create base of back-combed hair.

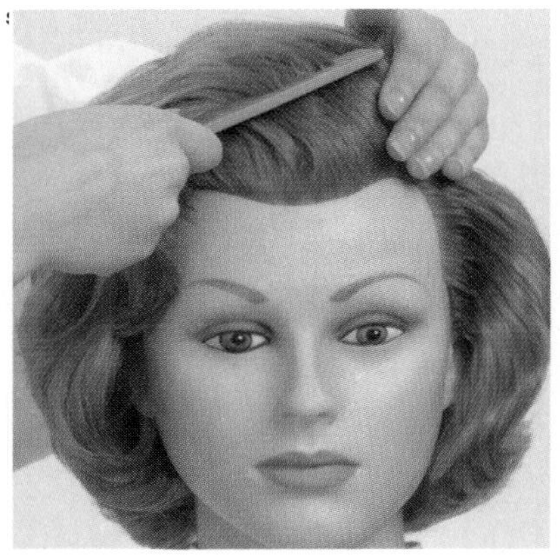

Figure 12–76 Hold brush at 45 degrees to hair.

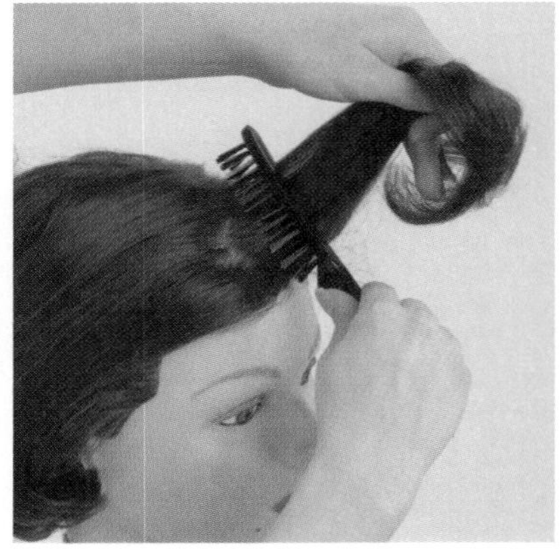

Figure 12–77 Roll brush.

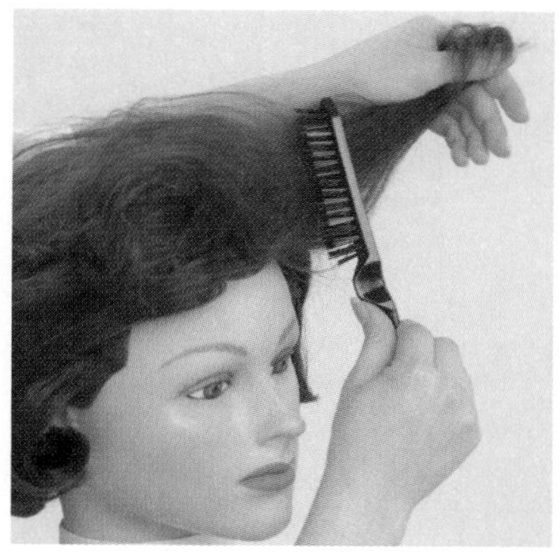

Figure 12-78a Remove brush.

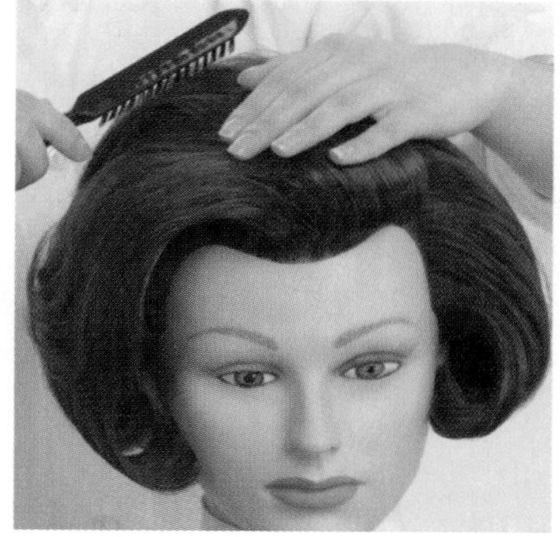

Figure 12-78b Finished style.

3. Repeat this procedure by moving the brush about ½ inch (1.25 cm) farther away from the scalp with each stroke until the desired volume has been achieved.

HAIR WRAPPING

The technique of wrapping hair is used to keep curly to extremely curly hair smooth and straight. It is similar to roller setting using very large rollers. Think of the head itself as a very large roller. Just as hair is wrapped around a roller to give it the shape of the roller, here you wrap the hair around the head so the hair takes on the shape of the head, although not much volume is attained because the hair at the scalp is not lifted up. If height is desired at the crown, you can place large rollers directly at the crown, with the remainder of the hair wrapped around the perimeter.

Wrapping can be done on wet or dry hair. On curly hair, wet wrapping is sufficient for a smooth, straight look. For very curly hair, you can press dry hair first and then wrap it.

BLOW-DRY STYLING

Blow-dry styling—the technique of drying and styling damp hair in one operation—has revolutionized the hairstyling world. Today's women desire hairstyles that require the least time and effort to maintain. The selection of

PROCEDURE 13

WRAPPING THE HAIR

Implements and Materials

- gel or silicone shine
- boar-bristle brush
- duckbill clips
- neck strip
- bobby pins

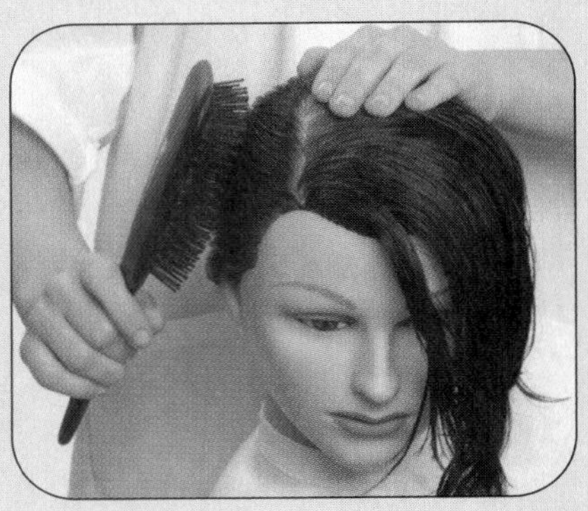

Figure 12-79 Wrap first section.

Procedure

1. If the hair is wet, a light gel can be applied before wrapping. If the hair is dry, a silicone shine product can be applied for a glossy comb-out.
2. Hold one hand at the top of the head. Using the brush in a pivot motion, wrap the hair on the outer perimeter of the head (Figure 12–79). Do not brush or push the hair to the back; the correct way is to always brush the hair clockwise around the head. Think of the head as a roller. Your job is to smooth the hair in a circular motion around it.
3. Use duckbill clips to keep the hair in place while wrapping (Figure 12–80).
4. Continue wrapping the hair in a clockwise direction around the head. Follow the brush with your hand, smoothing down the hair as you go along and keeping it tight to the head (Figure 12–81).

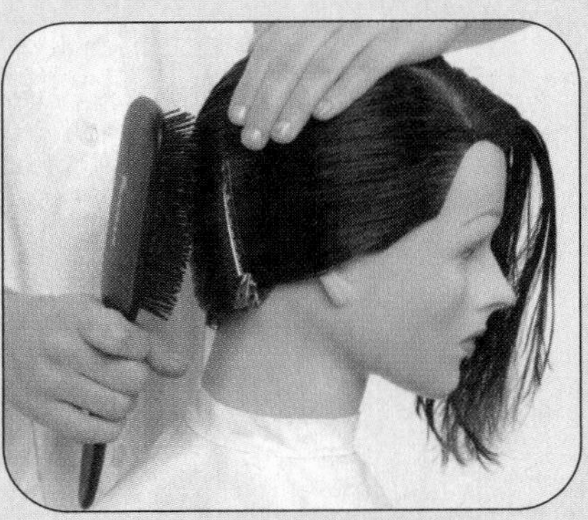

Figure 12-80 Hold wrapped hair with duckbill clips.

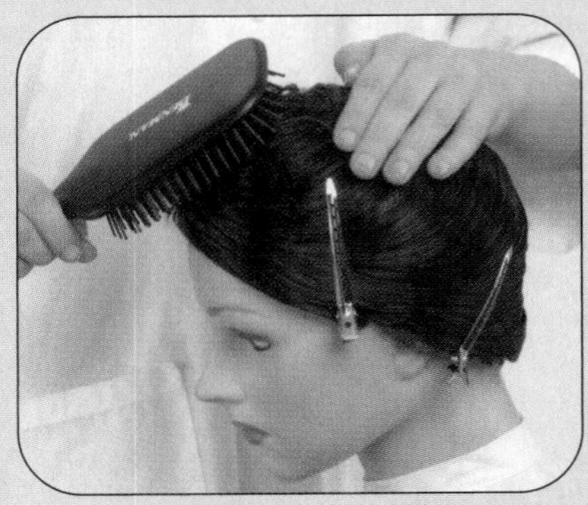

Figure 12-81 Continue wrapping hair.

12

5. When all the hair is wrapped, stretch a neck strip around the head so that it overlaps at the ends. Secure the wrapped strip with a bobby pin and remove the clips (Figure 12–82).
6. If you have been working on dry hair, leave the hair wrapped for about 15 minutes. If the hair was wet, place the client under a hooded dryer until the hair is completely dry, usually 45 minutes to one hour, depending on the hair length. The longer the hair is wrapped, the smoother it will be (Figure 12–83). 1

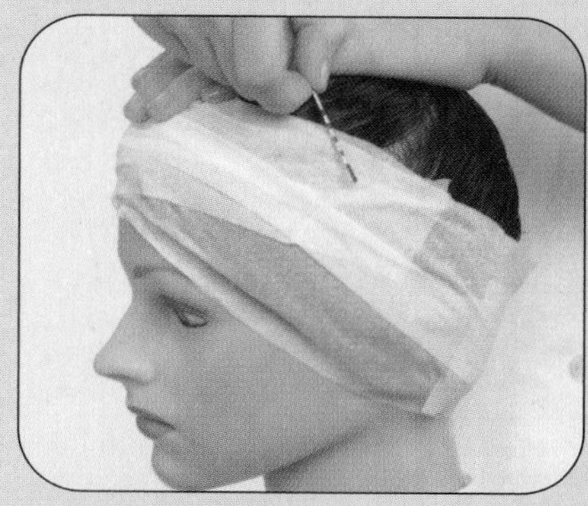

Figure 12–82 Wrap neck strip around hair.

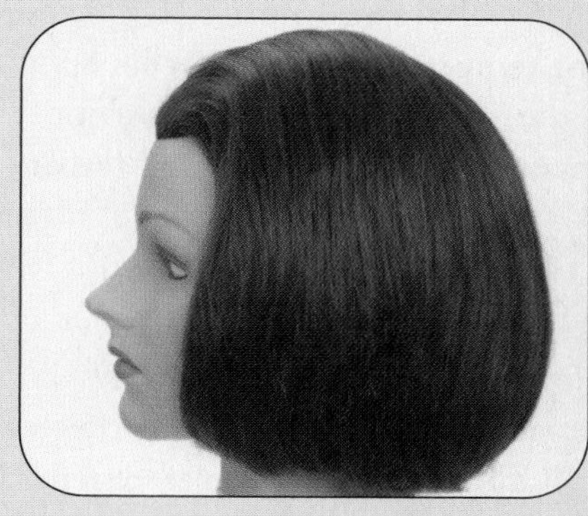

Figure 12–83 Finished style.

completed!

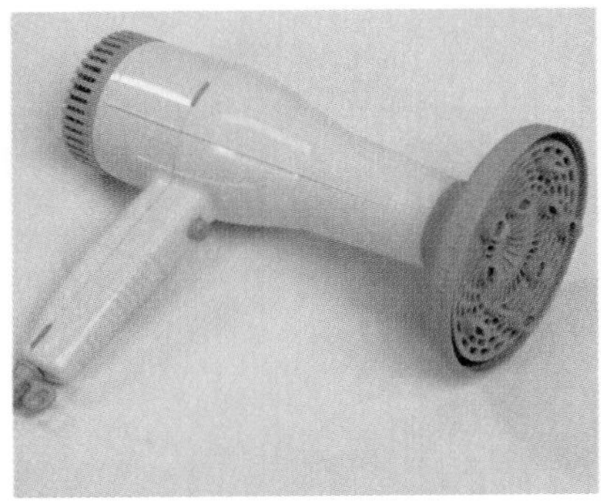

Figure 12-84 Blow-dryer and diffuser.

styling tools, techniques, and products must relate to the client's lifestyle. Is she capable of styling her own hair, and how much time will she have to do it? As the stylist, it is your responsibility to guide and educate the client through this process. To do so, you must first learn all about the tools and products available to you.

Remember, the first impression the client will have of the haircut you have performed will most likely be determined by the quality of the blow-dry. The haircut itself may be excellent, but if the blow-dry is weak, the client will perceive it as not being a good one or what she requested.

Tools for Blow-Dry Styling

The following are the basic tools used for blow-drying techniques.

The Blow-Dryer

A blow-dryer is an electrical device designed for drying and styling hair in a single service. Its main parts are a handle, a slotted nozzle, a small fan, a heating element, and speed/heat controls. Some also come with cooling buttons. The temperature control panel helps to produce a steady stream of air at the desired temperature. The blow-dryer's nozzle attachment, or **concentrator**, is a directional feature that can direct the air stream to any section of the hair more intensely. The **diffuser** attachment causes the air to flow more softly and helps to accentuate or keep textural definition (Figure 12–84).

To keep your blow-dryer as safe and effective as possible, make sure that it is always perfectly clean and free of dirt, grease, and hair before using. Dirt or hair in the device could cause extreme heat and hair burn. The air intake at the back of the dryer must be kept clear at all times. If this intake is covered and air cannot pass through freely, the dryer element could burn out.

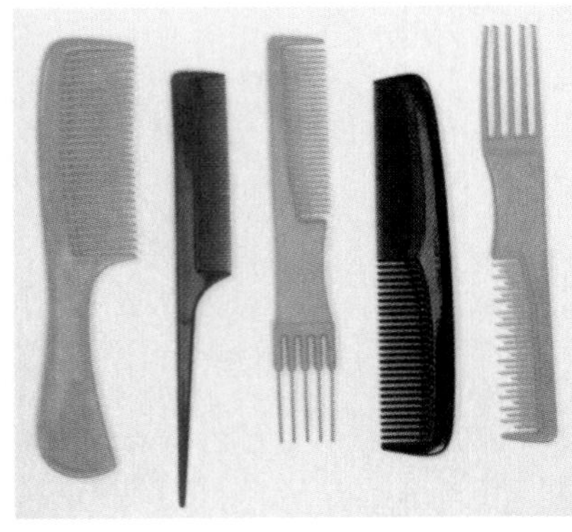

Figure 12-85 From left to right: wide-tooth comb, fine-tooth tail comb, styling comb with metal pins, finger wave comb, teasing comb.

Combs and Picks

Combs and picks are designed to distribute and part the hair. They come in a wide variety of sizes and shapes to adapt to many styling options (Figure 12–85). The length and spacing of the teeth may vary from one comb to another. Teeth that are closely spaced remove definition from the curl, thus creating a smooth surface, while widely spaced teeth shape larger sections of hair for more surface texture. Combs with picks at one end lift the hair away from the head.

Brushes

When choosing a styling brush, take into account the texture, length, and styling needs of the hair that you are working with. Brushes come in many sizes, shapes, and materials (Figure 12–86).

- *A classic styling brush* is a half-rounded rubber-based brush with smooth round-ended nylon quills, usually in either seven or nine rows. They are heat resistant and antistatic, ideal for smoothing and untangling all types of hair. While they are perfect for blow-drying precision haircuts where not too much volume is desired, they are less suitable for smooth classic

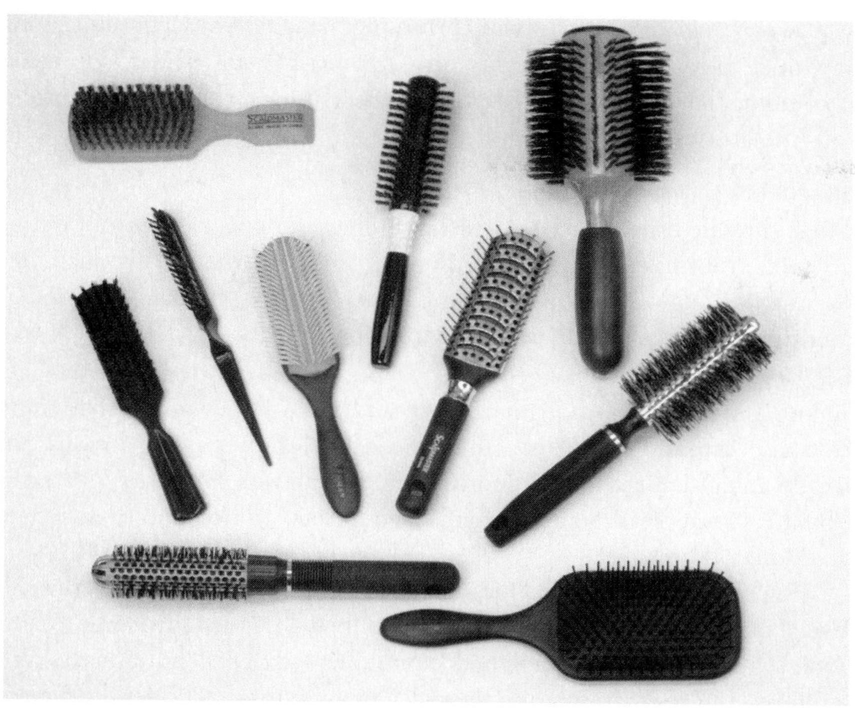

Figure 12–86 Brushes: paddle brush, grooming brush, teasing brush, classic plastic styling brush, vent brush, round brushes.

shapes with rounded edges. Excellent airflow through the brush is also a feature of the classic styling brush.

- *Paddle brushes*, with their large, flat bases, are well suited for mid- to longer-length hair. The best designs have ball-tipped nylon pins and staggered pin patterns that do not snag the hair.
- *Grooming brushes* are generally oval with pure natural bristles or quills of bristle and nylon mix. The boar bristles help distribute the scalp oils throughout the shaft of the hair, giving it shine. The nylon bristles stimulate the circulation of blood to the scalp. They are particularly useful for adding polish and shine to fine or normal hair and are great for combing out updos.
- *Vent brushes*, with their ventilated design, are used to speed up the blow-drying process, and are ideal for blow-drying fine hair and adding lift at the scalp.
- *Round brushes* come in different diameters. The client's hair should be able to wrap twice around the brush. Round brushes normally have natural bristles, sometimes with nylon mixed in for better grip. Smaller brushes add more curl, while larger brushes straighten the hair and bevel the ends of the hair. Large round brushes can also be used to lift the hair at the scalp. Some round brushes have metal cylinder bases so that the heat from the blow-dryer is transferred to the metal base, creating a stronger curl similar to ones produced with an electric roller. Always use the cooling button on the blow-dryer before releasing the section of hair.

- *A teasing brush* is a nylon styling brush that has a tail for sectioning, along with a narrow row of bristles. Teasing brushes are perfect for back-combing hair and then smoothing out the hair into a style, using the sides of the bristles.

Sectioning Clips

These clips are usually metal or plastic and have long prongs to hold wet or dry sections of hair in place. It is important to keep whatever wet hair you are not working on sectioned off in clips so that the wet hair does not sit over the dry hair, especially when drying long hair.

Styling Lotions

Styling lotions can be thought of as "liquid tools." They give a style more hold and can add shine and curl, or take curl away. Styling lotions can greatly enhance a style or, if poorly used, can ruin its overall look. That is why it is so important to understand how the hair will respond to each type of lotion.

With so many styling products on the market, the stylist must consider several questions before choosing one. First, how long does the style need to hold? Under what environmental conditions—dryness, humidity, wind, sun—will the client be wearing the style? You also must consider the type of hair—fine, coarse, straight, curly—when deciding on a product. Heavier products work by causing strands of hair to cling together, adding more pronounced definition, but they can also weigh the hair down, especially fine hair. Liquid styling products range from a light to very firm hold. Determine the amount of support desired and choose accordingly.

Foam or **mousse** is a light, airy, whipped styling product that resembles shaving foam. It builds moderate body and volume into the hair. Massage it into damp hair to highlight textural movement, or blow-dry it straight for styles in which body without texture is desired. Foam is good for fine hair because it does not weigh the hair down. It will hold for six to eight hours in dry conditions. Conditioning foams are excellent for drier, more porous hair.

Gel is a thickened styling preparation—firm-bodied and usually clear or transparent—that comes in a tube or bottle and probably has the strongest hold of all products, other than a finishing spritz or spray. It creates the strongest control for slicked or molded styles and distinct texture definition when spread with the fingers. When brushed out, it creates long-lasting body. Gel that produces the longest hold may overwhelm fine hair because of its high resin level. This is not a concern if fine hair is molded into the lines of the style and does not get brushed through when dry.

Similar in function to firm-hold gels, **liquid gels** or **texturizers** are lighter and more viscous, or liquid, in form. They allow for easy styling, defining, and molding. With brushing, they add volume and body to the style. Good for all hair types, they offer firmer, longer hold for fine hair with the least heaviness, and give a lighter, moderate hold to normal or coarse hair types.

When applied to damp hair that is wavy, curly, or extremely curly and then blow-dried, **straightening gels** relax the hair for a smooth, straight look, with the most hold in dry outdoor conditions. They counter frizzy

focus on ...retailing.

Styling products represent a natural retailing opportunity in the salon. As you style the client's hair, talk about what products you're using to achieve the desired look, and why. Demonstrate the uses and benefits of each product. Most clients are eager to learn any styling "secrets" you can share with them. Discussing products as you use them gives clients a reason to buy.

hair by coating the hair shaft and weighing it down. Of course, this is a temporary solution that will last only from shampoo to shampoo and may become undone in extremely humid conditions.

When sprayed into the base of fine, wet hair, **volumizers** add volume to the shape, especially at the base, when the hair is blow-dried. When a vent brush or round brush is used and the hair is not stretched too tightly around the brush, even more volume can be achieved. You may want to add a light gel or mousse to the rest of the hair for more hold, but be careful to avoid the base of the hair when applying.

Pomade, or **wax**, adds considerable weight to the hair by causing strands to join together, showing separation in the hair. Used on dry hair, this makes the hair very easy to mold. It allows greater manageability. But it should be used sparingly on fine hair because of the weight. As a man's grooming product, pomade is excellent on short hair.

Silicone shiners add gloss and sheen to the hair while creating textural definition. Nonoily silicone shine products are excellent for all hair types, either for applying before drying to provide lubrication and protection to the hair while blow-drying, or for finishing at the very end to add extra shine. Spray shiners, applied like hair spray, add shine without weight, so they are useful for all hair types.

Hair spray, or **finishing spray**, is applied in the form of a mist to hold a style in position. It is the most widely used hairstyling product. Available in a variety of holding strengths, in both aerosol or nonaerosol sprays, it is useful for all hair types and effective in dry or damp weather. Sprays generally may be easily combed or brushed through, as in a "working spray." Finishing spray is used for the firmest possible hold where the style will not be disturbed.

STYLING LONG HAIR

An **updo** is a hairstyle in which the hair is arranged up and off the shoulders and secured with implements such as hairpins, bobby pins, and elastics. Usually, clients request updos for special occasions such as weddings, proms, and evening events. Many stylists have a fear of putting hair up because they lack experience. They may find it overwhelming to look at a head of long, thick hair and create an elegant hairstyle that will last an evening. Like any other service in the salon, however, the more you do it, the better you will get at it. Once you start to practice the basics of hairstyling, updos will be a great creative outlet and you will look forward to performing this service for your clients.

Some popular updo styles are:

- the chignon: a true classic that has been popular for centuries. It is created out of a simple ponytail and can be dressed up with flowers or ornaments or kept simple. If the client's hair is very straight and silky, you will have

PROCEDURE 14

BLOW-DRY STYLING

Implements and Materials

- blow-dryer with attachments
- styling lotion
- wide-tooth comb
- round brush
- styling cape
- neck strip

Preparation for All Hair Types

1. After shampooing, return the client to the seated position and comb out any tangles in the hair. Remove excess moisture from the hair by blotting with a towel.
2. Place a clean neck strip on the client and drape with a cutting or styling cape.
3. Escort the client to the styling chair.

Procedures for Blow-Drying Different Hair Types and Lengths

To blow-dry short, layered, curly hair so as to produce a smooth and full finish, follow these steps.

1. Distribute styling product through the hair with your fingers, and comb through with a wide-tooth comb.
2. Using the comb, mold the hair into the desired shape while still wet (Figure 12–87).
3. For volume and lift, similar to that which you would get from a roller set, use a small round brush. Apply a mousse or spray volumizer at the base. Section and part the hair according to the size of the curl desired (Figure 12–88).

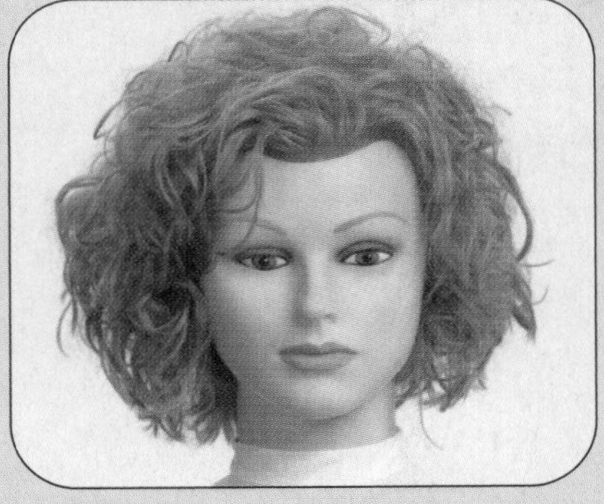

Figure 12–87 Mold the hair into shape it will take when dry.

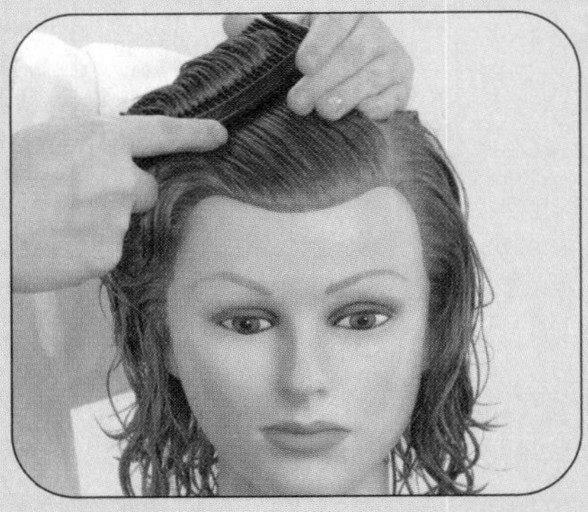

Figure 12–88 Section the hair for blow-drying.

4. Insert the round brush at the base of the curl. The degree of lift determines the type of volume you will achieve. Using the techniques you have learned in roller setting, dry each section either full base or half base. For maximum lift, insert the brush on base and direct the hair section up at a 125-degree angle (Figure 12–89). Roll the hair down to the base with medium tension (Figure 12–90). Direct the stream of air from the blow-dryer over the curl in a back-and-forth motion.
5. When the section is completely dry, press the cooling button and cool down the section to strengthen the curl formation.
6. Release the brush by unwinding the section from the brush. (Pulling it out could cause the hair to get tangled in the brush.) For less lift at the scalp, begin by holding the section at a 90- or 70-degree angle, following the same procedure (Figure 12–91). Make sure the scalp and hair are completely dry before combing out the style or the shape will not last. Finish with hair spray (Figure 12–92).

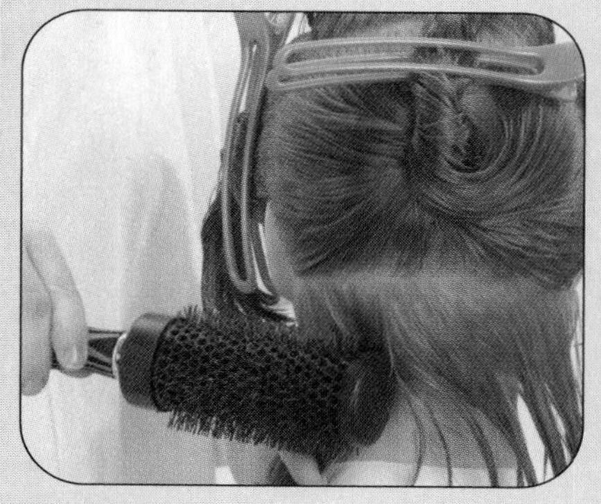

Figure 12–89 Direct the hair upward.

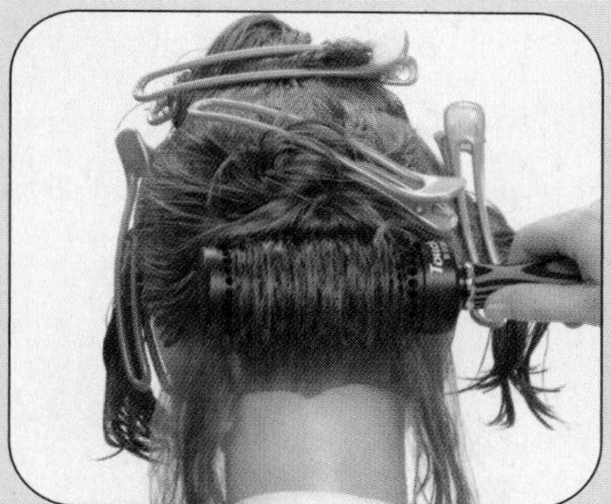

Figure 12–90 Roll the hair to the base.

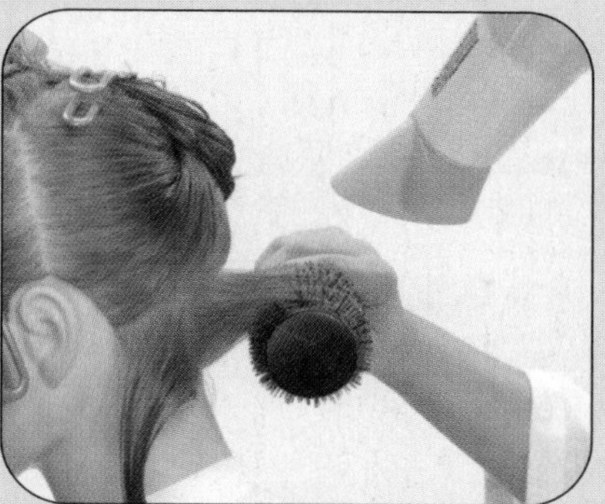

Figure 12–91 Full base section for blow-drying.

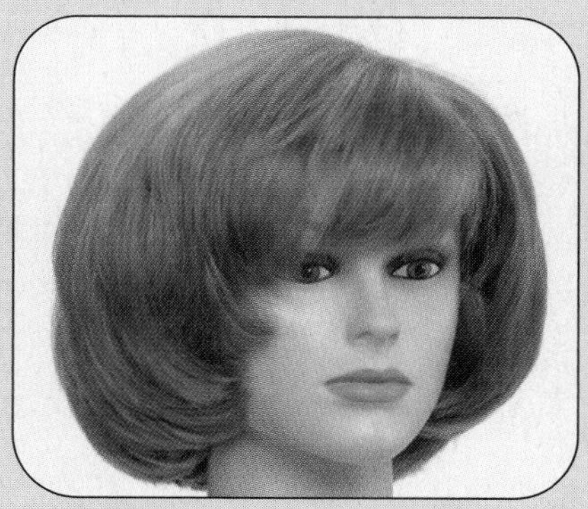

Figure 12–92 Finished style.

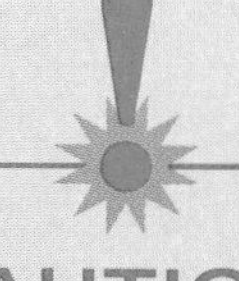

CAUTION

Never hold the blow-dryer too long in one place. Direct it from the scalp toward the ends of the hair. The hot air should flow in the direction in which the hair is wound; improper technique will rough up the hair cuticle and give the hair a frizzy appearance. Always direct the hot air away from the client's scalp to avoid scalp burns. Move the blow-dryer in a constant back-and-forth motion unless you are using the cooling button to cool a section. Because hair stretches easily when it is wet, partially towel-dry the hair before blow-drying, especially damaged or chemically treated hair. This is necessary if you are cutting the hair before you blow-dry it, as the hair will already be partially dry from the amount of time it takes to cut it.

completed!

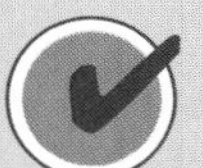

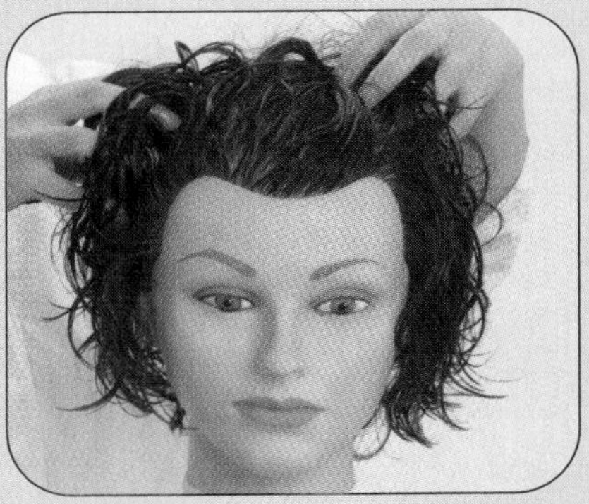

Figure 12-93 Comb hair into desired shape.

To blow-dry short, curly hair in its natural wave pattern, follow these steps.

1. Attach the diffuser to the blow-dryer.
2. Apply a liquid gel on the client's hair.
3. With a wide-tooth comb or your fingers, encourage the hair into the desired shape (Figure 12–93).
4. Diffuse the hair gently, pressing the diffuser on and off the hair without overmanipulating the hair, until each area of the head is dry (Figure 12–94).
5. To relax or soften the curl, slowly and gently run your fingers through the curl when the hair is almost dry, to give the curl a more open look.
6. For a tighter curl, scrunch the hair by placing your hand over a section of hair while it is being diffused, forming a fist with the hair in your hand (Figure 12–95). Using a pulsing motion, release and repeat until the section is dry.
7. For more shine, finish with a silicone spray or product to add the desired shine (Figure 12–96).

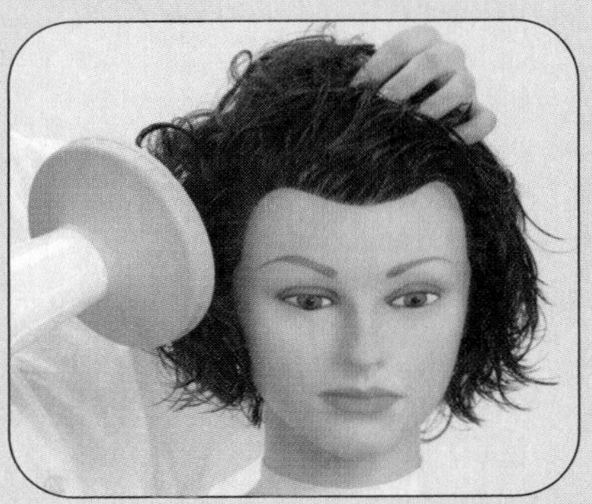

Figure 12-94 Hair being diffused.

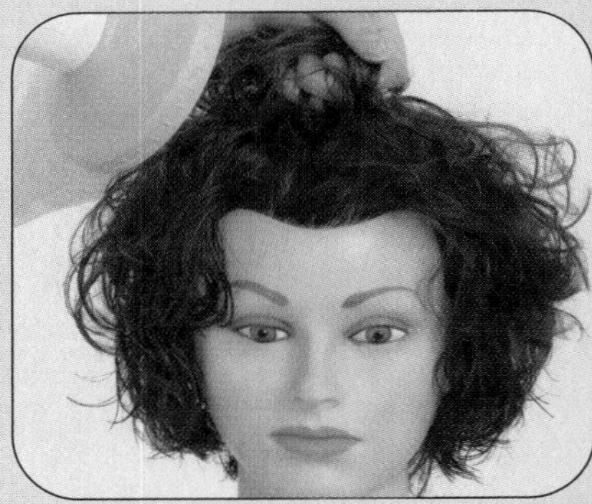

Figure 12-95 Scrunch the hair.

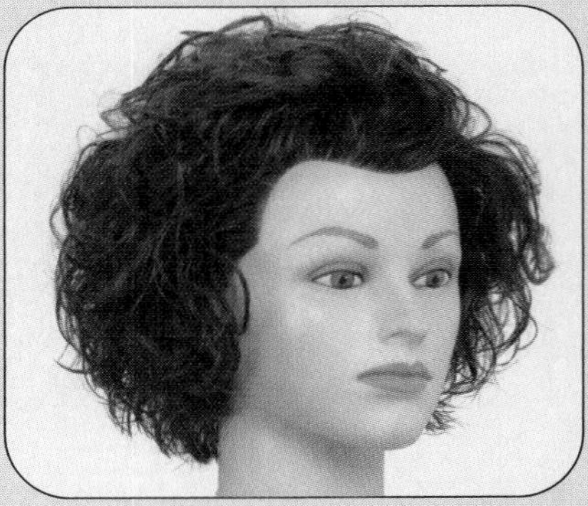

Figure 12-96 Finished hairstyle.

To diffuse long, curly to extremely curly hair in its natural wave pattern, use the steps below.

1. Apply a styling lotion or silicone shine product after towel-blotting hair.
2. For easier control, section the hair and work on one particular section at a time.
3. Attach the diffuser to the blow-dryer and diffuse the hair by letting the hair sit on top of the diffuser and pulsing the dryer toward the scalp and then away, repeating until the section is dry (Figure 12–97). Alternatively, gently run the section being dried through your fingers and bring the diffuser toward your hand (Figure 12–98).

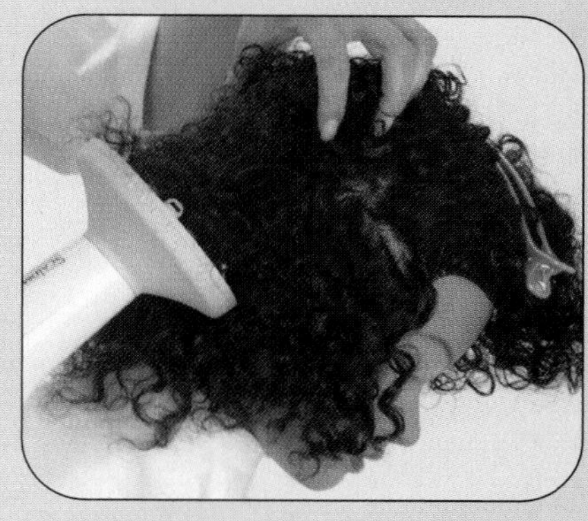

Figure 12–97 Using a diffuser.

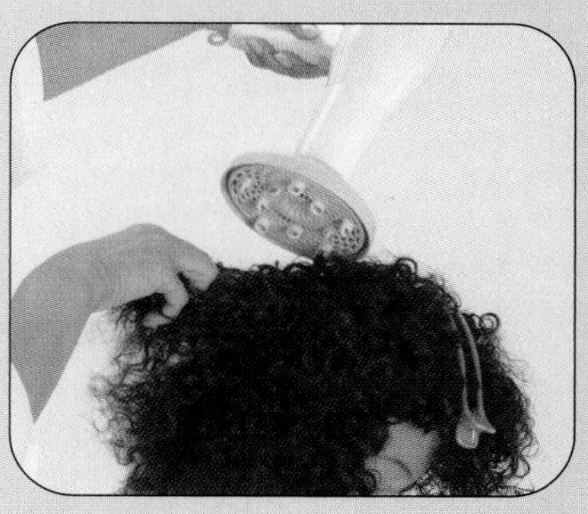

Figure 12–98 Another way to use a diffuser.

To blow-dry straight or wavy hair with maximum volume, use these steps.

1. Apply a mousse, a volumizing spray, or light-weight gel to dampen the hair.
2. Using a vent brush or classic styling brush, distribute the hair into the desired shape.
3. Build your shape from the bottom up, working from the nape up toward the crown. When you begin at the nape, hold the wet hair above the nape in a sectioning clip (Figure 12–99).
4. Insert the brush into the hair at the scalp. While turning the brush downward and away from the scalp, allow the brush to pick up a section of hair and begin drying. Direct the airflow towards the top of the brush, moving in the desired direction (Figure 12–100).

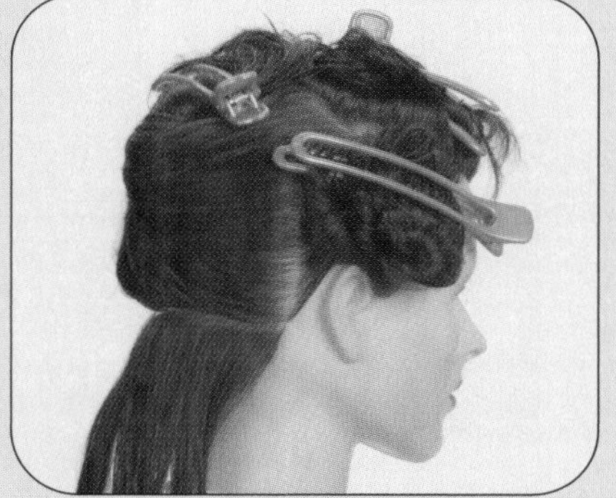

Figure 12–99 Clip hair above nape to begin drying.

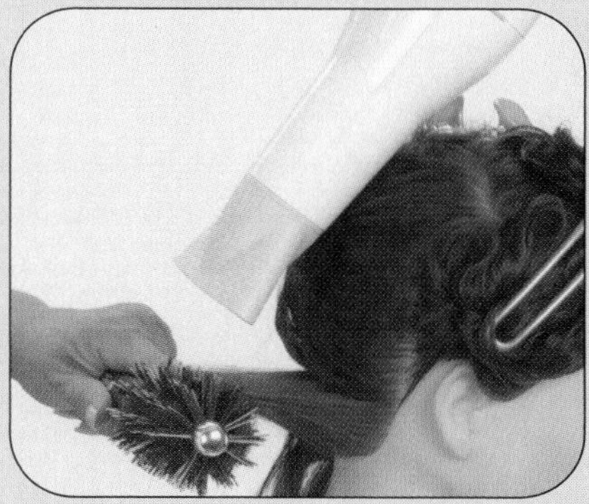

Figure 12–100 Lift the hair from the nape.

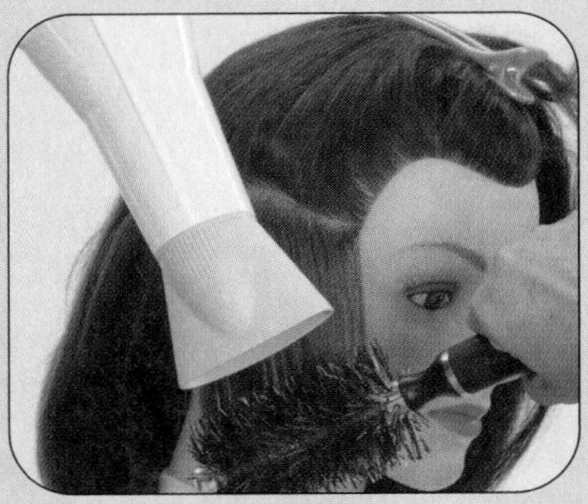

Figure 12–101 Brush hair in direction desired.

5. Work in sections, lifting and drying the sections, then brushing them in the design direction when they are completely dry. Repeat all over the head, directing the hair at the sides either away or forward (Figure 12–101). The fringe area could be dried either onto the forehead or away from the face.
6. Use an appropriate styling product to achieve the desired finish (Figure 12–102a and Figure 12–102b).

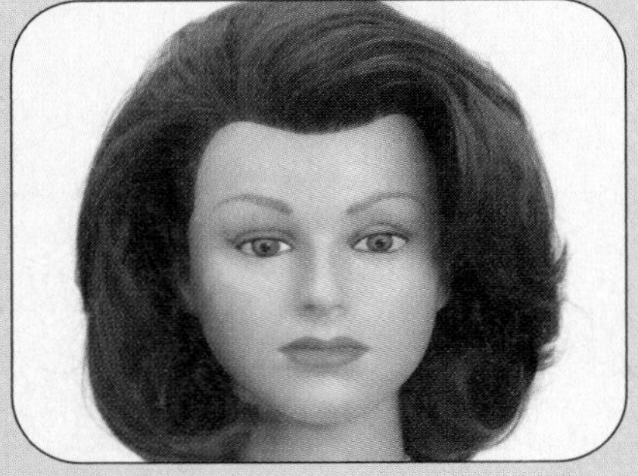

Figure 12–102a Finished style.

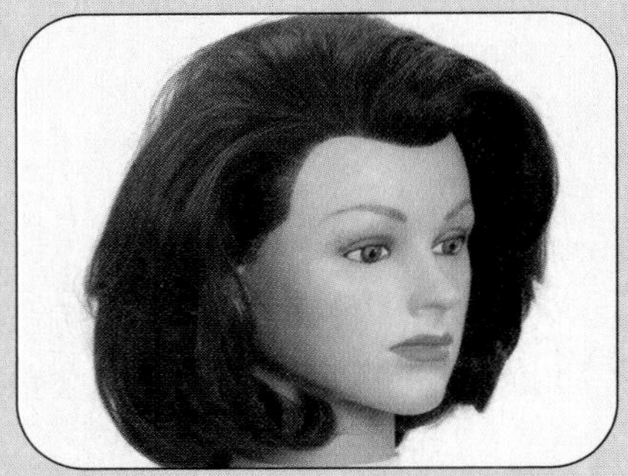

Figure 12–102 b.

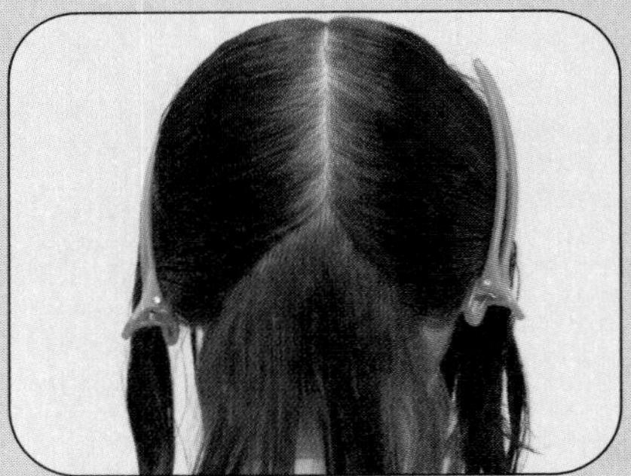

Figure 12–103 Hair sectioned for drying.

To blow-dry blunt or long layered, straight to wavy hair into a smooth straight style, follow these steps.

1. Attach the nozzle or concentrator attachment to the blow-dryer for more controlled styling. Part and section the hair so that only the section you are drying is not in clips. Apply a light gel (Figure 12–103).
2. Using 1-inch subsections, start your first section at the nape of the neck and use a classic styling brush to dry the hair straight and smooth. Place the brush under the first section and hold the hair low (Figure 12–104).
3. Follow the brush with the nozzle of the dryer while bending the ends of the hair in the preferred direction, either under or flipped outward. Continue using the same technique working up to the occipital area in 1-inch sections. To keep the shape flat and straight, continue using low elevation. For more lift and volume, hold the section straight out from the head or overdirect upward (Figure 12–105).
4. Work up to the crown, continuing to take 1-inch sections. On the longer sections toward the top of the crown, you could switch to a paddle brush, using the curve of the brush to add bend to the ends of the hair.
5. After each section is dried with heat, follow by using the cooling button on the blow-dryer to help set each section and to keep it smooth. For a fuller look, switch to a round brush.

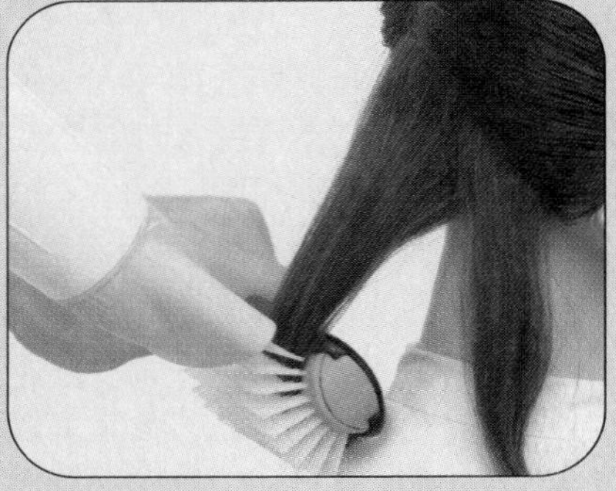

Figure 12–104 Hold the hair at low elevation.

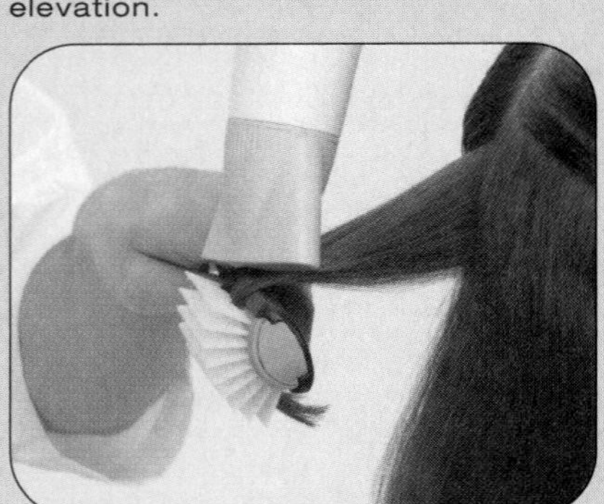

Figure 12–105 Hold the section straight out from the head.

6. Continue by subdividing the hair on the side and start with the section above the ear. Continue working in 1-inch sections. Hold at a low elevation and follow with the nozzle of the dryer facing toward the ends. Bend the ends under by turning the brush for a rounded edge, or outward for a flipped edge (Figure 12–106 and Figure 12–107).
7. Work in the same manner across the top. If there is a fringe, dry it in the desired direction. To dry the fringe straight and onto the forehead, point the nozzle of the dryer down over the fringe and dry it straight using your fingers or a classic styling brush to direct the hair (Figure 12–108).
8. To direct the fringe away from the face, brush the fringe back and push the hair slightly forward with the brush, creating a curved shaping (Figure 12–109 and Figure 12–110). Place the dryer on a slow setting and point the nozzle toward the brush. The fringe, when dry, will fall away from the face and slightly to the side, for a soft look (Figure 12–111a and Figure 12–111b).

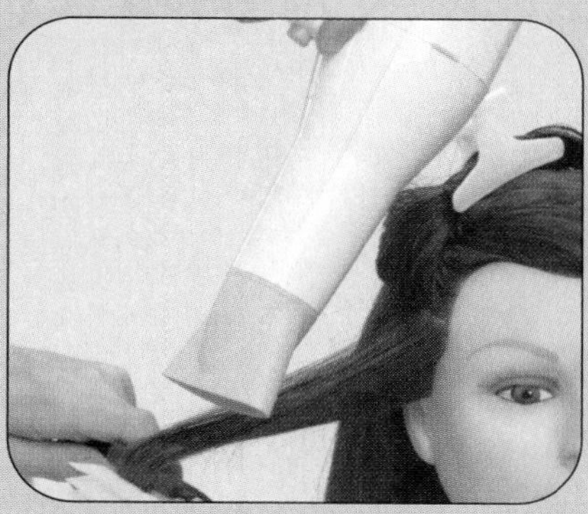

Figure 12-106 Side section turned under.

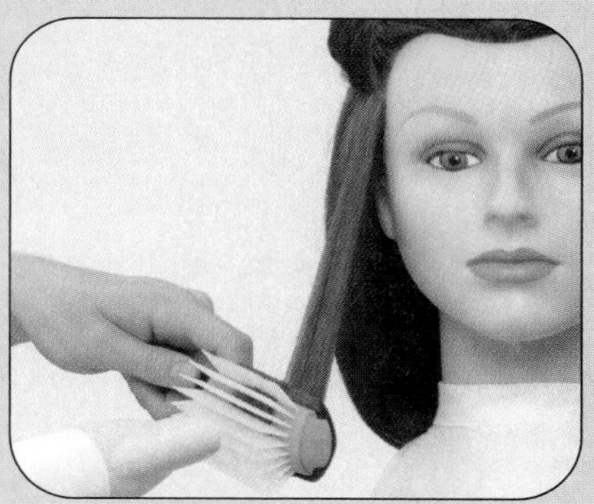

Figure 12-107 Side section flipped out.

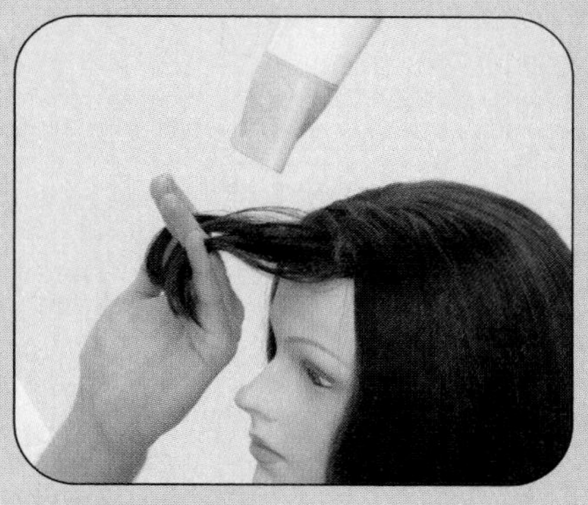

Figure 12-108 Dry fringe straight.

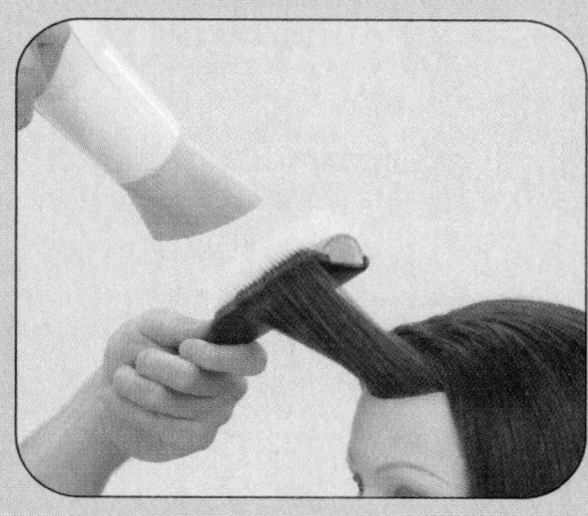

Figure 12-109 Brush fringe away.

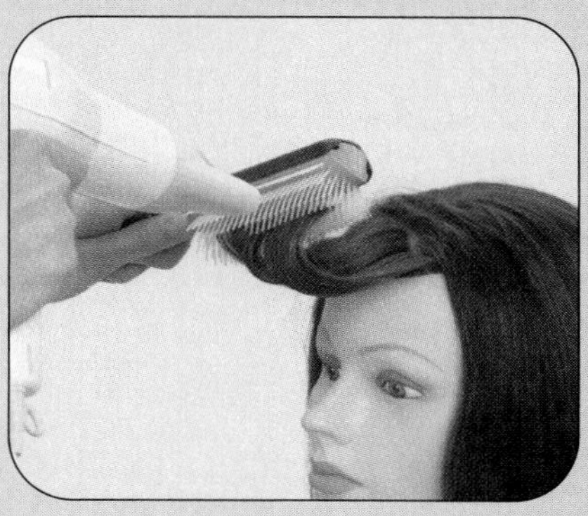

Figure 12-110 Curve section forward with nozzle facing section.

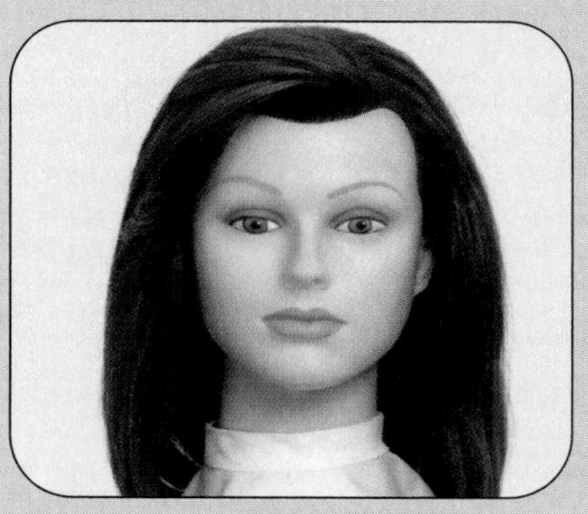

Figure 12-111a Finished style.

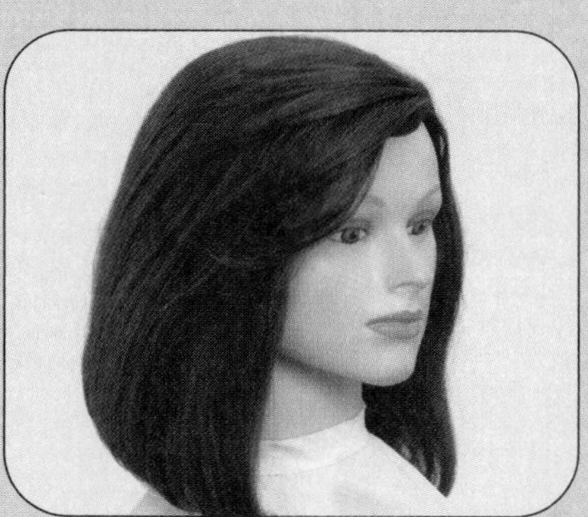

Figure 12-111b

To blow-dry curly hair into a straight style, follow the preceding procedure. You may want to apply a straightening gel and then use the largest round brush the hair length will allow. More tension will have to be applied to pull each 1-inch section straight. Be careful to keep the dryer moving in a back-and-forth motion at all times. If the hair is fragile or damaged, this method is not recommended. Consider an alternate method such as wrapping the hair.

Graduated haircuts have either long or short-layered interiors. To blow-dry graduated haircuts, use the same basic blow-drying techniques you have learned in the previous sections, choosing the technique that best suits the length of the hair you are working on.

Cleanup and Sanitation

1. Discard the neck strip.
2. Thoroughly clean brushes of any loose hair and disinfect them.
3. Clean the blow-dryer and remove any dust from the air intake area or filter.
4. Sanitize your workstation.
5. Wash your hands with soap and warm water.

completed!

to first set the hair for 10 minutes in electric rollers or the style will not last. If the hair is wavy to curly, blow-dry the hair straight. If it is extremely curly, you could press the hair first, or leave it natural for a textured-looking chignon.

- the basic French twist: this elegant, sleek look can go anywhere. If you are working on straight, fine hair, you may want to first set the hair in electric or Velcro rollers to give it more body.
- the classic French twist: the traditional way to style a French twist, mostly for special evening and black-tie events. The shape is much larger than the basic twist, and you can be more creative with the front area. When executing an updo, always inspect the shape you are building from every angle to make sure that it is well balanced and well proportioned.

CAUTION

Do not use electric vaporizing irons on pressed hair; the moisture could cause the hair to return to its natural extremely curly state.

Client Consultation

As always, consult with the client first to make sure you understand what she has in mind. Have on hand magazines that show a lot of updos, such as bridal magazines, or keep at your station a folder of pictures clipped from magazines that show the best current styles. If you are consulting with a bride, you might suggest that she come in for a trial run. That way, she can try several looks to see how they work with her headpiece. Take photographs so she can decide which style she likes best. It would be a good idea for you to have a copy of the photo so you can remember exactly what you did.

THERMAL HAIRSTYLING

Thermal waving (also called marcel waving) and **thermal curling** are methods of waving and curling straight or pressed hair using thermal irons and special manipulative techniques on dry hair. These irons, which can be either electrically heated or stove-heated, have been modernized so successfully that these methods of waving and curling hair are more popular than ever. Manipulative techniques are basically the same for electric irons or stove-heated irons.

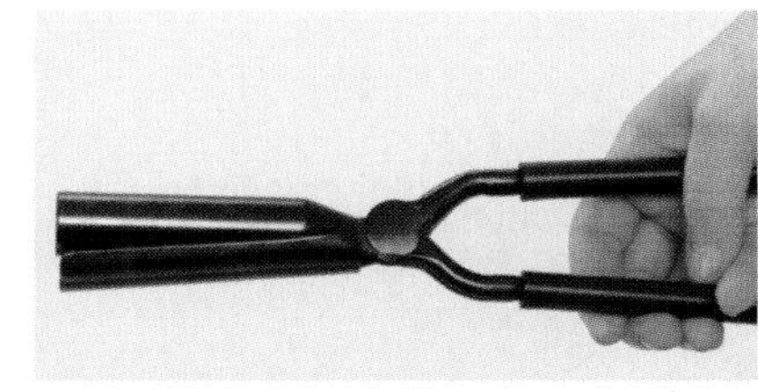

Figure 12–112 Conventional thermal (marcel) irons.

12

Thermal Irons

Thermal irons provide an even heat that is completely controlled by the stylist. The irons must be made of the best quality steel so that they hold an even temperature during the waving and curling process. The styling portion of the irons is composed of two parts: the **rod**, a perfectly round, solid steel prong; and the **shell**, also perfectly round with the inside grooved so that the rod can rest in it when the irons are closed. The edge of the shell nearest the stylist is called the inner edge; the one farthest from the stylist is called the outer edge.

Thermal irons come in a variety of styles, sizes, and weights, from small to jumbo, and are available in three different classifications.

1. Conventional (also called marcel) stove-heated (Figure 12–112).
2. Electric self-heated (Figure 12–113).
3. Electric self-heated, vaporizing.

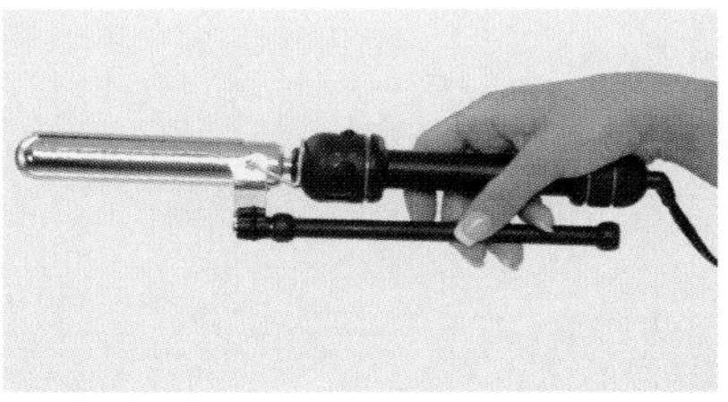

Figure 12–113 Electric thermal irons.

PROCEDURE 15

CHIGNON

Implements and Materials

- neck strip
- styling cape
- electric or Velcro rollers
- grooming or teasing brush
- bobby pins, hairpins
- elastics
- working hair spray
- finishing spray
- curling irons
- tail comb

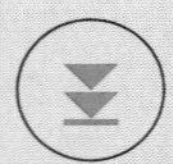

Here's a tip:

Performing an updo on hair that has been washed the previous day is often recommended. Freshly washed hair can be very slippery and difficult to work with. Many stylists also choose to set the hair in hot rollers prior to performing an updo. The curl allows the hair to be more easily manipulated into rolls or loops.

12

Preparation

1. Drape the client; shampoo and towel-dry the hair.
2. Redrape the client with a neck strip and styling cape.
3. Apply the appropriate styling product that will give the hair a lot of hold. Blow-dry the hair, smoothing it with a brush for a sleek finish.
4. Set hair in electric rollers or Velcro rollers, depending on the amount of curl (electric rollers) or volume (Velcro rollers) you may need.

Procedure

1. Using a grooming bristle brush, part the hair on whichever side you choose, and brush it into a low ponytail at the nape (Figure 12–114).
2. Secure the ponytail with an elastic rubber band, keeping the hair as smooth as possible. Use the side of the bristles on the brush to smooth the hair. An alternate method is to use elastics; this is kinder to the hair and keeps it smoother. Place two bobby pins onto the elastic and spread

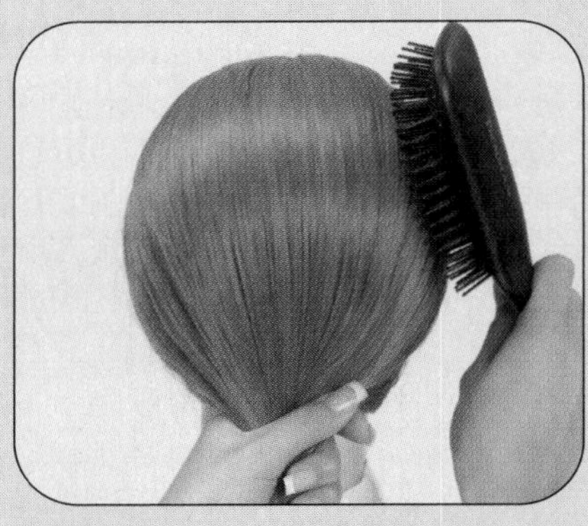

Figure 12–114 Brush hair into low ponytail.

them apart, one on each side (Figure 12–115). Place one bobby pin in the base of the ponytail. Stretch the elastic around the ponytail base. Place the second bobby pin in the base. Lock the two pins together (Figure 12–116).

3. Part a small section of hair from the underside of the ponytail, wrap it around the ponytail to cover the elastic, and secure with a bobby pin underneath (Figure 12–117).
4. Smooth out the ponytail and hold it with one hand, then begin back-brushing from underneath the ponytail with your other hand (Figure 12–118). Gently smooth out the ponytail after back-brushing, using the sides of the bristles.
5. Roll the hair under and toward the head to form the chignon (Figure 12–119). Secure on the left and right undersides of the roll with bobby pins (Figure 12–120).

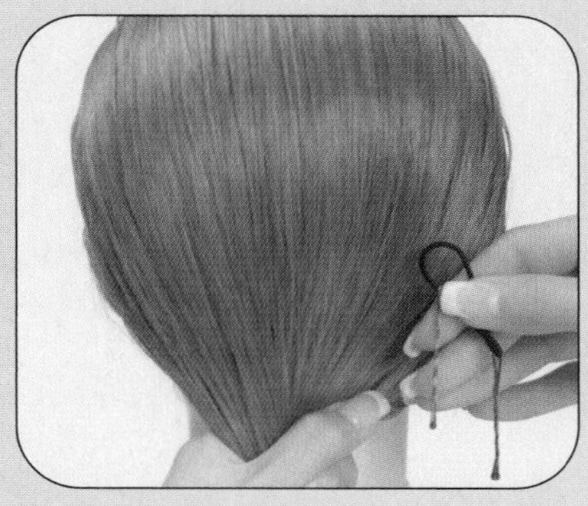

Figure 12–115 Elastic and bobby pins.

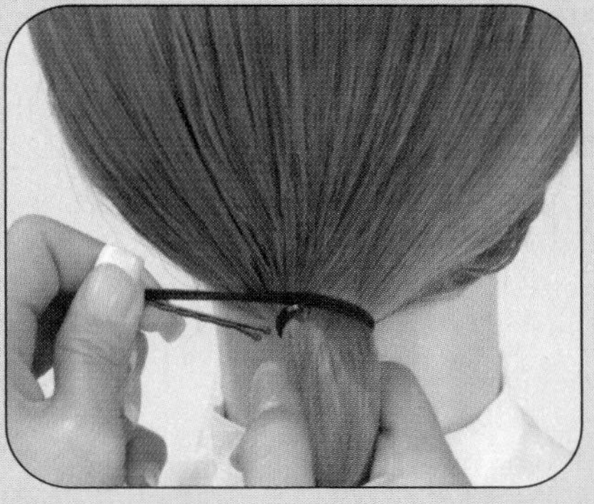

Figure 12–116 Lock bobby pins together around ponytail base.

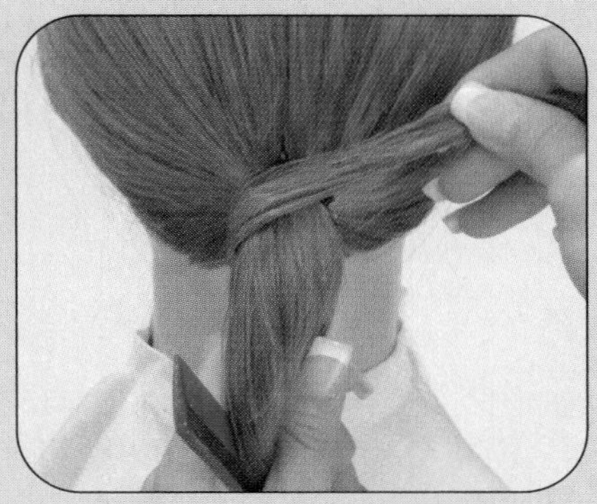

Figure 12–117 Pin wrapped section under.

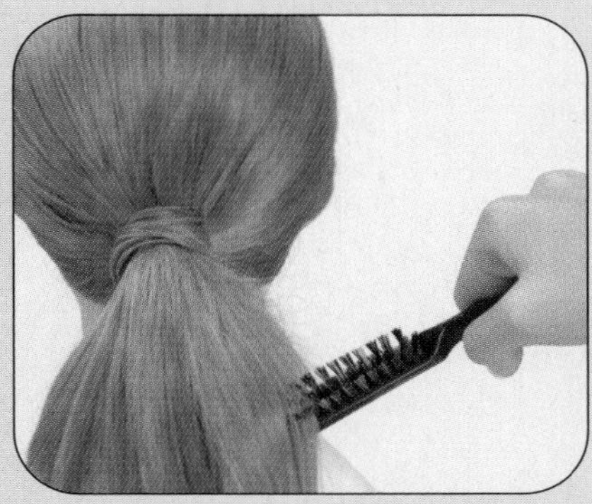

Figure 12–118 Back-brush the ponytail.

12

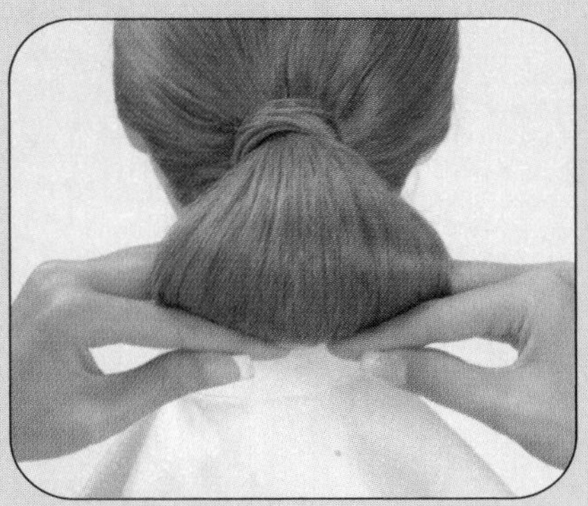

Figure 12–119 Roll the hair toward the head.

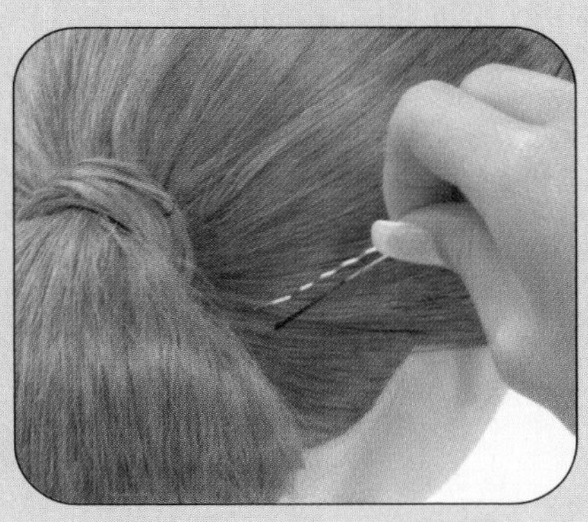

Figure 12–120 Pin the right side.

6. Fan out both sides by spreading the chignon with your fingers (Figure 12–121). Secure with hairpins, pinning close to the head. Use bobby pins if more hold is needed (Figure 12–122).
7. Finish with a strong finishing spray.
8. Add flowers or a hair ornament to dress up the chignon (Figure 12–123a and Figure 12-123b).

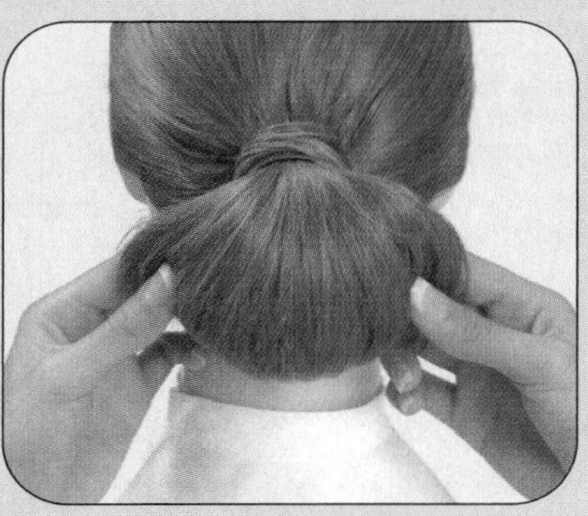

Figure 12–121 Spread out the sides.

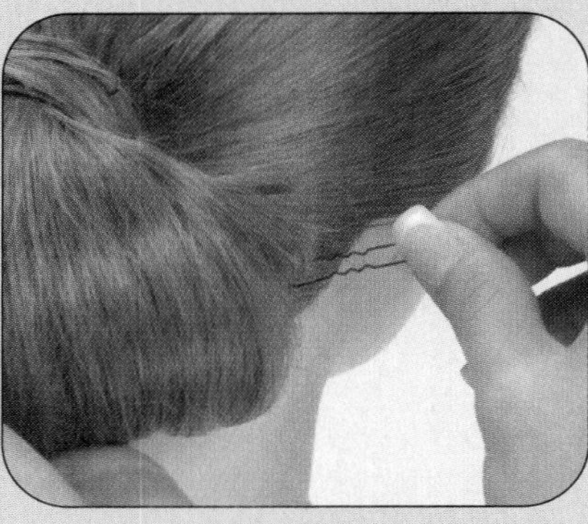

Figure 12–122 Pin the sides.

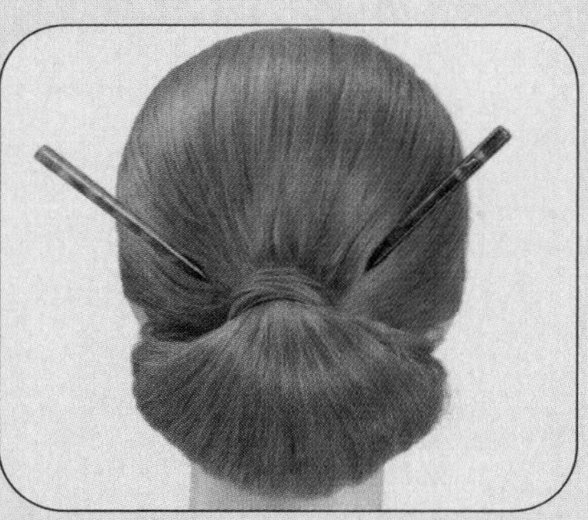

Figure 12–123a Finished chignon.

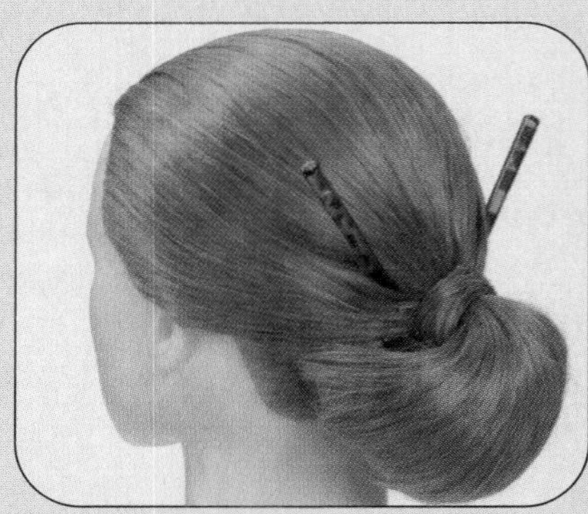

Figure 12–123b.

completed! 

PROCEDURE

BASIC FRENCH TWIST

Implements and Materials

Same as for Procedure 15—chignon.

Preparation

Same as for Procedure 15—chignon.

Procedure

1. Brush all the hair smoothly into a ponytail at the occipital bone (Figure 12–124).
2. With your free hand, reach in front of the hand that is holding the ponytail, with the thumb pointing down toward the client's nape (Figure 12–125).
3. Grab the ponytail with your thumb still pointing down and twist the hair in the direction in which your palm is facing, moving the hair inward and upward (Figure 12–126).

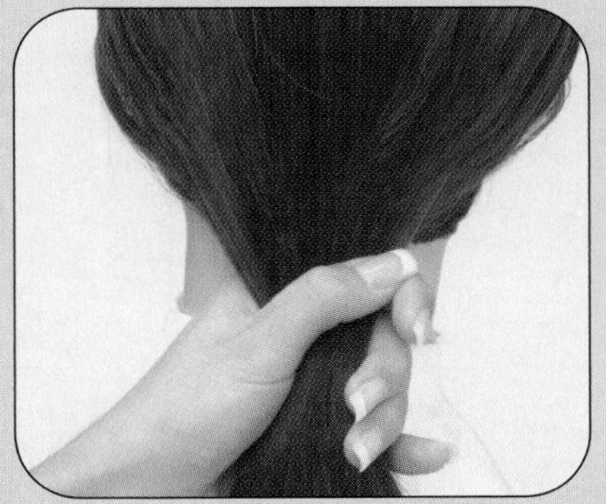

Figure 12–124 Brush hair out from the occipital.

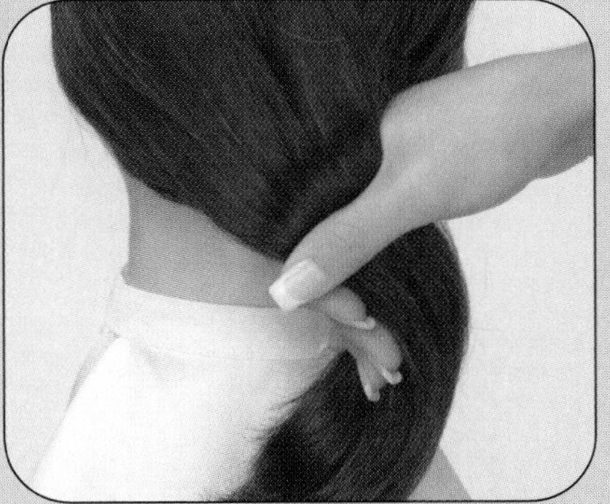

Figure 12–125 Reach over and grab the ponytail.

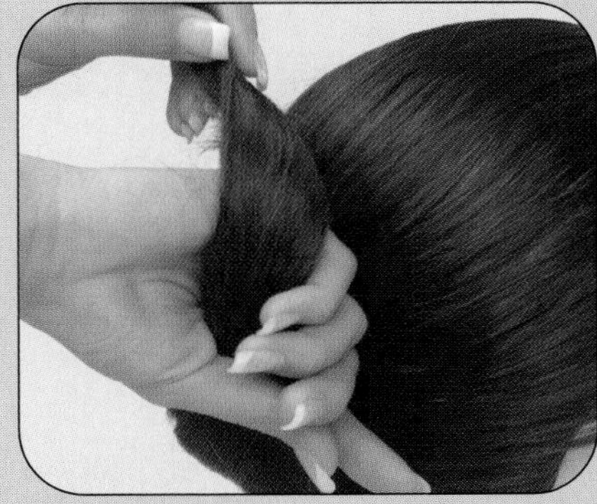

Figure 12–126 Twist the hair.

4. As you move toward the crown, twist the hair into a funnel shape and secure the twist with hairpins by pinning into the seam, making sure not to expose the pins (Figure 12–127a and Figure 12–127b).
5. Tuck the ends into the top of the funnel of the twist near the crown (Figure 12–128 and Figure 12-129).
6. For a less formal or younger look, let the hair ends fan out and fall loosely over the sides of the twist, instead of tucking them into the top of the twist. Another option is to form curls, loops, or knots with the hair at the top of the twist (Figure 12–130).

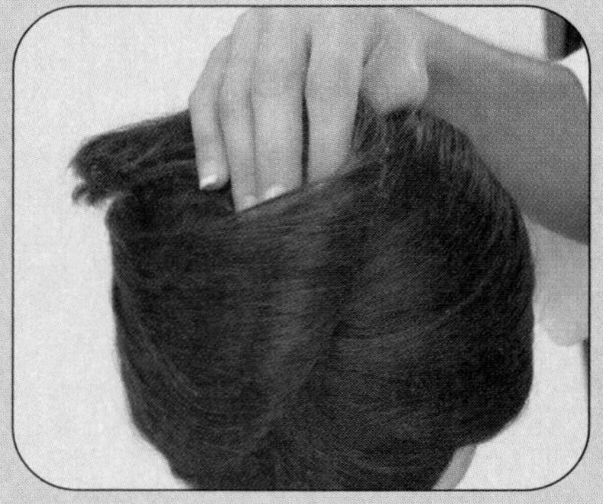

Figure 12–127a Create a funnel.

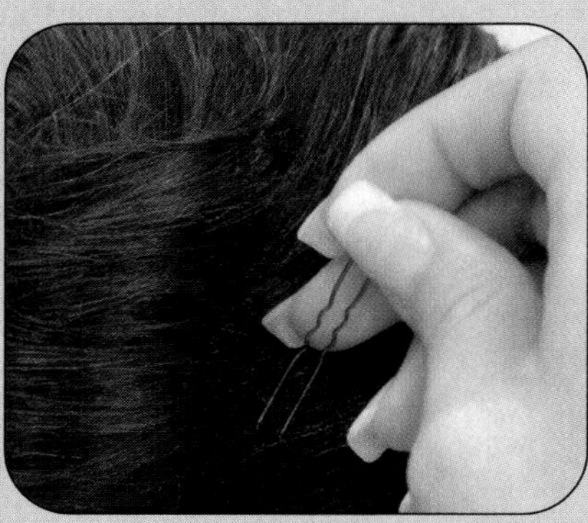

Figure 12–127b Pin into the seam.

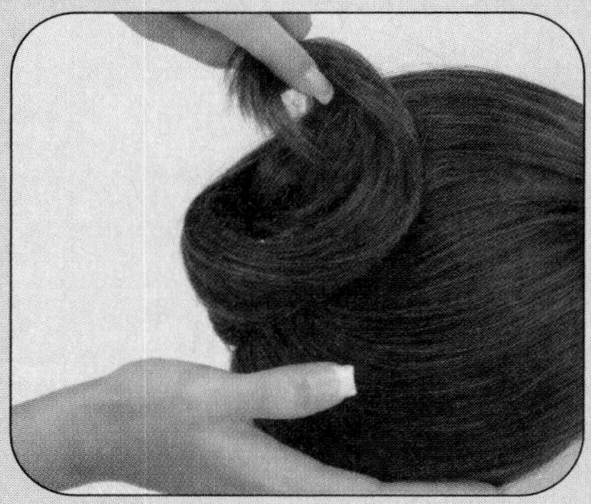

Figure 12–128 Tuck the ends into the top of the twist.

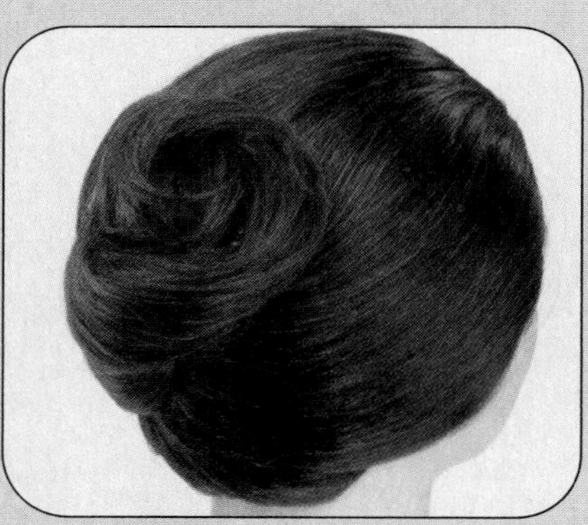

Figure 12–129 Completed basic French twist.

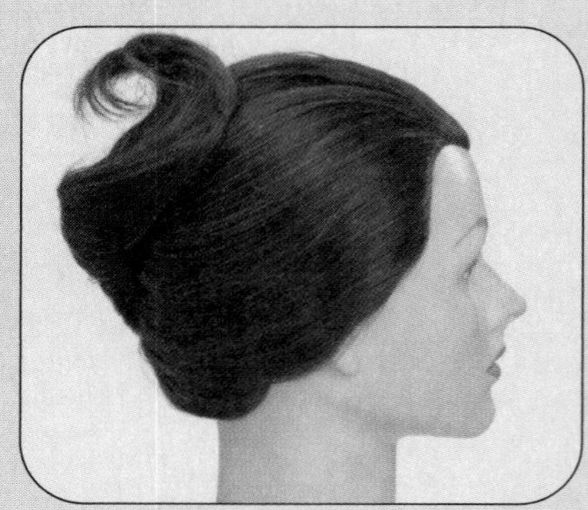

Figure 12–130 Option: form loops at the top of the twist.

completed!

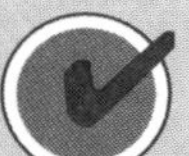

PROCEDURE

CLASSIC FRENCH TWIST

Implements and Materials

Same as for Procedure 15—chignon.

Preparation

Same as for Procedure 15—chignon. Set the hair with a wet set or, if you wish to save time, electric rollers or thermal irons.

Procedure

1. Section off the crown area and the two side sections (Figure 12–131).
2. Back-comb the entire back area, taking vertical sections (Figure 12–132).
3. Using the side bristles of a grooming brush or a teasing brush, gently smooth all the hair of the back section to one side of the head (in this example all the hair will move to the left). Hold the hair to that side by reaching over the client's head with your free hand.
4. Begin pinning the hair at the center of the nape, moving upward with bobby pins. Overlap the pins by criss-crossing them to lock into place. Repeat until you reach the back of the crown (Figure 12–133).

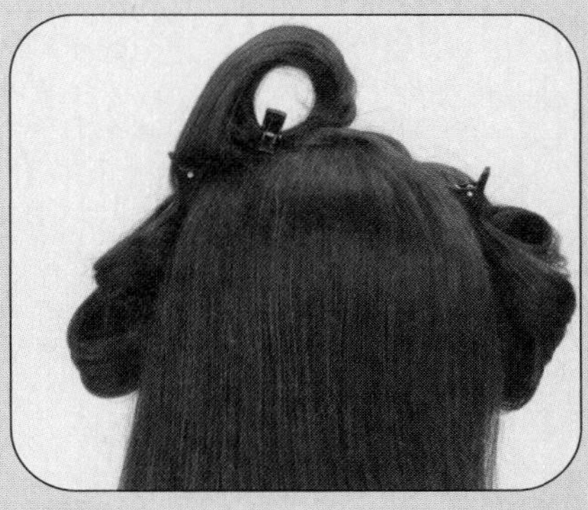

Figure 12–131 Sections.

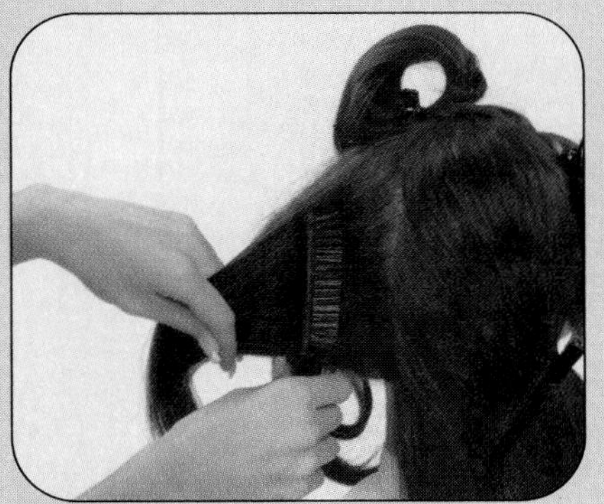

Figure 12–132 Back-comb vertical section.

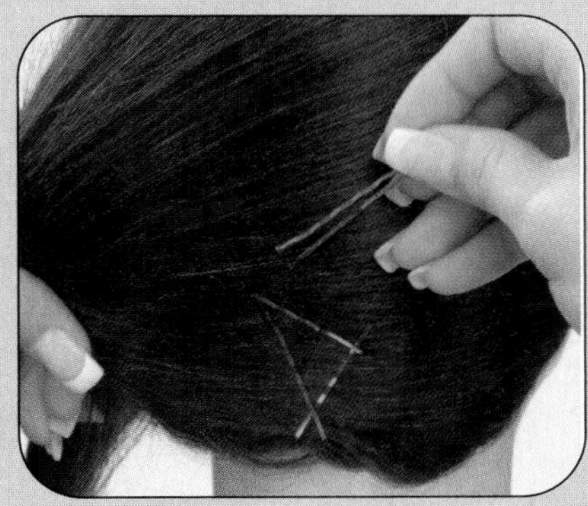

Figure 12–133 Criss-cross the bobby pins.

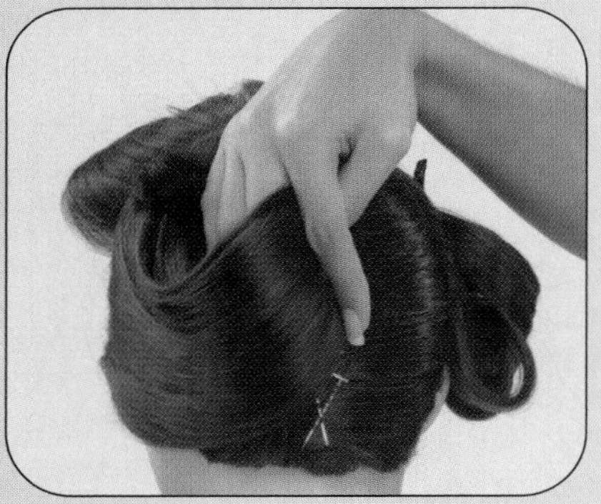

5. With the brush, bring the hair from the left side over the center line and twist from the center of the nape. Move upward and inward, tucking the ends into the fold as you move up, to create a funnel shape. Secure with hairpins into the seam as you move up, hiding the pins in the seam (Figure 12–134).
6. Tuck all the ends into the top of the twist and pin (Figure 12–135).
7. Move to a side section and lightly back-brush the section. Twist the section with the seam facing the back of the head, covering the part as you twist. Secure with a bobby pin at the top of the side section, leaving the ends out (Figure 12–136 and Figure 12–137).
8. Repeat on the other side.
9. Remove the sectioning clip from the top section. Make three subsections horizontally across the top of the head (Figure 12–138).
10. Beginning with the section closest to the back of the crown, slice out a subsection about a third of the width of the horizontal section (Figure 12–139).

Figure 12-134 Twist and pin the hair.

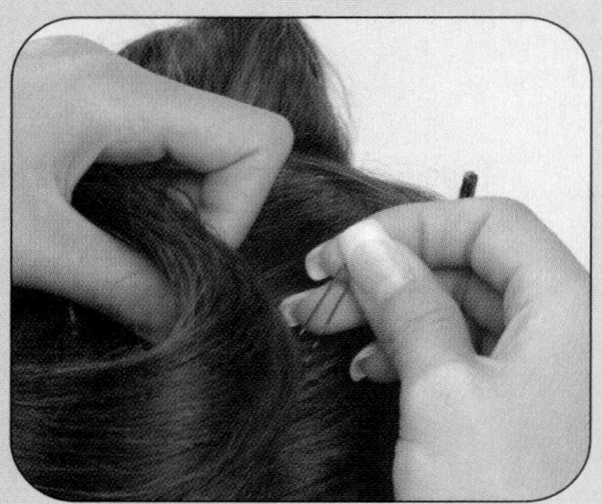

Figure 12-135 Completed center section.

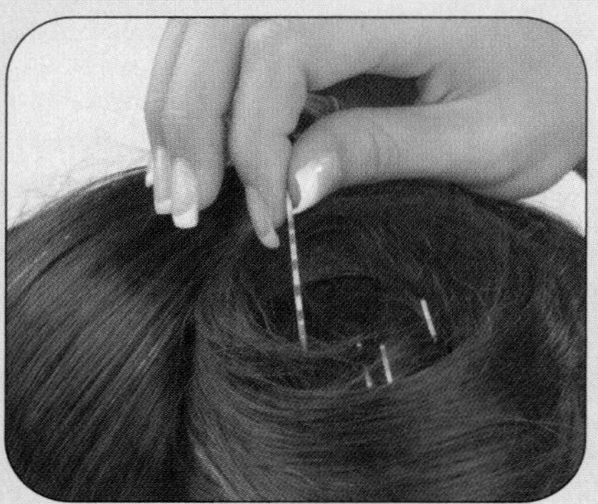

Figure 12-136 Twist the section.

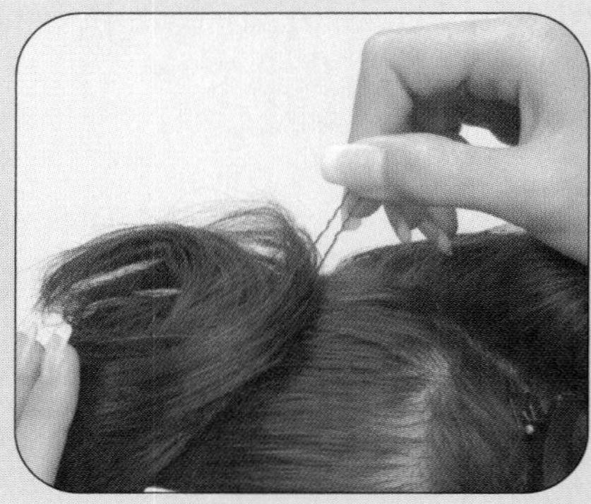

Figure 12-137 Pin the top.

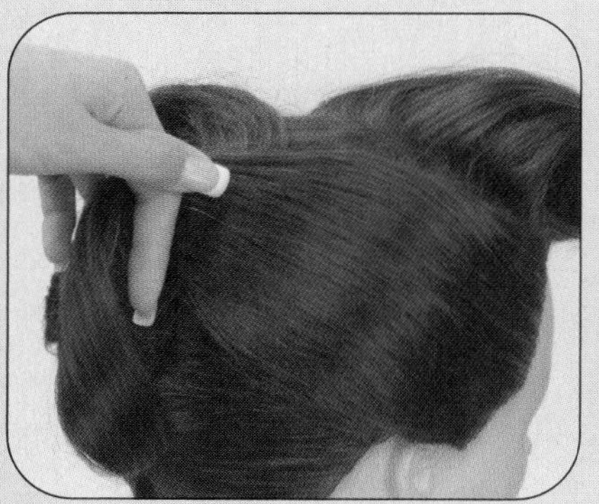

Figure 12-138 Subsections on top of the head.

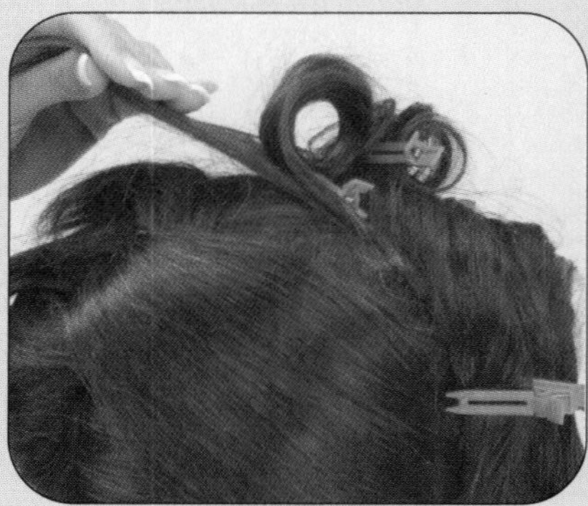

Figure 12-139 Hold out a third of the back section.

11. Back-brush and smooth the subsection, using the sides of the brush bristles. Loop the section over your fingers and secure at the base of the loop on the scalp with a bobby pin. Take care not to expose the pin (Figure 12–140).
12. Take the other two sections and form looped curls in the same manner. Pin the loops as close to the top of the twist as you can get, checking for balance and proportion.
13. Repeat with the center horizontal section, making two or three looped curls, depending on what the density of the hair will allow (Figure 12–141).
14. Go back to the side area, and with the hair remaining out from the side, twist, loop, and pin. Again, check in your mirror for balance and proportion.
15. Style the section in the front near the bangs as you wish. This section could also be brought back and added to the other looped curls if your client is comfortable with all her hair off her face, or sweep the hair loosely to the side and leave the ends hanging softly down. Here is where your design ability comes into play as you make the best design decision for your client (Figure 12–142, Figure 12–143a, and Figure 12–143b).
16. Spray with a firm-hold finishing spray, and check to make sure there are no exposed pins. 3

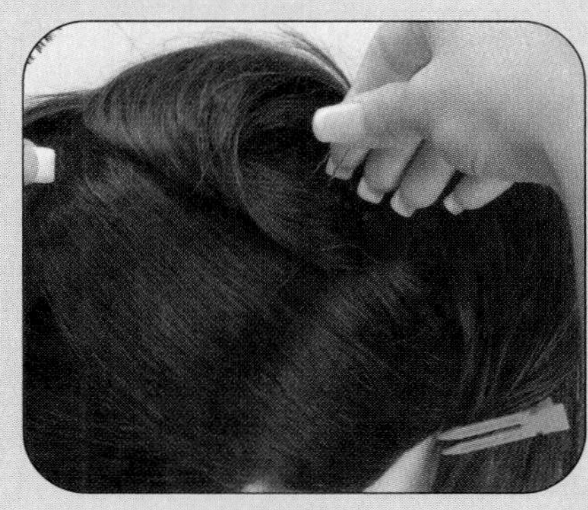

Figure 12–140 Loop hair over fingers.

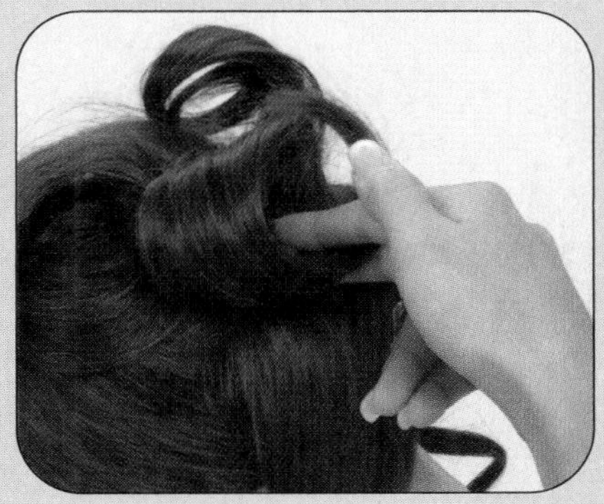

Figure 12–141 Loop the center section.

12

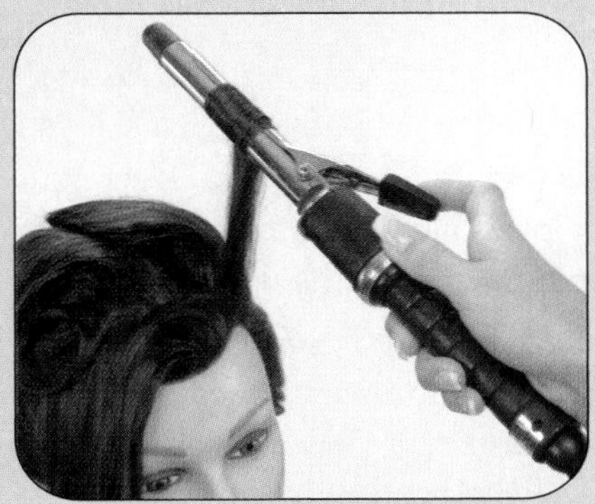

Figure 12–142 Front section curled back.

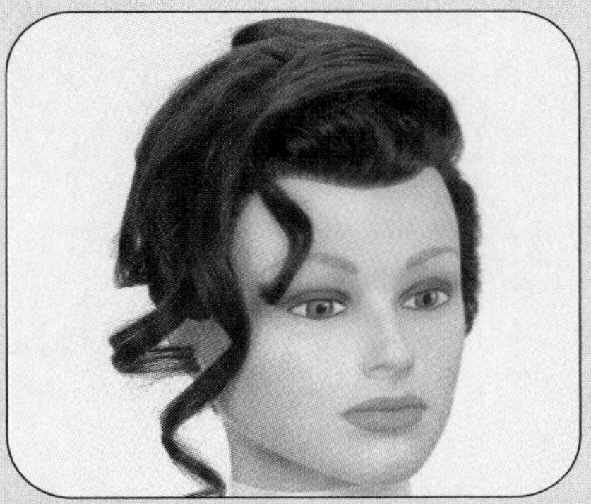

Figure 12–143a Finished classic French twist.

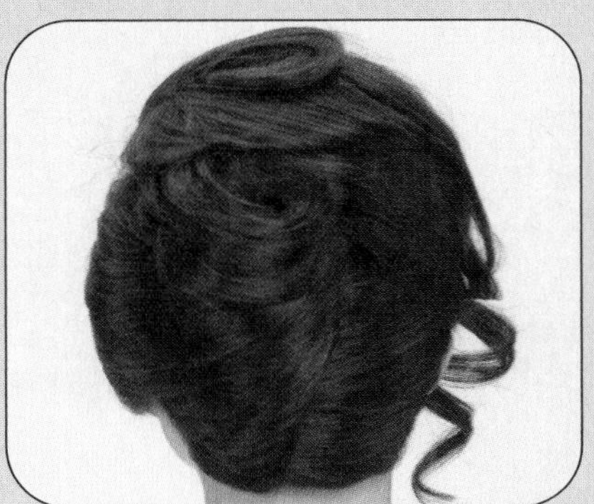

Figure 12–143b

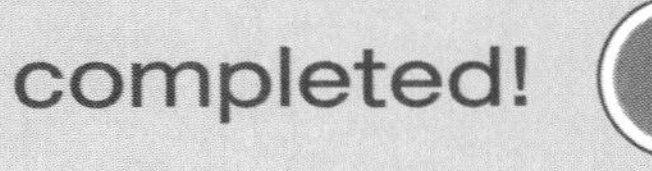

Figure 12–144 Testing the heat of thermal irons.

There is no one correct temperature used for the irons when thermal curling or thermal waving the hair. The temperature setting for irons depends on the texture of the hair, whether it is fine or coarse, or whether it has been lightened or tinted. Hair that has been lightened or tinted, as well as white hair, should be curled and waved with lukewarm irons. Coarse and gray hair, as a rule, can withstand more heat than fine hair.

Testing Thermal Irons

After heating the irons to the desired temperature, test them on a piece of tissue paper. Clamp the heated irons over the tissue and hold for five seconds. If the paper scorches or turns brown, the irons are too hot (Figure 12–144). Let them cool a bit before using. Overly hot irons can burn, scorch, or damage hair, and can discolor white hair. Remember that fine, lightened, or badly damaged hair withstands less heat than normal hair.

CAUTION

Do not use thermal irons on chemically straightened hair; to do so could cause breakage.

Care of Thermal Irons

Thermal irons should be kept clean and free from rust and carbon. To remove dirt or grease, wash the irons in a soap solution containing a few drops of ammonia. This cuts any oil and grease that might cling to the irons. Fine sandpaper, or steel wool with a little oil, helps to remove rust and carbon and polishes the irons. To make sure you get more movement, oil the joint of the irons.

Thermal irons are designed to hold heat in the most uniform manner. If you overheat the irons, however, in most cases they will be ruined.

Comb Used with Thermal Irons

The comb should be about 7 inches (17.5 cm) long, made of hard rubber or another nonflammable substance, and should have fine teeth. Fine teeth hold the hair more firmly than coarse teeth.

Hold the comb between the thumb and all four fingers of the left hand, with the index finger resting on the backbone of the comb for better control and one end of the comb resting against the outer edge of the palm. This position assures a strong hold and a firm movement (Figure 12–145).

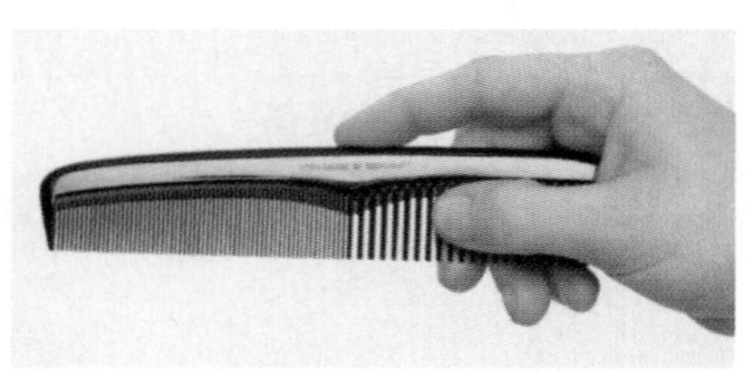

Figure 12–145 Holding the comb.

Manipulating Thermal Irons

Hold the irons in a comfortable position that gives you complete control. Grasp the handles of the irons in your right hand, or in the left hand if you are left-handed, far enough away from the joint to avoid the heat. Place your three middle fingers on the back of the lower handle, your little finger in front of the lower handle, and your thumb in front of the upper handle.

The best way to begin to practice manipulative techniques with thermal irons is by rolling the cold irons in your hand, first forward, then backward. This rolling movement should be done without any sway or motion in the arm; only the fingers are used as you roll the handles in either direction (Figure 12–146).

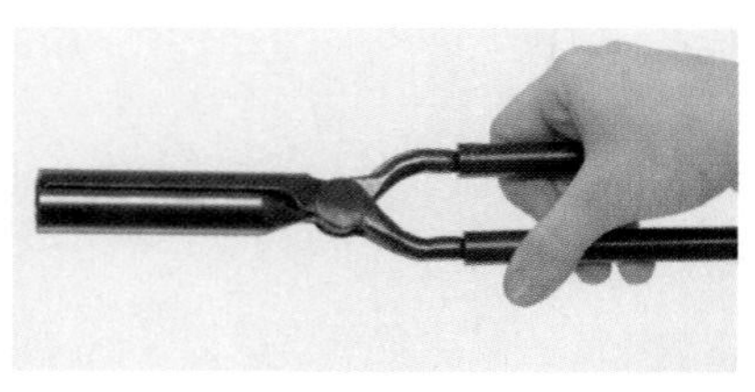

Figure 12–146 Rolling the irons.

PROCEDURE

THERMAL WAVING

Thermal waving requires no setting creams or lotions.

Implements and Materials

- shampoo
- styling cape and neck strip
- hard rubber comb (fine-toothed)
- conventional (marcel) or electric irons

Preparation

1. Shampoo the client's hair and dry it completely.
2. Drape the client for a dry hair service: Secure a neck strip around the client's neck. Place a cape over the neck strip and fasten it so that the cape does not touch the client's skin. Fold the uncovered portion of the neck strip down over the cape.
3. Heat the irons.

Procedure

Before beginning the waves, comb the hair in the general shape desired by the client. The natural growth will determine whether or not the first wave will be a left-going wave or a right-going wave. The procedure described here is for a left-going wave.

1. Comb the hair thoroughly, following its directional growth.
2. With the comb, pick up a strand of hair about 2 inches (5 cm) in width. Insert the irons in the hair with the groove facing upward (Figure 12–147).

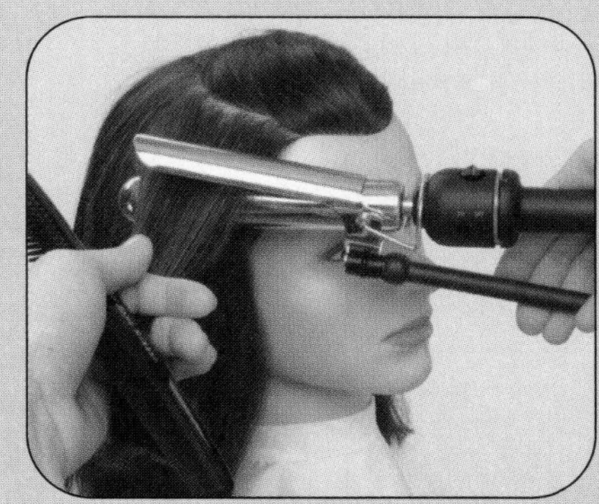

Figure 12–147 Insert irons in the hair.

12

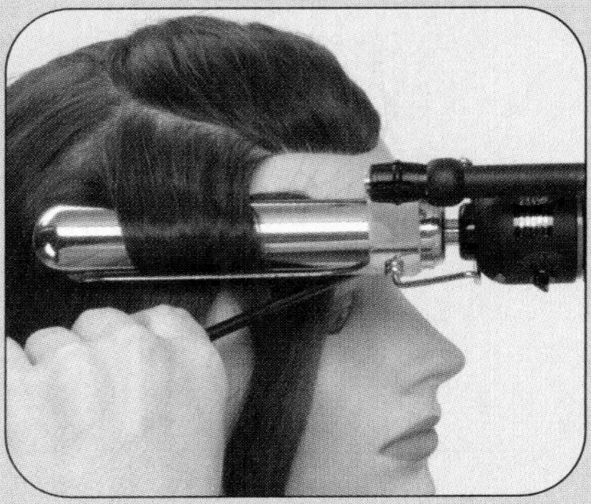

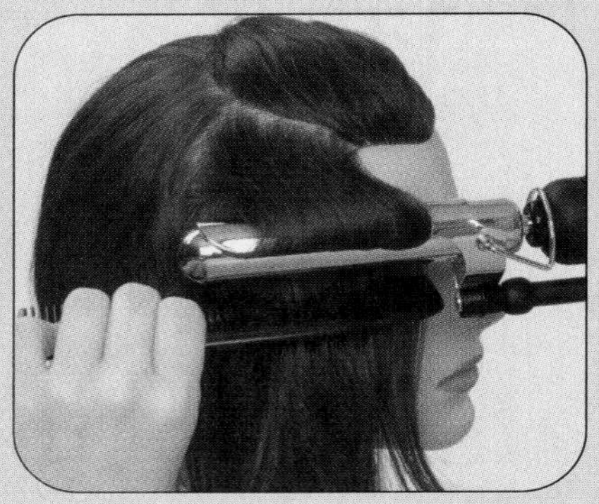

Figure 12–148 Direct the hair to the right with the comb.

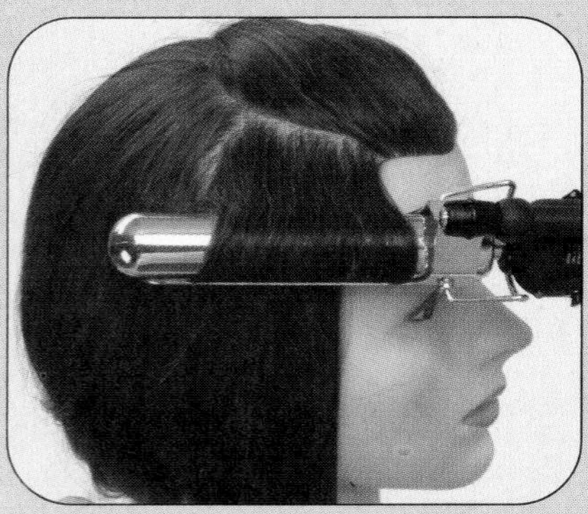

Figure 12–149 Roll irons one full turn forward.

3. Close the irons and give them a one-quarter turn forward (away from you). At the same time, draw the hair with the irons about 1/4 inch (.625 cm) to the left, and direct the hair 1/4 inch (.625 cm) to the right with the comb (Figure 12–148).
4. Roll the irons one full turn forward and away from you (Figure 12–149). In doing this, keep the hair uniform with the comb. You will find that the hair has rolled on a slight slant on the prong of the irons. Keep this position for a few seconds in order to allow the hair to become sufficiently heated throughout.
5. Reverse the movement by simply unrolling the hair from the irons and bringing it back into its first resting position (Figure 12–150). When this movement is completed, you will find the comb resting somewhat away from the irons.
6. Open the irons with your little finger and place them just below the ridge, or crest, by swinging the rod of the irons toward you and then closing them (Figure 12–151). The outer edge of the groove should be directly underneath the ridge just produced by the inner ridge.
7. Keeping the irons perfectly still, direct the hair with the comb upward about 1 inch (2.5 cm), thus forming the hair into a half circle (Figure 12–152). Remember that in order to perform step 7 properly, you do not move the comb from the position explained in step 6.
8. Without opening the irons, roll them one-half turn forward and away from you (Figure 12–153). In this movement, keep the comb perfectly still and unchanged.

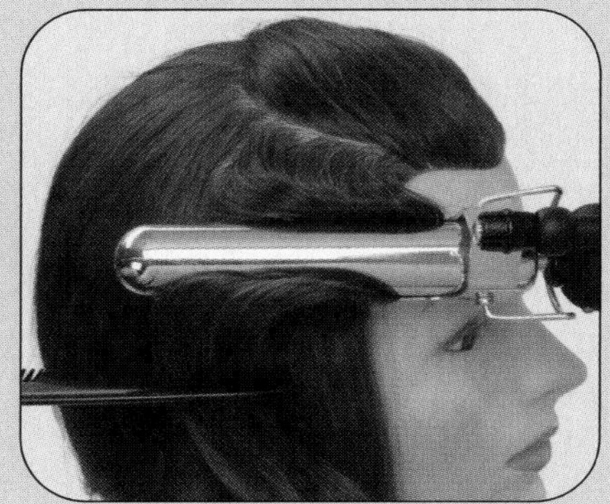

Figure 12–150 Reverse movement.

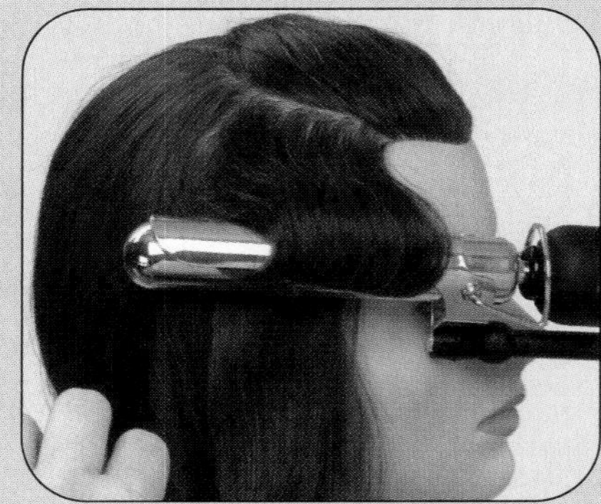

Figure 12–151 Start to form the curl.

Figure 12–152 Form the hair into a half circle.

9. Slide the irons down about 1 inch (2.5 cm) (Figure 12–154). This movement is accomplished by opening the irons slightly, gripping them loosely, and then sliding them down the strand.
10. After completing step 9, you will find the irons and comb in the correct position to make the second ridge. This is the beginning of a right-going wave, in which the hair is directed opposite to that of a left-going wave.
11. After completely waving one strand of hair, wave the next strand to match. Pick up the strand in the comb and include a small section of the waved strand to guide you as you form a new wave (Figure 12–155). When waving the second strand of hair, be sure to use comb and irons movements that are the same as those you used when waving the first strand of hair. This way, the waves will match.
12. Style and finish the hair as desired (Figure 12–156).

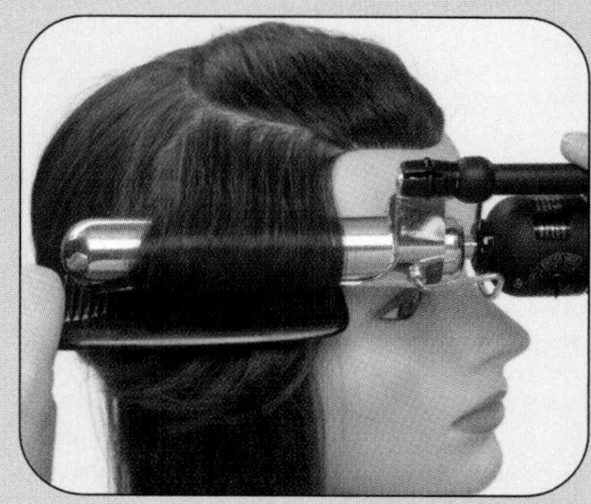

Figure 12–153 Roll irons one-half turn forward.

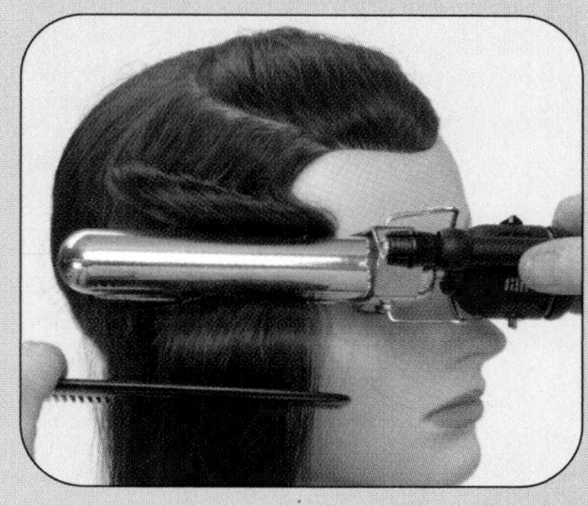

Figure 12–154 Slide irons down.

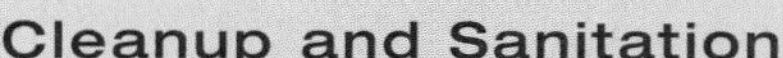

Cleanup and Sanitation

1. Discard the neck strip.
2. Disinfect combs and other implements.
3. Sanitize your workstation.
4. Wash your hands with soap and warm water.

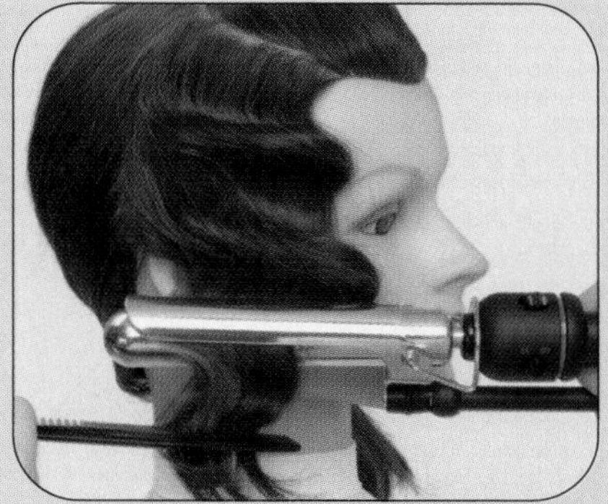

Figure 12–155 Matching the wave.

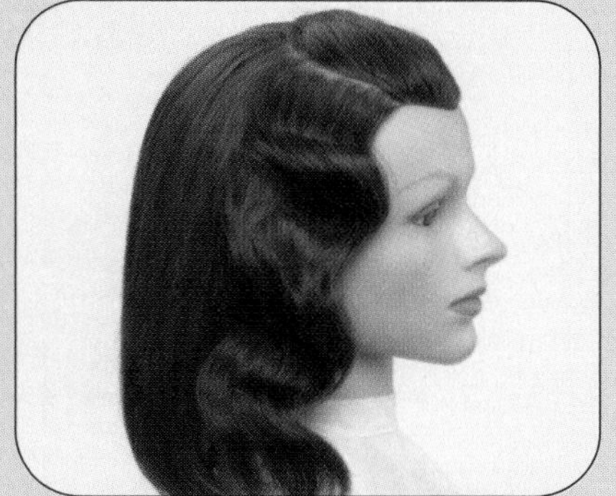

Figure 12–156 Finished thermal waved style.

completed!

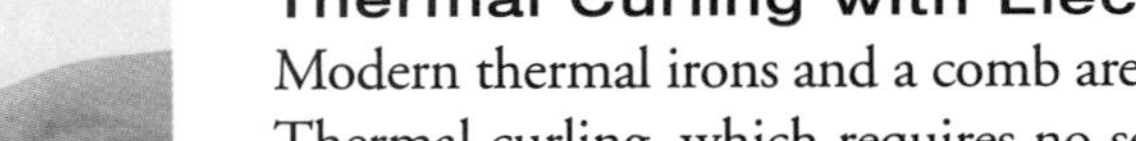

Figure 12-157 Use little finger to open clamp.

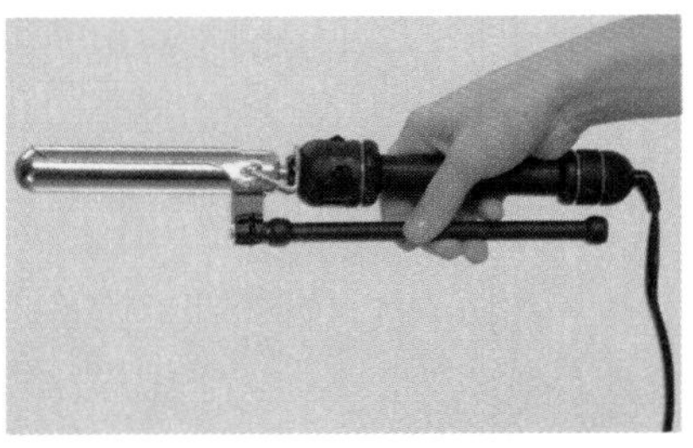

Figure 12-158 Use three middle fingers to close and manipulate irons.

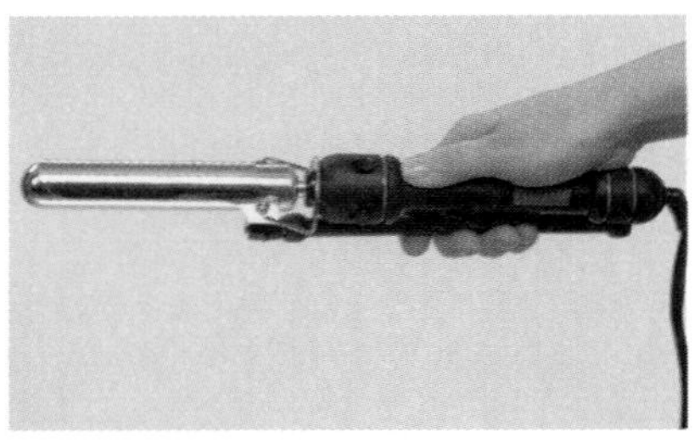

Figure 12-159 Shift thumb when manipulating irons.

Thermal Curling with Electric Thermal Irons

Modern thermal irons and a comb are all you need to give your client curls. Thermal curling, which requires no setting creams or lotions, may be used to great advantage on the following.

- *Straight hair.* Permits quick styling. Thermal curling eliminates working with wet hair and does away with the need for rollers and a long hair-drying process.
- *Pressed hair.* Permits styling the hair without the danger of its returning to its former extremely curly condition. Thermal curling prepares the hair for any desired style.
- *Wigs and hairpieces.* Presents a quick and effective method for their styling.

Curling Irons Manipulations

The following is a series of basic manipulative movements for using heated curling irons. Most other curling irons movements are variations of these basic movements (Figure 12–157, Figure 12–158, Figure 12–159, Figure 12–160, Figure 12–161, Figure 12–162, and Figure 12–163). Some stylists prefer to use just the little finger or the little finger plus the ring finger for this purpose. Either method is correct. The method of holding the irons is a matter of personal preference. Choose the one that gives you the greatest ease, comfort, and facility of movement.

If you want to get really good at using curling irons, the key is to practice manipulating them. Always remember to practice with cold irons, of course. The following four exercises are designed to help you learn the most effective ways to use your irons.

1. Since it is important to develop a smooth rotating movement, practice turning the irons while opening and closing them at regular intervals. Practice rotating the irons in both directions; that is, downward (toward you) and upward (away from you) (Figure 12–164).
2. Practice releasing the hair by opening and closing the irons in a quick, clicking movement.

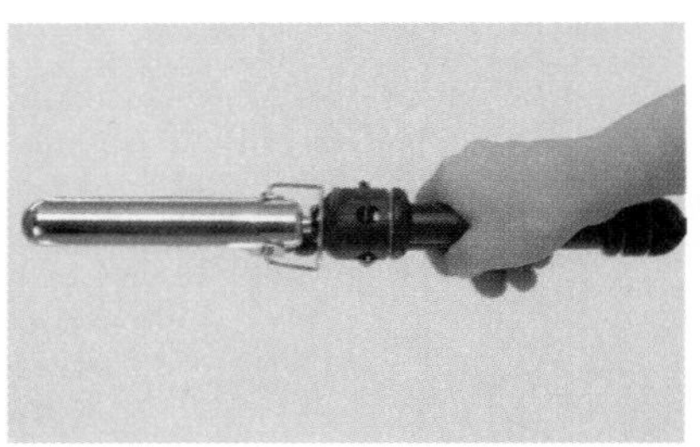

Figure 12-160 Close clamp and make a one-quarter turn downward.

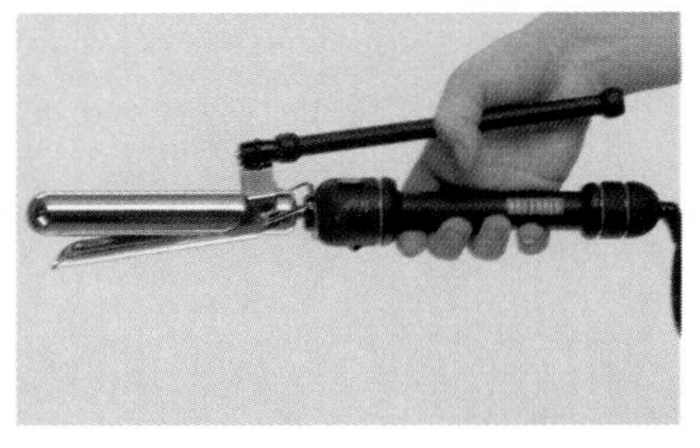

Figure 12-161 Irons have made a one-half turn. Use thumb to open clamp and relax hair tension.

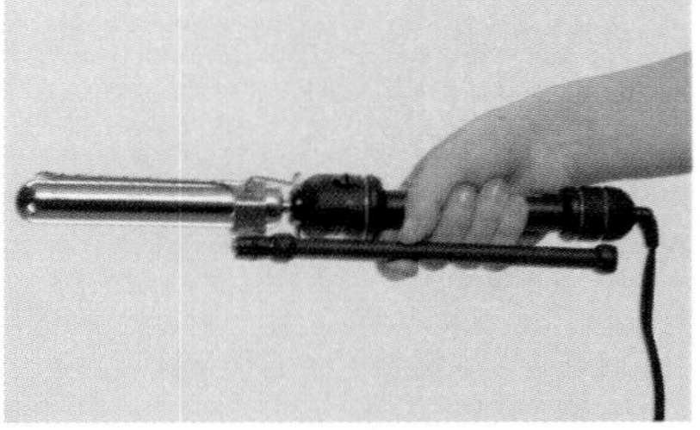

Figure 12-162 Rotate irons to three-quarters of a complete turn.

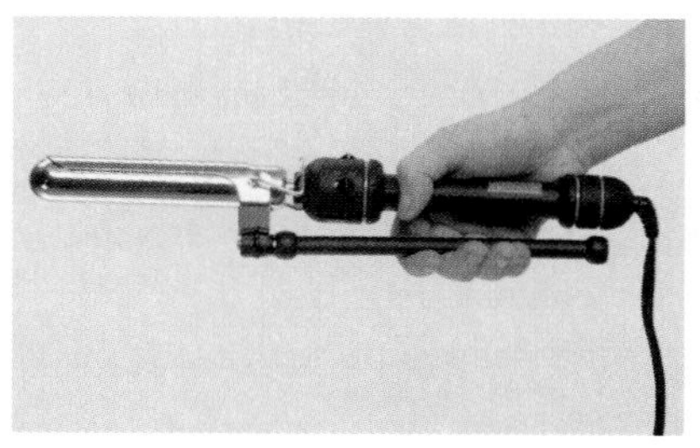
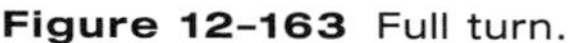

Figure 12–163 Full turn.

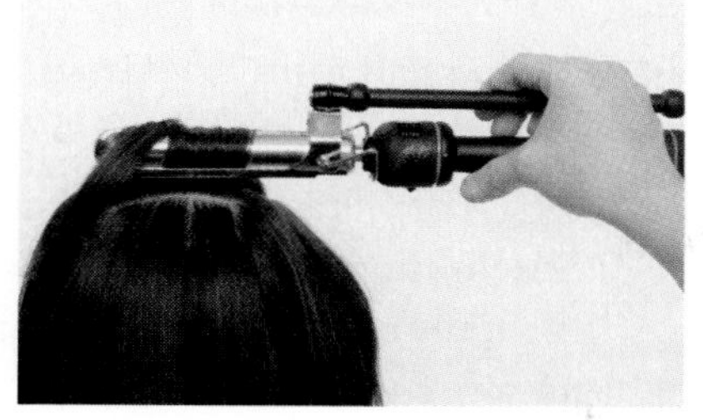

Figure 12–164 Rotate while opening and closing the irons.

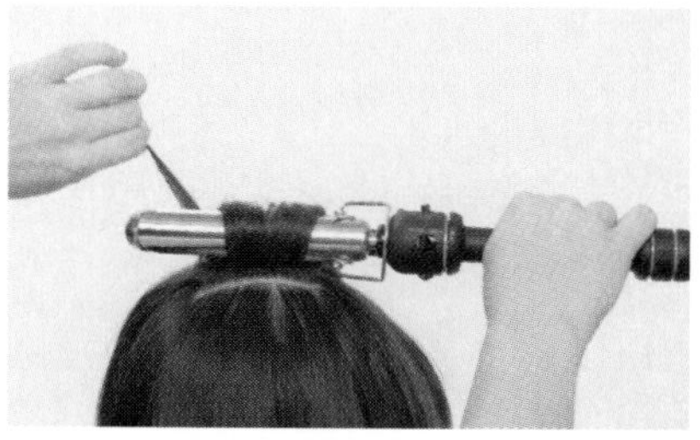

Figure 12–165 Guide hair strand into the center of curl while rotating irons

3. Practice guiding the hair strand into the center of the curl as you rotate the irons. This exercise will ensure that the end of the strand is firmly in the center of the curl (Figure 12–165).
4. Practice removing the curl from the irons by drawing the comb to the left and the rod to the right (Figure 12–166). Use the comb to protect the client's scalp from burns.

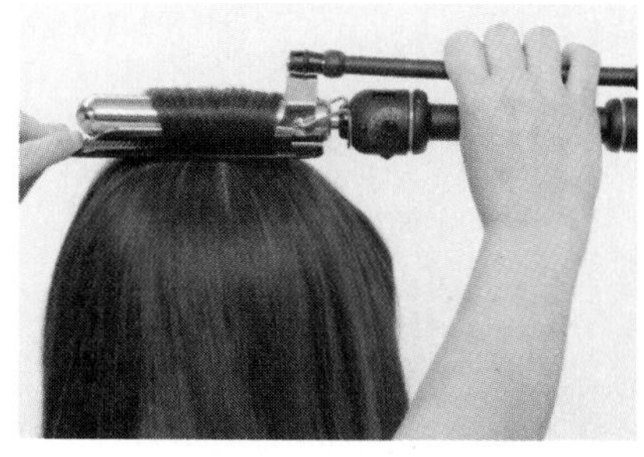

Figure 12–166 Remove curl using comb as guide.

CURLING SHORT HAIR

1. Shampoo and dry the hair. Divide the head into five sections. The first section about 2 ½ inches (6.25 cm) wide, extends from the center of the forehead to the nape of neck. Divide the two side panels in half, from the top parting to the neck, to create four additional sections.
2. Heat thermal irons (large or jumbo size).
3. Begin by sectioning and parting the base of each curl to match the size of the curl desired. It is important to consider hair length, density, and texture. The base is usually about 1-½ inches to 2 inches (3.75 cm to 5 cm) in width and ½ inch (1.25 cm) in depth.
4. After sectioning off the base, comb the hair smooth and straight out from the scalp. Loose hairs may result in an uneven and ragged curl.
5. After the irons have been heated to the desired temperature, pick up a strand of hair and comb it up smoothly. With the groove on top, insert the irons about 1 inch (2.5 cm) from the scalp and hold for a few seconds to form a base (Figure 12–167).
6. Hold the ends of the hair strand with your thumb and two fingers of your left hand (right hand if you are left handed), using a medium degree of tension. Turn the irons downward (toward you) with your right hand (Figure 12–168).
7. Open and close the irons rapidly as you turn, to prevent binding. Guide the ends of the strand into the center of the curl as you rotate the irons (Figure 12–169).
8. The result of this procedure will be a smooth, finished curl, with the ends firmly fixed in the center. Remove the irons from the curl (Figure 12–170).

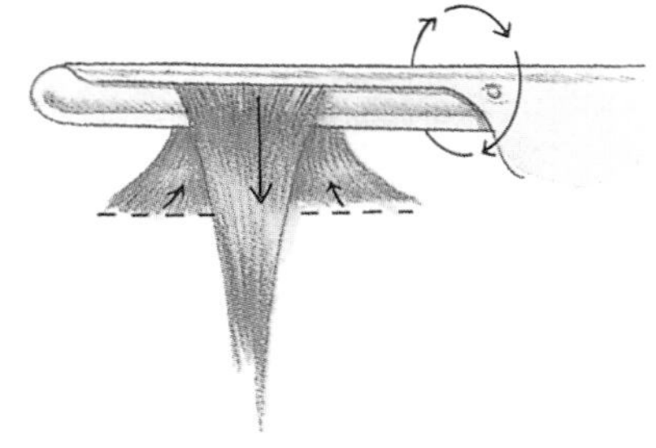

Figure 12–167 Form a base.

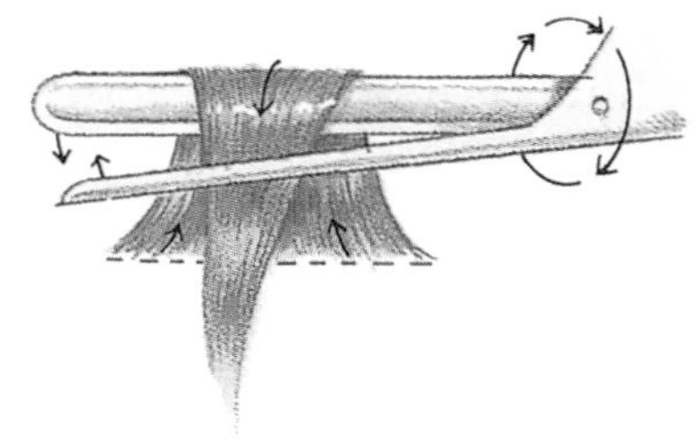

Figure 12–168 Turn irons

CURLING MEDIUM-LENGTH HAIR

1. Section and form the base of the curl as described for short hair.
2. Insert the hair into the open irons at the scalp. Pull the hair over the rod in the direction of the curl and close the shell. Hold irons in this position for about five seconds to heat the hair, and then slide the irons up to 1 inch (2.5 cm) from the scalp. The shell must be on top (Figure 12–171).
3. Turn the irons downward one-half revolution. Then pull the end of the strand over the rod to the left, directing the strand toward the center of the curl (Figure 12–172).
4. Complete the revolution of the irons, and continue directing the ends toward the center (Figure 12–173).
5. Make another complete revolution of the irons. The entire strand has now been curled with the exception of the ends. Enlarge the curl by opening the shell. Insert the ends of the curl into the opening created between the shell and the rod (Figure 12–174).
6. Close the shell and slide the irons toward the handles. This technique will move the ends of the strand into the center of the curl. Rotate the irons several times to even out the distribution of the hair in the curl (Figure 12–175).

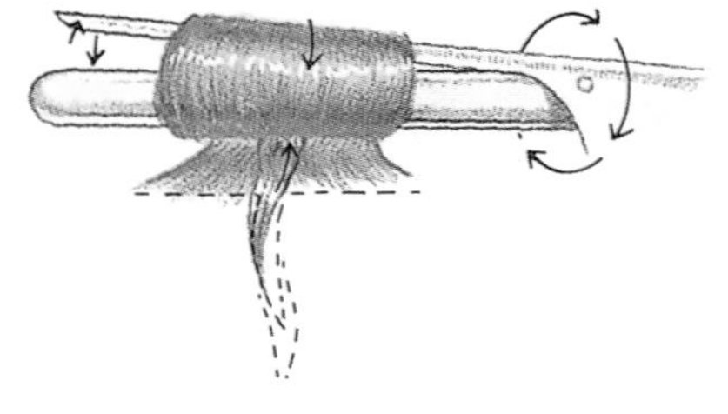

Figure 12-169 Rotate irons and guide ends of strand into center.

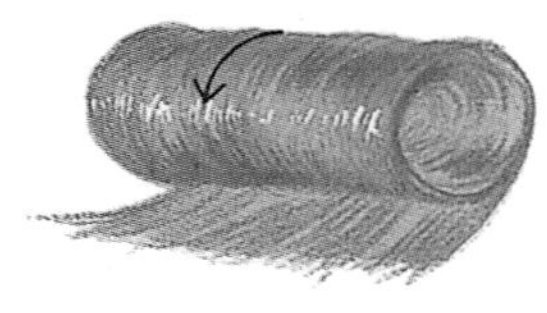

Figure 12-170 Finished curl.

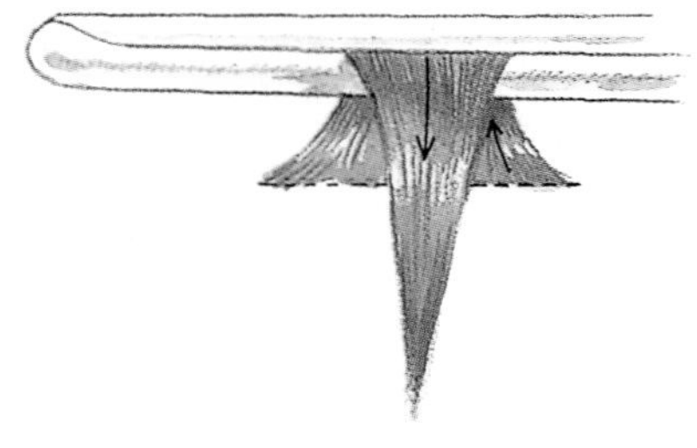

Figure 12-171 Insert hair into open irons at scalp.

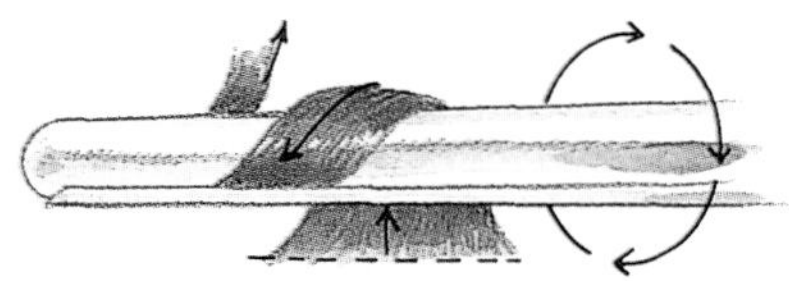

Figure 12-172 Turn irons downward one-half revolution.

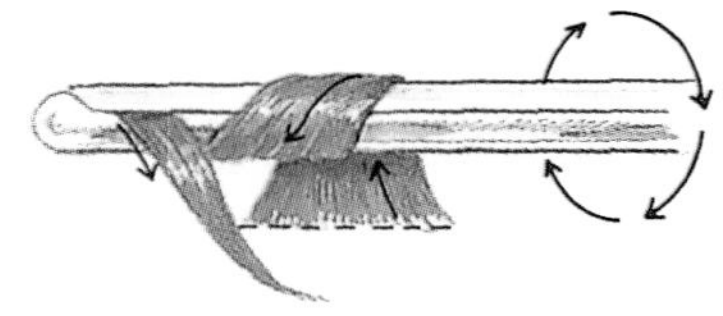

Figure 12-173 Complete revolution of irons.

7. When the curl is formed and the ends are freed from between the rod and the shell, make one complete revolution of the irons inside the curl. This smooths the ends and loosens the hair away from the irons. Use the comb to help remove the curl from the irons. Slowly draw the irons in one direction while drawing the hair in the opposite direction with the comb.

CAUTION

To protect the client during the curling process, use the comb between the scalp and the irons.

CURLING HAIR (USING TWO LOOPS OR "FIGURE 8")

1. Section and form the base of the curl as described for short hair.
2. Insert the hair into the open irons about 1 inch (2.5 cm) from the scalp. Pull the hair over the rod in the direction in which the curl is to move and close the shell. Hold the irons in this position for about five seconds, in order to heat the hair. Hold the strand of hair with a medium degree of tension (Figure 12–176).
3. Roll the irons under; click and roll them until the groove is facing you (Figure 12–177).
4. With the left hand, pick up the ends of the hair (Figure 12–178).
5. Continue to roll and click the irons, keeping them the same distance from the scalp (Figure 12–179).

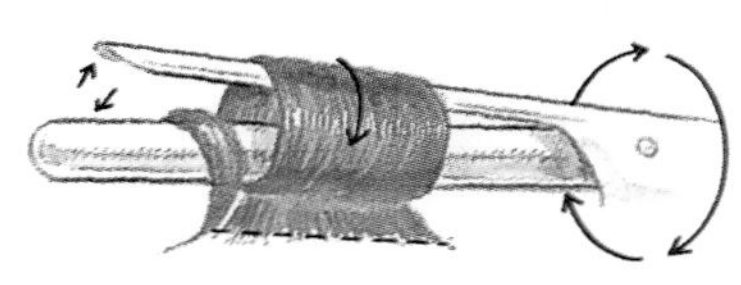
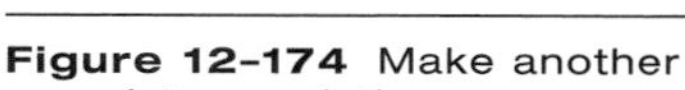

Figure 12–174 Make another complete revolution.

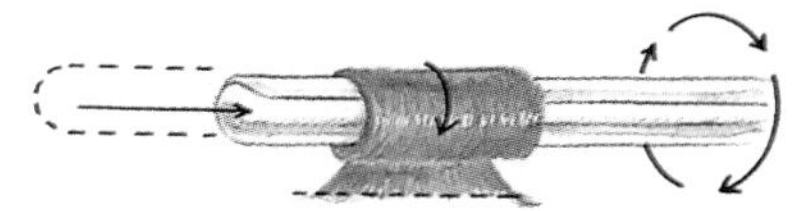

Figure 12–175 Close shell and slide irons toward handles.

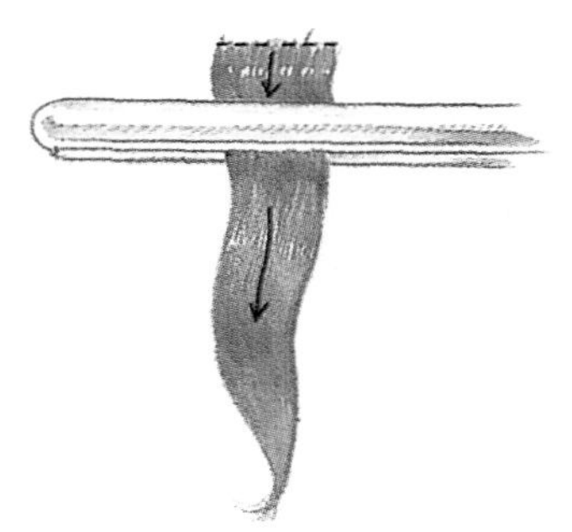

Figure 12–176 Insert hair 1 inch (2.5 cm) from scalp.

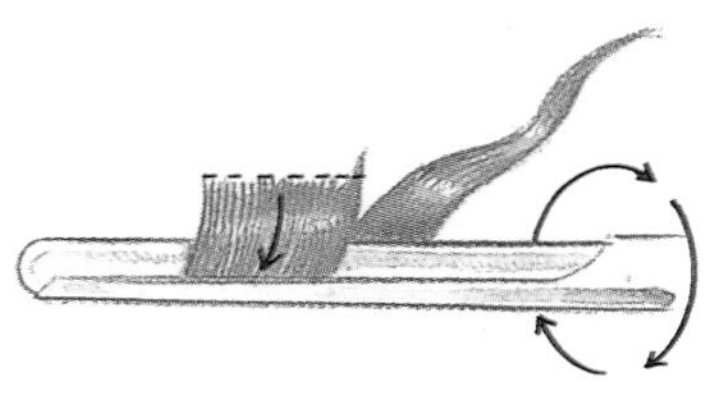

Figure 12–177 Roll irons under.

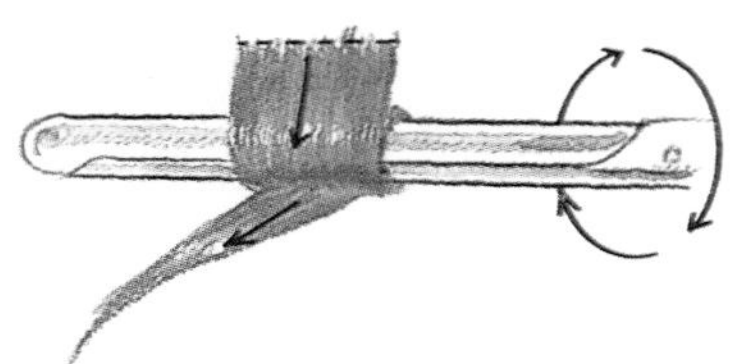

Figure 12–178 Pick up ends of hair.

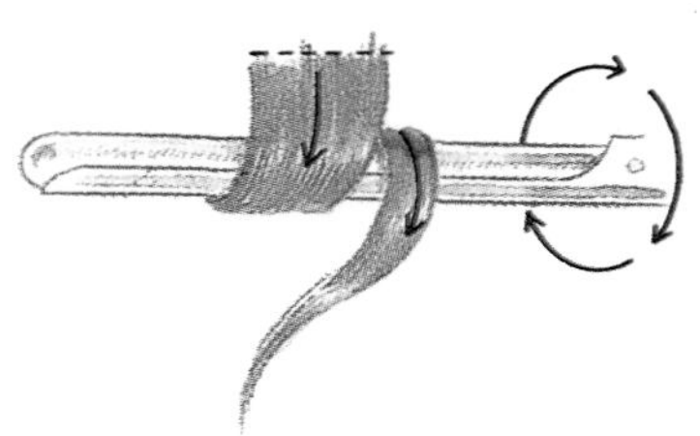

Figure 12–179 Continue to roll irons.

6. Draw the hair strand toward the tip of the irons (Figure 12–180).
7. Draw the strand a little to the right, and, at the same time, push the irons slightly to the left (Figure 12–181).
8. By pushing the irons forward and pushing the hair with the left hand, you will form two loops around the closed irons, with the ends of the strand extending out between the loops (Figure 12–182).
9. Roll under and click the irons until the ends of the hair disappear (Figure 12–183).
10. Rotate the irons several times to even out the distribution of the hair in the curl and to facilitate the movement of the curl off the irons.

Other Types of Curls

There are a number of other curls you can use for your styling purposes. The **spiral curl** is a method of curling the hair by winding a strand around the rod. It creates hanging curls suitable for medium to long hairstyles. To create a spiral curl, part the hair into as many sections as there will be curls and comb smooth. Insert the irons at an angle, with the bowl (groove) on top near the base of the strand, and rotate the irons until all the hair is wound. (Figure 12–184 and Figure 12–185). Hold the curl in this position for four to five seconds, and remove the irons in the usual manner (Figure 12–186 and Figure 12–187).

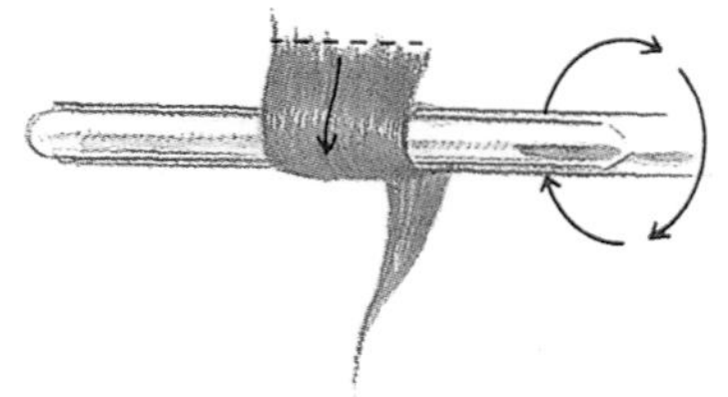

Figure 12-180 Draw hair strand toward the point of the irons.

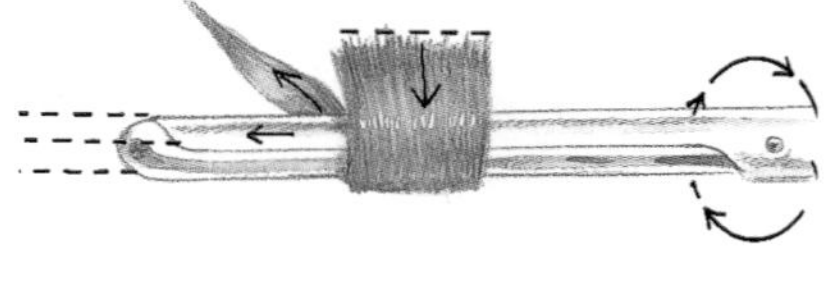

Figure 12-181 Draw strand right, push irons left.

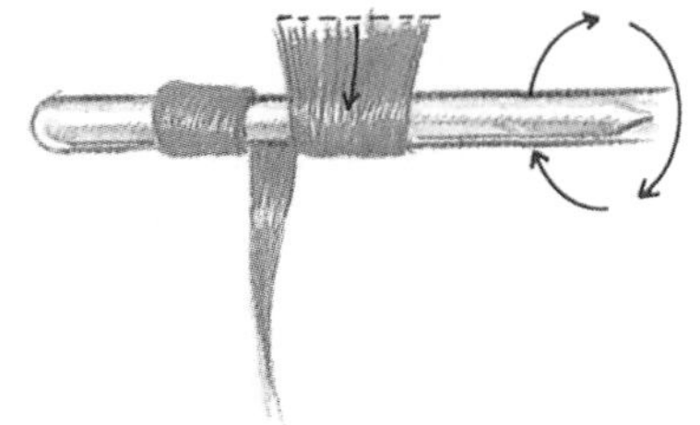

Figure 12-182 Form two loops around closed irons.

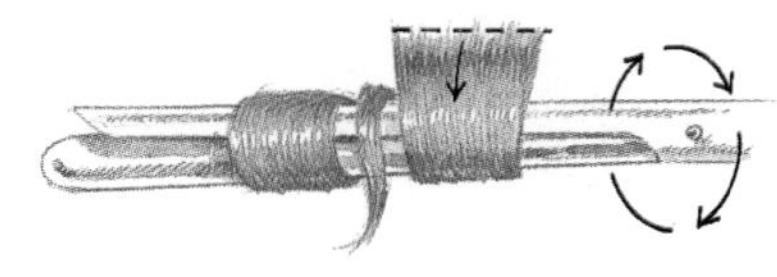

Figure 12-183 Roll irons until hair ends disappear.

End curls can be used to give a finished appearance to hair ends. Long, medium-length, or short hair may be styled with end curls. The hair ends can be turned under or over, as desired. The position of the curling irons and the direction of their movements will determine whether the end curls will turn under or over (Figure 12–188 and Figure 12–189).

Volume Thermal Iron Curls

Volume thermal iron curls are used to create volume or lift in a finished hairstyle. The degree of lift desired determines the type of volume curls to be used.

Volume-Base Thermal Curls

Volume-base curls provide maximum lift or volume, since the curl is placed very high on its base. Section off the base as described. Hold the curl strand at a 135-degree angle. Slide the irons over the strand about ½ inch (1.25 cm) from the scalp. Wrap the strand over the rod with medium tension. Maintain this position for approximately five seconds in order to heat the strand and set the base. Roll the curl in the usual manner and firmly place it forward and high on its base (Figure 12–190).

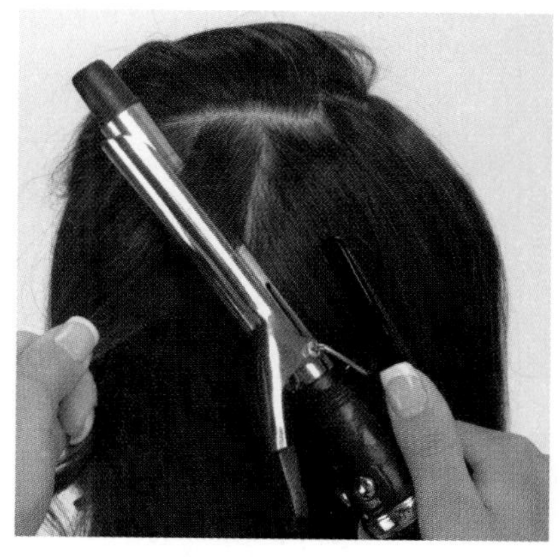

Figure 12–184 Insert irons at an angle.

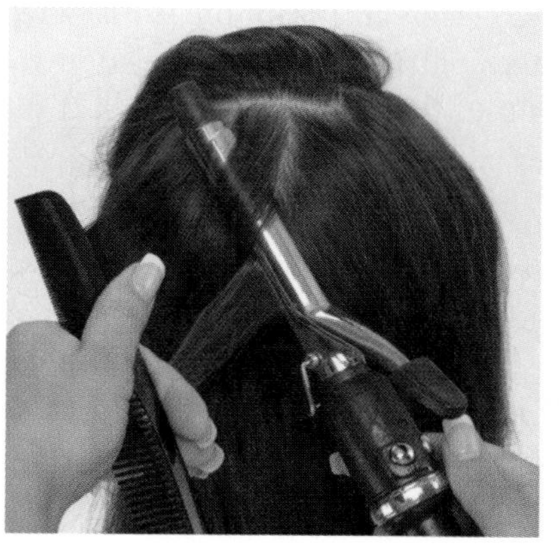

Figure 12–185 Rotate irons until hair is wound.

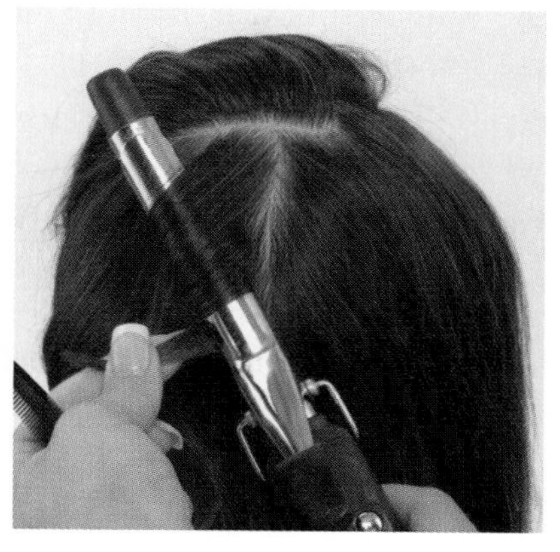

Figure 12–186 Hold curl in position.

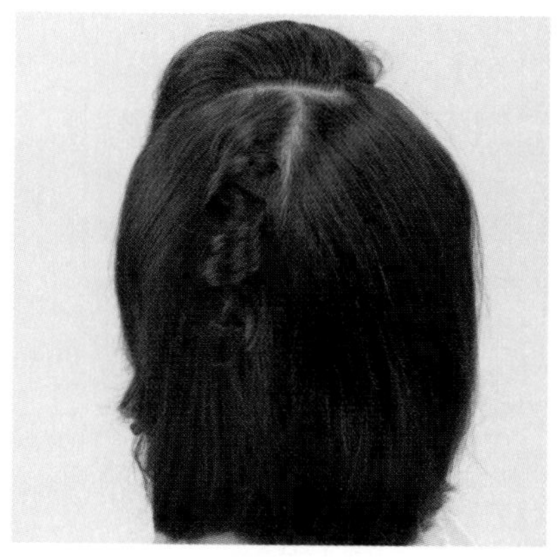

Figure 12–187 Finished curl.

12

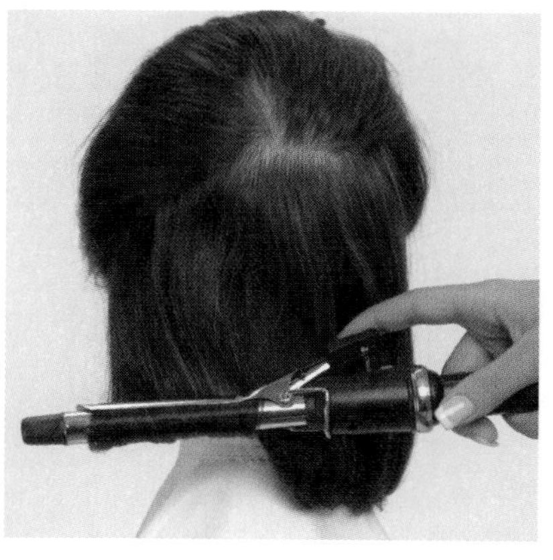

Figure 12–188 Turn irons under.

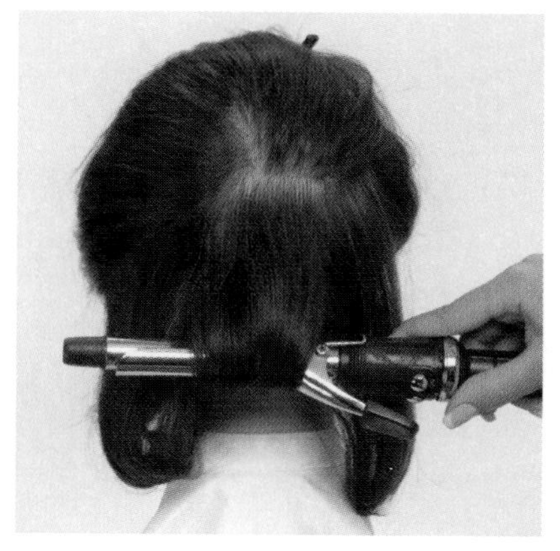

Figure 12–189 Turn irons over.

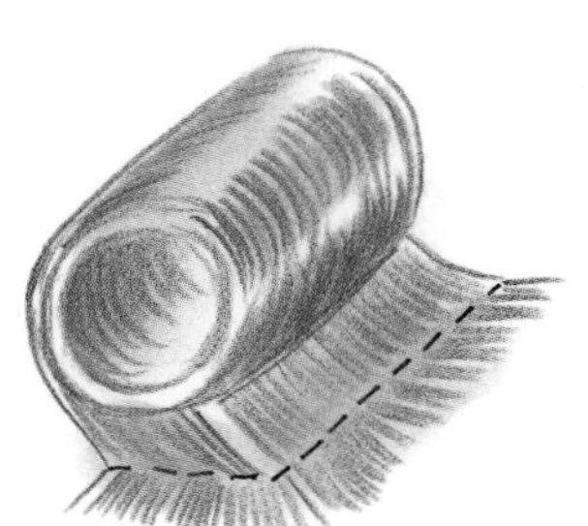

Figure 12–190 Volume-base curl.

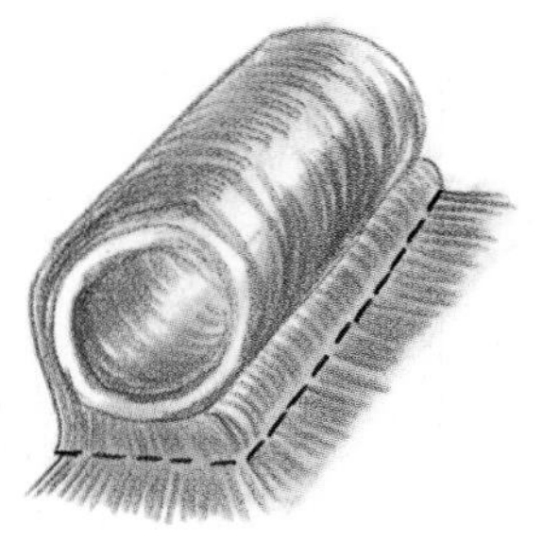

Figure 12–191 Full-base curl.

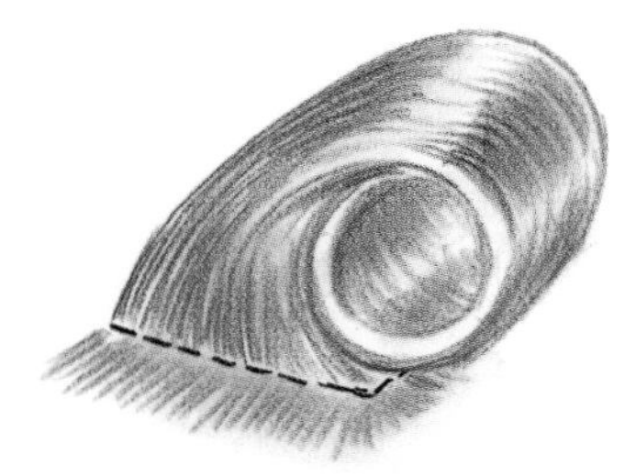

Figure 12–192 Half-base curl.

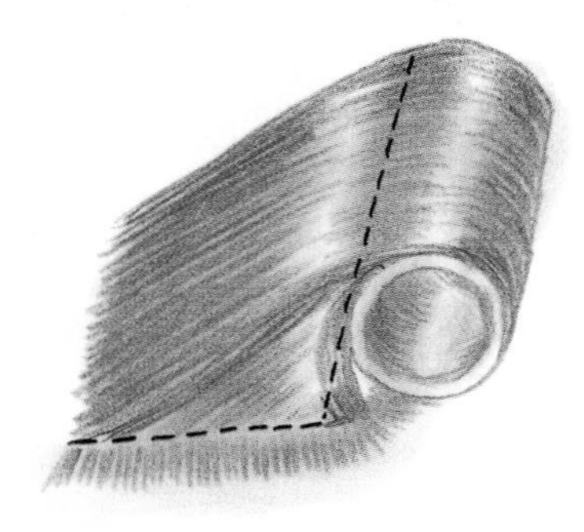

Figure 12–193 Off-base curl.

Full-Base Thermal Curls

Full-base curls provide a strong curl with full volume. Section off the base as described. Hold the hair strand at a 125-degree angle. Slide the irons over the hair strand about ½ inch (1.25 cm) from the scalp. Wrap the strand over the rod with medium tension. Maintain this position for about five seconds to heat the strand and set the base. Roll the curl in the usual manner, and place it firmly in the center of its base (Figure 12–191).

Half-Base Curls

Half-base curls provide a strong curl with moderate lift or volume. Section off the base as described. Hold the hair at a 90-degree angle. Slide irons over the hair strand about ½ inch (1.25 cm) from the scalp. Wrap the strand over the rod with medium tension. Maintain this position for about five seconds to heat the strand and set the base. Roll the curl in the usual manner, and place it half off its base (Figure 12–192).

Off-Base Curls

Off-base curls offer a curl option with only slight lift or volume. Section off the base as described previously, holding the hair at a 70-degree angle. Slide the irons over the hair strand about ½ inch (1.25 cm) from the scalp. Wrap the strand over the rod with medium tension. Maintain this position for about five seconds to heat the strand and set the base. Roll the curl in the usual manner, and place it completely off its base (Figure 12–193).

Finished Thermal Curl Settings

For best results when giving a thermal setting, clip each curl in place until the whole head is complete and ready for styling (Figure 12–194). Brush the hair, working up from the neckline and pushing the waves into place as you progress over the entire head. If the hairstyle is to be finished with curls, do the bottom curls last (Figure 12–195, Figure 12–196, and Figure 12–197). 5✓

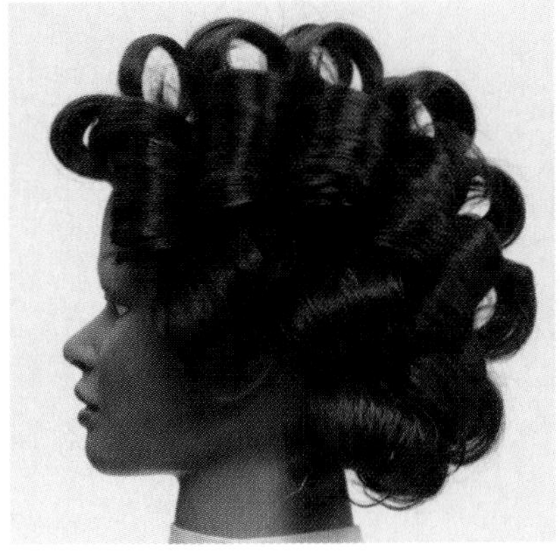

Figure 12–194 Completely curled head, side view.

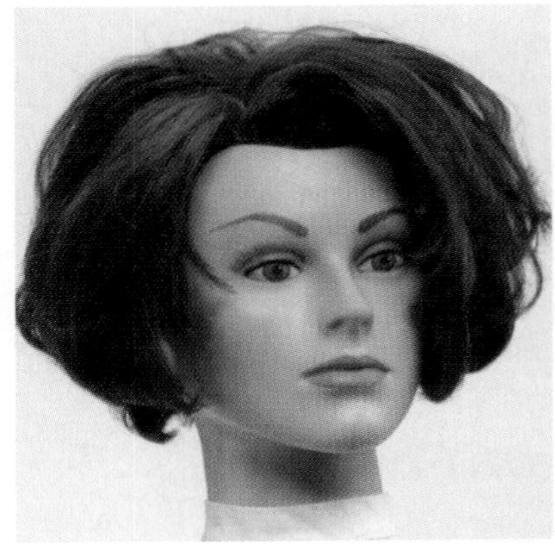

Figure 12–195 Finished thermal-curled short hairstyle.

Safety Measures

1. Use thermal irons only after receiving instruction in their use.
2. Keep thermal irons clean and oil the joint.
3. Do not overheat the irons, because this can damage the ability of the irons to hold heat uniformly.
4. Test the temperature of the irons on tissue paper before placing them on the hair. This will safeguard against burning the hair. Do not inhale the fumes of the irons because they are injurious to the lungs.
5. Do not place the hot irons near the face to test for temperature; a burn can result.
6. Handle thermal irons carefully to avoid burning yourself or the client.
7. Place hot irons in a safe place to cool. Do not leave them where someone might accidentally come into contact with them and be burned.
8. When heating the irons, do not place handles too close to the heater. Your hand might be burned when removing the irons.
9. Make sure the irons are properly balanced in the heater, or they might fall and be damaged or injure someone.
10. Use only hard rubber or nonflammable combs. Celluloid combs must not be used in thermal curling, as they are flammable.
11. Do not use metal combs; they can become hot and burn the scalp.
12. Do not use combs with broken teeth. They can break or split the hair or injure the scalp.
13. Place a comb between the scalp and the thermal irons when curling or waving hair to prevent burning the scalp.
14. The client's hair must be clean and completely dry to ensure a good thermal curl or wave.
15. If the hair is thick and bulky, thin and taper it first.
16. On lightened or tinted hair, use thermal irons only on lower settings.
17. Do not allow the hair ends to protrude over the irons; to do so will cause fishhooks (hair that is bent or folded)
18. Do not use vaporizing thermal irons on pressed hair because the hair will revert to its original extremely curly state.
19. Do not use thermal irons on chemically straightened hair because they might cause damage to the hair. They can be used on relaxed hair if the heat is controlled.
20. A first aid kit must always be kept available in case of an accident.

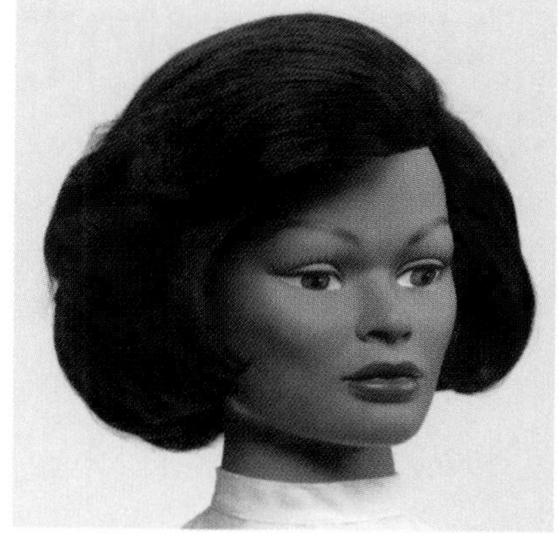

Figure 12–196 Finished thermal-curled medium-length hairstyle.

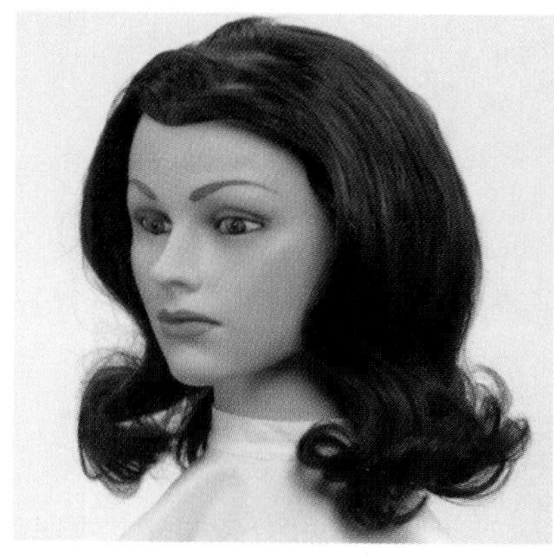

Figure 12–197 Finished thermal-curled long hairstyle.

insights

Holly Simon

After 19 years in the industry, freelance platform artist Holly Simon radiates fulfillment.

I always knew I was going to be in this field, ever since I was a little girl. As far back as I can remember, I was doing kids' hair in the bathroom and practicing on my sister and girlfriends. I went straight into beauty school after high school and then went straight into a job. I had the talent in my hands and I loved the work. To be able to meet so many different kinds of people—that's what I love.

I nurture every client into a friend. My clients bring me knowledge I couldn't learn from books. They give me recipes, hotel information—they even give me advice on raising my kids. I also love the work because it's such fun to turn a duckling into a swan. I can find beauty in anyone.

12

That's the challenge in this work—to keep yourself excited behind the chair. For me, every haircut is truly an individual way to express my creativity. It's not just a cookie cutter haircut; it's not just a trim. I'm giving them 100 percent of myself during the time they're here. And when you make one person happy, you get ten back—that's the secret of building a client base. But you have to be a great person on top of being a very good hairdresser. You have to be able to listen, to make people feel comfortable, and to be kind.

Continuing education, which is what I'm involved in as a platform artist, is also crucial. You use it to grow and to spread your wings. If you keep on learning and if you're a good person, you'll make it. You can even get beyond huge mistakes if you're honest and humble. Most mistakes are fixable, anyway. It's very rare that something so horrendous happens that you can't fix it with one more step. Usually something as simple as a filler or a deeper color, or even just a minute with a color remover, will do the trick. One thing that is not fixable, though: never cut a woman's bangs too short. That's a bad one!

It's such a great industry. And not just the glamour part. You can do little kids or you can work in a cancer ward making women feel good about themselves—there are so many ways to make other people happy. And we are in a profession where we will never lose our jobs. They have done research that shows that even in the midst of wars and depression, women will always have their hair done. Even with their last dollar. Because we have the talent and this awesome, awesome gift to bring out the beauty in someone.

THERMAL HAIR STRAIGHTENING (HAIR PRESSING)

Hair straightening, or pressing, is a popular service that is also very profitable in the salon. When properly done, **hair pressing** temporarily straightens extremely curly or unruly hair by means of a heated iron or comb. A pressing generally lasts until the hair is shampooed next. (Permanent hair straightening is covered in Chapter 15.) Hair pressing also prepares the hair for additional services, such as thermal roller curling and croquignole thermal curling (the two-loop or "Figure 8" technique). A good hair pressing leaves the hair in a natural and lustrous condition and is not at all harmful to the hair (Figure 12–198).

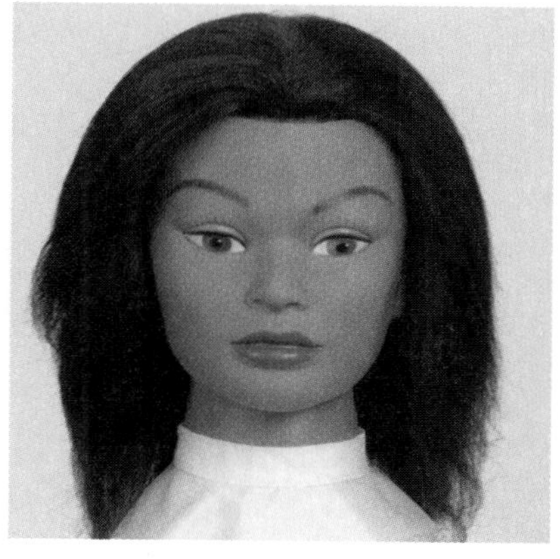

Figure 12-198 Pressed hairstyle.

There are three types of hair pressing.

1. **Soft press**, which removes about 50 to 60 percent of the curl, is accomplished by applying the thermal pressing comb once on each side of the hair.
2. **Medium press**, which removes about 60 to 75 percent of the curl, is accomplished by applying the thermal pressing comb once on each side of the hair, using slightly more pressure.
3. **Hard press**, which removes 100 percent of the curl, involves the application of the thermal pressing comb twice on each side of the hair. A hard press can also be done by first passing a hot curling iron through the hair. This is called a **double press**. 6

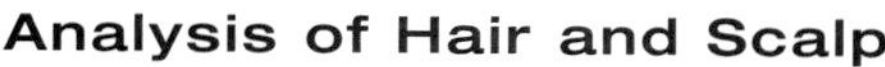

Analysis of Hair and Scalp

Before you press a client's hair, you will need to analyze the condition of the hair and scalp.

If the client's hair and scalp are not normal, you should give appropriate advice concerning corrective treatments. In the case of scalp abrasions, it is not the cosmetologist's job to diagnose the condition, but rather to advise the client to see a dermatologist. If the hair shows signs of neglect or abuse caused by faulty pressing, lightening, or tinting, recommend a series of conditioning treatments. Failure to correct dry and brittle hair can result in hair breakage during hair pressing. Burnt hair strands cannot be conditioned.

CAUTION

Under no circumstances should hair pressing be given to a client who has a scalp abrasion, a contagious scalp condition, a scalp injury, or chemically damaged hair. Chemically relaxed hair should not be pressed.

Remember to check your client's hair for elasticity and porosity. Under normal conditions, if a client's hair has good elasticity, it can be safely stretched to about 50 percent of its original length. If the porosity is normal, then the hair returns to its natural wave pattern when it is wet or moistened.

A careful analysis of the client's hair should cover the following points:

- wave pattern
- length
- texture (coarse, medium, fine, or very fine)
- feel (wiry, soft, or silky)

- elasticity
- shade (natural, faded, streaked, gray, tinted, lightened)
- condition (normal, brittle, dry, oily, damaged, or chemically treated)
- condition of scalp (normal, flexible, or tight)

It is important that the cosmetologist be able to recognize individual differences in hair texture, porosity, elasticity, and scalp flexibility. Guided by knowledge, the cosmetologist can determine how much pressure the hair and scalp can handle without breakage, hair loss, or burning from a pressing comb that may not be adjusted to the correct temperature.

Hair Texture

Variations in hair texture have to do with the diameter of the hair (coarse, medium, or fine) and the feel of the hair (wiry, soft, or silky). Touching the client's hair and asking specifically about hair characteristics will help you to determine the best way to treat a client's hair.

Coarse, extremely curly hair has qualities that make it difficult to press. Coarse hair has the greatest diameter, and during the pressing process it requires more heat and pressure than medium or fine hair.

Medium curly hair is the normal type of hair that cosmetologists deal with in the beauty salon. No special problem is presented by this type of hair, and it is the least resistant to hair pressing.

activity

Choose a partner and role-play a scene in which you must inform a client that you cannot work on his hair because of the condition of his hair or scalp. Read the following conversation for ideas.

Stylist: Hello, Mr. Richards. My name is Ben. I'll be cutting your hair today.

Mr. Richards: Hello, Ben. You can call me George.

Ben: OK, George. Have a seat in my chair and let's talk about what you'd like done today.

George: Fine. As you can see, I wear my hair fairly short. I like the style, but it needs some trimming. I last had a haircut four or five weeks ago.

Ben (examining the scalp): George, have you noticed any discomfort on your scalp lately?

George: As a matter of fact, yes, I have. Is there a problem?

Ben: Nothing that can't be easily fixed, I'm sure. I'm not qualified to make a diagnosis, but I do recommend that you see a dermatologist. Your scalp is very irritated and has abrasions in some spots. I'm concerned that combing your hair could make it worse. Why don't we reschedule your appointment? The dermatologist can probably recommend something that will control this problem very quickly.

George: I understand. Thanks for your advice. I had no idea it had gotten that bad.

Ben: My pleasure. Let's rebook that appointment.

Fine hair requires special care. To avoid hair breakage, less heat and pressure should be applied than for other hair textures. Whereas coarse and medium hair has three layers (cuticle, cortex, and medulla), fine hair has only two layers (cortex and cuticle)

Wiry, curly hair may be coarse, medium, or fine. It feels stiff, hard, and glassy. Because of the compact construction of the cuticle cells, it is very resistant to hair pressing and requires more heat and pressure than other types of hair.

Scalp Condition

The condition of the client's scalp can be classified as normal, tight, or flexible. It the scalp is normal, proceed with an analysis of the texture and elasticity of the hair. If the scalp is tight and the hair coarse, press the hair in the direction in which it grows to avoid injury to the scalp. The main difficulty with a flexible scalp is that the cosmetologist might not apply enough pressure to press the hair satisfactorily.

Record Card

Be sure to keep a record of the results of your hair and scalp analysis as well as all pressing treatments performed on a client. It is also a good idea to question the client about any lightener, tint, color restorer (metallic), or other chemical treatment that has been used on her hair. A release statement should be used for hair pressing, as with all services that might protect the stylist from responsibility for accidents or damages. See Figure 4–9 in Chapter 4 for an example of a release statement on the client consultation card.

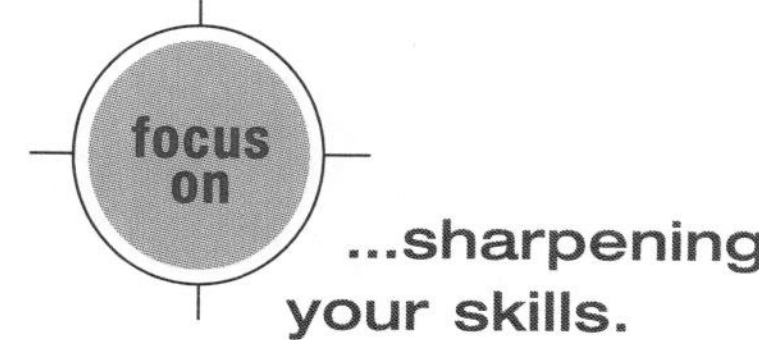

Once you become adept at the basic styles presented in this chapter, you will want to experiment and create your own styles. Each client's hair represents more possibilities for creativity. That is why having a mannequin at home to duplicate the looks you see in magazines is such an important part of your "continuing education." Trends change quickly, and you need to be current in your skills at all times.

Conditioning Treatments

Effective conditioning treatments involve special cosmetic preparations for the hair and scalp, thorough brushing, and scalp massage. Applying a conditioning treatment usually results in better hair pressing. The use of an infrared lamp is optional, depending on the type of treatment being given. Review Chapter 10 for suggested conditioning treatments, specifically Table 10–1.

A tight scalp can be made more flexible by the systematic use of scalp massage or hair brushing. The client benefits because there is better circulation of blood to the scalp.

Pressing Combs

There are two types of pressing combs: regular and electric. They should both be constructed of either good-quality stainless steel or brass. The handle is usually made of wood since wood does not readily absorb heat. The space between the teeth of the comb varies with the size and style of the comb. A comb with more space between the teeth produces a coarse or open-looking press, while a comb with less space produces a smoother press. Pressing combs vary in size. Some are short, to be used with short hair, while long combs are used with long hair.

It may be a good idea to temper a new pressing comb if it is made of brass. Tempering allows the brass to hold heat evenly along the entire length of the comb, which gives better results when used on your clients' hair. Another good reason to temper is to burn off any polish the manufacturer may have used to coat the comb. If the polish is not burned off, the comb may stick to the hair, causing scorching and breakage.

To temper a new pressing comb, place the comb in the heating appliance until it is extremely hot. Remove the comb and submerge or coat it in petroleum or pressing oil. Let it cool down naturally, then rinse under hot running water to remove the oil.

Heating the Comb

Depending on what they are made of, combs vary in their ability to accept and retain heat. Regular pressing combs may be heated on gas stoves or are heated electrically (Figure 12–199). While the comb is being heated, its teeth should face upward and the handle should be kept away from the fire. After heating the comb to the proper temperature, test it on a piece of light paper. If the paper becomes scorched, allow the comb to cool slightly before applying it to the hair.

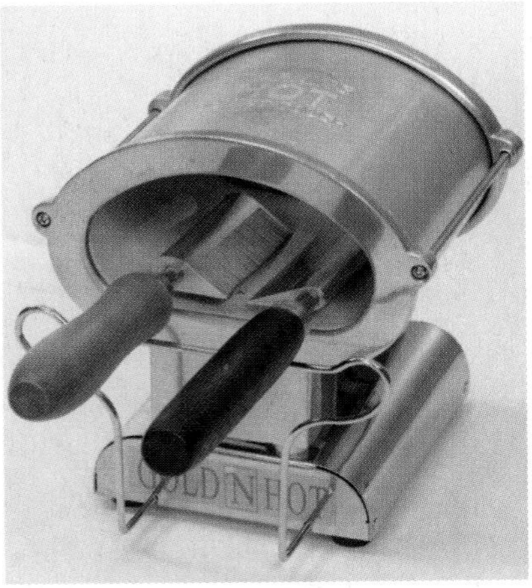

Figure 12-199 Electric heater for pressing combs.

Electric pressing combs are available in two forms. One comes with an "on" and "off" switch; the other is equipped with a thermostat that has a control switch indicating high or low degrees of heat.

There is also a straightening comb attachment that fits the nozzle of a standard hand-held dryer and is less damaging than an electric comb or an oven-heated comb.

Cleaning the Comb

The pressing comb will perform more efficiently if it is kept clean and free of carbon. Wipe the comb clean of loose hair, grease, and dust before and after every use. The intense heat keeps the comb sterile, once all loose hair or clinging dirt is removed.

Remove the carbon from the comb by rubbing the outside surface and between the teeth with a fine steel wool pad or fine sandpaper. Then place the metal portion of the comb in a hot baking soda solution for about one hour; rinse and dry. The metal will acquire a smooth and shiny appearance.

Pressing Oil or Cream

Prepare the hair for a hair pressing treatment by first applying pressing oil or cream. Both these products have the following effects:

- they make hair softer
- they prepare and condition hair for pressing
- they help prevent hair from burning or scorching
- they help prevent hair breakage
- they condition the hair after pressing
- they add sheen to pressed hair
- they help hair stay pressed longer

PROCEDURE

SOFT PRESSING FOR NORMAL CURLY HAIR

The following procedure is one of several ways to give a hair pressing treatment. Keep in mind that you can adjust the procedure according to the methods your instructor demonstrates.

Implements and Materials

- shampoo
- towels
- shampoo and styling capes
- neck strip
- pressing comb
- clips
- pressing oil or cream
- heating appliance (gas or electric heater or attachment)
- hairbrush and comb
- spatula
- pomade
- thermal irons

Preparation

1. Drape the client for shampooing.
2. Shampoo, rinse, and towel-dry the client's hair.
3. Drape the client for thermal styling, using a neck strip and styling cape.
4. Apply pressing oil or cream (some stylists prefer to apply pressing oil or cream to the hair after it has been completely dried) (Figure 12–200).
5. Dry hair thoroughly (blow-drying will leave the hair more manageable than hood drying).
6. Comb and divide the hair into four main sections and pin them up (Figure 12–201).

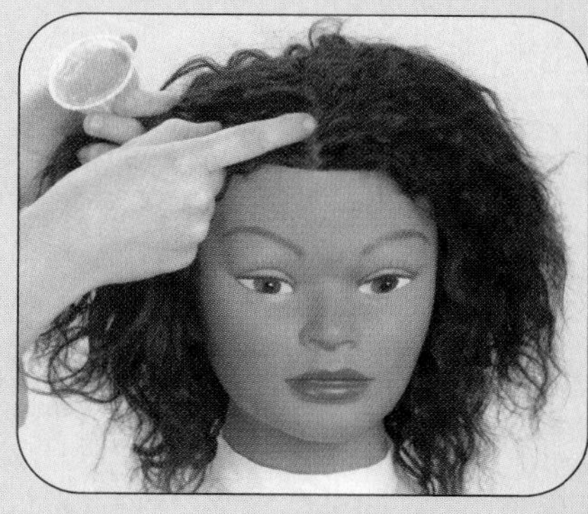

Figure 12-200 Apply pressing oil or cream to client's hair.

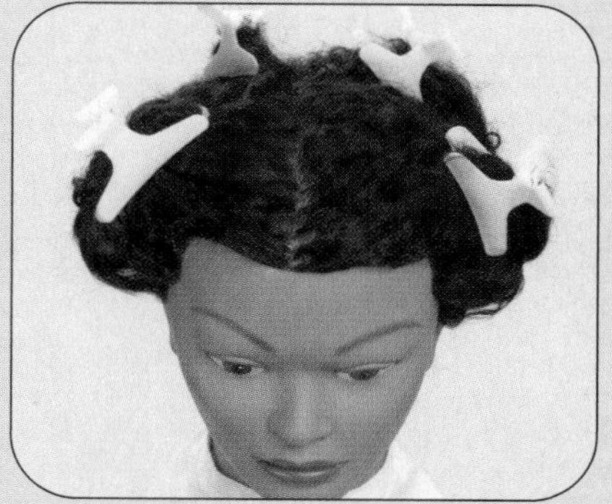

Figure 12-201 Divide hair into four sections.

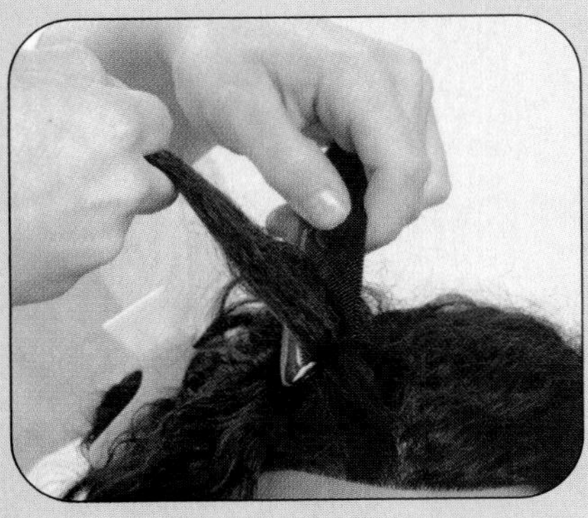

Figure 12-202 Unpin one section.

Procedure

1. Place the pressing comb in the heater.
2. Unpin one section of the hair at a time and subdivide into smaller partings. Beginning at the right side of the head, work from front to back (some stylists prefer to start at the back of the head and work forward) (Figure 12-202).
3. If necessary, apply pressing oil evenly and sparingly over the small hair sections.
4. Test the temperature of the heated pressing comb on a white cloth or white paper to determine heat intensity before you place it on the hair (Figure 12-203).
5. Lift the end of a small hair section with the index finger and thumb of the left hand and hold it upward, away from the scalp.
6. Holding the pressing comb in the right hand, insert the teeth of the comb into the top side of the hair section (Figure 12-204).
7. Draw out the pressing comb slightly; make a quick turn so that the hair strand wraps itself partly around the comb. The back rod of the comb actually does the pressing (Figure 12-205).

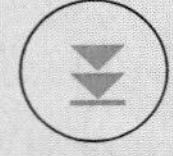

Here's a tip:

Subdivide the sections into 1-inch to 1 ½-inch (2.5 to 3.75 cm) partings, depending on the texture and density of the hair. For medium-textured hair of average density, use subsections of average size. For coarse hair with greater density, use smaller sections to ensure complete heat penetration and effectiveness. For thin or fine hair with sparse density, use larger sections.

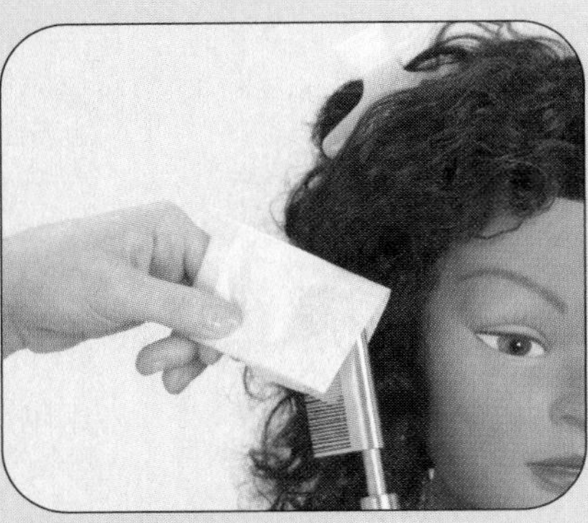

Figure 12-203 Test heated pressing comb.

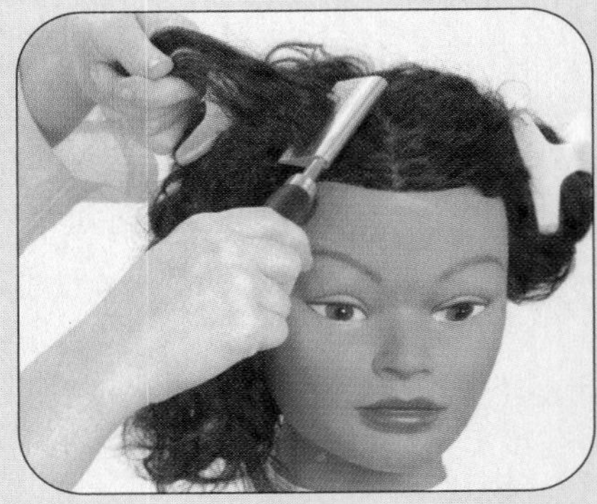

Figure 12-204 Insert comb into top side of hair section.

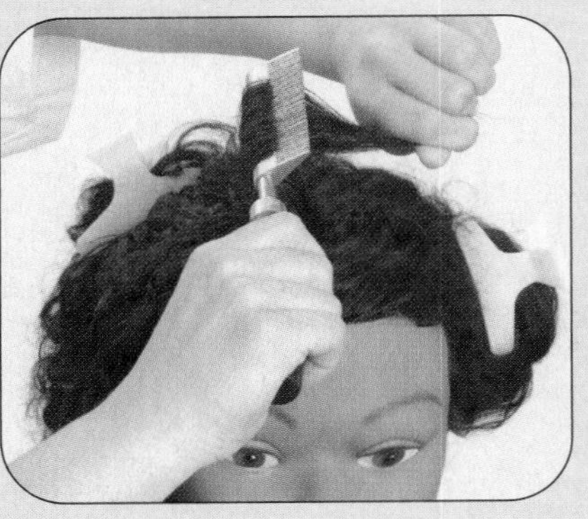

Figure 12-205 Press hair strand with back rod of comb.

8. Press the comb slowly through the hair strand until the ends of the hair pass through the teeth of the comb (Figure 12–206).
9. Bring each completed hair section over to the opposite side of the head (Figure 12–207).
10. Continue Steps 4 to 8 on both sections on the right side of the head; then do the same on both sections on the left side.
11. Apply a little pomade to the hair near the scalp and brush it through the hair. If desired, the hair can be curled with a curling iron at this time.
12. Style and comb the hair according to the client's wishes (Figure 12–208).

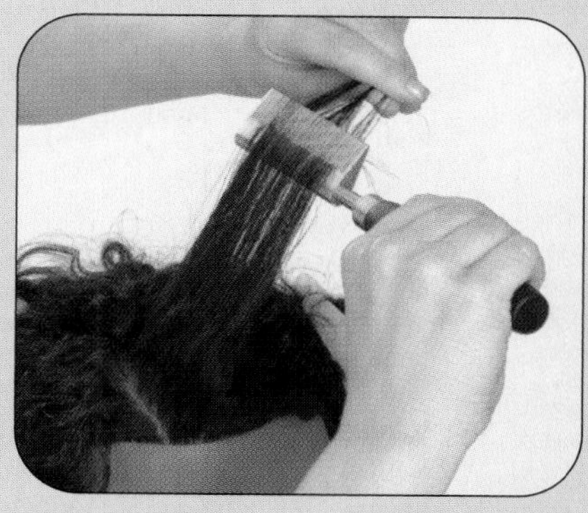

Figure 12-206 Bring pressing comb through ends of hair.

Cleanup and Sanitation

1. Discard disposable items. Disinfect brush and comb.
2. Clean the pressing comb according to the instructions on page 412.
3. Sanitize your workstation.
4. Wash hands with soap and warm water.

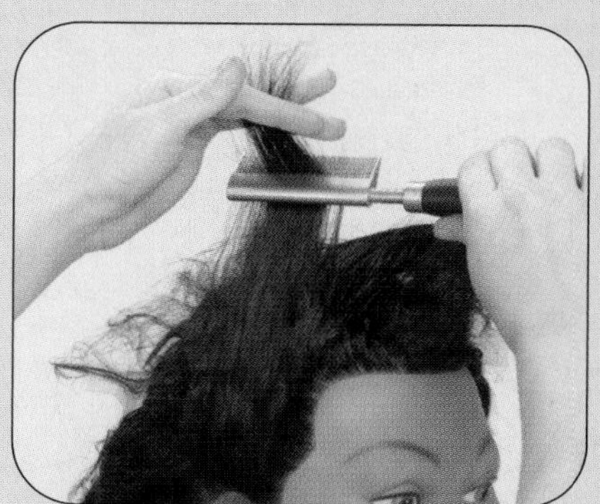

Figure 12-207 Bring finished section to one side.

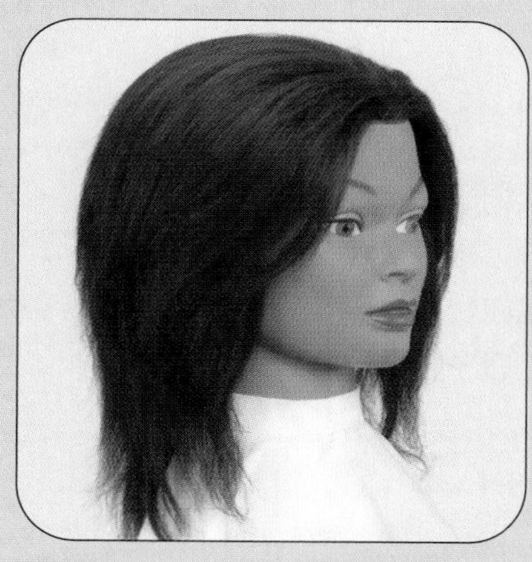

Figure 12-208 Finished pressed hairstyle.

completed!

Hard Press

A hard press is recommended when the results of a soft press are not satisfactory. The entire comb press procedure is repeated. Pressing oil should be added to hair strands only if necessary. A hard press is also known as a double-comb press.

Touch-Ups

Touch-ups are sometimes necessary when the hair becomes curly again due to perspiration, dampness, or other conditions. The process is the same as for the original pressing treatment, with the shampoo omitted. 7

Safety Precautions

The injuries that can occur in hair pressing are of two types.

1. Those that are the immediate results of hair pressing and that cause physical damage, such as burnt hair that breaks off, burnt scalp that causes either temporary or permanent loss of hair, and burns on the ears and neck that form scars.
2. Those that are not immediately evident but can later cause physical damage, such as a skin rash if the client is allergic to pressing oil or the breaking and shortening of the hair due to overly frequent hair pressings.

CAUTION

In case of a scalp burn, immediately apply 1 percent gentian violet jelly.

Good judgment should be used to avoid damage, with consideration always given to the texture of the hair and condition of the scalp. The client's safety is assured only when the stylist observes every precaution and is especially careful during the actual hair pressing. The stylist should avoid using the following:

- excessive heat or pressure on the hair and scalp
- too much pressing oil on the hair (it attracts dirt and makes the hair look greasy and artificial)
- perfumed pressing oil near the scalp if the client is allergic
- overly frequent hair pressing, which weakens the hair

Reminders and Hints on Soft Pressing

- Keep the comb clean and free from carbon at all times.
- Avoid overheating the pressing comb.
- Test the temperature of the heated comb on a white cloth or white paper before applying it to the hair.
- Adjust the temperature of the pressing comb to the texture and condition of the client's hair.
- Use the heated comb carefully to avoid burning the skin, scalp, or hair.
- Prevent the smoking or burning of hair during the pressing treatment by drying the hair completely after it is shampooed and avoiding excessive application of pressing oil over the hair.
- Use a moderately warm comb to press short hair on the temples and back of the neck. You may also use a temple comb, which is about half the size of a regular pressing comb.

Special Considerations

You should heed certain precautions and safeguards when dealing with the following special situations.

- *Pressing fine hair.* Follow the same procedure as for normal hair, being careful not to use a hot pressing comb or too much pressure. To avoid hair breakage, apply less pressure to the hair near the ends. After completely pressing the hair, style it.
- *Pressing short, fine hair.* Extra care must be taken at the hairline. When the hair is extra short, the pressing comb should not be too hot because the hair is fine and will burn easily; a hot comb can also cause accidental burns, which are very painful and can cause scars. In the event of an accidental burn, immediately apply one percent gentian violet jelly to the burn.
- *Pressing coarse hair.* Apply enough pressure so that the hair remains straightened.
- *Pressing tinted, lightened, or gray (unpigmented) hair.* This hair requires special care. Lightened or tinted hair might require conditioning treatments, depending on the extent to which it has been damaged. Gray hair may be particularly resistant. To obtain good results, use a moderately heated pressing comb applied with light pressure. Avoid excessive heat as discoloration or breakage can occur.

chapter glossary

back-brushing	technique used to build a soft cushion or mesh two or more curl patterns together for a uniform and smooth comb-out; also called ruffing
back-combing	combing small sections of hair from the ends toward the scalp, causing shorter hair to mat at the scalp and form a cushion or base; also called teasing, ratting, matting, or French lacing
barrel curls	pin curls with large center openings; are fastened to the head in a standing position on a rectangular base
base	the stationary, or nonmoving, foundation of a pin curl, which is the area closest to the scalp; the panel of hair on which a roller is placed
blow-dry styling	technique of drying and styling damp hair in one operation
carved curls	pin curls sliced from a shaping and formed without lifting the hair from the head
cascade or stand-up curls	pin curls fastened to the head in a standing position to allow the hair to flow upward and then downward
circle	the part of the pin curl that forms a complete circle; also, the hair that is wrapped around the roller
closed center curls	pin curls that produce waves that get smaller in size toward the end
curl	the hair that is wrapped around the roller; also called circle
concentrator	nozzle attachment of blow-dryer; directs the air stream to any section of the hair more intensely
diffuser	blow-dryer attachment that causes the air to flow more softly and helps to accentuate or keep textural definition
double press	technique of passing a hot curling iron through the hair before performing a hard press
finger waving	the process of shaping and directing the hair into in a pattern of "S"-shaped waves through the use of the fingers, combs, and waving lotion
foam or mousse	light, airy, whipped styling product that resembles shaving foam and builds moderate body and volume into the hair
full-base curls	thermal curls that sit in the center of their base; strong curls with full volume
full-stem curl	curl placed completely off the base; allows for the greatest mobility
gel	thickened styling preparation, firm-bodied and usually clear or transparent, that comes in a tube or bottle and has a strong hold
hair pressing	method of temporarily straightening extremely curly or unruly hair by means of a heated iron or comb
hair spray or finishing spray	styling product applied in the form of a mist to hold a style in position; available in a variety of holding strengths
half base	position of a curl or a roller one-half off its base, giving medium volume and movement
half-base curls	thermal curls placed half off their base; strong curls with moderate lift or volume
half-stem curl	curl (circle) placed half off the base; permits medium movement and gives good control to the hair
hard press	technique that removes 100 percent of the curl by applying the pressing comb twice on each side of the hair

liquid gel or texturizer	styling product that is lighter and more viscous than firm-hold gels, used for easy styling, defining, and molding
medium press	removing 60 percent to 75 percent of the curl by applying a thermal pressing comb once on each side of the hair using slightly more pressure than in the soft press
no-stem curl	curl placed directly on its base; produces a tight, firm, long-lasting curl and allows minimum mobility
off base	position of a curl or a roller completely off its base for maximum mobility and minimum volume
off-base curls	thermal curls placed completely off their base; have only slight lift or volume
on base	position of a curl or roller directly on its base for maximum volume; also called full base
open center curls	pin curls that produce even, smooth waves and uniform curls
pomade or wax	styling product that adds considerable weight to the hair by causing strands to join together, showing separation in the hair
ribboning	technique of forcing the hair between the thumb and the back of the comb to create tension
ridge curls	pin curls placed immediately behind or below a ridge to form a wave
rod	round, solid prong of a thermal iron
shaping	section of hair that is molded in a circular movement in preparation for the formation of curls
shell	part of thermal iron in which the rod rests when the irons are closed
silicone shiner	styling product that adds gloss and sheen to the hair while creating textural definition
skip waves	two rows of ridge curls, usually on the side of the head
soft press	pressing the hair to remove 50 to 60 percent of the curl by applying the thermal pressing comb once on each side of the hair
spiral curl	method of curling the hair by winding a strand around the rod
stem	the section of the pin curl, between the base and first arc (turn) of the circle, that gives the circle its direction and movement; the hair between the scalp and the first turn of the roller
straightening gel	styling product applied to damp hair that is wavy, curly, or extremely curly and then blow-dried; relaxes the hair for a smooth, straight look
thermal waving and curling	methods of waving and curling straight or pressed hair using thermal irons and special manipulative techniques on dry hair
updo	hairstyle in which the hair is arranged up and off the shoulders
volume-base curls	thermal curls placed very high on their base; provide maximum lift or volume
volumizer	styling product that adds volume to the shape, especially at the base, when the hair is blow-dried
waving lotion	type of hair gel that makes the hair pliable enough to keep it in place during the finger waving procedure

review questions

1. What is the purpose of finger waving?
2. What are the three parts of a pin curl?
3. Name the four pin curl bases and their uses.
4. Describe the three kinds of roller curl bases and the uses of each.
5. What is the purpose of back-combing and back-brushing?
6. How can you avoid burning the client's scalp during blow-drying?
7. List and describe the various styling lotions used in blow-dry styling.
8. How is volume achieved with thermal curls?
9. List at least 10 safety measures that must be followed when using thermal irons.
10. Name and describe the three types of hair presses.
11. How do you test the pressing comb before beginning a service?
12. What are the elements of a hair and scalp analysis prior to hair pressing?
13. Under what circumstances should hair not be pressed?
14. List at least four safety measures that must be followed when pressing the hair.

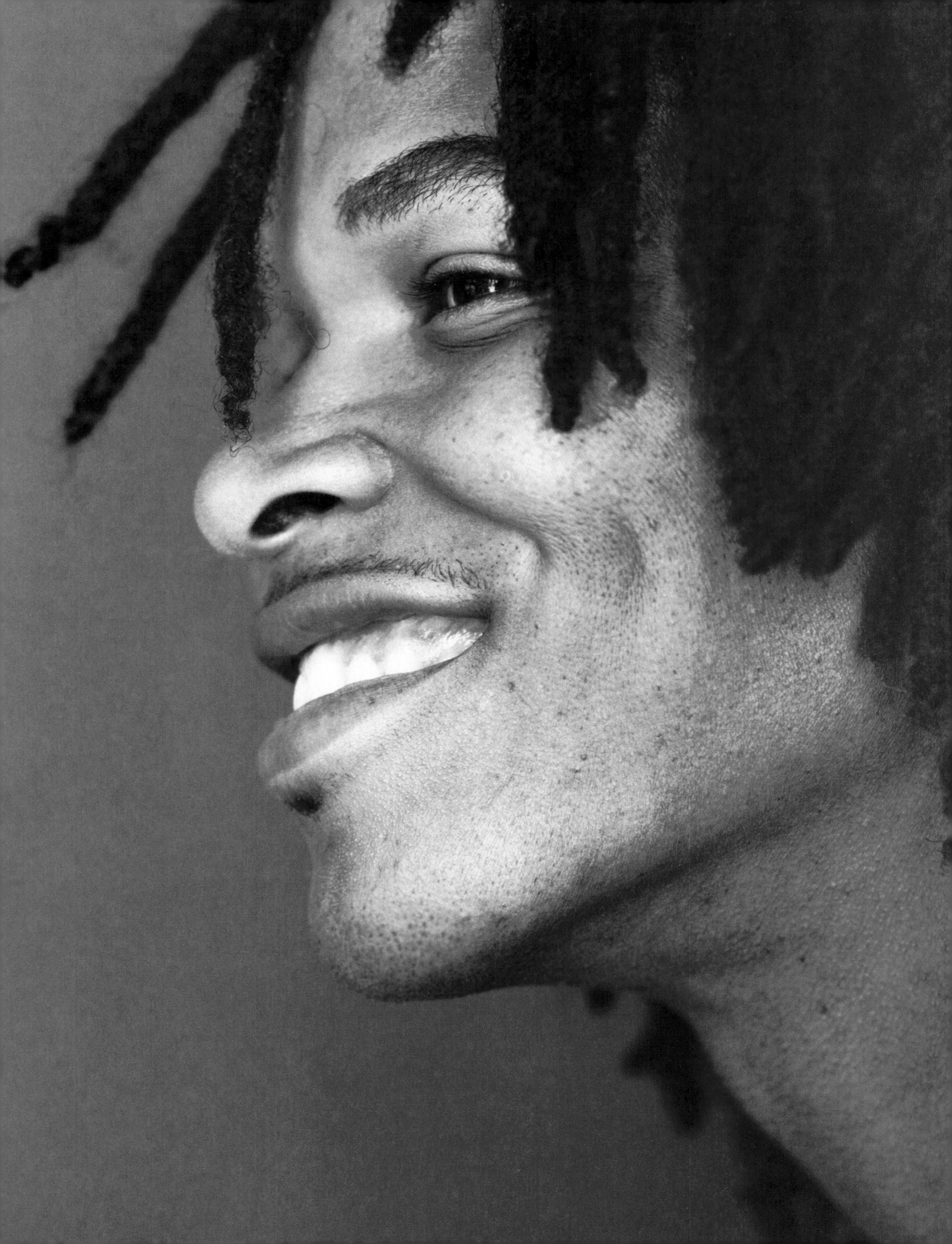

BRAIDING AND BRAID EXTENSIONS

Diane Carol Bailey

OWNER/ART DIRECTOR, TENDRILS NATURAL HAIR CARE SALON, BROOKLYN, NY

Chapter Outline

Learning Objectives

After completing this chapter, you should be able to:

1. **Perform a client consultation with respect to hair braiding.**
2. **Explain how to prepare the hair for braiding.**
3. **Demonstrate the procedures for the invisible braid, rope braid, and fishtail braid.**
4. **Demonstrate the procedures for single braids, with and without extensions.**
5. **Demonstrate the procedures for cornrowing, with and without extensions.**

National Skill Standards

This chapter provides you with the necessary information to master these National Industry Skill Standards for Entry-Level Cosmetologists.

Providing styling and finishing techniques to complete a hairstyle to the satisfaction of the client.

Providing nonsurgical hair additions.

Consulting with clients to determine their needs and preferences.

Key Terms

Page number indicates where in the chapter the term is used.

cornrows or canerows
pg. 441

fishtail braid
pg. 431

invisible or inverted braid
pg. 431

locks or dreadlocks
pg. 452

natural hairstyling
pg. 425

rope braid
pg. 431

single braids
pg. 441

visible braid
pg.431

The art of braiding has played an important role in many different cultures for thousands of years. From its origins in Africa to its widespread use today, hair braiding has always played a significant role in grooming and beauty practices.

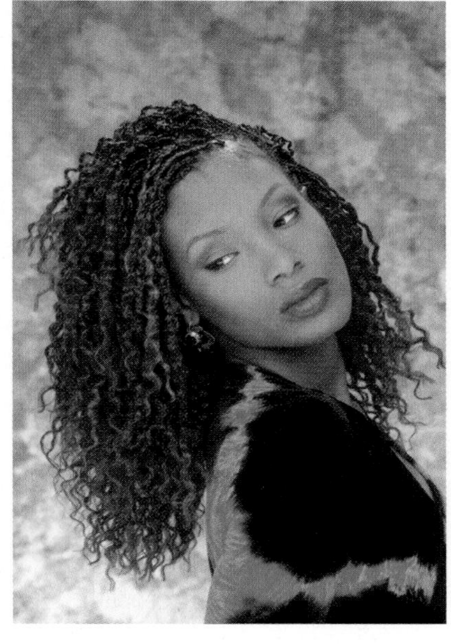

Figure 13-1 A contemporary braiding style.

In traditional cultures, the statement made by a person's braiding went beyond mere appearance or fashion. Different styles of braiding signified a person's social status within the community. The more important a person was, the more elaborate his or her braiding would be. Braiding patterns often indicated a woman's marital status as well. Unwed women wore different braiding styles than women who were married, were widows, or were expecting a child. Braiding styles distinguished one's tribe, age, economic status, occupation, geographic location, or religious and social standing. Today, braiding styles worn by individuals continue to communicate important signals about a person's self-esteem and self-image (Figure 13–1).

Hair braiding reached its peak of social and esthetic significance in Africa, where it has always been regarded as an art form to be handed down from generation to generation. Hair braiding can require an enormous investment of time; some styles can take an entire day, or even longer, to complete. Because braiding takes so much time, it was regarded in many African cultures as an opportunity for women to socialize and form bonds of trust.

Braiding salons have sprung up in many urban areas in the United States in recent years. These salons practice what is commonly known as **natural hairstyling**, which uses no chemicals or tints and does not alter the natural curl or coil pattern of the hair. While the origins of natural hairstyling are in African-American heritage, people of all races can appreciate its beauty and versatility. Natural hairstyling has brought a new and diverse approach to hair care.

FYI

Hair is referred to as "natural" or "virgin" if it has had no previous coloring or lightening treatments, chemicals, or physical abuse. Styles used in natural hairstyling include braid extensions, twists (two strands overlapped to form a "candy cane" effect), weaving, wrapping, and locks, also called African locks or dreadlocks. (Different states may define natural hairstyling in different ways.) For African-Americans, these styles are a proud acknowledgment of their cultural heritage. Their use is not limited to African-Americans, however. People today borrow and enjoy styles and traditions from many different cultures.

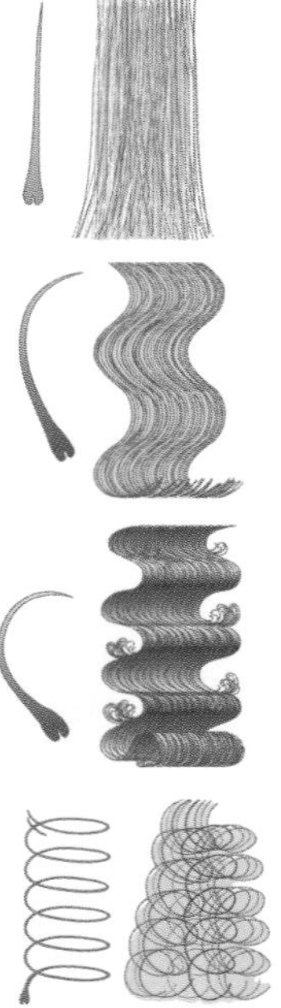

Figure 13–2 Wave pattern or coil configuration.

13

CLIENT CONSULTATION

Some braiding styles can take many hours, even days, to complete. The more complex styles should not be thought of as "disposable" hairdos to be casually washed away or brushed out. In fact, with proper care, a braiding pattern can last up to three months. The investment in time and money is high for both the client and the stylist. The last thing a stylist wishes to do is to spend hours on a braiding style and have the client reject it, demanding that all the braids be removed. The consultation is your opportunity to determine the client's needs and prevent dissatisfaction.

During the consultation, you will need to focus on your client's needs and expectations. Your first task is to build trust and confidence with your client. This will help make your client more expressive about the self-image he or she is hoping to project. Keep in mind the guidelines for client consultations set out in Chapter 4. Make sure you have a quiet spot where you can talk, take notes, and have pictures of styles on hand. Be friendly, be warm, and most of all, listen.

Fill out a client card during the initial consultation and update it each time the client returns. Note any scalp or hair problems, chemical history, and home-care products used.

Hair Analysis

During the consultation, when analyzing the condition of your client's hair, you must be particularly aware of the texture. When we talk about braiding and other natural hairstyling, texture refers to these three qualities.

1. *Diameter of the hair.* Whether the hair is coarse, medium, or fine.
2. *Feel.* Whether the hair feels oily, dry, hard, soft, smooth, coarse, or wiry.
3. *Wave pattern or coil configuration.* Whether the hair is straight, wavy, curly, or coiled (Figure 13–2).

With regard to the wave pattern, a coil is a very tight curl pattern. It is spiral in formation and, when lengthened or stretched, resembles a series of loops. For the purposes of this chapter, "textured hair" is hair with a tight coil pattern.

In addition to texture, take note of the hair's density and length, and to any areas where the hair is thinner, damaged, or broken. Check around the hairline. If the hair in this area is weak or damaged, certain braiding styles may be difficult to execute. Avoid styles that place direct tension on the hairline or partings along the hairline.

Facial Shapes

When you assist the client in choosing a braid style, an important consideration is to determine what best complements the client's most attractive features. During the consultation, you should first observe the facial structure and any distinct facial features of the client. You will need to understand and appreciate the distinct characteristics of different ethnic groups, all of whom have their own distinct facial characteristics. One is not "better" than another, and you should never impose your judgment where it does not belong.

As you learned in Chapter 9, part of your role as a hairstylist is to recognize different facial shapes and features, accentuate those that are attractive, and play down those that are less so. The following list offers a general description of flattering braid styles for these facial types and features.

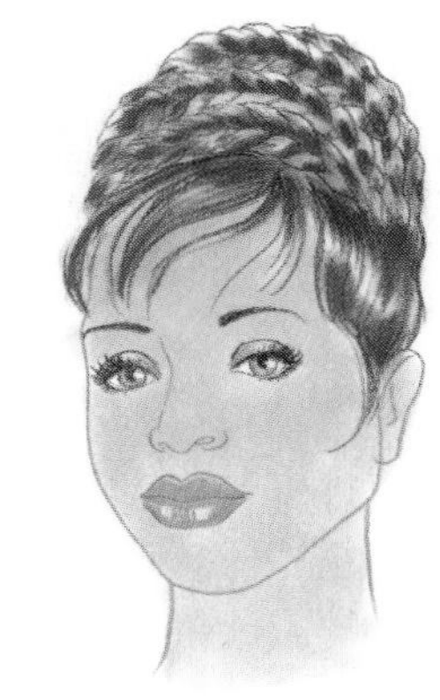

Figure 13-3 Round facial type.

- *Oval facial type.* Most braided styles are appropriate for this facial shape.
- *Round facial type.* When styling, add height to create the illusion of thinness. Updo braiding styles add length to the face. Asymmetrical styles that show the ears can also create a slenderizing look. Braided styles with waves or full curls frame the face and help to create balance (Figure 13–3).
- *Square facial type.* To create the illusion of length and to soften facial lines, choose full styles that frame the face around the forehead, temples, and jawline. Wisps of hair or a tapered fringe also help to soften angular lines.
- *Diamond facial type.* Create styles that are full around the forehead or jawline to help create a more oval appearance. Full bangs or partial bangs will help counter a narrow forehead. Keep braids close to the head along the cheekbones. Avoid updo styles and styles that move away from the cheeks or hairline (Figure 13–4).
- *Triangular (pear-shaped) facial type.* Soft fringes around the forehead will camouflage a small forehead without closing up the face. Styles that frame the cheekbones and are close to the ears or go behind the ears can reduce a wide chin line.
- *Inverted triangle (heart-shaped) facial type.* The goal is to minimize the width of the forehead by styling with partial bangs or wisps of hair and/or braids that frame the face. This will add fullness around the chin.
- *Oblong facial type.* Creating full styles can make the face appear shorter or wider. The fullness must not be overpowering. Soft, partial bangs or wisps of curls along the face can soften facial lines. Braids should be kept to a medium length. Avoid middle parts because they add length to a long, narrow face. 1

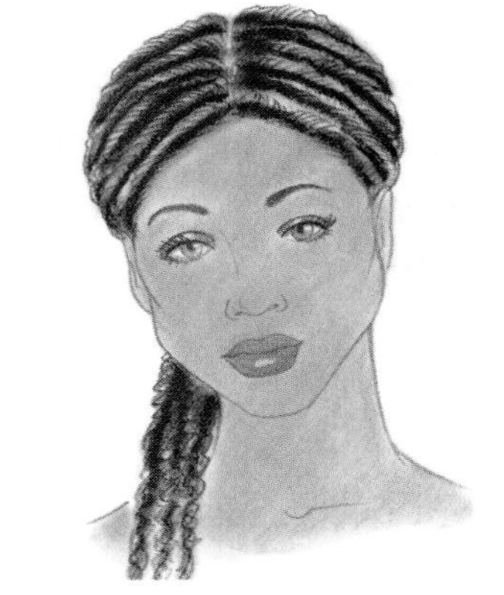

Figure 13-4 Diamond-shaped facial type.

13

UNDERSTANDING THE BASICS

Before we explore the various techniques of braiding, it is important that you have a good grasp of braiding basics. These include the tools you will

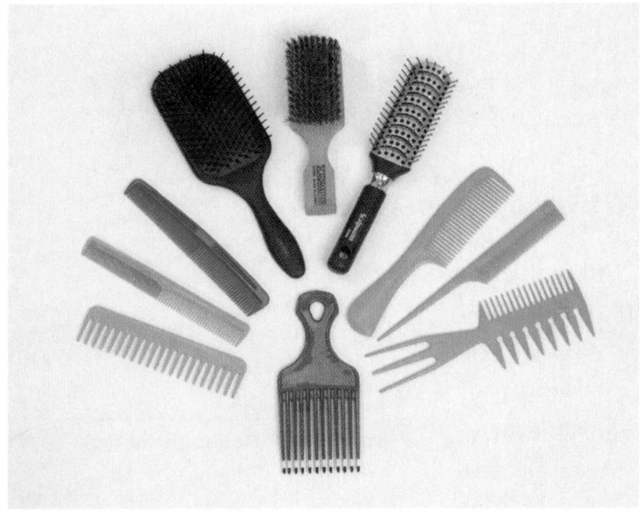

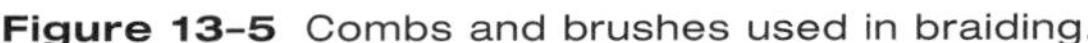

Figure 13–5 Combs and brushes used in braiding.

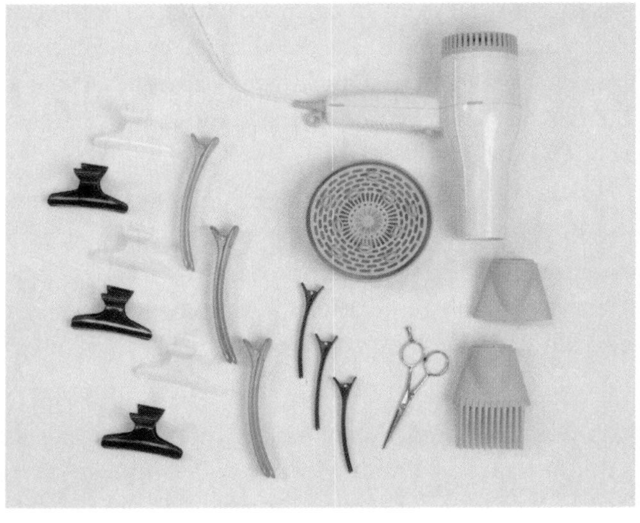

Figure 13–6 Clips, blow-dryer, diffuser, concentrator, pick nozzle, and scissors.

be using, the materials you will be working with, and the factors involved in styling wet and dry hair.

Tools for Braiding

An artist is as good as his tools, and hair artists who create elaborate braiding are artists indeed. Whether the hair is long, short, straight, or coiled, certain tools are essential in order to master the many different braiding styles (Figure 13–5 and Figure 13–6). These include the following.

- *Boar-bristle brush (natural hairbrush).* Best for stimulating the scalp as well as removing dirt and lint from locks. Nylon-bristle brushes are not as durable, and many snag hair. Soft nylon brushes may be an option for fine, soft hair around the hairline.
- *Square paddle brush.* Good for short textured hair and long straight hair. Flexible, antistatic rubber bristles bend and release tangles, knots, and snarls.
- *Vent brush.* Has a single or double row of teeth; useful, when used gently, to remove tangles on wet wavy or dry curly hair; excellent also on human hair extensions.
- *Wide-tooth comb.* Available in a variety of shapes and designs, these combs ply through hair with little snarling. The teeth, which range in width from medium to large, have long rounded tips to avoid scratching the scalp. The distance between the teeth is the most important feature of this comb; larger spacing allows textured hair to move between the rows of teeth with ease.
- *Tail comb.* Excellent for design parting, sectioning large segments of hair, and opening and removing braids.
- *Double-tooth comb.* Excellent on wet, curly hair; designed to minimize tangling and snarling.
- *Finishing comb.* Usually 8 to 10 inches in length, this is used while cutting and works well on fine or straight hair.

- *Cutting comb.* For cutting small sections. Should be used only after the hair is softened and elongated with a blow-dryer.
- *Pick with rounded teeth.* Useful for lifting and separating textured hair, this tool has long and widely-spaced teeth and is commonly made of metal, plastic, wood, or ivory.
- *Blow-dryer with pick nozzle.* Loosens the curl pattern in textured hair for braiding styles. Dries, stretches, and softens textured hair. Use hard plastic pick nozzles because metal attachments become too hot.
- *Diffuser.* Dries hair without disturbing the finished look and without removing moisture.
- *Five-inch scissors.* For creating shape and finished look, and for trimming fringes and excess extension material.
- *Long clips.* For separating hair into large sections.
- *Butterfly and small clips.* For separating hair into small or large sections.
- *Hood dryer.* Used to remove excess moisture before blow-drying hair. Eliminates excessive use of blow-drying and reduces direct heat on the hair.

Implements and materials you will need for extensions include the following.

- *Extension materials.* Kanekalon, nylon synthetic, rayon synthetic, human hair, yarn, lin, and yak.
- *Hackle.* A board of fine, upright nails through which human hair extensions are combed; used for detangling or blending colors and highlights.
- *Drawing board.* Flat leather pads with very close and fine teeth that sandwich the human hair extensions. The pads are weighed down with books, and the required amount of hair is extracted without loosening and disturbing the rest of the hair during the process of braiding.

Materials for Extensions

There is a wide variety of materials available for the purpose of extending hair. It is important to keep in mind that the materials you use will largely determine how successful and durable the extension will be. Though it may seem like a good idea to buy the least expensive product, in the long run, this may not prove to be the most economical solution, especially if you are buying in large quantities. You may get stuck with a lot of material that does not give you the results you desire. When buying a new product, buy in small quantities and test the fiber on a mannequin before using it on a client.

The following materials are most commonly used for hair extensions.

- *Human hair.* Human hair is, of course, the standard against which we compare all hair products, but human hair that is commercially sold is a confusing and somewhat mysterious product. Most of it is imported from Asia, and very little is known about how the hair is produced or processed. Some is imported from Europe and Africa. Although the label may say human hair, the buyer must be aware that there are disreputable dealers and wholesalers who misrepresent their product. Prepackaged human hair is generally less expensive than hair that is customized by a wholesaler. If a wholesaler is not available in your area, consider mail order.

- *Kanekalon.* A manufactured synthetic fiber of excellent quality, kanekalon has a texture similar to extremely curly or coiled hair types. It does not reflect light, which means it has less shine, but it comes in a variety of colors and is versatile and easy to match with natural hair colors. Durable, soft, and less inclined to tangle than other synthetics, kanekalon holds up to shampooing and styling. It costs more than most synthetics but is a better quality product. It feels smooth to both the client's scalp and your fingers and will not cut or damage natural hair as less expensive products might.
- *Nylon or rayon synthetic.* This product is less expensive than kanekalon and is available in varying qualities. It reflects light and leaves the hair very shiny. A drawback of nylon and rayon is that they have been known to cut or break the hair. Repeated shampooing will make these extensions less durable. They may also melt if high heat is applied.
- *Yarn.* Traditional yarn, such as that used to make sweaters and hats, is now being used to adorn hair. It can be made of cotton or a nylon blend and is very inexpensive and easy to find. Though it may expand when shampooing, it will not slip from the base, making it durable for braids. It is light, soft, and detangles easily. Unlike most synthetic fibers, it does not reflect any light and gives the braid a matte finish. Yarn is available in many colors; the most commonly used is black or brown. Be careful when choosing yarns, for some that appear jet black in the store show a blue or green tint in natural light.
- *Lin.* This beautiful wool fiber imported from Africa has a matte finish and comes only in black and brown. It is often used for Senegalese twists and "corkscrew" braid styles that are generally not shampooed. Lin comes on a roll and is used in any length and size. Keep in mind that this cottony fabric is very flammable.
- *Yak.* This strong fiber comes from the domestic ox found in the mountains of Tibet and Central Asia. Yak hair is shaved and processed to use alone or blended with human hair. A small mixture of yak with human hair helps to remove the manufactured shine.

Working with Wet or Dry Hair

In general, it is best to braid hair when it is dry. When hair is braided wet, it shrinks and recoils as it dries. This shrinkage may create excess pulling and tension. When the hair dries tightly around the braid, the tension can lead to breakage or hair loss from pulling or twisting. If you are using a style that requires your client's hair to be wet while being manipulated, you must allow for shrinkage, thereby avoiding any damage to the hair.

Long straight hair is best braided dry. This allows the hair to fall naturally, without tension. After you shampoo the client's hair, towel-blot it without rubbing, using several towels if necessary. Apply a leave-in conditioner to make combing the hair easier. Begin combing at the ends and gently work out the tangles while moving upward toward the scalp. Use a wide-tooth comb for this purpose. Then blow-dry the hair. Long straight hair can be slightly dampened with a spray bottle to keep layered or split ends in place. Pomades, gels, or lotions can be used to hold the hair in place for a finished look.

If the client washes her hair at home just before coming to the salon, this saves you both time. Brush the hair with a large paddle brush, beginning at the ends as you do with a comb.

Textured hair presents certain challenges when styling. It is very fragile both wet and dry. Most braiding styles require the hair to be dry; blow-drying is the most effective way to prepare the hair for the braiding service. Not only does blow-drying quickly dry the hair, but it softens it in the process, making it more manageable for combing and sectioning. It loosens and elongates the wave pattern while stretching the hair shaft length. This is great for short hair, allowing for easier "pick-up" and manipulation of the hair.

BRAIDING THE HAIR

Braiding styles can be broadly classified as visible and invisible. A **visible braid** is a three-strand braid that employs the underhand technique, in which strands of hair are woven under the center strand. An **invisible braid** or **inverted braid**, also a three-strand braid, is produced by overlapping the strands of hair on top of each other.

The following procedures will provide you with an overview of braiding styles commonly done in the salon, starting with the most basic and moving on to more complex styles, including braided extensions.

Invisible Braid

The invisible braid uses an overhand pick-up technique. It can be done on the scalp or off the scalp, with or without extensions. This style is ideal for long hair, but can also be executed successfully on hair that is layered. Layered hair must first be dampened slightly and gelled, however, to hold shorter strands in place. Procedure 21 demonstrates one braid down the back of the head.

Rope Braid

The **rope braid** (Procedure 22) is made with two strands that are twisted around each other. It can be done on hair that is all one length as well as on long, layered hair. Remember to add to both sides before you twist the right side over the left.

Fishtail Braid

The **fishtail braid** (Procedure 23) is a simple two-strand braid in which hair is picked up from the sides and added to the strands as they are crossed over each other. It is best done on dry, nonlayered hair that is at least shoulder length.

PROCEDURE

PREPARING TEXTURED HAIR FOR BRAIDING

Implements and Materials

- shampoo cape
- neck strip
- towels
- shampoo
- conditioner (protein or moisturizing)
- tail comb with large rounded teeth
- detangling solution (4 parts water to 1 part cream rinse or oil) in spray bottle
- butterfly clips
- blow-drying cream or lotion with oil or glycerine base

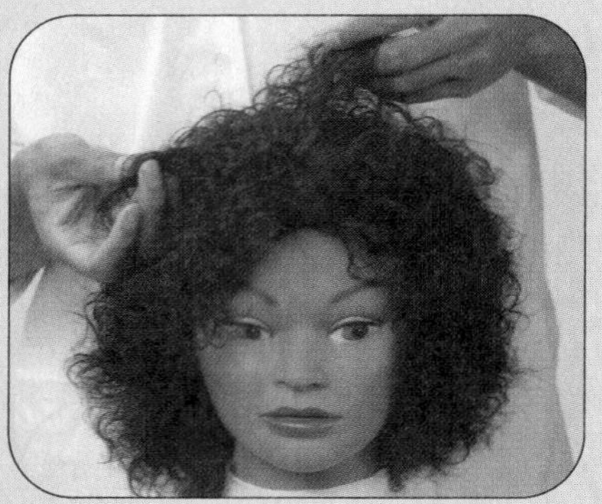

Figure 13–7 Scalp analysis.

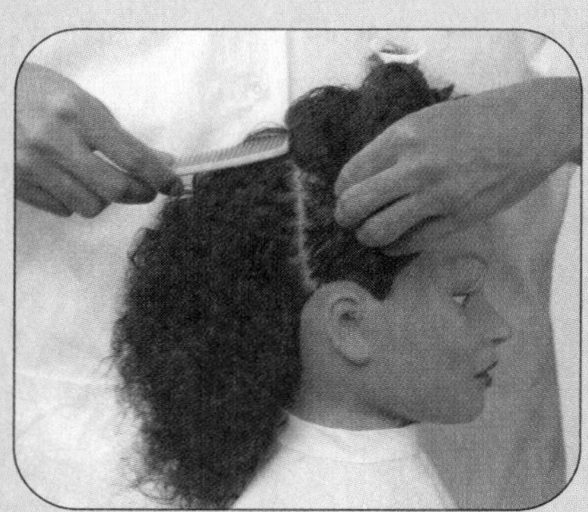

Figure 13–8 Part the hair across the crown.

Preparation

1. Wash your hands.
2. Perform a client consultation and hair and scalp analysis (Figure 13–7).
3. Drape the client for a shampoo. If necessary, comb and detangle the hair.
4. Shampoo, rinse, apply conditioner, and rinse thoroughly.
5. Gently towel-dry the hair.

Procedure

1. Part the damp hair from ear to ear across the crown. Use butterfly clips to separate the front section from the back section (Figure 13–8).
2. Part the back of the head into four to six sections. For thick textured hair, make more sections to allow for increased ease and control. For thinner hair, use fewer sections. The front half of the head, where the hair is less dense, can be sectioned in three or more sections. Separate the sections with clips.
3. Beginning on the left section in the back, start combing the ends of the hair first, working your way up to the base of the scalp. Lightly spray the section as you go along with detangling solution as needed. The combing movement should be fast and rhythmic, but not so much as to create tension on the scalp. It is better to use a picking motion to comb through the hair (Figure 13–9).

4. Once the hair is thoroughly combed, divide the section into two equal parts and twist them to the end to hold the section in place (Figure 13–10).
5. Repeat Steps 4 and 5 with the other sections of the hair until the entire head is sectioned.
6. Place the client under a medium heat hood dryer for 5 to 10 minutes to remove excess moisture.
7. Open one of the combed sections. Using your fingers, apply blow-drying cream to the hair from the scalp to the ends (Figure 13–11).
8. Using a pick nozzle attachment on the blow-dryer, hold the hair down and away from the client's head as you begin drying. Use a comb-out motion with the pick, always pointing the nozzle away from the client (Figure 13–12). As the ends relax and stretch, work the blow-dryer, with the heat blowing downward, toward the scalp. Blowing directly into the scalp can cause a burn. The hair is now ready to braid. (Figure13–13). 2 ✓

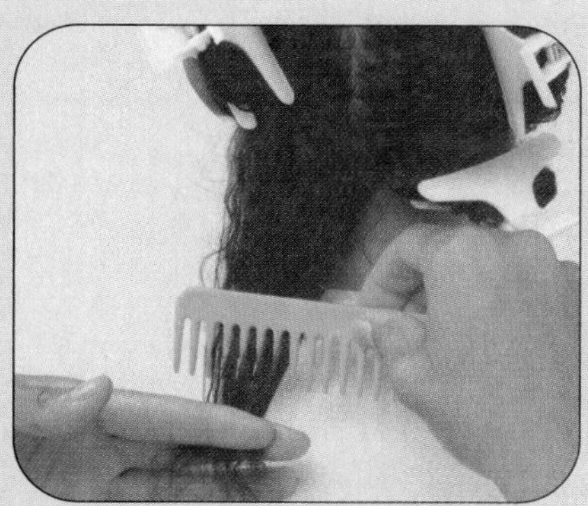

Figure 13-9 Comb the section.

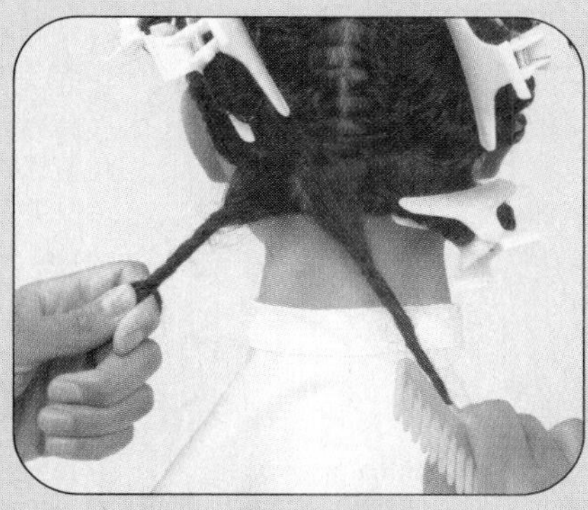

Figure 13-10 Twist the two parts of the section.

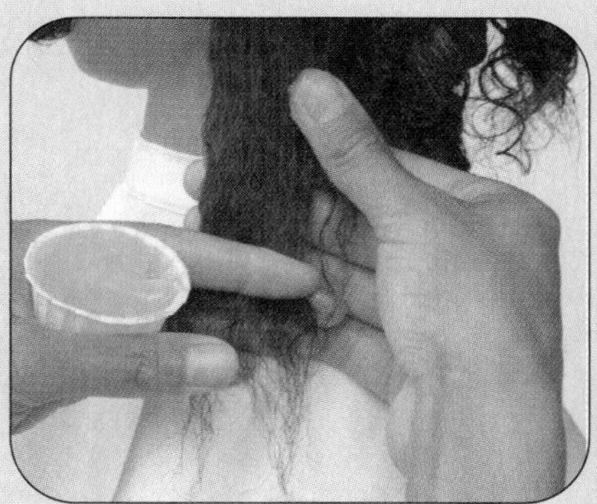

Figure 13-11 Apply blow-drying cream to hair.

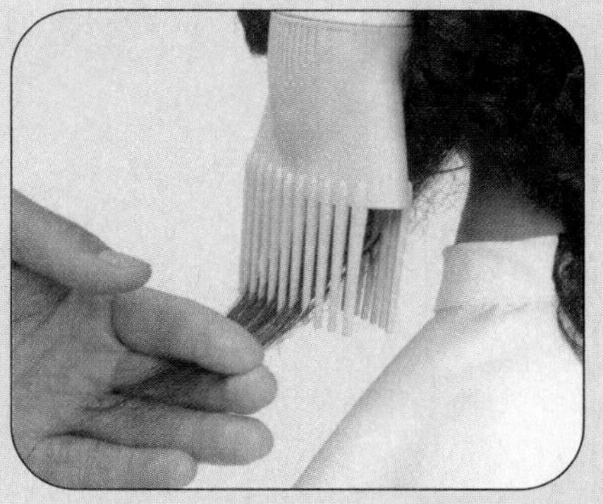

Figure 13-12 Blow-dry the section.

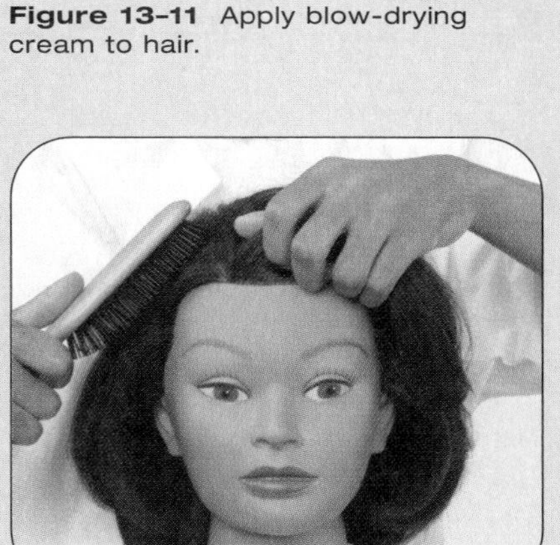

Figure 13-13 Hair prepared for braiding.

completed! 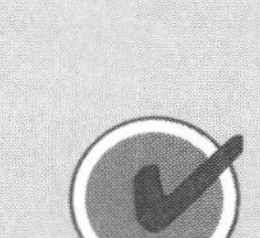

PROCEDURE 21

INVISIBLE BRAID

Implements and Materials

- styling cape
- neck strip
- rubber band or fabric-covered elastic
- tail comb

Preparation

Shampoo and condition the client's hair, then comb and blow-dry. If the client has shampooed at home, brush the hair with a paddle brush.

Procedure

1. At the crown of the head, take a triangular section of hair and place it in your left hand. Divide the section into three equal strands (Figure 13–14).
2. Place your fingers close to the scalp for a tight stitch. For a looser stitch, move away from the scalp. Cross the right strand over the center strand (Figure 13–15).
3. Cross the left strand over the center section and place it in your right hand.
4. Place all three strands in your left hand with your fingers separating the strands (Figure 13–16).
5. With your right hand, pick up a 1-inch (2.5-cm) section of hair on the right side. Add to the right strand in your left hand (Figure 13–17).

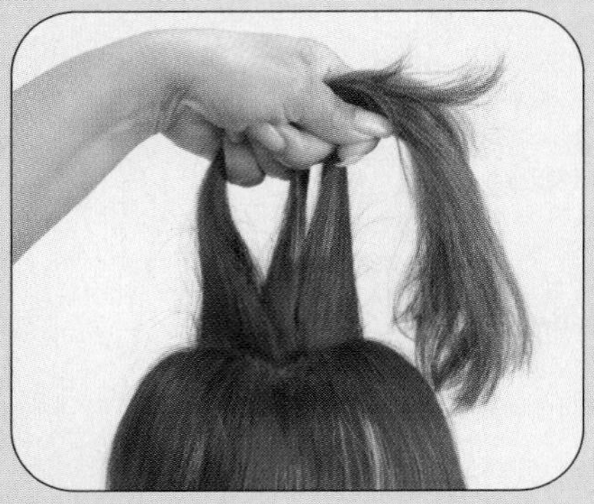

Figure 13–14 Divide section into three strands.

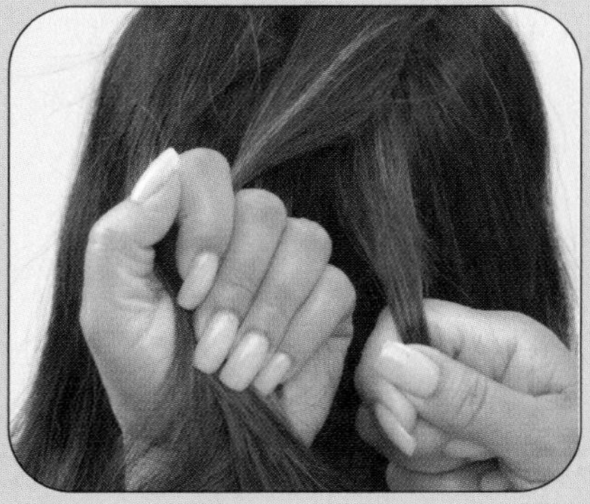

Figure 13–15 Cross right strand over center strand.

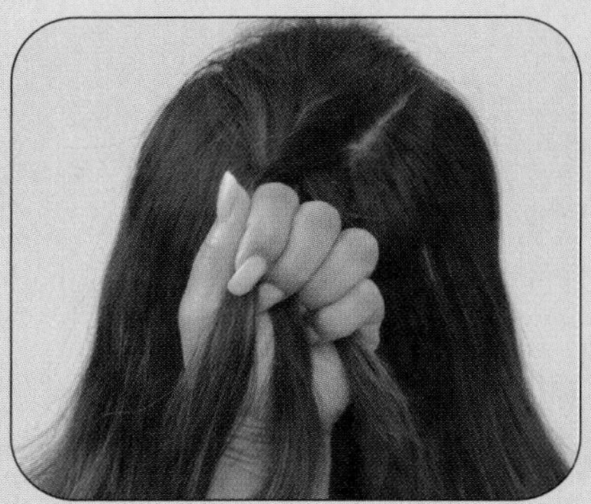

Figure 13–16 Place strands in left hand.

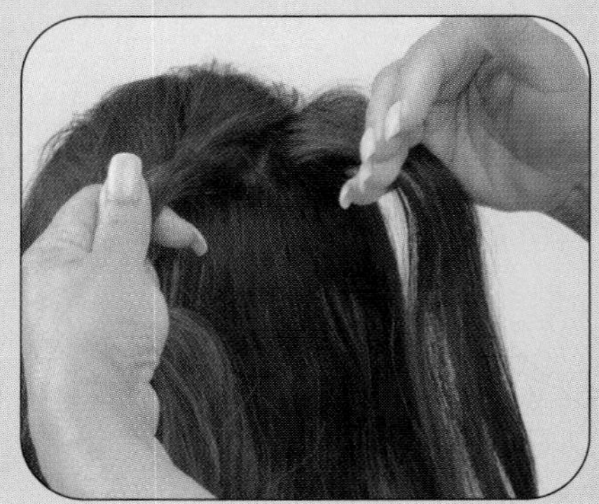

Figure 13–17 Add hair to the right strand

6. Take the combined strands in your right hand and cross them over the center strand. Place all the strands in your right hand (Figure 13–18).
7. With your left hand, pick up a 1-inch section on the left side. Add this section to the left outer strand in your right hand (Figure 13–19).
8. Take the combined strands and cross them over the center strand (Figure 13–20). Place all three sections in your left hand, pick up on the right side, and add to the outer strand (Figure 13–21).
9. Move down the head with alternating pick-up movements. Remember that the outer strands are added to and then crossed over the center. Continue these movements until the braid is complete. Secure the braid with a rubber band, then with a ribbon or other accessory for a finished style (Figure 13–22).

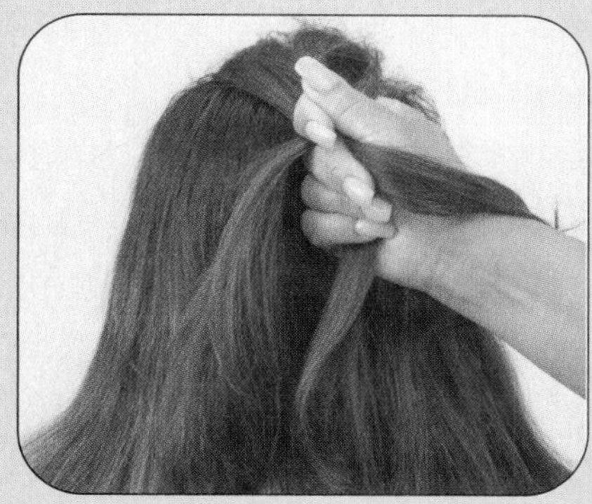

Figure 13-18 Place strands in right hand.

Cleanup and Sanitation

1. Disinfect all implements.
2. Place capes and towels in hamper for laundering.
3. Sanitize your workstation.
4. Wash your hands with soap and warm water.

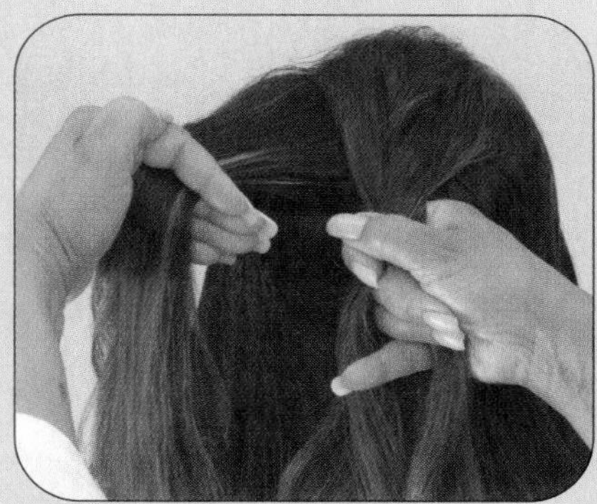

Figure 13-19 Add hair to outer right strand.

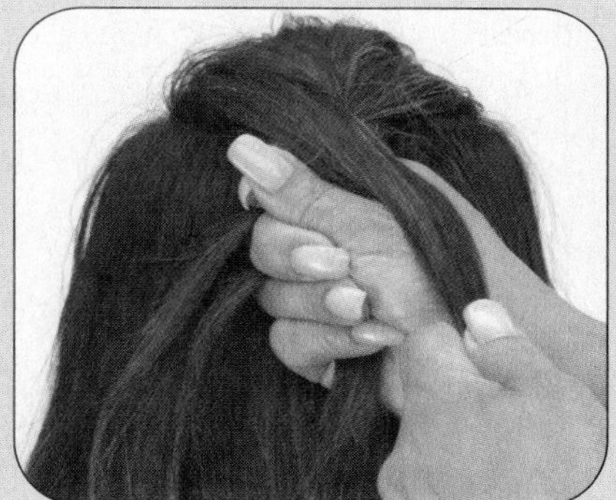

Figure 13-20 Cross combined strand over center strand.

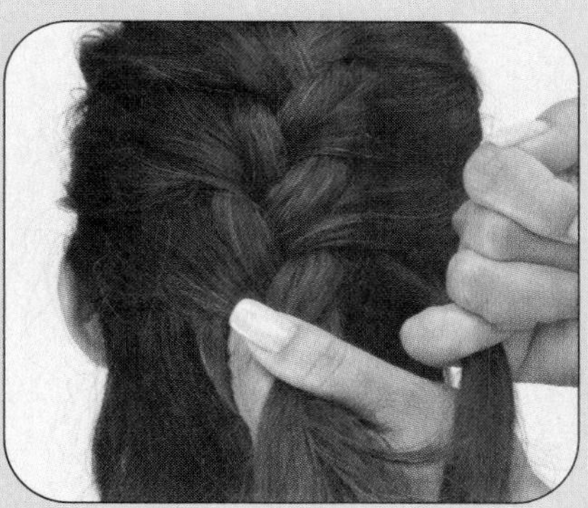

Figure 13-21 Add to outer right strand.

13

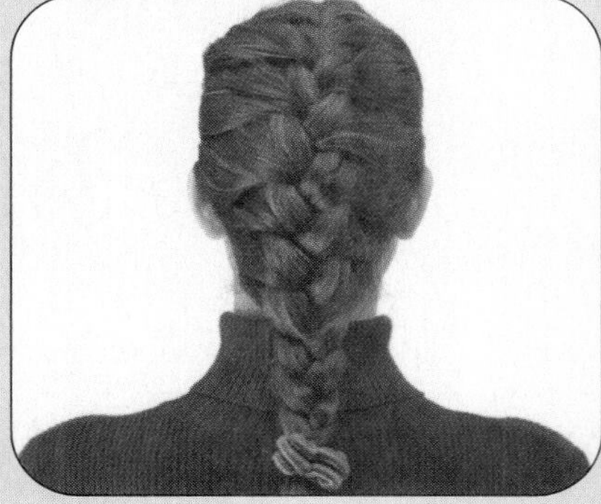

Figure 13-22 Finished invisible braid.

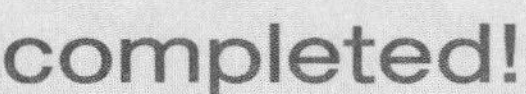

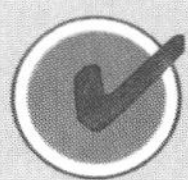

PROCEDURE

ROPE BRAID

Implements and Materials

Same as for Procedure 21 — invisible braid.

Preparation

Same as for Procedure 21 — invisible braid.

Procedure

1. Take a triangular section of hair from the front. If the client has a fringe, begin behind the fringe (Figure 13–23).
2. Divide the section into two equal strands. Cross the right strand over the left strand (Figure 13–24).
3. Place both strands in your right hand with your index finger in between and your palm facing upward (Figure 13–25).
4. Twist the left strand two times clockwise (toward the center) (Figure 13–26).

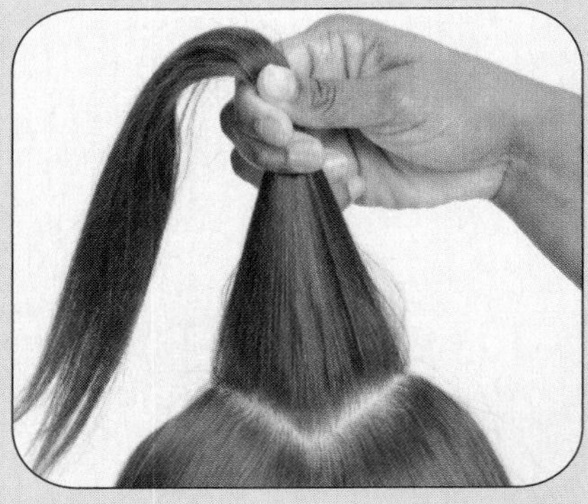

Figure 13-23 Take a triangular section of hair.

13

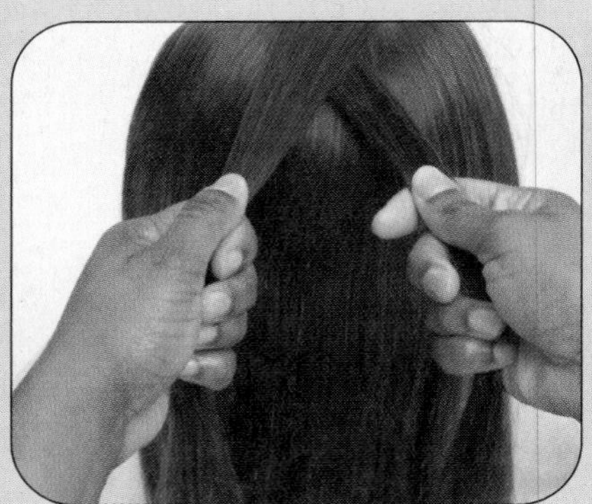

Figure 13-24 Cross the right strand over the left strand.

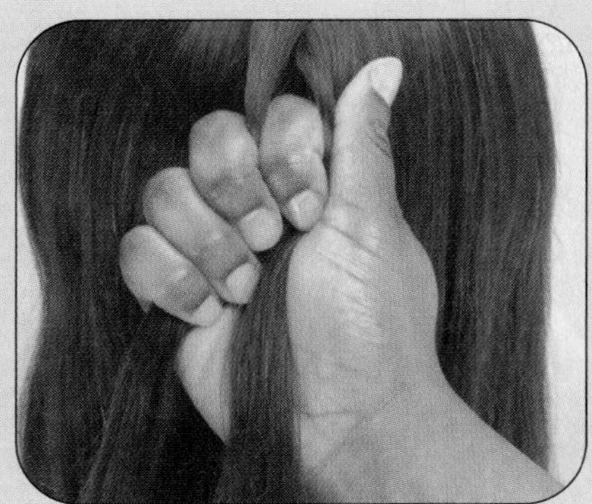

Figure 13-25 Place both strands in your right hand.

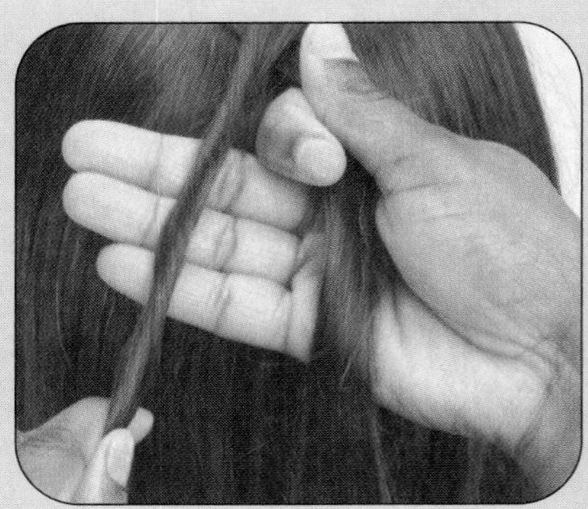

Figure 13-26 Twist left strand.

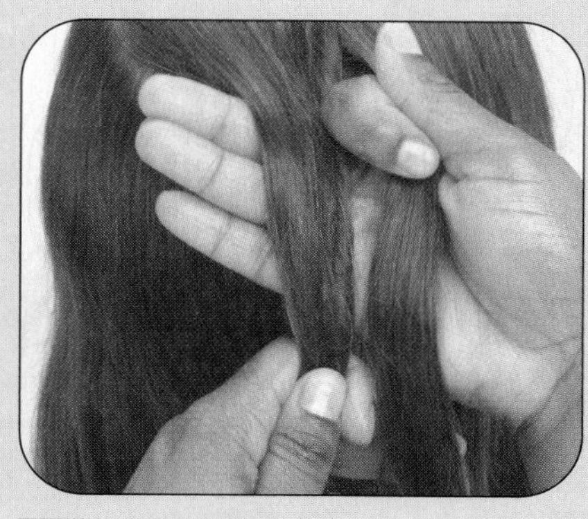

Figure 13–27 Add to left strand.

5. Pick up a 1-inch (2.5-cm) section from the left side. Add this section to the left strand (Figure 13–27).
6. Put both strands in your left hand with the index finger in between and your palm up (Figure 13–28).
7. Pick up a 1-inch section from the right side and add it to the right strand (Figure 13–29).
8. Put both strands in your right hand with your index finger in between and your palm up (Figure 13–30).
9. With your hand in this position, twist toward the left (counter-clockwise) until your palm is facing down (Figure 13–31).
10. Repeat Steps 3 through 9, working toward the nape until the style is done. Secure with a rubber band (Figure 13–32).

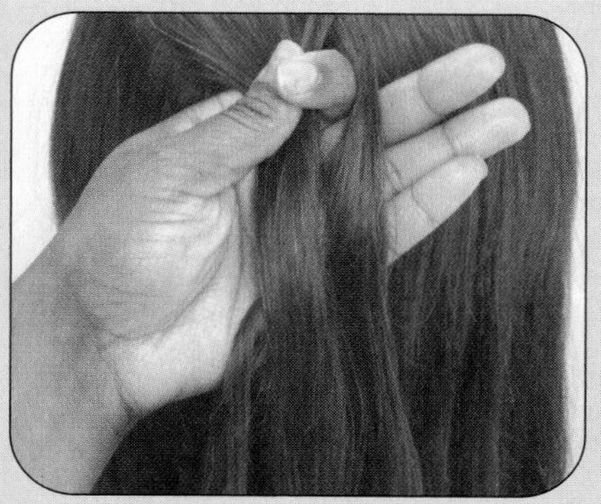

Figure 13–28 Put both strands in your left hand.

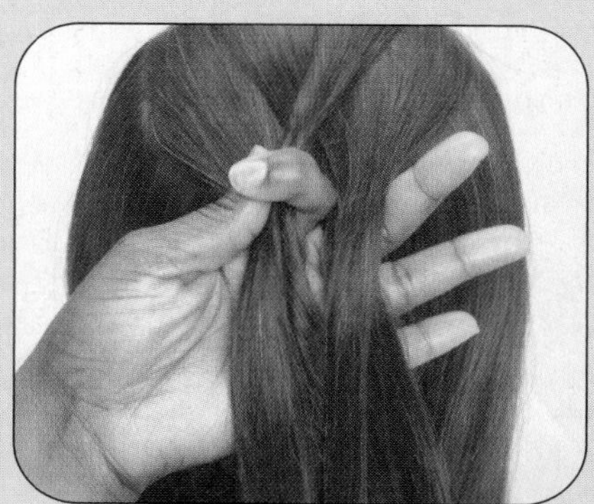

Figure 13–29 Add to the right strand.

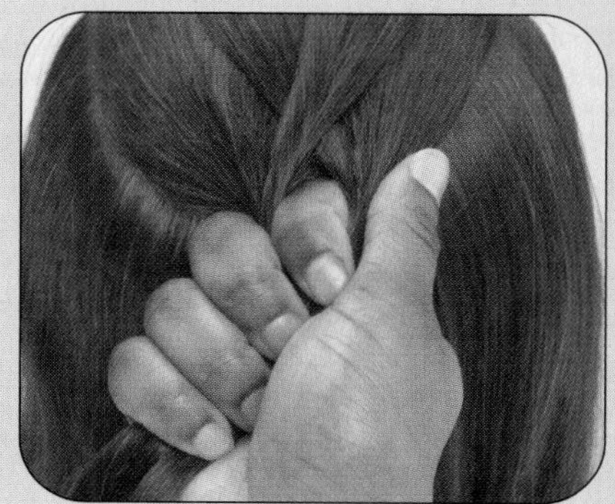

Figure 13–30 Put both strands in your right hand.

13

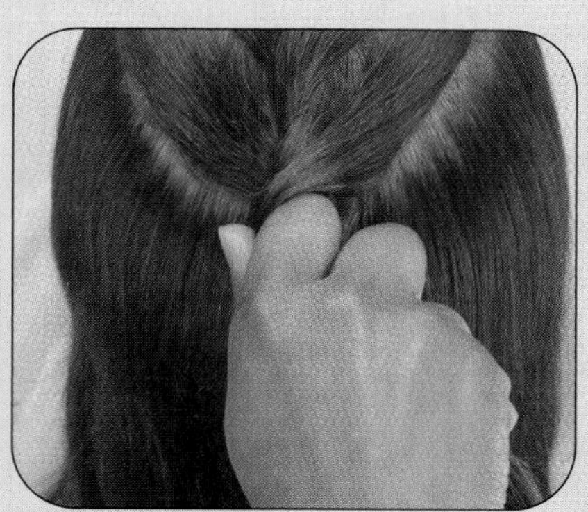

Figure 13–31 Twist hand toward the left.

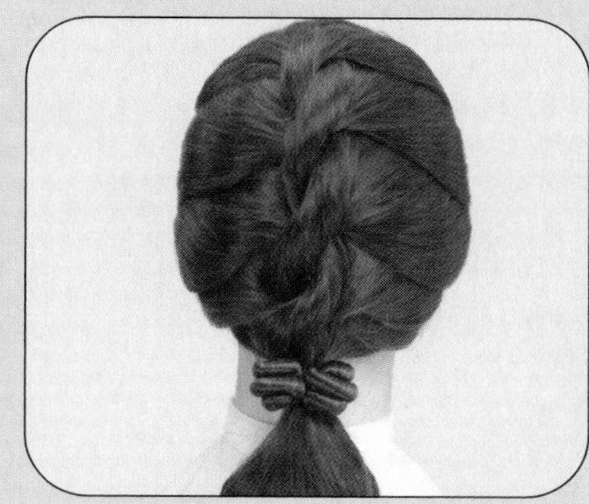

Figure 13–32 Finished rope braid.

11. When you run out of sections to pick up, another option is to create a rope ponytail with the remaining hair. Twist the left strand clockwise (to the right) two or three times. Place the strands in your right hand, index finger in between and palm up (Figure 13–33). Twist the palm down (counterclockwise), right strand over left (Figure 13–34). Repeat these steps until you reach the end of the hair. Secure ends with a rubber band (Figure 13–35).
12. Follow cleanup and sanitation procedures for Procedure 21 — invisible braid.

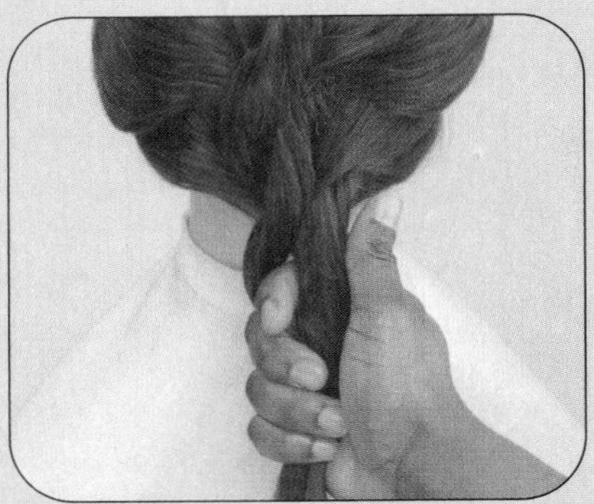

Figure 13-33 Place two strands in right hand.

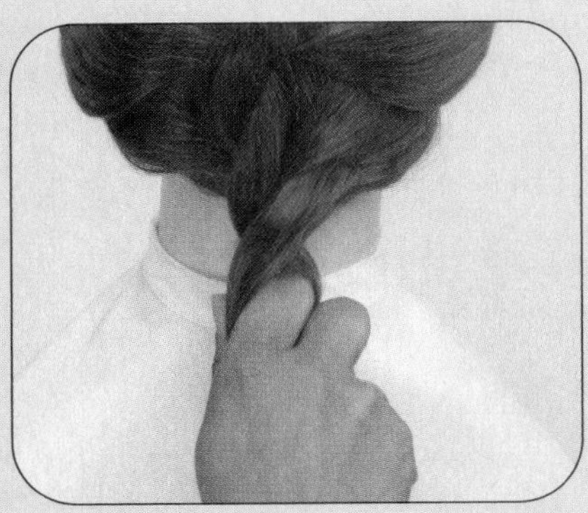

Figure 13-34 Twist hand counterclockwise.

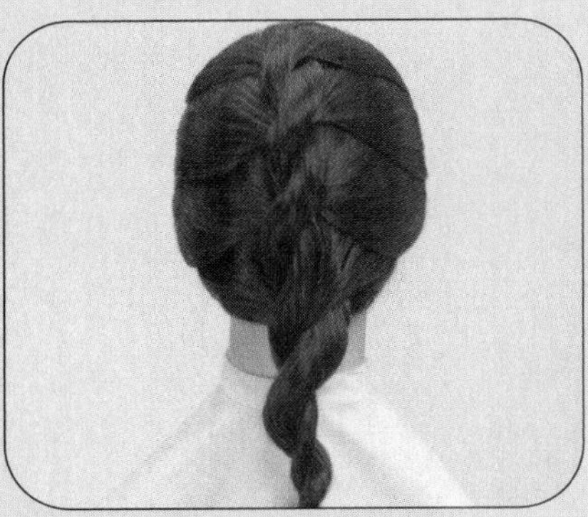

Figure 13-35 Finished rope ponytail.

13

completed!

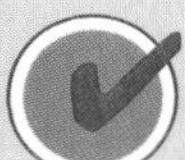

PROCEDURE

FISHTAIL BRAID

Implements and Materials

Same as for Procedure 21 — invisible braid.

Preparation

Same as for Procedure 21 — invisible braid.

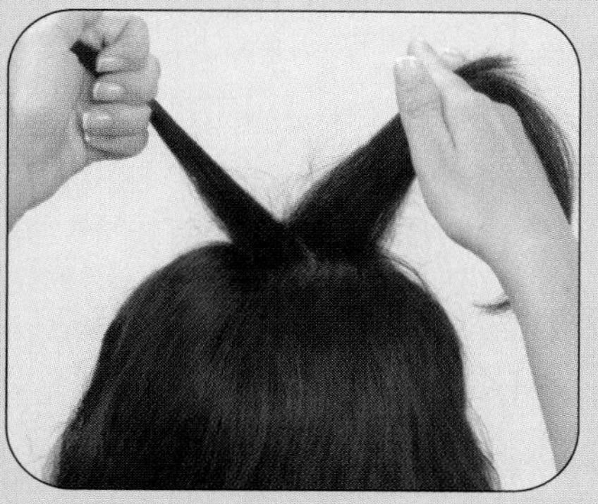

Figure 13–36 Divide section into two strands.

Procedure

1. Take a triangular section from the front. If the client has a fringe, begin behind the fringe. Divide this section into two strands (Figure 13–36).
2. Cross the right strand over the left strand (Figure 13–37). Place both strands in the right hand (Figure 13–38).
3. Pick up a 1-inch (2.5-cm) section on the left side. Cross this section over the left strand and add it to the right strand (Figure 13–39).

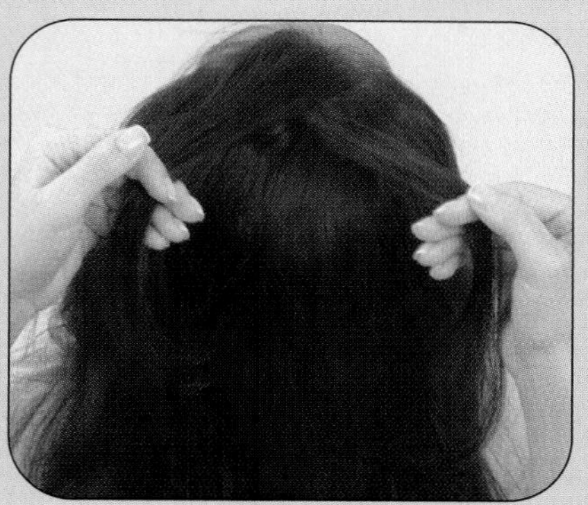

Figure 13–37 Cross right strand over left strand.

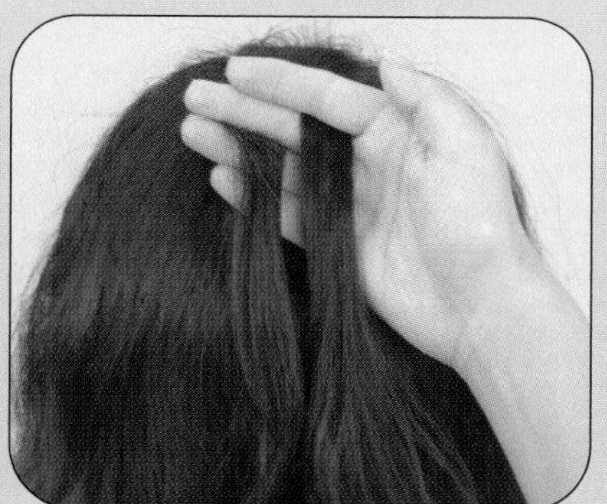

Figure 13–38 Place both strands in right hand.

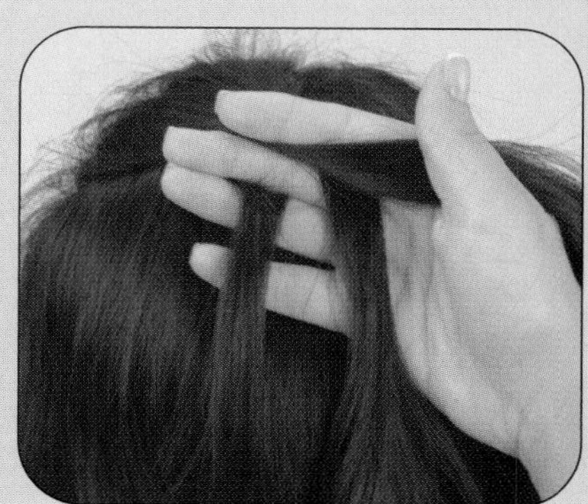

Figure 13–39 Add hair from the left side.

4. Put both strands in the left hand, index finger in between and palm up (Figure 13–40).
5. Pick up a 1-inch section on the right side. Cross this section over the right strand and add it to the left strand. You have now completed an "X" shape (Figure 13–41).
6. Put both strands in the right hand, as in Step 2 (Figure 13–42).
7. Repeat Steps 3 through 6, moving your hand down toward the nape with each new section picked up. When you run out of sections, secure the hair with a rubber band (Figure 13–43).
8. Follow cleanup and sanitation procedures for Procedure 21 — invisible braid. 3

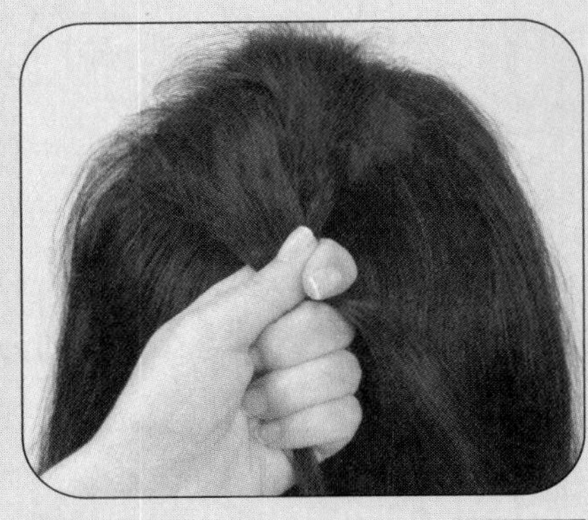

Figure 13–40 Put both strands in left hand.

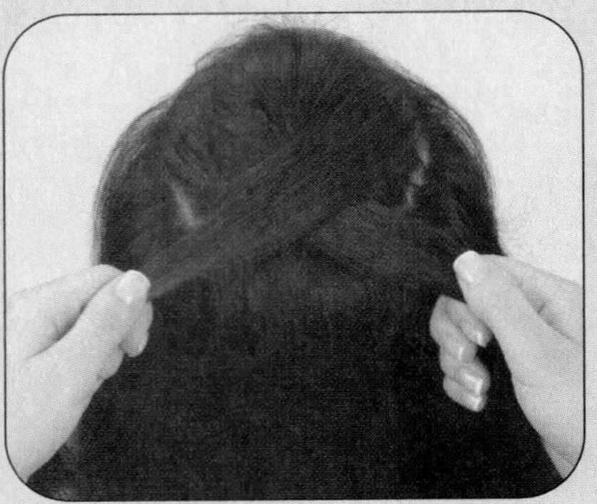

Figure 13–41 Add hair from the right side.

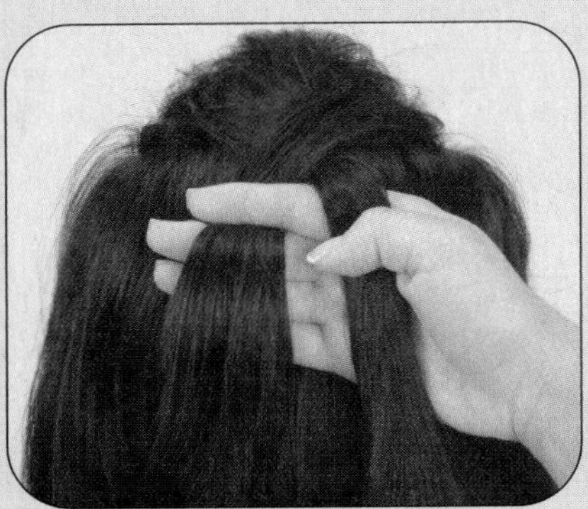

Figure 13–42 Put both strands in the right hand.

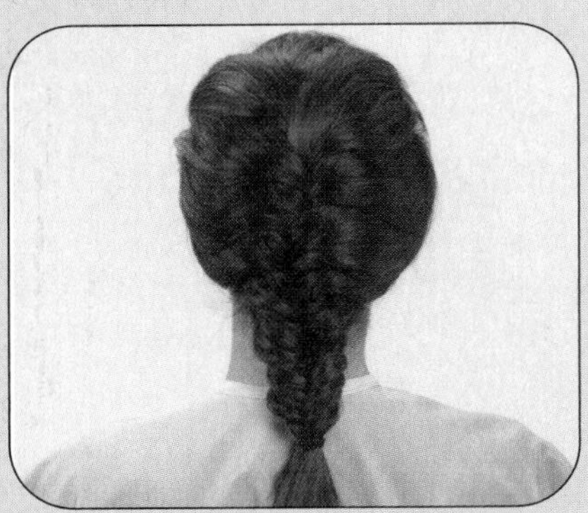

Figure 13–43 Finished fishtail braid.

13

completed! 

Single Braids

The terms **single braids**, box braids, and individual braids all refer to free-hanging braids, with or without extensions, that can be executed with either an underhand or overhand stitch. Single braids can be used with all hair textures and in a variety of ways. For instance, two or three single braids added to a ponytail or chignon can be a lovely evening look.

The partings or subsections for single braids can be square, triangular, or rectangular. The parting determines where the braid is placed and how it moves. Single braids can move in any direction. Make sure to braid in the direction you want them to go. As you are braiding, you are styling and shaping the finished look. The procedure for medium to large single braids done with an underhand stitch follows.

Extensions for single braids come in a wide range of sizes and lengths and are integrated into the natural hair using the three-strand underhand technique. Fiber for extensions can be selected from synthetic hair, yarn, or human hair; the selection is vital in determining the finished style. Braiding must be consistent and close together.

As part of the consultation step, open the package of extension fibers and show them to the client to verify that the color is correct. Remove the fibers from the package and, if necessary, cut them to the desired length. Place half the extension fibers in the bottom portion of the drawing board and "sandwich" them with the upper portion of board. To secure the hair extensions, place a heavy object on top of the board, such as a large book. This allows you to easily extract the appropriate amount of fibers for the braids. Hair extensions can also be separated and dispensed by a free-hand method.

Cornrows

The fundamentals of braiding start with the classic cornrow technique. **Cornrows**, also called **canerows**, are narrow rows of visible braids that lie close to the scalp. They are created with a three-strand, on-the-scalp braid technique. Consistent and even partings are the foundation of beautiful cornrows. Learning to create these partings requires patience and practice. Using a mannequin to practice will help develop your speed, accuracy, and finger and wrist dexterity.

Cornrows, which are worn by men, women, and children, can be braided on hair of various lengths and textures. For long straight hair, large cornrows are a fashionable and elegant hairstyle. Designer cornrows have become increasingly popular, with elaborate designs that demonstrate the stylist's skill and creative expression. The flat contoured styles can last several weeks when applied without extensions, and up to two months when applied with extensions.

Cornrows with Extensions (Feed-in Method)

Extensions can be applied to cornrows or individual braids with the feed-in method. In this method, the braid is built up strand by strand. Excess amounts of extension material can place too much weight on the fragile areas of the hairline and will tighten and pull the hair to leave an

PROCEDURE

SINGLE BRAIDS WITHOUT EXTENSIONS

Implements and Materials

Same as for Procedure 21 — invisible braid, with the following additions

- light essential oil
- butterfly clips
- small rubber bands (optional)
- oil sheen
- bobby pins

Preparation

Same as for Procedure 21 — invisible braid.

Procedure

1. Divide the hair in half by parting from ear to ear across the crown. Clip away the front section (Figure 13–44).
2. Based on the style that you and the client have selected, determine the size and direction of the base of the braid.
3. Part a diagonal section in the back of the head about 1 inch (2.5 cm) wide, taking into account the texture and length of the client's hair (Figure 13–45).
4. Divide the section into three even strands. Place your fingers close to the base. Cross the left strand under the center strand and then cross the right strand under.
5. Pass the outer strands under the center strands, moving down the braid to the end (Figure 13–46).

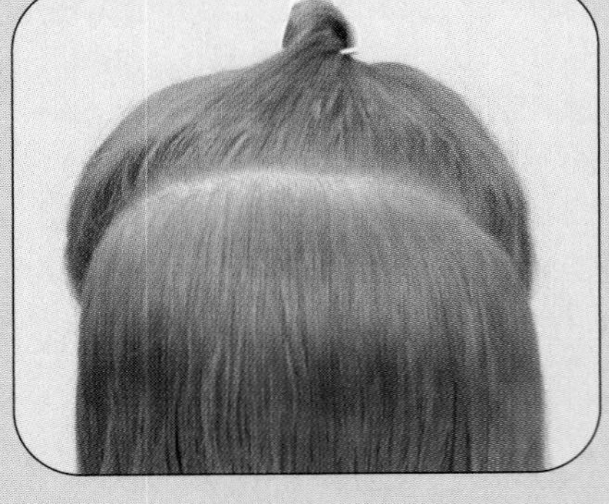

Figure 13–44 Divide hair into two main sections.

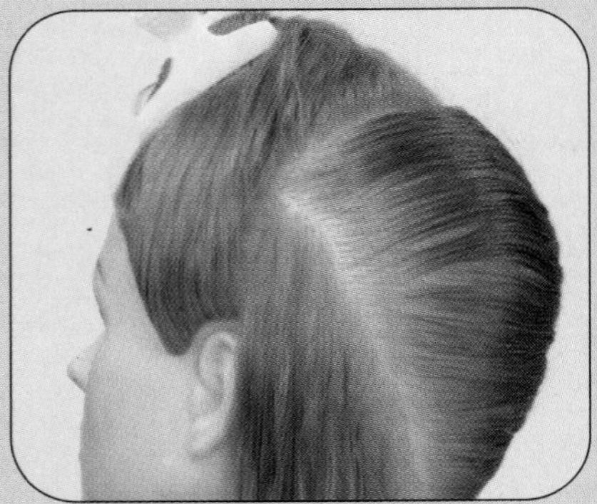

Figure 13–45 Part diagonal section.

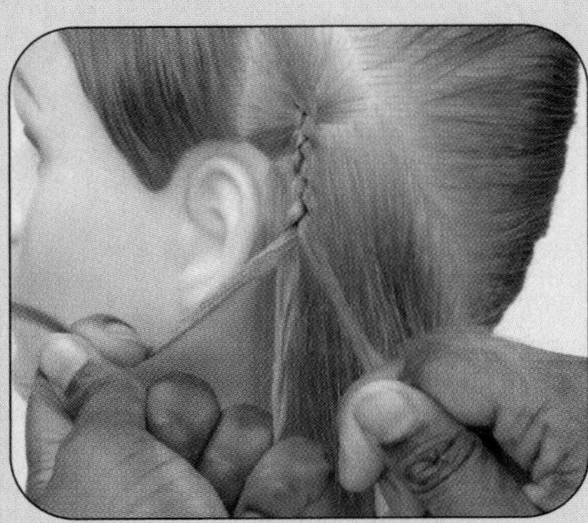

Figure 13–46 Braid the section with underhand stitch.

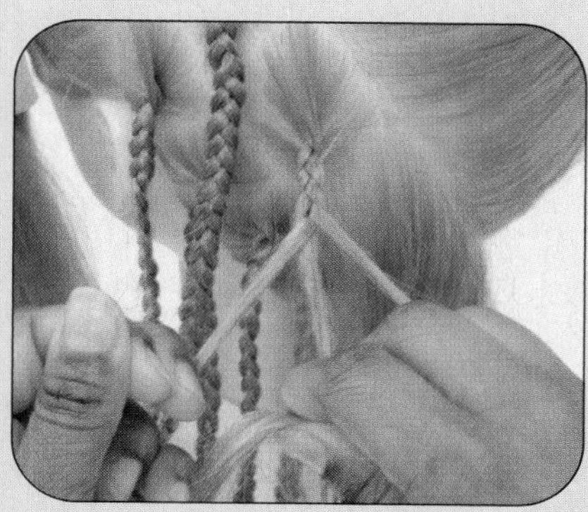

Figure 13–47 Braid the next section in the back.

6. Move to the next section. Repeat the braiding movement by passing the alternating outside strands under the center strand. Keep an even tension on all strands (Figure 13–47).
7. Repeat braiding procedure until the back is completed. Repeat in the front section (Figure 13–48).
8. Try to build up speed and accuracy to create straight and even braids. Rubber bands are optional to finish each braid (Figure 13–49).
9. Follow cleanup and sanitation procedures for Procedure 21 — invisible braid.

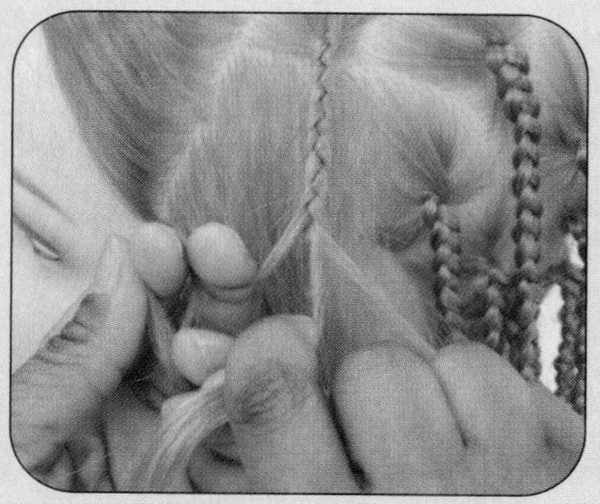

Figure 13–48 Braid the first section in the front.

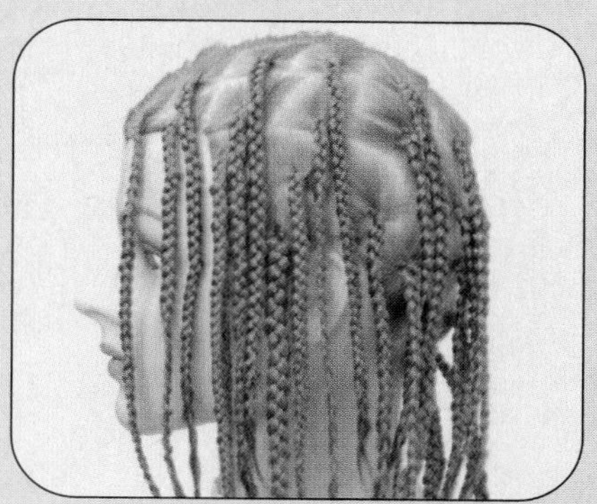

Figure 13–49 Finished single braids.

13

completed!

PROCEDURE 25

SINGLE BRAIDS WITH EXTENSIONS

Implements and Materials

Same as for Procedure 24 — single braids, with the following additions:

- extension fibers
- drawing board (optional)

Preparation

1. Shampoo, comb, and blow-dry the client's hair.
2. Prepare the extension fibers.

Procedure

13

1. Part the hair across the crown from ear to ear. Clip away the front section (Figure 13–50).
2. Part a diagonal section in the back of the head at about a 45-degree angle, from the ear to the nape of the neck. For a medium-size braid, this section can be from $^{1}/_{4}$ inch (.6 cm) to 1 inch (2.5 cm) wide, depending on the texture and length of the client's hair (Figure 13–51).
3. Using vertical parts to separate the base into subsections, create a diamond-shaped base (Figure 13–52).
4. Select the appropriate amount of extension fibers. It should always be proportional to the section to which it is being applied. For tapered ends, gently pull the extension fibers at both sides so that the ends are uneven. Then fold the fibers in half (Figure 13–53).

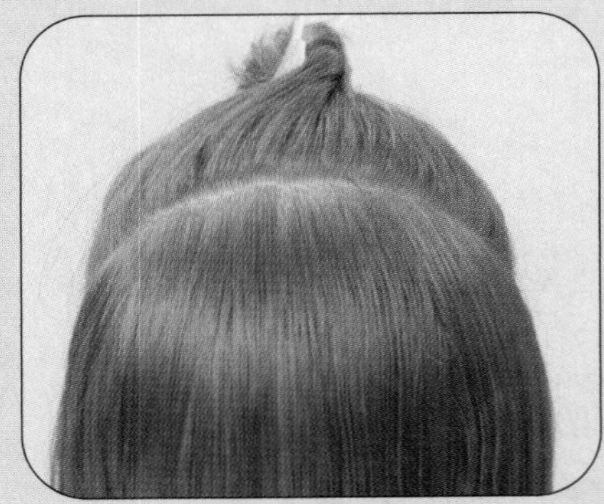

Figure 13–50 Part the hair across the crown.

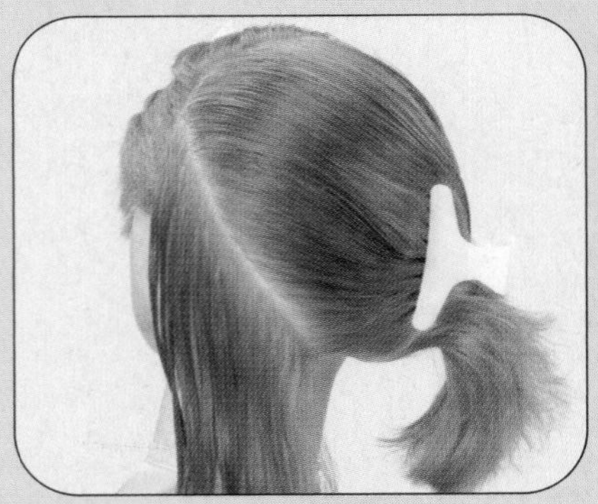

Figure 13–51 Part a diagonal section.

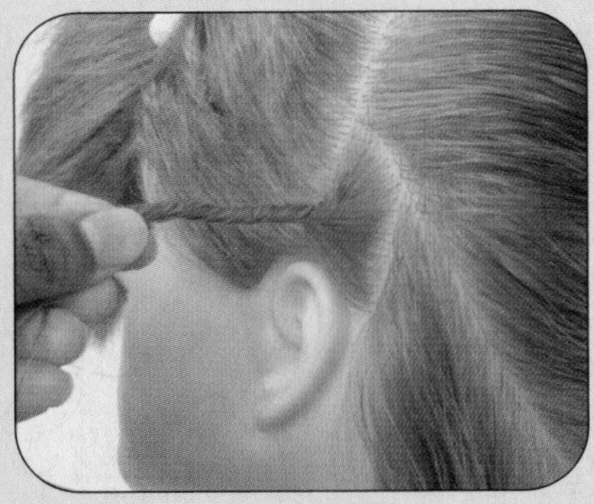

Figure 13–52 Create diamond-shaped base.

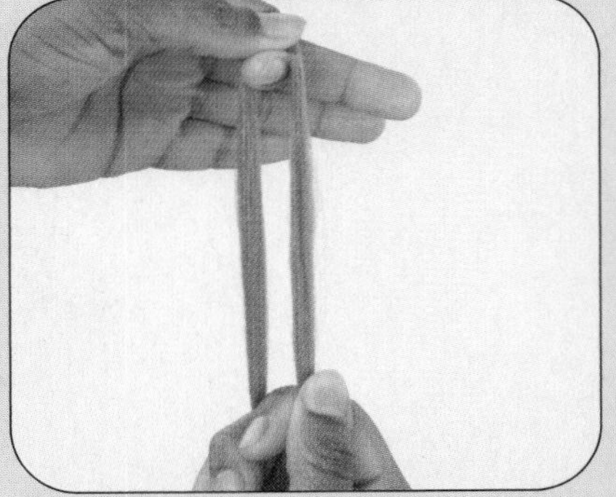

Figure 13–53 Fold extension fibers in half.

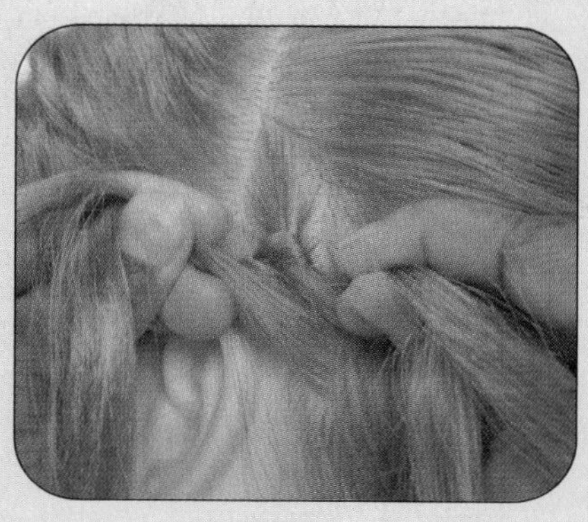

Figure 13–54 Place extension fibers on natural hair.

5. Divide the natural hair into three equal sections. Place the folded extension on top of the natural hair, on the outside and center portions of the braid (Figure 13–54).
6. Once the extension is in place, begin the underhand braiding movement. Remember that the outer stands should cross under the center strand. Each time you pass an outer strand under the center strand, bring the center strand over tightly so that the outside strand stays securely in the center. As you move down the braid, keep your fingers close to the stitch, so that the braid remains tight and straight (Figure 13–55).
7. Braid to the desired length.
8. The next section should be above the previous section on a diagonal part, moving toward the ear. After several sections have been completed, alternate the diagonal partings so that a V-shape pattern forms in the back of the head (Figure 13–56).
9. Once the back is finished, create a diagonal or horizontal parting above the ear in the front (Figure 13–57). As you get closer to the hairline, be aware of the amount of extension hair that is applied to the hairline.

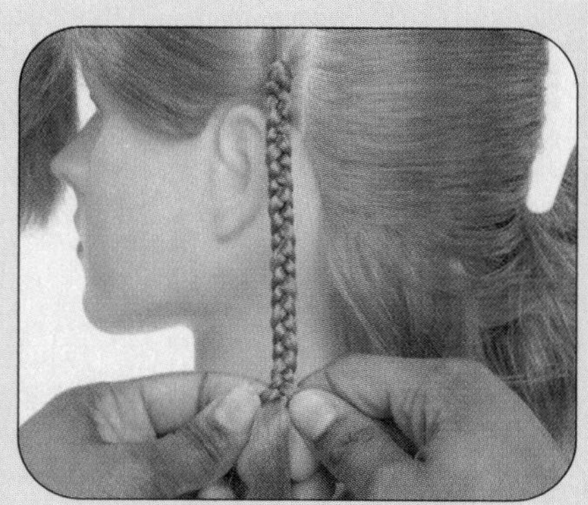

Figure 13–55 Braid the section.

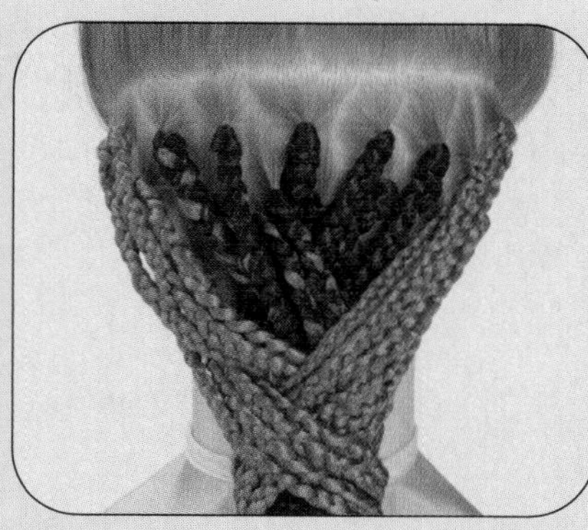

Figure 13–56 "V" pattern.

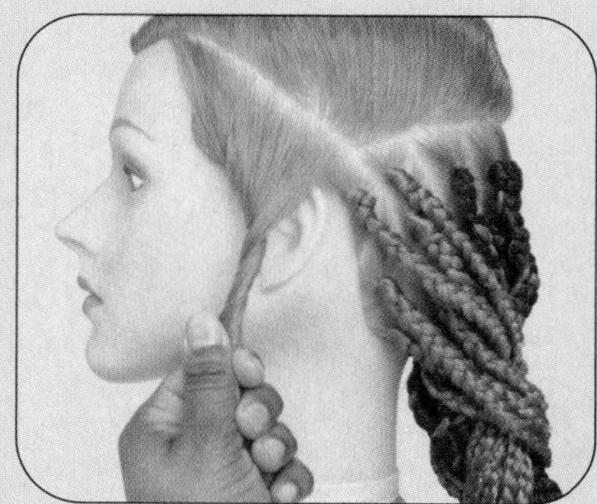

Figure 13–57 Create parting above the ear.

Do not add excessive amounts of fiber into a fragile hairline. The fiber should always be proportionate to the hair to which it is being applied (Figure 13–58 and Figure 13–59).

10. After the entire head has been braided, remove all loose hair ends from the braid shaft with scissors.
11. Finish the ends by spraying water to activate the wave in human hair extensions (Figure 13–60).
12. Follow cleanup and sanitation procedures for Procedure 21 — invisible braid. 4

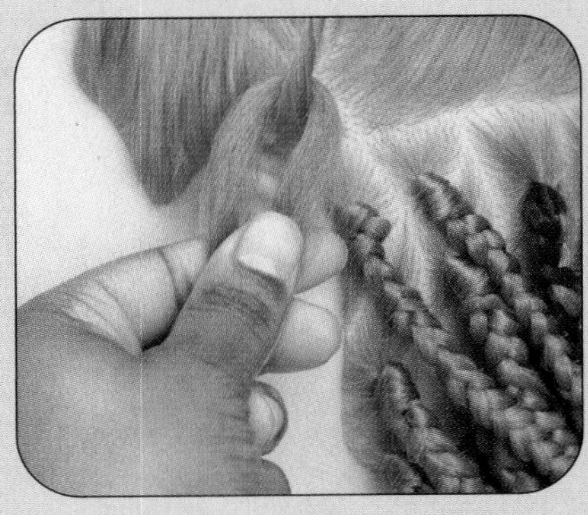

Figure 13–58 Work down the braid.

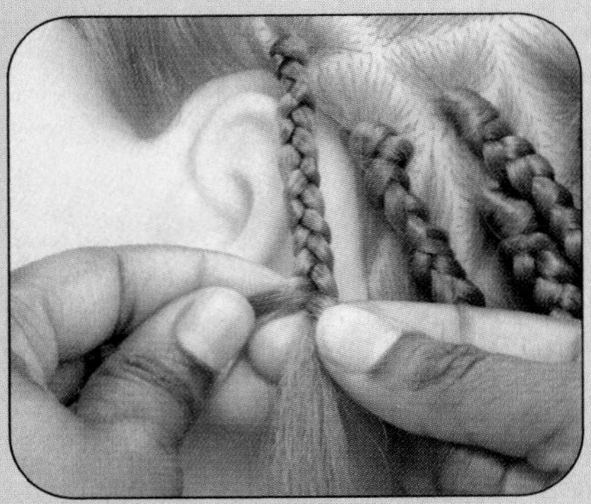

Figure 13–59 Add extension fibers.

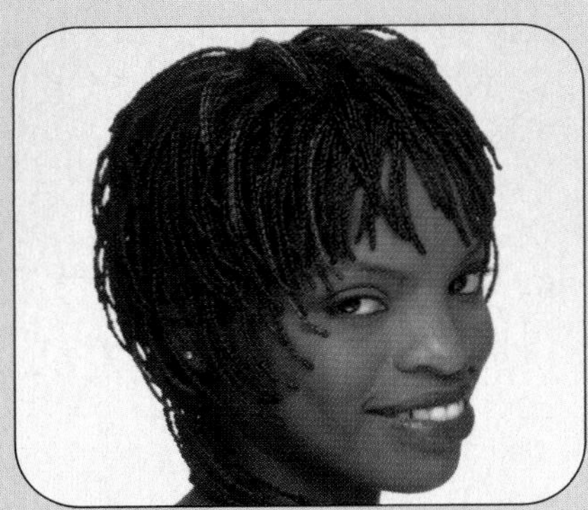

Figure 13–60 A finished style.

completed!

PROCEDURE

BASIC CORNROWS

Implements and Materials

Same as for Procedure 24 — single braids.

Preparation

Same as for Procedure 24 — single braids.

Procedure

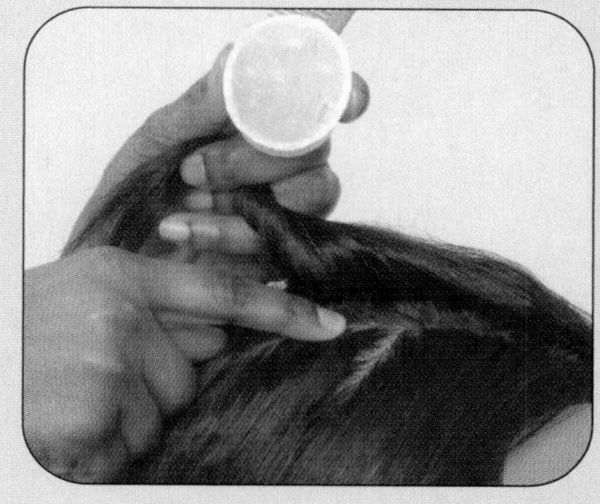

Figure 13–61 Massage essential oil through hair.

1. Depending on the style that has been selected, determine the correct size and direction of the cornrow base. With your tail comb, part the hair into 2-inch (5-cm) sections and apply a light essential oil to the scalp. Massage the oil throughout the scalp and hair (Figure 13–61).
2. To create a panel, start by taking two even partings to form a neat row for the cornrow base. With a tail comb, part the hair into a panel, using butterfly clips to keep the other hair pinned to either side (Figure 13–62).
3. Divide the panel into three even strands. To ensure consistency throughout the braid, make sure the strands are the same size. Place your fingers close to the base. Cross the left strand under the center strand (Figure 13–63).
4. Cross the right strand under the center strand. Passing the outer strands under the center strand this way creates the underhand cornrow braid (Figure 13–64).

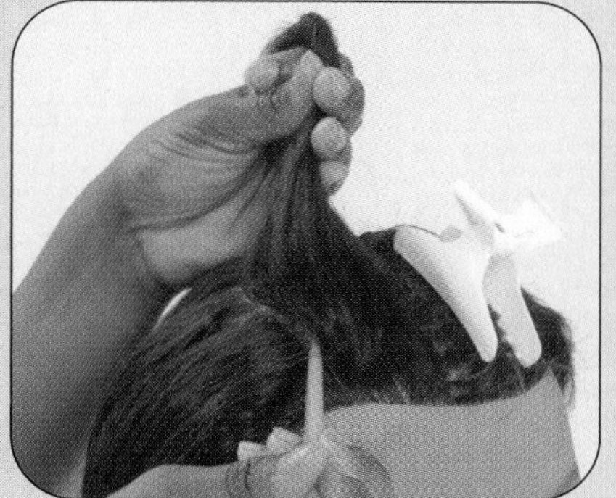

Figure 13–62 Part out a panel.

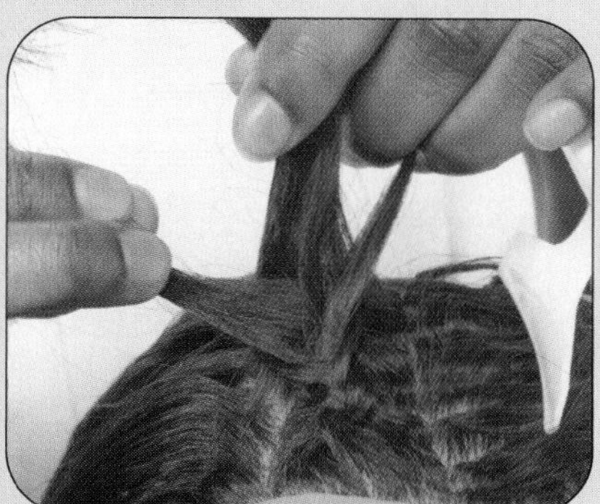

Figure 13–63 Pass left strand under center strand.

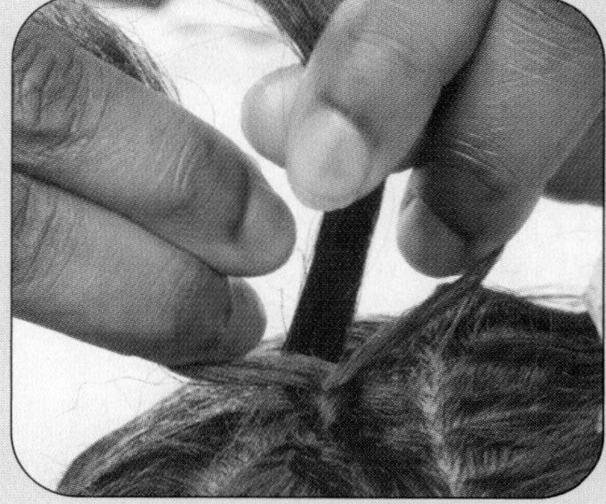

Figure 13–64 Pass right strand under center strand.

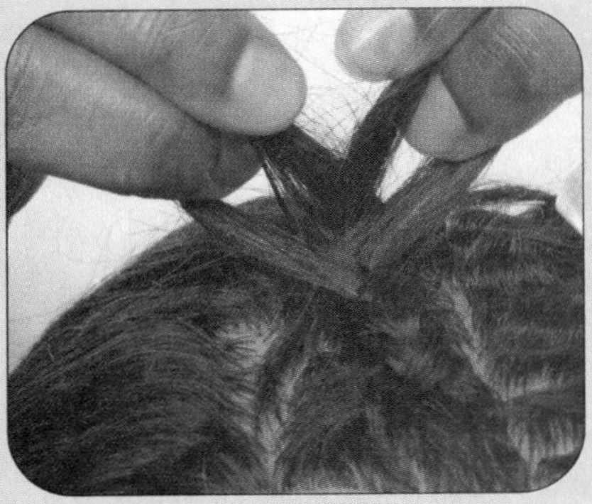

Figure 13-65 Add hair to left outer strand.

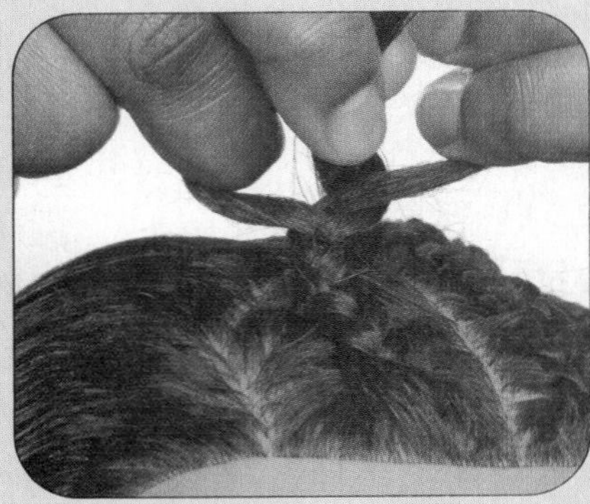

Figure 13-66 Add hair to right outer strand.

5. With each crossing under, or revolution, pick up from the base of the panel a new strand of equal size and add it to the outer strand before crossing it under the center strand (Figure 13–65).
6. As you move along the braid panel, pick up a strand from the scalp with each revolution and add it to the outer strand before crossing it under, alternating the side of the braid on which you pick up the hair (Figure 13–66).
7. As new strands are added, the braid will become fuller. Braid to the end.
8. Simply braiding to the ends can finish the cornrow; small rubber bands can be used to hold the ends in place (Figure 13–67). Other optional finishes, such as singeing, are considered advanced methods and require special training.
9. Braid the next panel in the same direction and in the same manner. Keep the partings clean and even (Figure 13–68).
10. Repeat until all the hair is braided. Apply oil sheen for a finished look (Figure 13–69).
11. Follow cleanup and sanitation procedures for Procedure 21 — invisible braid.

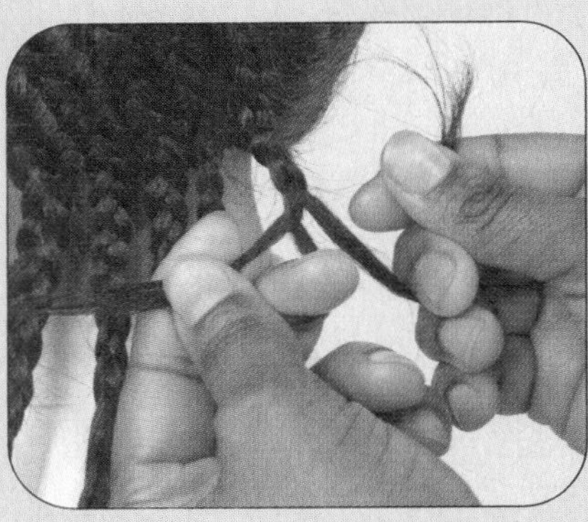

Figure 13-67 Braid cornrow to end.

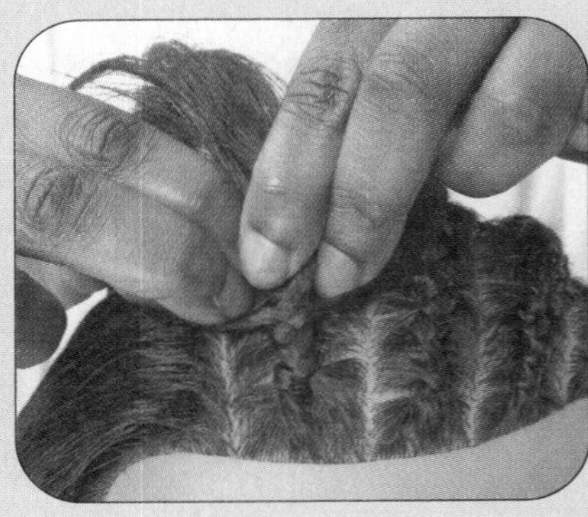

Figure 13-68 Braid next cornrow.

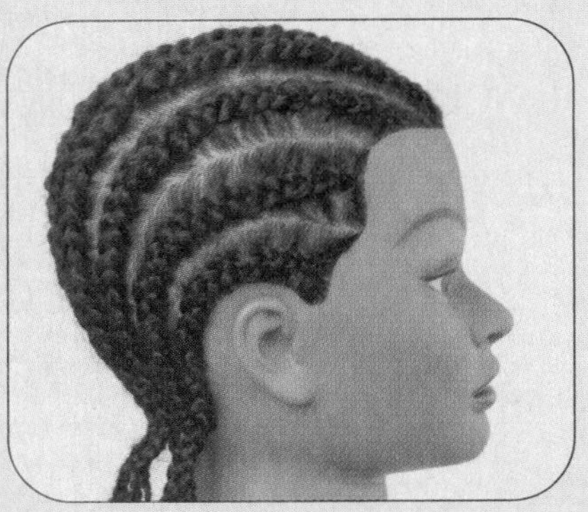

Figure 13-69 Finished cornrows.

completed! 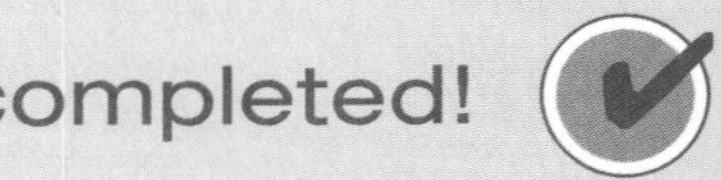

PROCEDURE

CORNROWS WITH EXTENSIONS

Implements and Materials

Same as for Procedure 25 — single braids with extensions.

Preparation

Same as for Procedure 25 — single braids with extensions.

Procedure

1. With your tail comb, part the hair into 2-inch (5-cm) sections and apply light essential oil to the scalp. Massage the oil throughout the scalp and hair.
2. Starting at the hairline, part off a cornrow base in the desired direction (Figure 13–70). No extension is added at the starting point. If the hair extension is required because of a thinning hairline, apply minute amounts, as small as 5 to 10 strands. Divide the natural hair into three equal strands.
3. With the first revolution, cross the outer strand under the center strand (Figure 13–71).
4. On the second revolution, the right strand crosses under the center strand. Pick up a small portion of natural hair and add it to the outer strand during the revolution (Figure 13–72).

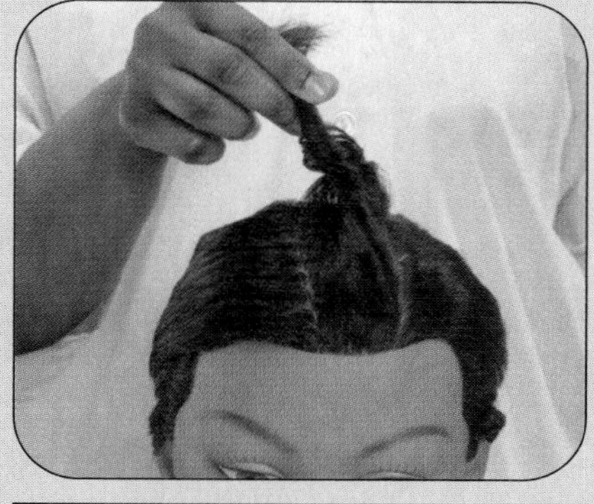

Figure 13–70 Part off cornrow base.

13

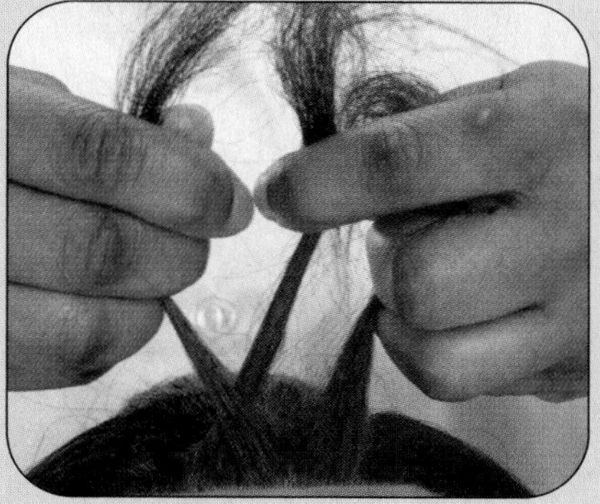

Figure 13–71 Cross outer strand under center strand.

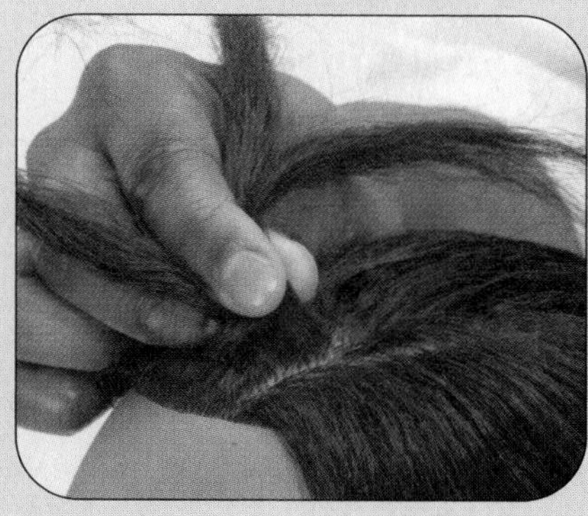

Figure 13–72 Add hair to outer strand.

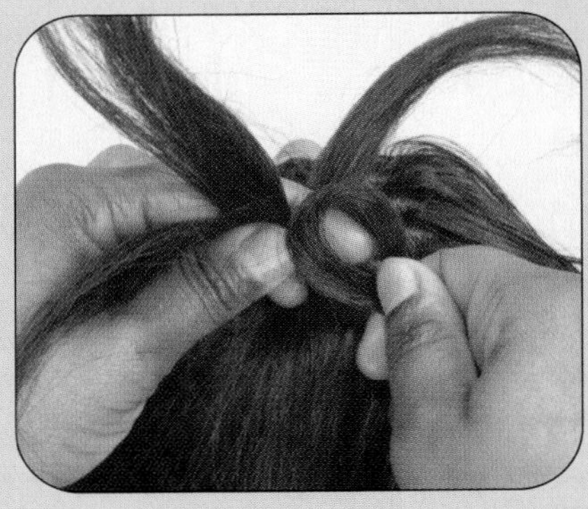

Figure 13-73 Tuck folded extension fibers into cornrow.

5. After a few revolutions and pick-ups of the natural hair, you can introduce small amounts of extension fiber, perhaps 10 to 20 fibers. To avoid bulk or knots, the amount of extension should be proportionately less than the size of the base. Fold the fibers in the middle and tuck the point in between two adjoining strands of natural hair (Figure 13–73). The folded fibers will form two portions, which are added to the center and outer strands before the next pick-up and revolution (Figure 13–74). Do not forget to continue picking up natural hair with each revolution in order to execute the cornrow (Figure 13–75 and Figure 13–76).
6. Repeat until all the hair is braided (Figure 13–77).
7. Follow cleanup and sanitation procedures for Procedure 21 — invisible braid.

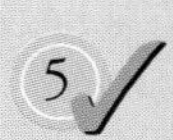

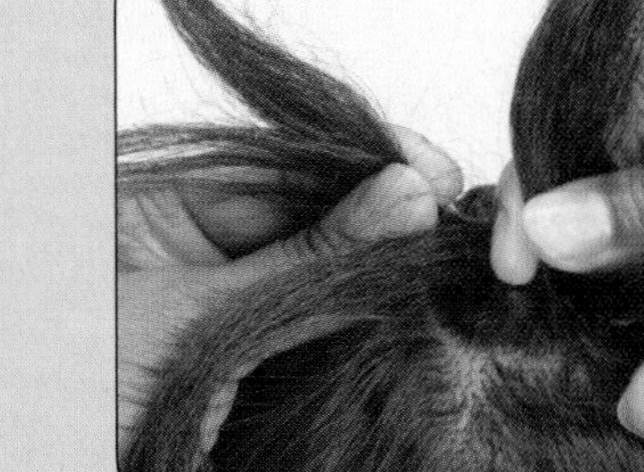

Figure 13-74 Add sides of extensions to center and outer strands.

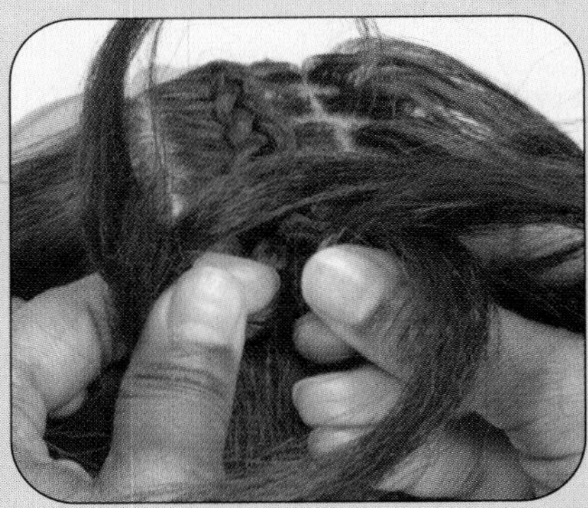

Figure 13-75 Pick up natural hair.

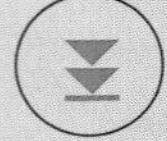

Here's a tip:

For a professional finish, always trim any ends that may stick up through the braid. Holding your scissors flat, move up the shaft as you trim, making sure that you avoid cutting into the braid.

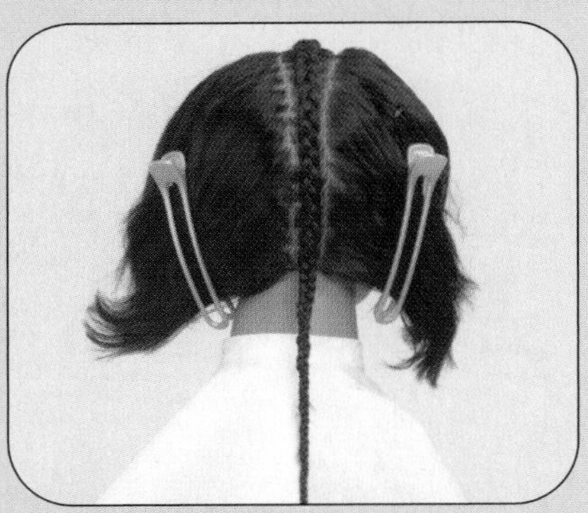

Figure 13-76 Braid to end of strand.

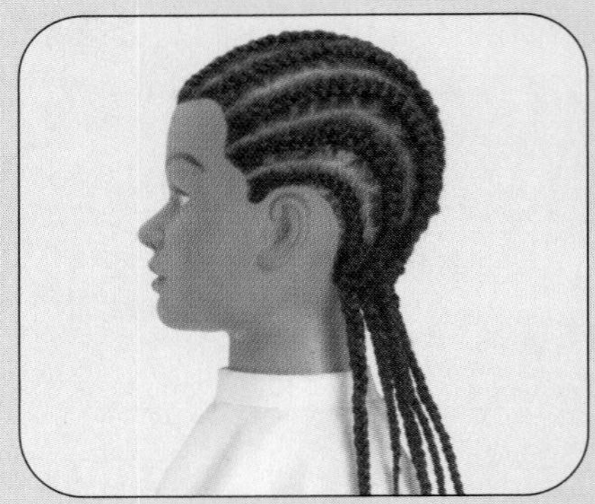

Figure 13-77 Finished style.

completed!

insights

Theo Perry

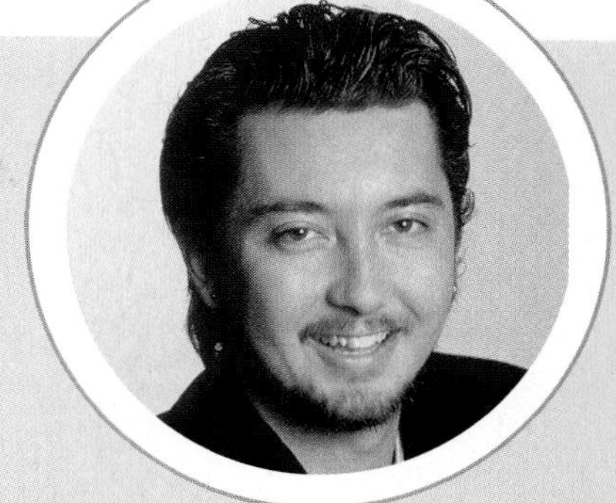

From an apprenticeship sweeping salon floors in Australia to being the National Artistic Technical Field Manager for L'Oreal Professional, Theo Perry has made it a point in his 14 years in the industry to explore all kinds of opportunities.

With this industry, the sky's the limit. There are so many fascinating avenues you can go down. You can travel, you can make a lot of money, you can become known and published. There are lots of different ways this industry can spiral. The greatest challenge for me was acknowledging that it couldn't be done overnight. I wanted it all to happen instantaneously. But I had to learn that it takes years to really master the art of hairdressing.

I did my apprenticeship in Australia, then came over and worked in a salon in Houston for three years. Then I went to L'Oreal. My focus for the first seven years was cutting and styling, and then I went into haircolor.

It's important in this industry to identify your needs. If I were a young hairdresser today looking for a salon to work for, I would sit back and study the business. I would identify my needs. Would it be education? Would it be eventually to have my own salon? I'm a strong believer in education as the cornerstone of everything we do. Being an educator is one of the fastest ways to learn. And I'm not talking about just learning hairdressing. Learning management skills, business skills, and marketing skills is also very, very important. Learning to communicate is vital.

Communication is challenging. One of the most beautiful things about working with a client is the fact that you develop this trusting relationship with an individual. You're basically guiding a person in a very, very precious moment in their lives. It is a very intimate profession. As a hairdresser, you have to learn never to overpromise anything. One of the greatest challenges we face continually as hairdressers is promising something we can't deliver—not due to a lack of talent, but to the condition of the hair or something like that.

To me, the basis of building up a loyal clientele is being in touch, listening, and being sensitive to the special events in their lives like anniversaries and birthdays where they might wish for a service. But, above all, it's about truth. It's what I call a thousand points of truth. You may be running late, for instance, and to be sensitive and to acknowledge that you are running ten minutes late is so important. Give your client a cup of tea or coffee, or tell her to go shopping and come back and you'll be ready. Be truthful and it will work. And when it works, this industry is so great. It's fun, you get to meet wonderful, caring, exciting people, you get to share ideas. It's an amazing network of individuals.

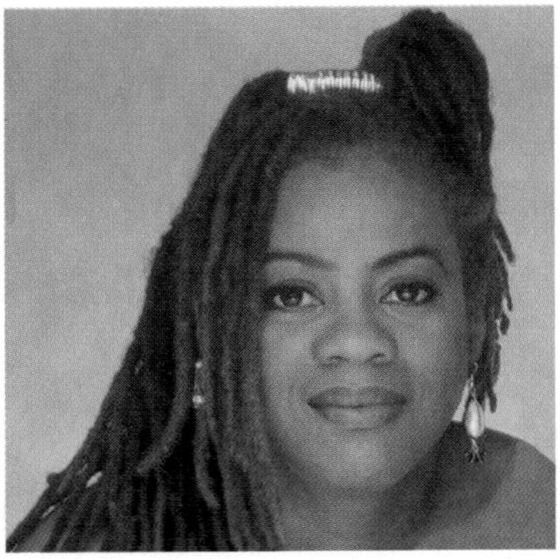

Figure 13–78 Locks.

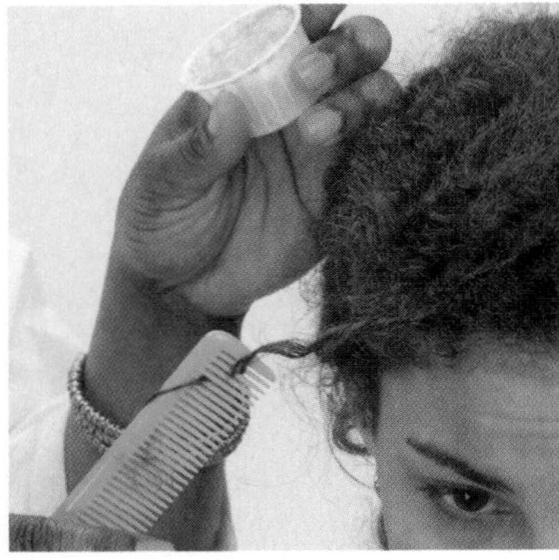

Figure 13–79 Spiral the hair with the comb.

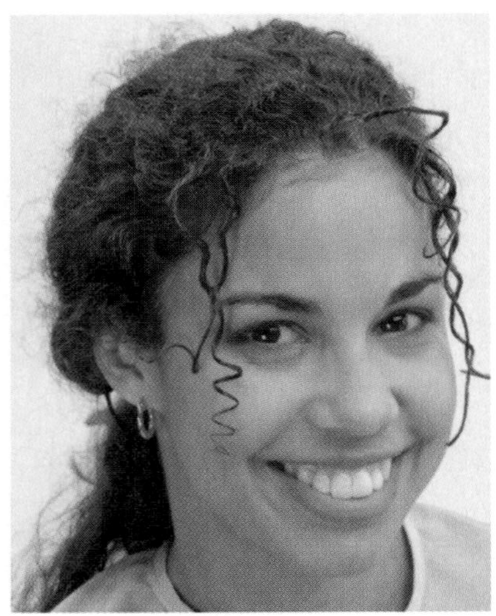

Figure 13–80 Finished coils.

unrealistic finished look. By properly applying the correct tension when using the feed-in method, the braid stylist can eliminate the artificial look and prevent breakage.

The traditional cornrow is flat, natural, and contoured to the scalp. The parting is important because it defines the finished style. The feed-in method creates a tapered or narrow base at the hairline. Small pieces or strips of extension hair are added to fill in the base, bringing the adjoining braids closer together. This technique takes longer to perform than traditional cornrowing. However, a cornrow achieved by the feed-in method will last longer, look more natural, and will not place excessive tension on the hairline. There are several different ways to start a cornrow and feed in extension pieces.

During the cornrow process, when picking up hair at the base, the hair directly underneath the previous revolution must be incorporated into the braid. The hair that you pick up must never come from another panel or be extended up into the braid from a lower part of the braid. The same is true when executing any braid technique. Overextending or misplacing the beginning of the extension leaves the hair exposed and unsupported, which can lead to breakage and hair loss in that area. This is particularly true when adding extensions at the hairline. If the extension is not made secure by two or three revolutions before picking up, it may shift away from the point of entry.

Locks

The ultimate in natural hair care is the textured richness offered by hair locking. **Locks**, also called **dreadlocks**, are natural textured hair that is intertwined and meshed together to form a single or separate network of hair. Hair locking is done without the use of chemicals. The hair locks in several slow phases, which can take from six months to a year depending on the length, density, and coil pattern of the hair (see Figure 13–78 and Table 13–1).

Locks are more than just a hairstyle; they are a cultural expression. There are several ways to cultivate locks, such as double twisting, wrapping with cord, coiling, braiding, or simply by not combing or brushing the lock. As demonstrated by the Rastafarians of Jamaica, leaving the hair to its own natural course will cause it to lock. Cultivated African locks have symmetry and balance.

The three basic methods of locking are as follows.

1. *The comb technique.* Particularly effective during the early stages of locking while the coil is still open, this method involves placing the comb at the base of the scalp and, with a rotating motion, spiraling the hair into a curl. With each revolution, the comb moves down until it reaches the end of the hair shaft. It offers a tight coil and is excellent on short (1-inch to 3-inch) hair (Figure 13–79 and Figure 13–80).

Phase	Characteristics
Phase 1 — Prelock Stage	Hair is soft and is coiled into spiral configurations. The coil is smooth and the end is open. The coil has a shiny or a glossy texture.
Phase 2 — Sprouting Stage	Hair begins to interlace and mesh. The separate units begin to "puff up" and expand in size. The units are no longer glossy or smooth.
Phase 3 — Growing Stage	A bulb can be felt at the end of each lock. Interlacing continues. Hair begins to regain length. Lock may still be frizzy, but also solid in some areas. Locks are closed at the ends, dense and dull, not reflecting any light.
Phase 4 — Maturation Stage	Lock is totally closed at the end. Hair is tightly meshed, giving the hair a rope-like cylinder shape, except where there is new growth at the base.
Phase 5 — Atrophy Stage	After several years of maturation, the lock may start to weaken or come apart at the ends.

Table 13-1 The Developmental Phases of Locks

2. *The palm roll.* This method is the gentlest on the hair and guides it through all the natural stages of locking. Palm rolling takes advantage of the hair's natural ability to coil. This method involves applying gel to dampened subsections, placing the portion of hair between the palms of both hands, and rolling in a clockwise or counterclockwise direction (Figure 13–81). With each revolution, as you move down the coil shaft, the entire coil is formed (Figure 13–82). Partings can be directional, horizontal, vertical, or bricklayered. Decorative designs and sculpting patterns are some of the creative options you can choose.
3. *Braids or extensions.* Another effective way to start locks involves sectioning the hair for the desired size lock and single braiding the hair to the end. Synthetic hair fiber, human hair fiber, or yarn can be added to a single braid to form a lock. After several weeks, the braid will grow away from the scalp, at which time the palm roll method can be used to cultivate the new growth to form a lock.

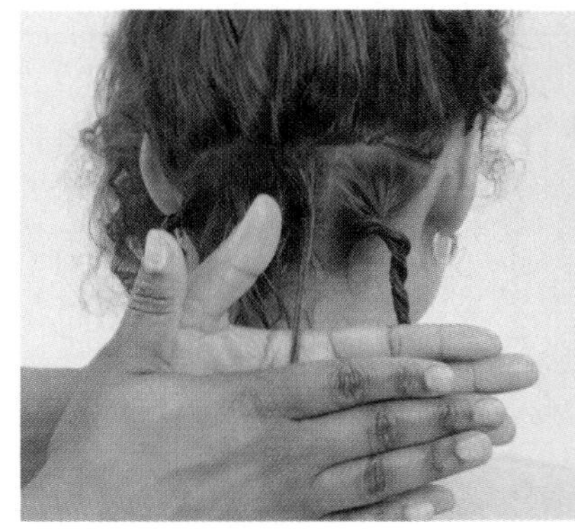

Figure 13-81 Roll the hair between the palms.

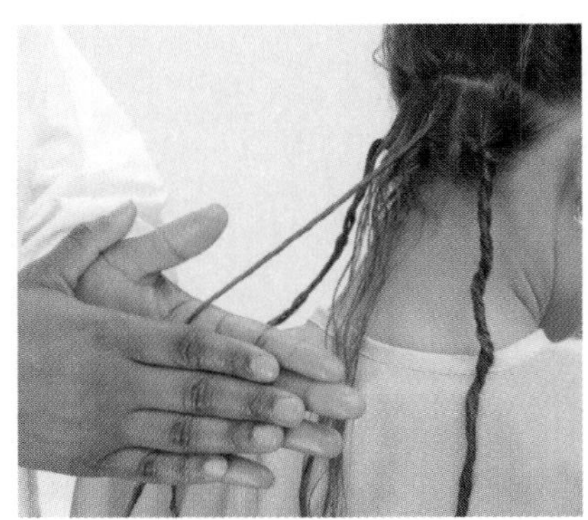

Figure 13-82 Roll down the coil shaft.

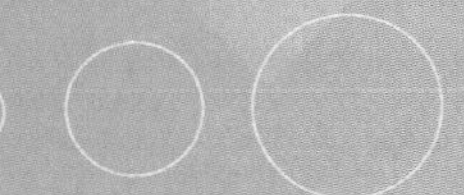

chapter glossary

cornrows or canerows	narrow rows of visible braids that lie close to the scalp; created with a three-strand, on-the-scalp braid technique
fishtail braid	simple two-strand braid in which hair is picked up from the sides and added to the strands as they are crossed over each other
invisible or inverted braid	three-strand braid produced by overlapping the strands of hair on top of each other
locks or dreadlocks	natural textured hair that is intertwined and meshed together to form a single or separate network of hair
natural hairstyling	hairstyling that uses no chemicals or tints and does not alter the natural curl or coil pattern of the hair
rope braid	braid made with two strands that are twisted around each other
single braids	free-hanging braids, with or without extensions, that can be executed either underhand or overhand; also called individual or box braids
visible braid	three-strand braid made by the underhand technique, in which the strands of hair are woven under the center strand

review questions

1. What is meant by "natural hairstyling"?
2. In the context of braiding, what are the three qualities that determine hair texture?
3. What is a coil?
4. What six materials are most commonly used for hair extensions?
5. Why does textured (extremely curly or coiled) hair require special preparation before braiding?
6. What is the difference between a visible and invisible braiding style?
7. Describe rope and fishtail braids.
8. Explain the basic procedure for creating single braids.
9. Explain the methods of cornrowing with and without extensions.
10. Name the three basic methods of hair locking.

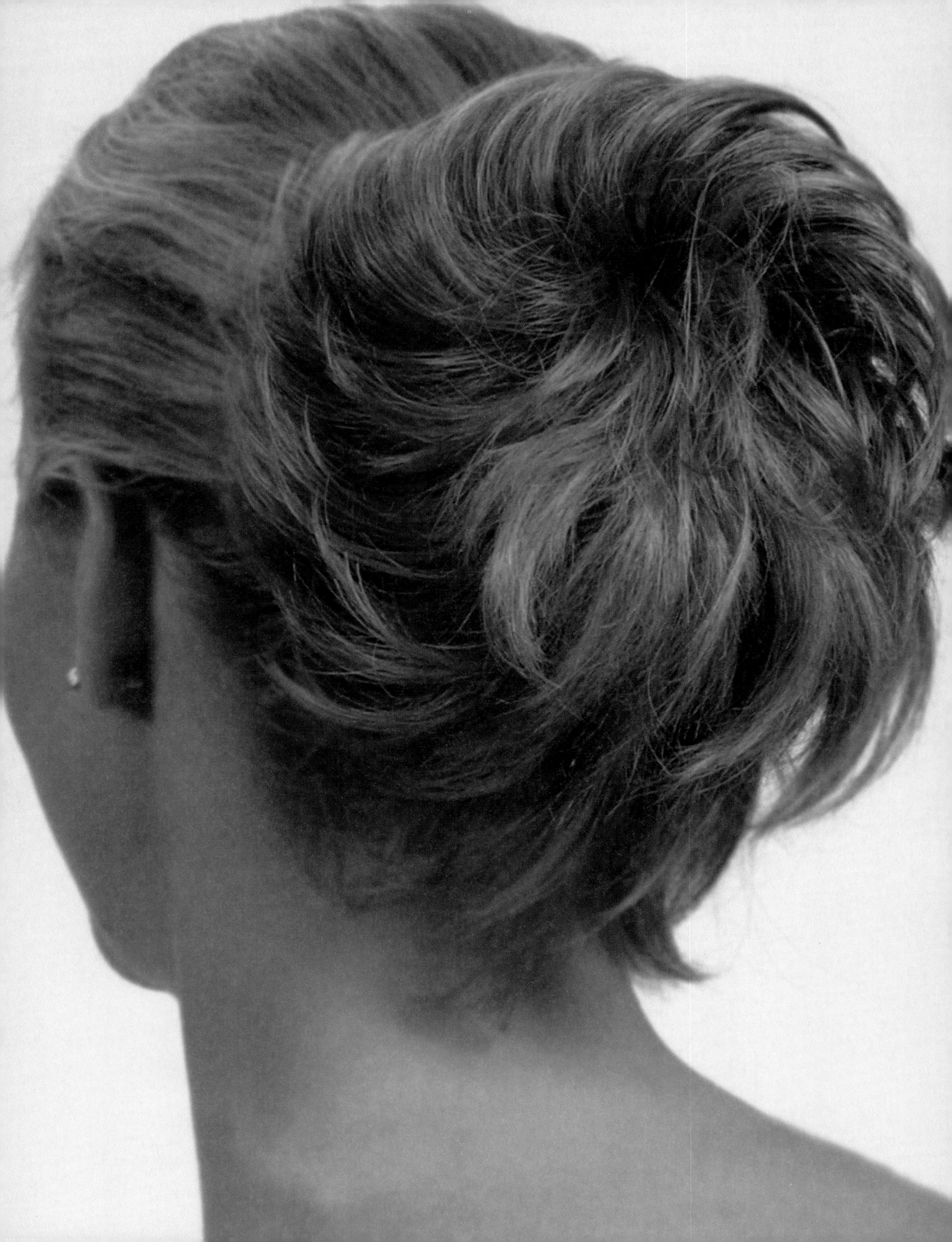

WIGS AND HAIR ENHANCEMENTS

Vivienne Mackinder

FREELANCE HAIRDRESSER FOR PRINT, RUNWAYS, AND SHOWS, NEW YORK CITY

Chapter Outline

The Consultation • Wigs • Hairpieces
Hair Extensions • Practice, Practice, Practice

Learning Objectives

After completing this chapter, you should be able to:

1. List the elements of a client consultation for wig services.
2. Explain the differences between human-hair and synthetic wigs.
3. Describe the two basic categories of wigs.
4. Demonstrate the procedure for taking wig measurements.
5. Demonstrate the procedure for putting on a wig.
6. Describe the various types of hairpieces and their uses.
7. Explain the various methods of attaching extensions.

National Skill Standards

This chapter provides you with the necessary information to master these National Industry Skill Standards for Entry-Level Cosmetologists.

Providing nonsurgical hair additions.

Consulting with clients to determine their needs and preferences.

Effectively marketing professional salon products.

Key Terms

Page number indicates where in the chapter the term is used.

block pg.465

bonding pg. 479

cap wigs pg. 464

capless wigs pg. 464

fusion pg. 480

hair extensions pg. 478

hairpiece pg. 462

hand-tied or hand-knotted wigs pg. 465

integration hairpiece pg. 475

machine-made wigs pg. 465

semi-hand-tied wigs pg. 465

toupee pg. 475

track and sew method pg. 478

turned hair pg. 464

wefts pg. 464

wig pg. 462

From the very beginning of recorded history, wigs have played an important role in the world of fashion. The ancient Egyptians shaved their heads with bronze razors and wore heavy black wigs to protect them from the sun. In ancient Rome, women wore wigs made from the prized blond hair of captured barbarians from the north. In Japan, the lacquered coiffures of the geishas were actually wigs. In 18th-century England, men wore wigs, called perukes, to indicate if they were in the army, the navy, or engaged in the practice of law.

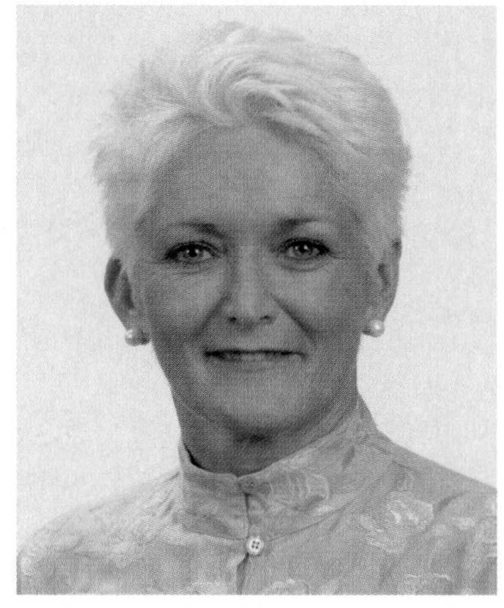

Figure 14–1 A client before fitting with a wig.

Wigs play a more important role than ever in today's fashion world. Models and celebrities who require a specific look for an assignment depend on hair additions to help them achieve that look. Specialists in hair additions and enhancements are increasingly in demand, working in runway and hair shows and on print and video shoots. Hair artists have adapted high-fashion concepts for the everyday needs of their clients (Figure 14–1 and Figure 14–2).

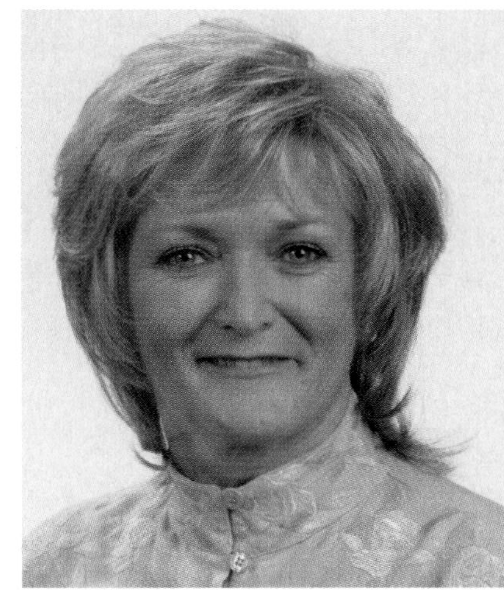

Figure 14–2 The same client, transformed.

Hair enhancements play an important role outside of fashion as well. For instance, would you find it personally gratifying to help a cancer patient who has suffered hair loss feel better about herself and her appearance? Perhaps you have a client who is going through premature hair loss and is feeling anxious about it. With the right knowledge and practice, you can use your skills in hair enhancement to bring a satisfying new dimension into the lives of many people.

THE CONSULTATION

focus on ...communication.

Always share styling tips with the client. This is a great way to build client trust and loyalty.

As with other salon services, the client consultation for wig services is designed to offer some degree of protection to both you and the client (Figure 14–3). Your client may have big dreams that he feels can be made into reality by a wig or hairpiece. It is important for both you and your client to remember that you are a stylist, not a magician. You can offer your client a makeover, but the results will always be bound by reality. This should be fully understood at the beginning. If it is not, it may lead to disappointment and frustration.

A wig service can also be a large financial and emotional investment for the client. Often, the decision to wear a wig comes about after the client has experienced hair loss. You will need to understand your client's motivation in seeking a wig service to make sure the client will be satisfied in the end.

Conduct your consultation with compassionate, "feeling" language. Make a person-to-person connection and convey a positive attitude. Keep in mind that regardless of the client's motivation for trying a hair enhancement—a social event, to cover up hair loss, or just for fun—the client is likely to feel a little nervous about it. Concerns may include how she looks, how her spouse will feel about it, whether people will know the hair is not the client's own, and how much money it will cost. The point of the consultation is to cut through the doubts and fears with genuine communication. Your best tool for achieving good communication is the Key Point Checklist (Figure 14–4). 1

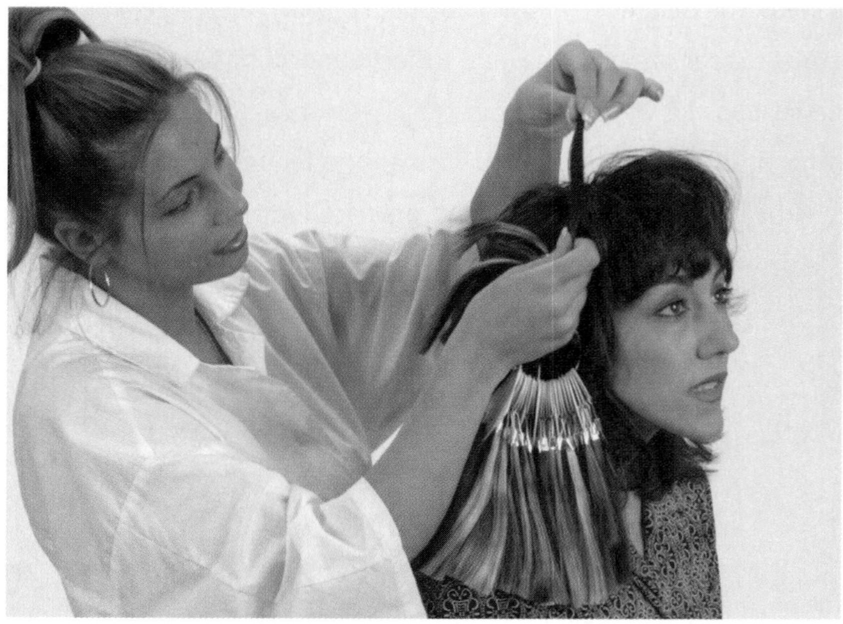

Figure 14-3 Client consultation.

Key Point Checklist

1. **Determining need and desire:**
   - Does your client intend to use the addition as a fashion accessory?
   - Will it be used in the context of a wedding, a prom, or some other special occasion?
   - Is the client seeking to create instant glamour for herself?
   - Will the primary purpose of the addition be to disguise thinning hair or hair loss due to illness?
   - Will the hair addition be used in the context of film work, TV, theater, fashion shows, or photo shoots?
2. **Matching the style with the client:**
   - Determine your client's personality type. The introverted client likes to "play it safe" with a style of hair addition that is natural and does not draw too much attention to itself. Her goal is to enhance what she already has. The extroverted client is bold and adventurous and may be looking for a change. She is drawn to the more stylized hair additions that pack a dramatic punch.
   - Consider your client's age. If she is young, she may want a playful style. If she is mature, she may prefer a more natural style.
   - Consider your client's personal image. Is it corporate? Trendy? Classic? Country? Glamorous? Cute? Athletic?
   - Take note of the client's job or career. If she works in a health club, for instance, she can get away with a look that would be out of place in a bank.
3. **Finding the right balance:**
   - Study your client's bone structure and body type. Step back and take a look at the big picture. Keep in mind the rule of classic proportions: the ratio of head size to body should be about 1 to 7. The added hair must not overwhelm the client, unless it is part of a theatrical look of some kind.
   - When adding hair, it is best to conduct your consultation with the client in her street clothes, not caped and gowned. Capes offer excellent protection when performing a service, but they can also camouflage the client's body type and can mask proportions. You want to make sure that the style you envision will work with the client's "look."
4. **Working with the client's hair type:**
   - You will need to determine hair texture in order to blend the artificial hair with the natural hair.
   - Be aware of natural hairlines and growth patterns, which will influence your choice of wig, hairpiece, or extensions.
   - The natural condition of the hair will determine how much of the real hair you decide to show and how much you decide to cover up.
   - Check the hair density. Does the client have a full head of hair and simply want an alternative look, or is the client's hair thinning and patchy?
5. **Selecting the appropriate hair addition:**
   - Among the hair addition options you will be bringing to your client's attention are wigs (human or synthetic, custom-made, or ready to wear), hair extensions (temporary, clip-in, or semipermanent), or hairpieces (falls, ponytails, switches, wiglets, braids, ponytail wraps, toupees).
   - Is the addition temporary or semipermanent? Does the client want to maintain the look through salon services or home maintenance? For how long will the client be wearing the wig? Are serious health issues involved that might determine the length of time the wig will be worn?
   - What environmental factors are involved? Consider humidity and exposure, for instance. You might suggest a synthetic hairpiece for a client in Florida, for example, because it won't frizz in high humidity. (The client would have to smooth her own hair down with gel first.)
   - Use a sample color ring to identify the correct color match for your client.
   - Have on hand various product photos and brochures from which your client can make a selection. It is also good to keep samples of the products themselves for your client to see and feel.
   - Will the wig or hairpiece need to be custom cut or colored?
6. **Budgetary concerns:**
   - What is the client's budget? This is often the biggest factor in choosing a product.
   - Using catalogs and price lists, be prepared to educate the client on the features and benefits of the various price points (high, medium, and low).
   - Establish salon service fees for custom cutting, coloring, and styling of hair additions.
7. **Other available creative options. Do not neglect to call your client's attention to the following services you can provide:**
   - Custom cutting.
   - Color, perming, setting, and styling of wigs, hairpieces, and extensions.
   - A styling maintenance program that will educate the client in the use of styling products.

Figure 14-4 Key Point Checklist.

WIGS

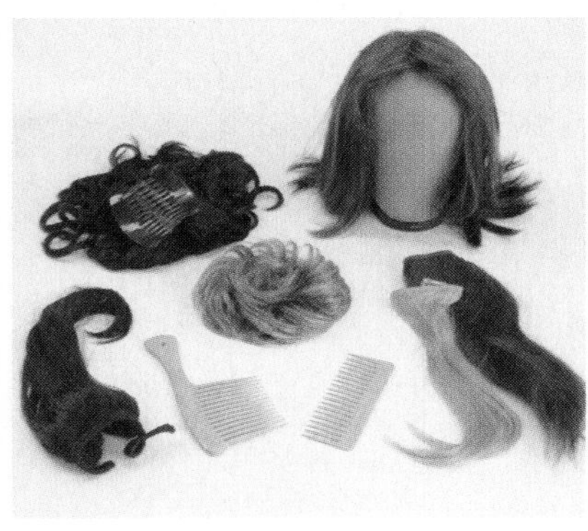

Figure 14-5 Wigs and hairpieces come in a wide range of styles and colors.

A **wig** can be defined as an artificial covering for the head consisting of a network of interwoven hair. When wearing a wig, the client's hair is completely concealed (100 percent coverage). If a hair addition does not fully cover the head, it is classified as a **hairpiece**, which is a small wig used to cover the top or crown of the head (Figure 14–5).

Human Hair versus Synthetic Hair

What is the fastest way to tell if a strand of hair is a synthetic product or real human hair? Pull the strand out of the wig or hairpiece and burn it with a match. Human hair will burn slowly, giving off a distinctive odor. A strand of synthetic fiber, on the other hand, will either "ball up" and melt, extinguishing itself (a characteristic of a synthetic like kanekalon), or will continue to flame and burn out very quickly (typical of polyester). In either case, it will not give off an odor.

How can you determine which is best for your client, real hair or synthetic? Both have their advantages and disadvantages.

Advantages of Human Hair Wigs

- A more realistic appearance than synthetic wigs.
- Greater durability.
- The same styling and maintenance requirements as natural hair. Human hair wigs can be custom colored to suit the client; they can be permed; and they tolerate heat from a blow-dryer, curling iron, or hot rollers.

Disadvantages of Human Hair Wigs

- Human hair reacts to the climate the way natural hair does. Depending on what type of hair it is, it may frizz or lose its curl in humid weather.
- After shampooing, the hair needs to be reset. This can be a challenge for the client who intends to maintain the wig at home.
- The color will oxidize, meaning that it will fade with exposure to light.
- The hair will break and split just like human hair if mistreated by harsh brushing, back-combing, or excessive use of heat.

Advantages of Synthetic Wigs

- Over the years, the technology of producing synthetic fibers has greatly improved. Wigs made of modacrylic are particularly strong and durable. Top-of-the-line synthetics like kanekalon, a modacrylic fiber, simulate protein-rich hair, with a natural lustrous look and feel. These synthetics are so realistic they can even fool stylists.
- Synthetic wigs are a great value. Not only are they very realistic, but they are also less expensive than real hair. Both style and texture are set into the hair. Ready-to-wear wigs are very easy for the client to maintain at home. Shampooing in cold water will not change the style; nor will exposure to extreme humidity.
- Most synthetic ready-to-wear wigs are cut according to the latest styles, with the cut, color, and texture already set. The only work you as the stylist may be required to do is some detailing or custom trimming.

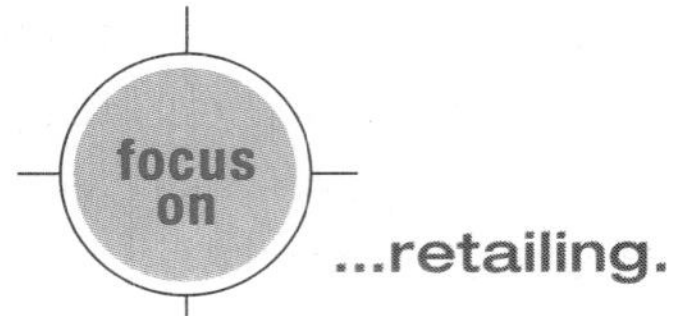

...retailing.

Retailing hair additions as well as home-care products can mean substantial additional income for you. To become an effective marketer, keep the following guidelines in mind:

- Make a cue card for yourself that lists the key points you should discuss with the client.
- Identify the client's needs.
- Explain why it would be worth it for the client to make the investment.
- Describe the features and benefits of the products you recommend.
- Discuss product performance and cost.
- Always believe in your recommendations and stand by your products.

- The colors are almost unlimited, ranging from natural to wild fantasy shades. Again, price is a factor here. The cheaper wigs tend to be more solid in color (less tone on tone) and the fiber is coarser (polyester-based). The high-end products are a mix of many shades, with highlights and lowlights for a natural effect.
- Synthetic colors will not fade or oxidize, even when exposed to long periods in the sun.

DRAWBACKS OF SYNTHETIC WIGS

- Synthetic hair cannot be exposed to extreme heat (curling irons, hot rollers, or the high heat of blow-dryers).
- Coloring synthetic fibers is not recommended, as traditional haircolor does not work on them.
- Sometimes, synthetic wigs are so shiny that they may not look natural. Also, if they are thick, they will look unnatural on a fine-haired client. Price has a lot to do with how natural a synthetic wig can look. 2

Quality and Cost

As you can see, both human hair wigs and synthetics have their pros and cons. The bottom line in both cases is that you get what you pay for. Ultimately, your success in working with any hair addition will be determined by the quality of the product itself. Do not be fooled by imitations. Cheap wigs may be great for "fun moments" or to practice cutting on, but in other situations they can look tacky and unattractive.

The most expensive wigs are those made of human hair. The price scale is as follows.

- *European hair* is at the top of the line. Virgin hair is the most costly; color-treated hair is second in cost.
- *Hair from India and Asia,* the two regions that provide most of the human hair commercially available, are next in cost. Indian hair is usually available in lengths from 12 inches to 16 inches. Asian hair is available in lengths of 12 inches to 28 inches. Indian hair is naturally wavy; Asian hair is naturally straight.
- *Human hair mixed with animal hair* is next. The animal hair may be angora, horse, yak, or sheep hair. Yak hair is taken from the animal's belly and is the purest of whites. Its natural color lends itself to adding fantasy colors, which attract the teen market. Mixed-hair products are often used in theatrical or fashion settings.

There are several important questions to ask when selecting a wig for the client.

- Is the wig made of human hair, animal hair, a mix of both, or is it synthetic?
- Is the hair colored or in its natural state (virgin hair)?
- If the hair is human hair, is it graded in terms of strength, elasticity, and porosity?

Here's a tip:

The key to working with a synthetic fiber wig is to pick a shape or style that suits your client, rather than trying to change the shape of the wig itself.

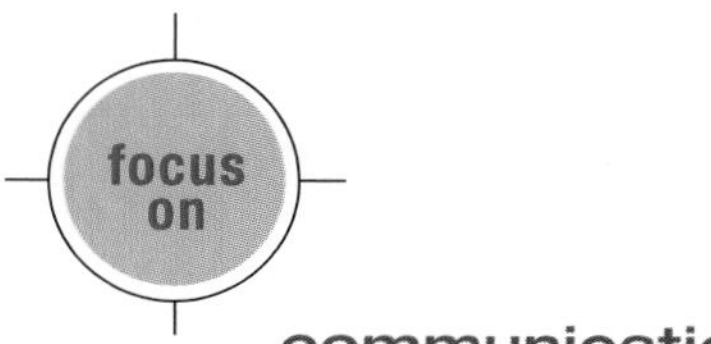

...communication.

To the average consumer, the "deals" at the local wig store may look good. But that apparent deal could be a mix of animal hair and human hair, and one washing could mat the wig into a big ball. Well-crafted wigs, such as those used in film work, might be valued at thousands of dollars. Your client will not necessarily need something so luxurious, but you must still pay attention to quality. As a professional, you must educate your client and recommend only well-made products. Remember, when you recommend something, you are putting your reputation on the line. And your reputation is precious.

Here's a tip:

If you are looking for wave and texture, buy Indian hair, which is naturally wavy. Chinese hair is naturally straight.

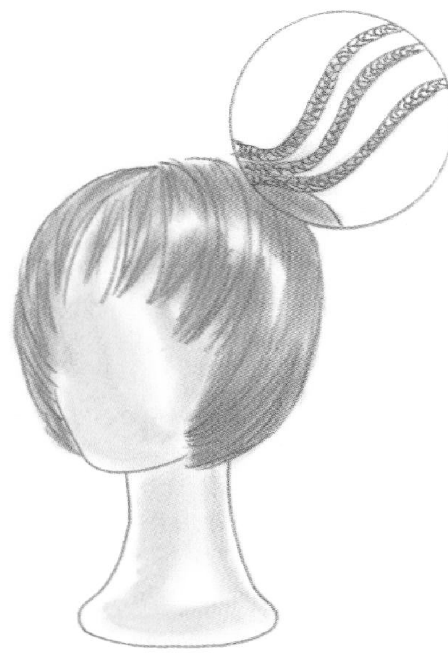

Figure 14–6 Turned hair.

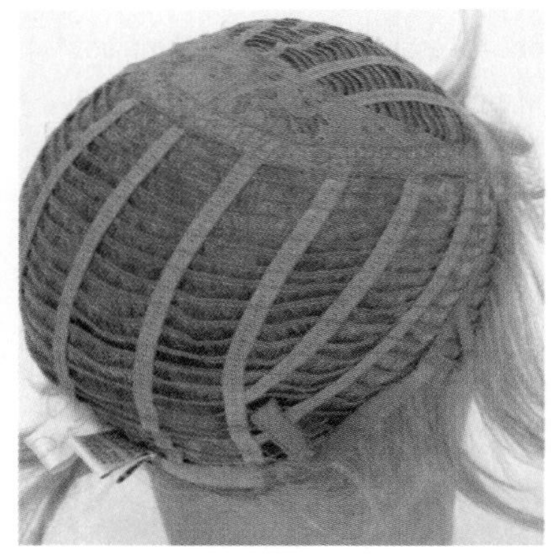

Figure 14–7 A capless wig.

14

- Is the cuticle intact? Cuticle-intact hair is more expensive, as the hair has been "turned." In **turned hair**, the root ends are arranged to prevent the hair from tangling. The root end of every hair strand is sewn into the base so that the cuticles of all hair strands slope in the same direction (Figure 14–6). The hair is in better condition and is much easier to work with. Turning is a tedious, time-consuming process that increases the cost of the hair.
- Is the hair fallen hair, meaning hair that has been shed from the head and perhaps gathered from a hairbrush, as opposed to hair that has been cut? Fallen hair is not turned roots to ends, and the cuticle is removed so that it will not lock and mat. This hair tends to be less expensive.
- Is the hair tangle-free? If the cuticle has been removed, this often means you cannot condition the hair, for it will tend to mat.
- What is the condition of the hair? Has it been bleached? Can it be colored? Has it been colored with metallic dye?
- Will the hair match the client's hair? Should you be blending to match?
- Can the hair be permed?
- If the client is going to maintain her hair at home, will the wig last a reasonable amount of time (four to six months if in continual use)?

Types of Wigs

There are two basic categories of wigs: cap and capless.

Cap wigs are constructed with an elasticized mesh-fiber base to which the hair is attached. They are made in several sizes and require special fittings. More often than not, cap wigs are hand-knotted. The front edge of a cap wig is made of a material that resembles the client's scalp, along with a lace extension and a wire support, used at the temples for a snug, secure fit. Hair is hand-tied under the net ("underknotted") to conceal the cap edge. The side and back edges contain wire supports, elastic, and hooks for a secure fit.

Capless wigs are machine-made. The hair (human or artificial) is woven into long strips called **wefts**. Rows of wefts are sewn to elastic strips in a circular pattern to fit the head shape. Capless wigs are more popular today than cap wigs as they are ready-to-wear and less expensive. The capless wig is a frame of connected wefts, and therefore there are open points. Compare a nylon stocking to a fishnet stocking: one has a closed framework (the cap wig), the other is open (capless). Due to the construction and airiness, capless wigs are extremely light and comfortable to wear (Figure 14–7).

In general, capless wigs or caps that allow the scalp to breathe are healthier, as they prevent excess perspiration. A cap wig is best for a client with extremely thin hair or no hair. If you put a capless wig on a bald client, her scalp will show through. 3

METHODS OF CONSTRUCTION

- **Hand-tied** or **hand-knotted wigs**. These wigs are made by inserting individual strands of hair into a mesh foundation and knotting them with a needle. Hand-tying is done particularly around the front hairline and the top of the head. These wigs have a natural, realistic look and are wonderful for styling. The hand-tied method most closely resembles actual human hair growth, with flexibility at the roots. There is no definite direction to the hair; it can be combed in almost any direction.
- **Semi-hand-tied wigs**. These wigs are constructed with a combination of synthetic hair and hand-tied human hair. Reasonably priced, they offer a natural appearance and good durability.
- **Machine-made wigs**. The least expensive option, these wigs are made by machine, not by hand. They are made by feeding wefts through a sewing machine, then sewing them together to form the base and shape of the wig. They have the disadvantage of the wefting direction, which restricts other styling options. Some hairstylists can become overcreative with this type of wig and cut it to a point of no return. Another aspect of these wigs is their "bounce back" quality. Even after shampooing, the style returns.

The artificial growth patterns of a wig are very important to be aware of. The wig construction will determine the direction in which you style the hair. The most flexible and versatile of all patterns is the hand-tied wig. Machine-made wigs are sewn in an exact direction, offering no versatility. If you like the style this is a good thing, but if you do not, you have a problem. Make sure you like the direction of the style and work within the framework.

Taking Wig Measurements

The creation of a custom-made wig begins with taking the client's measurements. Use a soft tape measure, keeping it close to the head without pressure.

Always keep a written record of the client's head measurements and forward a copy to the wig dealer or manufacturer. You should include precise specifications of hair shade, quality of hair, length of hair, and type of hair part and pattern.

If the wig is ready-to-wear, no measuring will be required, as it can be adjusted by tightening the straps or the elastic in the nape. Ready-to-wear are more common in the salon, largely because of the price difference. But every wig needs to be adjusted to the head and custom styled or trimmed to suit the client. 4

Blocking the Wig

A **block** is a head-shaped form, usually made of canvas-covered cork or Styrofoam, to which the wig is secured for fitting, cleaning, coloring, and styling. Canvas blocks are available in six sizes, from 20 inches (50 cm) to 22-½ inches (56.25 cm). The block is best attached to your work area with a swivel clamp, which allows for greater control.

PROCEDURE 28

TAKING WIG MEASUREMENTS

Implements and Materials

- styling cape
- neck strip
- boar-bristle brush
- duckbill clips
- cloth measuring tape

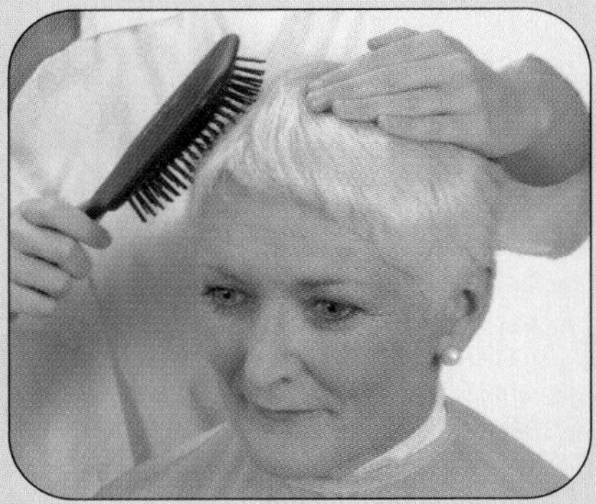

Figure 14-8 Brush hair down smoothly.

Preparation

1. Client consultation.
2. Drape the client for a dry hair service, with a styling cape and neck strip.
3. Brush the hair down smoothly and pin it as flatly and tightly to the scalp as possible (Figure 14–8).

Procedure

1. Measure the circumference of the head. Place the tape completely around the head, starting at the hairline at the middle of the forehead. Place the tape above the ears, around the back of the head, and return to the starting point (Figure 14–9).
2. Beginning from the hairline at the middle of the forehead, measure over the top to the nape of the neck. Bend the head back and measure to the point where the wig will ride on the base of the skull at the nape (Figure 14–10).

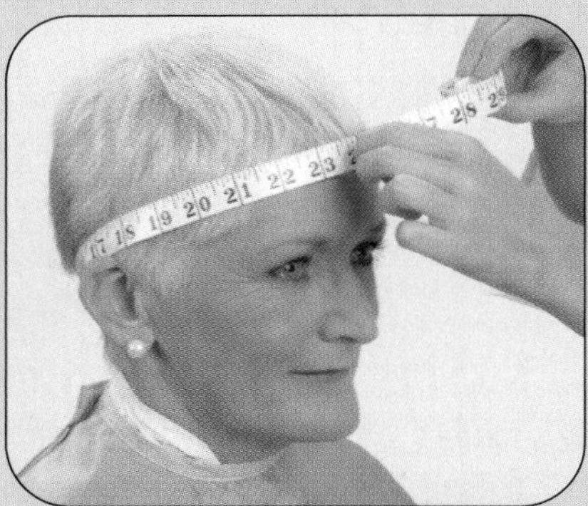

Figure 14-9 Measure circumference of head.

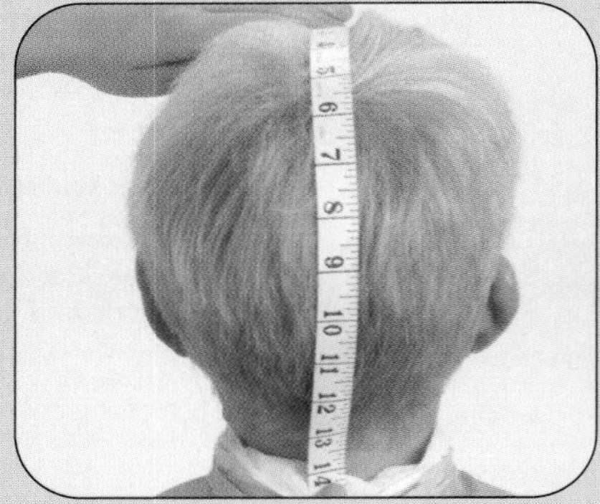

Figure 14-10 Measure from middle of front hairline to nape.

3. Measure from ear to ear, across the forehead (Figure 14–11).
4. Measure from ear to ear, over the top of the head (Figure 14–12).
5. Place the tape across the crown and measure from temple to temple (Figure 14–13).
6. Measure the width of the napeline, across the nape of the neck (Figure 14–14).

Cleanup and Sanitation

1. Disinfect all implements and store in appropriate containers.
2. Discard neck strip and place cape in hamper for laundering.
3. Sanitize your workstation.
4. Wash your hands with soap and warm water.

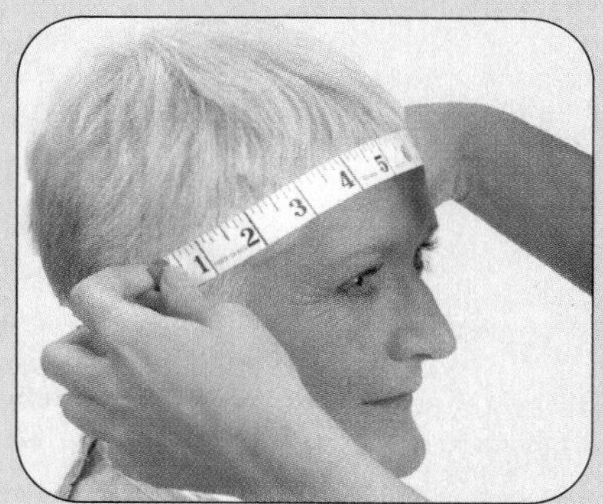

Figure 14-11 Measure across forehead.

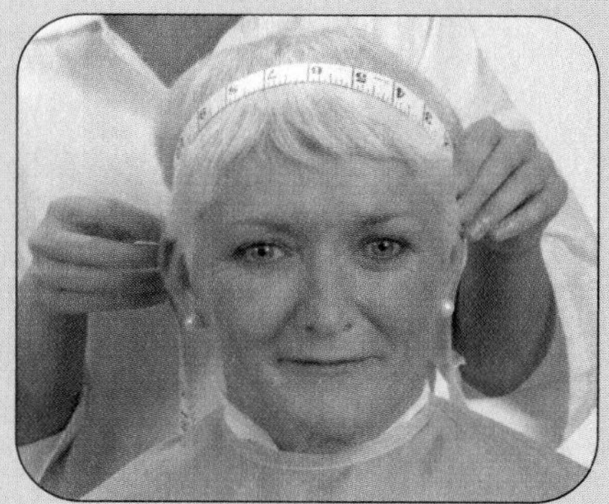

Figure 14-12 Measure top of head.

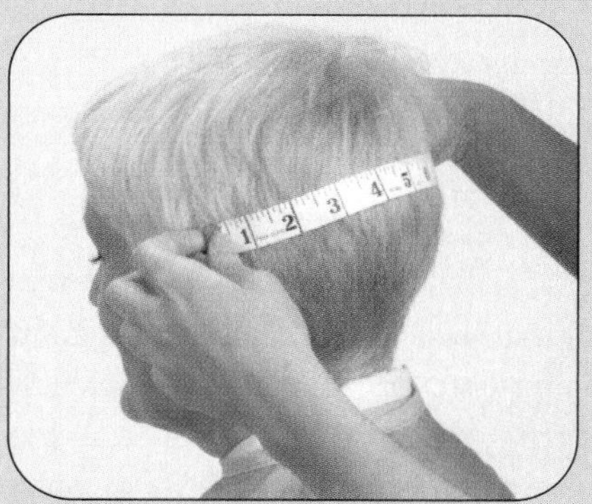

Figure 14-13 Measure from temple to temple.

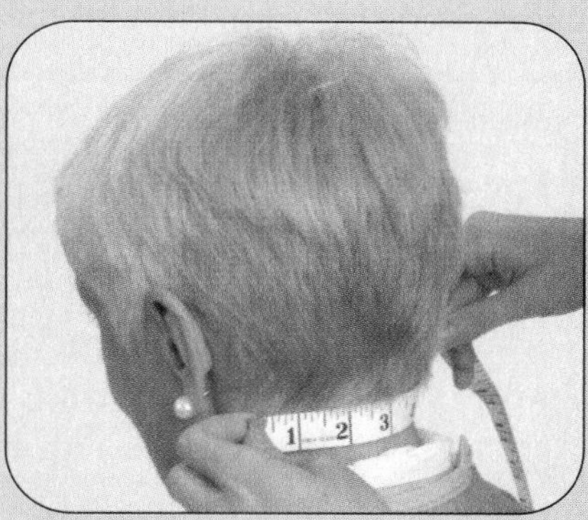

Figure 14-14 Measure width of napeline.

completed!

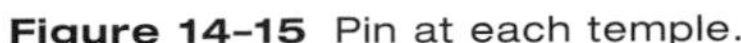

Figure 14–15 Pin at each temple.

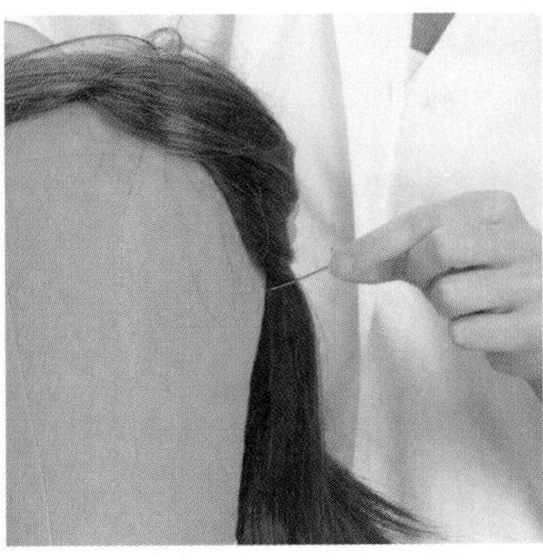

Figure 14–16 Pin above each ear.

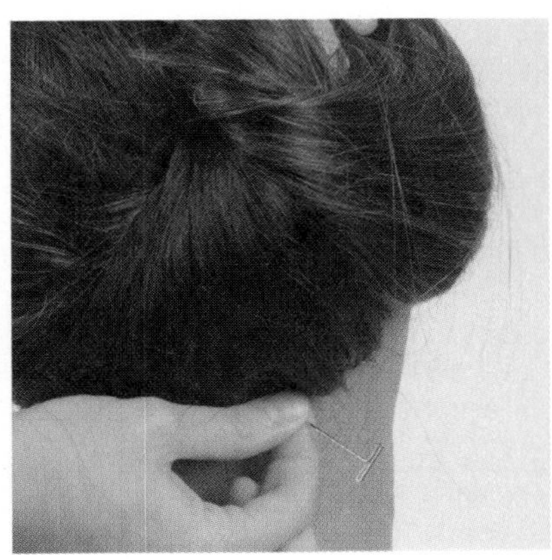

Figure 14–17 Pin each corner of the nape.

Always fit the wig to the right size block. Do not try to stretch a wig to fit it onto a block or allow a wig to hang loosely on a block that is too small. When mounting the wig on the block, pin it evenly with T-shaped pins at these points:

- the temples (use the seams of the block as a guide) (Figure 14–15)
- above each ear (Figure 14–16)
- each corner of the nape (Figure 14–17)

Putting on the Wig

One of the most important steps in the wig service has to do with instructing the client on how to put on the wig. Start by educating the client on the correct method for preparing her hair to receive the wig. The client's skill at securing her hair under the wig cap and making it flat and even will determine how well the wig sits on her head. Two methods for preparing the hair are the hair wrap and pin curls (Procedure 29).

Cleaning the Wig

To clean any wig, always follow the manufacturer's instructions. If shampooing is recommended, use a gentle shampoo, such as one you would use for color-treated hair. Avoid any harsh shampoos with a sulfur base, such as dandruff shampoos.

Cutting the Wig

When cutting a wig, generally your goal is to make the hair look more realistic. As you know, the hair on the human head has many lengths. Even when hair is cut to one length, internally there are various stages of hair growth. Hair that is one month old and hair that is years old all exist on the same head. The stylist should try to achieve this natural look within the wig. The most effective way to do this is to taper the ends when cutting the wig. The more solid the shape, the more unnatural the hair will look.

When cutting and trimming wigs, you can follow the basic methods of haircutting—blunt, layered, and graduated—using the same sectioning and elevations as on a real head of hair. Or you may do what many top stylists

PROCEDURE

PUTTING ON THE WIG

Implements and Materials

- styling cape and neck strip
- comb
- hairpins
- bobby pins
- wig cap
- wig

Preparation

1. Client consultation (Figure 14–18).
2. Drape the client for a dry hair service with a styling cape and neck strip.

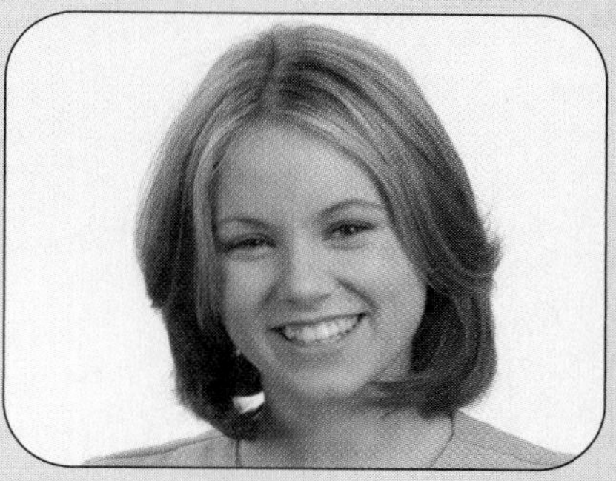

Figure 14–18 Client before draping.

Procedure for Pin Curls

1. Brush the hair smooth.
2. Take large sections of the hair and wrap them into flat pin curls, keeping the base of each pin curl as flat and smooth as possible (Figure 14–19 and Figure 14–20).

Procedure for Hair Wrap

1. Section off a large triangular section at the crown and pin this hair out of the way (Figure 14–21).
2. Taking small sections, brush the client's hair all around the head, as if you were setting the hair on a big roller, with the head as the roller (Figure 14–22).

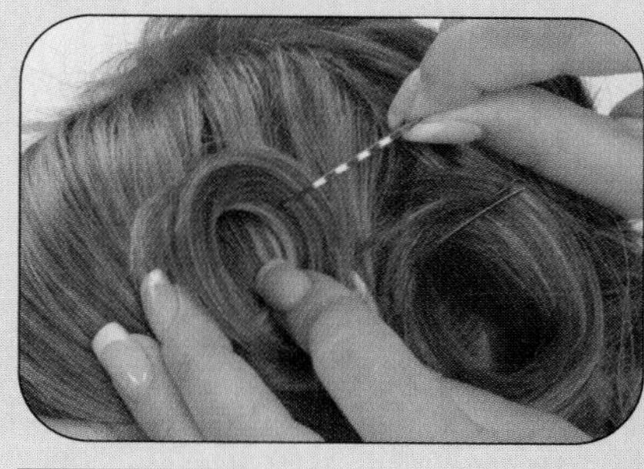

Figure 14–19 Arrange the hair in large pin curls.

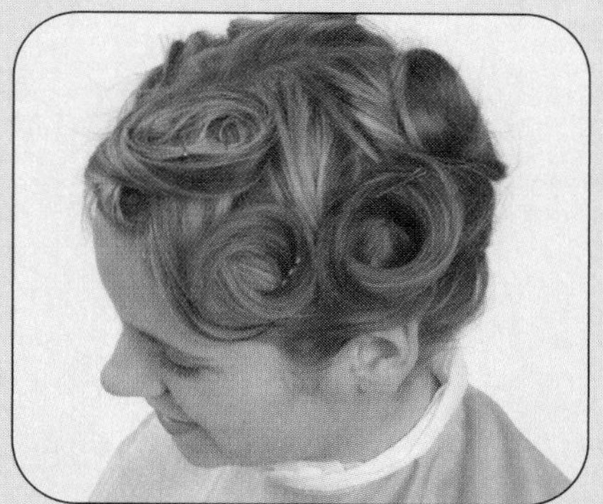

Figure 14–20 All the hair in pin curls.

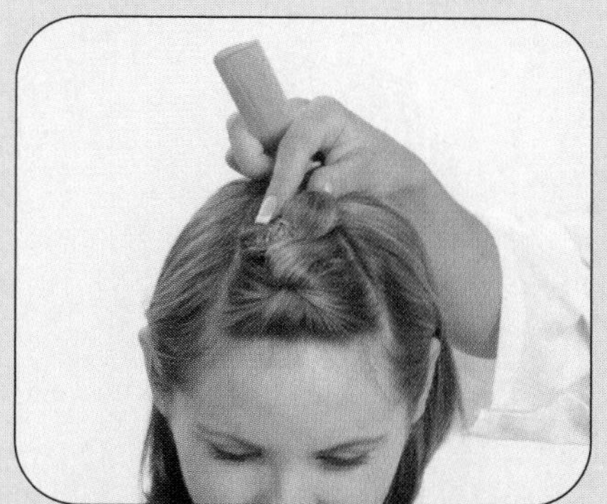

Figure 14–21 Section off triangle at crown.

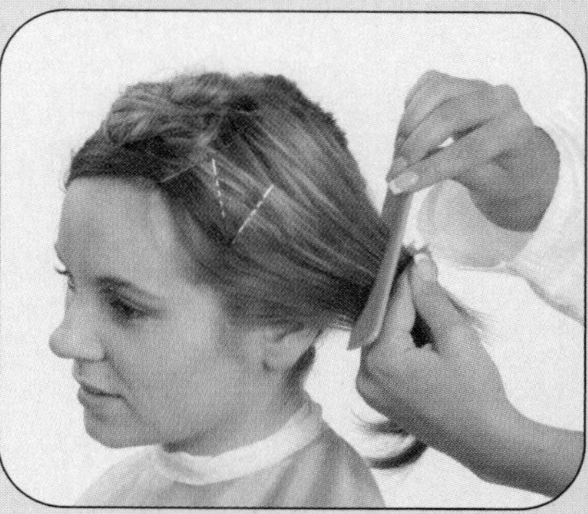

Figure 14–22 Wrap the hair around the head.

3. Pin the hair in place. You may pull a wig cap over the hair if desired. (Figure 14–23).

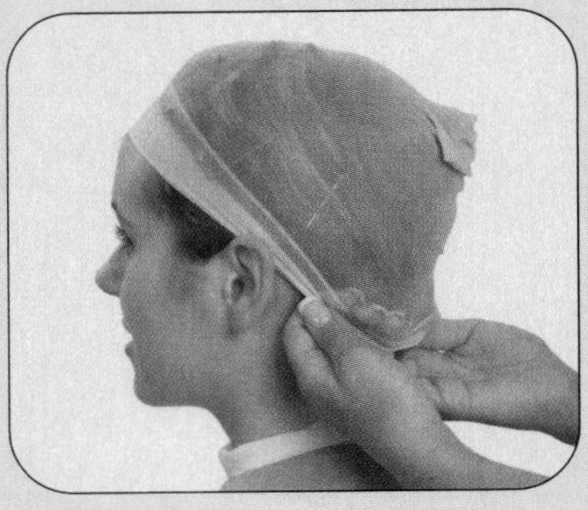

Figure 14-23 Wig cap over wrapped hair.

Procedure for Putting on the Wig

1. Holding the front of the wig against the forehead with one hand, use your other hand to gently slide the wig back onto the head (Figure 14–24).
2. Hold the edge in front of the ears and pull it down, making sure that the wig is sitting straight (Figure 14–25).
3. If the wig is loose, tighten it by adjusting the elastic and hooks at the nape. You may have to tighten it off the head and then refit it on the client (Figure 14–26 and Figure 14–27).
4. If the client has long or thick hair, you may need some extra pins to lock the wig deeper into place, as the client's hair could push the wig up. For clients with thin or short hair, additional pinning is not usually necessary.
5. Follow cleanup and sanitation procedures for Procedure 28 — measuring the wig.

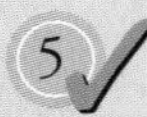

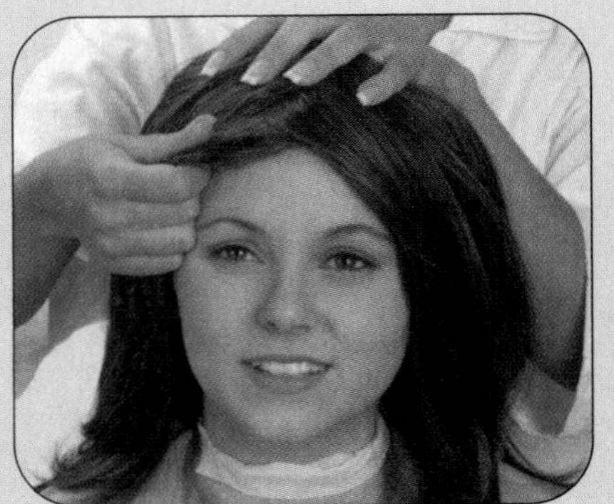

Figure 14-24 Pull the wig on front to back.

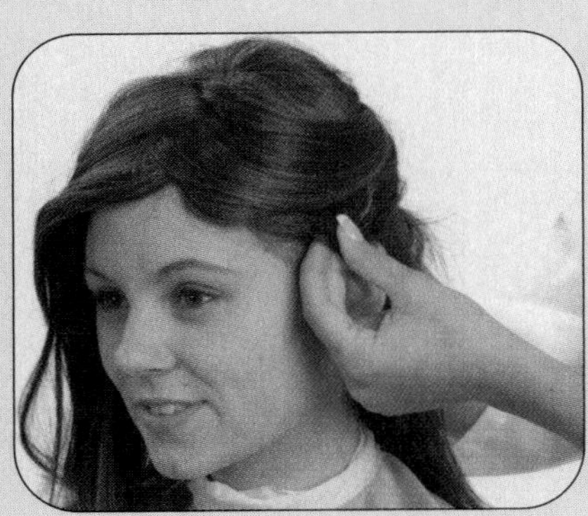

Figure 14-25 Pull the wig down at the sides.

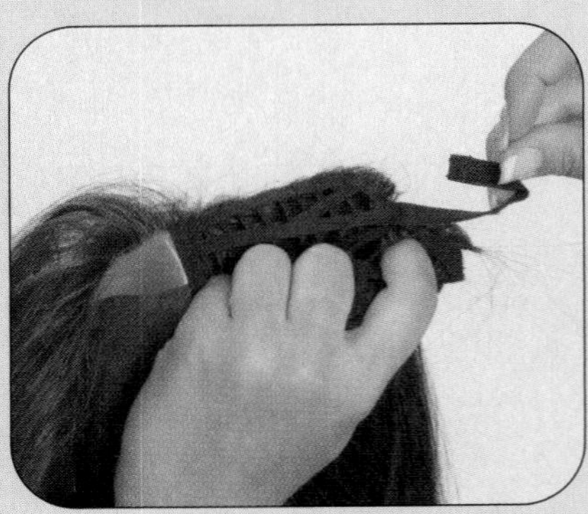

Figure 14-26 Tighten the wig off the client's head.

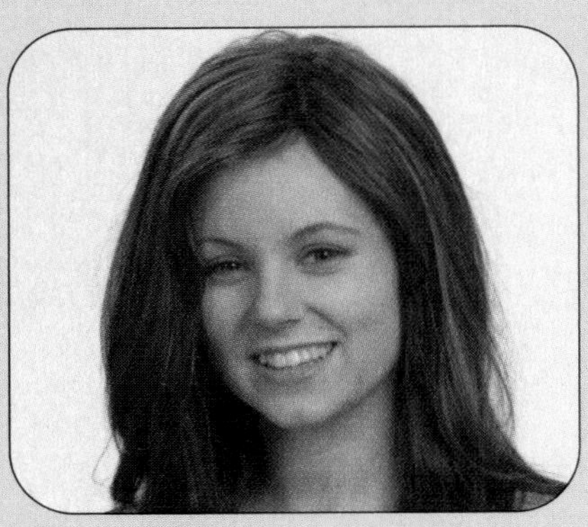

Figure 14-27 A well-fitted wig.

completed!

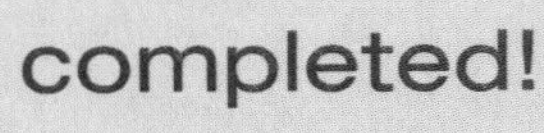

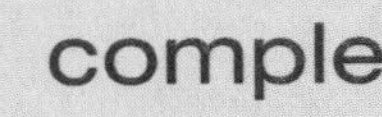

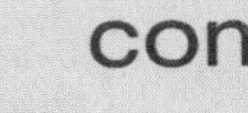

prefer to do, which is to cut free-form on dry hair. The wig should be placed on the block for cutting, but the comb-out and finishing should be done on the client's head.

Free-form cutting moves from longer to shorter lengths, always working toward the weight. Vertical sections create lightness. Diagonal sections create a rounder beveled edge. Horizontal sections build heavier weight (Figure 14–28, Figure 14–29, and Figure 14–30).

To use this visual approach, begin by cutting a small section and observe how the hair falls. Your next step will be based on how the hair responds. Draw a diagram of the silhouette or have handy a photo image for reference. These will work as a kind of blueprint for you to follow.

Free-form cutting is usually done on dry hair, which allows you to see more easily how the hair will fall. When the hair is wet, it can be hard to judge how the hair will lie.

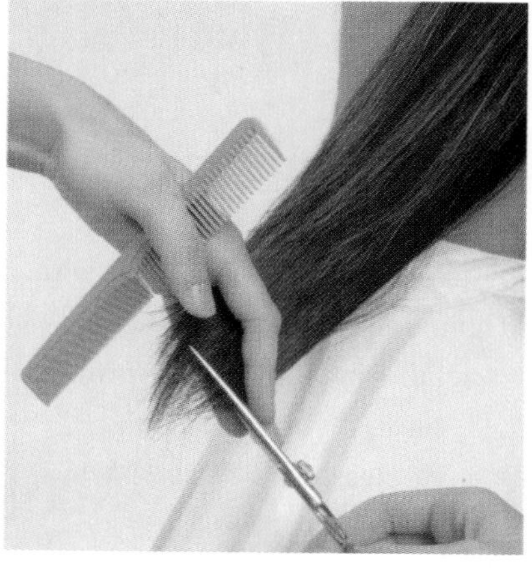

Figure 14-28 Free-form cutting with vertical sections.

Styling the Wig

Most of the hair you will be working with is chemically treated, so it needs to be handled gently. You will achieve the best styling results by following these guidelines.

- When using heat on human hair, always set the styling tool on low.
- Treat the hair gently and kindly; do not pull it or otherwise treat it carelessly.
- Traditionally, brushes made with natural boar-bristles have been regarded as the best for use on human hair. Their soft bristles are far preferable to sharp-edged synthetic bristles that can damage hair. Today, however, you will find many synthetic brushes that have smooth, rounded plastic teeth,

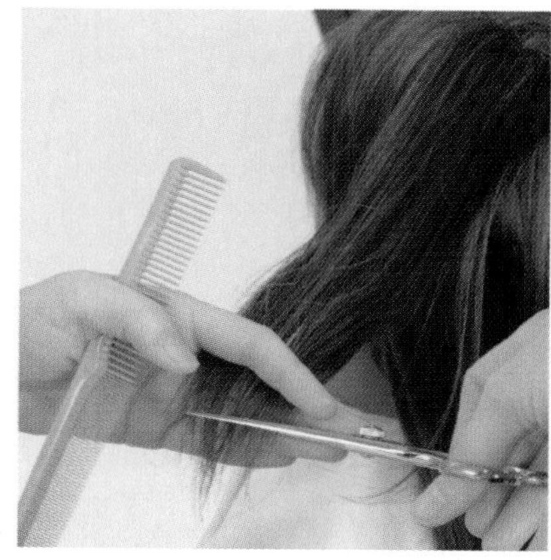

Figure 14-29 Free-form cutting with diagonal sections.

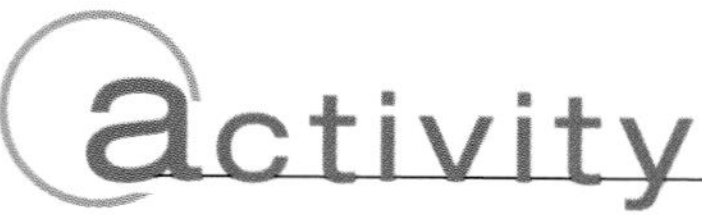

To practice wig-cutting, buy two inexpensive, ready-to-wear wigs in the same style. Take a photo for reference purposes. Draw a diagram of the sections, indicating how you are going to cut the wigs. This way, you can rehearse your plan before even picking up the scissors.

Begin your practice with the "shadow cut." Trim the wigs following the original design that has been precut into the wig, but cut the first wig wet. Then air-dry it and evaluate the style. Trim the second wig, following the same style, but this time cut it dry. Take photos of both results and evaluate the looks you have achieved with both dry and wet cutting.

What you may discover is that the wet cutting method was more controlled and technical, while the dry cutting method was freer and more abstract. Often, the more abstract method results in a cut that looks more realistic. What do you think? Repeat the above exercise with a razor, thinning scissors, and standard haircutting scissors using the tapering method only. Compare results.

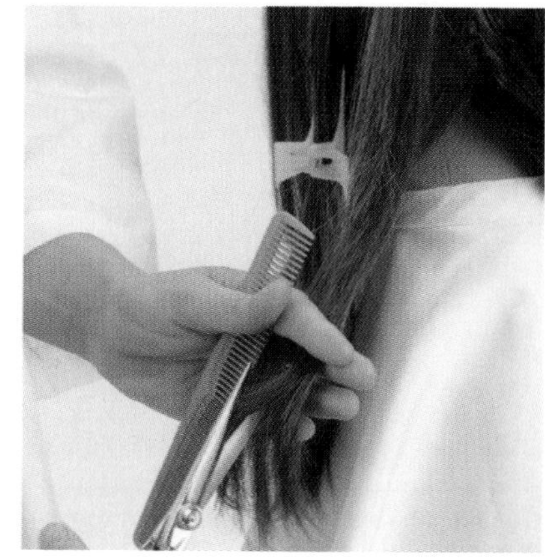

Figure 14-30 Free-form cutting with horizontal sections.

CAUTION

Harsh handling will damage wig hair. Unlike hair on the human head, wig hair will not grow back. If you treat a wig carelessly, it will have a short life.

more like a comb, and they are excellent and economical choices. Keep in mind that the key with any brush or comb is to be gentle, for hair can be easily damaged.

- Choose styling products that have been formulated for color-treated hair. These will work the best and are the kindest to human hair. Just remember that whatever you put into the hair will eventually have to be shampooed out.

Use a block for all your coloring, perming, setting, and basic cut outlining. The combing-out and finishing touches for most contemporary cuts should be completed on the client's head in order to achieve proper balance and personalization.

Remember that most clients come into the salon looking for a natural look. Making a wig look believable is very challenging, and to do it well is truly an art form. The areas that must appear the most convincing are the crown, the part, and the hairline. Sometimes, crowns and parts look more natural when they are flat to the head; other times it looks more natural to fluff up these areas and direct the emphasis away. This will be determined by the style. A general rule is to follow the direction of the knotting and weave, as preset by the wig maker. If you fight the direction, the results will look odd.

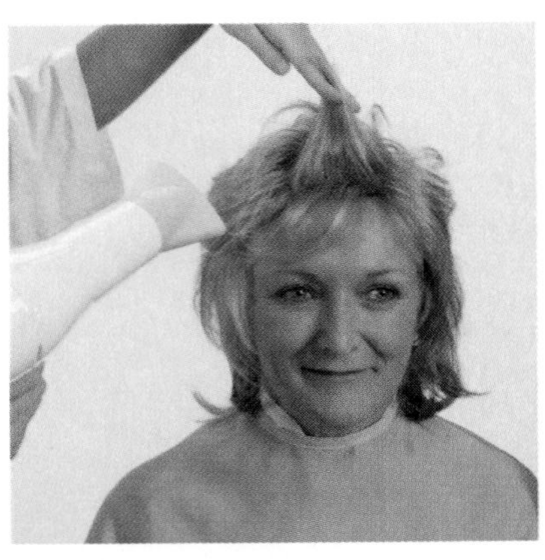

Figure 14–31 The wind test.

Styling Tips for the Hairline

- Back-comb gently around the hairline. The fluffy effect softens the hairline.
- Release the client's hair around the hairline and cut and blend it into the wig hair.
- The best test to gauge how realistic the wig looks is to use the "wind test." This test simulates the situation of a client walking outside with the wind blowing the hair off her face. Gently blow around the client's face with a blow-dryer set at cool and low and observe how the hairline looks. Does it seem realistic? If so, point out the results to the client, who may be feeling insecure about whether the wig looks natural enough (Figure 14–31).

14

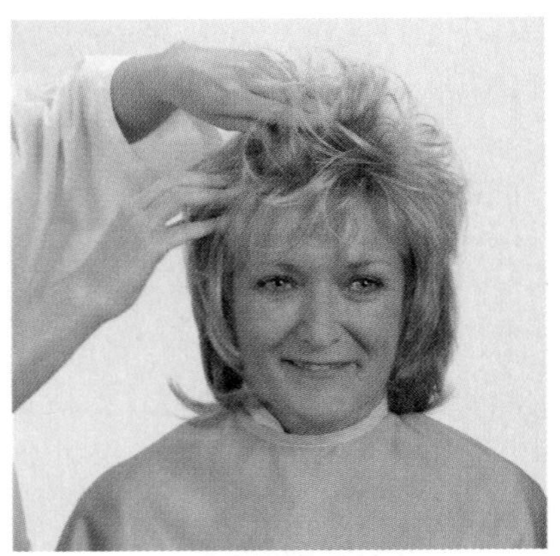

Figure 14–32 Style with the fingers for a natural look.

When styling a wig, do not try to make it look perfect. Little imperfections help achieve a realistic look. Use your hands rather than a brush for a more natural look (Figure 14–32). Do not plaster the hair down, which looks artificial.

The important thing to remember when you are styling a wig is that you must never lose sight of the big picture. Some stylists get overly involved in the wig, as if it is a creation that exists apart from the client. This is the wrong approach. An experienced and talented stylist works with the total person, not just the head. When you have finished styling the wig, step back and ask the client to stand up and walk around so that you can check for balance and proportion and make corrections accordingly.

Coloring Wigs and Extensions

All synthetic haircolors used for wigs and hairpieces are standardized according to the 70 colors on the haircolor ring used by wig and hairpiece manufacturers. The colors range from black to the palest blonde. As most commercially available hair originates from either India or China, the natural color level is 0, or black. It is very difficult to lift level 0 to level 10 (see Chapter 16 for a discussion of hair color levels). White yak hair is an excellent base to which you can add fantasy colors that appeal to the youth market.

If you are going to custom-color the hair, use hair that has been decolorized (bleached) through the lifting process, not with metallic dyes. Check with the manufacturer.

As in all disciplines, you must first learn the rules before you break any. Good colorists are not afraid to make mistakes, because they know how to correct them. The principles that guide the coloring of natural hair are applied as well to the art of coloring wigs and hair extensions.

First check to see if the cuticle is intact. Hair in which the cuticle is absent is very porous and will react to color in an extreme manner. Always strand-test the hair prior to full color application. Use semipermanent, demipermanent, glaze, rinse, or color mousse products. Use permanent haircolor on human hair wigs, unless the hair is porous, in which case semipermanent color will be the better choice (see Chapter 16 for descriptions and procedures).

When coloring a human hair wig or hairpiece, conduct regular color checks every 5 to 10 minutes. Remember that the hair that you are working on did not come from one head, but from many different heads, and can be unpredictable. It may be easier to color the client's hair to match a hairpiece than to color the piece itself.

Perming the Wig

If you want to perm a human hair wig hair to match the client's natural wave pattern, you need to know how the hair was colored. Was it decolorized (bleached) or dyed with metallic dye? Do not perm hair that has been colored with a metallic dye.

The permanent wave must be performed with the wig off the client's head. Cover the head form with plastic to protect it from the chemical solutions, pin the wig securely to the head form, and perm as you would a normal head of hair (see Chapter 15 for perming procedures).

CAUTION

Do not use oxidizing haircolor or haircolor with peroxide on hair that has been treated with metallic hair dye. If you do, the hair will swell and smoke, appearing to be boiling from the inside out.

HAIRPIECES

Hairpieces are another important area of hair additions. A hairpiece gives 20 to 70 percent coverage (Figure 14–33). Hairpieces sit on top of the client's hair and are usually attached by temporary methods (they are not worn at night during sleep).

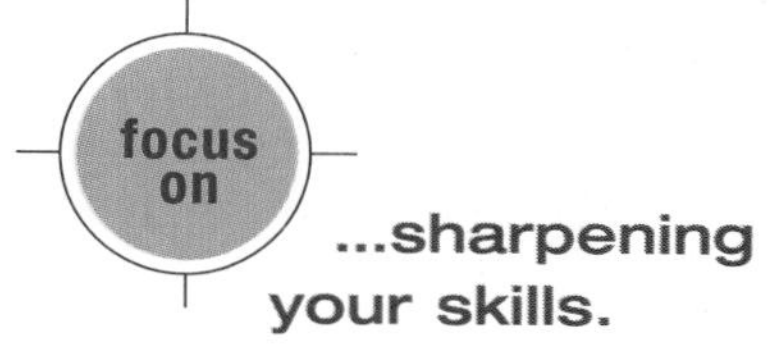

In 18th-century France, women wore towering hairdos complete with extensions and various apparatus like springs to adjust the height. Some of these coiffures were three feet high and had elaborate visual elements worked into them like ships or gardens. They were often untouched for weeks at a time. The bad news is that they sometimes attracted vermin! The moral of this story is not to get too swept up in current trends or passing fashions. Always be aware of the "good taste factor." Too much creativity can often backfire. Keep it simple, remember that less is more, and never let yourself get carried away.

insights

Claudia Tapp

A veteran with 27 years in the industry, Claudia Tapp, owner of a salon and spa in Palatine, Illinois, is a firm believer in continuing education.

To survive in this business, you have to always want to learn. That's the number-one rule. I see people who have been in this industry just a short time and have attained only a certain level of knowledge, and they think of themselves as being professionals. You know what? I've been in the business 27 years and I want to know more! I want to know everything I can know.

As a cosmetologist, you have to constantly set money aside to educate yourself. I find that people in my industry don't want to pay anything for education. People in every other profession have to pay a lot more money for their education than we do. If you don't spend any money on your education, then you'll get exactly what you pay for. You won't grow. You won't make money. You have to spend on your education in order to make money and become a professional.

I've always traveled for my education. I've always spent a lot of money on it. To me, it was a valuable investment. You have to make that kind of investment because the industry is always changing—not only in technique and styles, but also in terms of the kind of chemistry being used. I've seen tints from twenty years ago that are now totally different. The colors are more translucent. You don't have to spend a lot of time conditioning the hair after you do chemical processes because the chemicals themselves have been designed to condition the hair. And the same thing goes for perms. It's always changing.

You can't be bored in this industry. Plus there are the skills you need to learn, like salesmanship and psychology. Psychology is very important in this field. The hardest challenge is when you deal with people with unrealistic expectations. Or people who are basically not happy with themselves and are trying to project all their unhappiness on you, and you're supposed to solve their problems by doing some sort of remake on them. But there are courses on salesmanship and psychology, even for free, on the Internet.

If I were a young stylist today, I would look for a salon that is progressive, one where the owner believes strongly in education and recognizes that the salon has to move forward. In my salon, if I feel people are focused and career-oriented and look at this as a career profession, I pay for their education. It's a benefit to my salon to do so.

Many wig companies offer ready-to-wear, low-maintenance hairpieces that serve as an introduction to the world of wigs as well as a good retail item in the salon. Some hairpieces are easily blended into long hair, others into shorter hair. Some add natural-looking height or volume, while others add length. They can be placed just about anywhere on the head.

Temporary attachment methods include interlocking combs, flexible wire combs, elastic, claw clips, and even Velcro. In one versatile hairpiece, hair wefts are wrapped around elastic and resemble a cloth scrunchie. Some hairpieces are constructed on a weft base and are attached with a flexible comb that attaches around the front and nape. The one hairpiece that is attached by a semipermanent method is the integration hairpiece.

The client's hair can be prepared in a number of ways before the hairpiece is attached. It can be tied into a ponytail or bun or twisted into a French twist. It can be blended with the hairpiece or serve as a base for it.

Integration Hairpieces

An **integration hairpiece** has an opening in the base through which the client's own hair is pulled to blend with the hair (natural or synthetic) of the hairpiece. These hairpieces are a very lightweight, natural-looking product that add length and volume to the client's hair. If your client is wearing hair extensions and would like a change, the integration hairpiece can be a good alternative. It is also recommended for clients with thinning hair, but not for those with total hair loss, as the scalp is likely to show through (Figure 14–34 and Figure 14–35).

Toupees

While men are the typical customers for toupees, women can also wear these hairpieces. A **toupee** is a small wig used to cover the top and crown of the head. The fine net base is usually the most appropriate material for the client with severe hair loss. There are two ways to attach toupees: temporary (tape or clips) or semipermanent (weaving, tracks, adhesive, or sewing) (Figure 14–36 and Figure 14–37).

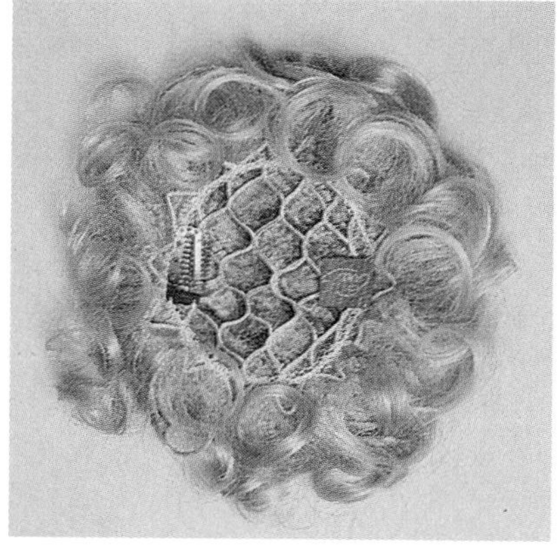

Figure 14–34 Integration hairpiece.

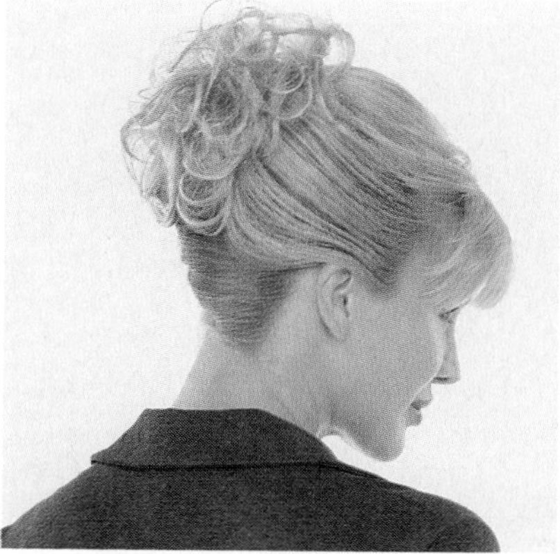

Figure 14–35 An integration hairpiece is easy to wear.

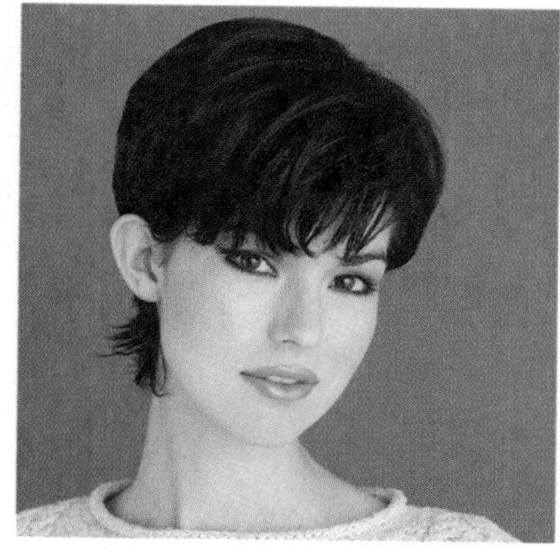

Figure 14–33 Hairpieces can look very natural.

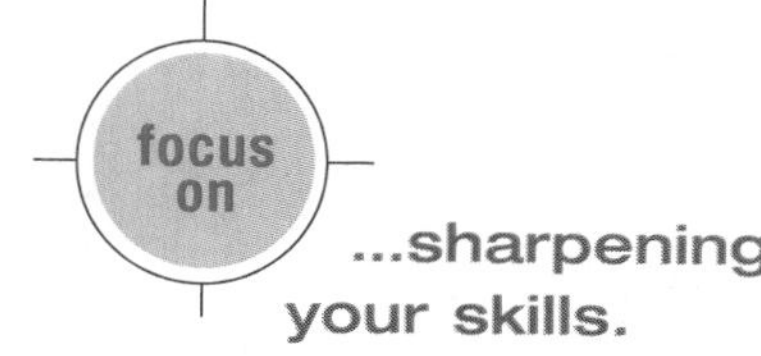

When it comes to hairpieces, there are many ways to go wrong. Too much hair on a small body frame will make the client look out of balance. An ill-fitting hairpiece may draw negative attention. It is easy to lose perspective when you are working with hairpieces. Too much focused concentration can get you into trouble and lead you to overwork the style. When you finally step back, you may discover that you have created an alarmingly large shape. Remember, less is more.

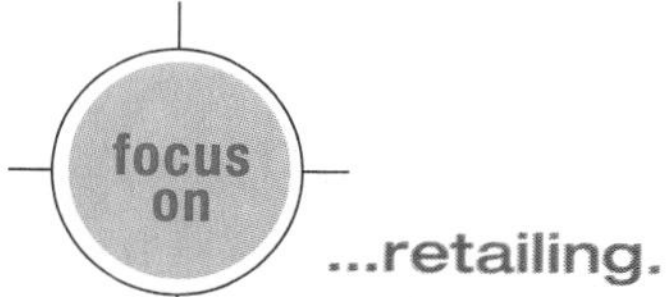

Hairpieces are a great retail product for the salon. They can be displayed in a fun, creative way, and because they are fairly easy to attach and remove, they almost sell themselves, particularly to younger, more adventurous clients.

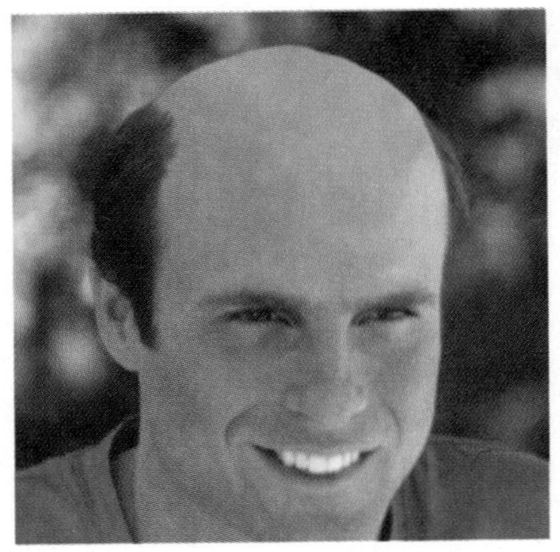

Figure 14-36 Male hair-enhancement client.

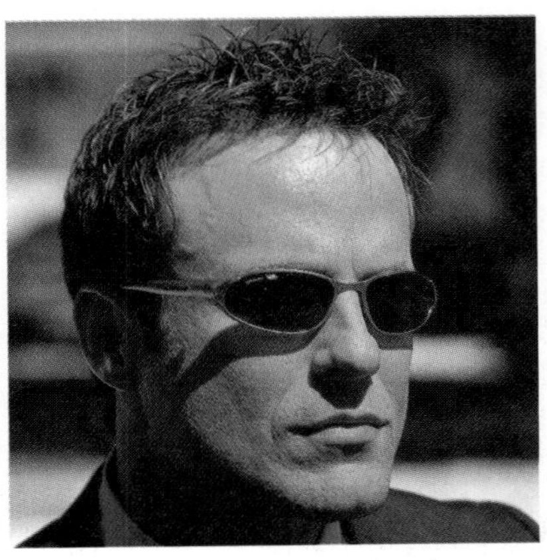

Figure 14-37 The same client fitted with a toupee.

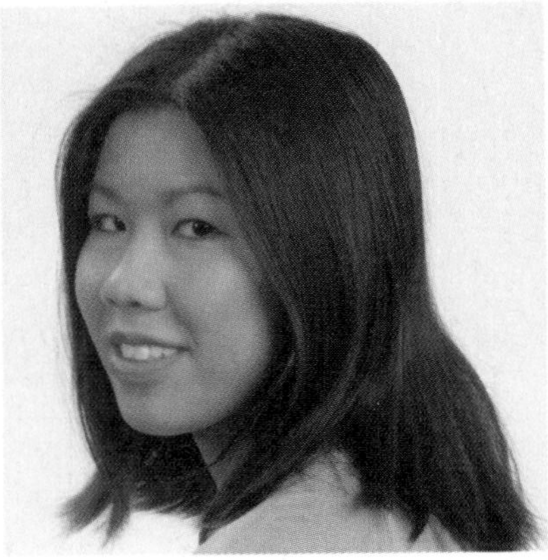

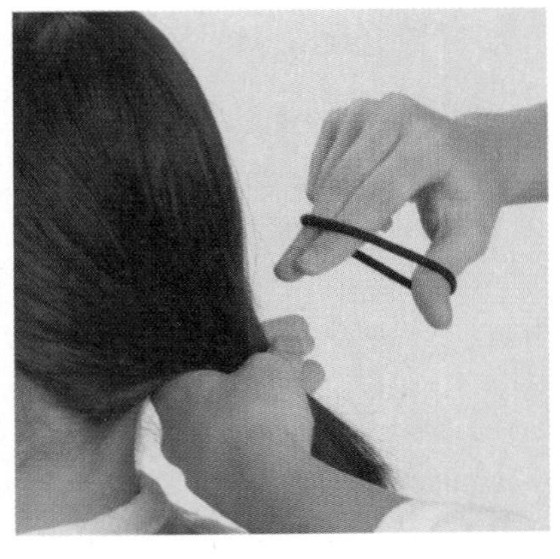

Figure 14-38 Client before fitting with a wraparound ponytail.

Most wearers of toupees prize the confidence gained from wearing an authentic-looking hairpiece and are prepared to pay a high price for it. The best toupees are custom designed. The top manufacturers offer in-depth instruction for those interested in learning this specialty service.

Fashion Hairpieces

Fashion hairpieces are a great salon product for special occasions or for use as fashion accessories. They are especially popular in the bridal business. These hairpieces vary in size and are constructed on a stiff net base. They are attached, on a temporary basis, with hairpins, clips, combs, bobby pins, or elastic. Three of these attachment methods are illustrated here.

- The wraparound ponytail is a long length of wefted hair that covers 10 to 20 percent of the head. It is used as a simple ponytail or in chignons. It is particularly useful for the client who can just get her own hair into a ponytail (Figure 14–38, Figure 14–39, Figure 14–40, Figure 14–41, and Figure 14–42).

Figure 14-39 Client's own ponytail.

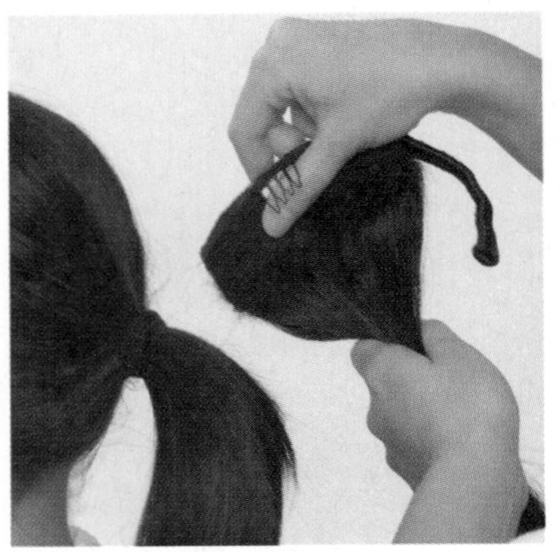

Figure 14-40 Attaching the hairpiece.

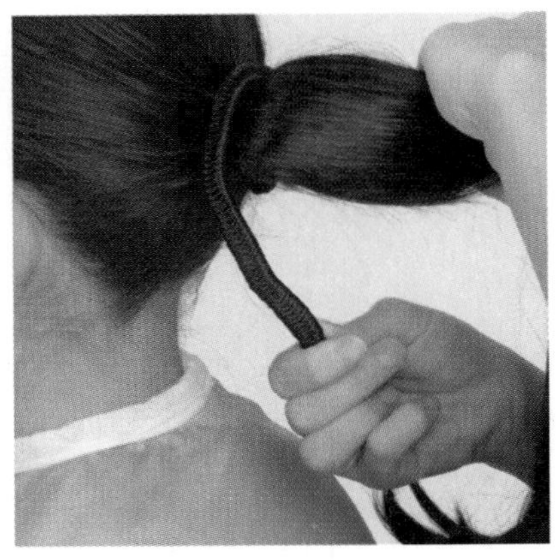

Figure 14-41 Wrapping the band around the ponytail base.

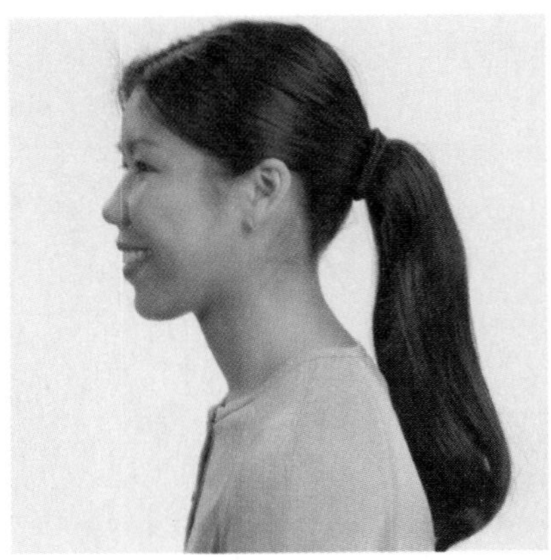

Figure 14-42 A "new," much longer ponytail.

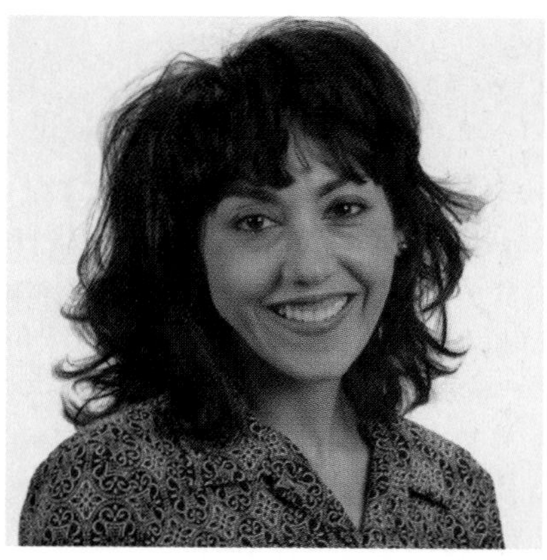

Figure 14-43 Client before fitting with comb-attached curls.

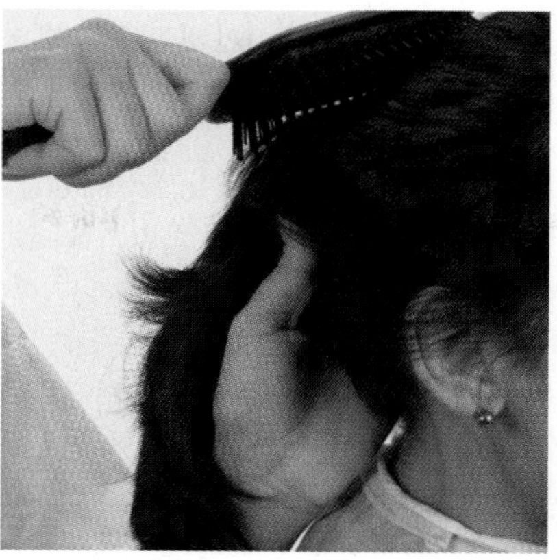

Figure 14-44 Brushing the client's hair into a ponytail.

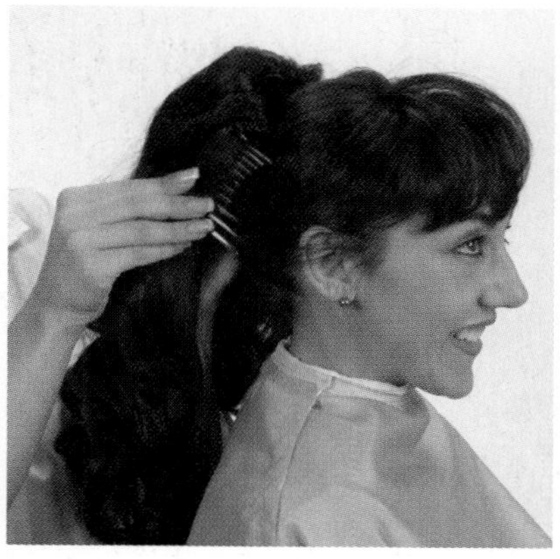

Figure 14-45 Attaching the combs.

- A cascade of curls is attached with combs (Figure 14–43, Figure 14–44, Figure 14–45, Figure 14–46, and Figure 14–47).
- A hair wrap is mounted on an elastic loop. It is further secured to the client's own hair with hairpins (Figure 14–48, Figure 14–49, Figure 14–50, and Figure 14–51).

In order to achieve a natural look, it is crucial that you blend the client's hair with the hairpiece. You must match up both the color and the wave pattern. If the client has naturally wavy hair, it may be wiser to find a wave pattern that matches her own. To match the color, use the color ring. The color selection of most lines of hairpieces is very broad and very easy to match to the client's hair. You cannot color the hairpiece, so any custom coloring to achieve a match must be performed on the client's hair. 6✓

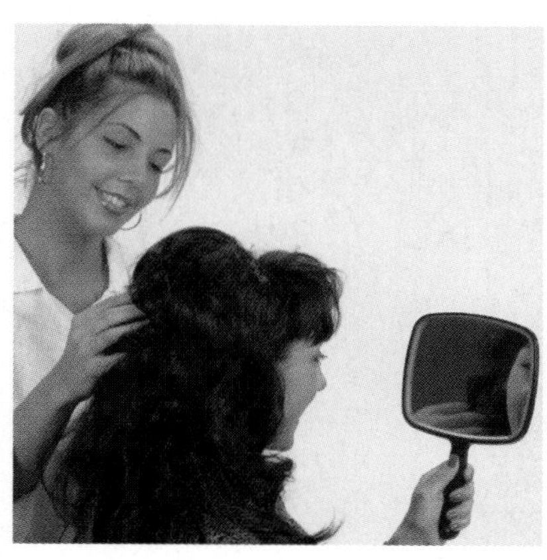

Figure 14-46 Adjusting the hairpiece.

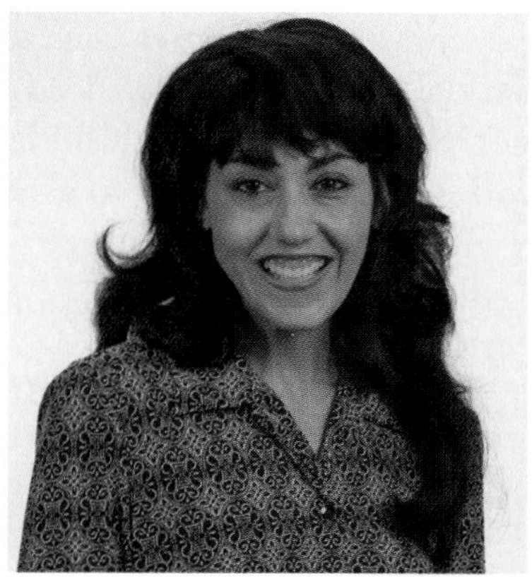

Figure 14-47 A cascade of curls.

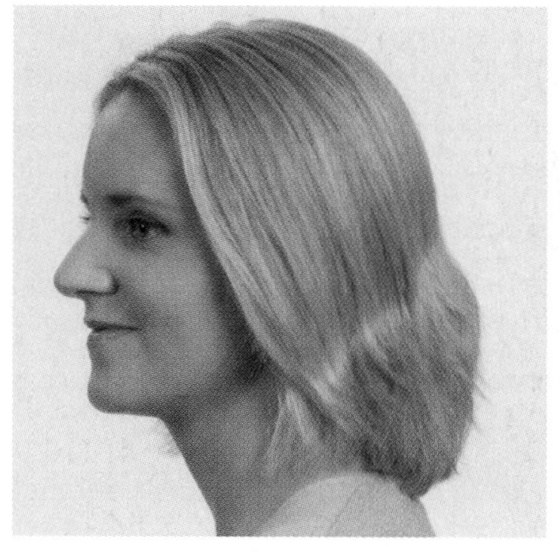

Figure 14-48 Client before fitting with a hair wrap.

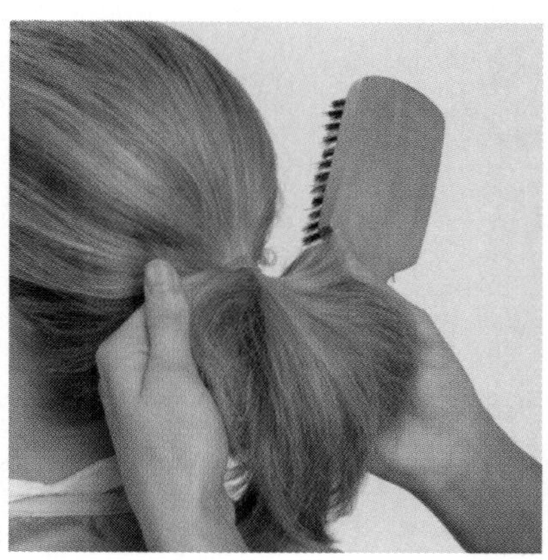

Figure 14-49 Brushing client's hair into a ponytail.

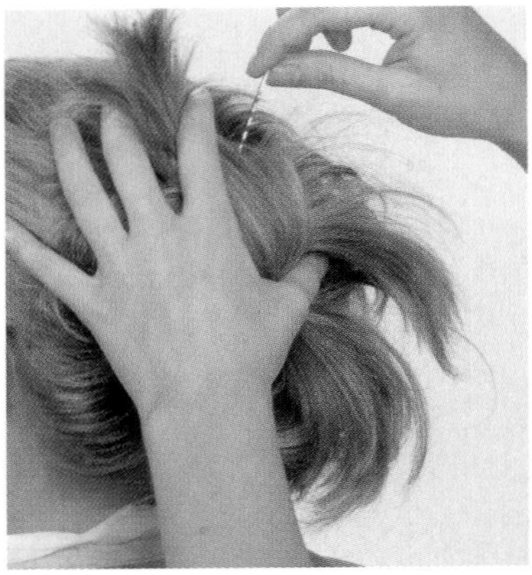

Figure 14–50 Securing the hairpiece with hairpins.

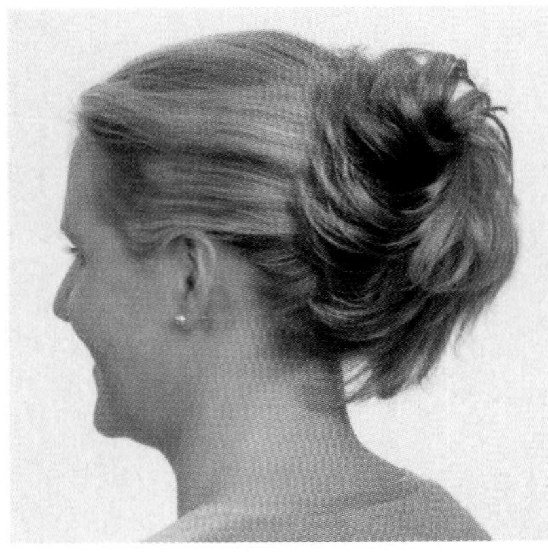

Figure 14–51 An easy, dressed-up look.

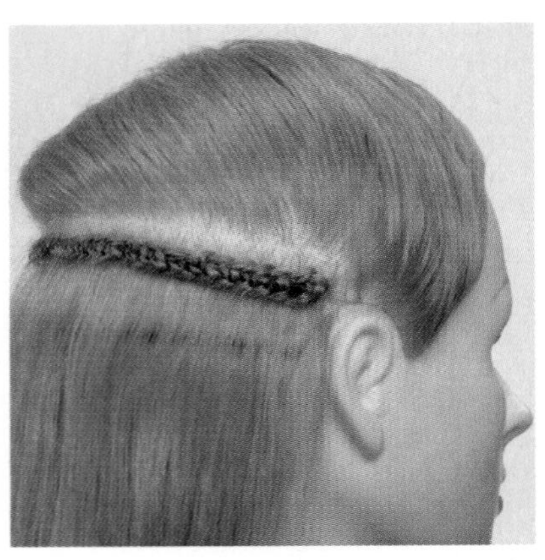

Figure 14–52 Cornrow track.

HAIR EXTENSIONS

Hair extensions are hair additions that are secured to the base of the client's natural hair in order to add length, volume, texture, or color. Extensions offer a greater blending of real and artificial hair than hairpieces. Extensions are also left in the hair for much longer periods and are not removed at nighttime. They are an increasingly popular salon service, not only for clients who are looking for something "different" but also for those suffering from hair loss.

Manufacturers generally offer training in the attachment of hair extensions, but there are certain general guidelines to keep in mind.

- Start by deciding whether you are adding length, thickness, or both.
- Know what final style you are striving for. Map out your desired style.
- As a general rule of thumb, stay 1 inch (2.5 cm) away from the hairline at the front, sides, and nape and 1 inch away from the part.
- With very thin hair, you must be careful that the base does not show through.
- Curly hair tends to expand and can give the illusion of being thicker than it really is. When working with curly hair, you will need to determine whether you are matching the curl or whether you wish to add another curl pattern to the hair.
- Straight thin hair and curly thin hair may have similar density, but curly hair will appear thicker. That means you may not need to put as many extensions in curly hair as in straight hair.

Track and Sew Attachment Method

In the **track and sew method**, hair extensions are secured at the base of the client's own hair by sewing. The hair is attached to an on-the-scalp braid, or cornrow, which serves as the track (Figure 14–52). The angle of the track determines how the hair will fall. You may position tracks horizontally, vertically, or diagonally, or along curved lines that follow the contours of the head.

Partings are determined according to the style you have chosen. The size of the sections is determined by the amount of hair that will be added to the head. Plan the tracks so that the ends of the braids will be hidden. It is best to position the tracks 1 inch (2.5 cm) behind the hairline to assure proper coverage.

When sewing the extension onto a track, use only a blunt, custom-designed needle, either straight or curved. These blunt ends will help avoid damage to the hair and will protect you and the client as well.

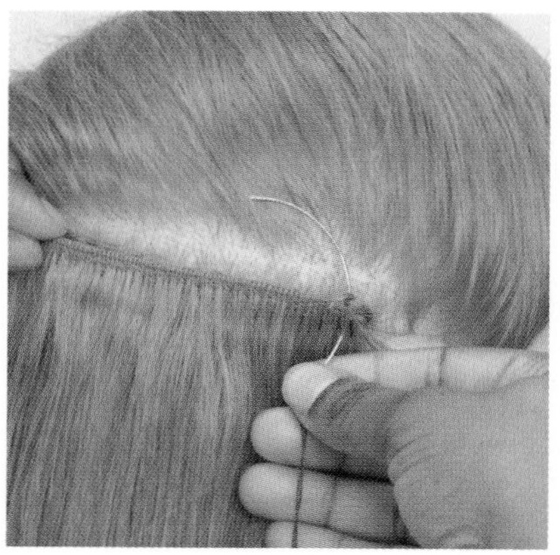

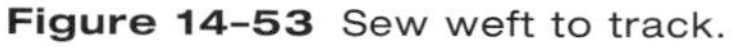

Figure 14-53 Sew weft to track.

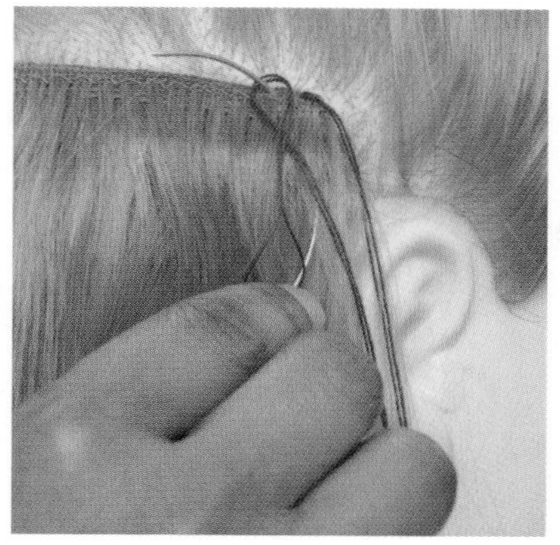

Figure 14-54 Wrap thread around needle.

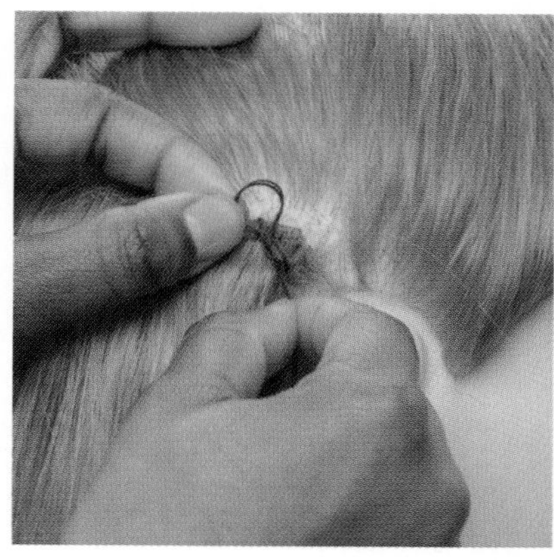

Figure 14-55 Form lock stitch.

Extensions can be sewn to the track using a variety of stitches.

- *Lock stitch.* Cut a length of thread double the length of the weft being sewn. Pass the needle through the weft to connect it to the track (Figure 14–53). Pull the thread through to create a loop. Pass the needle though the loop and wrap the thread around the needle (Figure 14–54). Pull the loop tight to form a lock stitch to secure the ends of the weft to the track (Figure 14–55). This stitch can also be used over the entire length of the track in evenly spaced stitches.
- *Double-lock stitch.* This stitch is much like the lock stitch, but the thread is wound around the needle twice to create the double lock. It is used in the same ways as the lock stitch.
- *Overcast stitch.* This simple, quick stitch can be used to secure the entire length of the weft to the track. Pass the needle under both the track and the weft, then bring it back over to make a new stitch (Figure 14–56). Moving along the track, repeat the stitch until you reach the end of the track. Complete with a lock stitch for security (Figure 14–57).

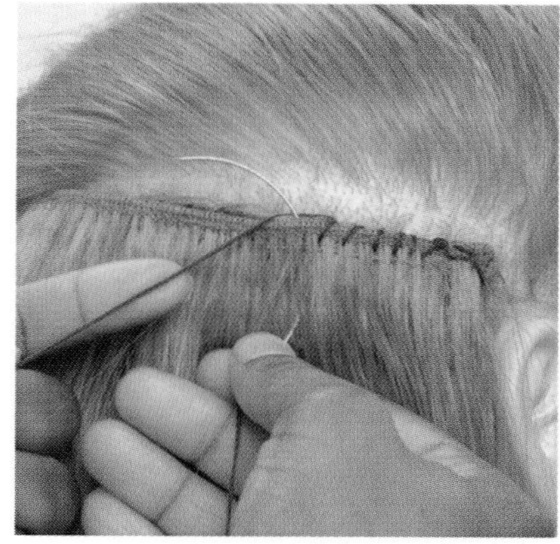

Figure 14-56 Finished overcast stitches.

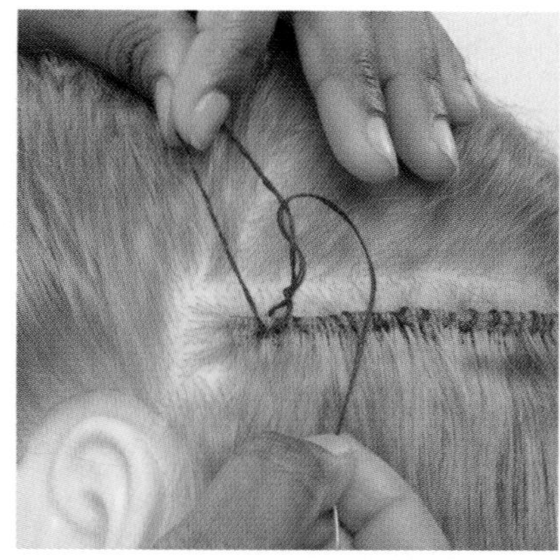

Figure 14-57 Completed line of overcast stitching.

Bonding Method

Bonding involves attaching hair wefts or single strands with an adhesive or a glue gun. This glue gun is not the kind available in crafts stores but a special tool created specifically for bonding.

Bonded hair sits snugly on the head and is fast to apply. There is, however, a certain degree of slippage. Generally, the bonding product lasts from two to four weeks, depending on factors such as the frequency of shampooing, the oiliness or dryness of the scalp, and the quality of the products used. This means that the client will need to be on a maintenance program that requires salon visits as often as every two weeks. One

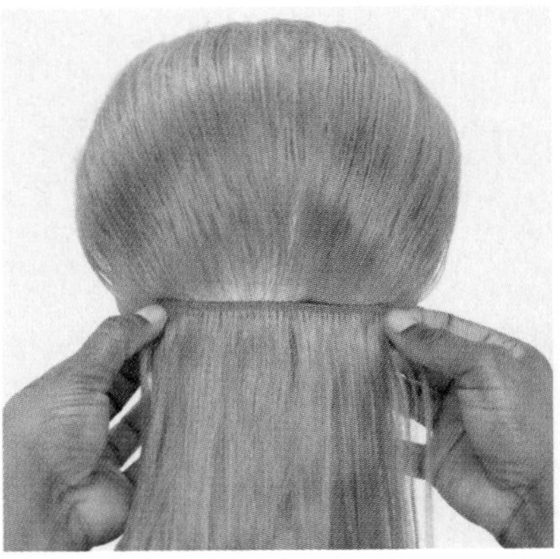

Figure 14-58 Measure weft against parting.

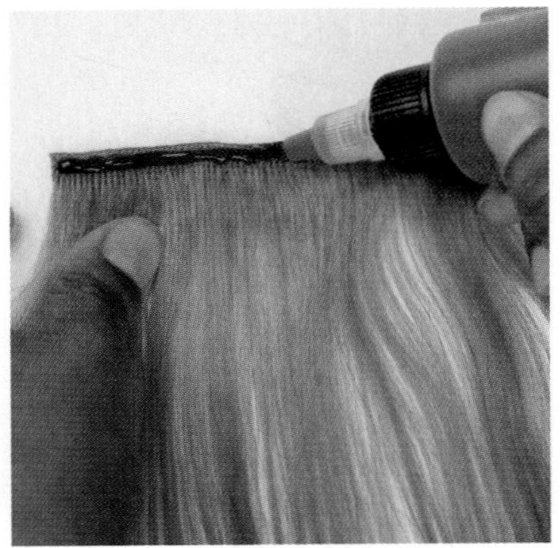

Figure 14-59 Apply adhesive to base of weft.

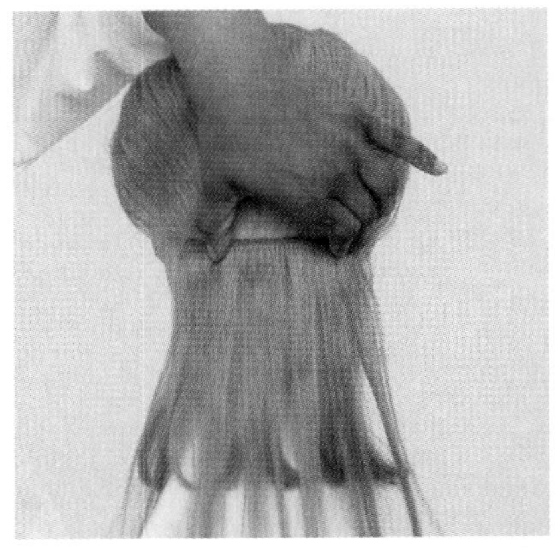

Figure 14-60 Press weft to parting.

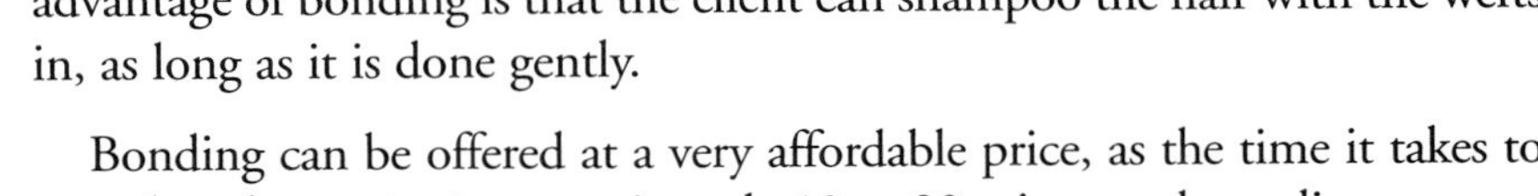

advantage of bonding is that the client can shampoo the hair with the wefts in, as long as it is done gently.

Bonding can be offered at a very affordable price, as the time it takes to complete the service is approximately 10 to 20 minutes, depending on your experience.

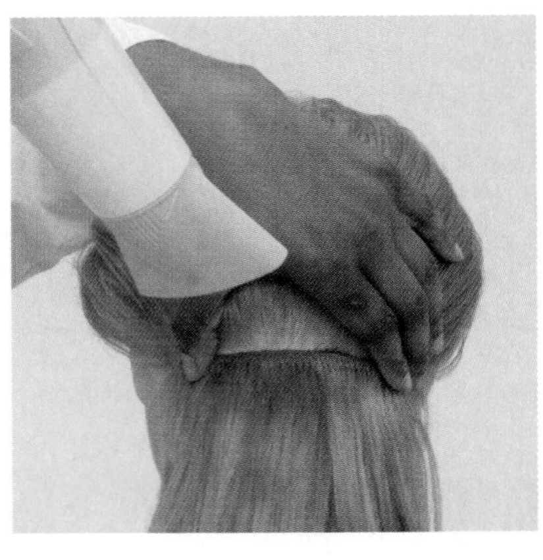

Figure 14-61 Using a blow-dryer can help seal the bond.

The bonding procedure generally begins by sectioning off the hair at the nape. Measure the first weft against the parting, 1/4 inch to 1/2 inch (.6 to 1.25 cm) from the hairline (Figure 14–58). Lay the weft on a flat surface and carefully apply adhesive along the base (Figure 14–59). Use a consistent amount of adhesive; too much will ooze on the head; too little will fail to adhere. Lightly press the weft against the clean parting (Figure 14–60). Hold for approximately 20 seconds, gently tugging to make sure that the weft has adhered. You may use a blow-dryer, set on low to medium heat, to help seal the bond (Figure 14–61). Proceed to the next section, working upward on the head, until the desired length and volume are achieved.

Care must be taken when bonding to avoid working too close to the crown or the parting, or the weft will show through. Working 1 inch (2.5 cm) away from the hairline will also keep the wefts from showing. Remember that hair is not a static material; it has a natural swing and it moves. When the wind blows, it should be the hairline that shows, not the wefts.

Bonded wefts are removed by dissolving the adhesive bond with oil or bond remover.

CAUTION

Some clients may have an allergic reaction to the ingredients in the bonding adhesive. Always perform a patch test prior to the application of these bonded extensions.

Fusion Method

In the **fusion** method of attaching extensions, extension hair is bonded to the client's own hair with a bonding material that is activated by the heat from a special tool. This method, while expensive, harmonizes with the client's natural hair with no uncomfortable and unattractive attachment sites. The bonds are light and comfortable to wear, and the hair moves like real hair and is easy to maintain (Figure 14–62). The attachment lasts up to four months, almost twice as long as other methods. Removal is quick and painless. The fusion method requires certification training.

Fusion may be the best choice for clients with fine, limp hair. Bonding and tracking can create bulk at the base, which is not a problem on hair with texture and fullness but may be too bulky and obvious with fine hair.

The fusion procedure involves wrapping a keratin-based strip around both the client's hair and the extension. The heating element is applied until the bonding agent has softened, and the bond is rolled between the fingers until both natural and added hair have ahered. 7

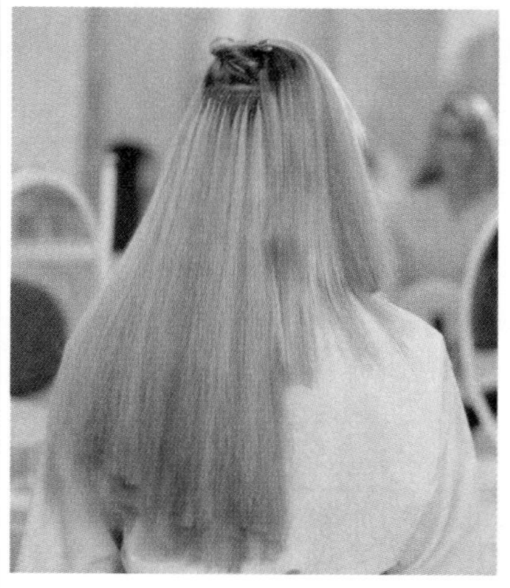

Figure 14-62 Fused extensions.

PRACTICE, PRACTICE, PRACTICE

Working with hair additions is one of the most exciting, challenging, and lucrative areas of cosmetology. But to become skilled at this work, you need to practice. The more you do, the better you will become. The better you become, the more you will be able to help people look good and feel good about themselves. There is a great satisfaction in being able to do that, particularly when working with people who have suffered the trauma of hair loss and who may have given up hope that they could look good again. When you see the smiles on their faces that your creativity and skill have put there, you will know that this is the area for you (Figure 14–63).

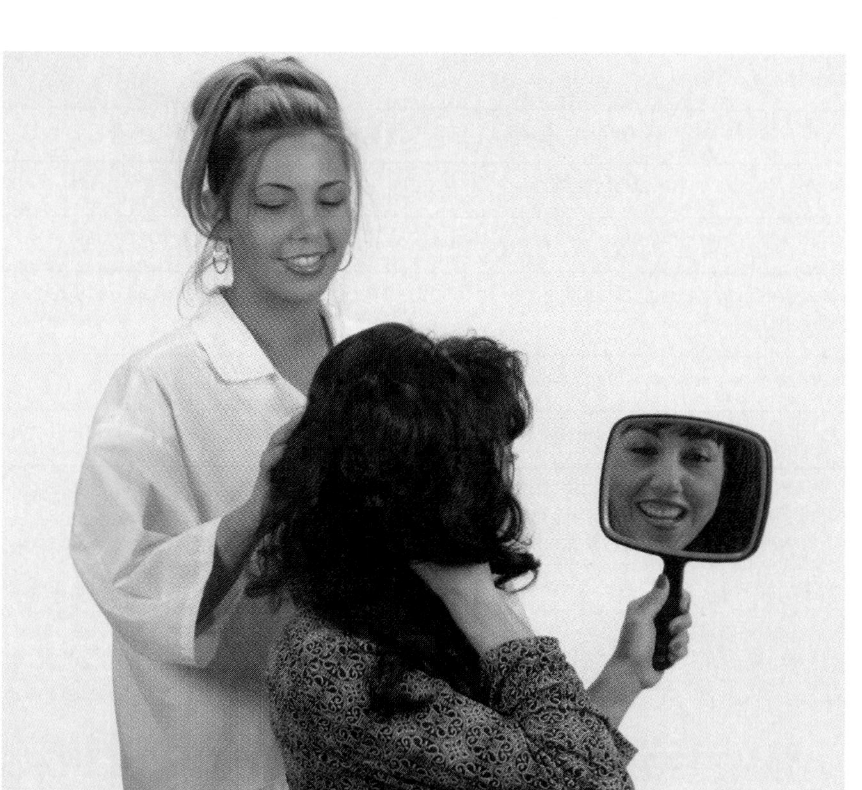

Figure 14-63 A wig specialist and her satisfied client.

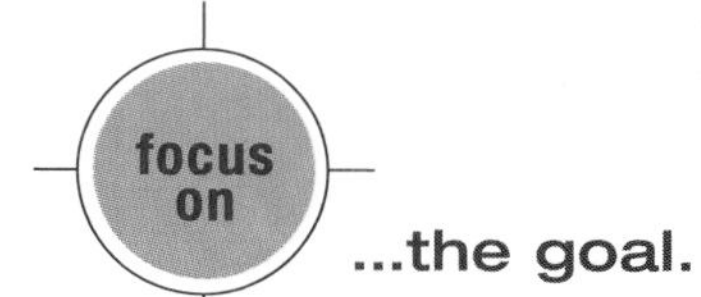

...the goal.

To be the best, work only with the best. Work with one or two companies that offer a good range of human and synthetic hair, high-quality products, good customer service, and first-rate support and product education through training, seminars, and videos. Always stick with companies that stand by their products.

chapter glossary

block	head-shaped form, usually made of canvas-covered cork or Styrofoam, to which the wig is secured for fitting, cleaning, coloring, and styling
bonding	method of attaching hair extensions in which hair wefts or single strands are attached with an adhesive or a glue gun
cap wigs	wigs consisting of elasticized mesh-fiber bases to which the hair is attached
capless wigs	machine-made wigs in which rows of wefts are sewn to elastic strips in a circular pattern to fit the head shape
fusion	method of attaching extensions in which extension hair is bonded to the client's own hair with a bonding material that is activated by heat from a special tool
hair extensions	hair additions that are secured to the base of the client's natural hair in order to add length, volume, texture, or color
hairpiece	small wig used to cover the top or crown of the head; add-on hair that is integrated with the client's own hair; toupee
hand-tied or hand-knotted wigs	wigs made by inserting individual strands of hair into mesh foundations and knotting them with a needle
integration hairpiece	hairpiece with an opening in the base through which the client's own hair is pulled to blend with the hair (natural or synthetic) of the hairpiece
machine-made wigs	wigs made by machine, not by hand, by feeding wefts through a sewing machine, then sewing them together to form the base and shape of the wigs
semi-hand-tied wigs	wigs constructed with a combination of synthetic hair and hand-tied human hair
toupee	small wig used to cover the top or crown of the head
track and sew method	attachment method in which hair extensions are secured at the base of the client's own hair by sewing
turned hair	wig hair in which the root end of every hair strand is sewn into the base so that the cuticles of all hair strands slope in the same direction
wefts	strips of human or artificial hair woven by hand or machine onto a thread
wig	artificial covering for the head consisting of a network of interwoven hair

review questions

1. List the seven key points you should cover in a client consultation for wig services.
2. Define wig, hairpiece, and hair extensions.
3. What are some advantages of human hair wigs? Of synthetic wigs?
4. Name and describe the two basic categories of wigs.
5. List the different measurements that must be taken when measuring a client for a wig.
6. List at least three guidelines for styling a wig.
7. What is an integration hairpiece?
8. Name at least three methods for attaching hairpieces.
9. Name three methods for attaching hair extensions.

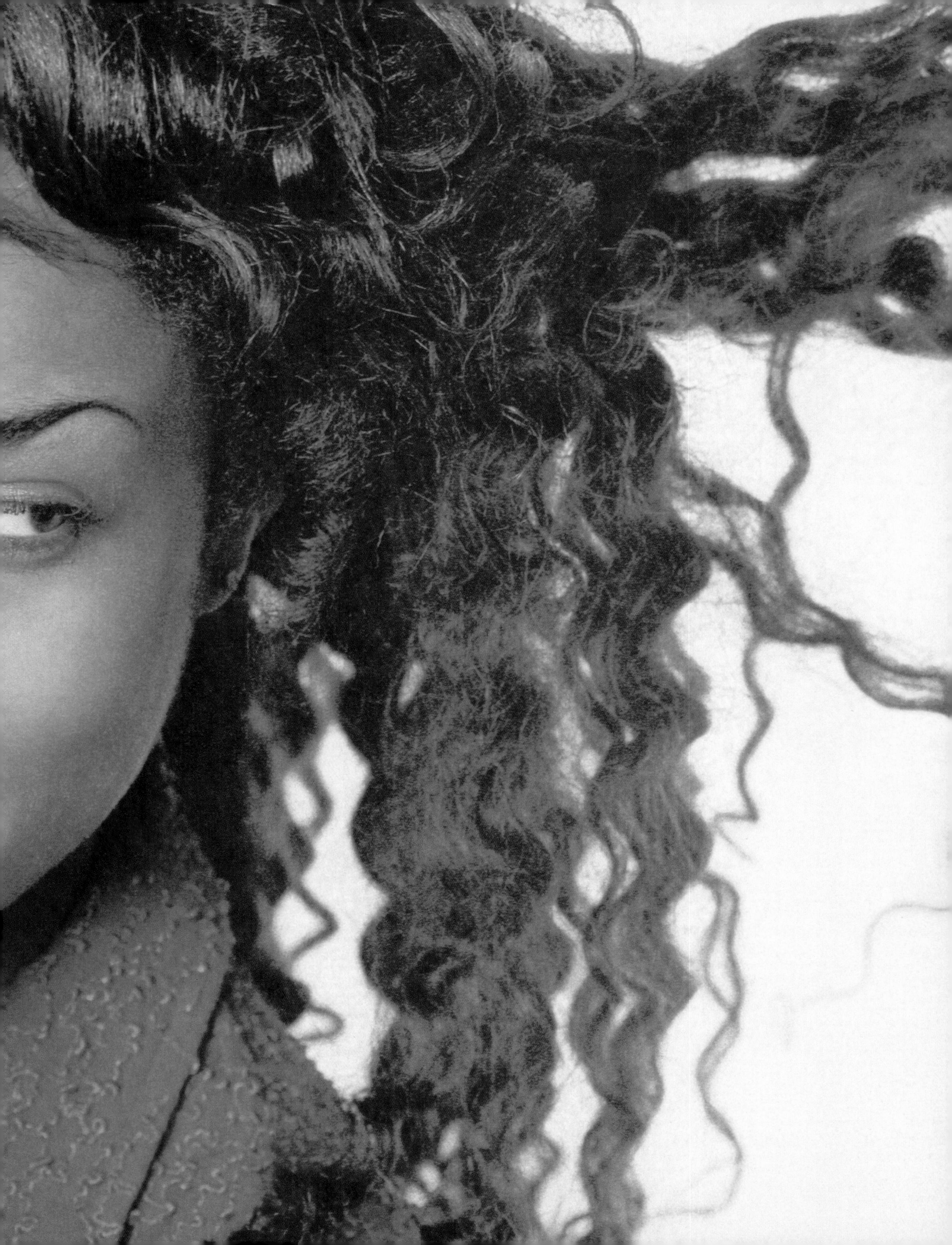

CHEMICAL TEXTURE SERVICES

John Halal

PRESIDENT, HONORS BEAUTY COLLEGE, INC., INDIANAPOLIS, IN

Chapter Outline

Learning Objectives

After completing this chapter, you should be able to:

1. **List the factors of a hair analysis for chemical texture services.**
2. **Explain the physical and chemical actions that take place during permanent waving.**
3. **List and describe the various types of permanent waving solutions.**
4. **Demonstrate basic wrapping procedures: straight set, curvature wrap, bricklay wrap, weave wrap, double tool wrap, and spiral wrap.**
5. **Describe the procedure for chemical hair relaxing.**
6. **Explain the basic procedure for a soft curl permanent.**

National Skill Standards

This chapter provides you with the necessary information to master these National Industry Skill Standards for Entry-Level Cosmetologists.

Performing hair relaxation and wave formation techniques in accordance with the manufacturers' directions.

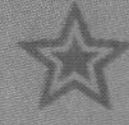

Consulting with clients to determine their needs and preferences.

Conducting services in a safe environment, taking measures to prevent the spread of infectious and contagious diseases.

Key Terms

Page number indicates where in the chapter the term is used.

acid-balanced waves
pg. 500

alkaline waves or cold waves
pg. 499

ammonia-free waves
pg. 501

ammonium thioglycolate (ATG)
pg. 499

base cream
pg. 528

base control
pg. 494

base direction
pg. 495

base relaxers
pg. 528

base sections
pg. 494

basic perm wrap
pg. 507

bookend wrap
pg. 498

bricklay perm wrap
pg. 507

chemical hair relaxing
pg. 525

chemical texture services
pg. 487

concave rods
pg. 496

croquignole perms
pg. 495

curvature perm wrap
pg. 507

disulfide bonds
pg. 489

double flat wrap
pg. 497

double tool (piggyback) technique
pg. 507

endothermic waves
pg. 501

end papers or end wraps
pg. 497

exothermic waves
pg. 500

glyceryl monothioglycolate (GMTG)
pg. 500

half-off-base placement
pg. 495

hydrogen bonds
pg. 489

hydoxide relaxers
pg. 526

lanthionization
pg. 526

low-pH waves
pg. 501

metal hydroxide relaxers
pg. 527

neutralization
pg. 504

no-base relaxers
pg. 528

normalizing solutions
pg. 529

off-base placement
pg. 495

on-base placement
pg. 494

peptide or end bonds
pg. 488

polypeptide chains
pg. 488

salt bonds
pg. 489

single flat wrap
pg. 498

soft curl permanents
pg. 539

spiral perms
pg. 496

spiral perm technique
pg. 507

straight rods
pg. 496

thioglycolic acid
pg. 498

thio relaxers
pg. 525

thio-free waves
pg. 501

true acid waves
pg. 500

weave technique
pg. 507

Chemical texture services cause a chemical change that permanently alters the natural wave pattern of the hair. Texture services can be used to curl and add volume to straight hair, straighten overly curly hair, or soften coarse, straight hair and make it more pliable and easier to work with. Texture services include permanent waving, soft curl permanents (also known as curl re-forming), and chemical hair relaxing. These services, continually being improved by new technologies, offer the client a variety of styling options that would not be possible otherwise (Figure 15–1).

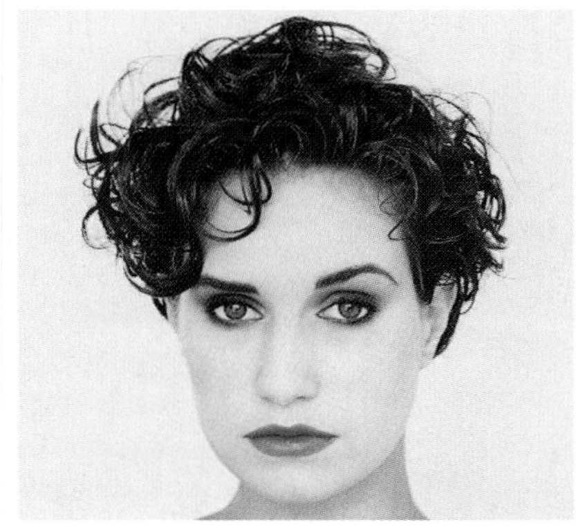

Figure 15–1 Permanent waving is one kind of texture service.

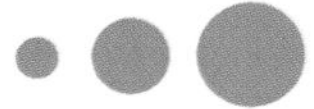

THE STRUCTURE OF HAIR

Although each distinct chemical texture service may use different chemicals and have different objectives and procedures, they all involve chemical and physical changes within the structure of the hair. Therefore, we need to begin by reviewing the structure of the hair and how chemicals can change that structure (refer to Chapter 8 for a more thorough discussion of hair structure).

The Cuticle

Starting from the outside in, we first encounter the cuticle, which is the tough outer layer of the hair (see Chapter 8). The cuticle surrounds the inner layers and protects the hair from damage. A strong, compact cuticle layer makes for resistant hair, meaning that the hair resists penetration and is difficult to service. Although the cuticle is not directly involved in chemical texture services, the chemicals must be able to penetrate through the cuticle in order to be effective (Figure 15–2).

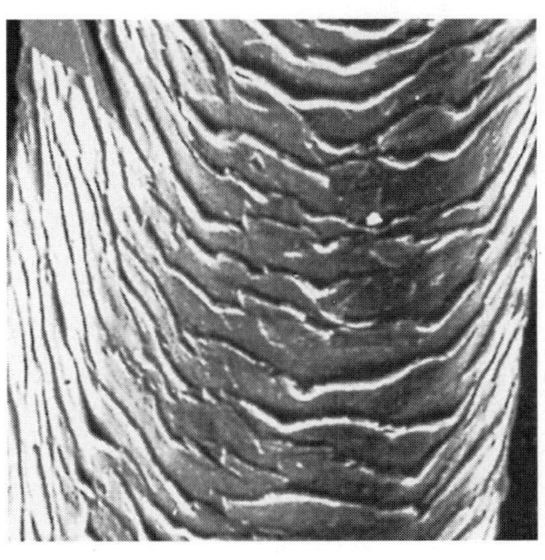

Figure 15–2 Normal cuticle.

Chemical hair texturizers offer you the ability to change the hair's natural curl pattern. These alkaline solutions soften and swell the hair, raising the cuticle and thereby permitting the solution to penetrate through the cuticle to its target within the cortex. Coarse, resistant hair with a strong, compact cuticle layer requires a texturizer, which is highly alkaline (high pH). A less alkaline (lower pH) solution is more suited to porous, damaged, or chemically treated hair.

The Cortex

The cortex is the middle layer of the hair, located directly beneath the cuticle layer. The polypeptide chains of the cortex are connected by end bonds and cross-linked by side bonds that form the fibers and structure of hair. These chemical bonds hold the hair in its natural wave pattern and are responsible for the incredible strength and elasticity of human hair. Breaking the side bonds of the cortex makes it possible to change the natural wave pattern of the hair.

Peptide Bonds (End Bonds)

The chemical bonds that join the amino acids are called **peptide** (PEP-tyd) bonds or **end bonds**. The peptide bonds, in turn, link together to form long chains of amino acids called **polypeptide chains**. Proteins are long, coiled, complex polypeptide chains made of many different amino acids linked together, end-to-end, like pop beads (Figure 15–3).

It is important to note that peptide bonds should not be broken during any salon service. Breaking the hair's peptide bonds causes the polypeptide chains to come apart and dramatically weakens the hair. If used incorrectly, chemical hair texturizers can break peptide bonds and cause hair breakage. Chemical hair texturizers must be used carefully.

Side Bonds

The cortex is made of millions of polypeptide chains cross-linked by three types of side bonds, or cross bonds: disulfide bonds, salt bonds, and hydrogen bonds. Altering these three types of side bonds is what makes wet setting, thermal styling, permanent waving, soft curl permanents, and chemical hair relaxing possible (Figure 15–4).

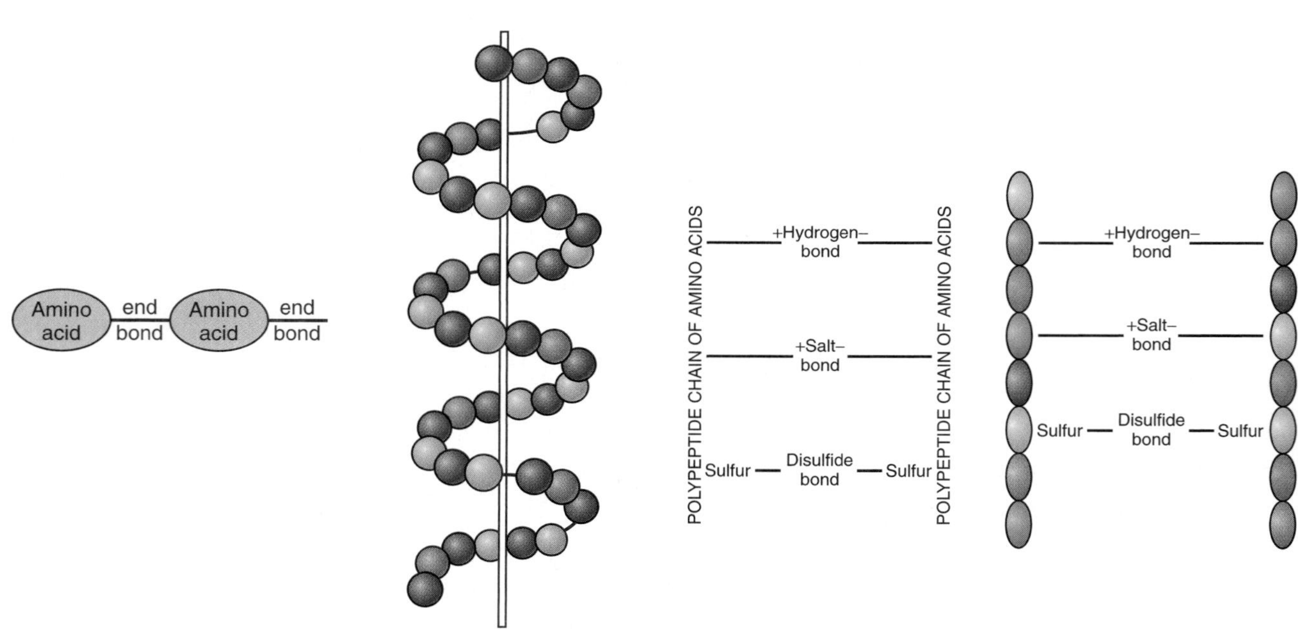

Figure 15–3 Peptide bonds.

Figure 15–4 Side bonds.

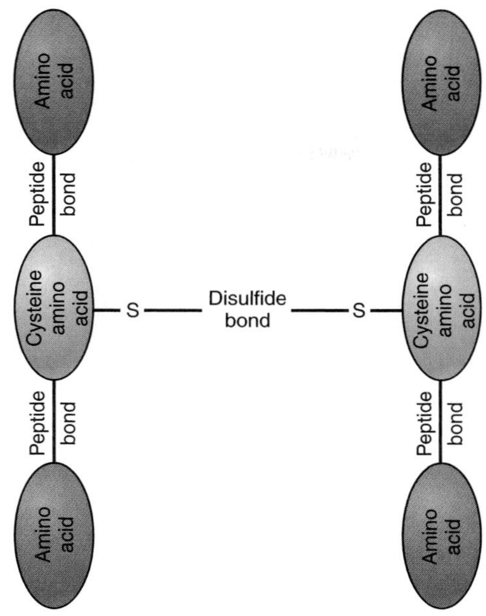

Figure 15–5 Disulfide bond.

Disulfide Bonds

Disulfide bonds are formed between two cysteine (SIS-tuh-een) amino acids, located on neighboring polypeptide chains. A disulfide bond joins a cysteine sulfur atom on one polypeptide chain with a second cysteine sulfur atom on a neighboring polypeptide chain to form cystine (SIS-teen), the oxidized form of cysteine. Disulfide bonds are weaker than peptide bonds, but are much stronger than hydrogen or salt bonds (Figure 15–5).

Disulfide bonds are strong chemical side bonds that are not broken by heat or water. Although there are far fewer disulfide bonds than hydrogen or salt bonds, disulfide bonds are the strongest of the three side bonds and account for about one-third of the hair's overall strength. The chemical and physical changes in disulfide bonds make permanent waving, soft curl permanents (curl re-forming), and chemical hair relaxing possible.

Salt Bonds (Side Bonds)

Salt bonds are relatively weak physical side bonds that are the result of an attraction between opposite electrical charges. Salt bonds are easily broken by changes in pH, as in permanent waving, and re-form when the pH returns to normal. Even though salt bonds are far weaker than disulfide bonds, the hair has so many salt bonds that they account for about one-third of the hair's total strength.

Hydrogen Bonds (Side Bonds)

Hydrogen bonds are relatively weak physical side bonds that are the result of an attraction between opposite electrical charges. Hydrogen bonds are easily broken by water, as in wet setting, or heat, as in thermal styling, and re-form as the hair dries or cools. Although individual hydrogen bonds are very weak, there are so many of them that they account for about one-third of the hair's total strength.

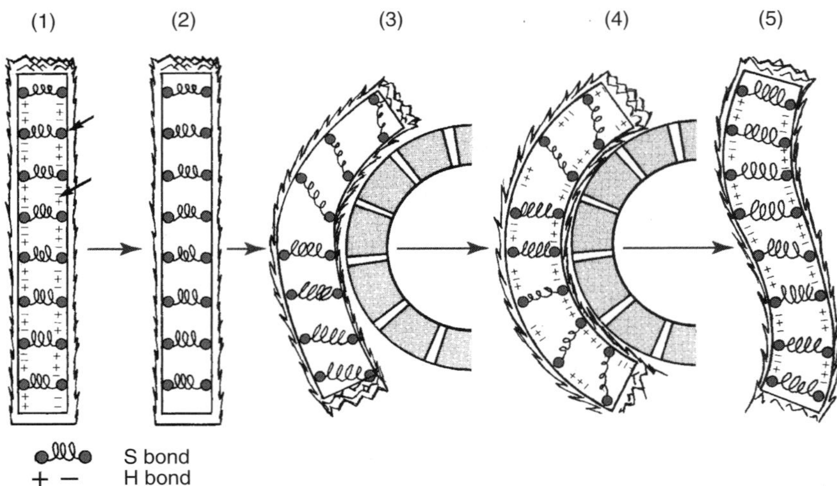

(1) **Straight hair** — showing position of H and S bonds.
(2) **Hair softened by water** — H bonds are broken.
(3) **Hair wound on rollers** — S bonds stretched into waved positions.
(4) **Hair after proper drying** — H bonds reformed into waved positions.
(5) **Hair after brushing out into set** — waves held only by H bonds. Hair is sprayed with moisture-repellent barrier.

Figure 15–6 Changes in hair cortex during wet setting.

A wet set is an example of a physical change that results from breaking and re-forming the hydrogen bonds within the hair. Wetting the hair breaks the hydrogen bonds and permits the hair to be stretched and wrapped on rollers. Drying the hair removes the water and re-forms the hydrogen bonds in their new shape. These changes are only temporary. As soon as the hair is wet or is exposed to high humidity, it will return to its original shape (Figure 15–6).

Thermal styling with hair dryers, curling irons, and pressing combs also breaks hydrogen bonds. These styles involve a physical change with temporary results. The hair returns to its original shape as soon as it is wet.

THE CLIENT CONSULTATION

The client consultation is one of the most important parts of a successful texture service. Before proceeding with any service, you must first determine exactly what the client expects and what is possible. No matter how advanced your technical skills are, nothing will compensate for a lack of communication between you and your client.

- Always greet your client by name and introduce yourself.
- Ask open-ended questions that allow you to find out why the client wants the texture service and what results are expected.

PERMANENT WAVE RECORD

Name .... Tel ....

Address...

City............................... State......... Zip ....

DESCRIPTION OF HAIR

Length	**Texture**	**Type**	**Porosity**	
□ short	□ coarse	□ normal	□ very porous	□ slightly porous
□ medium	□ medium	□ resistant	□ moderately porous	□ resistant
□ long	□ fine	□ tinted	□ normal	
		□ highlighted		
		□ bleached		

CONDITION

□ very good □ good □ fair □ poor □ dry □ oily

Tinted with ....

Previously permed with ....

TYPE OF PERM

□ alkaline □ acid □ body wave □ other...............................

No. of rods .... Lotion........... Strength...............

RESULTS

□ good □ poor □ too tight □ too loose

Date	Perm Used	Stylist	Date	Perm Used	Stylist

Figure 15–7 Permanent wave record.

- Look at pictures with your client to determine exactly what she wants.
- Ask about past texture services. Determine what the client liked and did not like.
- Ask how the client currently styles her hair and discuss any changes that would result from the texture service.
- Determine the finished hairstyle the client wants, considering the haircut and the degree of texture or relaxing that is needed.
- Evaluate the condition, texture, and wave pattern of the hair to make sure that the desired style is possible.
- Fill out a permanent wave record to document the condition of the hair and the desired outcome (Figure 15–7).

Client Records

Client records should include a complete evaluation of the length, texture, color, and condition of the hair prior to the service, and the results that are expected. Extra caution should be used to determine any previous problems or adverse reactions the client may have had in the past. This information must be reevaluated prior to each service since there may have been changes focus on . . . building your client base.

Accurate, detailed, systematic record-keeping is an essential part of successful chemical services. The importance of accurate records cannot be overemphasized. If you neglect to update your records, you may find yourself repeating past mistakes and eventually losing your client. If you make a habit of keeping good records, however, not only will you improve your technical skills, but you'll also build your client's trust and loyalty.

in the client's history or in the formulation of the product since it was last used (see Chapter 4).

Also include in your records the type of perm, the type and size of perm tools (rods), base direction, base control, wrapping technique, wrapping pattern, processing time, and the results achieved. Always remember to update your records and note any changes.

Client Release Form

Some schools and salons may require a client to sign a release form prior to receiving any chemical service. Although most release forms state that the school or salon is not responsible for any damages that may occur, they do not release the school or salon from all responsibility. Release forms do indicate that the client knew, before the chemical service was given, that there was a possibility of damage to the hair or an unexpected adverse reaction.

Scalp Analysis

An analysis of the scalp should always be performed prior to a chemical service. Look for cuts, scratches, or open sores. Do not proceed with the service if there are any skin abrasions or if there are any signs of scalp disease. Refer the client to a physician as necessary.

Hair Analysis

Hair is the fastest growing appendage on the human body. Anything that affects our general health also affects our hair. Diet, exercise, medications, and stress all affect hair growth. The quality of any permanent wave is directly related to the quality of the hair. All other things being equal, strong hair usually produces much stronger curls than weak hair.

Hair analysis is an essential part of a successful chemical hair service. A complete analysis will help you determine how the hair will react to the service and will help avoid most problems. The condition, texture, and wave pattern of the hair must be considered when selecting the type of relaxer, perm, the type and size of perm tool, and the wrapping method. The five most important factors to consider in hair analysis are texture, density, porosity, elasticity, and growth direction. Refer to Chapter 8 for a detailed discussion of these factors and how to test the hair for them.

Hair Texture

Hair texture describes the diameter of a single strand of hair and is classified as coarse, medium, or fine. Hair density differs not only from one individual to another but also from strand to strand on the same person's head. It is best determined by feeling a single, dry strand between the fingers. The three types of hair have the following characteristics.

- *Coarse hair* usually requires more processing than medium or fine hair and may also be more resistant to that processing. It is usually more difficult for permanent waving solutions to penetrate coarse hair.
- *Medium hair* is the most common hair texture. It is considered normal and does not pose any special problems or concerns.

- *Fine hair* is more fragile, easier to process, and more susceptible to damage from perm services than is coarse or medium hair. As a general rule, fine hair will process faster and more easily than medium or coarse hair.

Hair Density

Hair density measures the number of strands of hair on the head, indicating how thick or thin the hair is. Individuals with the same hair texture can have different densities. Some individuals with fine hair texture, characterized by each hair having a small diameter, may have high density, with many individual hairs per square inch. Others with coarse hair texture, characterized by each hair having a large diameter, may have low density, with few individual hairs per square inch.

Hair Porosity

Hair porosity is the ability of the hair to absorb moisture. The degree of porosity is directly related to the condition of the cuticle layer. Hair porosity is classified as resistant, normal, or porous.

- *Resistant hair* has a tight, compact cuticle layer that resists penetration. Chemical services performed on resistant hair require a more alkaline solution. A high pH raises the cuticle and permits uniform saturation and processing. Resistant hair also requires a slow and thorough application of perm solution to ensure complete saturation.
- *Hair with normal porosity* is neither resistant nor overly porous. Texture services performed on this type of hair will usually process as expected.
- *Overly porous hair* has a raised cuticle layer that easily absorbs solution. Chemical services performed on overly porous hair require a less alkaline solution than those performed on resistant hair. A lower pH minimizes swelling and helps prevent excessive damage to the hair.

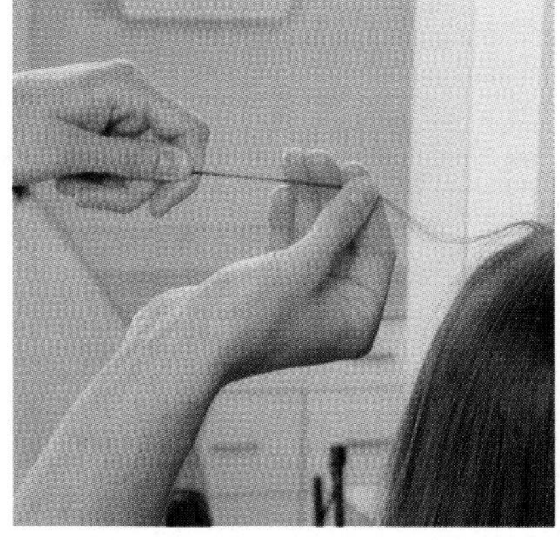

Figure 15–8 Elasticity test.

Hair Elasticity

Hair elasticity is an indication of the strength of the side bonds that hold the individual fibers of the hair in place. More than any other single factor, the elasticity of the hair determines its ability to hold curl. Hair elasticity is usually classified as normal or low (Figure 15–8).

- Wet hair with normal elasticity can stretch up to 50 percent of its original length and then return to that same length without breaking. Hair with normal elasticity usually holds the curl from wet sets and permanent waves.
- Wet hair with low elasticity does not return to its original length when stretched. Hair with low elasticity may not be able to hold the curl from wet sets and permanent waves.

Direction of Hair Growth

The individual growth direction of the hair causes hair streams, whorls, and cowlicks that influence the finished hairstyle and must be considered when selecting the base direction and wrapping pattern for each permanent wave. 1

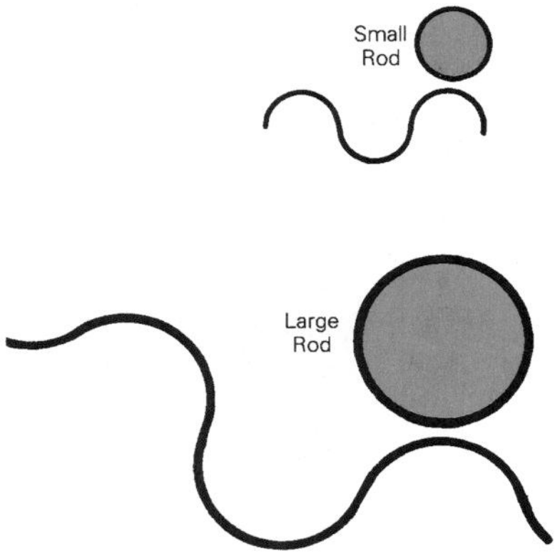

Small Rod

Large Rod

Figure 15–9 The size of the rod determines the size of the curl.

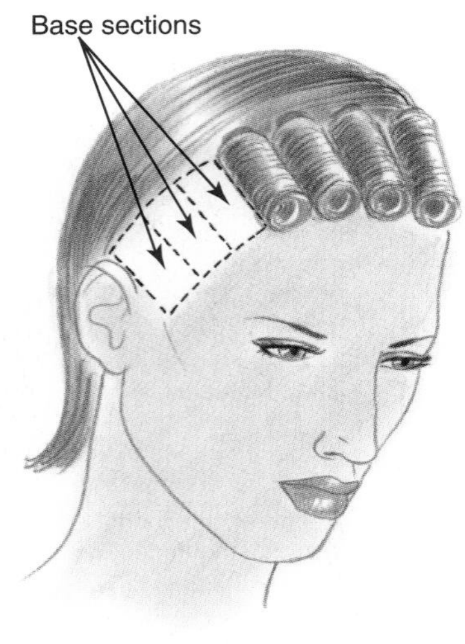

Figure 15–10 Base section.

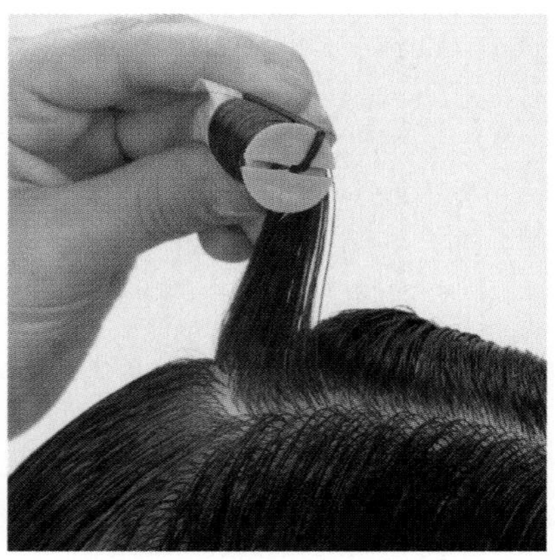

Figure 15–11 On-base placement.

PERMANENT WAVING

Permanent waving is a two-step process.

1. The first part of any perm is the physical change caused by wrapping the hair on the perm rods.
2. The second part involves the chemical changes caused by the permanent waving solution and the neutralizer.

The Perm Wrap

In permanent waving, the size, shape, and type of curl are determined by the size, shape, and type of tool used in wrapping the hair. Permanent waving solution, by itself, does not cause the hair to curl any more than water causes a wet set to curl. Permanent waving solution simply softens the hair, allowing it to conform to the shape in which it was wrapped. As long as a perm is processed correctly, what you wrap is what you get.

The first part of any permanent involves wrapping the hair in the desired shape. In a perm wrap, just as in a wet set, wetting the hair with water breaks the hydrogen bonds and permits the hair to be wrapped in the desired shape. A perm wrap is essentially a wet set on perm rods instead of rollers. The major difference between a wet set and a permanent wave is the type of side bonds that are broken. A wet set breaks hydrogen bonds. A permanent wave breaks disulfide bonds.

The size of the perm tool determines the size of the curl. Small tools produce small curls and large tools produce large curls (Figure 15–9). Wrapping the hair on small tools increases the tension, which increases the amount of curl. Although it is tension that produces the curl, too much tension, especially in one spot, can mark or break the hair. Keep the hair wet while wrapping, and always wrap with uniform, even tension.

Sectioning

All perm wraps begin by sectioning the hair into panels. The size, shape, and direction of these panels vary, based on the type of wrapping pattern and the type and size of the tool being used. Each panel is further divided into subsections called **base sections** (Figure 15–10). One tool is normally placed on each base section. The size of each base section is usually the length and width of the tool being used.

Base Control

Base control refers to the position of the tool in relation to its base section and is determined by the angle at which the hair is wrapped. Tools can be wrapped on base, half off base, or off base.

In **on-base placement**, the hair is wrapped at an angle 45 degrees beyond perpendicular to its base section. The tool is positioned on its base section (Figure 15–11).

Although on-base placement may result in greater volume at the scalp area, any increase in volume will be lost as soon as the hair begins to grow

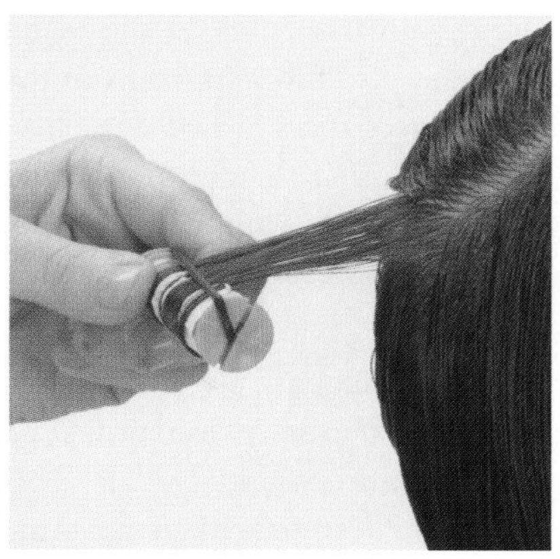

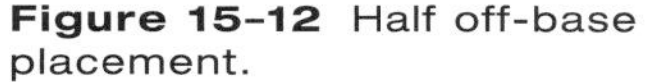

Figure 15–12 Half off-base placement.

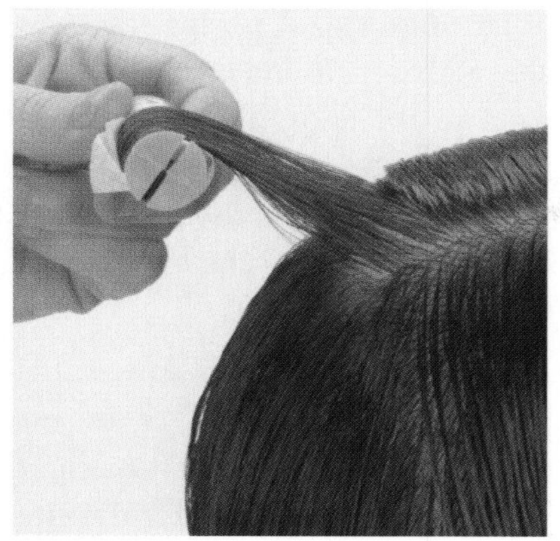

Figure 15–13 Off-base placement.

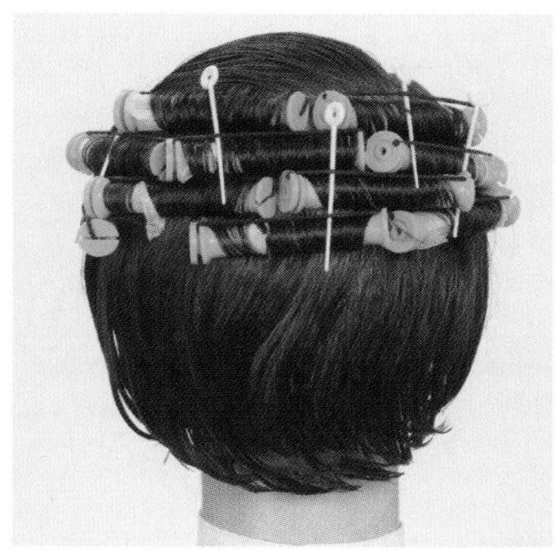

Figure 15–14 Horizontal base direction.

out. Caution should be used with on-base placement because of the additional stress and tension it places on the hair. Wrapping hair on base may damage or break the hair.

Half-off-base placement refers to wrapping the hair at an angle of 90 degrees (perpendicular) to its base section. The tool is positioned half off its base section (Figure 15–12). Half-off-base placement minimizes stress and tension on the hair.

Off-base placement refers to wrapping the hair at an angle 45 degrees below perpendicular to its base section. The tool is positioned completely off its base section (Figure 15–13). Off-base placement creates the least amount of volume and results in a curl pattern that begins farthest away from the scalp

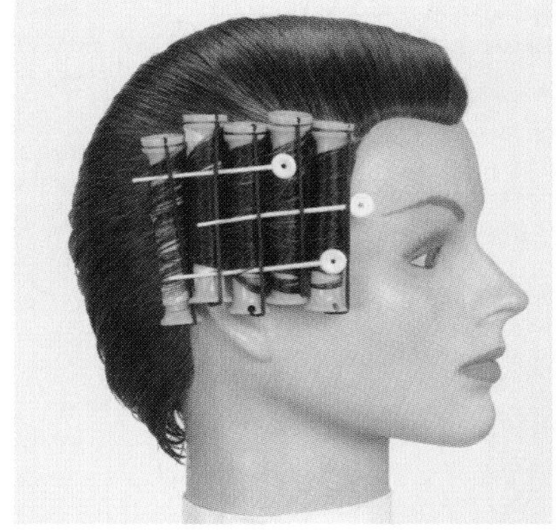

Figure 15–15 Vertical base direction.

Base Direction

Base direction refers to the angle at which the tool is positioned on the head: horizontally, vertically, or diagonally (Figure 15–14, Figure 15–15, and Figure 15–16).

Base direction also refers to the directional pattern in which the hair is wrapped. Although directional wraps can be wrapped backward, forward, or to one side, wrapping with the natural direction of hair growth causes the least amount of stress to the hair. Wrapping against the natural growth pattern causes excess stress that may damage or break the hair.

Wrapping Techniques

There are two basic methods of wrapping the hair around the perm tool: croquignole and spiral.

In **croquignole perms** (KROH-ken-yohl), the hair strands are wrapped from the ends to the scalp, in overlapping layers (Figure 15–17). Because the hair is wrapped at an angle perpendicular to the length of the tool, each new layer of hair is wrapped toward the scalp on top of the previous layer. This increases the effective size of the tool with each new overlapping layer and produces a tighter curl at the ends and a larger curl at the scalp. Longer, thicker hair increases this effect.

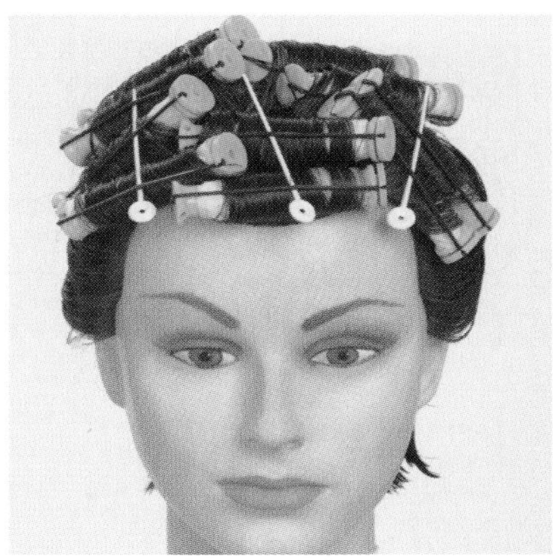

Figure 15–16 Diagonal base direction.

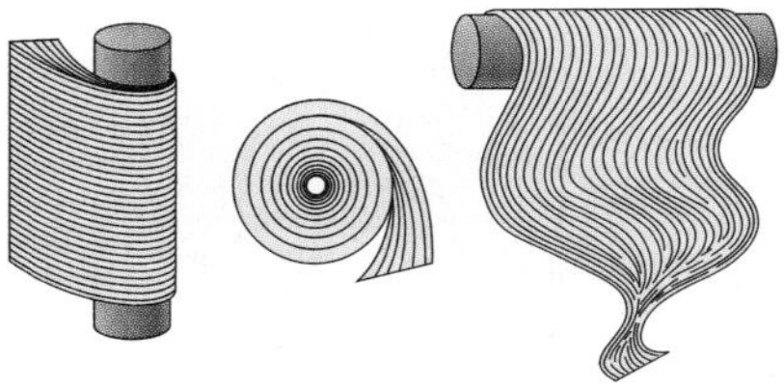

Figure 15-17 Croquignole perm wrap.

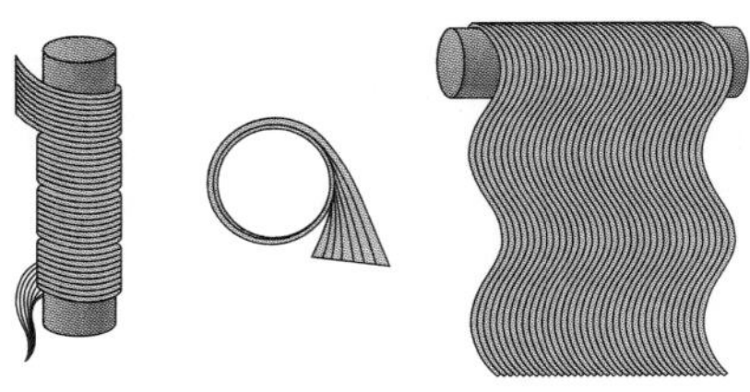

Figure 15-18 Spiral perm wrap.

In most **spiral perms**, the hair is wound from the ends to the scalp, although depending on the tools used, some may also be wrapped from the scalp to the ends. The difference should not affect the finished curl. In a spiral perm wrap, the hair is wrapped at an angle other than perpendicular to the length of the tool. The angle at which the hair is wrapped causes the hair to spiral along the length of the tool, like the grip on a tennis racquet (Figure 15–18).

Although the layers in a spiral perm wrap may partially overlap the preceding layers, as long as the angle remains constant, any overlap will be uniform along the length of the tool and the entire strand of hair. This wrapping technique causes the effective size of the tool to remain the same along the entire length of the strand, producing a uniform curl from the scalp to the ends. Longer, thicker hair will benefit the most from this effect.

Perm Tools

As we have noted, in permanent waving, the size of the tool determines the size of the curl. The shape and type of curl is determined by the shape and type of tool and the wrapping method. Selecting the correct perm tool and wrapping method is the key to creating a successful permanent. Perm tools come in a wide variety of sizes and shapes that can be combined with different wrapping methods to provide an exciting range of styling options.

Types of Rods

Concave rods are the most common type of perm rod. They are usually used with a croquignole wrapping technique. Concave rods have a smaller circumference in the center that increases to a larger circumference on the ends. They produce a tighter curl in the center and a looser, larger curl on either side of the strand (Figure 15–19).

Straight rods are also usually used with a croquignole wrapping technique. Since straight rods are equal in circumference along their entire length or curling area, they produce a uniform curl along the entire width of the strand (Figure 15–20).

Concave and straight rods come in different lengths. Since the length of

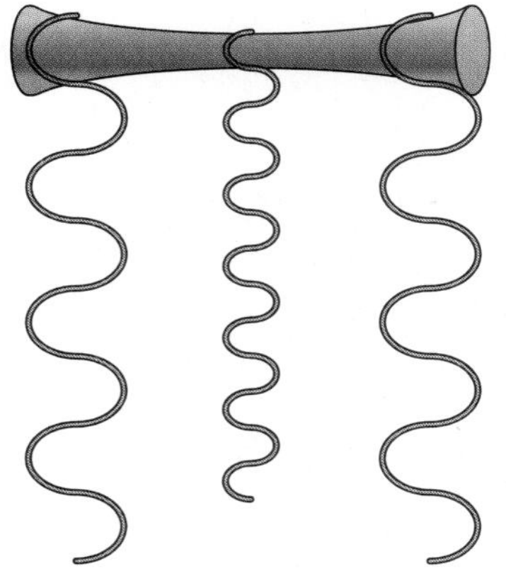

Figure 15-19 Concave rod and resulting curl.

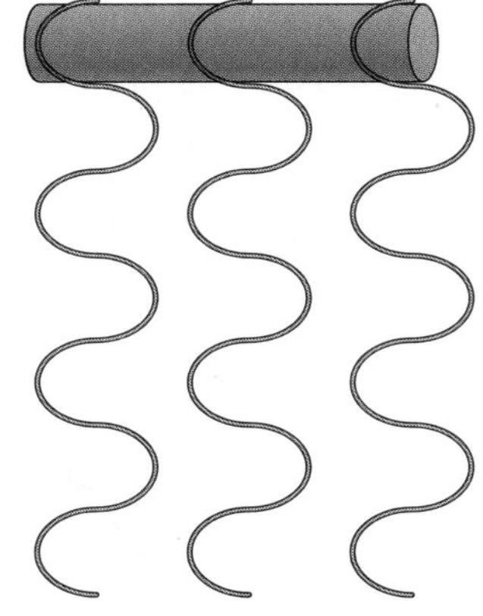

Figure 15-20 Straight rod and resulting curl.

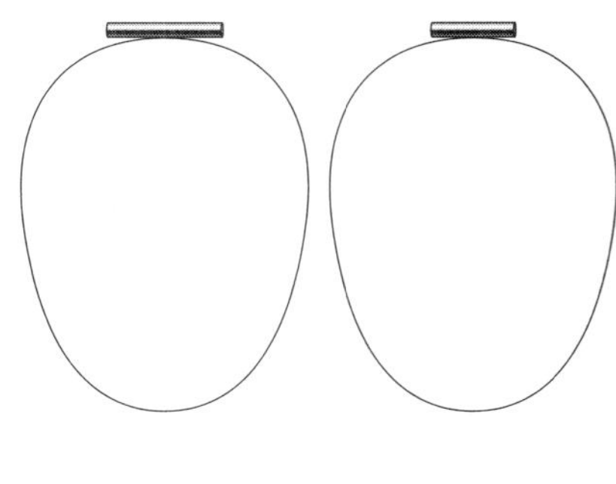

Figure 15-21 Long and short rods and the contours of the head.

the base section is usually the same length as the rod, fewer rods are required when using long rods. Long, straight rods can also be used with a spiral wrapping technique to produce spiral perms, as long as the length of the rod will accommodate the length of the hair.

Although more rods may be needed when using short rods, they fit closer to the rounded curvatures of the head. Short rods can also be used for wrapping small and awkward sections where long rods would not fit (Figure 15–21).

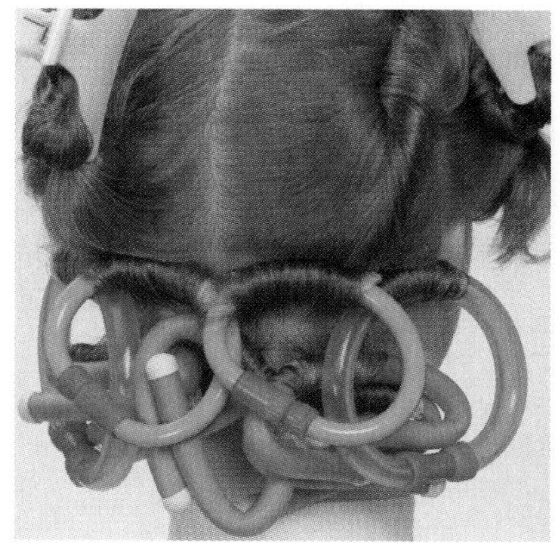

Figure 15-22 Soft bender rods and circle tools.

Other Perm Tools

Soft bender rods are usually about 12 inches long with a uniform diameter along the entire length. These soft foam rods have a stiff wire inside that permits them to be bent into almost any shape. Soft bender rods can be used with either a croquignole or spiral wrapping technique (Figure 15–22, Figure 15–23, and Figure 15–24).

The circle tool or loop rod is usually about 12 inches long with a uniform diameter along the entire length of the rod. The extra length of the circle tool is ideal for spiral wrapping on extremely long hair. After the hair is wrapped, the rod is secured by fastening the ends together to form a circle (Figure 15–25).

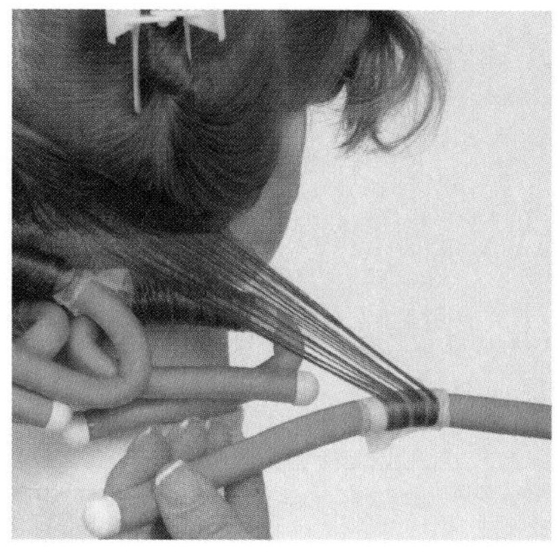

Figure 15-23 Croquignole wrapping with soft bender rods.

End Papers

End papers or end wraps are absorbent papers used to control the ends of the hair when wrapping and winding hair on the perm tools. End papers should extend beyond the ends of the hair to keep them smooth and straight and prevent "fishhooks." The most common end paper techniques are the double flat wrap, the single flat wrap, and the bookend single paper wrap.

- The **double flat wrap** uses two end papers, one placed under and one over the strand of hair being wrapped. Both papers extend past the hair ends. This wrap provides the most control over the hair ends and also helps keep them evenly distributed over the entire length of the tool (Figure 15–26).

15

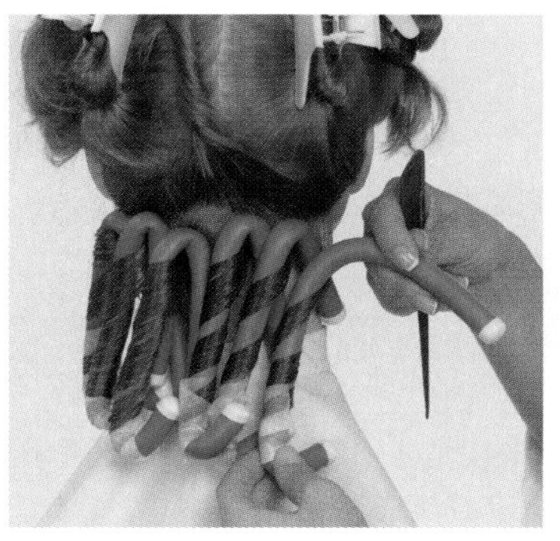

Figure 15-24 Spiral wrapping with soft bender rods.

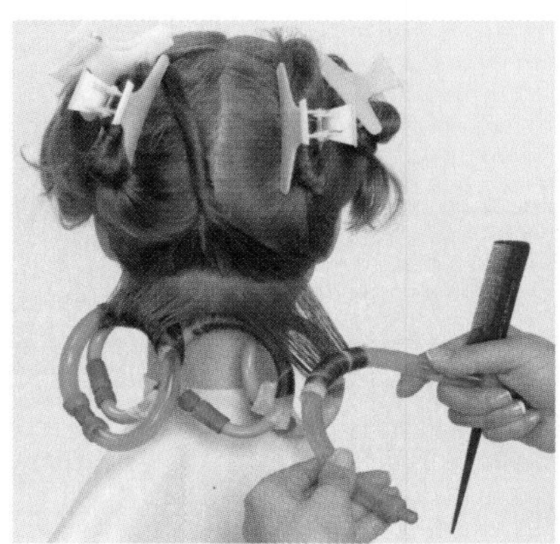

Figure 15-25 Circle tools.

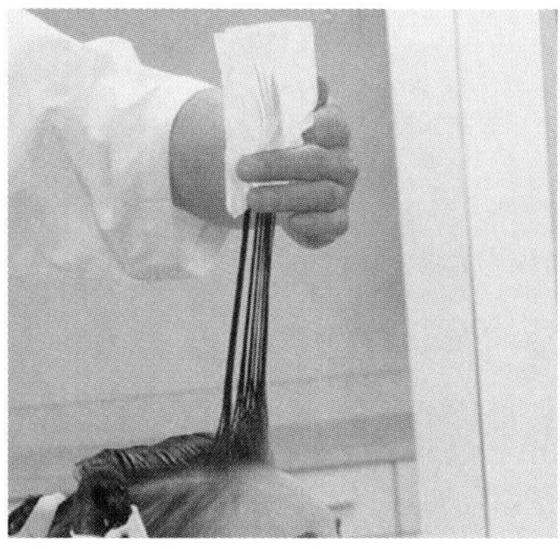

Figure 15-26 Double flat wrap.

- The **single flat wrap** is similar to the double flat wrap, but uses only one end paper, placed over the top of the strand of hair being wrapped (Figure 15–27).
- The **bookend wrap** uses one end paper folded in half over the hair ends like an envelope. Prefolded end papers are available, or you can fold a single large end paper and place it over the top and bottom of the hair so that it extends past the hair ends. The bookend wrap eliminates excess paper and can be used with short rods or with very short lengths of hair. Be careful to distribute the hair evenly over the entire length of the rod. Avoid bunching the ends together toward the center of the rod (Figure 15–28).

Figure 15-27 Single flat wrap.

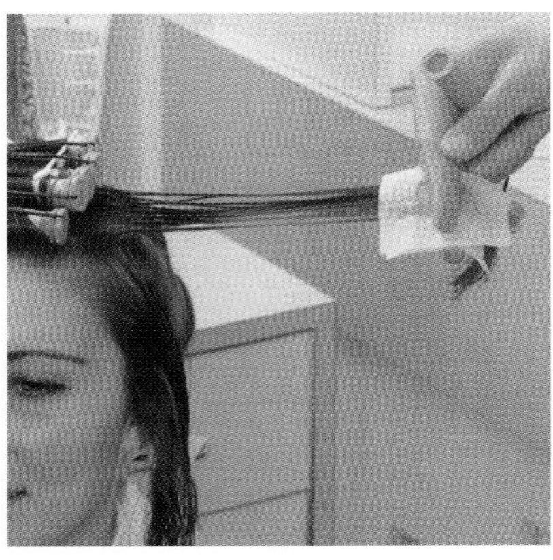

Figure 15-28 Bookend wrap.

The Chemistry of Permanent Waving

Alkaline permanent waving solution softens and swells the hair, which raises the cuticle and permits the solution to penetrate into the cortex. Figure 15–29 illustrates a hair saturated with alkaline permanent waving solution (pH 9.4) for five minutes. Note the swelling of the cuticle layer. In Figure 15–30, the same hair has been saturated with acid-balanced permanent waving solution (pH 7.5) for five minutes. Note that there is far less swelling of the cuticle layer. Once in the cortex, the waving solution breaks the disulfide bonds through a chemical reaction called reduction. A reduction reaction involves either the addition of hydrogen or the removal of oxygen (see Chapter 7). The reduction reaction in permanent waving is due to the addition of hydrogen.

In examining the reduction reaction more closely, we can see that a disulfide bond joins a sulfur atom on one polypeptide chain with a second sulfur atom on a neighboring polypeptide chain. Permanent waving solution breaks a disulfide bond by adding a hydrogen atom to each of the sulfur atoms in the disulfide bond. The sulfur atoms attach to the hydrogen from the permanent waving solution, breaking their attachment to each other (Figure 15–31). Once the disulfide bond is broken, the polypeptide chains are able to slip into their new curled shape.

The reducing agents used in permanent waving solutions are thiol (THY-ohl) compounds, commonly referred to simply as thio (THY-oh). **Thioglycolic acid** (thy-oh-GLY-kuh-lik) is the most common. It is a

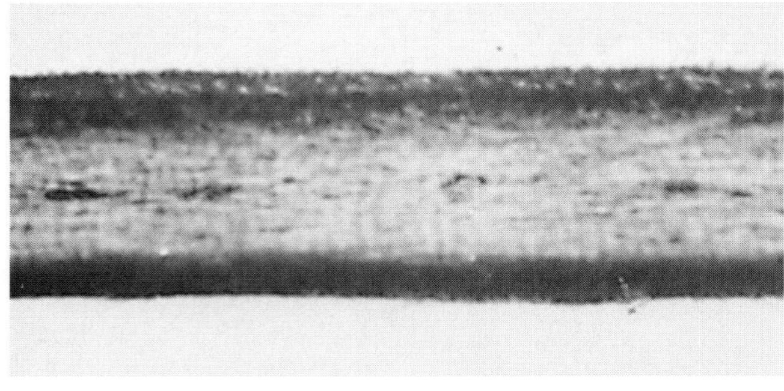

Figure 15-29 Hair saturated with alkaline solution.

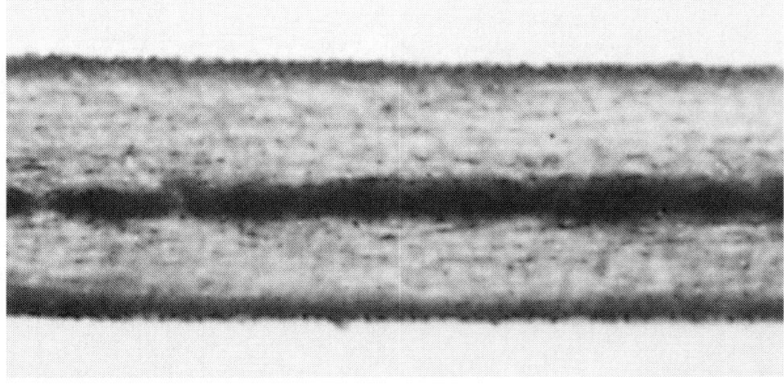

Figure 15-30 The same hair saturated with acid-balanced permanent waving solution.

colorless liquid with a strong unpleasant odor. Thioglycolic acid provides the hydrogen that causes the reduction reaction in permanent waving solutions.

The strength of the permanent waving solution is determined by the concentration of thio. Stronger perms have a higher concentration of thio with a greater number of hydrogen atoms. When more hydrogen atoms are available, more disulfide bonds are broken.

Thioglycolic acid is an acid, and since acids do not swell the hair or penetrate into the cortex, it is necessary for manufacturers to add an alkalizing agent. The addition of ammonia to thioglycolic acid produces a new chemical called **ammonium thioglycolate** (uh-MOH-nee-um thy-oh-GLY-kuh-layt) (ATG), which is alkaline. ATG is the main active ingredient or reducing agent in alkaline permanents.

The degree of alkalinity (pH) is a second factor in the overall strength of the permanent waving solution. Coarse hair with a strong, resistant cuticle layer may need the additional swelling and penetration that is provided by a more alkaline permanent waving solution.

By contrast, porous hair or hair with a damaged cuticle layer is easily penetrated and could be damaged by a highly alkaline permanent waving solution. The pH (alkalinity) of the perm solution should correspond to the resistance, strength, and porosity of the cuticle layer. 2

Types of Permanent Waves

A variety of permanent waves is available in salons today. Brief descriptions of the most commonly used perms follow.

Alkaline Waves or Cold Waves

The first **alkaline waves** (or cold waves) were developed in 1941 and relied on the same ATG that is still used in most alkaline waves today. Since alkaline waves process at room temperature without the addition of heat, they became commonly known as cold waves. Most alkaline waves have a pH between 9.0 and 9.6 (Figure 15–32).

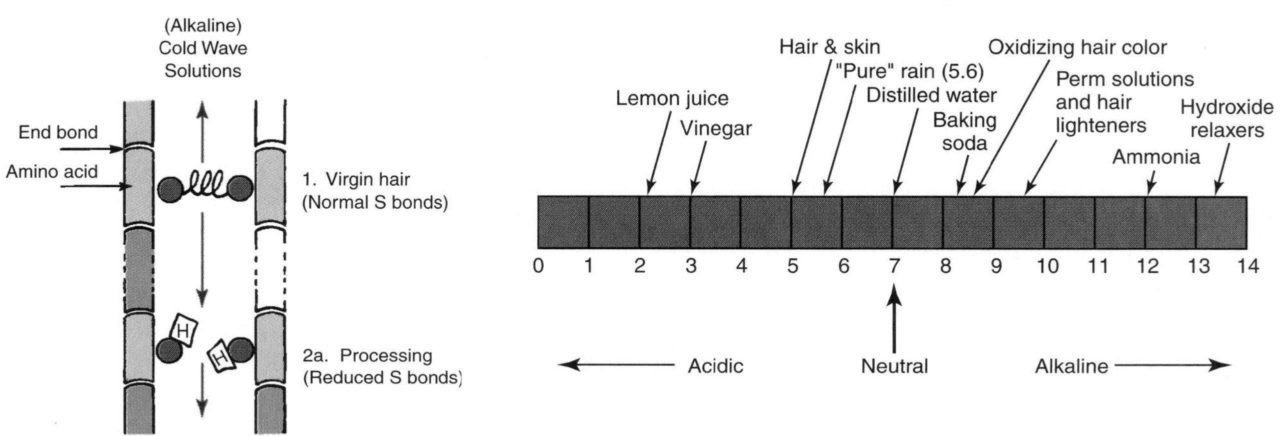

Figure 15-31 Reduction reaction of thio perms and relaxers.

Figure 15-32 pH scale of various perms.

True Acid Waves

The first **true acid waves** were introduced in the early 1970s. Most true acid waves have a pH between 4.5 and 7.0 and require heat to speed processing. **Glyceryl monothioglycolate** (GLIS-ur-il mon-oh-thy-oh-GLY-koh-layt) (GMTG) is the main active ingredient and is an acid, with a low pH. Although a lower pH tends to cause less damage to the hair, acid waves process more slowly, may require the added heat of a hair dryer, and do not usually produce as firm a curl as alkaline waves.

Since acidic solutions contract the hair, you may be wondering how a true acid wave, with a pH below 7.0, can cause the hair to swell. The average pH of hair is 5.0. So although a pH of 7.0 is neutral on the pH scale, a pH of 5.0 is neutral for hair. And since every step in the pH scale represents a tenfold change in pH, a pH of 7.0 is 100 times more alkaline than the pH of hair (see Chapter 7). Even pure water with a pH of 7.0 can damage the hair and cause it to swell.

Acid-Balanced Waves

In order to permit processing at room temperature and produce a firmer curl, the strength and pH of acid waves have increased steadily over the years. Most of the acid waves found in today's salons have a pH between 7.8 and 8.2, which means they are not really acidic. Modern acid waves are not true acid waves, but are actually **acid-balanced waves**. Because of their higher pH, they process at room temperature and do not require the added heat of a hair dryer. Modern acid waves also process more quickly and produce firmer curls than true acid waves.

CAUTION

Accidentally mixing the contents of the activator tube with the neutralizer instead of the permanent waving solution will cause a violent chemical reaction that can cause injury, especially to the eyes.

All acid waves have three separate components: permanent waving solution, activator, and neutralizer. The activator tube contains GMTG, which must be added to the permanent waving solution immediately before use.

Although GMTG is the primary reducing agent in all modern acid waves, it may not be the only reducing agent. Most of these waves also contain ATG, just like a cold wave. Although the low pH of acid waves may seem ideal, repeated exposure to GMTG is known to cause allergic sensitivity in both hairstylists and clients.

Exothermic Waves

An exothermic chemical reaction produces heat. **Exothermic waves** (ek-soh-THUR-mik) create an exothermic chemical reaction that heats up the solution and speeds up the processing.

All exothermic waves have three components: permanent waving solution, an activator, and a neutralizer. The permanent waving solution contains thio, just as in a cold wave. The activator contains an oxidizing agent (usually hydrogen peroxide) that must be added to the permanent waving solution immediately before use. Mixing an oxidizer with the permanent waving solution causes a rapid release of heat and an increase in the temperature of the solution. The increased temperature increases the rate of the chemical reaction, which shortens the processing time.

Endothermic Waves

An endothermic chemical reaction is one that absorbs heat from its surroundings. **Endothermic waves** (en-duh-THUR-mik) are activated by an outside heat source, usually a conventional hood-type hair dryer. Endothermic waves will not process properly at room temperature. Most true acid waves are endothermic and require the added heat of a hair dryer.

Ammonia-Free Waves

Ammonia-free waves use an ingredient that does not evaporate as readily as ammonia, so there is very little odor associated with their use. Aminomethylpropanol (uh-MEE-noh-meth-yl-pro-pan-all) (AMP), and monoethanolamine (mahn-oh-ETH-an-all-am-een) (MEA) are examples of alkanolamines that are used in permanent waving solutions as a substitute for ammonia. Even though these solutions may not smell as strong as ammonia, they can still be every bit as alkaline and just as damaging. Ammonia-free does not necessarily mean damage-free.

Thio-Free Waves

Thio-free waves use an ingredient other than ATG as the primary reducing agent. The most common thio-free waves rely on cysteamine (SIS-tee-uh-meen), or mercaptamine (mer-KAPT-uh-meen). Although these thio substitutes are not technically ATG, they are still thio compounds. Although thio-free is often marketed as damage-free, that is not necessarily true. At a high concentration, the reducing agents in thio-free waves can be just as damaging as thio.

CAUTION

The ingredients, strength, and pH of permanent wave solutions from different manufacturers may vary considerably, even within the same category. Always check the manufacturers' instructions and MSDS for accurate, detailed information.

Low-pH Waves

The use of sulfates, sulfites, and bisulfites presents an alternative to ATG known as **low-pH waves**. Sulfites work at a low pH and have been used in perms for years, but they have never been very popular. Permanents based on sulfites are very weak and do not provide a firm curl, especially on strong or resistant hair. Sulfite permanents are usually marketed as body waves or alternative waves. 3

Selecting the Right Type of Perm

It is extremely important to select the right type of perm for each client. Every client has hair with its own distinct texture and condition, so individual needs must always be addressed. After a thorough consultation, you should be able to determine which type of permanent is best suited to your client's hair type, condition, and desired results. Table 15–1 lists the most common types of permanent waves along with some of the advantages and disadvantages of each. These are only general guidelines.

Permanent Wave Processing

The strength of any permanent wave is based on the concentration of its reducing agent. In turn, the amount of processing is determined by the strength of the permanent waving solution. If weak permanent waving solution is used on coarse hair, there may not be enough hydrogen atoms to break the necessary number of disulfide bonds, no matter how long the

Perm Type	Active Ingredient	Process	Recommended Hair Type
alkaline/cold wave ph: 9.0 to 9.6	ammonium thioglycolate (ATG)	room temperature	coarse, thick, or resistant
exothermic wave ph: 9.0 to 9.6	ammonium thioglycolate (ATG)	exothermic	coarse, thick, or resistant
true acid wave ph: 4.5 to 7.0	glyceryl monothioglycolate (GMTG)	endothermic	extremely porous or very damaged hair
acid-balanced wave ph: 7.8 to 8.2	glyceryl monothioglycolate (GMTG)	room temperature	porous or damaged hair
ammonia-free wave ph: 7.0 to 9.6	monoethanolamine (MEA)/ aminomethylpropanol (AMP)	room temperature	porous to normal
thio-free wave ph: 7.0 to 9.6	mercaptamine/ cysteamine	room temperature	porous to normal
low-pH waves ph: 6.5 to 7.0	ammonium sulfite/ ammonium bisulfite	endothermic	normal, fine, or damaged

Table 15–1 Permanent Wave Categories

permanent processes. But the same weak solution may be exactly right for fine hair with fewer disulfide bonds. On the other hand, a strong solution, which releases many hydrogen atoms, may be perfect for coarse hair, but too damaging for fine hair. The amount of processing should be determined by the strength of the solution, not necessarily how long the perm processes.

In permanent waving, most of the processing takes place as soon as the solution penetrates the hair, within the first five to ten minutes. The additional processing time allows the polypeptide chains to shift into their new configuration (Figure 15–33).

Overprocessed Hair

If you find that your client's hair has been overprocessed, it probably happened within the first five to ten minutes of the service, and a weaker permanent waving solution should have been used. If the hair is not sufficiently processed after ten minutes, it may require a reapplication of solution. Resistant hair requires a stronger solution, and a more thorough saturation.

Thorough saturation of the hair is essential to proper processing in all permanent waves, but especially on resistant hair. Regardless of the strength or pH of the solution, resistant hair may not become completely saturated

Results	Advantages	Disadvantages
firm, strong curls	processes quickly at room temperature	unpleasant ammonia odor; may damage delicate hair
firm, strong curls	exothermic reaction causes solution to get hot	unpleasant ammonia odor; may damage delicate hair
soft, weak curls	low pH produces minimal swelling	requires heat from hair dryer; will not produce firm, strong curls
soft curls	minimal swelling; processes at room temperature	repeated exposure causes allergic sensitivity in clients and stylists
medium to fine curls	no unpleasant ammonia odor	overall strength varies with different manufacturers
medium to fine curls	may be gentler, depending on formula	overall strength varies with different manufacturers
weak curl or body wave	minimal swelling	requires heat from hair dryer; produces weak curls

with just one application of waving solution. You may need to apply the solution slowly and repeatedly until the hair is completely saturated.

A thorough saturation with stronger solution will break more disulfide bonds and process the hair more, but processing the hair more does not necessarily translate into more curl. A properly processed permanent wave should break and rebuild approximately 50 percent of the hair's disulfide

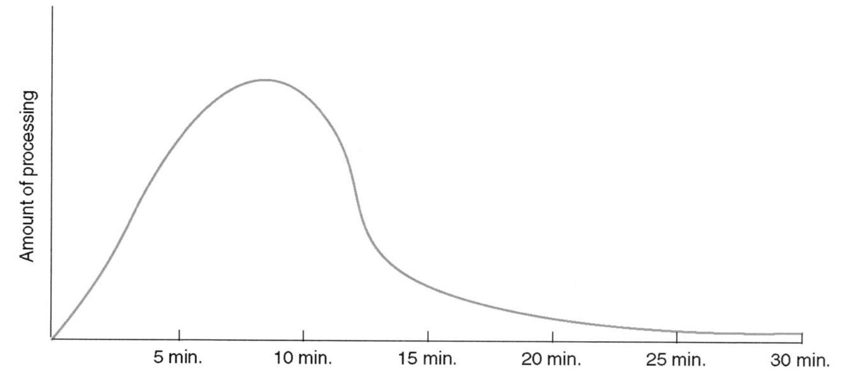

Figure 15–33 Processing time.

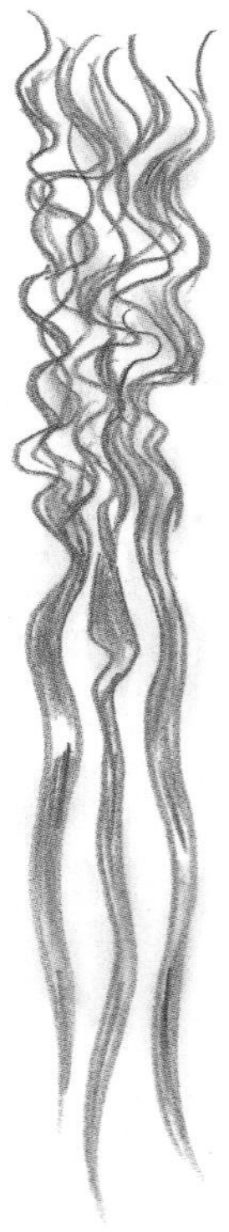

Figure 15–34 Overprocessed hair.

bonds. If too many disulfide bonds are broken, the hair may not have enough strength left to hold the desired curl. Weak hair equals a weak curl.

Contrary to what many believe, overprocessed hair does not necessarily mean hair that is overly curly. If too many disulfide bonds are broken, the hair will be too weak to hold a firm curl. Overprocessed hair usually has a weak curl or may even be completely straight. Since the hair at the scalp is usually stronger than the hair at the ends, overprocessed hair is usually curlier at the scalp and straighter at the ends (Figure 15–34). If the hair is overprocessed, processing it more will make it straighter.

Underprocessed Hair

Underprocessed hair is, as the name suggests, the exact opposite of overprocessed hair. If too few disulfide bonds are broken, the hair will not be sufficiently softened and will not be able to hold the desired curl. Underprocessed hair usually has a very weak curl, but it may also be straight. Since the hair at the scalp is usually stronger than the ends, underprocessed hair is usually straighter at the scalp and curlier at the ends (Figure 15–35). If the hair is underprocessed, processing it more will make it curlier.

Permanent Waving Neutralization

Neutralization is the process of stopping the action of a permanent wave solution and hardening the hair in its new form by the application of a chemical solution called the neutralizer. Neutralization performs two important functions.

1. It deactivates (neutralizes) any waving solution that remains in the hair.
2. It rebuilds the disulfide bonds that were broken by the waving solution.

The neutralizers used in permanent waving are oxidizers. In fact, the term neutralizer is not very accurate because the chemical reaction involved is actually oxidation. The most common neutralizer is hydrogen peroxide. Concentrations vary between 5 volume (1.5 percent) and 10 volume (3 percent).

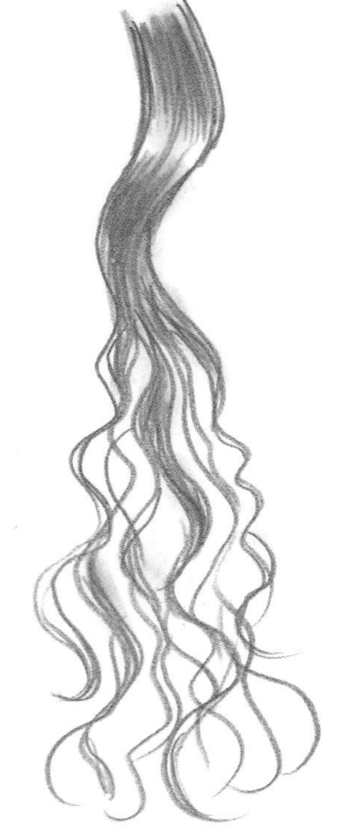

Figure 15–35 Underprocessed hair.

Neutralization: Stage One

The first function of permanent waving neutralization is the deactivation, or neutralization, of any waving lotion that remains in the hair after processing and rinsing. The chemical reaction involved is oxidation.

As we know, oxidation reactions can also lighten hair color, especially at an alkaline pH. To avoid scalp irritation and unwanted lightening of hair color, always rinse perm solution from the hair for at least five minutes before applying the neutralizer. After rinsing and before applying the neutralizer, the hair should be blotted with towels to remove as much moisture as possible. Blot each rod several times using dry towels. Excess water left in the hair prevents even saturation and dilutes the neutralizer.

Some manufacturers recommend the application of a preneutralizing conditioner after blotting and before application of the neutralizer. An acidic liquid protein conditioner can be applied to the hair and dried under a warm hair dryer for five minutes or more prior to neutralization. This added step is especially beneficial with very damaged hair because it strengthens the hair prior to neutralization. This step is optional, however. Always follow the manufacturers' directions and the procedures approved by your instructor.

Neutralization: Stage Two

As you have learned, waving solution breaks disulfide bonds by adding hydrogen atoms to the sulfur atoms in the disulfide bond. Neutralization rebuilds the disulfide bonds by removing those extra hydrogen atoms. The hydrogen atoms in the disulfide bonds are so strongly attracted to the oxygen in the neutralizer that they release their bond with the sulfur atoms and join with the oxygen (Figure 15–36). Each oxygen atom joins with two hydrogen atoms to rebuild one disulfide bond and make one molecule of water. The water is removed in the final rinse, and the disulfide bonds form in their new curled position.

When the neutralizer removes the extra hydrogen atoms, each sulfur atom forms a bond with its nearest neighboring sulfur atom. This is not the same pair that was originally bonded, but a newly created pair that is now closer together because of the physical forces involved in wrapping the hair around the perm rod. The strength of these newly formed disulfide bond pairs holds the hair in its new shape (Figure 15–37).

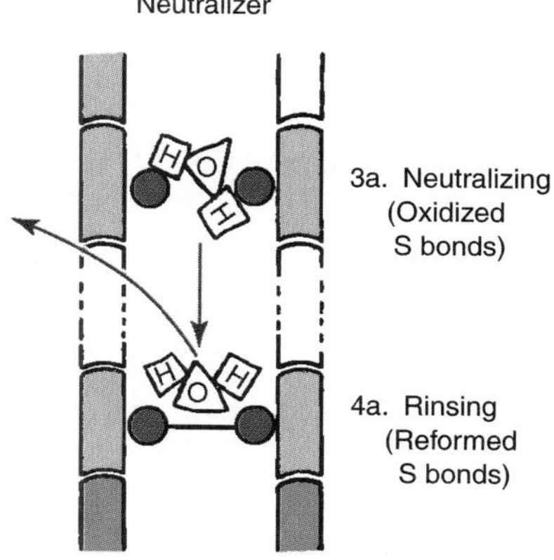

Figure 15-36 Oxidation reaction of thio neutralizers.

Post-Perm Hair Care

For a variety of reasons, most hairstylists have always recommended a three-day waiting period before shampooing freshly permed hair. Although some of their concerns may be valid, a properly neutralized perm is stable. The bonds in the hair are re-formed immediately, and there is no scientific basis for the standard three-day waiting period. Shampooing a properly processed permanent with the mild acid-balanced shampoos that are available today should not cause excessive relaxation or damage to the hair or scalp.

Most hairstylists have also recommended a three-day waiting period before performing haircolor services on freshly permed hair. Although there may be some concern about scalp irritation or excessive relaxation, a permanent is stable as soon as it has been properly neutralized. Unless there are signs of scalp irritation, modern demipermanent, deposit-only

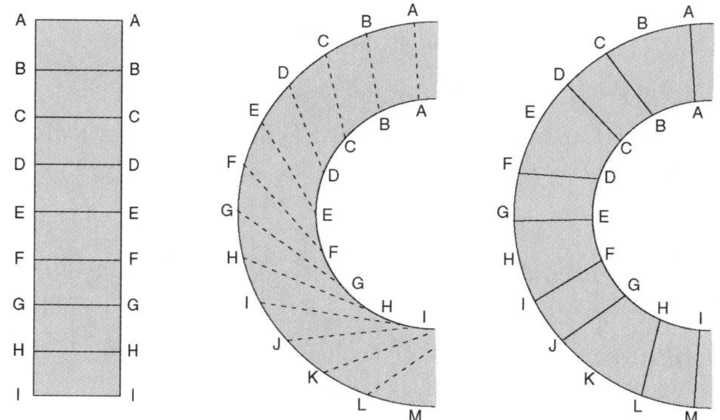

Figure 15-37 New disulfide pairs.

15

focus on ...retailing.

The permanent wave you give your client will not be as manageable or last as long without a proper at-home maintenance program. Your client depends on you for advice on how to care for the new permanent. Make sure you always explain different styling options and recommend the right professional retail products to use at home.

haircolors are safe to use on freshly permed hair. Always follow the manufacturers' directions and the procedures approved by your instructor.

Safety Precautions for Permanent Waving

- Always protect your client's clothing. Have the client change into a gown, use a waterproof shampoo cape, and double drape with towels to absorb accidental spills.
- Do not give a permanent to any client who has experienced an allergic reaction to a previous permanent.
- Do not save any opened, unused waving lotion or neutralizer. These lotions may change in strength and effectiveness if not used promptly.
- Do not dilute or add anything to the waving lotion or neutralizer unless specified in the manufacturers' directions.
- Keep waving lotion out of the client's eyes and away from the client's skin. In case of accidental exposure, rinse thoroughly with cool water.
- Always follow the manufacturers' directions.
- Wear gloves when applying solutions.
- Immediately replace cotton or towels that have become wet with solution.
- Always examine the scalp before the perm service. Do not proceed if there are any skin abrasions or any signs of scalp disease.
- Do not perm hair that is excessively damaged or shows signs of breakage.
- Do not attempt to perm hair that has been previously treated with hydroxide relaxers.
- Always perform a test for metallic salts if there is a possibility that metallic haircolor was used on the hair previously.
- Always apply protective barrier cream around the client's hairline and ears prior to applying permanent waving solution.
- The hair should be given reconditioning treatments until the condition improves and the damaged hair can be cut off.

15

Metallic Salts

Some home haircoloring products contain metallic salts that are not compatible with permanent waving. Metallic salts leave a coating on the hair that may cause uneven curls, severe discoloration, or hair breakage.

Metallic salts are commonly found in men's haircolors that are sold for home use. Haircolor restorers and progressive haircolors that darken the hair gradually with repeated applications are the most likely to contain metallic salts. If you suspect that metallic salts may be present on the hair, perform the following test.

In a glass or plastic bowl, mix 1 ounce of 20 volume peroxide with 20 drops of 28 percent ammonia. Immerse at least 20 strands of hair in the solution for 30 minutes. If metallic salts are not present, the hair will lighten slightly and you may proceed with the service. If metallic salts are present, the hair will lighten rapidly. The solution may get hot and give off an unpleasant odor, indicating that you should not proceed with the service.

PERMANENT WAVING PROCEDURES

Let us now turn to the basic perm procedures. The information presented earlier in the chapter on sectioning, base control, base direction, perm tools, wrapping techniques, and wrapping patterns should be used with the following procedures. These basic wrapping methods may be combined in different ways to create a wide variety of specialized perm wraps that provide an unlimited number of styling options.

The **basic perm wrap** is also called a straight set wrap. In this wrapping pattern, all the tools within a panel move in the same direction and are positioned on equal-size bases. All base sections are horizontal, with the same length and width as the perm tool. The base control is half off base (Figure 15–38).

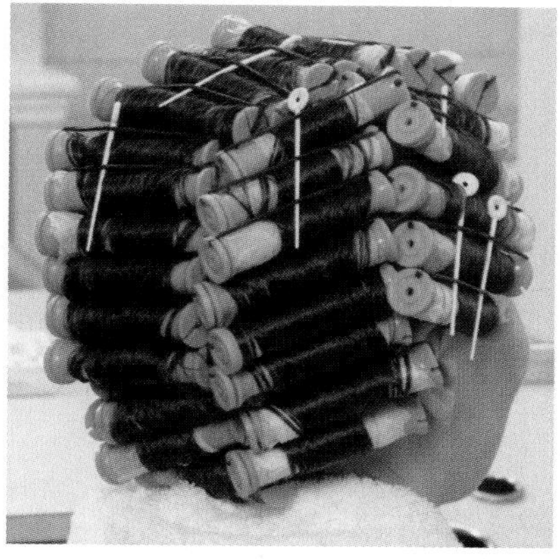

Figure 15-38 Basic perm wrapping pattern.

In the **curvature perm wrap**, the movement curves within sectioned-out panels. Partings and bases radiate throughout the panels to follow the curvature of the head. This wrapping pattern uses pie-shaped base sections in the curvature areas (Figure 15–39).

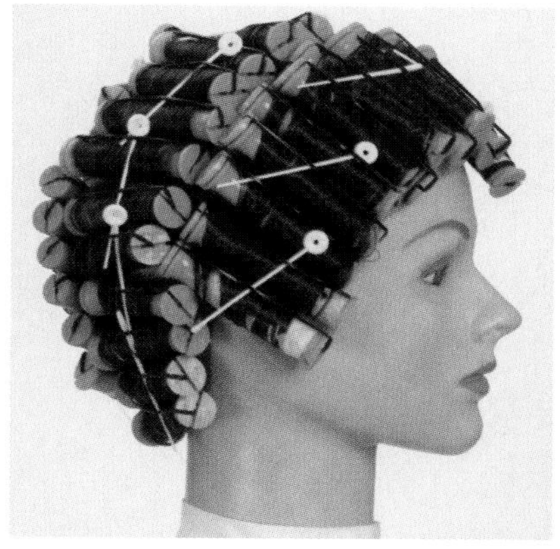

Figure 15-39 Curvature perm wrapping pattern.

The **bricklay perm wrap** is similar to the actual technique of bricklaying. Base sections are offset from each other row by row, to prevent noticeable splits and to blend the flow of the hair. Different bricklay patterns use different starting points (front hairline, occipital area, and crown), and these starting points affect the directional flow of the hair. The bricklay perm wrap can be used with different combinations of sectioning, base control, base direction, wrapping techniques, and perm tools (Figure 15–40).

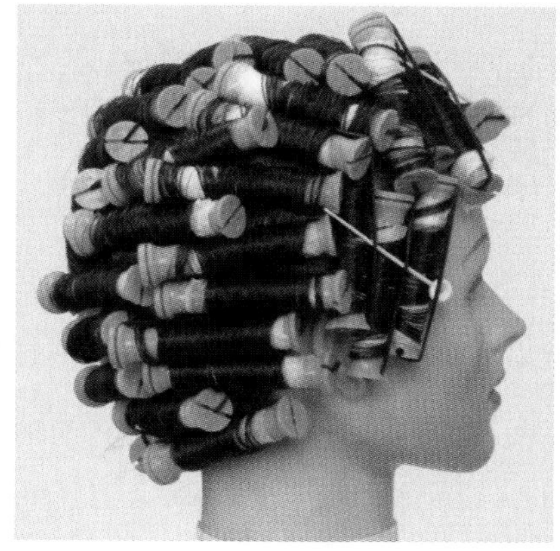

Figure 15-40 Bricklay perm wrapping pattern.

The **weave technique** uses zigzag partings to divide base areas. It can be used throughout the entire perm wrap or can be kept to selected areas. This technique is very effective for blending between perm rods with opposite base directions. It can also be used to create a smooth transition from the rolled areas into the unrolled areas of a partial perm. The weave technique can be used with a variety of base directions, wrapping patterns, and perm tools (Figure 15–41).

The **double tool technique** is also called a **piggyback wrap** because two tools are used for one strand of hair, one on top of the other. The lower half of the strand is wrapped around one tool, and then the upper half of the same strand is wrapped around a second tool and stacked on top of the first (Figure 15–42).

The double tool technique doubles the number of tools used. Using more tools increases the amount of curl in the finished perm, making this technique especially effective on long hair. Tools with different diameters may be used to create different effects. This technique can also be used with a variety of base directions, wrapping patterns, and perm tools.

Unlike other techniques that are performed at an angle perpendicular to the length of the tool, the **spiral perm technique,** also called a spiral perm wrap is done at an angle that causes the hair to spiral along the length of the tool, like the grip on a tennis racquet (see Figure 15–18). Although the

insights

Floyd Kenyatta

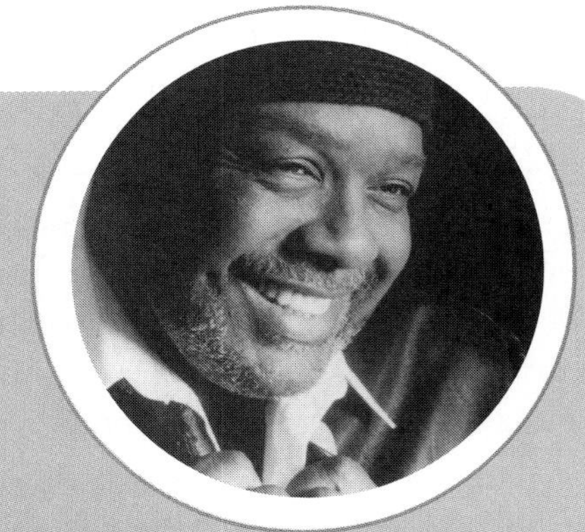

Working in the beauty industry is about working with people. Motivating and managing people is the specialty of Floyd Kenyatta, Global Ambassador for John Paul Mitchell Systems and CEO of Kenta Salon Designs.

I entered the industry in 1969. My father, a minister, suggested that I find some kind of work that would allow me to be my own boss, so I had that in the back of my mind. Then I was working at a Playboy Club in Manhattan and one of the bunnies told me how her boyfriend, who owned a beauty school, made a lot of money. I liked the idea of being in a nice, clean environment like that and working with women, because I love women, and so I made up my mind.

But getting through beauty school was my greatest challenge. It's supposed to be a six-month course, but it took me two years because I was working to put myself through school.

I haven't worked behind the chair since 1984. I still own salons, but what I really love is education. I am a motivational speaker and have trained 800 educators for John Paul Mitchell Systems.

The greatest fulfillment I have found is in having the knowledge and the power to transform people. There's nothing more exciting than seeing the tears of joy running down the face of a person who's so delighted with the new image you have created for her. One thing you must realize about styling is that lots of times, clients come to you for an uplift, and that uplift starts with your ability to make them feel good about themselves mentally. Being the best hairdresser is not just about giving the best haircut. Being the best is about being the strongest in natural people skills.

When it comes to managing, the most challenging thing is to develop your people skills to the point where you are sharp enough to identify the type of person you need to stay away from. I believe in the philosophy that you cannot shine a pair of sneakers. You cannot motivate a cabbage. You have to be able to evaluate people quickly so you know if it's worthwhile to invest your time and energy in trying to make them be an asset for you. And you have to be an asset to yourself.

If I were a young stylist starting out today, I would look for a salon that offers continuous education. Cosmetology school prepares you for the state board. Once you pass your state board, then you find out what the real world is all about.

layers in a spiral perm may partially overlap as they go along, as long as the angle remains constant, any overlap will be uniform along the length of the tool and the entire stand of hair. Since the effective size of the tool remains constant along the entire strand of hair, this technique produces a uniform curl from the scalp to the ends. Longer, thicker hair will benefit most from this effect (Figure 15–43).

The spiral wrapping technique can be used with a variety of base sections, base directions, and wrapping patterns. Base sections may be either horizontal or vertical and do not affect the finished curl. Conventional rods, bendable soft foam rods, and the circle tool can all be used for this technique, depending on the length of the hair.

The implements and materials and the procedures for preparation, processing, and cleanup are the same for all perms, as described in the Basic Perm Wrap.

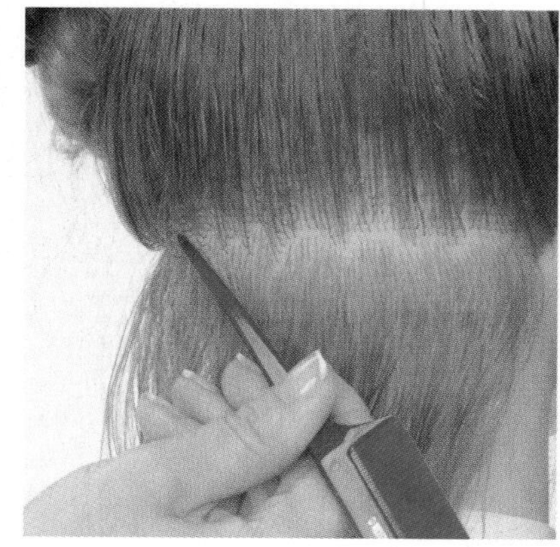

Figure 15-41 Weave technique.

Preliminary Test Curls

Taking preliminary test curls helps you predict how your client's hair will react to a perm. It is advisable to take preliminary test curls if the hair is damaged or if there is any uncertainty about the results. Preliminary test curls provide the following information:

- correct processing time for optimal curl development
- results you can expect from the type of perm solution you have selected
- curl results for the tool size and wrapping technique you are planning to use

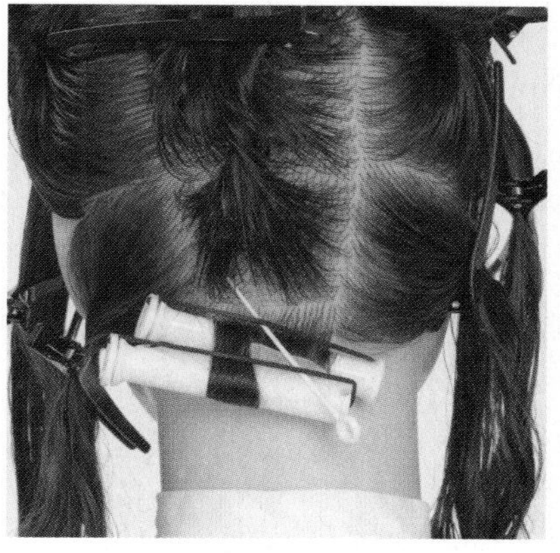

Figure 15-42 Double tool perm technique.

Partial Perms

If your client wants a perm but does not wish for the entire head of hair to be curled, a partial perm may be the answer. Partial perms also allow you to give a perm when some of the hair is too short to roll on tools. Partial perms can be used for:

- male and female clients who have long hair on the top and crown, but very short hair with tapered sides and nape.
- clients who only need volume and lift in certain areas.
- clients who desire a hairstyle with curls along the perimeter but a smooth, sleek crown.

Partial perms rely on the same techniques and wrapping patterns as those used with other perms, but there are some additional considerations.

- In order to make a smooth transition from the rolled section to the unrolled section, use a larger tool for the last tool next to an unrolled section.
- Applying waving lotion to unrolled hair may straighten it or make it difficult to style. To protect the unrolled hair, apply a protective barrier cream to the unrolled section before applying the waving lotion.

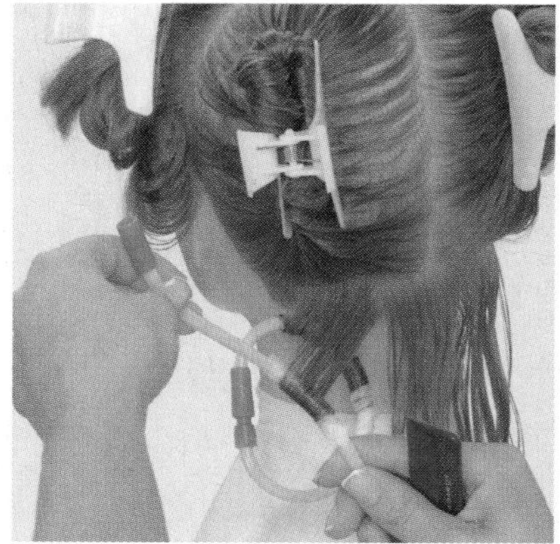

Figure 15-43 Spiral perm technique.

PROCEDURE

BASIC PERM

Implements and Materials

The following is a general list of the implements and materials used in permanent waving.

- perm solution
- neutralizer
- acid-balanced shampoo (optional)
- preneutralizing conditioner (optional)
- conditioner (optional)
- protective barrier cream
- applicator bottles
- perm tools
- shampoo cape
- towels
- neutralizing bib
- roll cotton
- plastic clips for sectioning
- styling comb
- plastic rattail comb
- end papers
- roller picks (optional)
- spray bottle
- disposable gloves
- timer

Preparation for All Perms

1. Wash your hands.
2. Conduct a client consultation and evaluation. Fill out the client's perm record. Note any changes in the client's history (Figure 15–44).
3. Perform an analysis of the client's hair and scalp.
4. Have the client change into a gown and remove eyeglasses, earrings, and necklace.
5. Drape the client for shampoo.
6. Gently shampoo and towel-dry hair. Avoid irritating the client's scalp.
7. Perform a preliminary test curl procedure.

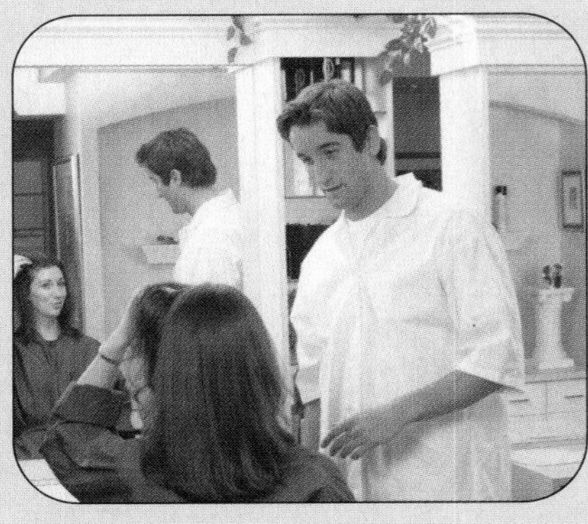

Figure 15–44 Client consultation.

Procedure for Preliminary Test Curls

1. Wrap one tool in each different area of the head (the top, the side, and the nape) (Figure 15–45).
2. Wrap a coil of cotton around each tool.
3. Apply waving lotion to the wrapped curls. Do not allow waving lotion to come into contact with unwrapped hair (Figure 15–46).
4. Set a timer and process according to the manufacturer's directions.
5. Check each test curl frequently for proper curl development. Unfasten the tool and unwind the curl about 1 ½ turns of the tool. Do not allow the hair to become loose or completely unwound. Gently move the tool toward the scalp to encourage the hair to fall loosely into the wave pattern.
6. Curl development is complete when a firm and definite "S" is formed that reflects the size of the tool used. Different hair textures will have slightly different "S" formations. The wave pattern for fine, thin hair may be weak, with little definition. The wave pattern for coarse, thick hair is usually stronger and better defined (Figure 15–47).
7. When the curl has been formed, rinse thoroughly with warm water for at least five minutes, blot thoroughly, apply neutralizer, and process according to the manufacturer's directions. Gently dry the hair and evaluate the results. Do not proceed with the permanent if the test curls are extremely damaged or overprocessed. If the test curl resuts are satisfactory, proceed with the perm, but *DO NOT re-perm these preliminary test curls.*

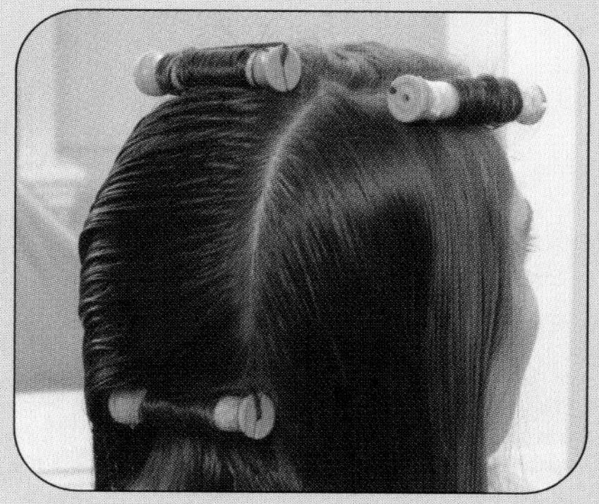

Figure 15–45 Wrap rods in three areas of the head.

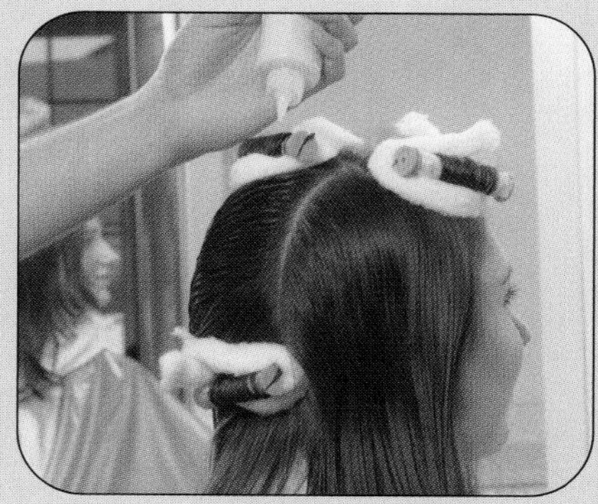

Figure 15–46 Apply waving lotion to test curls.

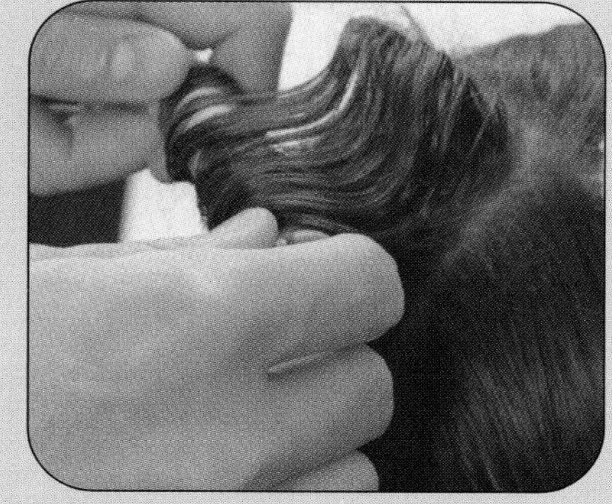

Figure 15–47 S formation.

15

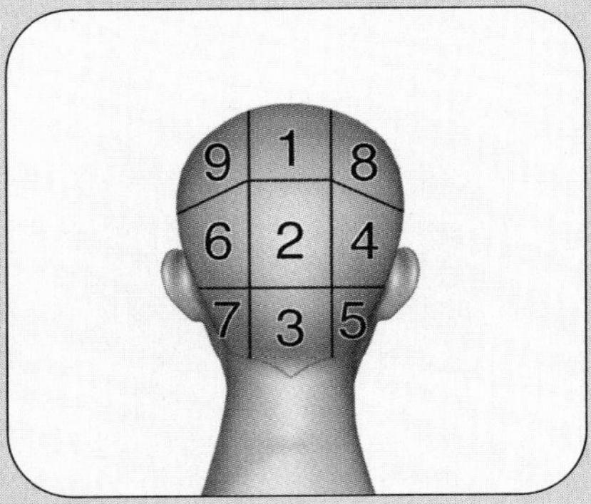

Figure 15-48a Wrapping pattern.

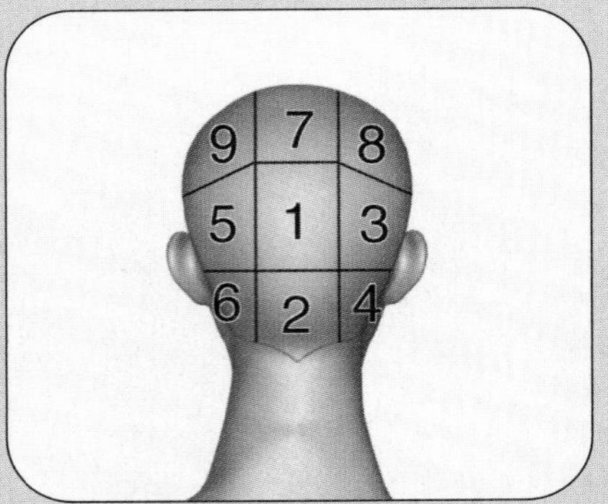

Figure 15-48b Alternate wrapping pattern.

Procedure for Basic Perm Wrap (Straight Set Wrap)

1. Divide the hair into nine panels (Figure 15-48a and Figure 15-48b). Use the length of the tool to measure the width of the panels. Remember to keep the hair wet as you wrap.
2. Begin wrapping at the front hairline or crown. Make a horizontal parting the same size as the tool. Using two end papers, roll the hair down to the scalp in the direction of hair growth and position the tool half-off base (Figure 15-49). The band should be smooth, not twisted, and should be fastened straight across the top of the tool (Figure 15-50). Excessive tension may cause band marks or hair breakage. Continue wrapping the remainder of the first panel using the same technique (Figure 15-51). *Option*: Insert roller picks to stabilize the tools. Although roller picks may be used to eliminate any tension caused by the band, they will not compensate for a poorly wrapped perm. If roller picks are not used correctly, they can cause the same damage as the incorrect placement of the rubber band.
3. Continue wrapping the remaining eight panels in numerical order, holding the hair at a 90-degree angle (Figure 15-52).

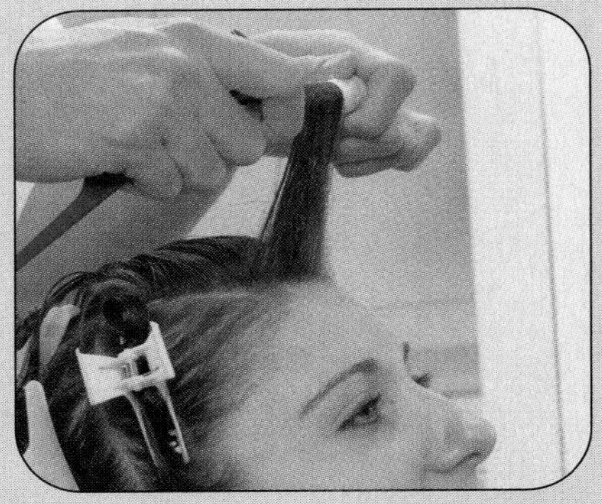

Figure 15-49 Roll the hair down to the scalp.

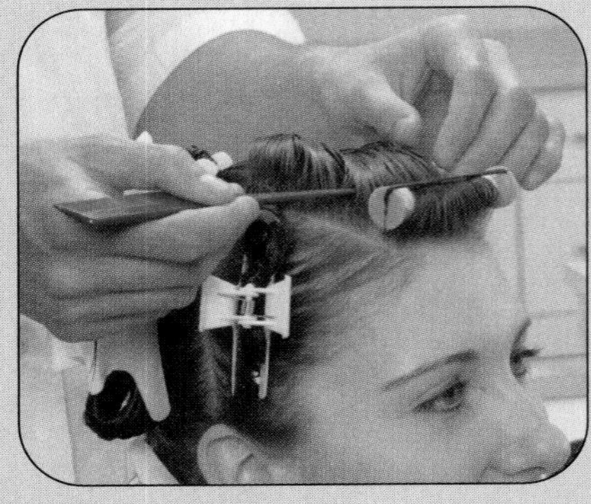

Figure 15-50 Position rod half off base.

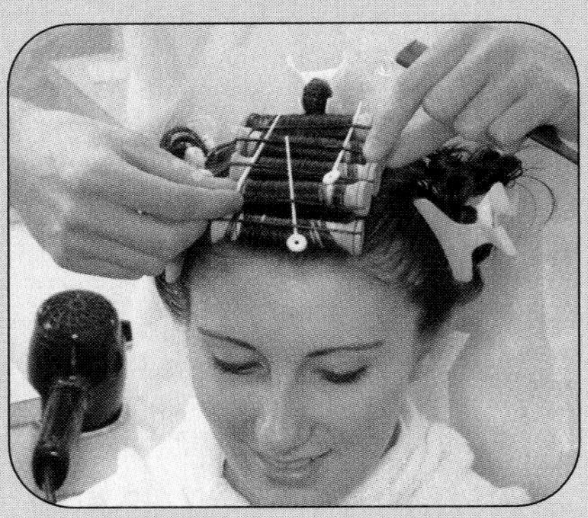

Figure 15-51 Finished first panel.

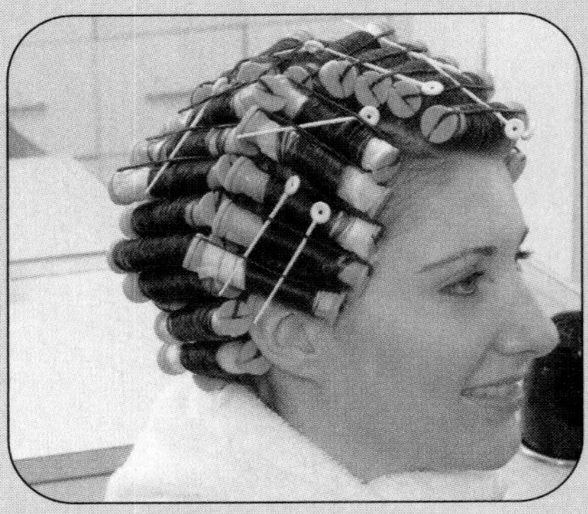

Figure 15-52 Completed basic perm wrap.

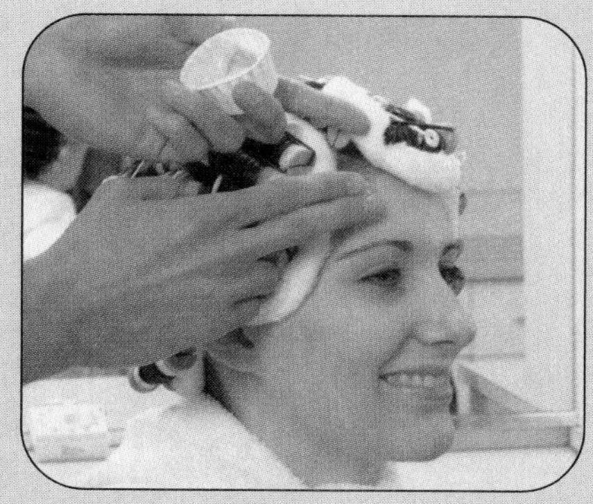

Figure 15-53 Apply base cream and cotton.

Procedure for Processing Permanents

1. Apply protective barrier cream to the hairline and the ears. Apply roll cotton around the entire hairline and offer the client a towel to blot any drips (Figure 15–53).
2. Slowly and carefully apply the perm solution with a bottle to the hair on each tool. Ask the client to lean forward while you apply solution to the back area, and then ask the client to lean back as you apply solution to the front and sides. Avoid splashing and dripping. Continue to apply the solution slowly until each tool is completely saturated (Figure 15–54).
3. If a plastic cap is used, punch a few holes in the cap and cover all the hair completely. Do not allow the plastic cap to touch the client's skin (Figure 15–55).
4. Check cotton and towels. If they are saturated with solution, replace them.
5. Process according to the manufacturer's directions. Processing time varies according to the strength of the solution, the hair type and condition, and the desired results. Processing usually takes less than 20 minutes at room temperature.
6. Check frequently for curl development. Unwind the tool and check the "S" pattern formation described in the preliminary test curl procedure (Figure 15–56).
7. When processing is completed, rinse the hair thoroughly for at least five minutes, then towel-blot the hair on each tool to remove any excess moisture (Figure 15–57 and Figure 15–58). Another option that some manufacturers recommend is to apply a preneutralizing conditioner to the hair, after rinsing and blotting and before applying the neutralizer. Remember, though, that this step is optional. Always follow the manufacturers' directions and the procedures approved by your instructor.

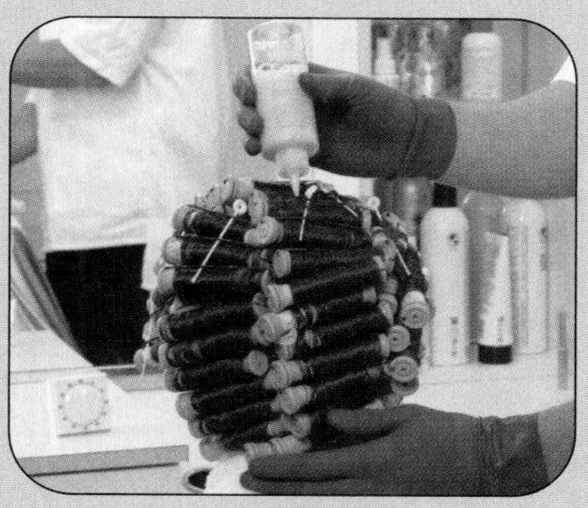

Figure 15-54 Apply perm solution.

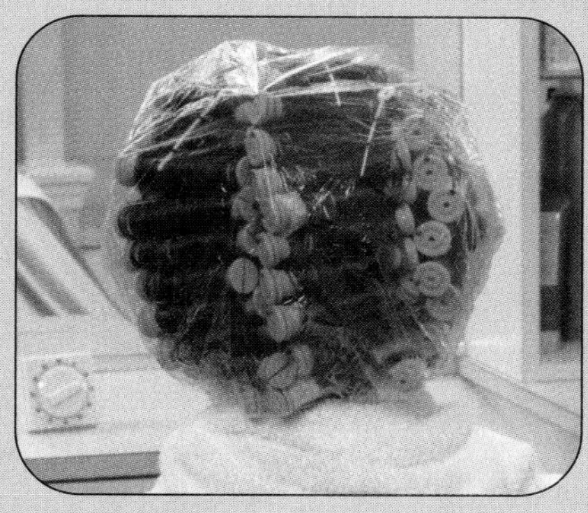

Figure 15-55 Cover head with plastic cap.

15

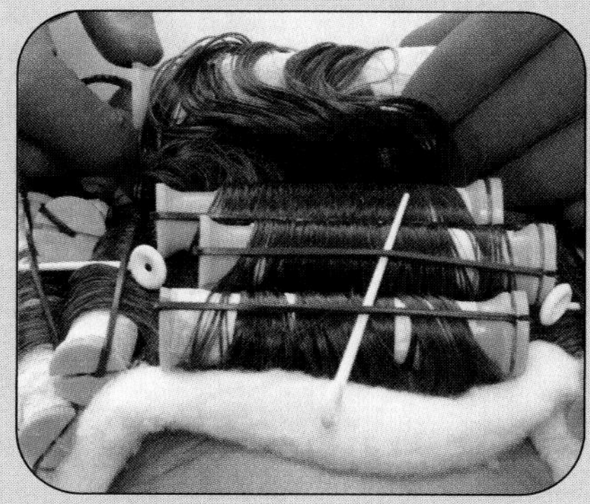

Figure 15-56 Take a test curl.

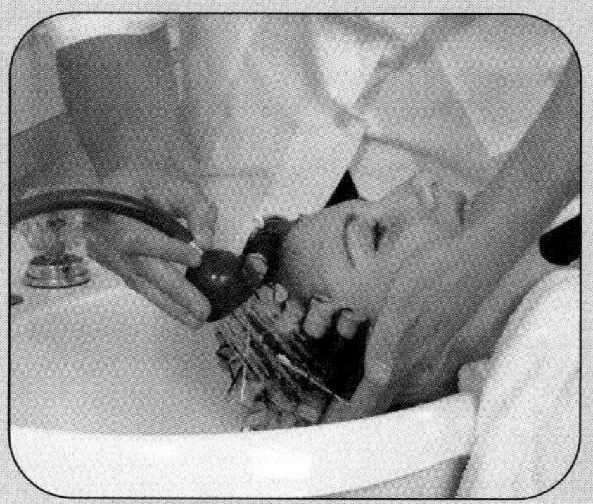

Figure 15-57 Rinse waving solution from hair.

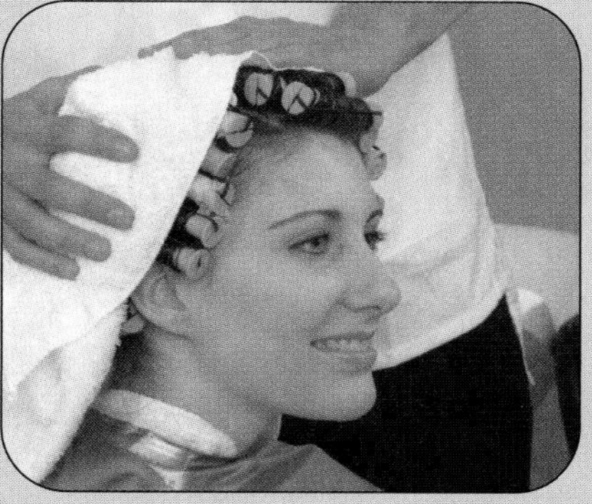

Figure 15-58 Towel-blot the hair.

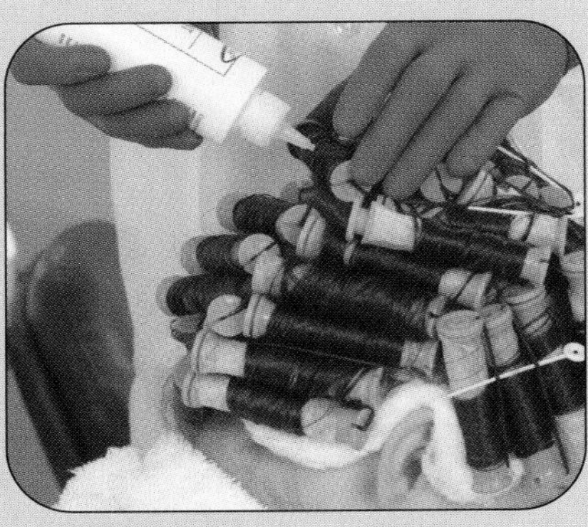

Figure 15–59 Apply neutralizer.

8. Apply the neutralizer slowly and carefully to the hair on each tool. Ask the client to lean forward while you apply solution to the back area, then to lean back as you apply solution to the front and sides. Avoid splashing and dripping. Continue to apply the neutralizer until each tool is completely saturated (Figure 15–59).
9. Set a timer for the amount of time specified by the manufacturer. After processing, remove the tools and work the remaining neutralizer through the hair gently with your hands.
10. Rinse thoroughly. It is optional, at this point, to also shampoo and condition. Always follow the manufacturers' directions and the procedures approved by your instructor.
11. Style the hair as desired (Figure 15–60).

Cleanup and Sanitation

1. Discard disposable supplies in appropriate receptacles.
2. Sanitize implements and store according to sanitation requirements.
3. Clean, sanitize, and prepare your workstation for the next service.
4. Wash your hands thoroughly with soap and warm water.
5. Complete the client record.

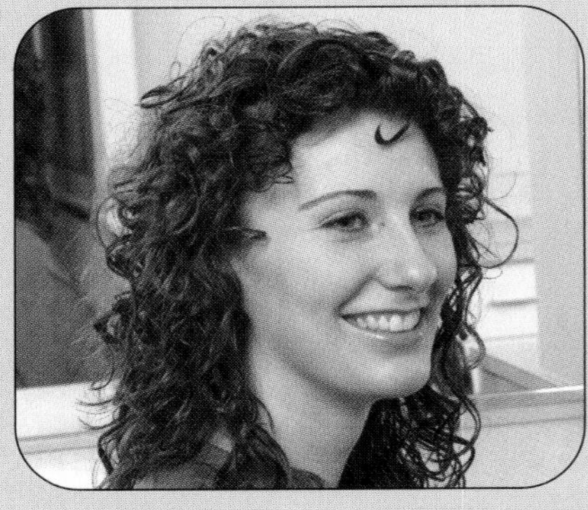

Figure 15–60 Styled basic perm.

completed! 

PROCEDURE

CURVATURE PERM WRAP

Implements and Materials

Same as for Procedure 30—basic perm.

Preparation

Same as for Procedure 30—basic perm.

Procedure

1. Begin sectioning at the front hairline on one side of the part. Comb the hair in the direction of growth, then section out individual panels to match the length of the rod (Figure 15–61).
2. Alternate from side to side as you section out all the curvature panels over the entire head. Sectioning the panels in advance creates a road map that provides direction and gives continuity to the wrapping pattern (Figure 15–62).
3. Begin wrapping the first panel at the front hairline, on one side of the part. Comb out a base section the same width as the diameter of the rod. The base direction should point away from the face. Hold the hair at a 90-degree angle to the head. Using two end papers, roll the hair down to the scalp and position the rod half-off base (Figure 15–63).

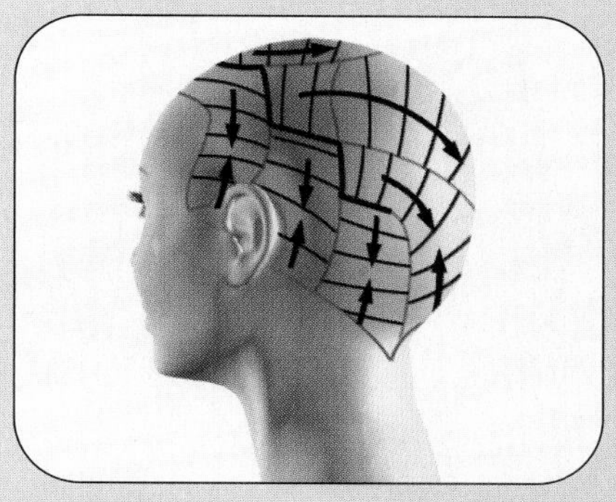

Figure 15-61 Sectioning diagram for curvature wrap.

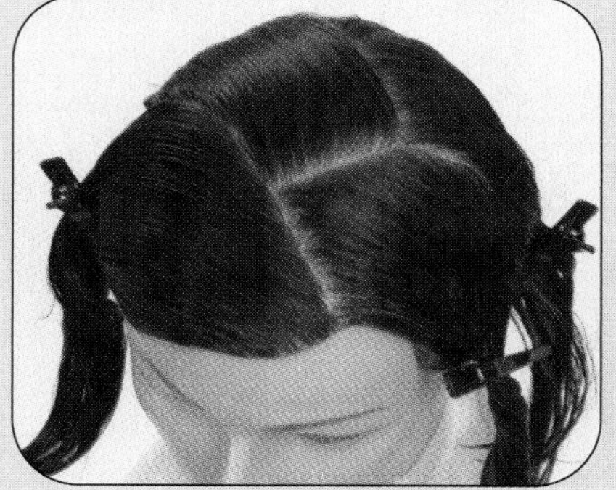

Figure 15-62 Section all the panels.

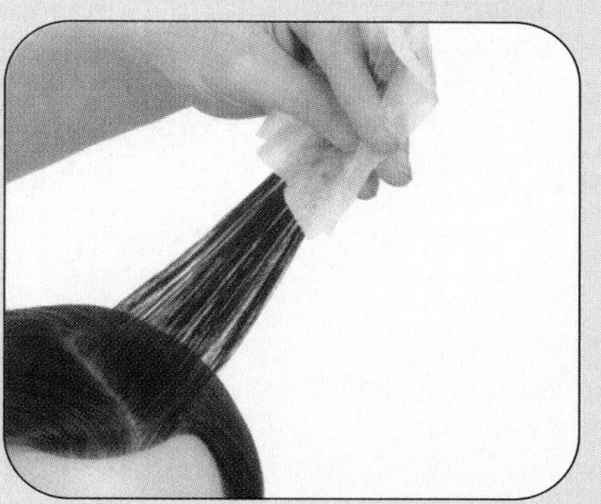

Figure 15-63 Wrap first rod at front hairline.

15

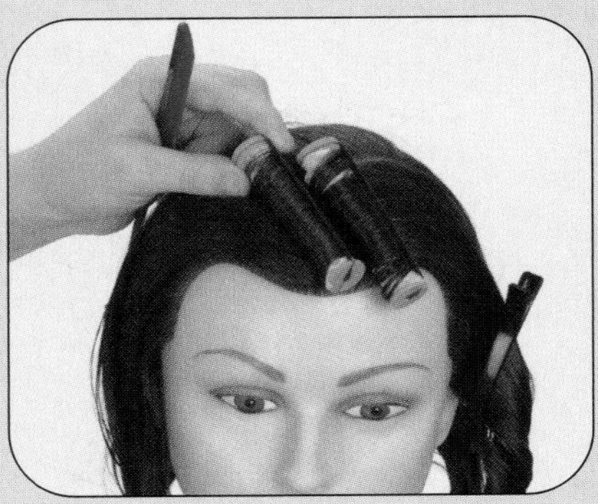

Figure 15-64 Wrap second rod.

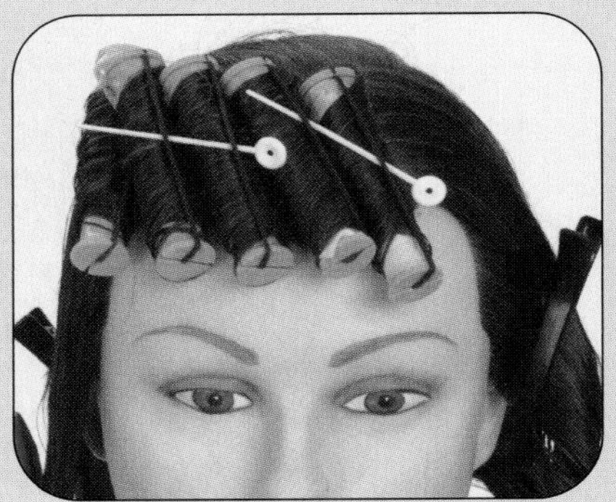

Figure 15-65 Picks can be used to stabilize the rods.

4. The remaining base sections in the panel should be wider on the outside of the panel (the side farthest away from the face). Continue wrapping the rest of the rods in the panel, alternating rod diameters (Figure 15–64). *Option*: Insert picks to stabilize the rods and to eliminate any tension caused by the band (Figure 15–65).
5. When you reach the last rod at the hairline, comb the hair flat at the base and change the base direction. Direct the rod up and toward the base, keeping the base area flat (Figure 15–66).
6. Continue with panel two, which is the front panel on the other side of the part. Repeat the same procedure as on the first panel (Figure 15–67).
7. Continue with the third panel, which is the panel behind and next to the first panel. Repeat the same procedure until you reach the last two rods at the hairline. Comb the hair flat at the base and change the base direction. Direct the last two rods up and toward the base, keeping the base area flat (Figure 15–68).
8. Continue with the fourth panel, on the opposite side of the head, behind and next to the second panel. Repeat the same procedure you used with the third panel.

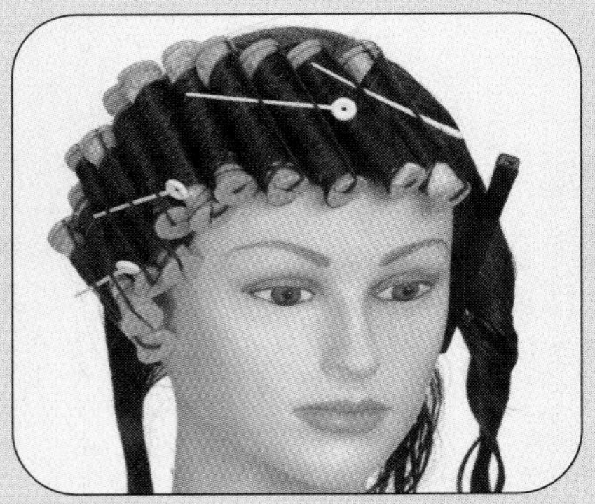

Figure 15-66 Wrap last rod in panel.

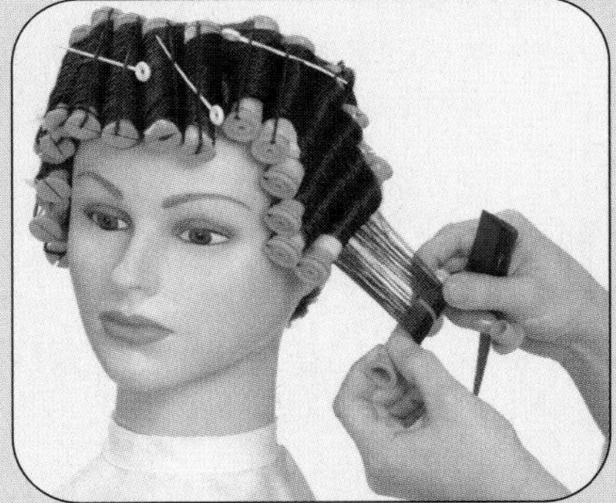

Figure 15-67 The second panel.

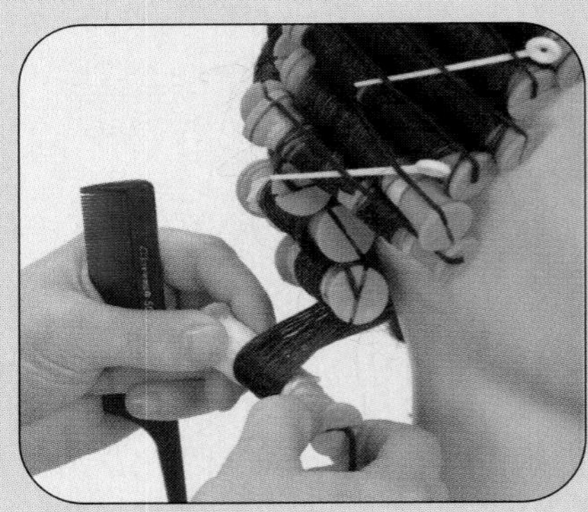

Figure 15-68 The third panel.

9. Follow the same procedure with the fifth panel. The base direction should remain consistent with the pattern already established. The base direction in the back flows around and contours to the perimeter hairline area.
10. All panels should fit the curvature of the head and should blend into the surrounding panels (Figure 15–69).
11. Process and style the hair (Figure 15–70).
12. Follow cleanup and sanitation procedures for Procedure 30—basic perm.

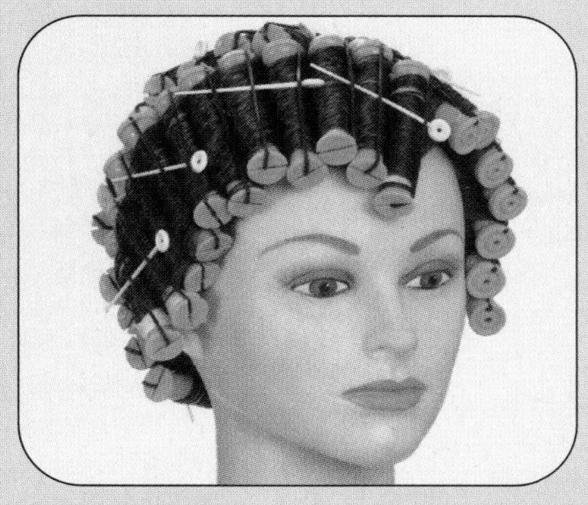

Figure 15-69 Finish wrapping all panels.

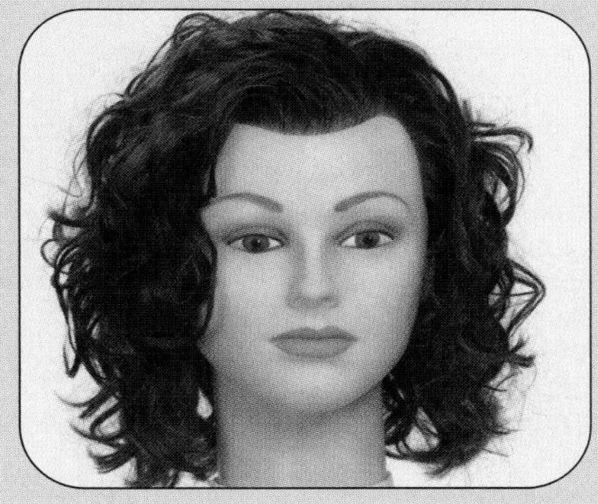

Figure 15-70 Finished and styled curvature perm.

completed!

PROCEDURE

BRICKLAY PERM WRAP

Implements and Materials

Same as for Procedure 30—basic perm.

Preparation

Same as for Procedure 30—basic perm.

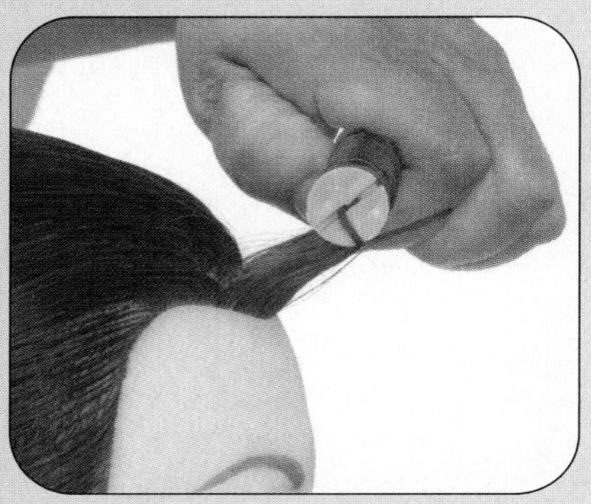

Figure 15-71 Wrap first rod.

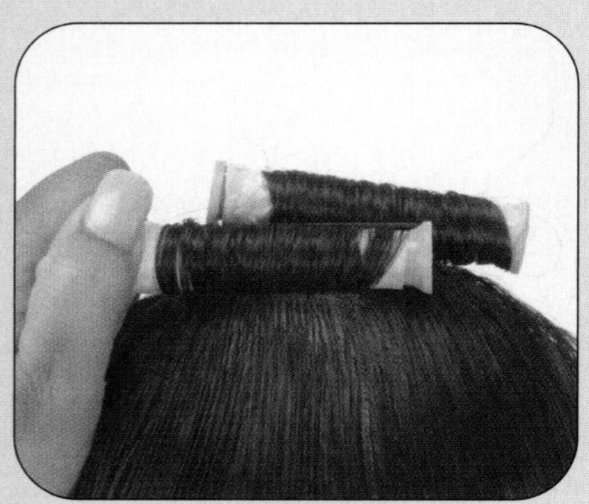

Figure 15-72 Wrap second rod in second row.

Procedure

1. Begin by parting out a base section parallel to the front hairline that is the length and width of the rod being used. The base direction is back, away from the face. Hold the hair at a 90-degree angle to the head. Using two end papers, roll the hair down to the scalp and position the rod half-off base (Figure 15–71).
2. In the second row directly behind the first rod, part out two base sections for two rods offset from the center of the first rod. Hold the hair at a 90-degree angle to the head. Using two end papers, roll the hair down to the scalp and position the rods half-off-base (Figure 15–72). *Option*: Insert picks to stabilize rods and eliminate any tension caused by the band.
3. Begin the third row by parting out a base section at the point where the two rods meet in the previous row. This same pattern is used throughout the entire wrap (Figure 15–73).
4. Continue to part out rows that radiate around the curve of the head through the crown area. Extend rows around and down to the side hairline, parting out base sections at the center of the point where the two tools meet in the previous row (Figure 15–74).

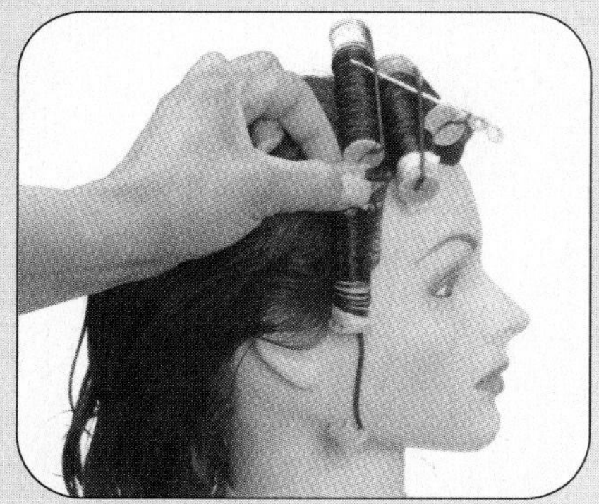

Figure 15-73 Third row.

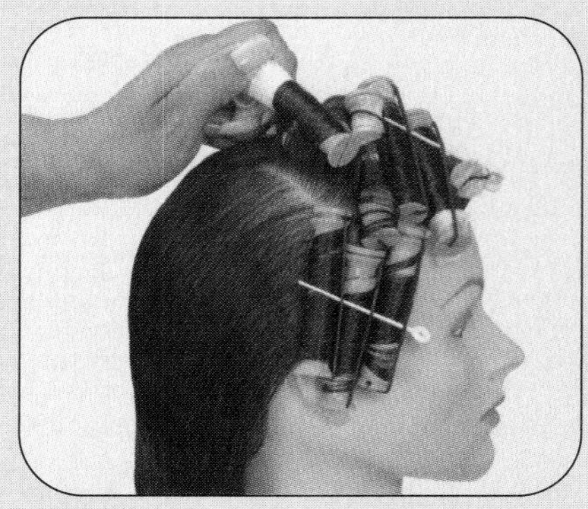

Figure 15-74 Side hairline.

5. Stop the curving rows after you have finished wrapping the crown area. Part out horizontal sections throughout the back of the head and continue with the bricklay pattern. You may need to change the length of the rods from row to row to maintain the pattern (Figure 15–75).
6. Process and style the hair (Figure 15–76).
7. Follow cleanup and sanitation procedures for Procedure 30—basic perm.

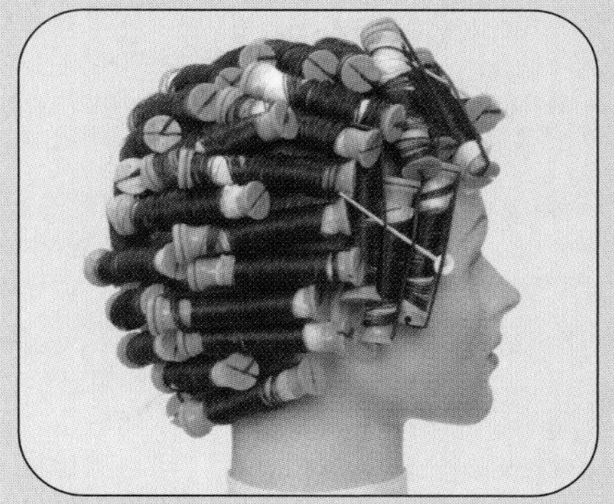

Figure 15–75 Completed bricklay wrap.

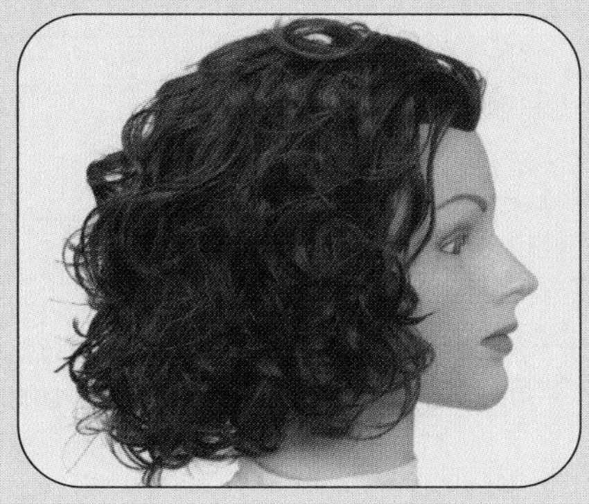

Figure 15–76 Finished and styled bricklay perm.

completed!

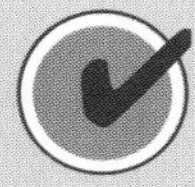

PROCEDURE

WEAVE TECHNIQUE

The weave technique can be used with any of the wrapping patterns in this chapter.

Implements and Materials

Same as for Procedure 30—basic perm.

Preparation

Same as for Procedure 30—basic perm.

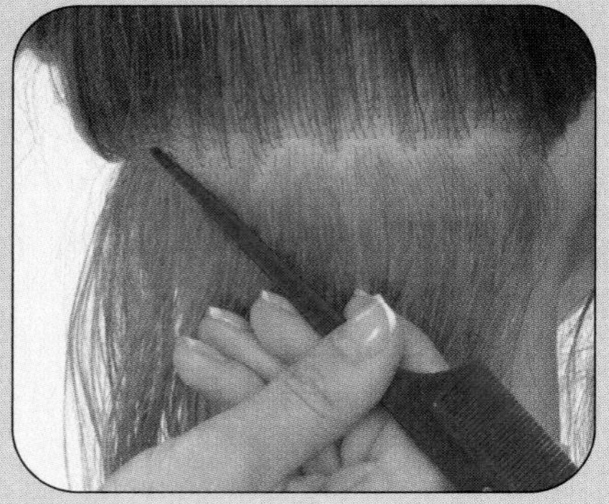

Figure 15–77 Make zigzag parting in base section.

Procedure

1. Part out one base section the same size as two rods. Comb the entire base section at a 90-degree angle to the head and use a rattail comb to make a zigzag parting along the length of the base section (Figure 15–77).
2. Using two end papers, roll half of the strand down to the scalp (Figure 15–78). Comb the remaining half of the base section at a 90-degree angle, use two end papers, and roll the strand down to the scalp (Figure 15–79). *Option*: Secure the rods and insert picks to stabilize the rods and to eliminate any tension caused by the band.
3. Continue with the same procedure in any sections where the effect is desired (Figure 15–80).
4. After processing and styling, follow cleanup and sanitation procedures for basic perm.

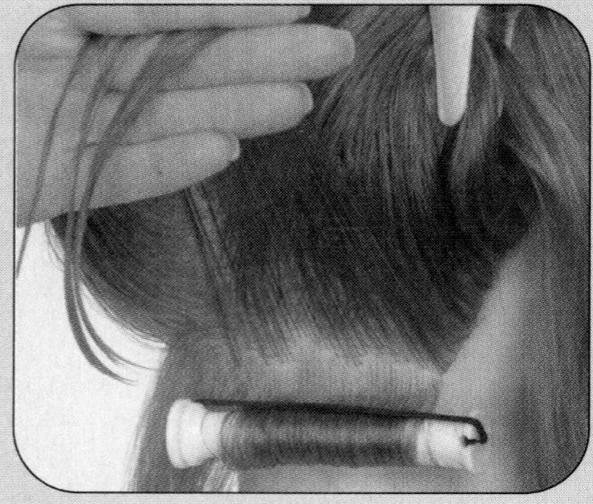

Figure 15–78 Wrap the first rod.

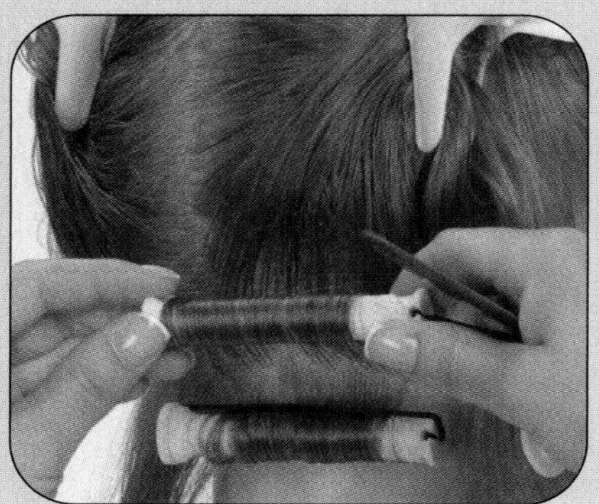

Figure 15–79 Wrap the second rod.

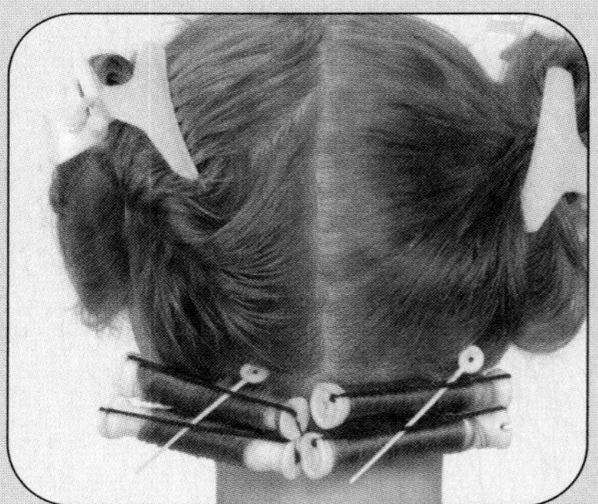

Figure 15–80 Finished weave technique.

completed!

PROCEDURE

DOUBLE TOOL (PIGGYBACK) TECHNIQUE

The double tool (piggyback) technique can be used with any of the wrapping patterns in this chapter.

Implements and Materials

Same as for Procedure 30—basic perm.

Preparation

Same as for Procedure 30—basic perm.

Procedure

1. Begin by placing the base rod in the middle of the strand. Wrap the end of the strand one revolution around the rod while holding it to one side (Figure 15–81). Roll the rod to the base area, letting the loose ends follow as you roll (Figure 15–82). *Option*: Insert picks to stabilize the rods and to eliminate any tension caused by the band.
2. Place two end papers on the ends of the strand and position a rod to roll from the ends toward the base area (Figure 15–83). Secure the end rod on top of the base rod (Figure 15–84).

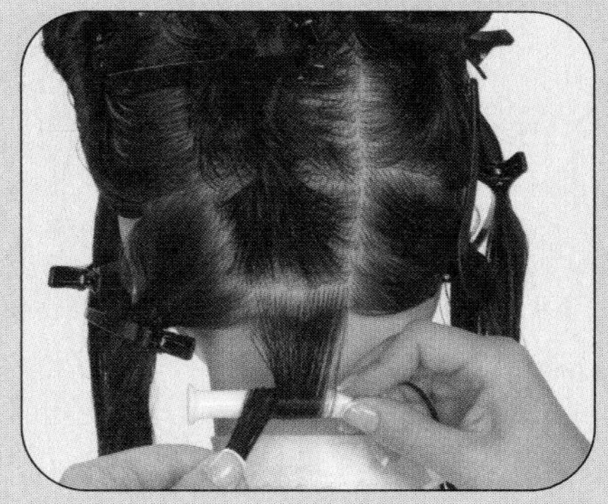

Figure 15-81 Wrap the end of the strand.

15

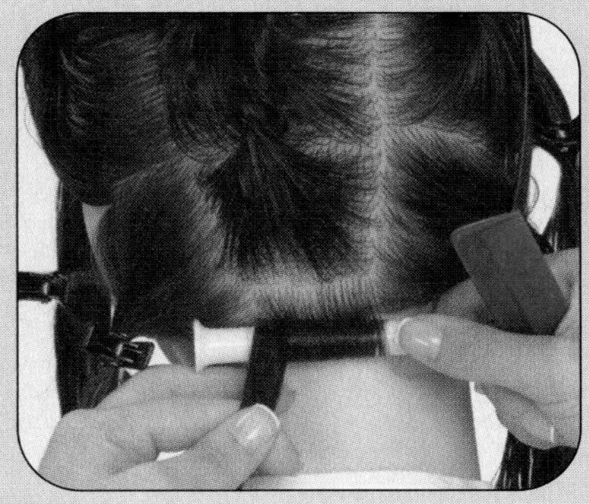

Figure 15-82 Secure rod.

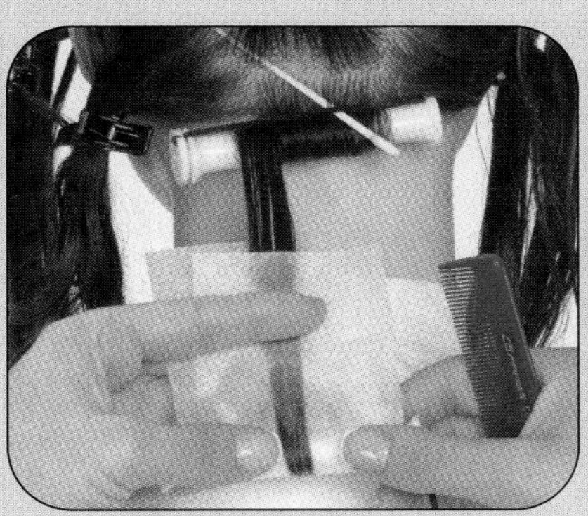

Figure 15-83 Wrap second rod on hair ends.

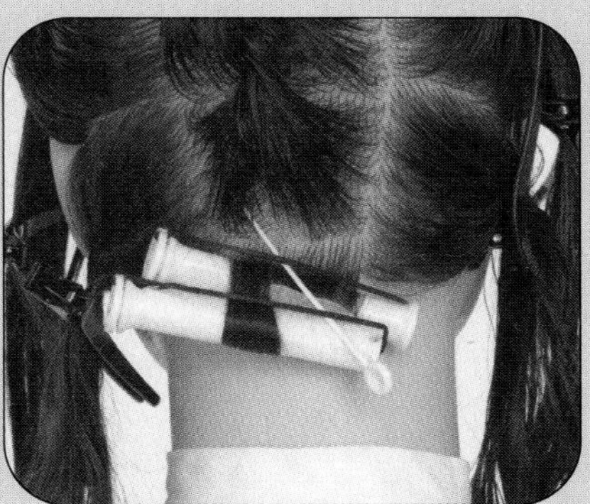

Figure 15-84 Secure end rod on base rod.

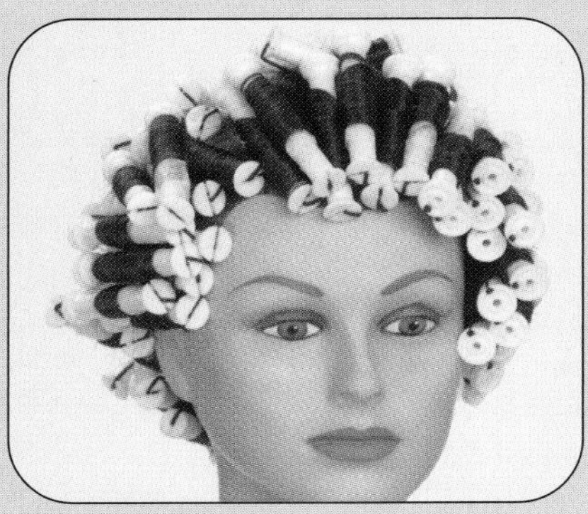

Figure 15-85a Completed double-tool wrap.

3. Depending on the length and size of the rods, it may be possible to roll as many as three end strands together on the same end rod.
4. Continue with the same procedure in any sections where the effect is desired (Figure 15-85a).
5. Process and style the hair (Figure 15-85b).
6. Follow cleanup and sanitation procedures for Procedure 30—basic perm.

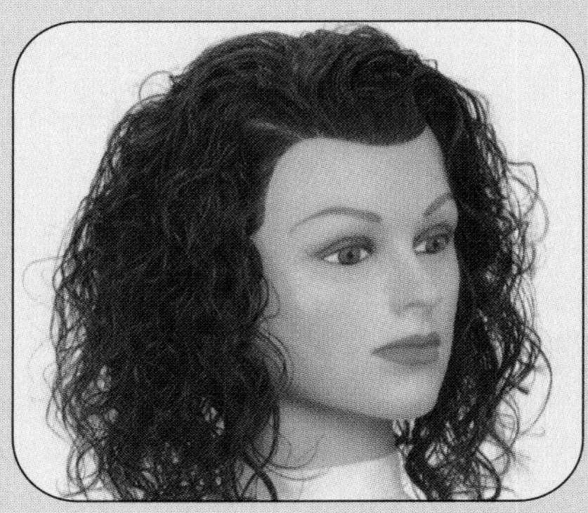

Figure 15-85b Finished and styled double-tool perm.

15

completed! 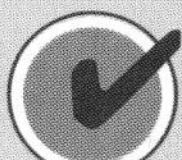

PROCEDURE

SPIRAL PERM TECHNIQUE

Implements and Materials

Same as for Procedure 30—basic perm.

Preparation

Same as for Procedure 30—basic perm.

Procedure

1. Part the hair into four panels, from the center of the front hairline to the center of the nape and from ear to ear. Section out a fifth panel from ear to ear in the nape area (Figure 15–86).
2. Section out the first row along the hairline in the nape area. Comb the remainder of the hair up and secure it out of the way.
3. Part out the first base section on one side of the first row. Hold the hair at a 90-degree angle to the head. Using one or two end papers, begin wrapping at one end of the tool. Starting the wrap from the right or left side of the tool will orient the curl in that direction (Figure 15–87).
4. Roll the first two full turns at a 90-degree angle to the tool to secure the ends of the hair, and then start spiraling the hair on the tool by changing the angle to an angle other than 90 degrees (Figure 15–88). Continue to spiral the hair toward the other end of the tool. Roll the hair down to the scalp, position the tool half off base, and secure it by fastening the ends of the tool together (Figure 15–89).

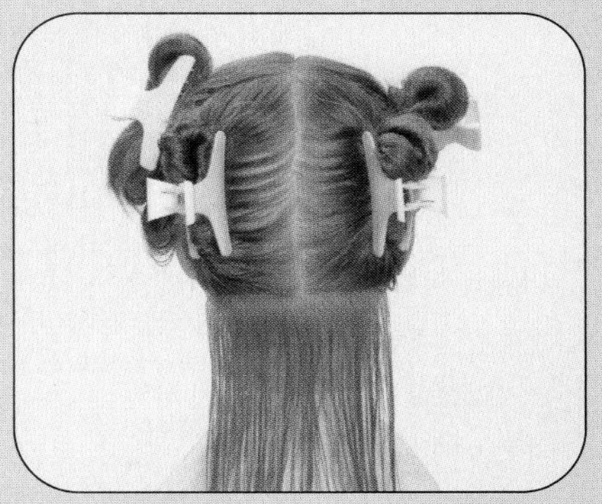

Figure 15-86 Part hair into four sections.

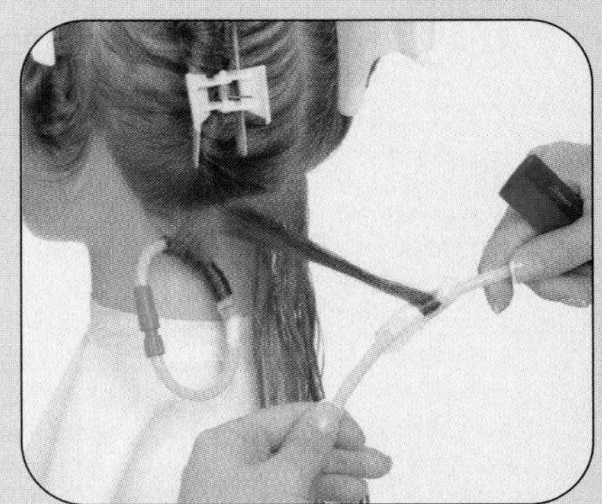

Figure 15-87 Wrap the first two turns.

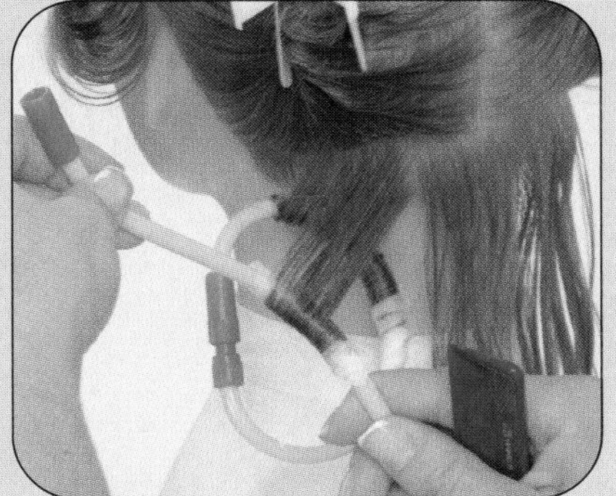

Figure 15-88 Wrap the same tool at an angle.

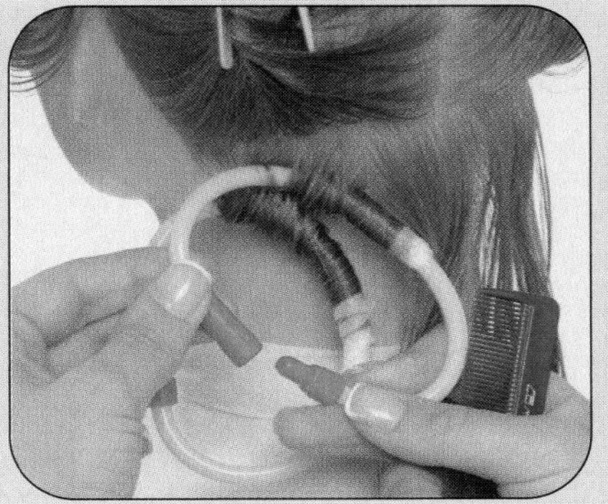

Figure 15-89 Fasten ends of tool together.

15

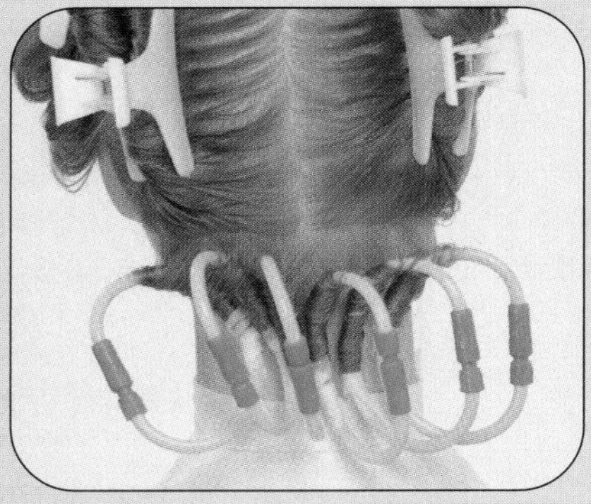

Figure 15-90 Completed first row.

5. Continue wrapping with the same technique, in the same direction, until the first row is completed (Figure 15-90).
6. Section out the second row above and parallel to the first row. Comb the remainder of the hair up and secure it to keep it out of the way.
7. Begin wrapping at the opposite side from the side where the first row began, and move in the direction opposite the direction established in the first row (Figure 15-91).
8. Follow the same procedure to wrap the second row but begin wrapping each tool at the opposite end established in the first row. Continue wrapping with the same technique, in the same direction, until the second row is completed (Figure 15-92).
9. Section out the third row above and parallel to the second row. Follow the same wrapping procedure, alternating the rows from left to right as you move up the head. This will alternate the orientation of the curl throughout the head (Figure 15-93).
10. Process and style the hair (Figure 15-94).
11. After processing and styling, follow cleanup and sanitation procedures for Procedure 30—basic perm.

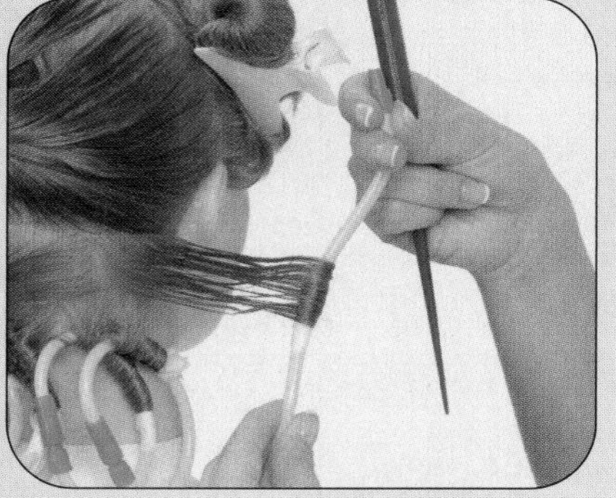

Figure 15-91 Begin second row.

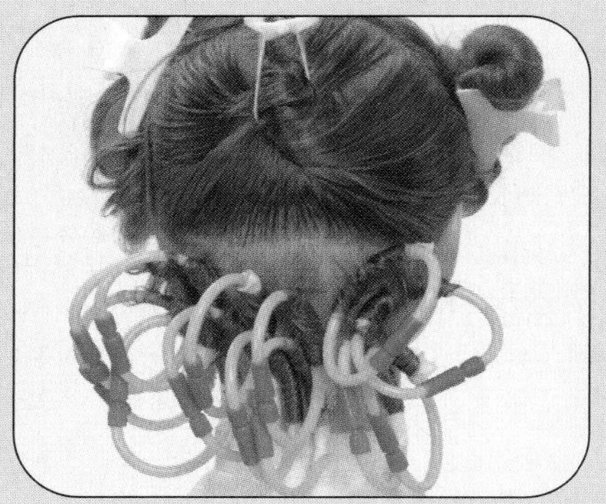

Figure 15-92 Second row.

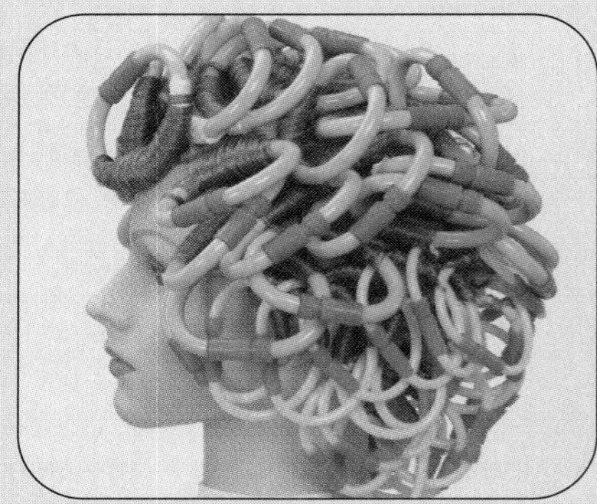

Figure 15-93 Completed spiral wrap.

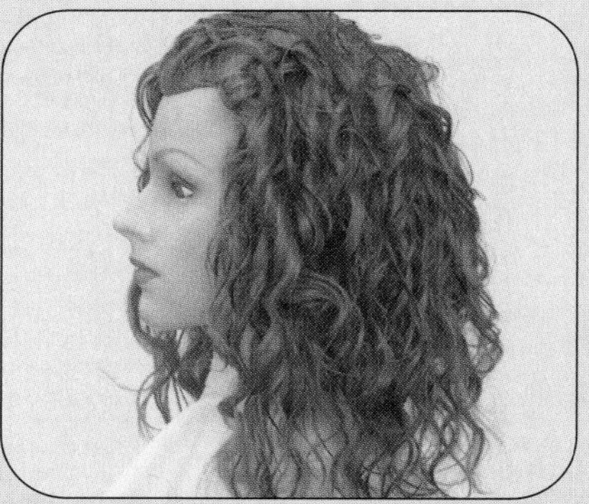

Figure 15-94 Finished styled spiral perm.

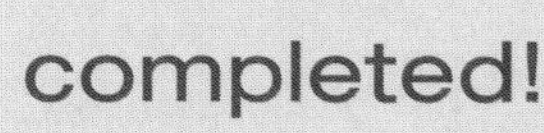

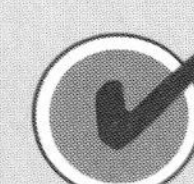

Perms for Men

Do not assume that perms are only for women. Many male clients are looking for the added texture, fullness, style, and low maintenance that only a perm can provide. Perms help thin hair look fuller, make straight or coarse hair more manageable, and help control stubborn cowlicks. Although men's and women's hairstyles may be different, the techniques for permanent waving are essentially the same.

CHEMICAL HAIR RELAXERS

Chemical hair relaxing is the process of rearranging the basic structure of extremely curly hair into a straight form. Whereas permanent waving curls straight hair, chemical hair relaxing straightens curly hair (Figure 15–95). Other than their objectives being so different, the two services are very similar. In fact, the chemistry of thio relaxers and permanent waving is exactly the same. And even though the chemistry of hydroxide relaxers and permanent waving may be different, all relaxers and all permanents change the shape of the hair by breaking disulfide bonds.

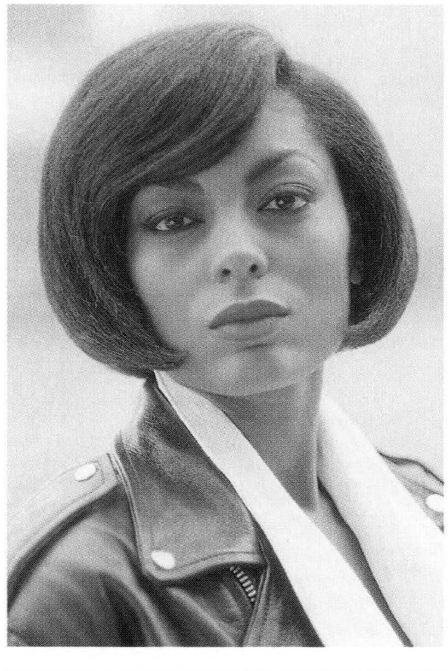

Figure 15-95 Relaxed hair.

The two most common types of chemical hair relaxers are thio (ATG) and hydroxide.

CAUTION

Relaxers are characterized by an extremely high alkalinity and can literally melt or dissolve hair if used incorrectly. Most relaxers contain the same ingredients used in depilatories (products used for temporary hair removal).

Extremely Curly Hair

Extremely curly hair exists in all races. That means anyone of any race, or mixed race, can have extremely curly hair. It is also true that, within races, individuals can have hair with different degrees of curliness.

Extremely curly hair grows in long twisted spirals, or coils. Cross-sections are highly elliptical and vary in shape and thickness along their lengths. Compared to straight or wavy hair, which tends to possess a fairly regular and uniform diameter along a single strand, extremely curly hair is irregular, exhibiting varying diameters along a single strand.

The thinnest and weakest sections of the hair strands are located at their twists. These sections are also bent at an extremely sharp angle and will be stretched the most during relaxing. A chain is only as strong as its weakest link, and hair is only as strong as its weakest section. Hair breaks at its weakest point. Extremely curly hair usually breaks at the twists because of the inherent weakness in that section and the extra physical force that is required to straighten it.

Thio Relaxers

Thio (AGT) is the same reducing agent that is used in permanent waving. **Thio relaxers** usually have a pH above 10 and a higher concentration of ATG than is used in permanent waving. Thio relaxers are also thicker, with a higher viscosity that is more suitable for application as a relaxer.

Thio relaxers break disulfide bonds and soften hair, just as in permanents. After enough bonds are broken, the hair is straightened into its new shape and the relaxer is rinsed from the hair. Blotting comes next, followed by a neutralizer. The chemical reactions of thio relaxers are identical to those in permanent waving.

Thio Neutralization

The neutralizer used with thio relaxers is an oxidizing agent, usually hydrogen peroxide, just as in permanents. The oxidation reaction caused by the neutralizer rebuilds the disulfide bonds that were broken by the thio relaxer.

Hydroxide Relaxers

The hydroxide ion is the active ingredient in all **hydroxide relaxers**. Sodium hydroxide, potassium hydroxide, lithium hydroxide, and guanidine hydroxide are all types of hydroxide relaxers. All hydroxide relaxers are very strong alkalis that can swell the hair up to twice its normal diameter.

Hydroxide relaxers are not compatible with thio relaxers because they use a different chemistry. Thio relaxers have a pH of about 10 and use thio to break the disulfide bonds. Although the high pH of a thio relaxer swells the hair, thio breaks the disulfide bonds. Hydroxide relaxers have an even higher pH. The average pH of the hair is 5.0 and many hydroxide relaxers have a pH over 13.0. Since each step in the pH scale represents a tenfold change in concentration, a pH of 13.0 is 100 million (100,000,000) times more alkaline than a pH of 5.0 (Figure 15–96) (see Chapter 7).

Hydroxide relaxers break disulfide bonds differently than in the reduction reaction of thio relaxers. Hydroxide relaxers remove one atom of sulfur from a disulfide bond, converting it into a lanthionine bond by a process called **lanthionization** (lan-thee-oh-ny-ZAY-shun). Disulfide bonds contain two sulfur atoms. Lanthionine bonds contain only one sulfur atom. The disulfide bonds that are broken by hydroxide relaxers are broken permanently and can never be re-formed.

Hydroxide Neutralization

Unlike thio neutralization, the neutralization of hydroxide relaxers does not involve oxidation. The deactivation (neutralization) of hydroxide relaxers neutralizes the alkaline residues left in the hair by the relaxer. The pH of hydroxide relaxers is so high that the hair remains at an extremely high pH, even after thorough rinsing. Although rinsing is important, rinsing alone does not deactivate the relaxer or restore the normal acidic pH of the hair and scalp.

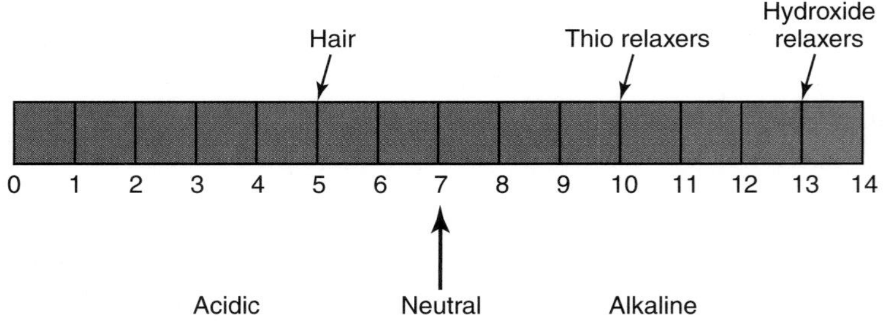

Figure 15-96 pH of thio and hydroxide relaxers.

As we know from Chapter 7, acids neutralize alkalis. Therefore, the application of an acid-balanced shampoo or a normalizing lotion neutralizes any remaining hydroxide ions to lower the pH of the hair and scalp. Some neutralizing shampoos intended for use after hydroxide relaxers have a built-in pH indicator that changes color to indicate when the pH of the hair has returned to normal.

Since the disulfide bonds that have been broken by hydroxide relaxers cannot be re-formed by oxidation, application of a neutralizer that contains an oxidizing agent will not rebuild the disulfide bonds and will only damage the hair. 5 ✓

Types of Hydroxide Relaxers

Metal hydroxide relaxers are ionic compounds formed by a metal—sodium (Na), potassium (K), or lithium (Li)—which is combined with oxygen (O) and hydrogen (H). Metal hydroxide relaxers include sodium hydroxide (NaOH), potassium hydroxide (KOH), and lithium hydroxide (LiOH). Although calcium hydroxide (CaOH) is sometimes added to hydroxide relaxers, it is not used by itself to relax hair.

All metal hydroxide relaxers contain only one component and are used exactly as they are packaged in the container, without mixing. The hydroxide ion is the active ingredient in all hydroxide relaxers. There is no significant difference in the performance of these metal hydroxide relaxers.

Sodium hydroxide (NaOH) relaxers are commonly called lye relaxers. Sodium hydroxide is the oldest and still the most common type of chemical hair relaxer. Sodium hydroxide is also known as lye or caustic soda. Sodium hydroxide is the same chemical that is used in drain cleaners and chemical hair depilatories.

Lithium hydroxide (LiOH) and potassium hydroxide (KOH) relaxers are often advertised and sold as "no mix–no lye" relaxers. Although technically they are not lye, their chemistry is identical and there is very little difference in their performance.

CAUTION

Application of a thio relaxer or thio permanent on hair that has been treated with a hydroxide relaxer will not properly relax or curl the hair and may cause extreme damage. Hair that has been treated with hydroxide relaxers is unfit for thio relaxers or soft curl permanents.

Guanidine Hydroxide Relaxers

Guanidine (GWAN-ih-deen) hydroxide relaxers are usually advertised and sold as "no lye" relaxers. Although technically they are not lye, the hydroxide ion is still the active ingredient. Guanidine hydroxide relaxers contain two components that must be mixed immediately prior to use.

They straighten hair completely with much less scalp irritation than other hydroxide relaxers. Most guanidine hydroxide relaxers are recommended for sensitive scalps and are sold over-the-counter for home use. Although they reduce scalp irritation, they do not reduce hair damage. They swell the hair slightly more than other hydroxide relaxers and are also more drying, especially after repeated applications.

Low-pH Relaxers

Sulfites and bisulfites are sometimes used as low-pH hair relaxers. The most commonly used are ammonium sulfite and ammonium bisulfite. Sulfites are marketed as mild alternative relaxers. They are compatible with thio relaxers, but not compatible with hydroxide relaxers. They do not completely straighten extremely curly hair. Low-pH relaxers are intended for use on color-treated, damaged, or fine hair. (See Table 15–2 for a summary of the types and uses of relaxers.)

Base and No-base Relaxers

Hydroxide relaxers are usually sold in base and no-base formulas. **Base cream** is an oily cream used to protect the skin and scalp during hair relaxing. **Base relaxers** require the application of base cream to the entire scalp prior to the application of the relaxer.

No-base relaxers do not require application of a protective base. They contain a base cream that is designed to melt at body temperature. As the relaxer is applied, body heat causes the base to melt and settle out onto the scalp in a thin, oily, protective coating. No-base relaxers are simply an improvement on the protection that is provided by the oils in all hydroxide relaxers. For added protection, base cream may be applied to the entire hairline and around the ears, even with no-base relaxers.

Relaxer Strengths

Most chemical hair relaxers are available in three different strengths: mild, regular, and super. The difference in strength of hydroxide relaxers is due to the concentration of hydroxide.

- Mild strength relaxers are formulated for fine, color-treated, or damaged hair.
- Regular strength relaxers are intended for normal hair texture with a medium natural curl.
- Super strength relaxers should be used for maximum straightening on coarse hair that is extremely curly.

Active Ingredient	pH	Marketed As	Advantages	Disadvantages
sodium hydroxide	12.5–13.5	no-mix lye relaxer	very effective for extremely curly hair	may cause scalp irritation and damage the hair
lithium hydroxide and potassium hydroxide	12.5–13.5	no-mix lye relaxer	very effective for extremely curly hair	may cause scalp irritation and damage the hair
guanidine hydroxide	13–13.5	no-lye relaxer	causes less skin irritation than other hydroxide relaxers	more drying to hair with repeated use
ammonium thioglycolate	9.6–10.0	thio relaxer, no-lye relaxer	compatible with soft curl permanents	strong, unpleasant ammonia smell
ammonium sulfite/ammonium bisulfite	6.5–8.5	low-pH relaxer, no-lye relaxer	less damaging to hair	does not relax extremely curly hair sufficiently

Table 15–2 Selecting the Correct Relaxer

CHEMICAL HAIR RELAXING PROCEDURES

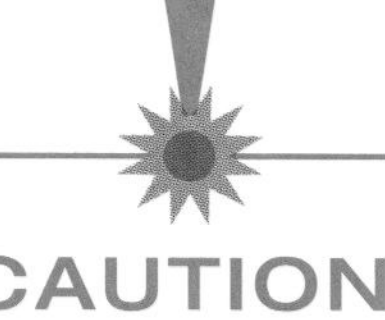

CAUTION

Make sure the client has not had haircoloring containing metallic salts, such as gradual or progressive haircolors, before applying either thio or hydroxide relaxers to the hair. Extreme damage or breakage can occur.

Many of the steps for applying thio and hydroxide relaxers are the same, but they do differ in some ways.

Hydroxide Relaxer Procedures

Some of the steps for hydroxide relaxers are different from those for thio relaxers. The procedure below should be used for all hydroxide relaxers. Although all hyroxide relaxers follow the same procedure, different application methods are used for virgin relaxers and retouch relaxers.

- A *virgin relaxer* application should be used for hair that has not had previous chemical texture services. Since the scalp area and the porous ends will usually process more quickly than the middle of the strand, the application for a virgin relaxer starts ¼ inch (.6 cm) to ½ inch (1.25 cm) away from the scalp and includes the entire strand, up to the porous ends. To avoid overprocessing and scalp irritation, do not apply relaxer to the hair closest to the scalp or to the ends until the last few minutes of processing.
- A *retouch relaxer* application should be used for hair that has had previous chemical texture services. The application for a retouch relaxer starts ¼ inch to ½ inch away from the scalp and includes only the new growth. To avoid overprocessing and scalp irritation, do not apply relaxer to the hair closest to the scalp until the last few minutes of processing. In order to avoid breakage of the previously relaxed hair, apply cream conditioner over the hair that received the earlier treatment. Avoid overlapping on the previously relaxed hair unless it requires additional strengthening. If the previously relaxed hair requires additional straightening, relaxer may be applied for the last few minutes of processing.

Option: Some manufacturers recommend the use of a normalizing solution after rinsing out the relaxer and prior to shampooing. **Normalizing solutions** are conditioners with an acidic pH that condition the hair and restore the natural pH prior to shampooing.

Periodic Strand Testing

Periodic strand testing during processing will help to tell you when the hair is sufficiently relaxed. After the relaxer is applied, stretch the strands to see how fast the natural curls are being removed. You may also smooth and press the strand to the scalp using the back of the comb or your finger. If the strand remains smooth, it is sufficiently relaxed. If the curl returns, continue processing. Processing time will vary according to the strength of the tool, the hair type and condition, and the results you are looking for (Figure 15–97 and Figure 15–98).

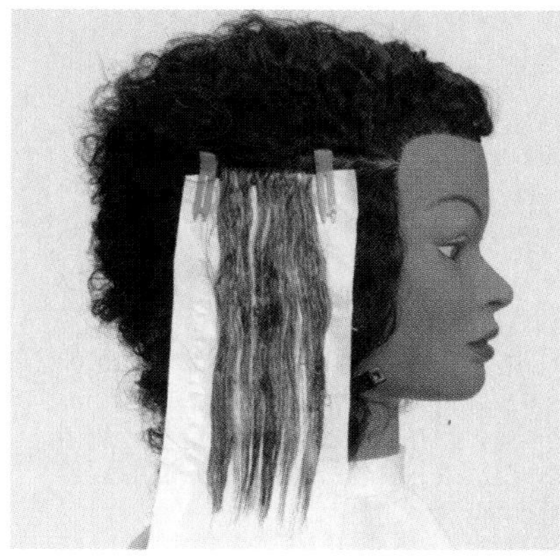

Figure 15–97 Sufficiently relaxed strand.

15

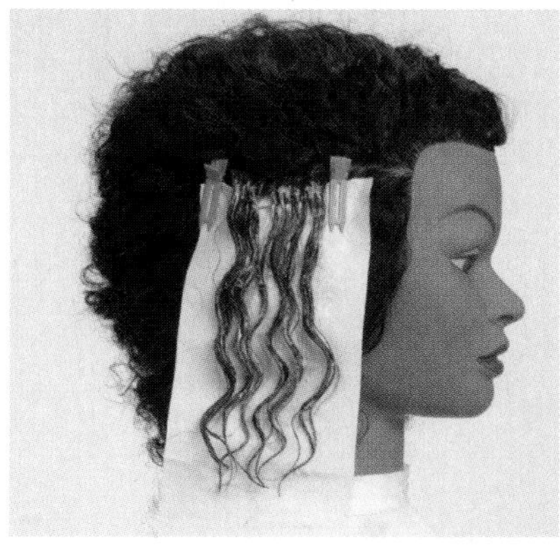

Figure 15–98 Insufficiently relaxed strand.

PROCEDURE

RELAXING WITH HYDROXIDE RELAXER

Implements and Materials

- hydroxide relaxer
- hydroxide neutralizer
- protective base cream
- acid-balanced shampoo
- conditioner
- bowl and applicator brush
- shampoo cape
- towels
- plastic clips
- styling comb
- plastic rattail comb
- spray bottle
- disposable gloves
- timer

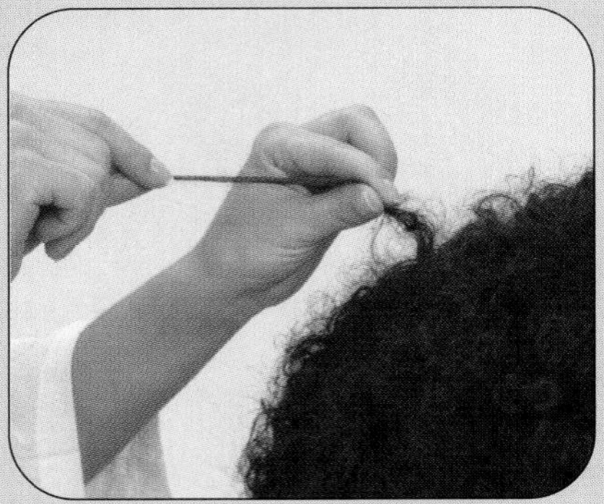

Figure 15-99 Hair analysis.

Preparation

1. Wash your hands.
2. Perform an analysis of the hair and scalp (Figure 15–99). Perform tests for porosity and elasticity (see page 212, Chapter 8).
3. Complete the client consultation. Fill out the client relaxer record. Note any changes in the client's history.
4. Have the client change into a gown and remove eyeglasses, earrings, and necklace. Drape the client with a shampoo cape and two towels. To avoid scalp irritation, do not shampoo the hair prior to a hydroxide relaxer.

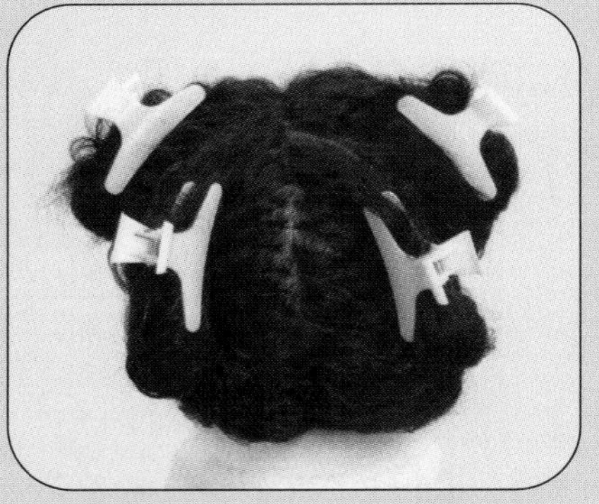

Figure 15-100 Four sections.

Procedure for Applying Virgin Hydroxide Relaxers

1. Part the hair into four sections, from the center of the front hairline to the center of the nape, and from ear to ear. Clip the sections up to keep them out of the way (Figure 15–100).

2. Apply protective base cream to the hairline and ears. *Option*: Take ¼ to ½-inch (.6 to 1.25 cm) horizontal partings and apply a protective base cream to the entire scalp. (Always follow the manufacturers' directions and the procedures approved by your instructor) (Figure 15–101).

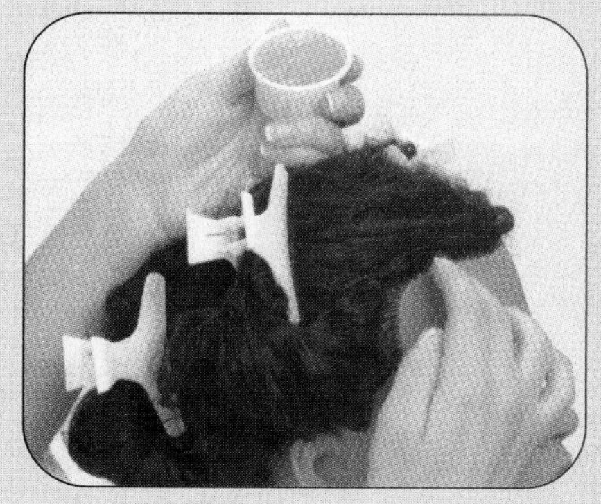

Figure 15-101 Apply protective base cream.

3. Wear gloves on both hands. Begin application in the most resistant area, usually at the back of the head. Make ¼-inch to ½-inch horizontal partings and apply the relaxer to the top of the strand first (Figure 15–102), then to the underside (Figure 15–103). Apply the relaxer with an applicator bottle, brush, or the back of a rattail comb. Apply relaxer ¼ inch to ½ inch away from the scalp and up to the porous ends. To avoid scalp irritation, do not allow the relaxer to touch the scalp until the last few minutes of processing.

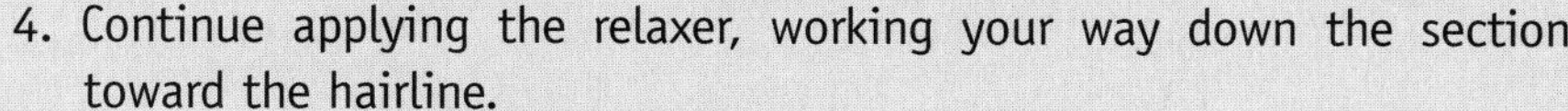

4. Continue applying the relaxer, working your way down the section toward the hairline.

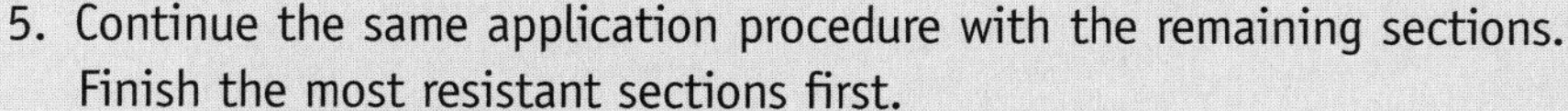

5. Continue the same application procedure with the remaining sections. Finish the most resistant sections first.
6. After the relaxer has been applied to all sections, use the back of the comb or your hands to smooth each section (Figure 15–104).
7. Process according to the manufacturer's directions. Perform periodic strand tests. Processing usually takes less than 20 minutes at room temperature.
8. During the last few minutes of processing, work the relaxer down to the scalp and through the ends of the hair, using additional relaxer as needed (Figure 15–105). Carefully comb and smooth all sections.

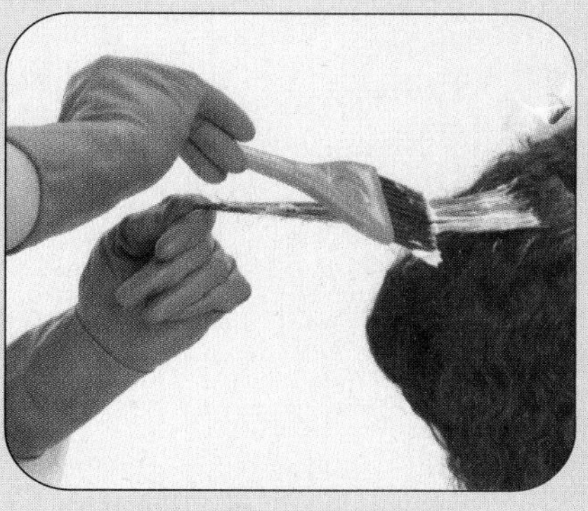

Figure 15-102 Apply relaxer to top side of strand.

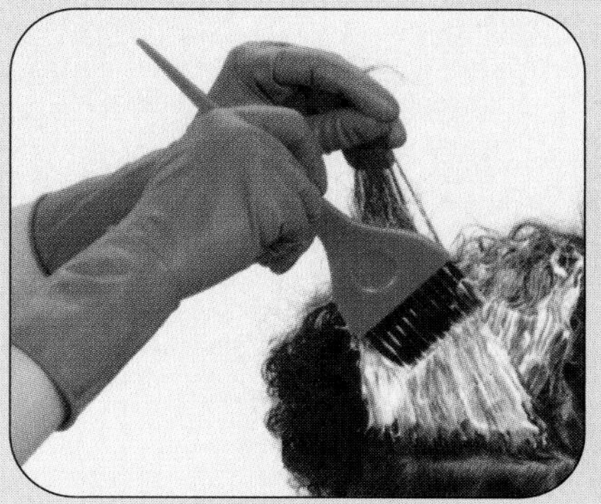

Figure 15-103 Apply relaxer to underside of strand.

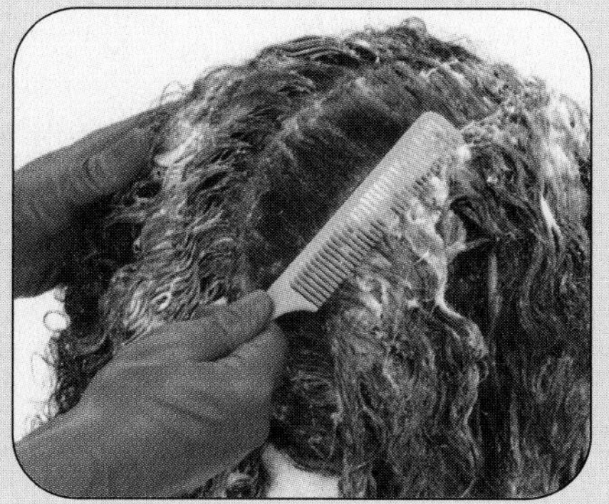

Figure 15-104 Smooth section with back of comb.

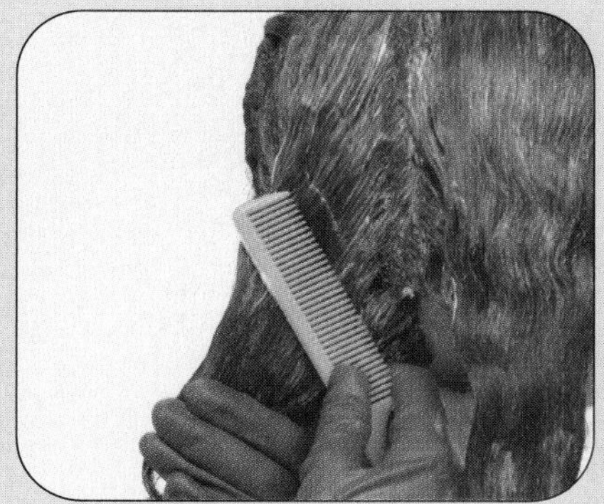

Figure 15-105 Work relaxer down to scalp.

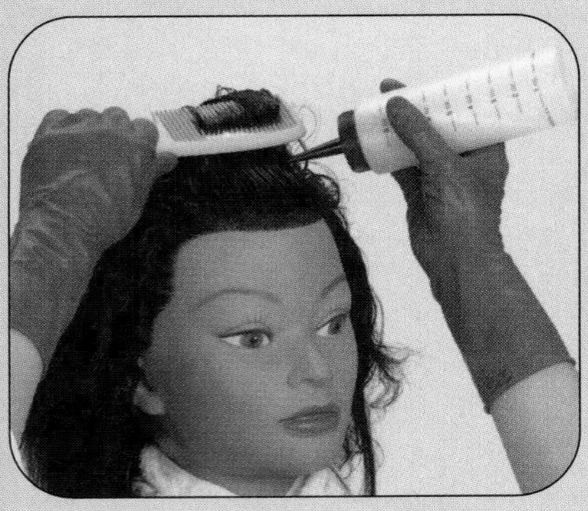
Figure 15–106 Apply neutralizer.

9. Rinse thoroughly with warm water to remove all traces of the relaxer.

Neutralization Procedure

1. *Optional step*: Apply the normalizing solution and comb it through to the ends of the hair (Figure 15–106). Leave it on for approximately five minutes and then rinse thoroughly. Always follow the manufacturers' directions and the procedures approved by your instructor.
2. Shampoo at least three times with an acid-balanced neutralizing shampoo. It is essential that all traces of the relaxer be removed from the hair. *Option*: If you are using a neutralizing shampoo with a color indicator, a change in color will indicate when all traces of the relaxer are removed and the natural pH of the hair and scalp has been restored.

---

3. Rinse thoroughly, condition, and style as desired (Figure 15–107).

Cleanup and Sanitation for All Relaxers

1. Discard disposable supplies in appropriate receptacles.
2. Disinfect implements and store according to sanitation requirements.
3. Clean, sanitize, and prepare your workstation for the next service.
4. Wash your hands with warm soap and water.
5. Complete the client record.

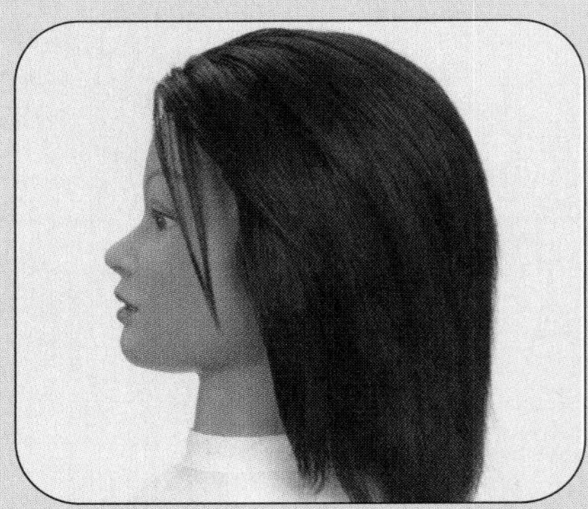
Figure 15–107 Finished relaxed style.

completed!

PROCEDURE

HYDROXIDE RELAXER RETOUCH

Implements and Materials

Same as for Procedure 36—relaxing with hydroxide relaxer.

Preparation

Same as for Procedure 36—relaxing with hydroxide relaxer.

Procedure

1. Do not shampoo the hair. Divide the hair into four sections, from the center of the front hairline to the center of the nape, and from ear to ear. Clip sections up to keep them out of the way.
2. Wear gloves on both hands. Apply a protective base cream to the hairline and ears. *Option*: Take ¼-inch to ½-inch horizontal (.6 to 1.25 cm) partings and apply base cream to the entire scalp (Figure 15–108).
3. Begin application of the relaxer in the most resistant area, usually at the back of the head. Make ¼-inch to ½-inch horizontal partings and apply the relaxer to the top of the strand. Apply the relaxer ¼ inch to ½ inch away from the scalp and only to new growth. Do not allow the relaxer to touch the scalp until the last few minutes of processing. To avoid overprocessing or breakage, do not overlap the relaxer onto the previously relaxed hair (Figure 15–109).
4. Continue applying the relaxer, using the same procedure and working your way down the section toward the hairline.

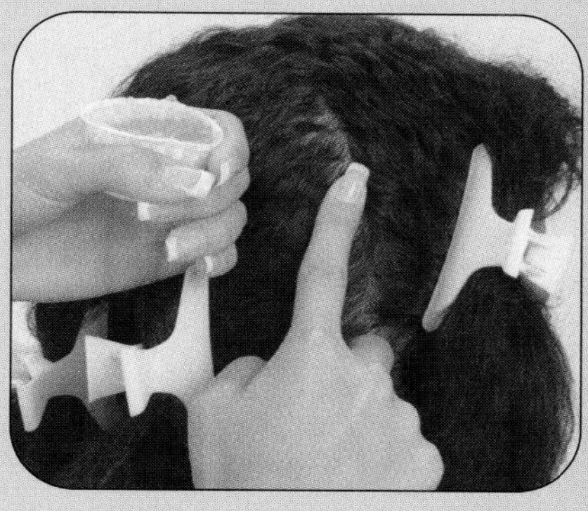

Figure 15–108 Apply base cream.

15

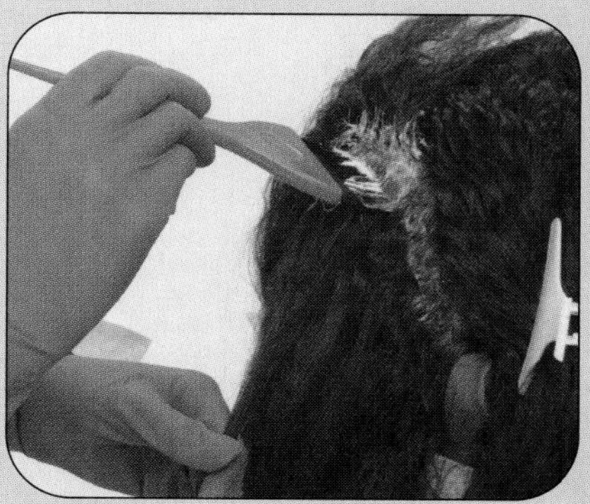

Figure 15–109 Apply relaxer to new growth.

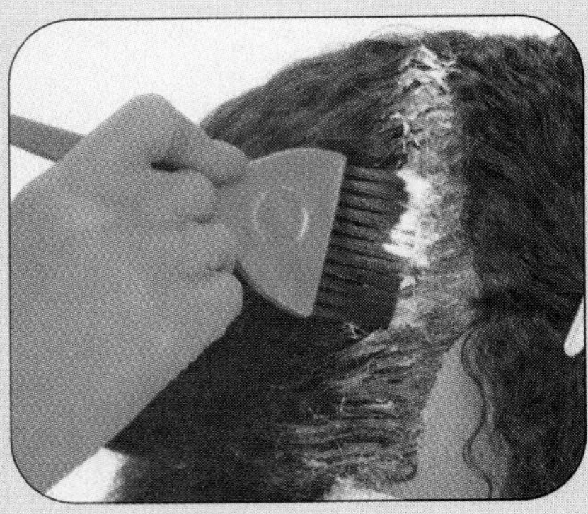

Figure 15–110 Continue applying relaxer.

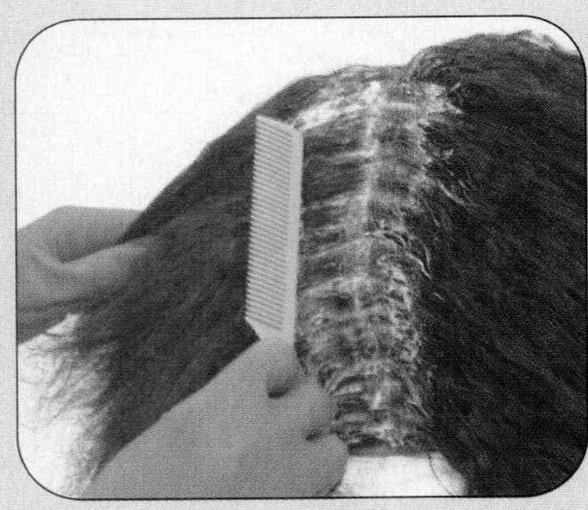

Figure 15–111 Smooth section with back of comb.

5. Continue the same application procedure with the remaining sections, finishing the most resistant sections first (Figure 15–110).
6. After the relaxer has been applied to all sections, use the back of the comb or your hands to smooth each section (Figure 15–111).
7. Process according to the manufacturer's directions. Perform periodic strand tests. Processing usually takes less than 20 minutes at room temperature.
8. During the last few minutes of processing, work the relaxer down to the scalp.
9. If the ends of the hair need additional relaxing, work the relaxer through to the ends for the last few minutes of processing (Figure 15–112).
10. Rinse thoroughly with warm water to remove all traces of the relaxer.
11. Follow virgin hydroxide neutralizing procedure. Style the hair as desired.
12. Follow cleanup and sanitation procedures for Procedure 36—relaxing with hydroxide relaxer.

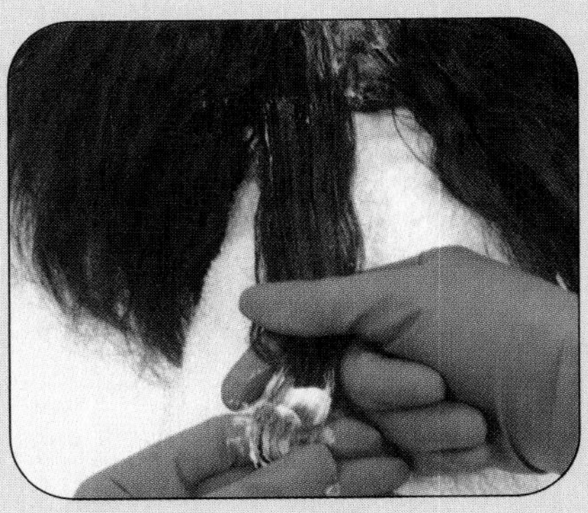

Figure 15–112 Work relaxer through hair ends.

completed!

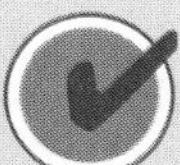

PROCEDURE

RELAXING WITH THIO RELAXER

Implements and Materials

Use the same implements and materials as for Procedure 36—hydroxide relaxer, but use thio relaxer, normalizing lotion, and neutralizing shampoo (with color indicator).

Preparation

Follow the same preparation steps as for Procedure 36—hydroxide relaxer. A light shampoo is optional. Do not forget to perform an analysis of the client's hair and scalp. Test the hair for elasticity and porosity in several areas of the head. If the hair has poor elasticity, do not perform a relaxer service.

Procedure for Virgin Thio Relaxer

Follow the same application procedure as for Procedure 36—hydroxide relaxer.

Neutralization Procedure for Thio Relaxers

1. Blot excess water from the hair. Apply thio neutralizer in ¼ to ½-inch (.6 to 1.25 cm) sections throughout the hair, and smooth with your hands or the back of the comb.
2. Process the neutralizer according to the manufacturer's directions.
3. Rinse thoroughly, shampoo, condition, and style.

Cleanup and Sanitation

Follow the same cleanup and sanitation procedure as for Procedure 36—hydroxide relaxer.

Procedure for Thio Relaxer Retouch

1. Follow the preparation and application procedures for Procedure 37—hydroxide relaxer retouch. A shampoo prior to relaxer application is optional.
2. Follow the virgin thio relaxer neutralizing and cleanup procedures from Procedure 37.

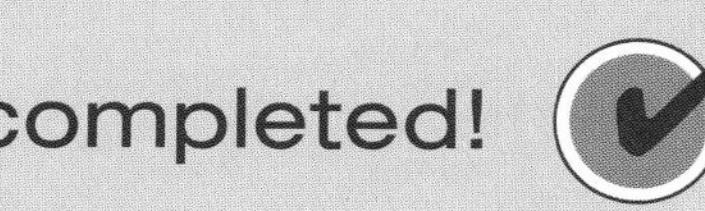

Thio Relaxer Procedures

The application steps for thio relaxers are the same as those for hydroxide relaxers, although the neutralization procedure is different. Relaxer may be applied with bowl and brush, applicator bottle, or the back of a rattail comb. Although all thio relaxers follow the same procedure, different application methods are used for virgin relaxers and retouch relaxers.

SOFT CURL PERMANENTS (CURL RE-FORMING)

Soft curl permanents (curl re-forming) do not straighten the hair; they simply make the existing curl larger and looser. A soft curl permanent may also be called a Jheri curl or simply a curl. It is a combination of a thio relaxer and a thio permanent that is wrapped on large tools. Soft curl permanents use ATG and oxidation neutralizers, just as thio permanent waves do.

Soft Curl Permanent Procedure

A soft curl permanent is actually two services. Extremely curly hair must be relaxed with a thio relaxer (curl rearranger) before it is wrapped on tools. All base sections should be horizontal, with the same length and width as the perm tool. The base direction should be in the direction of hair growth. The base control should be half off base.

Once it is wrapped on large tools, it is then processed with a second thio solution (curl booster). After processing, the hair is rinsed, blotted, and neutralized, just as with any other permanent.

Safety Precautions for Hair Relaxing

- Perform a thorough hair analysis and client consultation prior to the service.
- Examine the scalp for abrasions. Do not proceed with the service if redness, swelling, or skin lesions are present.
- Keep accurate and detailed client records of the services performed and the results achieved.
- Have the client sign a release statement that indicates that the client understands the possible risks involved in the service.
- Do not apply a hydroxide relaxer on hair that has been previously treated with a thio relaxer.

- Do not apply a thio relaxer on hair that has been previously treated with a hydroxide relaxer.
- Do not chemically relax hair that has been treated with a metallic dye.
- Do not relax overly damaged hair. Suggest instead a series of reconstruction treatments.
- Do not shampoo the client prior to the application of a hydroxide relaxer.
- The client's hair and scalp must be completely dry and free from perspiration prior to the application of a hydroxide relaxer.
- Apply a protective base cream to avoid scalp irritation.
- Wear gloves during the relaxer application.
- Protect the client's eyes.
- If any solution accidentally gets into the client's eye, flush the eye immediately with cool water and refer the client to a doctor.
- Do not allow chemical relaxers to accidentally come into contact with the client's ears, scalp, or skin.
- Perform periodic strand tests to see how fast the natural curls are being removed.
- Avoid scratching the scalp with your comb or fingernails.
- Do not allow the application of a relaxer retouch to overlap onto previously relaxed hair.
- Never use a strong relaxer on fine or damaged hair. It may cause breakage.
- Do not attempt to remove more than 80 percent of the natural curl.
- Thoroughly rinse the chemical relaxer from the hair. Failure to rinse properly can cause excessive skin irritation and hair breakage.
- Use a normalizing lotion to restore the hair and scalp to their normal acidic pH.
- Use a neutralizing shampoo with a color indicator to guarantee that the hair and scalp have been restored to their normal acidic pH.
- Use a conditioner and wide-tooth comb to eliminate excessive stretching when combing out tangles.
- Do not use hot irons or excessive heat on chemically relaxed hair.

Performing texture services involves using powerful chemicals, which must be handled with the utmost caution. If you act responsibly and perfect your techniques, your services will be in great demand.

PROCEDURE

SOFT CURL PERMANENT

Implements and Supplies for Soft Curl Perms

- thio cream relaxer (curl rearranger)
- thio curl booster
- preneutralizing conditioner (optional)
- thio neutralizer
- protective base cream
- acid-balanced shampoo
- conditioner
- plastic or glass bowl
- applicator brush
- applicator bottles
- shampoo cape
- neutralizing bib
- disposable gloves
- roll cotton
- towels
- plastic clips
- styling comb
- plastic tail comb
- perm tools
- end papers
- spray bottle
- timer

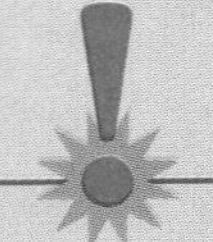

CAUTION

Hair that has been treated with hydroxide relaxers must not be treated with thio relaxers or soft curl permanents.

Preparation

1. Wash your hands.
2. Perform a client consultation, including an analysis of the client's hair and scalp. Note results in the client record.
3. Have the client change into a gown and remove eyeglasses, earrings, and necklace. Drape the client with a shampoo cape and two towels. *Option*: Shampoo the hair gently and towel-dry. Avoid any irritating scalp manipulations.

Procedure

1. Follow Procedure 36 — applying virgin hydroxide relaxer.
2. After rinsing the hair, part it into nine panels. Use the length of the rod to measure the width of the panels (Figure 15–113).

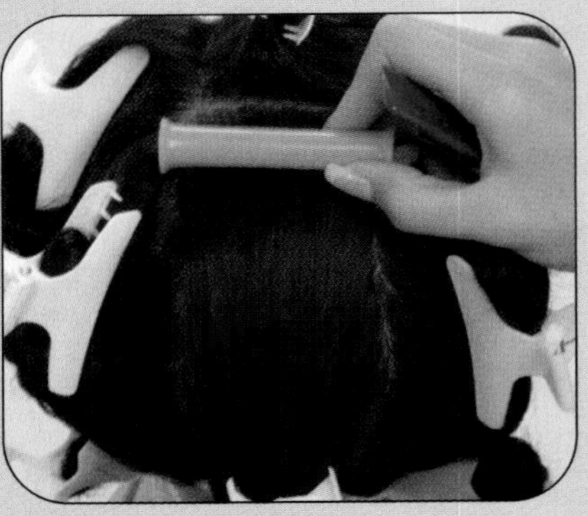

Figure 15–113 Measure panel width.

3. Wear gloves on both hands and begin wrapping at the most resistant area. Apply and distribute the thio curl booster to each panel as you wrap the hair (Figure 15–114). Make a horizontal parting the same size as the rod. Hold the hair at a 90-degree angle to the head. Using two end papers, roll the hair down to the scalp and position the rod half-off base (Figure 15–115). *Option*: Insert roller picks to stabilize the rods and eliminate any tension caused by the band.
4. Continue wrapping the remainder of the first panel using the same technique.
5. Continue wrapping the remaining eight panels in numerical order using the same technique (Figure 15–116).
6. Place cotton around the hairline and neck and apply thio curl booster to all the curls until they are completely saturated (Figure 15–117).
7. If a plastic cap is used, punch a few holes in the cap and cover all the hair completely. Do not allow the plastic cap to touch the client's skin (Figure 15–118).
8. Check cotton and towels. If they are saturated with solution, replace them.
9. Process according to manufacturers' directions. Processing time will vary according to the strength of the product, the hair type and condition, and desired results. Processing usually takes less than 20 minutes at room temperature.

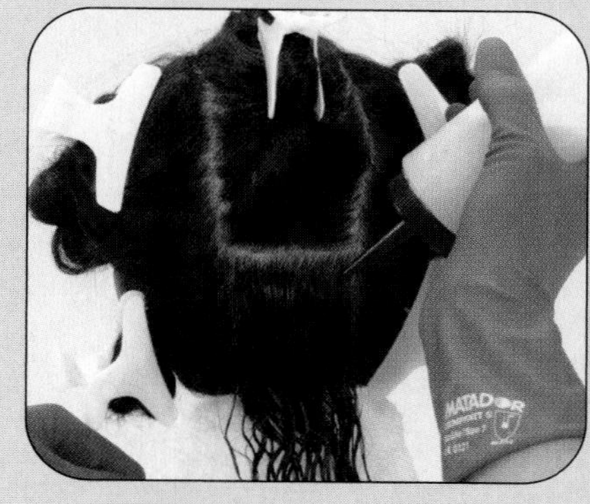

Figure 15–114 Apply thio curl booster.

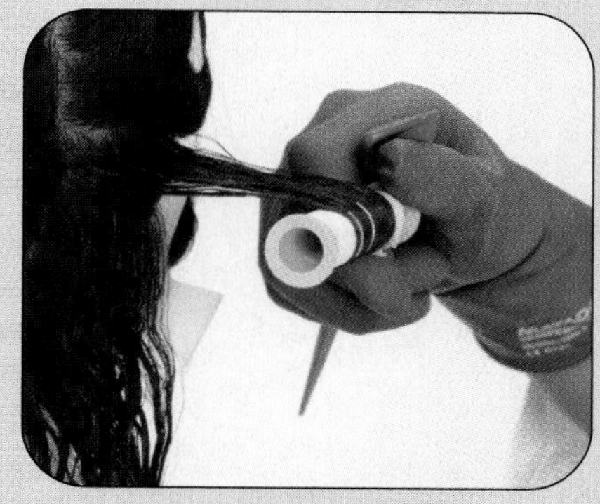

Figure 15–115 Roll hair down to scalp.

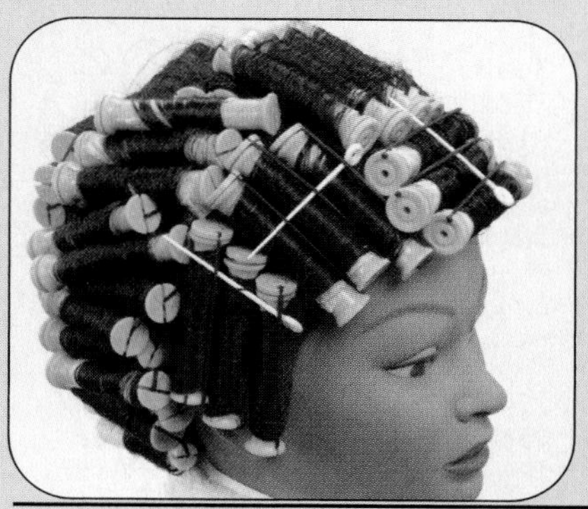

Figure 15–116 Wrap last panel.

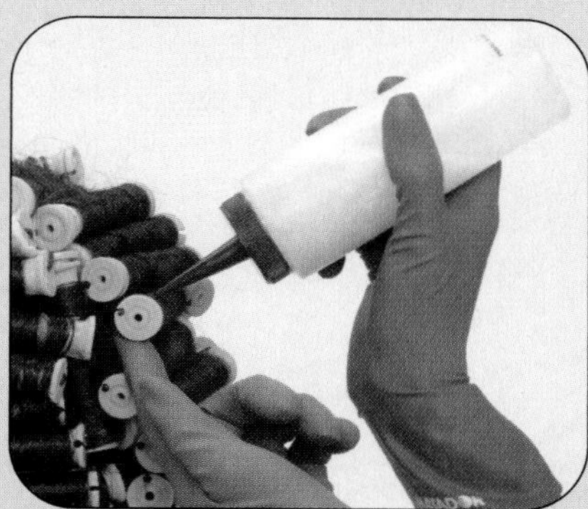

Figure 15–117 Saturate rods with thio booster lotion.

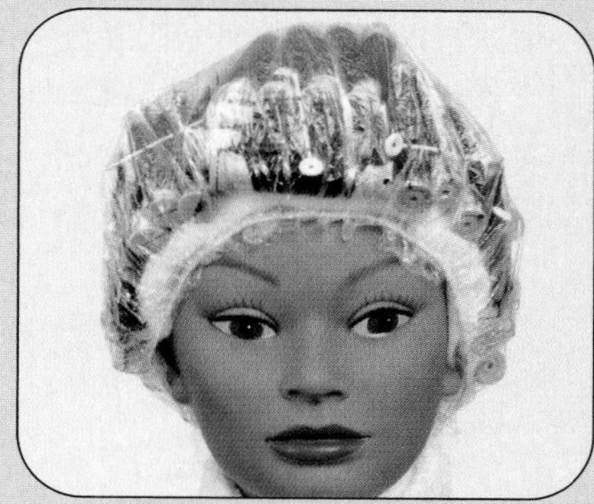

Figure 15–118 Process with plastic cap.

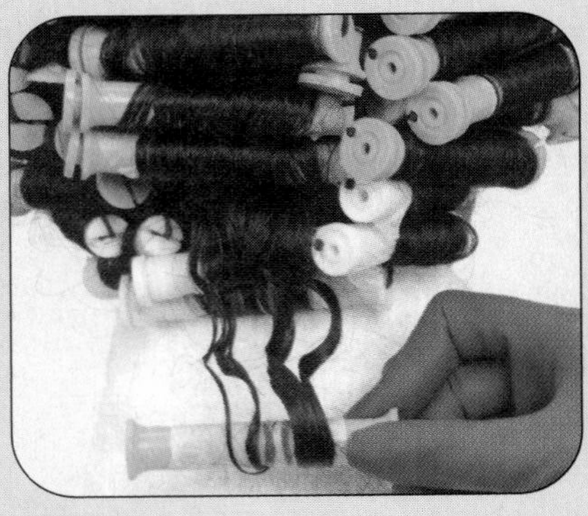

Figure 15-119 Take test curl.

10. Check for proper curl development (Figure 15–119).
11. When processing is completed, rinse the hair thoroughly, for at least five minutes. Then towel-blot the hair on each tool to remove excess moisture. *Option*: Apply preneutralizing conditioner according to the manufacturers' directions. Always follow the manufacturers' directions and the procedures approved by your instructor.
12. Apply the neutralizer slowly and carefully to the hair on each tool. Avoid splashing and dripping. Make sure each rod is completely saturated.
13. Set a timer and neutralize according to the manufacturers' directions. Remove the rods, distribute the remaining neutralizer through the ends of the hair, and rinse thoroughly. *Option*: Shampoo and condition. Always follow the manufacturer's directions and the procedures approved by your instructor.

6

14. Style the hair as desired (Figure 15–120).

Cleanup and Sanitation

1. Discard all disposable supplies in appropriate receptacles.
2. Disinfect implements and store according to sanitation requirements.
3. Clean, sanitize, and prepare your workstation for the next service.
4. Wash your hands with soap and warm water.
5. Complete the client record.

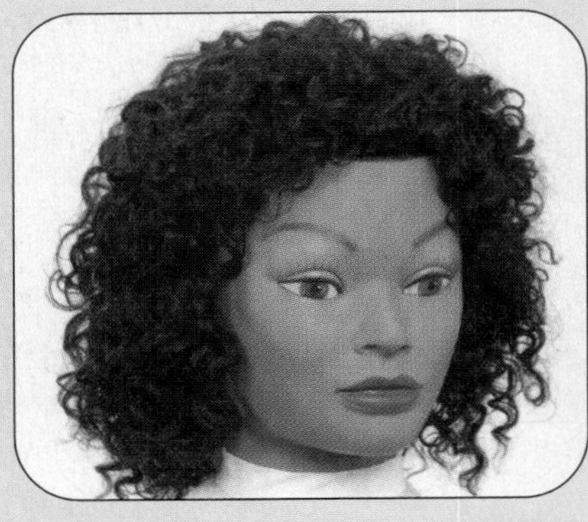

Figure 15-120 Finished soft curl permanent.

15

completed! 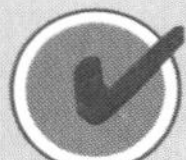

chapter glossary

acid-balanced waves	perm with a pH between 7.8 and 8.2 that process at room temperature and do not require the added heat of a hair dryer; process more quickly and produce firmer curls than true acid waves
alkaline waves or cold waves	permanent waves that process at room temperature without the addition of heat; most alkaline waves have a pH between 9.0 and 9.6
ammonia-free waves	perms that use an ingredient that does not evaporate as readily as ammonia, so there is very little odor associated with their use
ammonium thioglycolate (ATG)	main active ingredient or reducing agent in alkaline permanents
base cream	oily cream used to protect the skin and scalp during hair relaxing
base control	the position of the tool in relation to its base section, determined by the angle at which the hair is wrapped
base direction	the angle at which the tool is positioned on the head (horizontally, vertically, or diagonally); also, the directional pattern in which the hair is wrapped
base relaxers	relaxers that require the application of base cream to the entire scalp prior to the application of the relaxer
base sections	subsections of panels into which hair is divided for perm wrapping; one tool is normally placed on each base section
basic perm wrap	perm wrap in which all the tools within a panel move in the same direction and are positioned on equal-size bases; all base sections are horizontal, with the same length and width as the perm tool
bookend wrap	perm wrap in which one end paper is folded in half over the hair ends like an envelope
bricklay perm wrap	perm wrap similar to actual technique of bricklaying; base sections are offset from each other row by row
chemical hair relaxing	process of rearranging the basic structure of extremely curly hair into a straight form
chemical texture services	hair services that cause a chemical change that permanently alters the natural wave pattern of the hair
concave rods	perm rods that have a smaller circumference in the center that increases to a larger circumference on the ends
croquignole perms	perms in which the hair strands are wrapped from the ends to the scalp, in overlapping layers
curvature perm wrap	perm wrap in which partings and bases radiate throughout the panels to follow the curvature of the head
disulfide bonds	side bonds between the polypeptide chains in the cortex; join cysteine sulfur atom on one polypeptide chain with cysteine sulfur atoms on neighboring polypeptide chains to form cystine, the oxidized form of cysteine
double flat wrap	perm wrap in which one end paper is placed under, and one paper over, the strand of hair being wrapped
double tool (piggyback) technique	perm wrap in which two tools are used for one strand of hair, one on top of the other
endothermic waves	perm activated by an outside heat source, usually a conventional hood-type hair dryer
end papers or end wraps	absorbent papers used to control the ends of the hair when wrapping and winding hair on perm tools
exothermic waves	perm that creates an exothermic chemical reaction that heats up the solution and speeds up the processing
glyceryl monothio-glycolate (GMTG)	main active ingredient in true acid and acid-balanced waving lotions that effectively reduces the pH

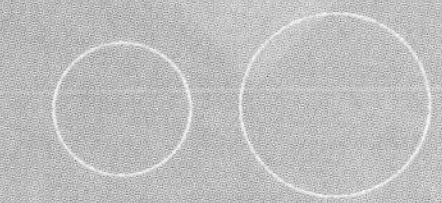

chapter glossary *(continued)*

half-off-base placement	base control in which the hair is wrapped at an angle of 90 degrees (perpendicular) to its base section and the tool is positioned half off its base section
hydrogen bonds	relatively weak physical side bonds that are the result of an attraction between opposite electrical charges; easily broken by water, as in wet setting, or heat, as in thermal styling, and re-form as the hair dries or cools
hydroxide relaxers	relaxers with a very high pH, sometimes over 13
lanthionization	process by which hydroxide relaxers permanently straighten hair; lanthionization breaks the hair's disulfide bonds during processing and converts them to lanthionine bonds when the relaxer is rinsed from the hair
low-pH waves	perms that work at a low pH and use sulfates, sulfites, and bisulfites as an alternative to ammonium thioglycolate
metal hydroxide relaxers	ionic compounds formed by a metal (sodium, potassium, or lithium) combined with oxygen and hydrogen
neutralization	process of stopping the action of a permanent wave solution and hardening the hair in its new form by the application of a chemical solution called the neutralizer
no-base relaxers	relaxers that do not require application of a protective base
normalizing solutions	conditioners with an acidic pH that condition the hair and restore the natural pH prior to shampooing
off-base placement	base control in which the hair is wrapped at an angle 45 degrees below perpendicular to its base section and the tool is positioned completely off its base section
on-base placement	base control in which the hair is wrapped at an angle 45 degrees beyond perpendicular to its base section and the tool is positioned on its base section
peptide or end bonds	chemical bonds that join amino acids together
polypeptide chains	amino acid chains joined together by peptide bonds
salt bonds	relatively weak physical side bonds that are the result of an attraction between opposite electrical charges; are easily broken by changes in pH, as in permanent waving, and re-form when the pH returns to normal
single flat wrap	perm wrap that is similar to double flat wrap but uses only one end paper, placed over the top of the strand of hair being wrapped
soft curl permanents	combination of thio relaxers and thio permanents that are wrapped on large tools; used to make existing curl larger and looser
spiral perms	perms in which the hair is wrapped at an angle other than perpendicular to the length of the tool; depending on the tool, the hair may be wound from the scalp toward the ends or from the ends toward the scalp
spiral perm technique	perm wrap done at an angle that causes the hair to spiral along the length of the tool; particularly effective on longer, thicker hair
straight rods	perm rods that are equal in circumference along their entire length or curling area
thioglycolic acid	colorless liquid with a strong, unpleasant odor; provides the hydrogen that causes the reduction reaction in permanent waving solutions
thio relaxers	relaxers that usually have a pH above 10 and a higher concentration of ammonium thioglycolate than is used in permanent waving

thio-free waves	perm that uses an ingredient other than ammonium thioglycolate as the primary reducing agent
true acid waves	perms that have a pH between 4.5 and 7.0 and require heat to speed processing; process more slowly than alkaline waves and do not usually produce as firm a curl
weave technique	wrapping technique that uses zigzag partings to divide base areas

review questions

1. What is the difference between end bonds and side bonds?
2. Describe the three different types of side bonds.
3. How do different hair texture services—wet sets, thermal styling, thio permanents and relaxers, and hydroxide relaxers—change side bonds?
4. What is the difference between a croquignole and a spiral perm wrap?
5. How does the reduction reaction of thio waving solution work?
6. What is the function of thio neutralizer?
7. List and describe the eight major types of permanent waving solutions.
8. Explain the procedure for a soft curl permanent.
9. What is lanthionization?
10. What is the major difference between thio and hydroxide relaxers?
11. What is the difference between thio and hydroxide neutralizers?
12. List at least 10 safety precautions for permanent waving, soft curl permanents, and chemical hair relaxers.

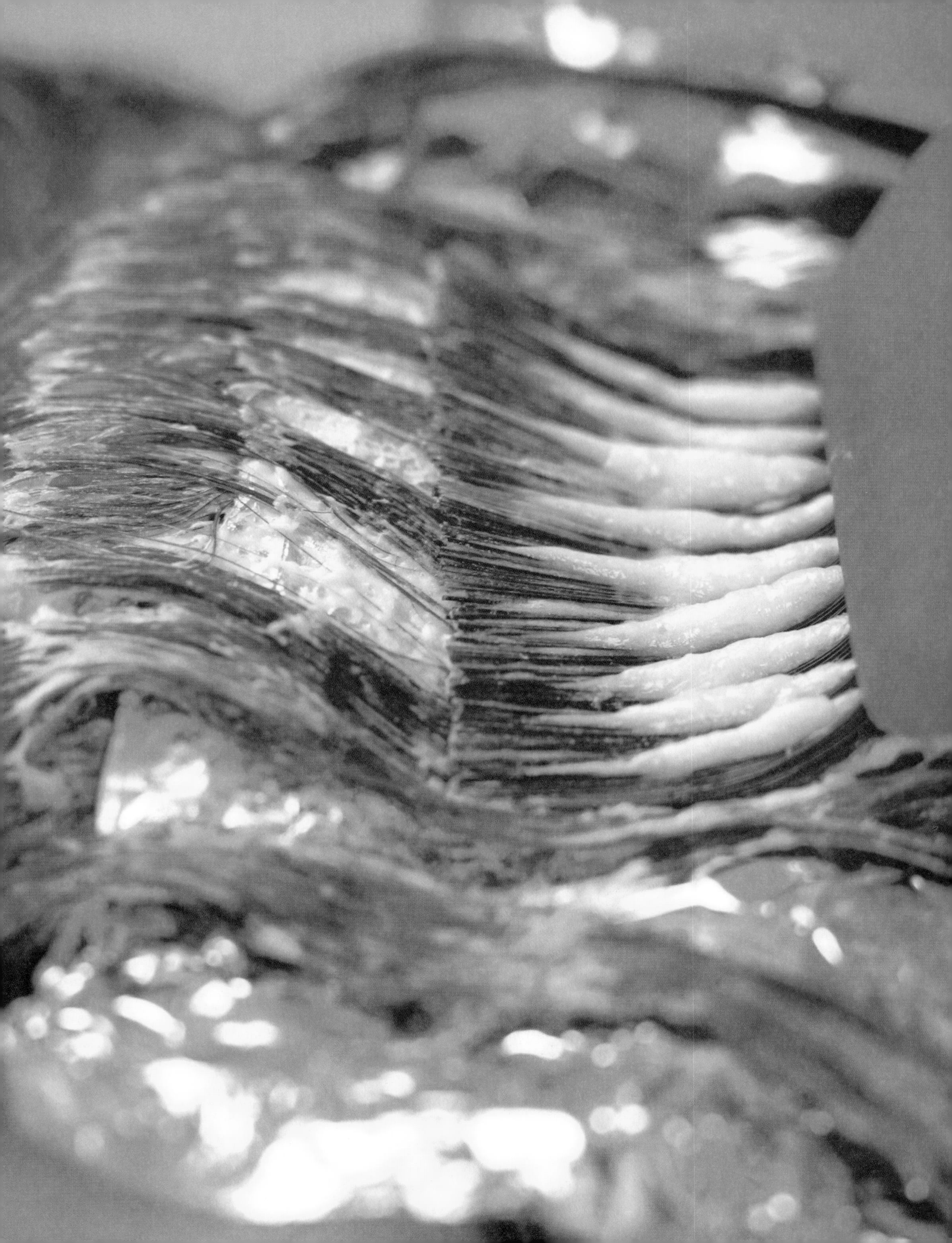

HAIRCOLORING

Colleen Hennessey
PROFESSIONAL HAIRCOLOR CONSULTANT

Chapter Outline

Why People Color Their Hair • Color Theory
Hair Facts • The Level System • Types of Haircolor
Consultation • Haircolor Application Procedures
Lightening Techniques • Special Effects Haircoloring
Special Problems in Haircolor/Corrective Coloring
Salon Menu of Services • Haircoloring Safety Precautions

Learning Objectives

After completing this chapter, you should be able to:

1. Identify the principles of color theory and relate them to haircolor.
2. Explain level and tone and their role in formulating haircolor.
3. List the four basic categories of haircolor, explain their chemical effect on the hair, and give examples of their use.
4. Explain the action of hair lighteners.
5. Demonstrate the application techniques for
   a) temporary colors,
   b) semipermanent colors,
   c) permanent colors, and
   d) lighteners.
6. Demonstrate special effects haircoloring techniques.

National Skill Standards

This chapter provides you with the necessary information to master these National Industry Skill Standards for Entry-Level Cosmetologists.

Conducting a color service in accordance with a client's needs or expectations.

Consulting with clients to determine their needs and preferences.

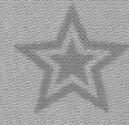
Using a variety of salon products while providing client services.

Conducting services in a safe environment, taking measures to prevent the spread of infectious and contagious disease.

Key Terms

Page number indicates where in the chapter the term is used.

activator pg. 575
aniline derivative pg. 555
balayage or free-form technique pg. 585
base color pg. 552
booking time pg. 596
cap technique pg. 584
color fillers pg. 593
color or tint removers pg. 595
complementary colors pg. 549
conditioner filler pg. 593
contributing pigment pg. 551
demipermanent color pg. 555
developer pg. 555
double-process haircoloring pg. 571
filler pg. 593
foil technique pg. 584
foundation pg. 580
glaze pg. 597
hair color pg. 548
haircolor pg. 548
hair lightening pg. 553
highlighting pg. 580
highlighting shampoos pg. 589
highlighting shampoo tints pg. 589
intensity pg. 552
Law of Color pg. 548
level pg. 551
Level System pg. 551
lighteners pg. 557
line of demarcation pg. 572
metallic or gradual haircolors pg. 556
mixed melanin pg. 551
natural or vegetable haircolors pg. 556
new growth pg. 576
off-the-scalp lighteners pg. 575
on-the-scalp lighteners pg. 575
patch test pg. 563
permanent haircolor pg. 555
prelightening pg. 564
presoftening pg. 592
primary colors pg. 548
resistant pg. 592
reverse highlighting or lowlighting pg. 580
secondary color pg. 549
semipermanent haircolor pg. 554
single-process haircoloring pg. 571
slicing pg. 585
soap cap pg. 596
special effects haircoloring pg. 580
temporary haircolor pg. 554
tertiary color pg. 549
tone or tonality pg. 551
toners pg. 558
virgin application pg. 571
volume pg. 555
weaving pg. 585

One of the most creative, challenging, and popular salon services is haircoloring. It also has the potential for being one of the most lucrative areas in which a stylist can choose to work. You will probably find that most of your clients, at some time or another, will color their hair. They may want to enhance or change their hair color or cover gray. Clients who have their hair colored usually visit the salon every four to twelve weeks. These are the kinds of "regulars" you want among your client base (Figure 16–1).

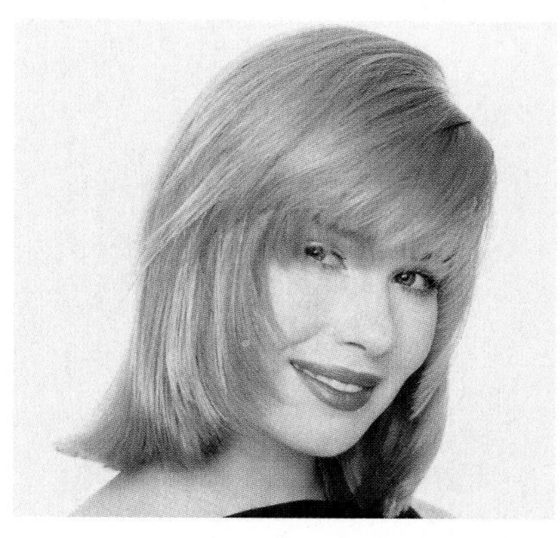

Figure 16–1 Haircoloring is a popular salon service.

Haircoloring is both a science and an art. A skilled haircolorist needs to become an expert in the following processes:

- depositing color on natural hair color
- depositing color on previously colored hair
- depositing color on hair that has been lightened
- lightening and depositing color in one step

You have reason to be excited about working in the area of haircoloring. It is artistic, adventurous, and in great demand. Color is an area of tremendous growth in the salon. If you fully understand both the theory and practical aspects of haircolor, you will have the opportunity to build a significant and loyal client base and earn a higher income. Statistics show that clients who have haircuts only stay with their stylist for an average of two years, while clients who receive color services stay with their stylist for eight years. Once a stylist demonstrates the ability to skillfully color a client's hair, the client will generally remain loyal.

WHY PEOPLE COLOR THEIR HAIR

It is important to have an understanding of what motivates people to color their hair. This information, which should come out of the client consultation, will help you determine which products and haircolor services are appropriate for your client. A few common reasons clients color their hair include the following:

- to cover up or blend gray (unpigmented) hair (Figure 16–2)
- to enhance an existing haircolor
- to create a fashion statement or a statement of self-expression
- to correct unwanted tones in hair from environmental exposure such as sun or chlorine
- to accentuate a particular haircut

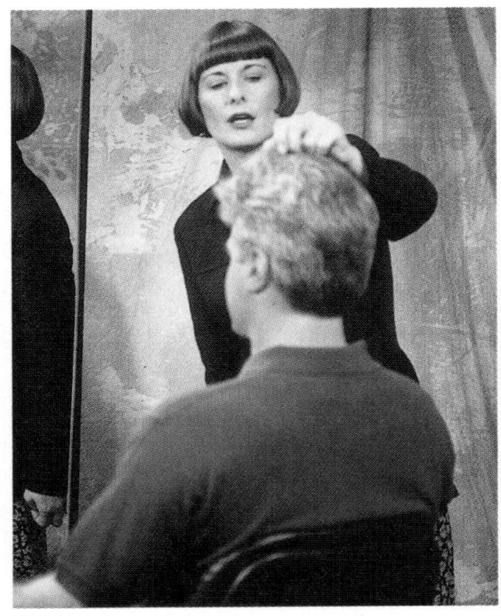

Figure 16-2 Many clients choose to cover or blend gray hair.

Many people experiment with haircoloring. When a client turns to you for advice and service, you need to have a thorough understanding of the hair structure and how haircoloring products affect it. As a trained professional, you will learn which shades of color are most flattering on your clients and which products and techniques will achieve the desired look.

NOTE: **Haircolor** (one word) is a professional, industry-coined term referring to artificial haircolor products and services. **Hair color** (two words) is the color of hair created by nature. For example, you might say of a client, "Mrs. Bailey's natural hair color is brown."

COLOR THEORY

Color is a form of light energy. All the colors we can see are contained in the visible spectrum of light (see Chapter 7). Before you attempt to apply haircoloring products, it is important to have a good general understanding of how colors work together.

The Law of Color

The **Law of Color** is a system for understanding color relationships. When combining colors, you will always get the same result from the same combination. Equal parts of red and blue mixed together always make violet. Equal parts of blue and yellow always make green. Equal parts of red and yellow always make orange. This system is called the Law of Color because these relationships have been tested over and over and have proven to be true. The color wheels that appear on this page and page 549 will help you understand these color relationships.

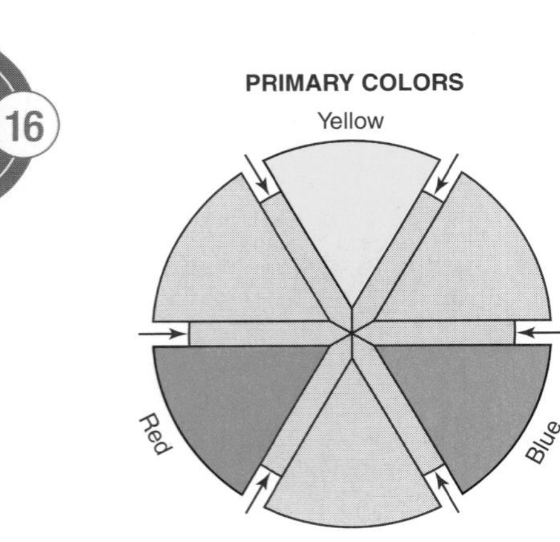

Figure 16-3 Primary colors.

Primary Colors

Primary colors are pure or fundamental colors that cannot be achieved from a mixture. The primary colors are blue, red, and yellow. All colors are created from these three primaries. Colors with a predominance of blue are cool-toned colors, and colors with a predominance of red are warm-toned colors (Figure 16–3).

Blue is the darkest of the primary colors and is the only cool primary color. In addition to coolness, blue also brings depth or darkness to any color to which it is added.

Red is the medium primary color. Red added to blue-based colors will cause them to appear lighter. Red added to yellow colors will cause them to become darker.

Yellow is the lightest of the primary colors. When you add yellow to other colors, the resulting color is lighter and brighter in appearance.

When all three primary colors are present in equal proportions, the resulting color is black. It is helpful to think of hair colors in terms of their relative proportions of primary colors. Neutral brown, for example, has the primary colors in the following proportions: blue—B, red—RR, yellow—YYY.

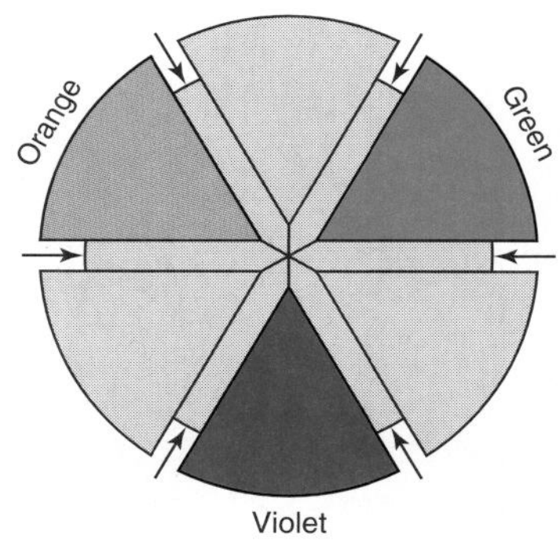

Figure 16–4 Secondary colors.

Secondary Colors

A **secondary color** is a color obtained by mixing equal parts of two primary colors. The secondary colors are green, orange, and violet. Green is an equal combination of blue and yellow. Orange is an equal combination of red and yellow. Violet is an equal combination of blue and red (Figure 16–4).

Tertiary Colors

A **tertiary color** is an intermediate color achieved by mixing a secondary color and its neighboring primary color on the color wheel in equal amounts. The tertiary colors include blue-green, blue-violet, red-violet, red-orange, yellow-orange, and yellow-green. Natural-looking haircolor is made up of a combination of primary and secondary colors (Figure 16–5).

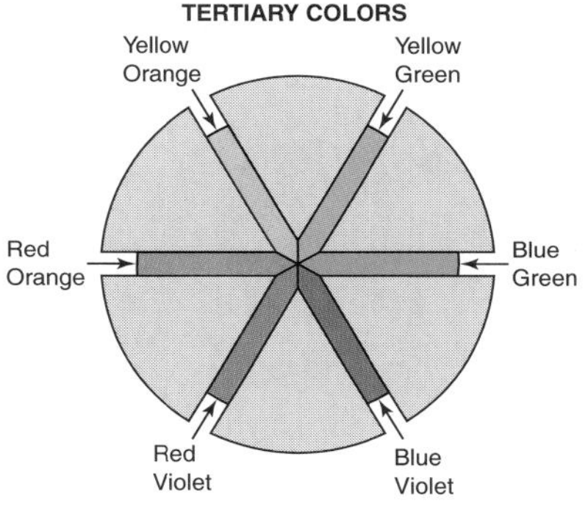

Figure 16–5 Tertiary colors.

Complementary Colors

Complementary colors are a primary and secondary color positioned opposite each other on the color wheel. Complementary colors include blue and orange, red and green, and yellow and violet.

Complementary colors neutralize each other (Figure 16–7). When formulating haircolor, you will find that it is often your goal to emphasize or distract from skin tones or eye color. You may also want to neutralize or refine unwanted tones in the hair. Understanding complementary colors will help you choose the appropriate tone to accomplish that goal. 1

activity

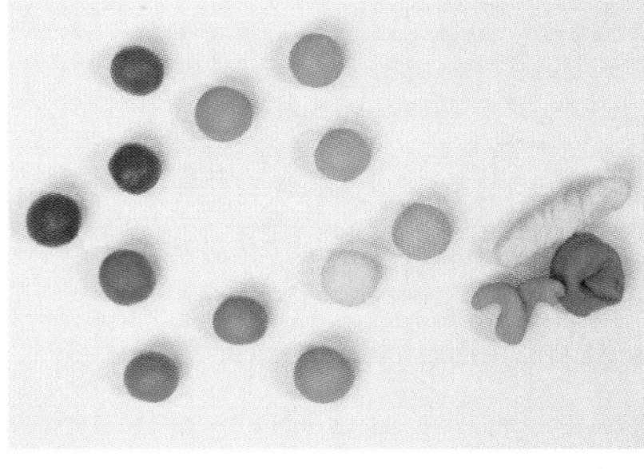

Figure 16–6 Creating the color wheel with clay.

Using modeling clay that represents the three primary colors—red, blue, and yellow—create secondary and tertiary colors. You will see that if you mix red clay with yellow clay in equal proportions, you will get orange. If you mix red clay with the orange clay you created, what is the result? What happens if you change the proportion of each color? The combinations are endless (Figure 16–6).

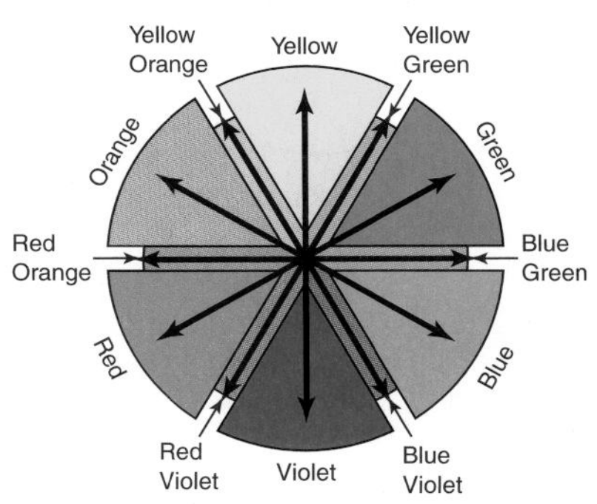

Figure 16–7 Complementary colors neutralize each other.

HAIR FACTS

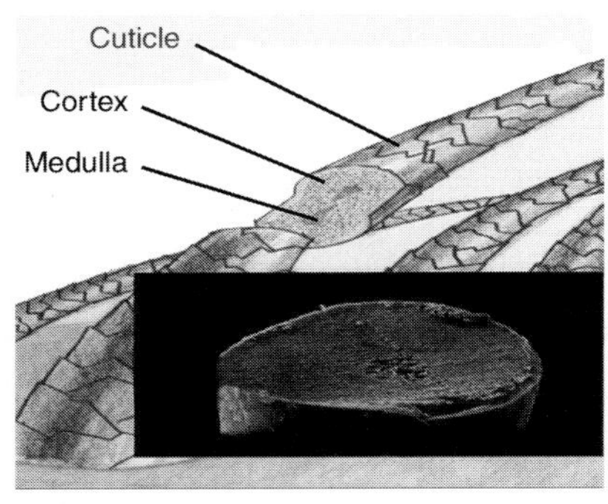

Figure 16-8 A cross-section of the hair shaft.

The structure of a client's hair is a determining factor in choosing which haircolor to use. The hair structure will also affect the quality and ultimate success of the haircolor service. Some haircolor products may cause a dramatic change in the structure of the hair while others cause relatively little change. Knowing how products affect the hair will allow you to make the best product choices for your client.

Hair Structure

The structure of hair is discussed in depth in Chapter 8. Let us do a quick review here. The hair is composed of three main parts (Figure 16–8).

- The cuticle is the outermost layer of the hair. It protects the interior cortex layer and contributes to 20 percent of the overall strength of the hair.
- The cortex is the middle layer and gives the hair strength and elasticity. A healthy cortex contributes about 80 percent to the overall strength of the hair. It contains the natural pigment called melanin, which determines if we are blondes, brunettes, or redheads. Melanin granules are scattered between the cortex cells like chips in a chocolate chip cookie.
- The medulla is the innermost layer. It is sometimes absent from the hair and plays a very minor role in the haircoloring process.

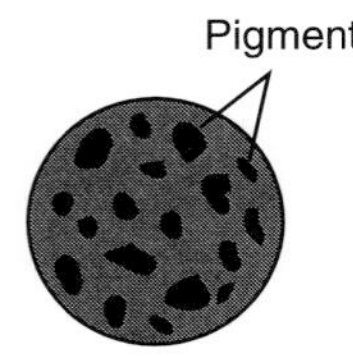

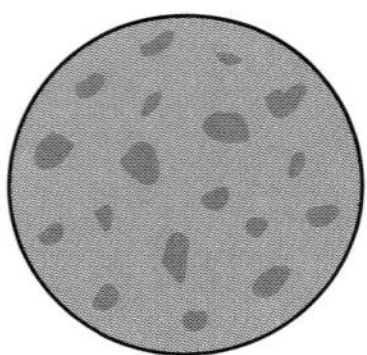

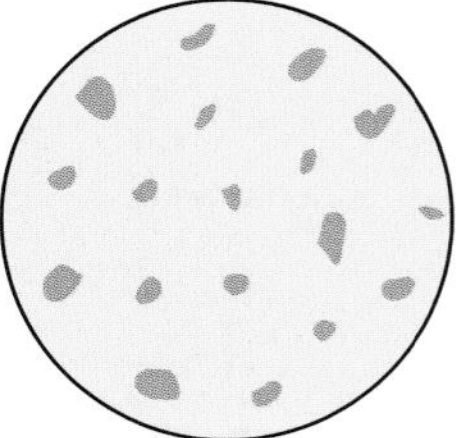

Figure 16-9 Melanin distribution according to hair texture.

Texture

Hair texture is determined by the diameter of the individual hair strand. Large, medium, and small diameter hair strands translate into coarse, medium, and fine hair textures, respectively. Melanin is distributed differently within the different textures. The melanin granules in fine hair are grouped more tightly, so the hair takes color faster and can look darker. Medium-textured hair has an average response to haircolor products. Coarse-textured hair has a larger diameter and can take longer to process (Figure 16–9).

Density

Another aspect of hair that plays a role in haircoloring is density. Hair density, the number of hairs per square inch, can range from thin to thick. Density must be taken into account when applying haircolor to assure proper coverage.

Porosity

Porosity is the ability to absorb liquid. Porous hair accepts haircolor faster and permits darker color than less porous hair. There are different degrees of porosity:

- *Low porosity.* The cuticle is tight; the hair is resistant, which means it is difficult for moisture or chemicals to penetrate, and requires a longer processing time.
- *Average porosity.* The cuticle is slightly raised; the hair is normal and processes in an average amount of time.

- *High porosity.* The cuticle is lifted; the hair is overporous and takes color quickly; color also tends to fade quickly.

Let us review the test for porosity from Chapter 8. Take a strand of several hairs from four different areas of the head: the front hairline, the temple, the crown, and the nape. Hold the strand securely with one hand and slide the thumb and forefinger of the other hand from the ends to the scalp. If the hair feels smooth and the cuticle is compact, dense, and hard, it has low porosity. If you can feel a slight roughness, it has average porosity. If the hair feels very rough, dry, or breaks, it has high porosity.

Natural Hair Color

Learning to identify a client's natural color is the most important step in becoming a good colorist. Natural hair color ranges from black to dark brown to red, and from dark blonde to light blonde. Hair color is unique to each individual; no two people have exactly the same color.

As you learned in Chapter 8, there are two types of melanin in the cortex:

- eumelanin is the melanin that gives black and brown color to hair
- pheomelanin is the melanin found in red hair. Very dark hair and most brunettes contain this pigment. Blonde hair contains a small amount of pheomelanin

Natural hair color can be a combination of both types of melanin. This is called **mixed melanin.**

Contributing pigment is the pigment that lies under the natural hair color and must be taken into consideration when you select a haircolor. Generally, when you lighten natural hair color, you expose contributing pigment (see page 558). The foundation of haircoloring is based on modifying this pigment with haircolor products to create new pigment.

THE LEVEL SYSTEM

Level is the unit of measurement used to identify the lightness or darkness of a color; it is sometimes referred to as value or depth. Colorists use the **Level System** to analyze the lightness or darkness of a hair color (Figure 16–10). Haircolor levels are arranged on a scale of 1 to 10, with 1 being the darkest and 10 being the lightest. The names for the natural hair color levels may vary from manufacturer to manufacturer. What is important is to be able to identify the degrees of lightness to darkness at each level.

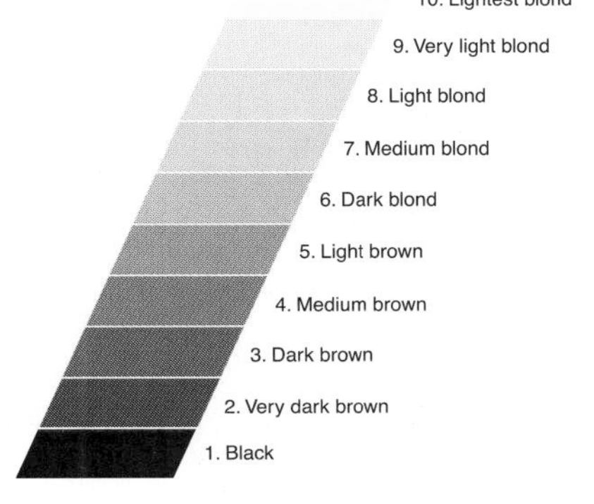

Figure 16–10 Natural hair color levels.

Tone and Intensity

The term **tone**, or **tonality**, is used to describe the warmth or coolness of a color. Reds, oranges, and yellows are all warm tones, as are auburn, copper, gold, bronze, or honey. The cool tones are blue, green, and violet. Descriptive haircolor names in the cool range include ash, drab, smoky, or platinum.

Figure 16–11 Manufacturers' swatches are a useful tool.

Intensity refers to the strength of a color tone. Intensity is described as mild, medium, or strong. Strawberry blonde, copper brown, and bright orange are various intensities of red shades.

Artificial haircolors are developed from the primary and secondary colors that form base colors. A **base color** is the predominant tonality of an existing color. The base color influences the final color result. For example, a violet base color will deliver cool results and will help minimize unwanted yellow tones. A blue base color will provide the coolest result and will help minimize orange tones in the hair. A red-orange base will create the kind of bright, warm results clients are looking for when they say they wish to be redheads. Gold bases create beautiful gold haircolor, from brunettes to light blondes. These are just a few examples of how base colors work.

Identifying Natural Level and Tone

Identifying natural levels is the first step in performing a haircolor service. One of the most valuable tools to help you with your work is the color wheel. Haircolor swatch books provide a visual representation as well (Figure 16–11).

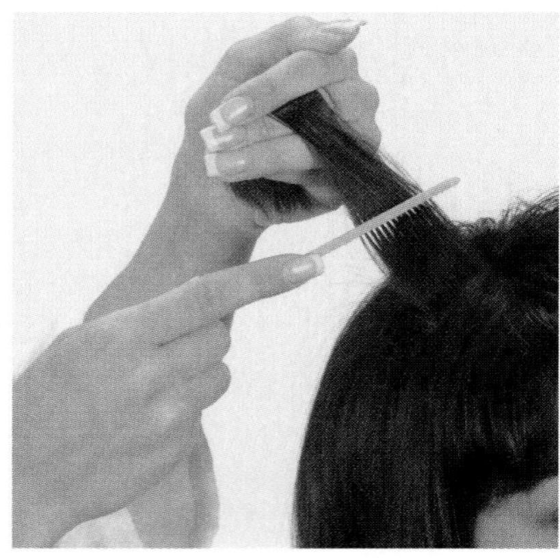

Figure 16–12 Take a 1/2" square section in the crown.

To determine natural level, perform the following four steps.

1. Take a ½-inch square section in the crown area and hold it up from the scalp, allowing light to pass through (Figure 16–12).
2. Using the natural level finder swatches provided by the manufacturer, select a swatch that you think matches the section of hair and place it against the hair. Remember, you are trying to determine depth level (darkness or lightness). Do not part or hold the hair flat against the scalp; that will give you an incorrect reading, as the hair will appear darker (Figure 16–13).
3. Move the swatch from the scalp area along the hair strand.
4. Determine the natural hair color level.

Gray Hair

Gray hair is normally associated with aging, although heredity is also a contributing factor. Even though the loss of pigment increases as a person ages, few people ever become completely white-haired. Most retain a certain

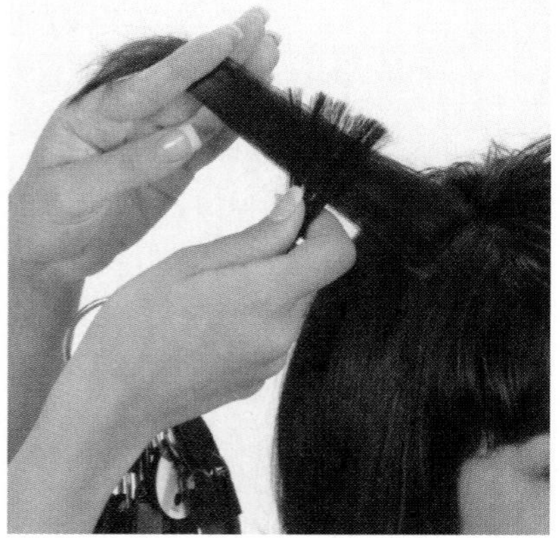

Figure 16–13 Hold the color swatch against the hair strand.

activity

The missing primary color in this activity is what you would use to neutralize the unwanted tone. Find the missing primary to neutralize the following:

Tone	Missing Primary
Orange	?
Green	?
Violet	?

(Answers: blue, red, yellow)

Percentage of Gray Hair	Characteristics
30%	More pigmented than gray hair
50%	Even mixture of gray and pigmented hair
70 to 90%	More gray than pigmented; most of remaining pigment is located in the back of the head
100%	Virtually no pigmented hair; tends to look white

Table 16–1 Determining the Percentage of Gray Hair

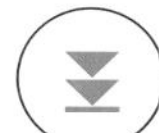

Here's a tip:

The question of light is critical in analyzing hair color. You may wish to rely on natural light, even walking out of doors with a client to make your analysis. Artificial light affects your perception of natural hair color, particularly fluorescent light, which can distort color drastically.

percentage of pigmented hair. The gray can be solid or blended throughout the head, as in "salt and pepper hair" (see Table 16–1).

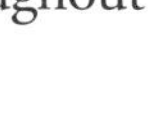

Gray hair requires special attention in formulating haircolor (this will be discussed later in the chapter).

TYPES OF HAIRCOLOR

Haircoloring products generally fall into four categories: temporary, semipermanent, demipermanent, and permanent. All these haircolor products, except for temporary color, require a patch test before application to determine if the client is allergic to the product (see page 563 for procedure). Lighteners, metallic haircolors, and natural colors will also be discussed in this chapter. Each of these categories has a unique chemical composition, which, in turn, affects the final color result and how long it will last.

First, let us discuss the process of **hair lightening**, often referred to as "bleaching" or "decolorizing," which is a chemical process involving the diffusion of the natural color pigment or artificial color from the hair. This process is central to both permanent haircolor and hair lighteners.

All permanent haircolor products and lighteners contain both a developer, or oxidizing agent, and an alkalizing ingredient as part of their composition (see Chapter 7). The role of the alkalizing ingredient—ammonia or an ammonia substitute—is to:

- raise the cuticle of the hair fiber so the tint (permanent color) can penetrate

- facilitate the formation of tints within the hair fiber (also referred to as the "oxidation reaction")
- bring about the lightening action of peroxide

When the tint containing the alkalizing ingredient is combined with the developer (usually hydrogen peroxide), the peroxide becomes alkaline and diffuses, or breaks up, through the hair fiber, entering the cortex, where the melanin is located. The lightening occurs when the alkaline peroxide breaks up the melanin and replaces it with new color.

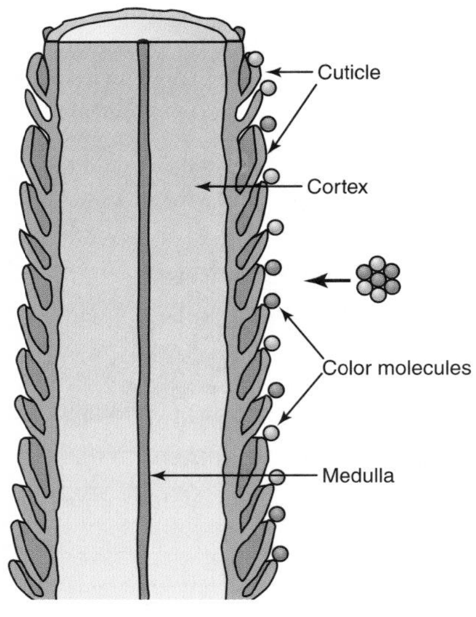

Figure 16-14 Action of temporary haircolor.

Temporary Haircolor

For individuals who wish to use a subtle neutralizer for yellowing hair or to neutralize unwanted tones, **temporary haircolor** would be a good choice. The pigment molecules in temporary color are large and, therefore, do not penetrate the cuticle layer, allowing only a coating action that may be removed by shampooing (Figure 16–14). Temporary haircolor makes only a physical change, not a chemical change, in the hair shaft, and no patch test is required.

Temporary haircolors are available in a variety of colors and products:

- color rinses applied weekly to shampooed hair to add color; the hair is styled dry
- colored mousses and gels used for slight color and for dramatic effects
- hair mascara used for dramatic effects
- spray-on haircolor that is easy to apply, used for special effects
- color-enhancing shampoos used to brighten, impart slight color, and eliminate unwanted tones

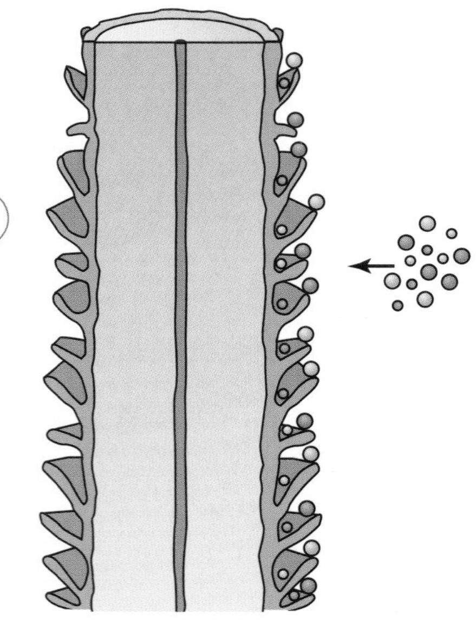

Figure 16-15 Action of semipermanent haircolor.

Semipermanent Haircolor

Semipermanent haircolor is haircolor formulated to last through several shampoos, depending on the hair's porosity. The pigment molecules are small enough to partially penetrate the hair shaft and stain the cuticle layer, but they are also small enough to diffuse out of the hair during shampooing and thus fade with each shampoo. It lasts only six to eight weeks. It does not lighten the hair, so there is no significant color change, and it does not require maintenance of new growth. It is formulated without ammonia and is generally as gentle to the hair as shampoo, but it does require a patch test before application (Figure 16–15).

Many semipermanent colors can be used right out of the bottle. Others require the addition of an activator prior to application. This activator develops the color pigments within the formula and helps to swell the cortex and open the cuticle for color penetration.

Some semipermanent colors come packaged with an after-rinse. The rinse helps prevent fading to a lighter color as well as fading off-tone and leaves the hair soft, pliable, and easy to comb. Whether or not the product you select is packaged this way, it is always a good idea to finish your service with a mild conditioning rinse.

Demipermanent Haircolor

Demipermanent haircolor (also called deposit-only haircolor and referred to as semipermanent by some manufacturers) is similar in nature to semipermanent haircolor but is longer lasting. It is formulated to deposit but not lift (lighten) color. It has a smaller tint molecule and therefore is able to penetrate the hair shaft. This formula generally imparts vivid color results. Demipermanent haircolors are ideal for covering unpigmented hair, refreshing faded permanent color, depositing tonal changes without lift, corrective coloring, and reverse highlighting.

By their very nature, demipermanent or deposit-only haircolors darken the natural hair color when applied (Figure 16–16). They cause little or no damage to the hair and are generally positioned as gentle and mild due to their low ammonia or no-ammonia formula. In recent years, demipermanent products have been used exclusively on the middle of the hair shaft to the ends after permanent color has been applied to the base area. This fights the buildup effect that can occur on previously colored hair and is also less aggressive, resulting in less damage.

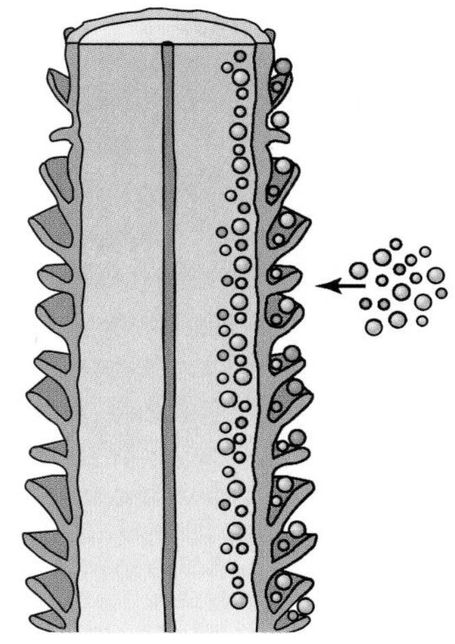

Figure 16–16 Action of demipermanent haircolor.

Demipermanent haircolor is available as a gel, cream, or liquid. It requires a patch test.

Permanent Haircolor

Permanent haircolor is mixed with a developer (hydrogen peroxide) and remains in the hair shaft until the new growth of hair occurs. It is used to match, lighten, and cover gray hair. Permanent haircolor products generally contain ammonia, oxidative tints, and peroxide. They require a patch test.

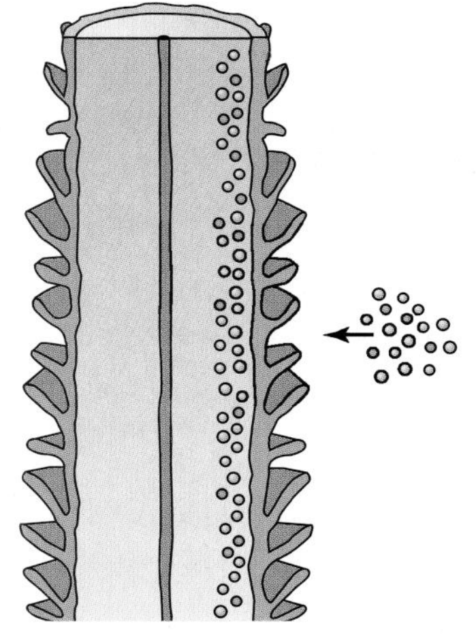

Figure 16–17 Action of permanent haircolors.

The tint formula contains uncolored dye precursors, which are very small compounds that can diffuse into the hair shaft. These dye precursors, also referred to as **aniline derivatives**, combine with hydrogen peroxide to form larger, permanent tint molecules. These molecules are trapped within the cortex of the hair and cannot be shampooed out (Figure 16–17 and Figure 16–18). This is why these products are considered permanent.

16

Permanent haircoloring products are regarded as the best products for covering gray hair. They simultaneously remove natural pigment from the pigmented hair through the action of lightening while adding artificial color to both the gray and the pigmented hair. The action of simultaneously removing and adding color, blending gray and nongray hair uniformly, results in a natural-looking color. Table 16–2 provides a brief review of the four haircolor categories. 3✓

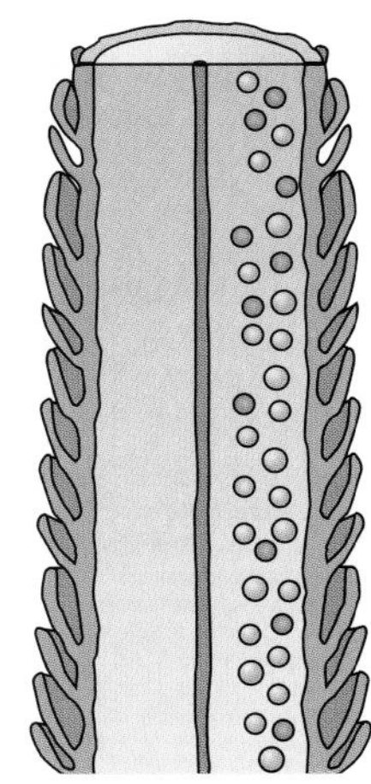

Figure 16–18 Permanent haircolor molecules inside the cortex.

Hydrogen Peroxide Developers

A **developer** is an oxidizing agent that, when mixed with an oxidative haircolor, supplies the necessary oxygen gas to develop color molecules and create a change in hair color. Developers, also called oxidizing agents or catalysts, have a pH between 2.5 and 4.5. Although there are a number of developers on the market, hydrogen peroxide (H_2O_2) is the one most commonly used in haircolor.

Volume is the measure of the potential oxidation of varying strengths of hydrogen peroxide. The lower the volume, the less lift is achieved; the higher

Category	Uses
Temporary color	Creates fun, bold results that easily shampoo from the hair Neutralizes yellow hair
Semipermanent color	Introduces a client to haircolor services Adds subtle color results Tones prelightened hair
Demipermanent color	Blends gray hair Enhances natural color Tones prelightened hair Refreshes faded colorFiller in color correction
Permanent haircolor	Changes existing haircolor Covers gray Creates bright or natural-looking haircolor changes

Table 16–2 Review of Haircolor Categories and Their Uses

the volume, the greater the lifting action. The majority of permanent haircolor products use 10, 20, 30, or 40 volume hydrogen peroxide for proper color development (see Table 16–3). Store peroxide in a cool, dark, dry place.

16

Natural and Metallic Haircolors

A group of haircolors that are not generally used in the salon but that you should be familiar with are natural, or vegetable, haircolors and metallic haircolors, also referred to gradual colors.

Natural Haircolors

Natural or **vegetable haircolors** such as henna are natural colors obtained from the leaves or bark of plants. There is no lightening of natural hair color with this process, the color result tends to be weak, and the process tends to be lengthy and messy. Also, shade ranges are limited; for instance, henna is usually available only in black, chestnut, and auburn tones. Finally, when the client who has used natural haircolors comes to the salon for chemical haircoloring services, she may be distressed to find out that many of these chemical products cannot be applied over natural hair colors.

Metallic Haircolor

Metallic haircolors, also called **gradual colors**, contain metal salts and change hair color gradually by progressive buildup and exposure to air, creating a dull, metallic appearance. These products require daily

Volume	When to Use
10 Volume	When less lightening is desired to enhance a client's natural hair color
20 Volume	The standard volume; used to achieve most results with permanent haircolor and used for complete gray coverage
30 Volume	Used for additional lift with permanent haircolor
40 Volume	Used with most high-lift colors to provide maximum lift in a one-step color service

Table 16-3 Hydrogen Peroxide Volume and Uses

application and historically have been marketed to men. The main problem with this type of haircolor is that the shades can appear unnatural. The limited shade range is also a drawback. Compound dyes are a combination of metallic colors and a vegetable tint. They are also not used professionally.

Lighteners

Lighteners are the chemical compounds that lighten hair by dispersing, dissolving, and decolorizing the natural hair pigment. As soon as hydrogen peroxide is mixed into the lightener formula, it begins to release oxygen. This process, known as oxidation, occurs within the cortex of the hair shaft.

Hair lighteners are used to create a blonde shade that is not achievable with permanent haircolor and to achieve the following:

- lighten the hair prior to application of a color; to create the final color
- lighten hair to a particular shade
- brighten and lighten an existing shade
- lighten only certain parts of the hair
- lighten dark natural or color-treated levels

The Decolorizing Process

The hair goes through different stages of color as it lightens (Figure 16–19). The amount of change depends on how much pigment the hair has, the strength of the lightening product, and the length of time it is processed.

During the process of decolorizing, natural hair can go through as many as 10 stages (Figure 16–20).

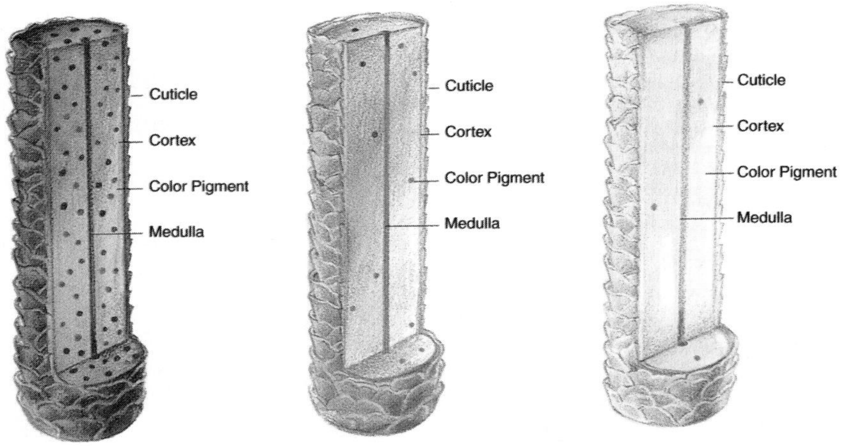

Figure 16–19 Hair lighteners diffuse pigment.

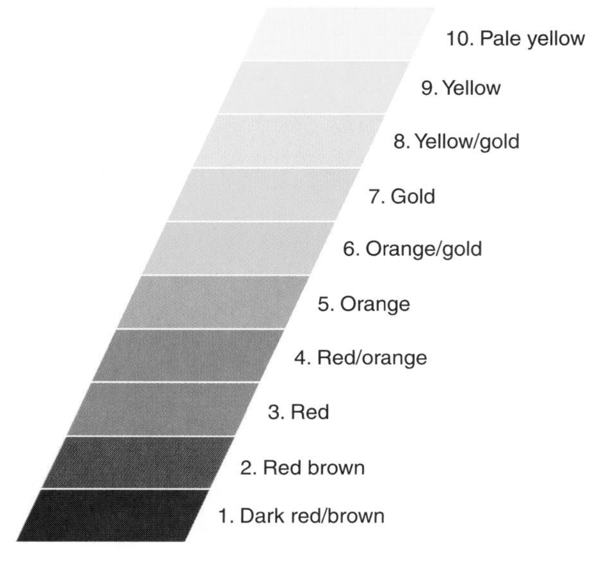

Figure 16–20 Ten degrees of decolorization.

CONTRIBUTION OF UNDERLYING PIGMENT

Decolorizing the hair's natural melanin pigment allows the colorist to create the exact degree of contributing pigment needed for the final result. First, the hair is decolorized to the appropriate level. Then the new color is applied to deposit the desired color. The natural pigment that remains in the hair contributes to the artificial color that is added. Lightening the hair to the correct stage is essential to a beautiful, controlled, final haircoloring result.

Toners are semipermanent, demipermanent, and permanent haircolor products that are used primarily on prelightened hair to achieve pale and delicate colors. They are applied to the lightest degree of contributing pigment that remains after the decolorizing process.

CAUTION

It is often difficult to lighten dark hair to a very pale blonde without extreme damage to the hair. The client should be alerted to the danger before proceeding with the service.

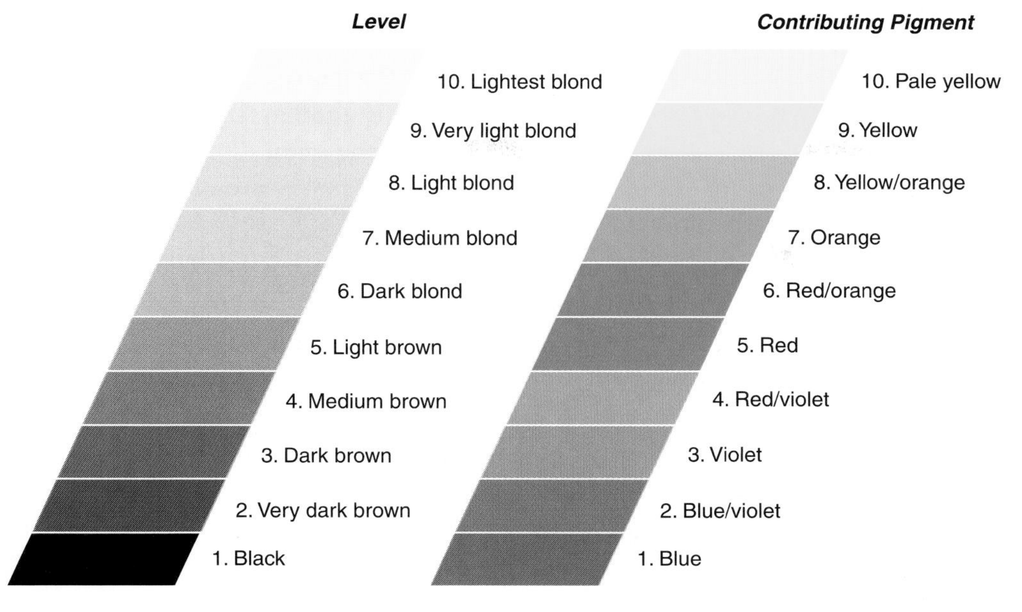

Figure 16–21 Contributing pigment (undertones).

Not all hair will go through all 10 degrees of decolorization. Each natural hair color starts the decolorization process at a different stage. Remember, the goal is to create the correct degree of contributing pigment as the foundation for the final haircolor result (Figure 16–21).

The hair is never safely lifted past the pale yellow stage to white with lightener. The extreme diffusion of color necessary to give hair a white appearance causes excessive damage to the hair strand. The result is that wet hair feels "mushy" and will stretch without returning to its original length. When dry, the hair is harsh and brittle. Such hair often suffers breakage and will not accept a toner properly. However, this does not mean that only those born with blonde hair can be white-blondes. The baby-blonde look can be achieved by lightening to pale yellow and neutralizing the unwanted undertone (contributing pigment) with a toner. 4 ✓

CONSULTATION

A haircolor consultation is the most critical part of the color service. The consultation is the first important step in establishing a relationship with your client. During the consultation, your client will communicate what she is looking for in a haircolor service. You will be listening carefully, taking in all the information so that you can make an appropriate haircolor recommendation. Allowing sufficient time for the consultation is the single most reliable way to help ensure a client's satisfaction (Figure 16–22).

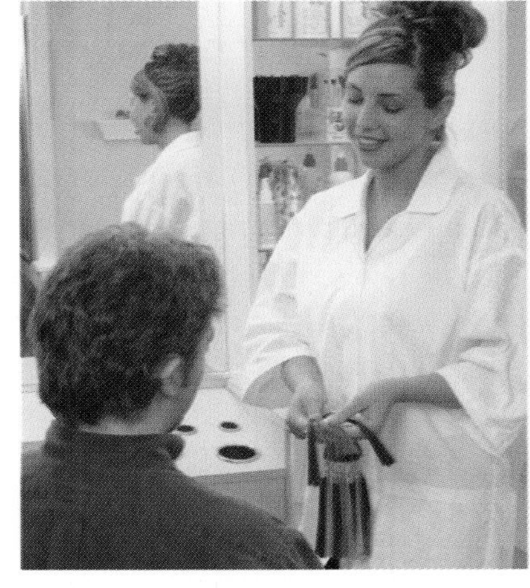

Figure 16–22 A client consultation should precede every haircolor service.

16

CAUTION

Medications can affect hair color. In the consultation, determine if the client is taking any medications. Medical treatments for conditions such as diabetes, high blood pressure, and thyroid problems will all affect the outcome of color and most chemical services. Discuss this with your instructor for more information.

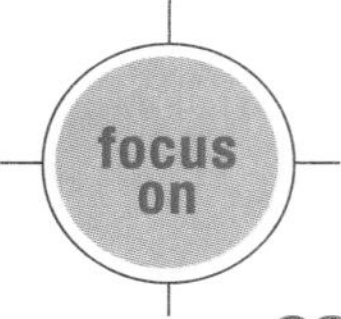

...communication.

Using descriptive language to discuss products and services with your clients is an important part of the communication process. It also helps you sell.

- Use persuasive language in discussing haircolor (for example, "soft, buttery blonde," "rich chocolate brown," "spicy, coppery red").
- Avoid words that can be interpreted negatively like "bleached," "frosted," and "roots."
- Use positive "mood" words to convey the benefits to your client (for example, "healthy-looking," "richer," "natural-looking," "subtle").

Begin the consultation in an area with proper lighting so you can accurately assess the client's hair. If possible, the walls should be white or neutral. Include the following steps in the consultation.

1. Book 15 minutes extra for the consultation. Introduce yourself to the client and welcome him to the salon. Offer a beverage. During this time with a new client, make sure there are no interruptions.
2. Have the client fill out an information card (see Chapter 4). This allows you to compile a hair history and to note what type of color service he is looking for. Pay attention to the client's skin and eye color, condition and length of the hair, and amount of gray hair.
3. Look at the client directly. Do not look at him through the mirror. Ask him what he is thinking about doing with his hair color. Ask leading questions. Let him talk. Keep him on track by discussing the recent history of his hair (over the past six months). Your questions might include:
   - Are you looking for a temporary or permanent change?
   - Do you want color all over or just a few highlights?
   - Do you see yourself with a more conservative or dramatic type of color?
   - Have you seen so-and-so's hair? (For instance, a TV celebrity.) That color would look great on you.
   - Would you like to add shine to your hair?
4. Recommend at least two different haircolor options. Show pictures of different ranges of colors, from brunette to blonde, red, and highlighted colors.
5. Review the procedure and application technique, the maintenance involved, and the cost of the service and follow-up maintenance. Sometimes, several steps may be necessary to obtain a haircolor result. A client may love a certain haircolor, but may not be able to afford it. Have a more economical back-up solution ready.
6. Be honest and do not promise the world. If you are faced with a corrective situation, let the client know what you can do today and how many visits it will take to achieve what he is looking for.
7. Gain approval from the client.
8. Start the haircolor service.
9. Follow through during the service by educating and informing the client about home care, products, and rebooking. Let the client know what type of shampoo and conditioner is needed to maintain the color. Let him know how many weeks it will be before he needs to come back for another service.
10. Fill out the client's haircolor record (Figure 16–23).

HAIRCOLOR RECORD

Name ______________________ Tel. ______________________

Address ______________________ City ______________________

Patch Test: ☐ Negative ☐ Positive Date ______________________

Eye Color ______________________ Skin Tone ______________________

DESCRIPTION OF HAIR

Form	**Length**	**Texture**	**Density**	**Porosity**	
☐ straight	☐ short	☐ coarse	☐ sparse	☐ very porous	☐ resistant
☐ wavy	☐ medium	☐ medium	☐ moderate	☐ porous	☐ very resistant
☐ curly	☐ long	☐ fine	☐ thick	☐ normal	☐ perm. waved

Natural hair color ______________________

Level (1-10) Tone (Warm, Cool, etc.) Intensity (Mild, Medium, Strong)

Scalp Condition

☐ normal ☐ dry ☐ oily ☐ sensitive

Condition

☐ normal ☐ dry ☐ oily ☐ faded ☐ streaked (uneven)

% unpigmented ______________________ Distribution of unpigmented ______________________

Previously lightened with ______________________ for ______________________ (time)

Previously tinted with ______________________ for ______________________ (time)

☐ original hair sample enclosed ☐ original hair sample not enclosed

Desired hair color ______________________

Level (1-10) Tone (Warm, Cool, etc.) Intensity (Mild, Medium, Strong)

CORRECTIVE TREATMENTS

Color filler used ______________________ Conditioning treatments with ______________________

HAIR TINTING PROCESS

whole head ______________________ retouch inches (cm) ______________________ shade desired ______________________

formula: (color/lightener) ______________________ application technique ______________________

Results: ☐ good ☐ poor ☐ too light ☐ too dark ☐ streaked

Comments: ______________________

Date	**Operator**	**Price**	**Date**	**Operator**	**Price**

Figure 16–23 Haircolor Record.

16

Release Statement

A release statement is used by many salons when providing chemical services. Its purpose is to explain to clients that if their hair is in questionable condition, it may not withstand the requested chemical treatment. It also asks that clients provide more information about any prior chemical experimentation that may affect the current color selection and its end result.

To some degree, the release statement is designed to protect the school or salon owner from responsibility for accidents or damages and is required for most malpractice insurance. Take note, however, that a release statement is not a legally binding contract and will not clear the cosmetologist of responsibility for what may happen to a client's hair (Figure 16–24).

RELEASE FORM

I, the undersigned, ____

(name)

residing at ____

(street, address)

____

(city, state and zip)

about to receive services in the Clinical Department of

____

and having been advised that the services shall be performed by either students, graduate students, and/or instructors of the school, in consideration of the nominal charge for such services, hereby release the school, its students, graduate students, instructors, agents, representatives, and/or employees, from any and all claims arising out of and in any way connected with the performance of these services.

The Proprietor Is Not Responsible for Personal Property

Signed ____

Date ____

Witnessed ____

THIS RELEASE FORM MUST BE SIGNED BY THE PARENT OR GUARDIAN IF THE CLIENT BEING SERVED IS UNDER 18 YEARS OF AGE.

Figure 16–24 Release Form.

Patch Test

When working with haircolor, you will have to determine whether your clients have any allergies or sensitivities to the mixture. To identify an allergy in a client, the U.S. Federal Food, Drug, and Cosmetic Act prescribes that a **patch test**, also called a predisposition test, be given 24 to 48 hours prior to an application of an aniline tint or toner. The tint used for the patch test must be the same type as the tint that will be used for the haircolor service and the same color (that is, if someone is having their hair colored with 5BR by a particular manufacturer, for instance, use the 5BR shade in the patch test). The following procedure for patch tests should be closely followed:

CAUTION

A patch test must be given before coloring the hair with an aniline derivative product. Aniline derivative tints must never be used on the eyelashes or eyebrows. To do so may cause blindness.

Performing a Patch Test

1. Select the test area. Behind the ear or on the inside of the elbow are good choices.
2. Using a mild soap, cleanse and dry an area about the size of a quarter (Figure 16–25).
3. Mix a small amount of product according to the manufacturer's directions (Figure 16–26).
4. Apply to the test area with a sterile cotton swab (Figure 16–27).
5. Leave undisturbed for 24 hours.
6. Examine the test area. If there are no signs of redness or irritation, you can proceed with the color service.
7. Log the results on the client information card.

A negative skin test will show no sign of inflammation and indicates that the color may be safely applied. A positive result will show redness and a slight rash or welt. A client with these symptoms is allergic, and under no circumstances should she receive a haircolor service with the substance tested.

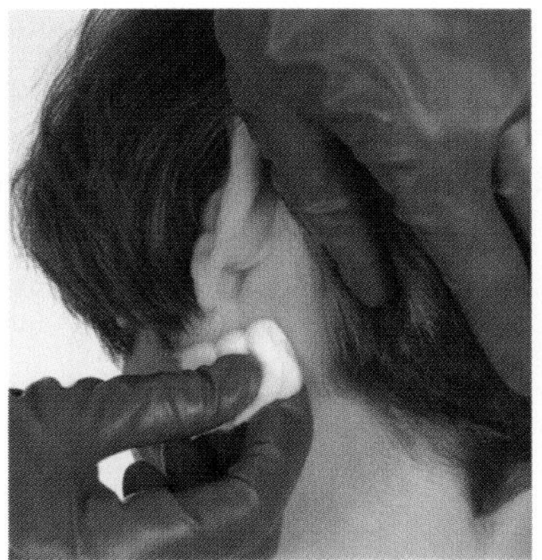

Figure 16-25 Clean patch area.

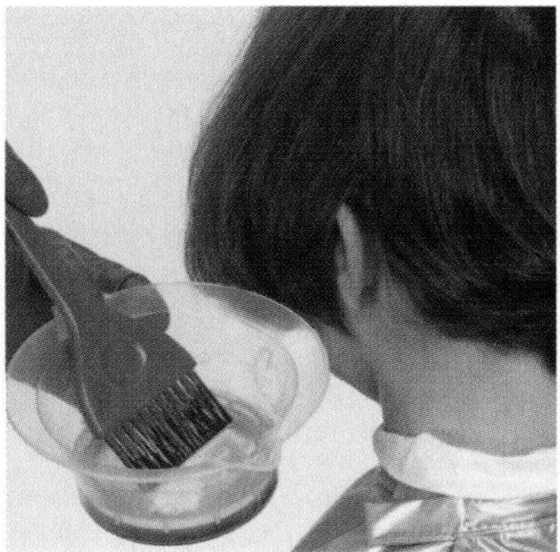

Figure 16-26 Mix tint and peroxide.

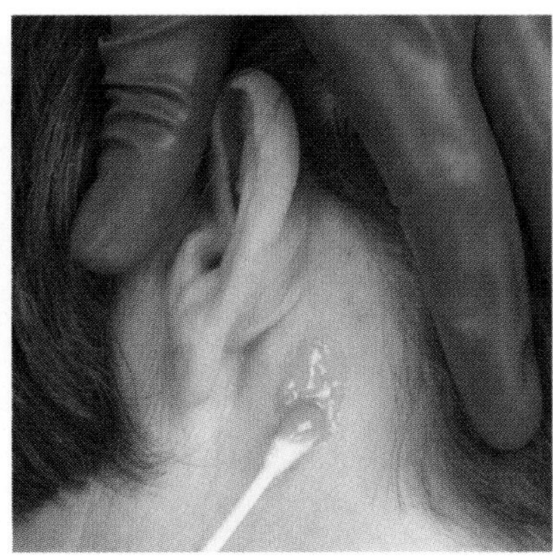

Figure 16-27 Apply tint mixture.

HAIRCOLOR APPLICATION PROCEDURES

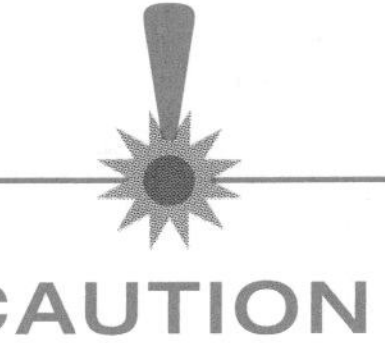

CAUTION

Always perform a patch test before applying semipermanent color. Semipermanent tints contain aniline derivatives to which some people may be sensitive or allergic. If the patch test proves negative, you may proceed, but follow the manufacturers' directions carefully.

To ensure successful results when performing haircoloring services, the colorist must follow a prescribed procedure. A clearly defined system makes for the greatest efficiency and the safest and most satisfactory results. Without such a plan, the work will take longer, results will be uneven, and mistakes may be made.

Preliminary Strand Test

Once you have created a color formula for your client, try it out first on a small strand of hair. This preliminary strand test will tell you how the hair will react to the formula and how long the formula should be left on the hair. The strand test is performed after the client is prepared for the coloring service.

Temporary Colors

There are many methods of applying a temporary color, depending on the product used. Your instructor will help you interpret each manufacturer's directions. One method of applying color rinse is outlined in Procedure 44. To apply gels, mousses, foams, or sprays, return the client to your work area after shampooing and apply color according to manufacturers' directions.

Semipermanent Haircolors

Semipermanent colors lack the strong oxidizers necessary to lift; they deposit color and do no substantial lifting. When selecting a semipermanent color, remember that color applied on top of color always creates a darker color.

The porosity of the hair will determine how well these products "take." Due to their depositing nature, semipermanent colors may also build up on the hair ends with each application. A strand test will determine your formula and processing time before each service.

16

Demipermanent (Deposit-only) Haircolor

The application procedure for a demipermanent haircolor is similar to that of a semipermanent color, since neither color alters the hair's natural melanin or produces lift. Follow the manufacturer's guidelines for application and processing time for the product you have selected.

Gray (unpigmented) hair presents special challenges when formulating demipermanent haircolor. As there is no lift, the resulting depth of color when covering gray hair may appear too extreme unless you allow for some brightness in your formulation. It is usually not advisable to color gray hair one even shade, since natural hair color has different depths and tonalities that give it the added life that gray hair is lacking.

Hair that has previously received a color service will have a greater degree of porosity, which must also be taken into account when formulating and applying a demipermanent haircolor.

Permanent Haircolor

Permanent haircolor applications are classified as either single-process or double-process.

PROCEDURE

PRELIMINARY STRAND TEST

Implements and Materials

- tint cape
- plastic clips
- glass or plastic mixing bowl
- spray water bottle
- shampoo
- towels
- color brushes
- protective gloves
- aluminum foil or plastic wrap
- client record card
- selected tint
- tint brush or bottle
- hydrogen peroxide developer

Procedure

1. Client consultation. Perform a scalp and hair analysis.
2. Drape the client. Drape the client to protect her skin and clothing.
3. Part off a ½-inch (1.25-cm) square strand of hair in the lower crown. Using plastic clips as necessary, fasten other hair out of the way.
4. Place the strand over the foil or plastic wrap and apply the mixture. Follow the application method for the color procedure you will be using (Figure 16–28 and Figure 16–29).
5. Check the development at 5-minute intervals until the desired color has been achieved (Figure 16–30). Note the timing on the record card.

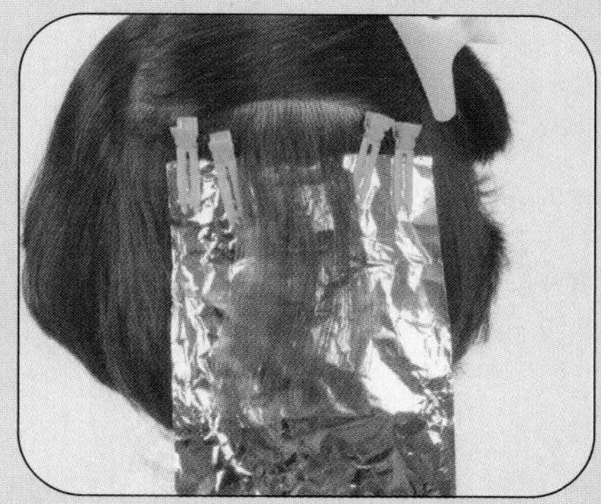

Figure 16–28 Place the test strand over foil.

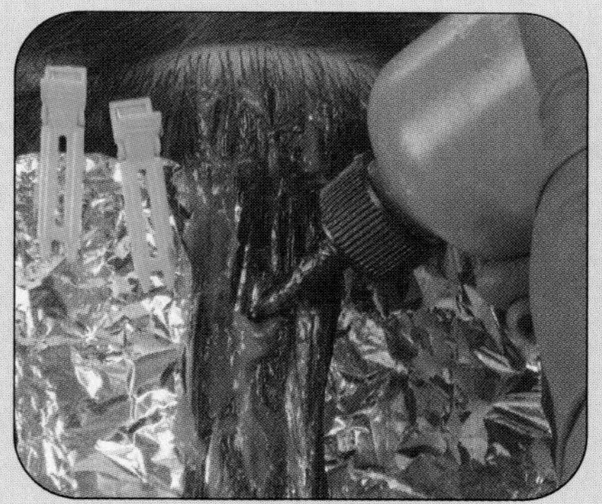

Figure 16–29 Apply tint to strand.

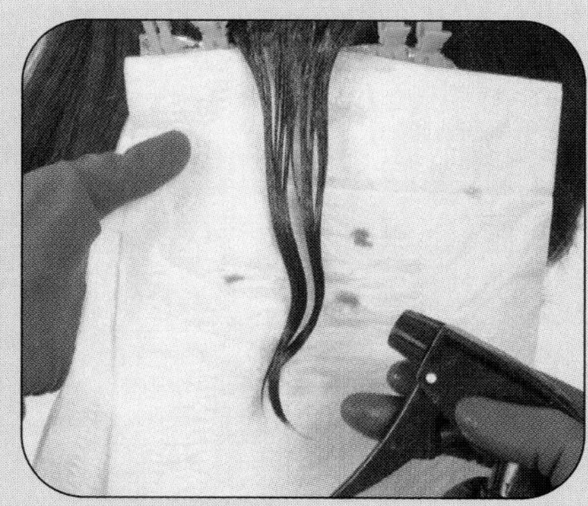

Figure 16–30 Check strand.

6. When satisfactory color has developed, remove the protective foil or plastic wrap. Place a towel under the strand, mist it thoroughly with water, add shampoo, and massage through (Figure 16–31). Rinse by spraying with water. Dry the strand with the towel and observe results.
7. Adjust the formula, the timing, or the application method as necessary and proceed with the color service.

CAUTION

Operator dermatitis, although rare, involves the same types of negative reactions to chemicals as those a client may experience. Since a colorist's hands are in contact with chemical solutions repeatedly during an average day, it is important to take proper precautions. Protect yourself from allergic reactions by wearing gloves until the haircolor product is completely removed from the client's hair.

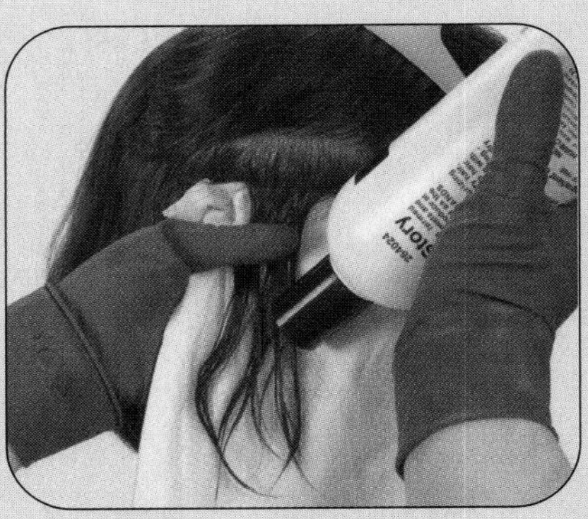

Figure 16–31 Shampoo strand.

completed! 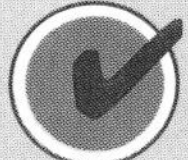

PROCEDURE

TEMPORARY HAIRCOLOR APPLICATION

Implements and Materials

- shampoo cape
- towels
- protective gloves
- comb
- applicator bottle (optional)
- temporary haircolor product
- shampoo
- record card
- gloves
- timer

Preparation

1. Perform a client consultation (Figure 16–32).
2. Ask the client to remove any jewelry and keep it in a safe place.
3. Drape the client for a haircoloring service. Slide a towel down from the back of the client's head and place lengthwise across the client's shoulders. Cross the ends of the towel beneath the chin and place the cape over the towel. Fasten the cape in the back. Fold the towel over the top of the cape and secure in front.
4. Shampoo and towel-dry the hair.

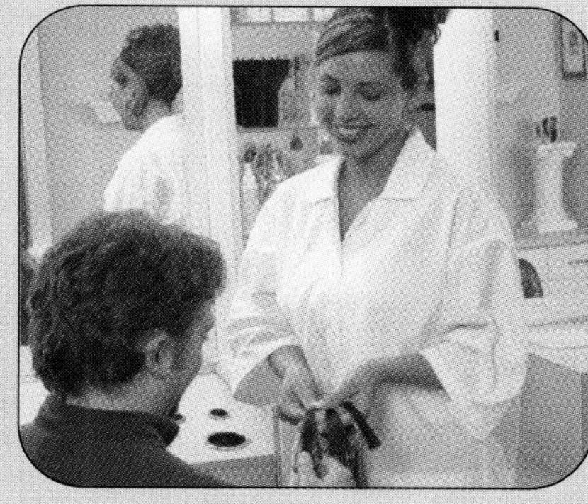

Figure 16-32 Client consultation.

Procedure

1. Make sure the client is comfortably reclined at the shampoo bowl. Put on the gloves. Use an applicator bottle as directed by your instructor. Shake the product thoroughly to blend any pigments that may have settled. Apply the color and work it around the entire head (Figure 16–33).

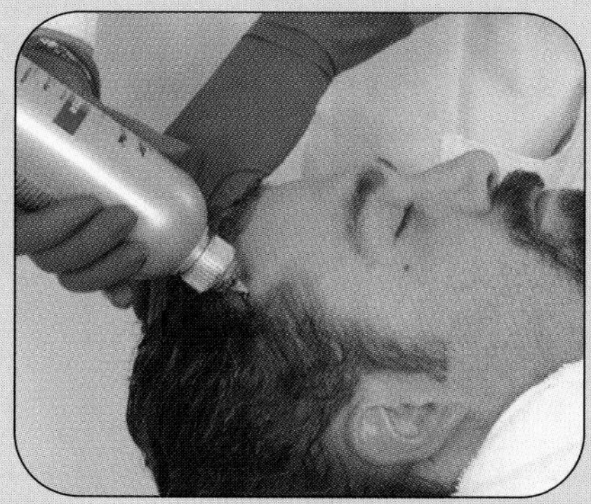

Figure 16-33 Apply color rinse at the shampoo bowl.

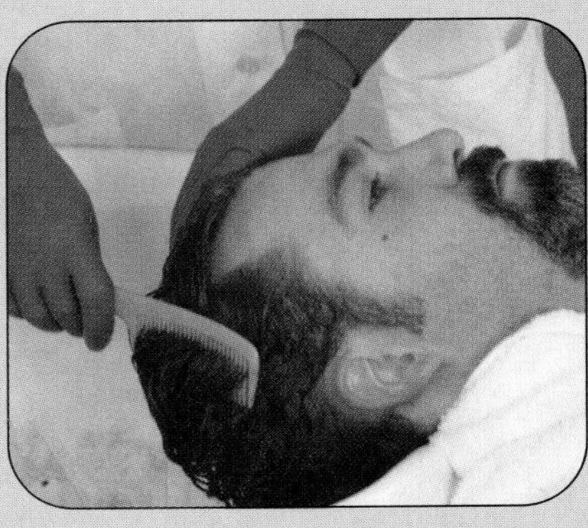

Figure 16–34 Blend color rinse through the hair.

2. Blend the color with a comb, applying more color as necessary (Figure 16–34).
3. Do not rinse the hair. Towel-blot excess product.
4. Proceed with styling (Figure 16–35).

Cleanup and Sanitation

1. Discard all disposable supplies and materials.
2. Close containers, wipe them off, and store in the proper place.
3. Sanitize implements, cape, and your workstation.
4. Wash your hands with soap and warm water.
5. Record results on a record card and file it away.

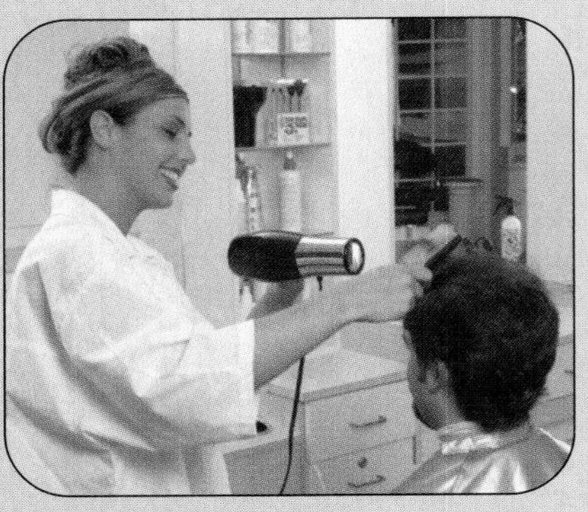

Figure 16–35 Style the hair.

completed!

PROCEDURE

SEMIPERMANENT HAIRCOLOR APPLICATION

Implements and Materials

- applicator bottle or brush
- towels
- plastic cap (optional)
- plastic clips
- tint cape
- cotton
- protective cream
- protective gloves
- shampoo
- record card
- comb
- color chart
- selected color
- conditioner
- timer

Preparation

1. Perform a preliminary patch test 24 hours before the service. Proceed only if the test is negative.
2. Client consultation. Thoroughly analyze the hair and scalp. Record the results on the client's record card.
3. Ask the client to remove all jewelry and store it in a safe place. Drape the client for the haircolor service.
4. Apply protective cream around the hairline and over the ears (Figure 16–36).
5. Perform a strand test. Record the results on the client's card.

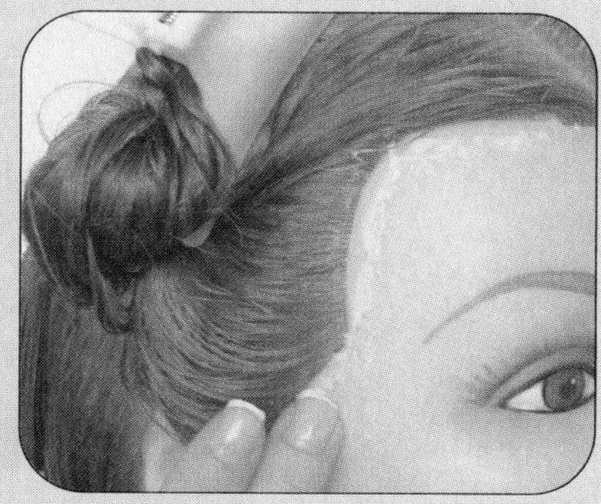

Figure 16-36 Apply protective cream.

16

Procedure

1. Shampoo the client's hair with mild shampoo, if required. Towel-dry the hair.
2. Part the hair into four sections. Put on protective gloves.
3. Working with ¼-inch to ½-inch (.6-cm to 1.25-cm) subsections, apply semipermanent color to the entire hair shaft. Start near the scalp and gently work the color through the ends. Apply with a bottle or brush, depending on the consistency of the color and your instructor's directions (Figure 16–37).

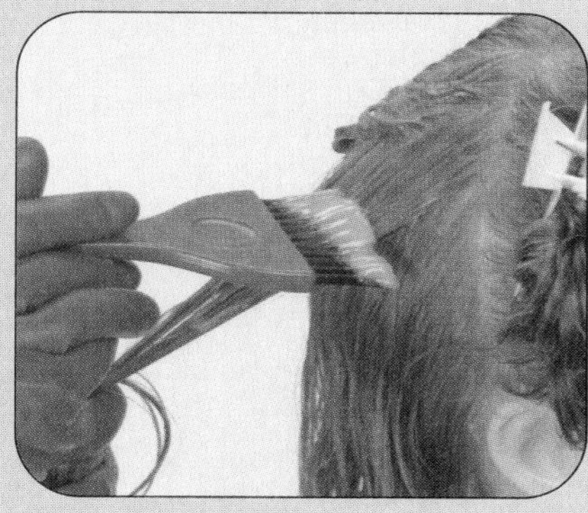

Figure 16-37 Apply semipermanent color.

Do not perform any haircoloring service if the client has abrasions or inflammations on the scalp. Do not brush the hair.

4. Pile the hair loosely on top of the head (Figure 16–38).
5. Follow the manufacturer's directions with regard to process options. Some colors require the use of a plastic cap (Figure 16–39).
6. Process according to your strand test results.
7. Follow the timing instructions provided by the manufacturer. When the color has developed, wet the client's hair with warm water and lather.
8. Rinse well, then shampoo. Finish with conditioner.
9. Rinse and towel-blot the hair. Style as desired (Figure 16–40).

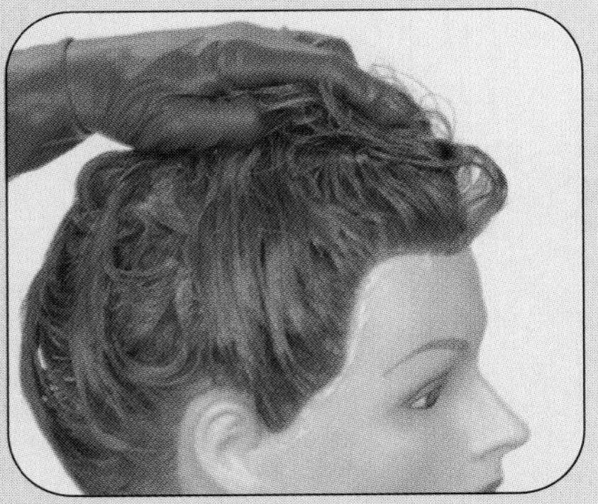

Figure 16-38 Pile the hair on the head.

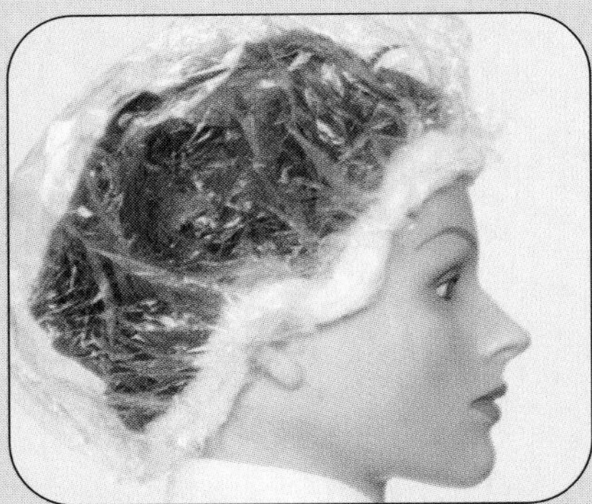

Figure 16-39 Use a plastic cover if required.

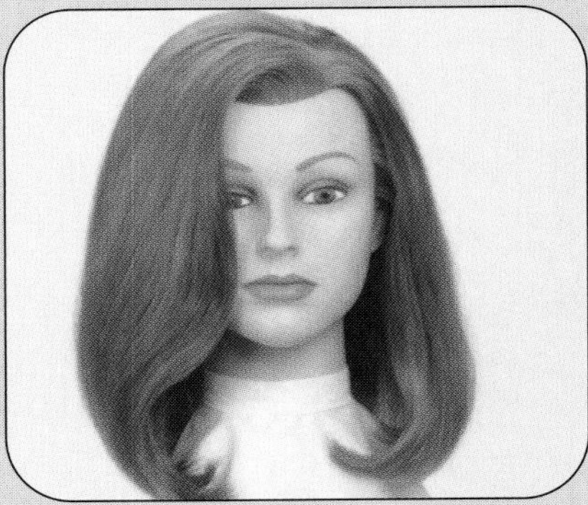

Figure 16-40 Finished styled hair.

Cleanup and Sanitation

1. Perform cleanup and sanitation as in procedure for temporary color rinse.
2. In addition, rinse plastic bottles, bowls, and brushes, and disinfect according to your state's regulations.
3. Complete the record card and file it away.

completed!

Single-process haircoloring is a process that lightens and colors the hair in a single application. Examples of single-process coloring are virgin tint applications and tint retouch applications. A **virgin application** refers to the first time the hair is tinted. Prelightening or presoftening (see page 592) is not required with these applications.

Single-process tints usually contain a lightening agent, a shampoo, an aniline derivative tint, and an alkalizing agent to activate the added peroxide. Most color is formulated to be used with 20 volume peroxide. When other volumes of peroxide are used, the color results will be altered.

Double-process coloring, also known as double-application tinting and two-step coloring, is a technique requiring two separate procedures in which the hair is prelightened before the depositing color is applied. Prelightening lifts or lightens the natural pigments, preliminary to the application of toner. Because the lightening action and the color deposit are independently controlled, a wider range of haircolor possibilities is opened up.

Formulation

There are four basic questions that must always be asked when formulating a haircolor.

1. What is the natural level? Is there any gray hair? (Review the steps to evaluate level and tone, page 552.)
2. What is the client's desired level and tone?
3. Are contributing pigments (undertones) revealed?
4. What colors should be mixed to get the desired result?

The combination of the shade selected and the volume of hydrogen peroxide determines the lifting ability of a haircolor. Always remember to formulate with both lift and deposit in mind, in order to achieve the proper balance for the desired end result. A higher lifting formula, however, may not have enough depositing tonality to subdue the warmth of a client's natural contributing pigment. The volume of hydrogen peroxide mixed with the haircolor product will also influence the lift and deposit.

Mixing Permanent Colors

Your method of mixing permanent colors is determined by the type of application you are using. Permanent color is applied by either the applicator bottle or bowl-and-brush method (always follow the manufacturers' directions) (Figure 16–41).

- *Applicator bottle.* Be sure that the applicator bottle is large enough to hold both the color product and developer, with enough air space to shake the bottle until the mixture is thoroughly blended. For a 1:1 ratio, pour 1 ounce of the developer into the bottle, add 1 ounce of the color, put the top on the bottle, and shake gently. For a 2:1 ratio, pour 2 ounces of the developer into the bottle, add 1 ounce of color, and mix. This ratio is for most permanent high-lift blonde colors.
- *Brush and bowl.* Use a nonmetallic mixing bowl. Measure the developer into the bowl. Add the color or colors you have selected in the

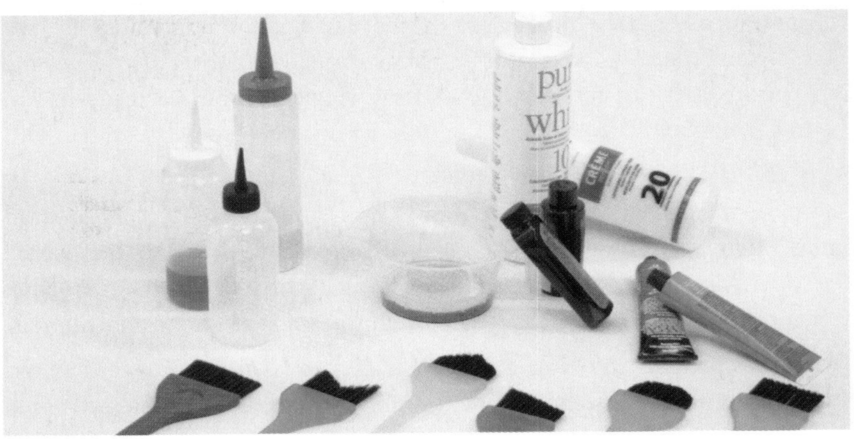

Figure 16–41 Haircolor can be mixed in an applicator bottle or a bowl.

appropriate proportions. Using a tint applicator brush, stir the mixture until it is thoroughly blended. A creamy consistency is best for control during application.

Single-Process Tint Retouch

As the hair grows, you will need to retouch it to keep it looking attractive and to avoid a two-toned effect. Follow the same preparation steps as for the virgin single-process procedure, including a consultation and patch test. Then follow this procedure.

1. Apply tint to the new growth only, being careful not to overlap on previously tinted hair. Overlapping can cause breakage and can create a sign of roots or a **line of demarcation**, which is the visible line separating colored hair from new growth.
2. Process color according to your analysis and strand test results.
3. To refresh faded ends, formulate a demipermanent color for the ends to match the regrowth, or rinse the color through to the ends. Then shampoo.

Double-Process Color

If the client asks for a dramatically lighter color, the hair has to first be prelightened. Also, to achieve pale or cool colors, it is sometimes more efficient to use a double-process application. By first decolorizing the hair with a lightener and then using a separate product to add the desired tonality, you will have more control over the coloring process.

You may find that the contributing pigment of the hair will work for you in a double-process coloring application. By prelightening the hair to the desired degree of decolorization, you can create a perfect foundation for longer-lasting red colors that avoid muddiness and stay true to tone.

The prelightener is applied in the same manner as for a regular hair lightening treatment (see the following section). Once the prelightening has reached the desired shade, the hair is lightly shampooed, acidified, and towel dried. After a strand test has been taken, the color is then applied in the usual manner.

PROCEDURE

SINGLE-PROCESS COLOR FOR VIRGIN HAIR

Implements and Materials

Use the list of implements and materials under Procedure 42—semipermanent color—and add the following:

- plastic or glass bowl and applicator brush or applicator bottle
- selected permanent haircolor
- hydrogen peroxide

Preparation

Same as preparation for Procedure 42—semipermanent color, including patch test.

Procedure

1. Part dry hair into four sections (Figure 16–42).
2. Apply protective cream to the hairline and ears.
3. Prepare the tint formula for either bottle or brush application.
4. Begin in the section where the color change will be greatest or where the hair is most resistant, usually the hairline and temple areas. Part off a ¼-inch (.6-cm) subsection with the applicator (Figure 16–43).
5. Lift the subsection and apply color to the midshaft area. Stay at least ½ inch (1.25 cm) from the scalp, and do not go through the porous ends (Figure 16–44).

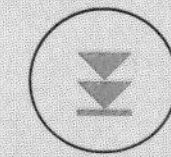

Here's a tip:

The hair at the scalp processes faster due to body heat. For this reason, the color is applied in the scalp area only after being applied to the shaft. Your strand test will determine the application procedure and timing for even color development.

16

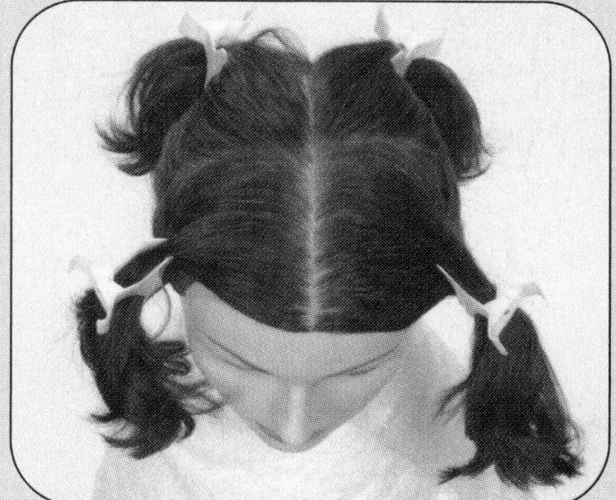

Figure 16-42 Section the hair.

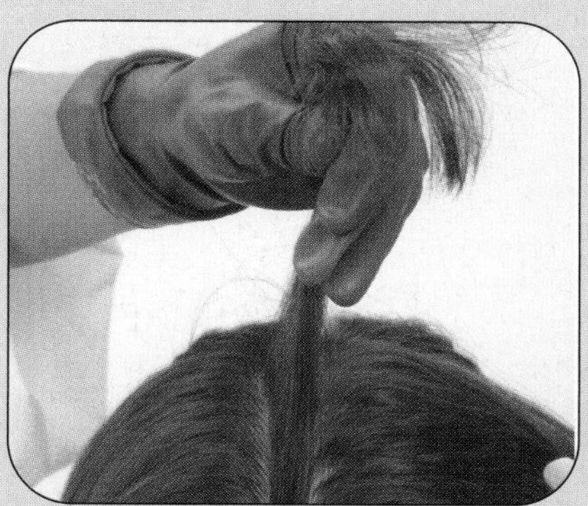

Figure 16-43 Part out a subsection.

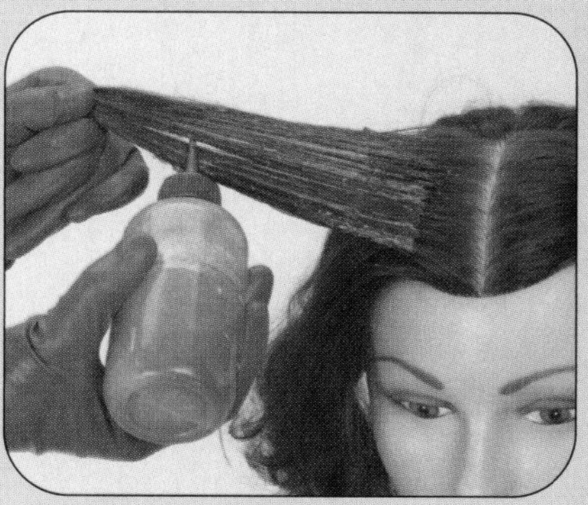

Figure 16-44 Apply color to subsection.

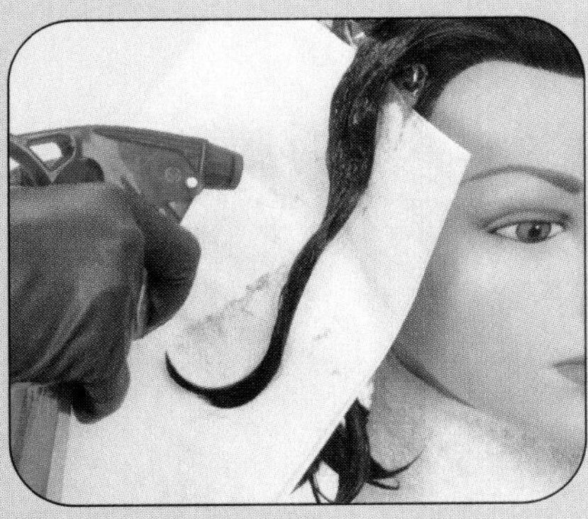

Figure 16–45 Perform strand test.

6. Process according to the strand test results. Check for color development by removing color as described in the strand test procedure (Figure 16–45).
7. Apply color to the hair at the scalp (Figure 16–46).
8. Pull the color through onto the hair ends (Figure 16–47).
9. Lightly rinse with lukewarm water. Massage color into a lather and rinse thoroughly.
10. Remove any stains around the hairline with shampoo or stain remover. Use a towel to gently remove stains.
11. Shampoo the hair. Condition as needed.
12. Towel-dry and style the hair (Figure 16–48).
13. Perform cleanup and sanitation as in procedure for semipermanent haircolor application.
14. Complete the client's record card and file it away.
15. Follow cleanup and sanitation procedures for Procedure 42—semipermanent color. 5✓

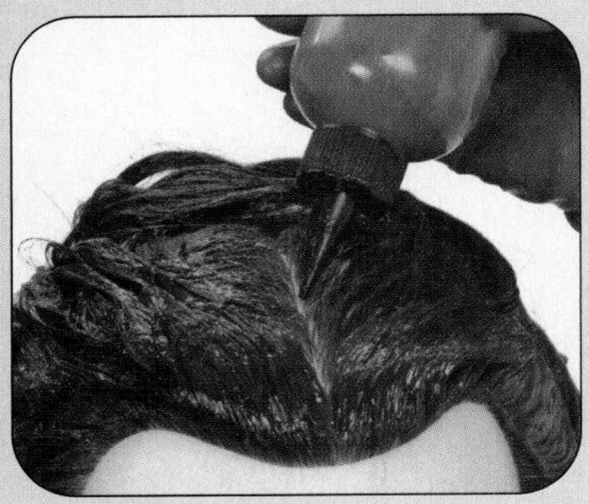

Figure 16–46 Apply color to hair at scalp.

16

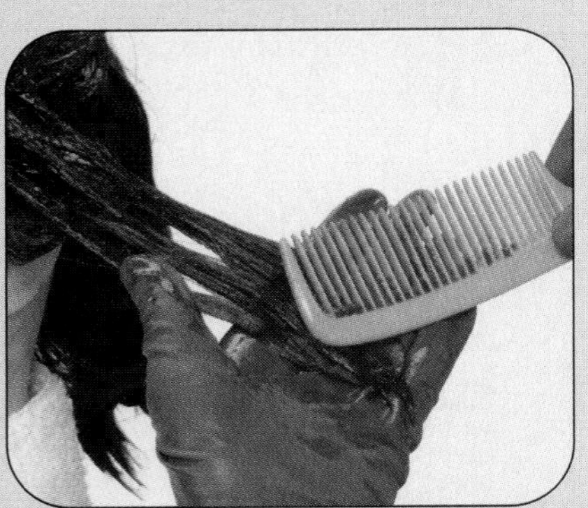

Figure 16–47 Blend color to hair ends.

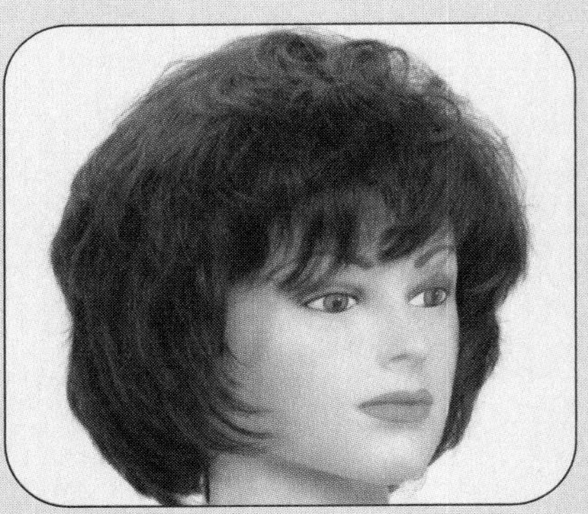

Figure 16–48 Styled hair.

completed! 

LIGHTENING TECHNIQUES

Colorists can choose from three forms of lighteners: oil, cream, and powder. Oil and cream lighteners are considered **on-the-scalp lighteners**, which can be used directly on the scalp. Powder lighteners are **off-the-scalp lighteners**, which cannot be used directly on the scalp. Each type has its unique abilities, chemical characteristics, and formulation procedures.

On-the-Scalp Lighteners

Cream and oil lighteners are the most popular type of lighteners because they are easy to apply. Oil lighteners are the mildest type, appropriate when only one or two levels of color lift are desired. Because they are so mild, they are also used professionally to lighten dark facial and body hair.

Cream lighteners are strong enough to do blonding, but gentle enough to be used on the scalp. They have the following beneficial features:

- they contain conditioning agents that give some protection to the hair and scalp
- thickeners give more control during application
- because cream lighteners do not run or drip, overlapping is prevented during retouching services

Cream lighteners may be mixed with activators (sometimes called boosters, protinators, or accelerators) in the form of dry crystals. An **activator** is an oxidizer added to hydrogen peroxide to increase its chemical action, in this case its lifting power. The greater the number of activators, the greater the strength of the formula. Up to three activators can be used for on-the-scalp applications, and up to four for off-the-scalp applications.

Off-the-Scalp Lighteners

Powder lightener is a strong, fast-acting lightener in powdered form. Like cream lightener, it is strong enough to do blonding. However, powder lightener should not be applied directly to the scalp.

Powder lighteners, which are also called quick lighteners, contain oxygen-releasing boosters for quicker and stronger action. They may dry out more quickly than other types of lighteners, but they do not run or drip. Most powder lighteners expand and spread out as processing continues and should not be used for retouch services.

Time Factors

Processing time for lightening is affected by several factors.

- The darker the natural hair color, the more melanin it has. The more melanin it has, the longer it takes to lighten the color.
- The amount of time needed to lighten the natural color is also influenced by the porosity. Porous hair of the same color level will lighten faster than hair that is nonporous, because the bleaching agent can enter the cortex more rapidly.

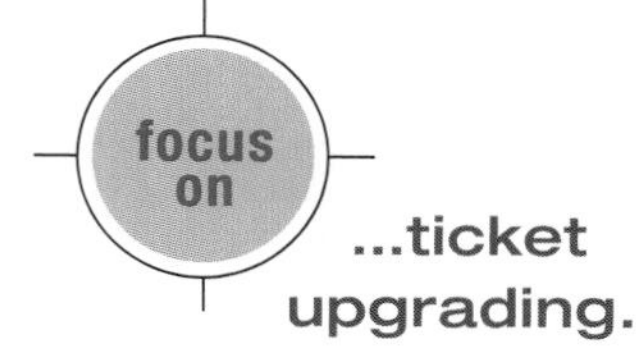

...ticket upgrading.

Getting your clients interested in haircoloring can be done in indirect as well as direct ways:

- Wear color in your hair. As a professional hairstylist, you should be an example of what those products can do.
- Display haircolor-related materials at your work station. These could be swatches, pictures of great haircoloring you clip out of magazines, and so forth.
- Suggest haircolor to almost every client and see every client as a potential user of your services.

CAUTION

Powder lighteners are used exclusively for off-the-scalp applications and special effects, such as foil-wrapped weaving, highlighting with plastic caps, and hair painting.

- Tone also influences the length of time necessary to lighten the natural hair color. The greater the percentage of red reflected in the natural color, the more difficult it is to achieve the pale, delicate shades of blonde. Ash blondes are especially difficult to achieve because the melanin must be diffused sufficiently to alter both the level and tone of the hair.
- The strength of the product also affects the speed and amount of lightening. The stronger lighteners attain the pale shades in the fastest time.
- Heat, too, leads to quicker lightening. But the stages of lightening must be carefully observed to avoid excessive lift that could lead to the diffusion of so much natural pigment that the desired toner shade may not develop properly in the hair shaft. When this occurs, the toner shade may "grab" the base color, giving the hair an ashy, unpigmented tone.

Perform a preliminary strand test prior to lightening to determine the process time, the condition of the hair after lightening, and the end results. Watch the strand carefully for its reaction to the lightening mixture and for any discoloration or breakage. Reconditioning may be required prior to toning. If the color and condition are good, you can proceed with the lightening. Carefully record all data on the client's record card.

If the test shows the hair is not light enough, increase the strength of the mixture and/or increase the processing time. If the hair strand is too light, decrease the strength of the mixture and/or decrease the processing time.

A patch test must be taken 24 hours prior to the application of a toner containing aniline derivatives. To save the client time, the strand test for lightening can be done on the same day as the patch test.

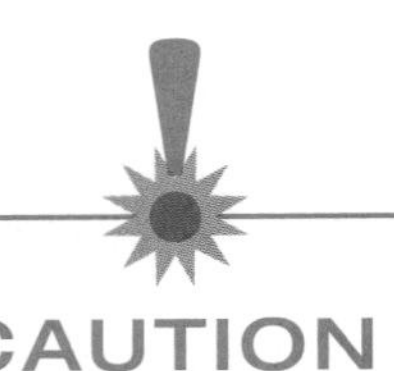

CAUTION

When heat is used in conjunction with lightening chemicals, it softens the hair but can also make it more fragile. Excessive heat will cause the motion of the molecules to become so great that damage can occur as cuticle layers are removed and cortical bonds are destroyed. Therefore, extreme caution must always be exercised when using heat.

Lightener Retouch

As the hair grows, dark, **new growth** will become very obvious. The new growth, or regrowth, is the part of the hair shaft between the scalp and the hair that has previously received treatment. In each case, lighten the new growth first. The procedure for a lightener retouch is the same as that for lightening a virgin head of hair, except that the mixture is applied only to the new growth of hair. A cream lightener is generally used for a lightener retouch because its consistency helps prevent overlapping of previously lightened hair. This overlapping can cause severe breakage and lines of demarcation. Also, cream lighteners are gentler on the scalp.

Always consult the client's record card for information about which lightener formulas have been used in the past, timing, and other matters.

Toners

Toners are used primarily on prelightened hair to achieve pale, delicate colors. They require a double-process application. The first process is the application of the lightener; the second process is the application of the toner.

PROCEDURE

LIGHTENING VIRGIN HAIR

Implements and Materials

- towels
- comb
- protective gloves
- plastic clips
- tint cape
- plastic or glass bowl
- shampoo
- peroxide
- acid or finishing rinse
- cotton
- record card
- applicator bottle or brush
- lightener
- timer
- protective cream

Preparation

Follow the same preparation steps as for Procedure 42—semipermanent color — including a patch test. Carefully analyze the hair and record all information on the client card (Figure 16–49).

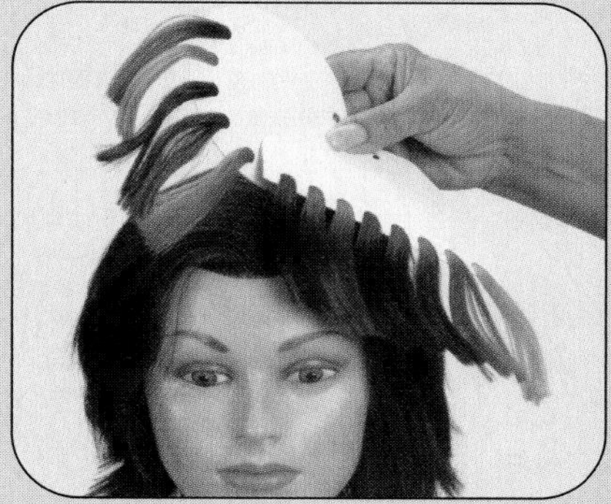

Figure 16-49 Perform a consultation and scalp analysis.

16

Procedure

1. Divide dry hair into four sections.
2. Apply a protective cream around the hairline and over the ears.
3. Put on protective gloves.
4. Prepare the lightening formula and use it immediately to prevent deterioration.
5. Apply the lightener. Begin the application where the hair seems resistant or especially dark, usually at the back of the head. Use ⅛-inch (.3-cm) partings to apply the lightener. Start ½ inch (1.25 cm) from the scalp and extend the lightener up to, but not through, the porous ends. Apply the lightener to the top and underside of the subsection in quick, rhythmic movements (Figure 16–50).

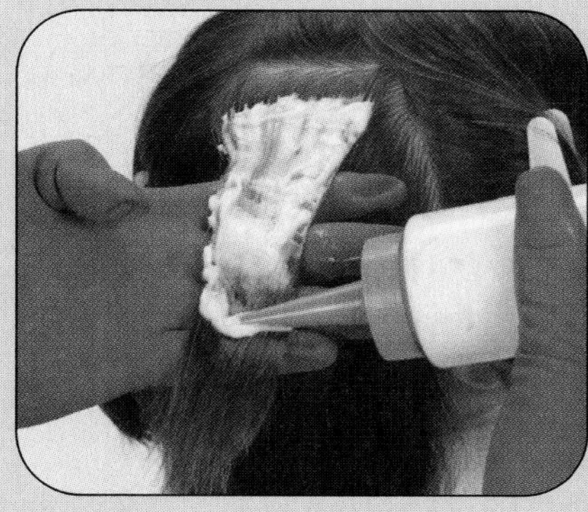

Figure 16-50 Apply lightener to top and underside of subsection.

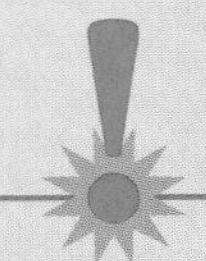

CAUTION

In all procedures requiring the use of a towel to check for lightening level, make sure that the towel is damp. Blot—do not rub—the strand. Rubbing could cause a roughening of the cuticle, giving a false reading for the entire process.

6. Place strips of cotton at the scalp area along the parts to prevent the lightener from touching the base of the hair (Figure 16–51). Complete all four sections in this manner (Figure 16–52).
7. Continue to apply the lightener. Double-check the application, adding more lightener if necessary. Do not comb the lightener through the hair. Keep the lightener moist during development by reapplying as the mixture dries on the hair.
8. Check for lightening action about 15 minutes before the time indicated by the preliminary strand test. Spray a hair strand with a water bottle and remove the lightener with a damp towel (Figure 16–53). Examine the strand. If the strand is not light enough, reapply the mixture and continue testing frequently until the desired level is reached.
9. Remove the cotton from the scalp area. Apply the lightener to the hair near the scalp with a ⅛-inch (.3-cm) parting (Figure 16–54). Prepare fresh lightener. Process and perform your strand test until the entire shaft has reached the desired stage.
10. Rinse the hair thoroughly with tepid water. Shampoo gently and condition as needed, keeping your hands under the hair to avoid tangling.
11. Neutralize the alkalinity of the hair with a conditioner. Recondition if necessary.
12. Towel-dry the hair, or dry it completely under a cool dryer if the manufacturer requires it.

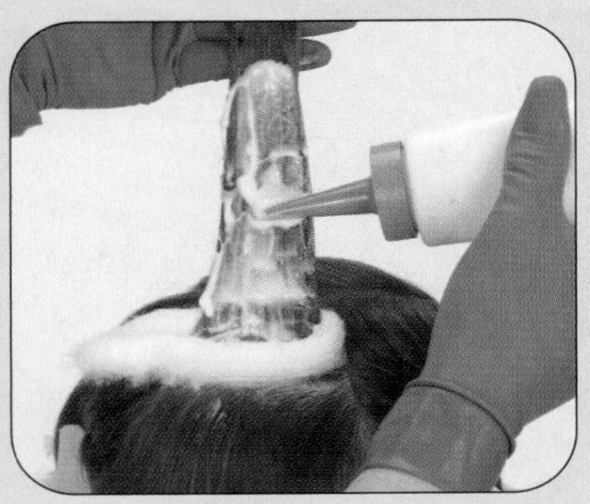

Figure 16–51 Place cotton strips at scalp.

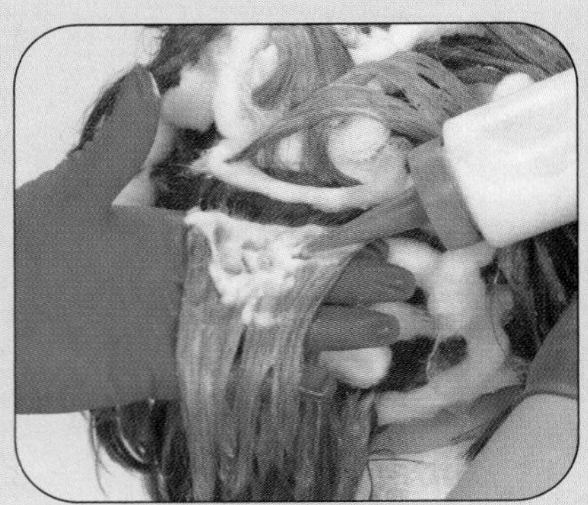

Figure 16–52 Complete lightener application.

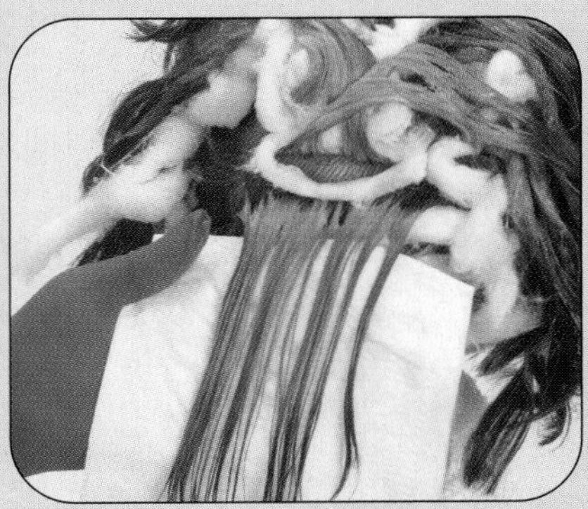

Figure 16–53 Mist the strand with water.

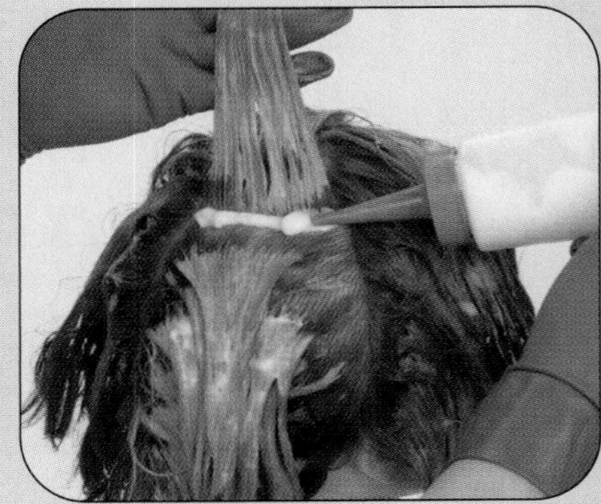

Figure 16–54 Apply lightener at scalp.

13. Examine the scalp for any abrasions. Analyze the condition of the hair (Figure 16–55).
14. Proceed with a toner application if desired (Procedure 45).
15. Perform cleanup and sanitation as in Procedure 42— semipermanent haircolor application.

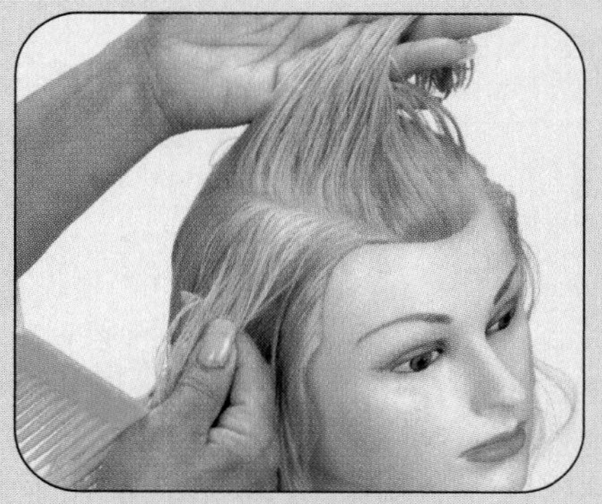

Figure 16-55 Examine the hair.

16

completed!

After the hair goes through the 10 stages of decolorizing, the color that is left in the hair is known as its **foundation**. It is essential that you achieve the correct foundation in order to create the degree of porosity required for proper toner development.

Manufacturers of toners generally include literature with their products that recommends the foundation necessary to achieve the color you desire. As a general rule, the paler the color you are seeking, the lighter a foundation you will need. It is important to follow the literature closely and to understand that overlightened hair will "grab" the base color of the toner. Underlightened hair, on the other hand, will appear to have more red, yellow, or orange than the intended color.

It is not advisable to prelighten past the pale yellow stage. This will create overporous hair that will have inadequate amounts of natural pigment left in the cortex for the toner to bond to. Refer to the Law of Color to select a toner that will neutralize or tone the prelightened hair to the desired shade.

Preliminary Toner Application

Administer a patch test for allergies or other sensitivities 24 hours before the toner application. To save time, a strand test may be given on the same day as the patch test. Proceed with the application only if the patch test results are negative and the hair is in good condition.

For your protection, wear gloves throughout the application. Your speed and accuracy are both important factors in the application and will determine, to a large extent, whether or not you get good color results. The procedure for applying low or nonperoxide toners may vary. Check with your instructor for directions.

SPECIAL EFFECTS HAIRCOLORING

Special effects haircoloring refers to any technique that involves partial lightening or coloring. Coloring for special effects can be thought of as a pure fashion technique. It is a versatile and exciting haircoloring service.

One way you can create special effects is by strategically placing light and dark colors in the hair. **Highlighting** involves coloring some of the hair strands lighter than the natural color to add the illusion of sheen and depth; highlights do not generally contrast strongly with the natural color. Light colors cause an area to advance toward the eye, to appear larger, and to make details more visible. **Reverse highlighting** or **lowlighting** is the technique of coloring strands of hair darker than the natural color. Contrasting dark areas recede, appear smaller, and make detail less visible.

PROCEDURE

TONER APPLICATION

Implements and Materials

- towels
- tail comb
- protective gloves
- plastic clips
- tint cape
- plastic or glass bowl
- shampoo
- peroxide
- acid or finishing rinse
- cotton
- protective cream
- record card
- toner
- applicator bottle or brush
- timer

Preparation

1. Prelighten the hair to the desired stage of decolorization.
2. Shampoo the hair lightly, rinse, and towel-dry. Condition as necessary.
3. Select the desired toner shade.
4. Apply protective cream around the hairline and over the ears.
5. Take a strand test and record the results on the client's record card.
6. If using an oxidative toner, mix the toner and the developer in a nonmetallic bowl or bottle, following the manufacturer's directions (Figure 16–56).

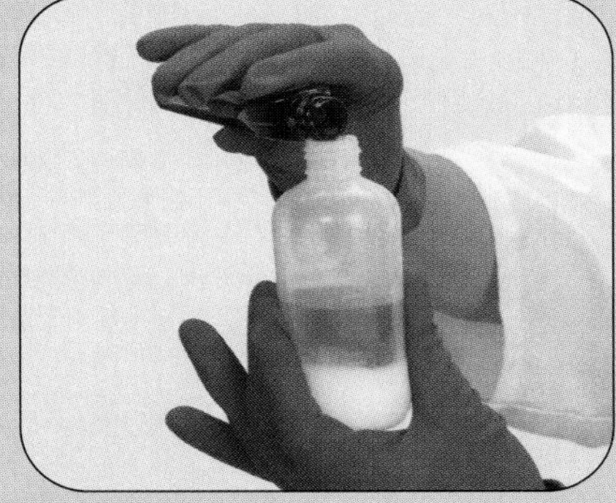

Figure 16–56 Mix toner.

Procedure

1. Part the hair into four equal sections, using the end of the tail comb or tint brush. Avoid scratching the scalp.
2. At the crown of one of the back sections, part off ¼-inch (.6-cm) partings and apply the toner from the scalp up to, but not including, the porous ends (Figure 16–57).

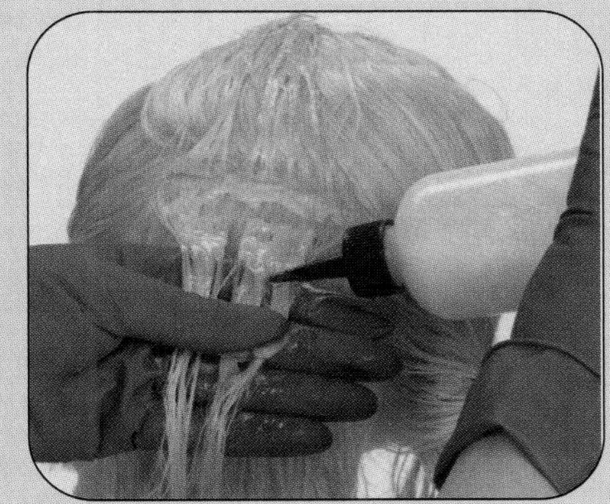

Figure 16–57 Apply toner.

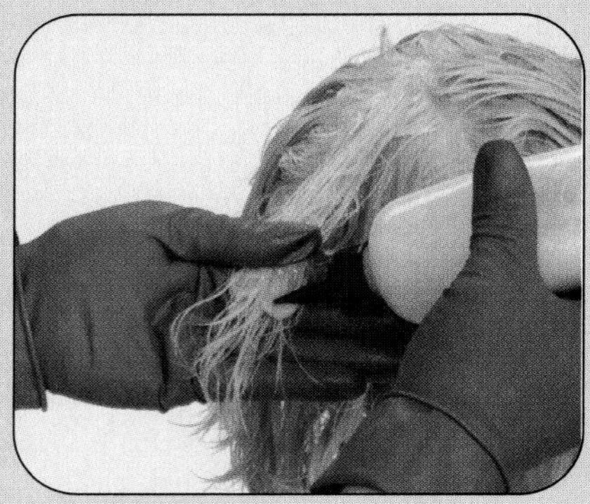

Figure 16-58 Work toner through hair ends.

3. Take a strand test. If it indicates proper color development, gently work the toner through the ends of the hair, using a brush or your fingers (Figure 16–58).
4. If necessary for coverage, apply additional toner to the hair and blend it in. Leave the hair loosely piled to permit air circulation or cover the hair with a cap if required.
5. Time the procedure according to your strand test. Check frequently until the desired shade has been reached evenly throughout the shaft and ends.
6. Remove the toner by wetting the hair and massaging the toner into a lather.
7. Rinse, shampoo gently, and rinse well again.
8. Apply conditioner to close the cuticle, lower the pH, and help prevent fading.
9. Remove any toner stains from the skin, hairline, and neck.
10. Style as desired. Use caution to avoid stretching the hair (Figure 16–59).
11. Perform cleanup and sanitation as in Procedure 42—semipermanent color. 5

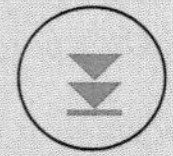

Here's a tip . . .

Do not bring the toner mixture down through the porous ends of the hair until the end of the procedure, and then only if you are planning to change the tonal value or you are correcting significant fading. To do so will only make the hair even more porous and more susceptible to continued fading.

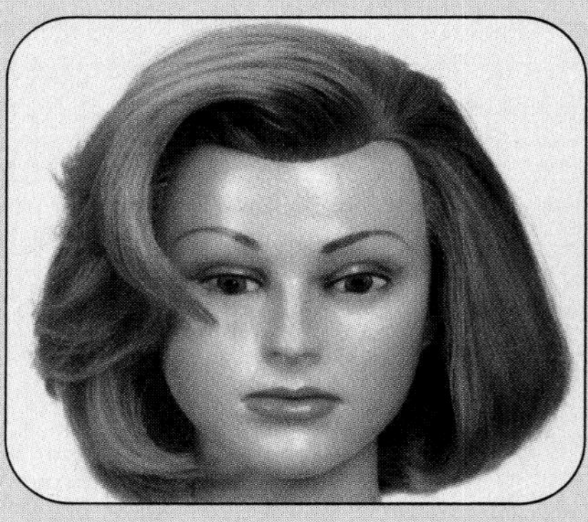

Figure 16-59 Styled hair.

completed!

insights

Rudy Gomez

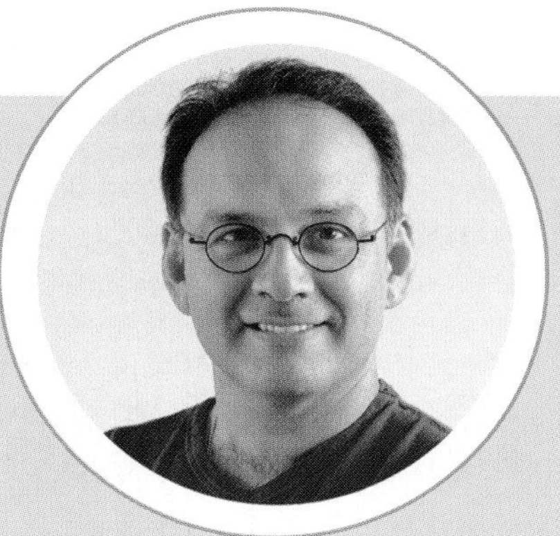

Owner and president of Salon Sa Bel, Rudi has overcome adversities and has been able to sustain a satisfying and rewarding career in cosmetology.

I was an art major in college. In my fourth year, I dropped out and got a job with a sign company. I wound up meeting Horst Rechelbacher, who started Aveda. I was working on a sign for one of his salons and was noticing what a fun atmosphere it was. I thought to myself, I can do that. So I went to him and said I wanted to go to his school, and he gave me a scholarship with the understanding that I would work for him when I was done. I worked for Aveda and the Horst and Friends Salon for several years.

It became clear to me that if I wanted to be successful, I needed to learn the finer elements of building a clientele. I've always been one to look for a mentor, and fortunately I hooked in early with someone who helped me with people skills. I've worked with incredible hairdressers who weren't busy because they hadn't developed their people skills. Anyone who comes out of cosmetology school today should find someone in the business who's a busy stylist and should study that person to find out what he or she is doing right. It usually has to do with a lot more than how that person cuts hair.

I think the secret to success as a stylist is an understanding that there is a great deal of honor in being of service.

You're not an artist;

you're a craftsperson creating for others. You need to change your thinking from believing that you're an artist to believing that you're going to do whatever is necessary and possible to make your client happy when she leaves you. That might mean coming in early, or leaving late, or coming in on your day off. That's what it takes to get your clients to understand that you want to provide the best thing for them. You don't have to bend over backwards. To capture clients, rather than take them in off the street, cut their hair, and say good-bye, you have to give the impression that you have a long-term interest in their image and in them.

One of the most important people skills that a stylist can possess is the ability to convince a client that when she comes in she has your total, undivided attention. The other thing is to develop the skill of active listening—that's very, very important.

Just remember that you can do whatever it is that you set out to do. Five years ago I suffered a stroke, at the age of 37. I had a torn artery in my brain. I nearly died, and my recovery took a long time. I had to relearn everything: how to write my name, how to walk, how to cut hair. But I managed. I was motivated, because I knew what a great life I had. I enjoy coming to work every day and feel blessed.

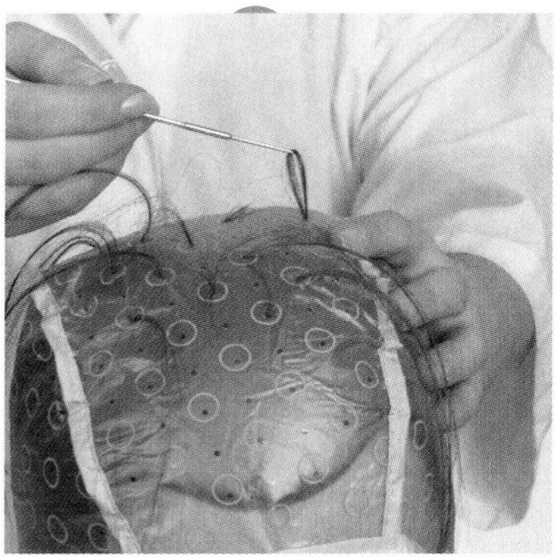

Figure 16-60 Draw strands through holes in cap.

As you begin to expand your knowledge of haircoloring and lightening and develop your technical ability, you will become more creative. Your instructor will help you master the basic techniques, but the rest is up to you. The possibilities are limited only by your imagination and your client's willingness to go along with your ideas.

There are several methods for achieving highlights. The three most frequently used techniques are:

- cap technique.
- foil technique.
- balayage or free-form technique.

Cap Technique

The **cap technique** involves pulling clean strands of hair through a perforated cap with a thin plastic or metal hook, then combing them to remove tangles (Figure 16–60). The number of strands pulled through determines the degree of highlighting or lowlighting you can achieve. When only a small number of strands are pulled through, the result will be a subtle look. A more noticeable effect is achieved if many strands are pulled through, and the effect is even more dramatic if larger strands of hair are pulled through the holes and colored.

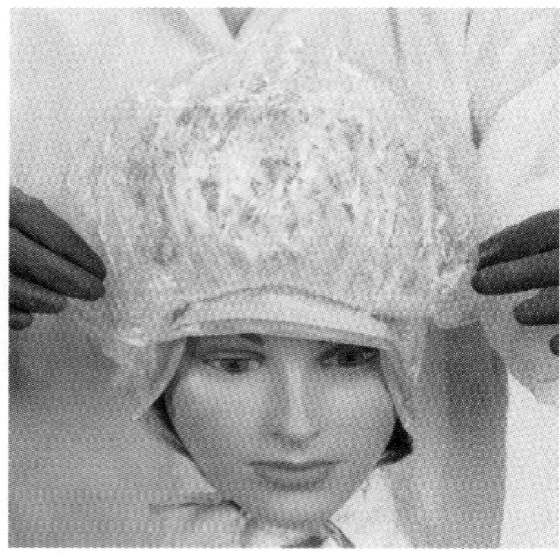

Figure 16-61 Cover loosely with a plastic cap.

For highlighting, the hair is usually lightened with a bleach product or high-lifting color, beginning in the area that is most resistant. The lightener is removed by thorough rinsing, then shampooing. After towel-blotting and conditioning (if necessary), the lightened hair can be toned, if desired (Figure 16–61 and Figure 16–62).

Foil Technique

The **foil technique** involves coloring selected strands of hair by slicing or weaving out sections, placing them on foil or plastic wrap, applying lightener or color, and sealing them in the foil or plastic wrap (Figure 16–63). You can also apply permanent haircolor to the strands to create softer, more natural-looking highlights, for instance, red for red highlights.

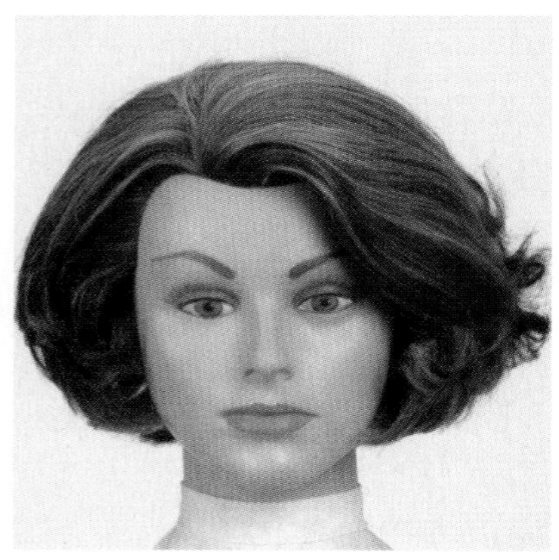

Figure 16-62 Styled hair.

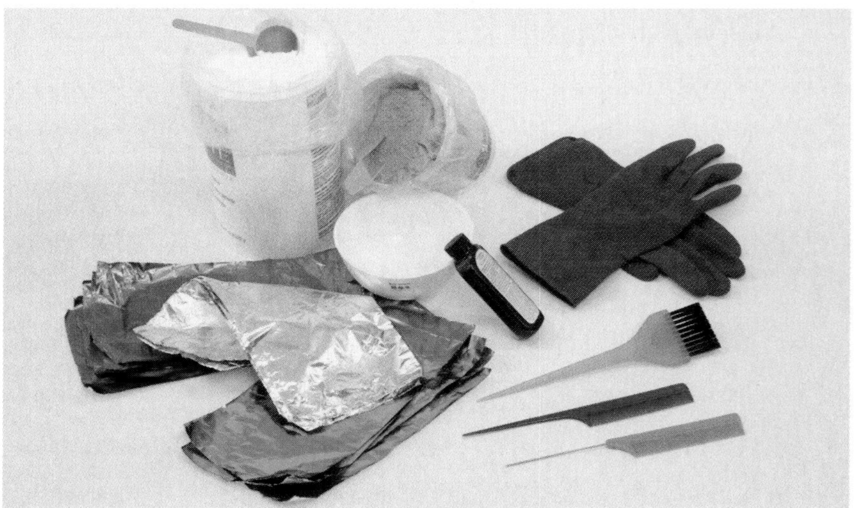

Figure 16-63 Lightening tools.

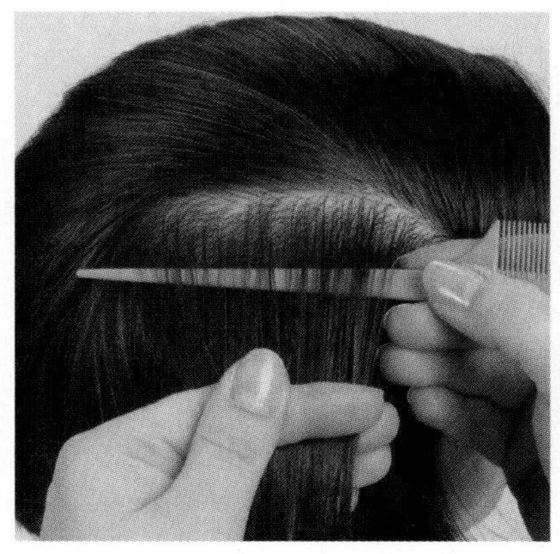

Figure 16–64 Slicing.

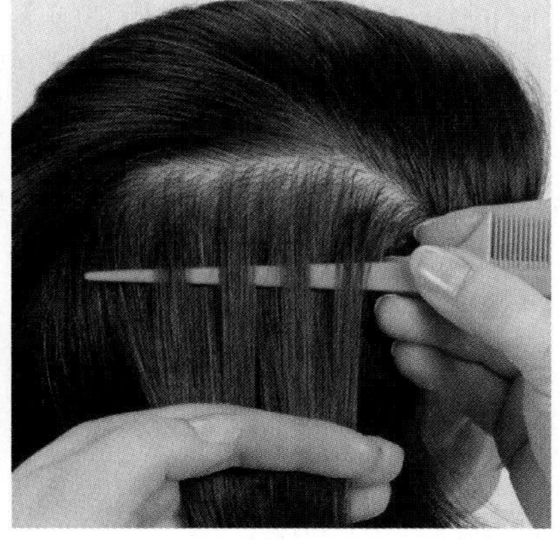

Figure 16–65 Weaving.

Placing foil in the hair is an art. It takes practice and discipline. To make it easier, start by working to create clean section blocks on the head. Once you have perfected this, you will fully understand the difference between a slice parting and a weave parting. **Slicing** involves taking a narrow, 1/8-inch (.3 cm) section of hair by making a straight part at the scalp, positioning the hair over the foil, and applying lightener or color (Figure 16–64). In **weaving**, selected strands are picked up from a narrow section of hair with a zigzag motion of the comb, and lightener or color is applied only to these strands (Figure 16–65).

There are many patterns in which foil can be placed in the hair. There are face-frame, half-head, three-quarter head, and full-head wrapping patterns that produce different highlights in different portions of the head. The procedure for a full-head highlight follows on p. 586.

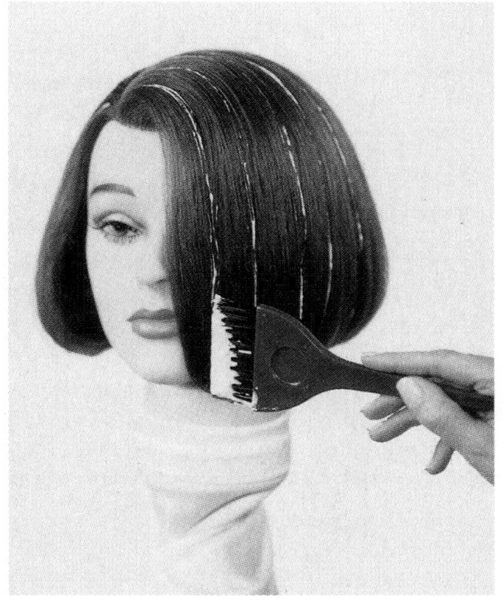

Figure 16–66 Balayage technique.

Balayage Technique

The **balayage or free-form technique** involves the painting of a lightener (usually powder lightener) directly onto clean, styled hair. The lightener is applied with a tint brush or a tail comb from base to ends around the head (Figure 16–66). The effects are extremely subtle and are used to draw attention to the surface of the hair (Figure 16–67).

16

Toning Overhighlighted and Dimensionally Colored Hair

When the hair is decolorized to the desired level during a highlighting service, the use of a toner may not be necessary. However, if a cool tonality is desired, then you will want to use a toner to cancel out any undesirable yellow contributing pigment.

When using a toner on highlighted hair, it is important to consider not only the varying degrees of porosity in the hair, but also the difference in pigmentation created by the lightening process from strand to strand. An oxidative toner would impart color to the highlighted strands, but it might also affect the natural, or pigmented, hair, causing a slight amount of lift. The result may be an uneven tonality, with the underlying warmth brought out by the oxidative color. Strand test to ensure best results.

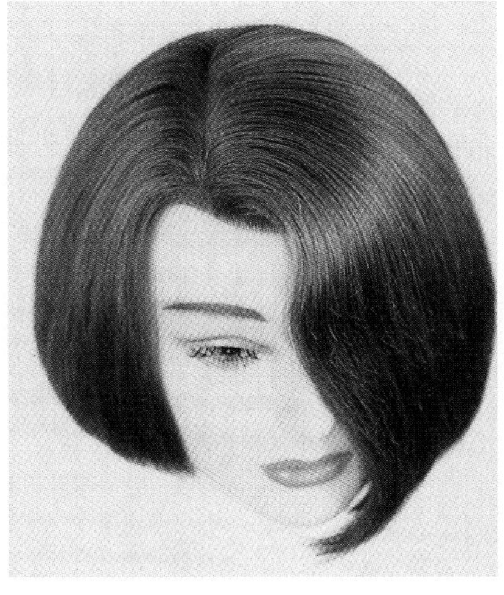

Figure 16–67 Finished hair.

To avoid affecting the untreated hair, choose from the following options:

- A nonoxidative toner, which contains no ammonia, requires no developer

PROCEDURE 46

SPECIAL EFFECTS HAIRCOLORING WITH FOIL

Implements and Materials

- tint cape
- towel
- foil
- gloves
- plastic clips
- bowl/brushes
- tail comb
- brush
- lightener
- record card
- applicator bottle

Preparation

Follow the same preparation steps as for Procedure 44 — lightening virgin hair — and include a patch test (if toner will be applied) and a strand test. Carefully analyze the hair and record all information on the client's card.

Procedure

1. With a tail comb, take a slice of hair at the lower crown area of the head (Figure 16–68).
2. Place a piece of foil under the slice of hair (Figure 16–69).
3. Holding the hair taut, brush on the lightener, from the upper edge of the foil to the hair ends (Figure 16–70).

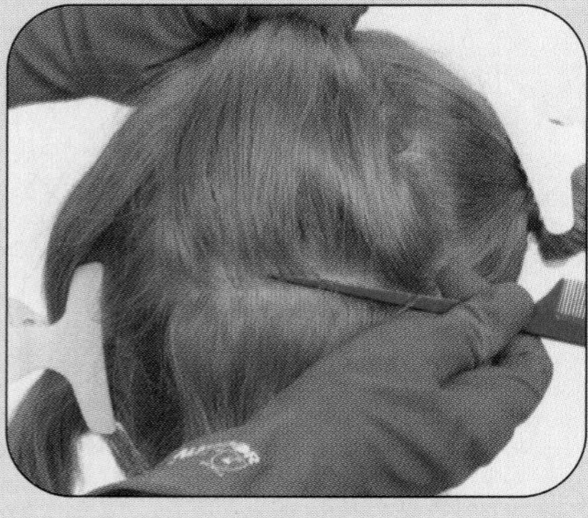

Figure 16–68 Slice of hair.

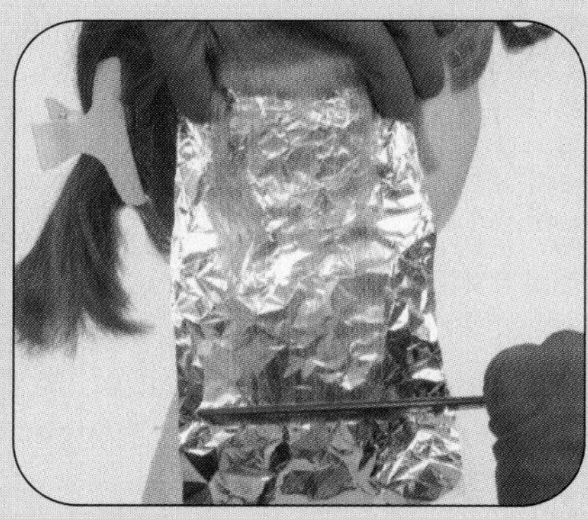

Figure 16–69 Place foil under hair.

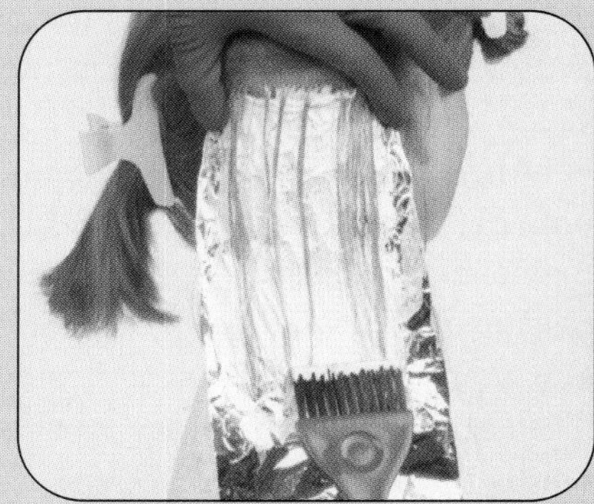

Figure 16–70 Brush lightener onto hair.

4. Fold the foil in half until the ends meet (Figure 16–71).
5. Fold the right side of the foil in halfway, using the comb to crease it (Figure 16–72). Then fold the left side of the foil in halfway (Figure 16–73).
6. Clip the foil upward (Figure 16–74).
7. Take a ¾-inch (1.8-cm) subsection in between foils. Clip this hair up and out of the way (Figure 16–75). (Note the contrast in size between the foiled and unfoiled subsections.)
8. Continue working down the back center of the head until the section is complete.
9. Once the section is complete, release the clipped-up foils (Figure 16–76).
10. Working around the head into the side area, divide it into two smaller sections (Figure 16–77).

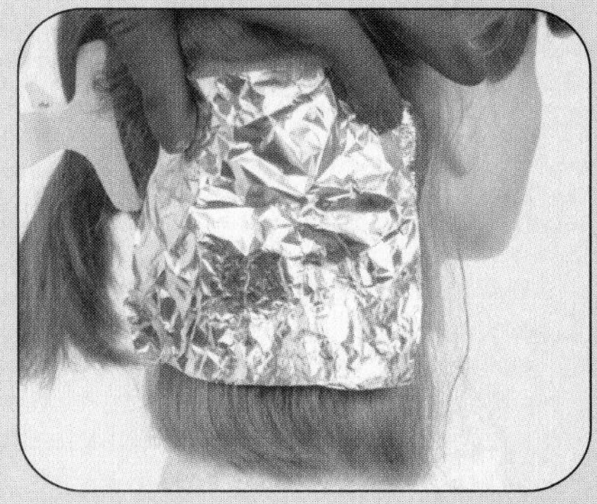

Figure 16–71 Fold foil in half.

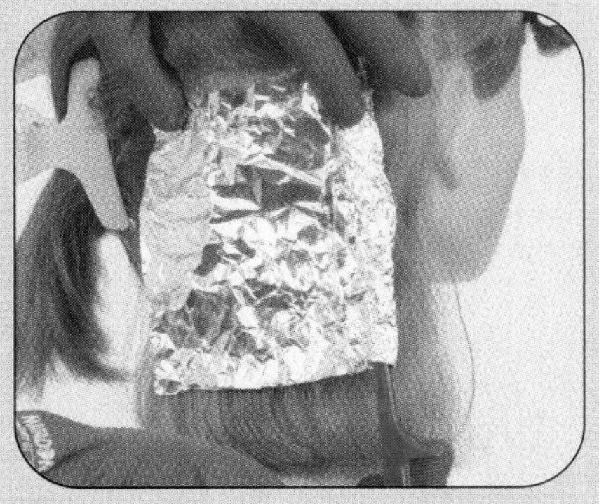

Figure 16–72 Fold right side of foil.

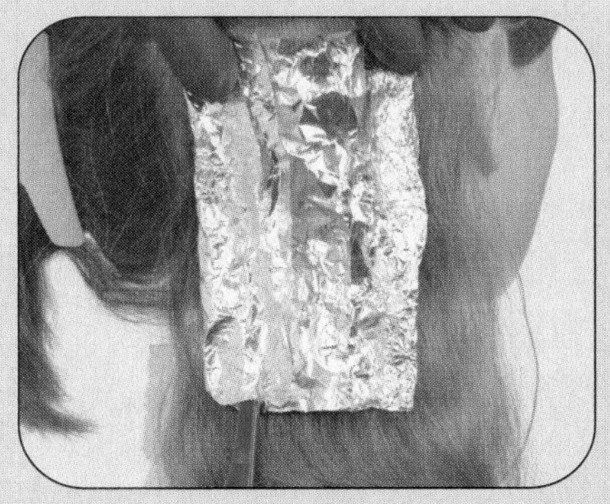

Figure 16–73 Fold left side of foil.

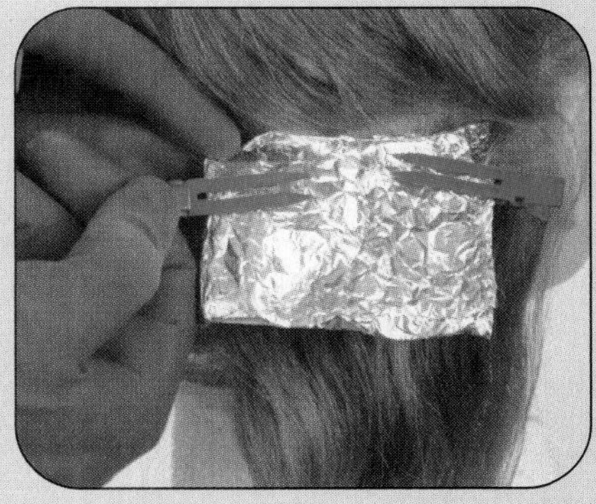

Figure 16–74 Clip foil up.

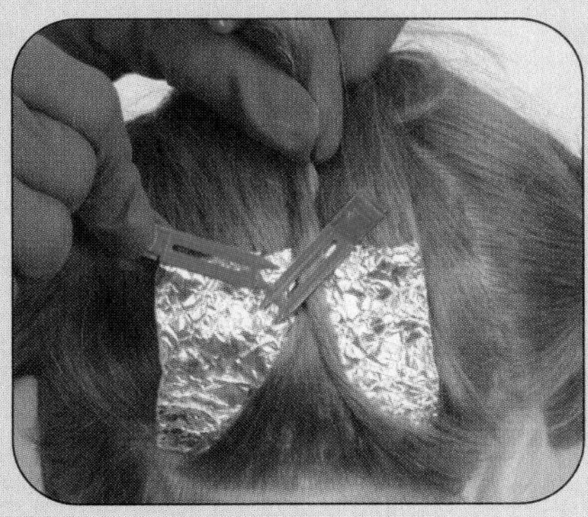

Figure 16–75 Subsection between foils.

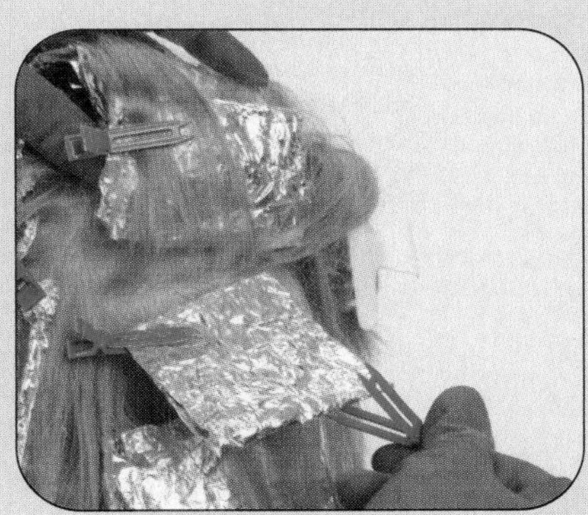

Figure 16–76 Release the foils.

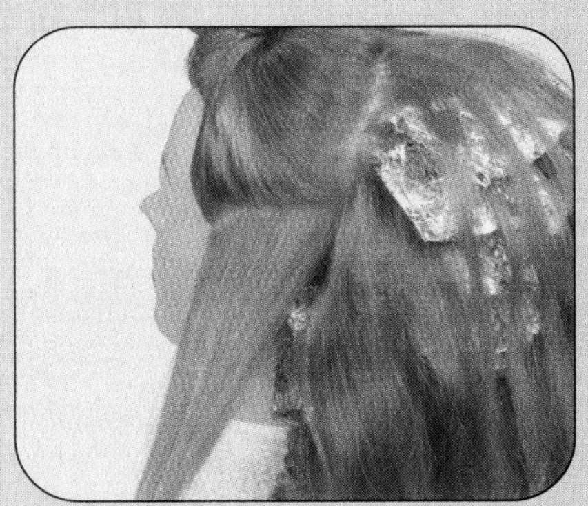

Figure 16–77 Divide side panels.

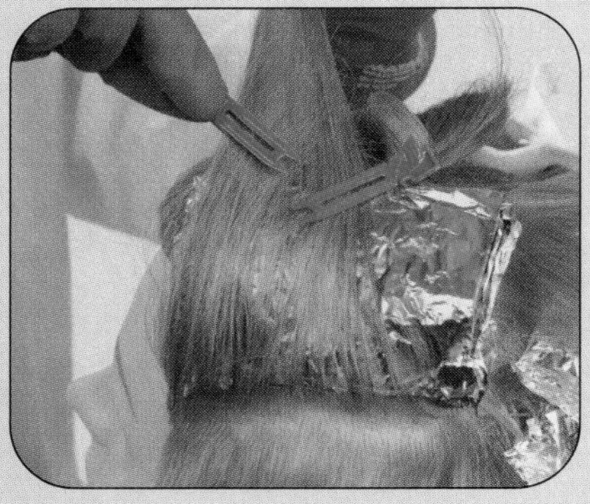

Figure 16-78 Work down the sides.

11. Working down the side, bring fine slices of hair into the foil and apply lightener to the hair. Clip up the foil (Figure 16–78).
12. Move to the other side of the head and complete the matching sections.
13. Move to the top of the head. Take a fine slice of hair off the top of a large section, place it on the foil, and apply lightener (Figure 16–79).
14. Part out a larger section, and then take a fine slice from the top of this section. Apply lightener (Figure 16–80).
15. Continue toward the front until the last foil is placed (Figure 16–81).
16. Allow the lightener to process according to the strand test. Check the foils to see if you've achieved the desired lightness (Figure 16–82).
17. Remove the foils one at a time at the shampoo area. Rinse the hair immediately to prevent the color from affecting the untreated hair.
18. Apply haircolor glaze to the hair, from base to ends (Figure 16–83).
19. Work the glaze into the hair to make sure it is completely saturated. Process up to 20 minutes.
20. Rinse the hair. Shampoo and condition.
21. Style the hair as desired (Figure 16–84).
22. Perform cleanup and sanitation as in Procedure 42— semipermanent color.

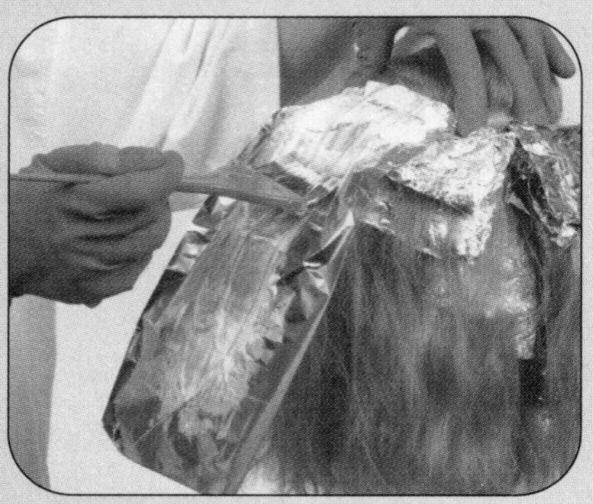

Figure 16-79 Work on top of head.

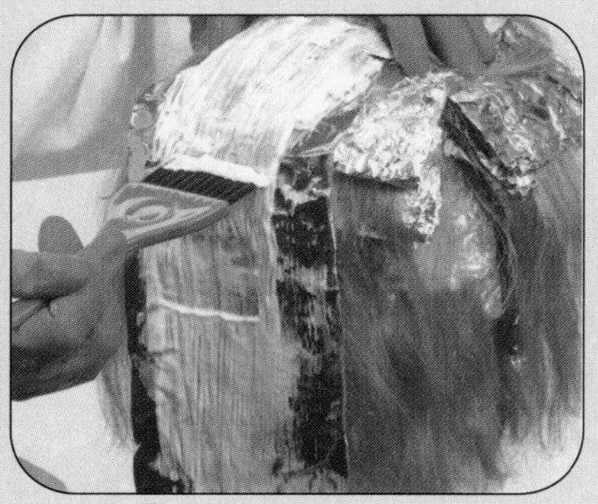

Figure 16-80 Apply lightener.

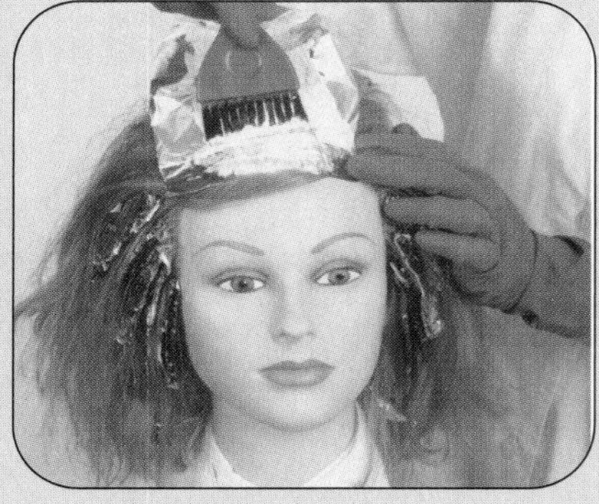

Figure 16-81 Last foil in front.

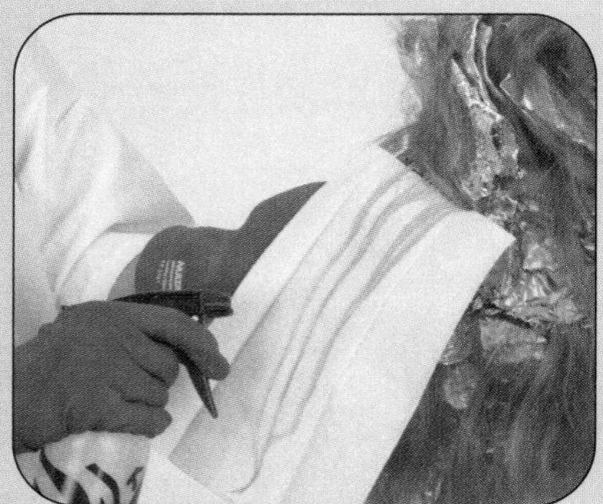

Figure 16-82 Check a subsection for proper processing.

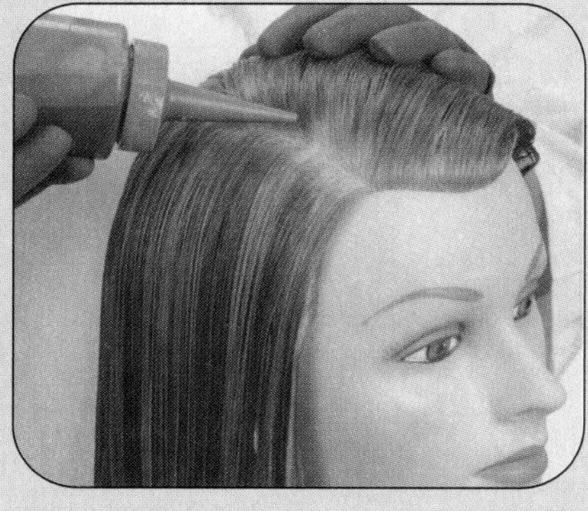

Figure 16-83 Apply glaze.

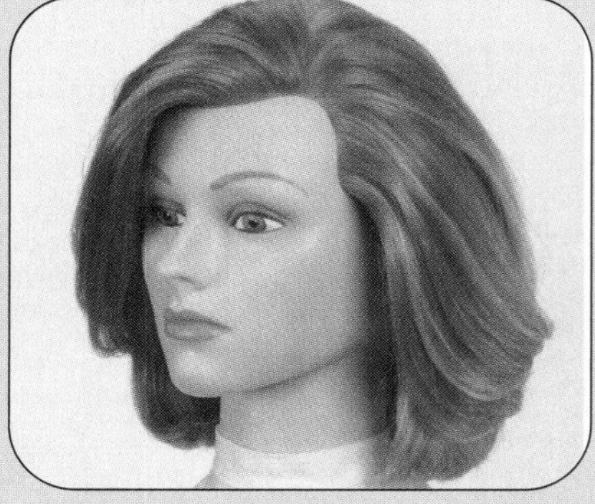

Figure 16-84 Styled hair.

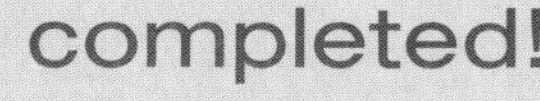

(thus producing no lift of the natural hair color), and is gentle on the scalp and hair.

- Semipermanent color may be used to deposit tonality without lift. Not all colors are delicate enough to avoid overpowering the prelightened hair. Always check the manufacturers' color chart for the base color of your chosen toner. This way you can make sure that when the toner combines with the contributing pigment in the hair you will have the exact tonality you want.
- A demipermanent haircolor, which is a deposit-only color without ammonia, can also be used to recolor hair. It will not further decolorize, but is longer lasting than temporary or semipermanent toner.

Highlighting Shampoos

Highlighting shampoo tints are prepared by combining permanent haircolor, hydrogen peroxide, and shampoo. They are used when a very slight change in hair shade is desired, or when the client's hair processes very rapidly. These tints highlight the hair's natural color in a single application. A patch test is required 24 hours prior to application.

Highlighting shampoos are a mixture of shampoo and hydrogen peroxide. The natural color is slightly lightened. No patch test is required. Follow manufacturers' directions. 6 ✓

SPECIAL PROBLEMS IN HAIRCOLOR/CORRECTIVE COLORING

Each haircoloring service is unique and, in the same vein, can present unique problems. To give each haircoloring service a good start, the colorist must factor in sufficient time for a complete consultation with the client and the careful analysis of the client's hair. Strand tests must be taken to ensure satisfactory final results. But even the most skilled colorist will occasionally have a problem that none of the above could predict. This may be due to the particular structure or condition of the client's hair. The good news, however, is that most haircoloring problems can be resolved or corrected if the colorist just stays calm.

Gray Hair: Challenges and Solutions

Gray, white, and salt-and-pepper hair all have characteristics that present unique coloring challenges. For instance, gray hair can turn orange if the lightener used is not processed long enough. A great many salon coloring services, however, will successfully cover or enhance gray hair if used correctly (Figure 16–85 and Figure 16–86).

Yellowed Hair

A problem that can occur with gray hair is the yellow cast caused by a variety of factors. Smoking, medication, exposure to the sun, and, to a lesser

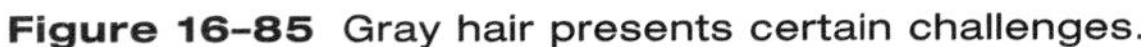

Figure 16-85 Gray hair presents certain challenges.

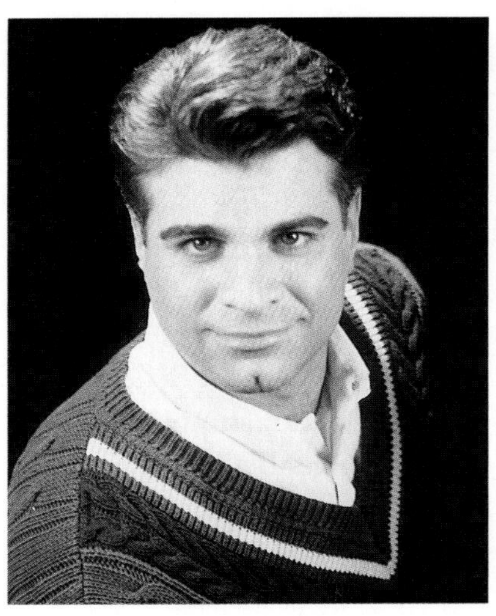

Figure 16-86 Many haircolor options cover gray successfully.

degree, hair sprays and styling aids can all cause the hair to turn yellow. Lightener and tint removers will help remove yellow discoloration.

Undesired yellow can often be overpowered by the artificial pigments deposited by violet-based colors of an equal or darker level than the yellow.

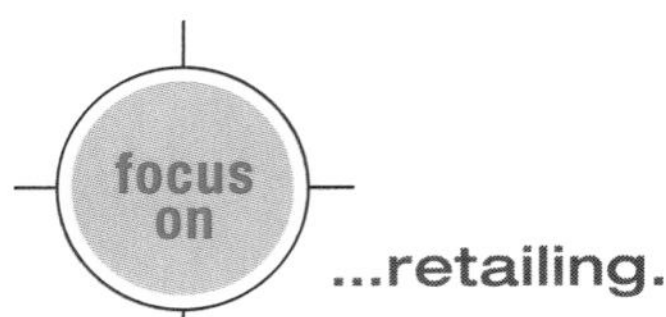

...retailing.

How can you increase your salary as a colorist? Sell retail! Let's say you recommend one or two products, such as a color shampoo and conditioner, to each haircoloring client. (Of course, you will only recommend those products that are truly beneficial for their hair type and condition.) Figure an average of $15 per client, 5 clients a day, 5 days a week. That's $375 per week. Many stylists and colorists make even more than that selling retail products. Selling is a boon to your budget and a service to your clients.

Formulating for Gray Hair

Gray hair basically accepts the level of the color applied. However, Level 9 or lighter shades may not give complete coverage because of the small percentage of artificial pigment formulated into these shades. Generally, formulations from Levels 6, 7, or 8 will give better coverage and can be used to create pastel and blonde tones if desired.

For those clients who are 80 to 100 percent gray, a haircolor within the blonde range is generally more flattering than a darker shade. This lighter level of artificial color may be selected to give a warm or cool finished product, depending on the client's skin tone, eye color, and personal preference.

Another factor to consider when coloring low percentages of gray or salt-and-pepper hair to a darker level is that color on color will always make a darker color. The addition of dark artificial pigment to the natural pigment results in a color that the eye perceives as darker. For this reason, when attempting to cover the unpigmented hair in a salt-and-pepper head, a shade lighter than the naturally dark hair is recommended.

For the purposes of a strand test, a manufacturer's product color chart can be used in conjunction with the following formulation charts (Table 16-4 and Table 16-5) to select a color tonality within the proper level.

The gray hair formulation tables provide general guidelines, but there are other, more subjective considerations to take into account such as the client's personality, personal preferences, and the amount of gray hair and its location. You will note that in the tables there are no tones given in the formulations, only levels of haircoloring and various techniques.

Percentage of Gray Hair	Formulation
90–100%	Desired level
70–90%	Equal parts desired and one level lighter
50–70%	one level lighter than desired level
30–50%	Equal parts one level lighter and two levels lighter
10–30%	two levels lighter than desired level

Table 16-4 Semipermanent/Demipermanent Color Formulation for Gray Hair

Also note that in the table there are no accommodations made for the location of the gray hair. The chart is designed so the section that indicates 30 percent unpigmented presumes that the gray hair is equally distributed throughout the entire head. If, for instance, the majority of the 30 percent gray hair is located in the front section of the head, that section would be considered 80 percent gray with the back portion containing just a sprinkling of gray hair. In that instance, you would have to determine what

Percentage of Gray Hair	Formulation
90–100%	Desired level
70–90%	two parts desired level and one part lighter level
50–70%	Equal parts desired and lighter level
30–50%	two parts lighter level and one part desired level
10–30%	one level lighter

Table 16-5 Permanent Color Formulation for Gray Hair

formulation would best suit the client: formulating for 80 percent gray or the sprinkling of gray. If the gray hair around the face is what the client sees, then you would be well advised to formulate for the 80 percent unpigmented hair. The section of hair that surrounds the face is what influences the client's self-perception.

There are many techniques to help you solve your haircolor challenges. The more techniques that you have at your disposal, the greater latitude you will have. Remember that your knowledge and your techniques are your tools for successful haircoloring. There is no final destination when it comes to learning haircolor. The learning curve keeps going in a journey that never ends, but that is filled with fascinating places to visit.

focus on ...building your client base.

- Be as knowledgeable about haircolor as you can be. Maintain your skills through continuous education.
- Be honest when recommending color options to your client. That means including information on maintenance, costs, and other such issues.
- Keep up to date with celebrity hair trends, because your clients will be asking for them.
- Maintain a positive and excited attitude about your work and convey your confidence and enthusiasm to your client.

Presoftening

Occasionally, gray hair is so resistant that even when formulation, application, and time are correct, you will find that the coverage is not satisfactory. In such cases, presoftening becomes necessary. **Presoftening** is the process of treating gray or very resistant hair to allow for better penetration of color by opening the cuticle. It is a double-application haircoloring service. A presoftener is applied, processed, and removed. Then the tint is applied.

Presoftening is also effective on pigmented resistant hair, but care must be taken to leave the presoftening mixture on the hair only long enough to help open the cuticle, making the hair porous enough to accept the color. Otherwise, you may create more underlying warmth than desired and will have to compensate for this added warmth in your color selection and formulation for deposit.

To presoften hair, mix the product according to the manufacturer's directions. Apply it with a brush or bottle in the most resistant areas first. Process at room temperature for 5 to 20 minutes. Wipe the color gently with a cloth or paper towel to remove. Next, apply the desired level and tone of the color to achieve your end results.

Rules for Effective Color Correction

Sometimes, the color may not come out as expected. This can seem disastrous, for your client and for you. It need not be, however. Problems can be corrected. Keep the following guidelines in mind.

1. Do not panic.
2. Establish the true problem.
3. Establish what caused the problem.
4. Establish the most suitable remedy.
5. Always take one step at a time.
6. Never guarantee an exact result.
7. Always strand test for accuracy.

Damaged Hair

Blow-drying, wind, harsh shampoos, and chemical services all take their toll on the condition of the hair. Coating compounds such as hair sprays, styling agents, and some conditioners can also damage the hair in that they can lead to diminished color penetration.

Hair is considered damaged when it has one or more of the following characteristics:

- rough texture
- overporous condition
- brittle and dry to the touch
- susceptible to breakage
- no elasticity
- becomes spongy and matted when wet
- color fades or absorbs too rapidly

Any of these hair conditions will create problems during a tinting, lightening, permanent waving, or hair relaxing treatment. Therefore, damaged hair should receive reconditioning treatments prior to, and after the application of, these chemical processes. When dealing with damaged hair:

- use a penetrating conditioner that can deposit protein, oils, and moisture-rich ingredients.
- complete each chemical service by normalizing the pH with a finishing rinse. This will restore the cuticle's protective capacity.
- postpone any further chemical service until the hair is reconditioned If the hair is still unresponsive after a conditioning treatment.
- schedule the client for between-service conditioning.
- recommend retail products for use at home to prepare for the next service.

Fillers

Fillers are specialized preparations designed to help equalize porosity and deposit a base color in one application. They can be either a ready-made manufacturers' preparation or a mixture of tint and conditioner that your instructor can help you prepare. There are two types of fillers: conditioner fillers and color fillers.

Conditioner fillers are used to recondition damaged, overly porous hair. They can be applied in a separate procedure or immediately prior to color application. The conditioner and the color are then working at the same time.

Color fillers are often demipermanent color products that are used when there is doubt as to whether the color result will be an even shade. Using color fillers has several advantages:

- deposits color to faded ends and hair shaft
- helps hair to hold color
- prevents streaking and dull appearance
- prevents off-color results
- produces more uniform, natural-looking color in a tint
- produces uniform color when doing a tint back

Selecting the Correct Color Filler

To obtain satisfactory results, select the color filler that will replace the missing primary color in your formulation. Always remember that all three primaries—red, blue, and yellow—must be present for natural-looking haircolor. If you have blonde (yellow) hair, for example, that is being tinted back to an ash (yellow and blue) brown, you will need to use an orange-red filler so that the end result will be correct.

Color fillers may be applied directly from their containers to damaged hair prior to tinting. They may also be added to the tint and applied to damaged ends.

Fading Reds

Fading is a common problem with color-treated red hair. With every shampoo, blow-dry, permanent wave, and exposure to sun, chlorine, or salt water, the artificial pigment within the hair shaft continues to oxidize and fade.

Use of a lower volume of hydrogen peroxide can prevent excessive fading and brassiness. If the desired depth of red is of the same or deeper level than the natural color, the hue can be achieved through deposit without excessive lift. This technique can be particularly useful in achieving and retaining the violet-based reds.

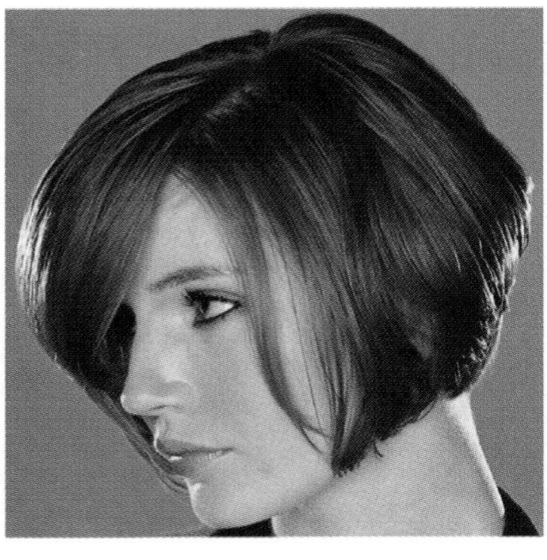

Figure 16–87 Vibrant red hair.

For warmer or brighter (red-orange or gold) reds on darker natural levels, prelightening before application of your tint can have its advantages. The lightening process naturally brings out the warm contributing pigment, which serves as the ideal foundation for a vibrant red color (Figure 16–87). Care must be taken, however, to avoid overlightening the hair, which will create the opposite effect than you desire, leaving the hair dull, flat, and with a lifeless color tonality.

When you are retouching with a red-based tint, the formula you are using to create the correct amount of lift at the new growth may produce too much lift if it is pulled through the ends to refresh the color. Your reds will last longer if you create them using a separate formula with a deposit-only haircolor product applied to the midshaft and ends. Your selection should correspond in tone and level to the formula used on the new growth. Strand testing will point you toward the correct color choice.

Tips for Reds

- Use a low-volume hydrogen peroxide.
- Prelighten darker hair to achieve brighter, warmer reds.
- Make sure you formulate correctly to achieve the proper intensity of red.
- When performing a retouch, always use permanent color on the new growth and refresh the ends with a deposit-only color.

Correcting Brassiness and Other Unwanted Tones in the Hair

As the artificial pigment fades, brassy red, orange, or gold notes may become apparent. The natural tendency of the client will be to request more frequent retouches. Scheduling retouches at closer and closer intervals causes greater porosity and diffusion of the natural pigment, leaving the hair even brassier than before as the tint once again fades. And so a never-ending cycle begins.

Your first step in camouflaging excessive brassiness in either natural or tinted hair is to analyze it. Are the brassy notes red, yellow, or orange? Locate the particular shade on the color wheel and use the complementary color to neutralize it. A number of options exist for solving the problem. Temporary rinses, a soap cap during retouches (see p. 596), fillers, and semipermanent or demipermanent colors of a neutralizing shade can all be effective in correcting brassiness, depending on the situation. Your instructor will guide you in recommending the appropriate treatment for the situation.

CAUTION

When performing a tint removal service, never leave the client unattended, as lightening may occur quite rapidly.

Tint Removal

Sometimes, it is necessary to remove all or part of the color from the hair in order to achieve the desired color. The client may want to change to a lighter shade or the present haircolor may have been a mistake. Occasionally, color builds up or processes too dark because of formulation error.

Prepared commercial products designed to remove artificial pigment from the hair are known as **color** or **tint removers**. Color removers are not generally sold for use by nonprofessionals because the process is too complex. Therefore, color removing should be seen as a professional service that can bring new clients into the salon.

Color removers may contain ingredients that are designed to diffuse pigment, both natural and artificial, and are sometimes mixed with hydrogen peroxide. Others have the option of being mixed with distilled water to create a milder color remover. Always follow the individual manufacturer's directions.

Tint Back to Natural Color

Clients who have been either tinting or lightening will often want to return to their natural shade. However, the effects of sun, chlorinated pool water, or prior chemical services can alter the hair color.

Each tinting procedure to return the client's hair to its natural color must be handled as a unique problem. Porous hair will absorb color quickly and process darker and cooler than expected. It may also fade faster than normal. The natural pigment may be so diffused that it will not accept color at all. Check the hair for its natural color next to the scalp. Carefully record all observations and treatments on the client's record card.

After wearing the hair lighter than its natural color for any length of time, your client may not realize how drastic a change it will be to return to the natural color. Discuss options such as reverse highlighting or selection of a color one or two levels lighter than her natural color. Either of these options will enable you to gradually add more depth to your client's hair. A strand test will be essential to ensure desired results.

The key to a successful tint back to natural may be the use of a filler to even out the porosity and to achieve color correction. You will want to create a formulation with enough warmth to prevent drab, unnatural-looking color in the finished product. Demipermanent, deposit-only color is a great choice.

CAUTION

Sometimes, the hair is so overporous that there are insufficient protein bonds and natural melanin left within the cortex for the artificial pigment to attach to. The hair may look "gun-metal gray," and this lighter-than-expected result is a real danger sign. Hair that is this porous is very fragile and may be close to the breaking point.

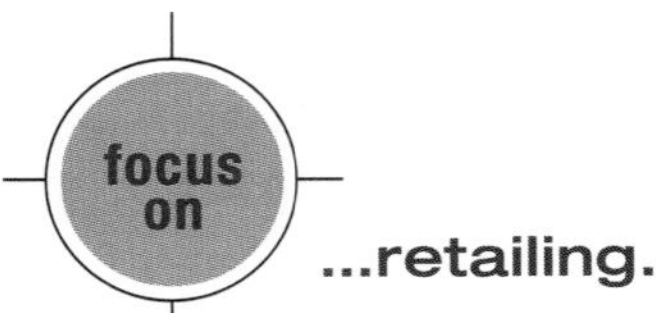

...retailing.

Offer the client the opportunity to purchase high-quality salon products to help prevent color fading at home.

A **soap cap** is a combination of equal parts of prepared tint and shampoo and is applied to the hair like a regular shampoo. It is used in conjunction with a tint back to natural if the tint does not exactly match the natural color. A quick soap cap will break the line of demarcation. A patch test should be administered 24 hours prior to the service. Proceed only if results are negative.

SALON MENU OF SERVICES

As a salon professional you will, of course, need to become fully familiar with the way color services are identified, listed, and described. It is also important to have a sense of how much time should be scheduled for performing these various services. This is known as the **booking time**. Keep in mind that all new clients will need an extra 15 minutes for consultation. Junior colorists will also need more time to perform these services. As you become more experienced, your speed will automatically build and you can reduce your booking times.

Here is an example of how a salon might present their color services in a brochure (Figure 16–88).

- *Single-process color and/or color enhancement.* This service is performed when a client wants to lighten the hair, cover up gray hair, or enhance the natural haircolor. It usually processes for 20 to 45 minutes, depending on the situation. Time between appointments is generally four to six weeks.

HAIRCOLOR SERVICES	
Full Highlight	$00 and up
Partial Highlight	$00 and up
Permanent Color	$00 and up
Semipermanent	$00 and up
Lighten and Tone	$00 and up
Deep Conditioner	$00
Correction Color	As Quoted

Figure 16–88 Salon menu.

- *Single-process retouch color with a glaze.* A single process with glaze involves two steps. In the first step, the first color is applied to the base area, or new growth, and is processed for 30 to 45 minutes. The second step involves the **glaze** (demipermanent, also known as overlay), which is a nonammonia color that adds shine and tone to the hair. After the first color is rinsed out, the glaze is applied at the shampoo bowl and is processed for 10 to 15 minutes. The time between appointments is generally four to six weeks.
- *Double-process color.* Clients who wish to be very blonde all over require this service. The hair is prelightened first, then toned with a toner or glaze. This process can take anywhere from 45 to 90 minutes. The time between appointments is generally four to five weeks.
- *Double-process retouch.* In this process, only the base regrowth area is lightened with a lightener and then the entire head is toned or glazed to refresh the color. Time between appointments is generally four to five weeks.
- *Dimensional haircolor.* In this service, popularly referred to as highlighting, strands of hair are isolated with foil or free-hand painting to create dimension or a variety of different colors in the hair. Dimensional haircolor services include:
- *Face-frame highlight.* In this service, which is an easy way to introduce a client to highlighting, the face is framed with foils from ear to ear. A glaze is included to add tone and shine to both the new highlights and the existing hair. Processing time is 30 minutes. Time between appointments is generally 8 to 12 weeks.
- *Half-head highlight.* Foils are placed on the sides and top of the head. A glaze is included to add tone and shine to the new highlights and existing color. Processing time is 30 to 45 minutes. Time between appointments is generally 8 to 12 weeks.
- *Three-quarter-head highlight.* Foils are placed on the sides, top, and back of the head to the occipital bone. A glaze is included. Processing time is 45 minutes to one hour. Time between appointments is generally 8 to 12 weeks.
- *Full-head highlight.* Foils are placed all over the head. A glaze is included. Processing time is from one hour to one hour and fifteen minutes. Time between appointments is generally 8 to 12 weeks.
- *Special effects highlighting* (also known as creative color techniques). Includes any highlighting service that is not described above, such as tone on tone, reverse highlighting, and scrunching. A consultation is recommended, and the price is determined at that time.
- *Corrective color.* This includes color situations that require special attention over a series of visits. A consultation is advised to determine the time and cost involved.

HAIRCOLORING SAFETY PRECAUTIONS

- Give a patch test 24 hours prior to any application of aniline derivative. Apply a tint only if the patch test is negative.
- Do not apply tint if abrasions are present.
- Do not apply tint if a metallic or compound tint is present.
- Do not brush the hair prior to applying color.
- Always read and follow all of the manufacturers' directions.
- Use sanitized applicator bottles, brushes, combs, and towels.
- Protect your client's clothing with proper draping.
- Perform a strand test for color, breakage, and/or discoloration.
- Use an applicator bottle or bowl (glass or plastic) for mixing the tint.
- Do not mix tint before you are ready to use it; discard leftover tint.
- Wear gloves to protect your hands.
- Do not permit the color to come in contact with the client's eyes.
- Do not overlap during a tint retouch.
- Use a mild shampoo. An alkaline or harsh shampoo will strip the color.
- Always wash hands before and after serving a client.

Your haircoloring work offers you the opportunity to exercise your creative impulses and can bring great pleasure to your clients (Figure 16–89). Enjoy your work, but, most of all, enjoy and appreciate all the learning you need to do, now and in the future.

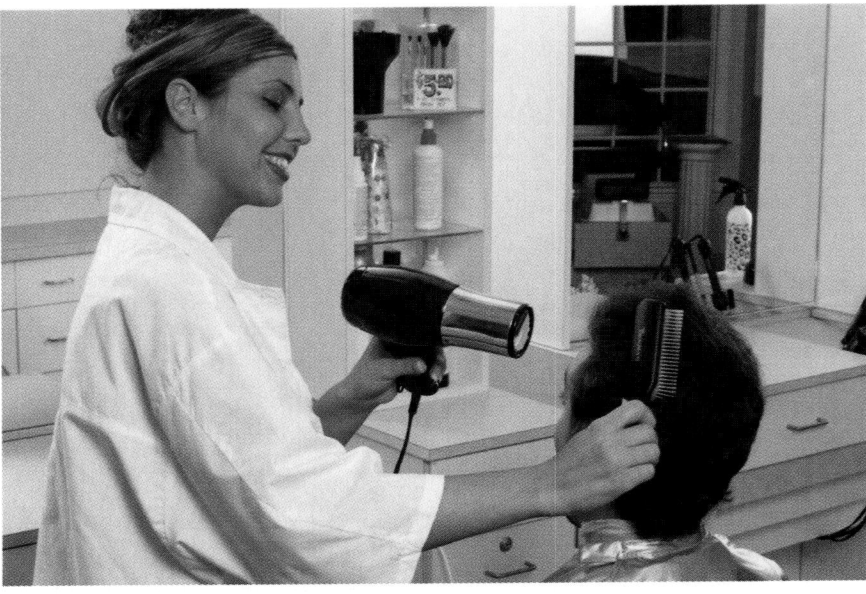

Figure 16–89 A haircolor specialist has both skill and creativity.

chapter glossary

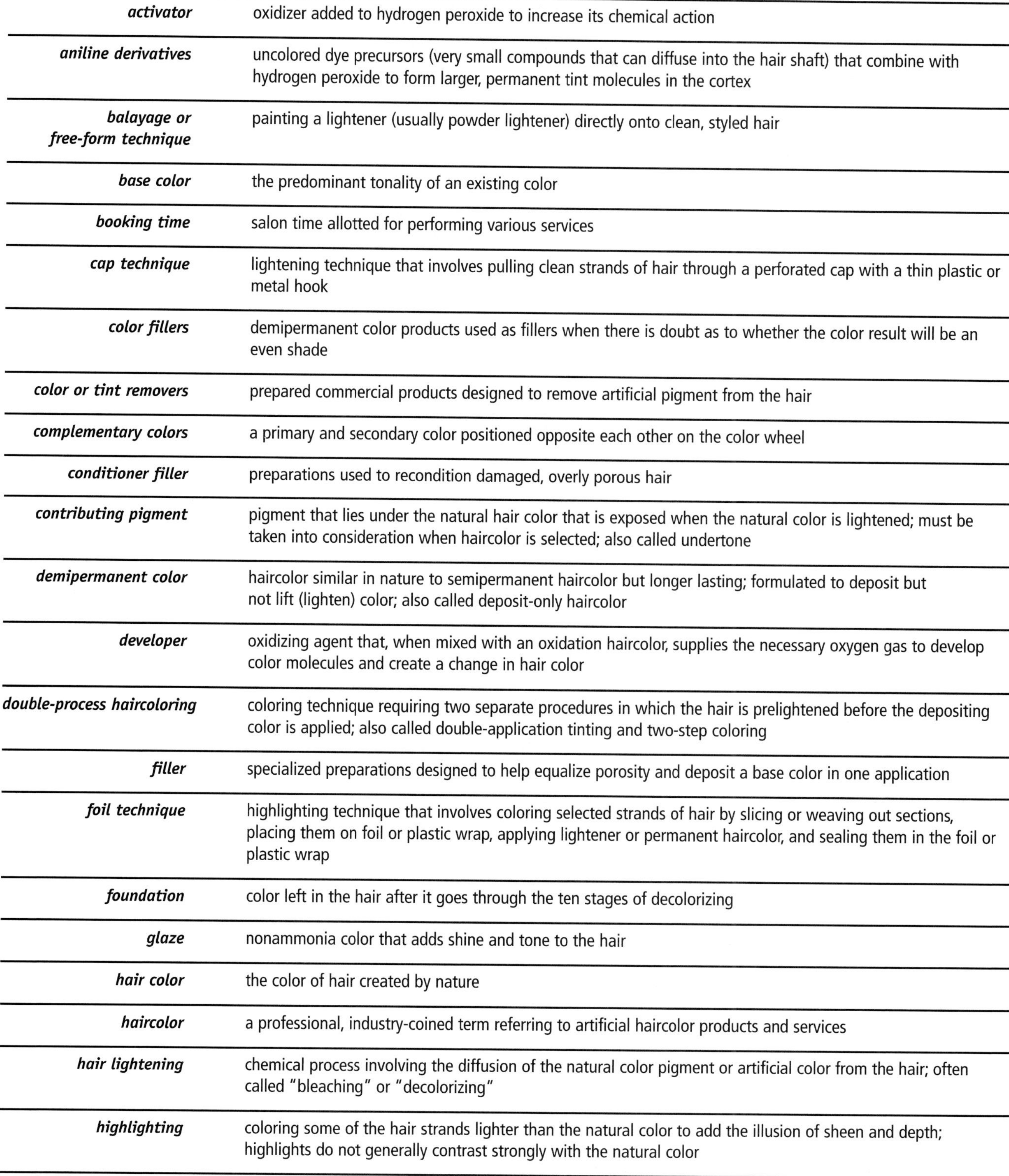

activator	oxidizer added to hydrogen peroxide to increase its chemical action
aniline derivatives	uncolored dye precursors (very small compounds that can diffuse into the hair shaft) that combine with hydrogen peroxide to form larger, permanent tint molecules in the cortex
balayage or free-form technique	painting a lightener (usually powder lightener) directly onto clean, styled hair
base color	the predominant tonality of an existing color
booking time	salon time allotted for performing various services
cap technique	lightening technique that involves pulling clean strands of hair through a perforated cap with a thin plastic or metal hook
color fillers	demipermanent color products used as fillers when there is doubt as to whether the color result will be an even shade
color or tint removers	prepared commercial products designed to remove artificial pigment from the hair
complementary colors	a primary and secondary color positioned opposite each other on the color wheel
conditioner filler	preparations used to recondition damaged, overly porous hair
contributing pigment	pigment that lies under the natural hair color that is exposed when the natural color is lightened; must be taken into consideration when haircolor is selected; also called undertone
demipermanent color	haircolor similar in nature to semipermanent haircolor but longer lasting; formulated to deposit but not lift (lighten) color; also called deposit-only haircolor
developer	oxidizing agent that, when mixed with an oxidation haircolor, supplies the necessary oxygen gas to develop color molecules and create a change in hair color
double-process haircoloring	coloring technique requiring two separate procedures in which the hair is prelightened before the depositing color is applied; also called double-application tinting and two-step coloring
filler	specialized preparations designed to help equalize porosity and deposit a base color in one application
foil technique	highlighting technique that involves coloring selected strands of hair by slicing or weaving out sections, placing them on foil or plastic wrap, applying lightener or permanent haircolor, and sealing them in the foil or plastic wrap
foundation	color left in the hair after it goes through the ten stages of decolorizing
glaze	nonammonia color that adds shine and tone to the hair
hair color	the color of hair created by nature
haircolor	a professional, industry-coined term referring to artificial haircolor products and services
hair lightening	chemical process involving the diffusion of the natural color pigment or artificial color from the hair; often called "bleaching" or "decolorizing"
highlighting	coloring some of the hair strands lighter than the natural color to add the illusion of sheen and depth; highlights do not generally contrast strongly with the natural color

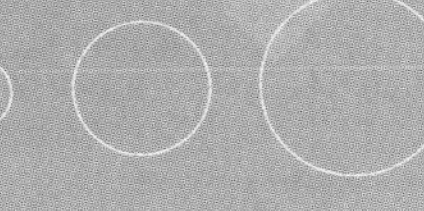

chapter glossary *(continued)*

highlighting shampoos	mixtures of shampoo and hydrogen peroxide; used to slightly lighten natural hair color
highlighting shampoo tints	permanent haircolors mixed with hydrogen peroxide and shampoo; used when a very slight change in hair shade is desired, or when the client's hair processes very rapidly
intensity	strength of a color tone; described as mild, medium, or strong
Law of Color	system for understanding color relationships
level	unit of measurement used to identify the lightness or darkness of a color; sometimes referred to as value or depth
Level System	system colorists use to analyze the lightness or darkness of a hair color
lighteners	chemical compounds that lighten hair by dispersing, dissolving, and decolorizing the natural hair pigment
line of demarcation	visible line separating colored hair from new growth
metallic or gradual haircolors	haircolors containing metal salts that change hair color gradually by progressive buildup and exposure to air, creating a dull, metallic appearance
mixed melanin	combination of eumelanin and pheomelanin often found in natural haircolor
natural or vegetable haircolors	natural colors, such as henna, obtained from the leaves or bark of plants
new growth	the part of the hair shaft between the scalp and the hair that has previously received treatment; also called regrowth
off-the-scalp lighteners	lighteners that cannot be used directly on the scalp
on-the-scalp lighteners	lighteners that can be used directly on the scalp
patch test	test for identifying a possible allergy in a client, required by Federal Food, Drug, and Cosmetic Act; also called predisposition test
permanent haircolor	haircolor that is mixed with a developer (hydrogen peroxide) and remains in the hair shaft until the new growth of hair occurs
prelightening	the first step of double-process haircoloring, used to lift or lighten the natural pigment, preliminary to the application of toner
presoftening	process of treating gray or very resistant hair to allow for better penetration of color
primary colors	pure or fundamental colors that cannot be achieved from a mixture
resistant	characteristic of some hair types that makes penetration by moisture or chemicals difficult
reverse highlighting or lowlighting	technique of coloring strands of hair darker than the natural color
secondary color	color obtained by mixing equal parts of two primary colors

semipermanent haircolor	haircolor formulated to last through several shampoos; partially penetrates the hair shaft and stains the cuticle layer, slowly fading with each shampoo
single-process haircoloring	process that lightens and colors the hair in a single application
slicing	coloring technique that involves taking a narrow, 1/8-inch (.3 cm) section of hair by making a straight part at the scalp, positioning the hair over the foil, and applying lightener or color
soap cap	combination of equal parts of prepared tint and shampoo applied to the hair like a regular shampoo
special effects haircoloring	any technique that involves partial lightening or coloring
temporary haircolor	nonpermanent color whose large pigment molecules prevent penetration of the cuticle layer, allowing only a coating action that may be removed by shampooing
tertiary color	intermediate color achieved by mixing a secondary color and its neighboring primary color on the color wheel in equal amounts
tone or tonality	term used to describe the warmth or coolness of a color
toners	semipermanent, demipermanent, and permanent haircolor products that are used primarily on prelightened hair to achieve pale and delicate colors
virgin application	the first time the hair is tinted
volume	the measure of the potential oxidation of varying strengths of hydrogen peroxide; the higher the volume, the greater the lifting action
weaving	coloring technique in which selected strands are picked up from a narrow section of hair with a zigzag motion of the comb, and lightener or color is applied only to these strands

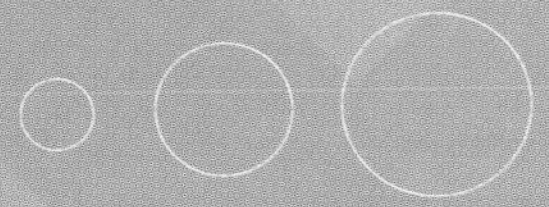

review questions

1. List the primary, secondary, and tertiary colors.
2. Name the two types of melanin.
3. Define level, tone, and intensity.
4. What are the classifications of haircolor? Briefly describe each one.
5. Why is a patch test important?
6. What is a strand test?
7. What is the role of ammonia in a haircolor formula?
8. What is the role of hydrogen peroxide in a haircolor formula?
9. What are the four key questions you ask when formulating a haircolor?
10. Explain the procedure for a single-process tint.
11. What are the two processes involved in double-process haircoloring?
12. What are three forms of hair lightener?
13. What are the three most commonly used methods for highlighting?
14. What are fillers, and for what purpose are they used?
15. List at least 10 safety precautions to follow during the haircolor process.

part 4

SKIN CARE

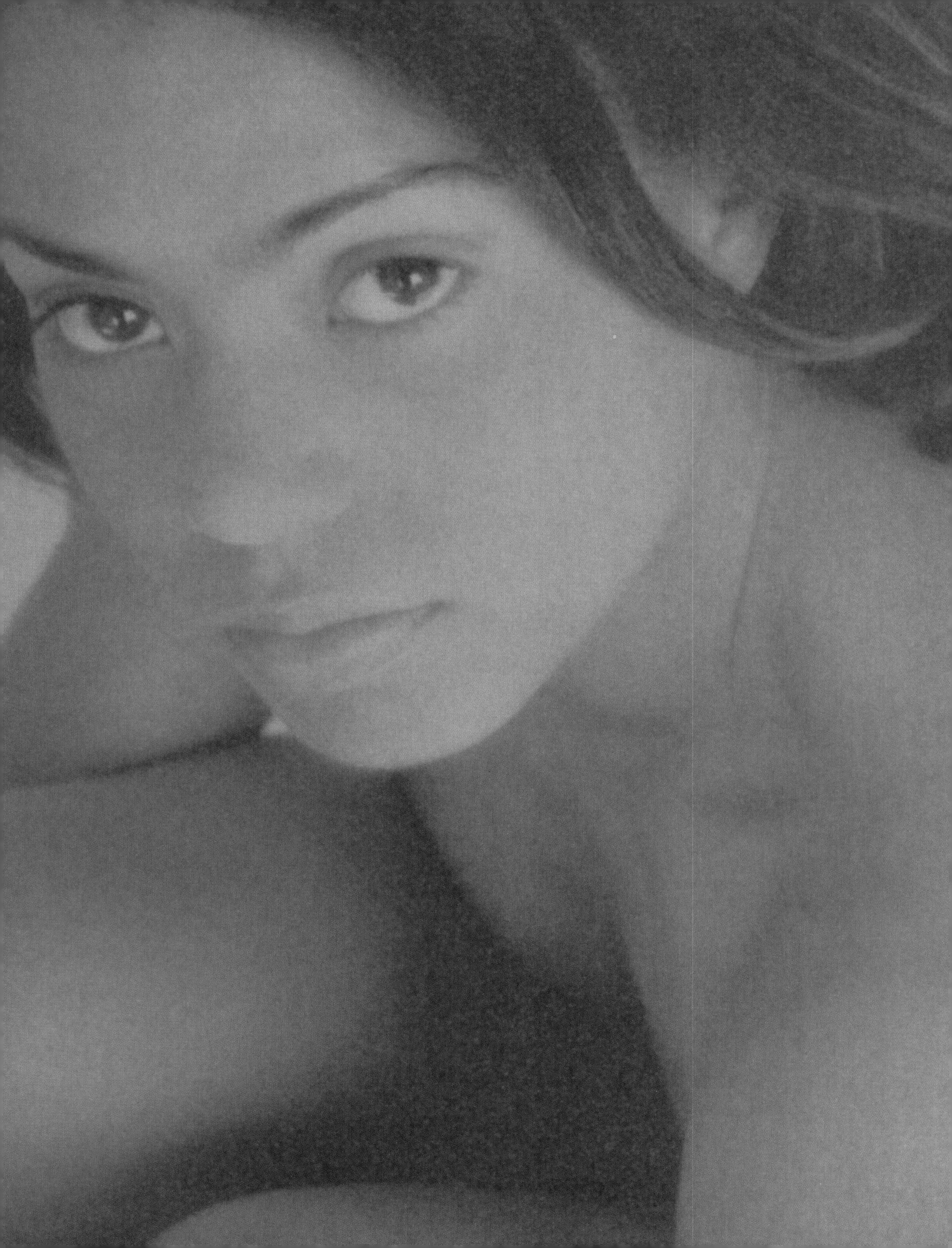

HISTOLOGY OF THE SKIN

Aly Evirs
ESTHETICS INSTRUCTOR AND FREELANCE EDUCATOR

Chapter Outline

Learning Objectives

After completing this chapter, you should be able to:

1. Describe the structure and composition of the skin.
2. List the functions of the skin.
3. Describe the aging process and the factors that influence aging of the skin.
4. Define important terms relating to skin disorders.
5. Discuss which skin disorders may be handled in the salon and which should be referred to a physician.

National Skill Standards

This chapter provides you with the necessary information to master these National Industry Skill Standards for Entry-Level Cosmetologists.

Providing basic skin care services.

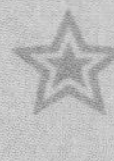
Conducting services in a safe environment, and taking measures to prevent the spread of infectious and contagious disease.

Using appropriate methods to ensure personal health and well-being.

Key Terms

Page number indicates where in the chapter the term is used.

acne pg. 620
albinism pg. 622
anhidrosis pg. 620
asteatosis pg. 620
basal cell carcinoma pg. 623
bromhidrosis pg. 620
bulla (plural: bullae) pg. 617
chloasma pg. 622
collagen pg. 611
comedone pg. 620
crust pg. 619
cyst pg. 618
dermatitis pg. 621
dermatitis venenata pg. 621
dermatologist pg. 607
dermatology pg. 607
dermis pg. 609
eczema pg. 621
elastin pg. 611
epidermis pg. 607
esthetician pg. 607
excoriation pg. 619
fissure pg. 619
fundus pg. 612
herpes simplex pg. 621
hyperhidrosis pg. 621
hypertrophy pg. 622
keloid pg. 619
keratin pg. 608
keratoma pg. 622
lentigenes pg. 622
lesion pg. 617
leukoderma pg. 622
macule (plural: maculae) pg. 618
malignant melanoma pg. 623
melanin pg. 610
melanocytes pg. 609
milia pg. 620
miliaria rubra pg. 621
mole pg. 622
nevus pg. 622
papillary layer pg. 609
papule pg. 618
psoriasis pg. 621
pustule pg. 618
reticular layer pg. 609
retinoic acid pg. 624
rosacea pg. 620
scale pg. 619
scar or cicatrix pg. 619
sebaceous glands pg. 612
seborrhea pg. 620
skin tag pg. 623
squamous cell carcinoma pg. 623
stain pg. 622
steatoma pg. 620
stratum corneum pg. 608
stratum germinativum pg. 608
stratum granulosum pg. 608
stratum lucidum pg. 608
subcutaneous tissue pg. 610
sudoriferous glands pg. 612
tactile corpuscles pg. 609
tan pg. 622
tubercle pg. 618
tumor pg. 618
ulcer pg. 620
verruca pg. 623
vesicle pg. 619
vitiligo pg. 622
wheal pg. 619

Clear, glowing skin is one of the hallmarks of beauty, and consumers' desire to have such skin has created a multibillion-dollar industry of skin care products. Many of your clients will be hoping for the kind of beautiful skin they see on models in magazines and on television and will likely call on you as a consultant in their quest. It is important for you to be familiar with the range of skin care products available, but, even more important, you need to know about the natural structure of the skin. A cosmetologist who has a thorough understanding of the skin, its structure, and its functions is in a better position to give clients professional advice on scalp, facial, and hand care.

ANATOMY OF THE SKIN

The medical branch of science that deals with the study of skin and its nature, structure, functions, diseases, and treatment is called **dermatology**. A **dermatologist** is a physician engaged in the science of treating the skin, its structures, functions, and diseases. An **esthetician** is a specialist in the cleansing, preservation of health, and beautification of the skin and body.

The skin is the largest and one of the most important organs of the body. Healthy skin is slightly moist, soft, and flexible with a texture (feel and appearance) that ideally is smooth and fine-grained. Healthy skin possesses a slightly acid reaction with good immunity responses to organisms that touch or try to enter it. Appendages of the skin include hair, nails, and sweat and oil glands.

Skin varies in thickness. It is thinnest on the eyelids and thickest on the palms and soles. Continued pressure on any part of the skin can cause it to thicken and develop into a callus. The skin of the scalp is constructed similarly to the skin elsewhere on the human body, but the scalp has larger and deeper hair follicles to accommodate the longer hair of the head.

The skin is composed of two main divisions: the epidermis and the dermis (Figure 17–1).

The **epidermis** (ep-uh-DUR-mis) is the outermost layer of the skin. This layer is also called the cuticle (KYOO-tih-kul) or scarf skin. It is the thinnest layer of skin and forms a protective covering for the body. It contains no

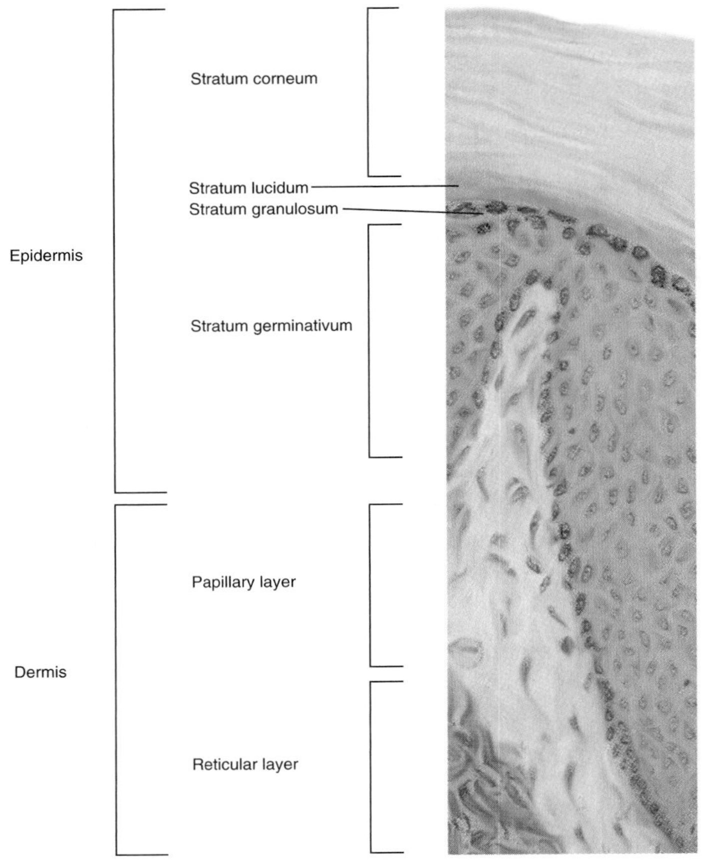

Epidermis

Stratum corneum

Stratum lucidum

Stratum granulosum

Stratum germinativum

Dermis

Papillary layer

Reticular layer

Figure 17–1 The layers of the skin.

blood vessels, but has many small nerve endings. The epidermis is made up of the following layers:

- The **stratum corneum** (STRAT-um KOR-nee-um), or horny layer, is the outer layer of the epidermis. Its scale-like cells are continually being shed and replaced by cells coming to the surface from underneath. These cells are made up of **keratin**, a fiber protein that is also the principal component of hair and nails. The cells combine with a thin layer of oil to help make the stratum corneum a protective, waterproof layer.
- The **stratum lucidum** (LOO-sih-dum) is the clear, transparent layer under the stratum corneum; it consists of small cells through which light can pass.
- The **stratum granulosum** (gran-yoo-LOH-sum), or granular layer, consists of cells that look like distinct granules. These cells are almost dead and are pushed to the surface to replace cells that are shed from the stratum corneum.
- The **stratum germinativum** (jer-mih-nah-TIV-um), formerly known as the stratum mucosum (myoo-KOH-sum) and also referred to as the basal or Malpighian layer, is the deepest layer of the epidermis. It is composed of several layers of different-shaped cells. The deepest layer is responsible for the growth of the epidermis. It also contains a dark skin pigment,

called melanin, which protects the sensitive cells below from the destructive effects of excessive ultraviolet rays of the sun or those from an ultraviolet lamp. These special cells are called **melanocytes** (muh-LAN-uh-syts). They produce melanin, which determines skin color.

The **dermis** (DUR-mis) is the underlying or inner layer of the skin. It is also called the derma, corium (KOH-ree-um), cutis (KYOO-tis), or true skin. This highly sensitive layer of connective tissue is about 25 times thicker than the epidermis. Within its structure, there are numerous blood vessels, lymph vessels, nerves, sweat glands, oil glands, and hair follicles, as well as arrector pili muscles (small muscles that work in connection with the hair follicles) and papillae (small cone-shaped projections of elastic tissue that point upward into the epidermis). The dermis is made up of two layers: the papillary or superficial layer, and the reticular or deeper layer (Figure 17–2).

- The **papillary layer** (PAP-uh-lair-ee) is the outer layer of the dermis, directly beneath the epidermis. Here you will find the dermal papillae (puh-PIL-eye), which are small, cone-shaped elevations at the bottom of the hair follicles. Some papillae contain looped capillaries and others contain small structures called **tactile corpuscles** (TAK-tile KOR-pus-uls), with nerve endings that are sensitive to touch and pressure. This layer also contains some melanin.
- The **reticular layer** (ruh-TIK-yuh-lur) is the deeper layer of the dermis that supplies the skin with oxygen and nutrients. It contains the following structures within its network:
    - fat cells
    - blood vessels
    - lymph vessels
    - oil glands
    - sweat glands
    - hair follicles
    - arrector pili muscles

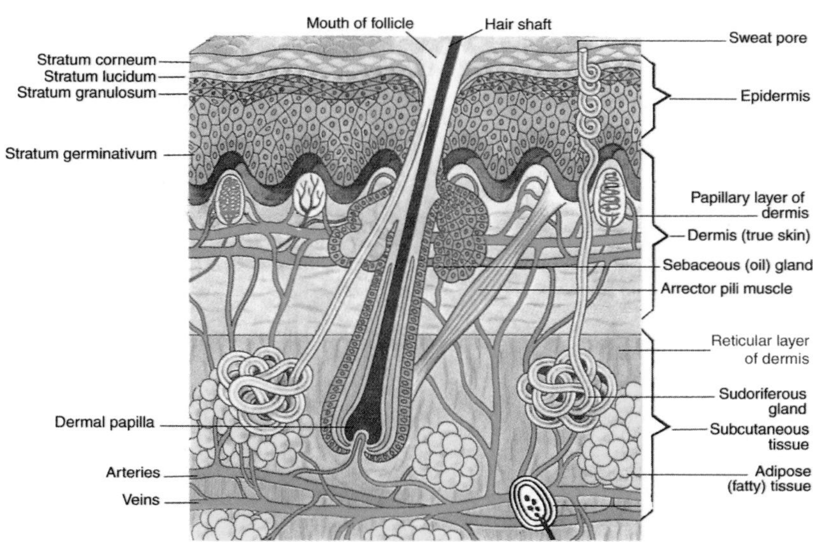

Figure 17–2 Structures of the skin.

Subcutaneous tissue (sub-kyoo-TAY-nee-us) is a fatty layer found below the dermis that some specialists regard as a continuation of the dermis. This tissue is also called adipose (AD-uh-pohs) or subcutis (sub-KYOO-tis) tissue and varies in thickness according to the age, sex, and general health of the individual. It gives smoothness and contour to the body, contains fats for use as energy, and also acts as a protective cushion for the outer skin.

How the Skin Is Nourished

Blood and lymph, the clear fluids of the body that resemble blood plasma but contain only colorless corpuscles, supply nourishment to the skin. As they circulate through the skin, the blood and lymph contribute essential materials for growth, nourishment, and repair of the skin, hair, and nails. Networks of arteries and lymph vessels in the subcutaneous tissue send their smaller branches to hair papillae, hair follicles, and skin glands (see Chapter 6).

Nerves of the Skin

The skin contains the surface endings of the following nerve fibers:

- *Motor nerve fibers*, which are distributed to the arrector pili muscles attached to the hair follicles. These muscles can cause goose bumps when a person is frightened or cold.
- *Sensory nerve fibers*, which react to heat, cold, touch, pressure, and pain. These sensory receptors send messages to the brain.
- *Secretory nerve fibers*, which are distributed to the sweat and oil glands of the skin. Secretory nerves, which are part of the autonomic nervous system, regulate the excretion of perspiration from the sweat glands and control the flow of sebum (a fatty or oily secretion of the sebaceous glands) to the surface of the skin (see Chapter 6).

Sense of Touch

The papillary layer of the dermis houses the nerve endings that provide the body with the sense of touch. These nerve endings register basic sensations such as touch, pain, heat, cold, and pressure. Nerve endings are most abundant in the fingertips. Complex sensations, such as vibrations, seem to depend on the sensitivity of a combination of these nerve endings.

Skin Color

The color of the skin, whether fair, medium, or dark, depends, in part, on the blood supply to the skin but primarily on **melanin**, the tiny grains of pigment (coloring matter) deposited in the stratum germinativum of the epidermis and the papillary layers of the dermis. The color of pigment varies from person to person. The distinctive color of the skin is a hereditary trait and varies among races and nationalities. Dark skin contains more melanin; light skin contains less (Figure 17–3).

Melanin protects sensitive cells against strong light rays. A sun protection factor (SPF) should be used to help the melanin in the skin protect it from burning.

Strength and Flexibility of the Skin

The skin gets its strength, form, and flexibility from two specific structures composed of flexible protein fibers found within the dermis. These two

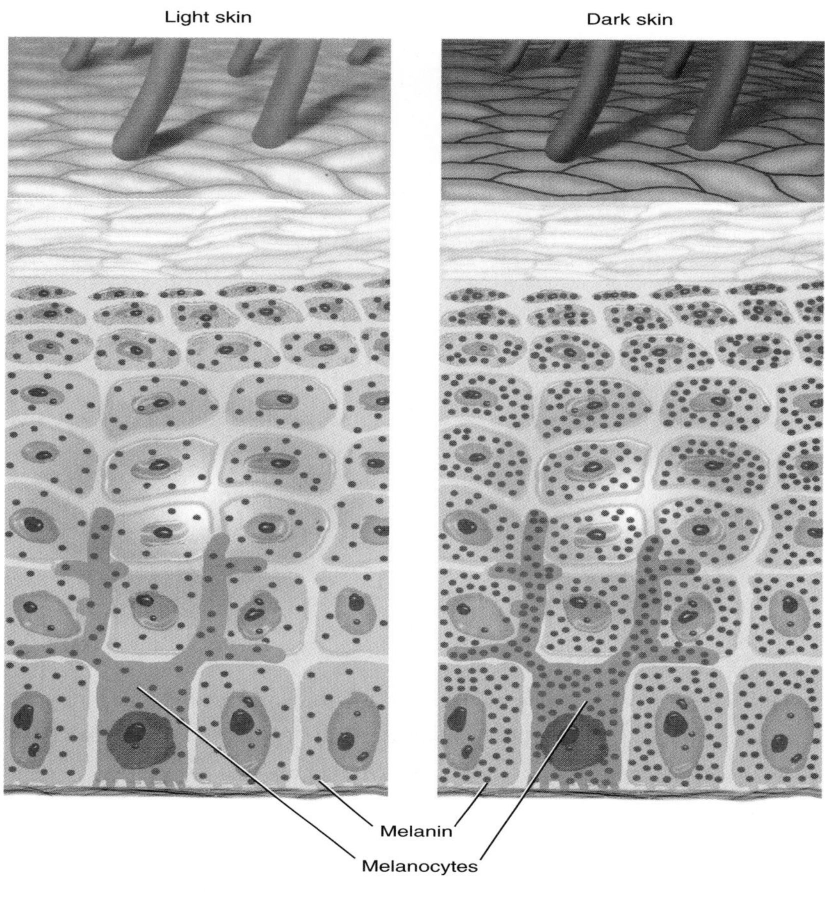

Figure 17–3 Melanocytes in the epidermis produce melanin.

structures, which make up 70 percent of the dermis, are called collagen and elastin.

Collagen is a fibrous protein that gives the skin form and strength. This fiber makes up a large portion of the dermis and helps give structural support to the skin by holding together all the structures found in this layer. When collagen fibers are healthy, they allow the skin to stretch and contract as necessary. If collagen fibers become weakened, due to a lack of moisture in the skin, environmental damage, or frequent changes in weight, the skin will begin to lose its tone and suppleness. Wrinkles and sagging are often the result of collagen fibers losing their strength.

Collagen fibers are interwoven with **elastin**, a protein base similar to collagen that forms elastic tissue. This fiber gives the skin its flexibility and elasticity. Elastin helps the skin regain its shape, even after being repeatedly stretched or expanded.

Both of these fibers are important to the overall health and appearance of the skin. As we age, these fibers naturally weaken, causing the kind of wrinkling and sagging mentioned above. Keeping the skin healthy, moisturized, and free of disease will slow the weakening process and help keep the skin looking young longer.

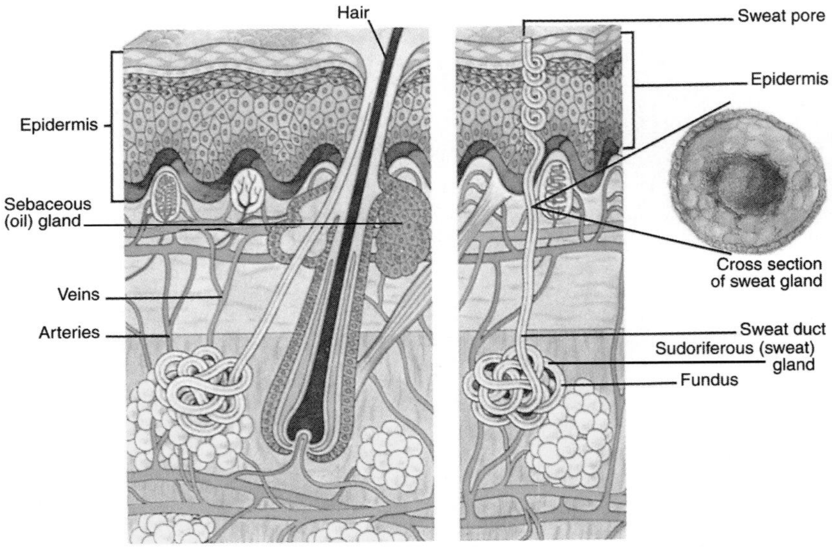

Figure 17–4 Sweat gland and oil gland.

Glands of the Skin

The skin contains two types of duct glands that extract materials from the blood to form new substances: the **sudoriferous glands** (sood-uh-RIF-uh-rus) or **sweat glands**, and the **sebaceous glands** (sih-BAY-shus) or **oil glands** (Figure 17–4).

Sudoriferous (Sweat) Glands

The sudoriferous or sweat glands, which excrete sweat from the skin, consist of a coiled base, or **fundus** (FUN-dus), and a tube-like duct that ends at the skin surface to form the sweat pore. Practically all parts of the body are supplied with sweat glands, which are more numerous on the palms, soles, forehead, and in the armpits.

The sweat glands regulate body temperature and help to eliminate waste products from the body. Their activity is greatly increased by heat, exercise, emotions, and certain drugs.

The excretion of sweat is controlled by the nervous system. Normally, one to two pints of liquids containing salts are eliminated daily through sweat pores in the skin.

Sebaceous (Oil) Glands

The sebaceous or oil glands of the skin are connected to the hair follicles. They consist of little sacs with ducts that open into the follicles. They secrete sebum, a fatty or oily secretion that lubricates the skin and preserves the softness of the hair. With the exception of the palms and soles, these glands are found in all parts of the body, particularly in the face and scalp, where they are larger.

Ordinarily, sebum flows through the oil ducts leading to the mouths of the hair follicles. However, when the sebum hardens and the duct becomes clogged, a blackhead is formed. 1

insights

Kimberley Comiskey

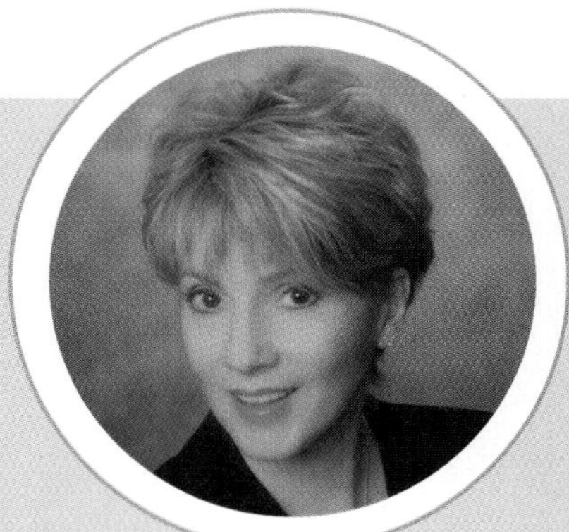

The founder of a highly successful day spa outside of Albany, New York, Kimberley Comiskey sometimes feels she is living a dream come true.

I had to overcome a lot of resistance from my grandparents and parents when I decided to go to beauty school. They sent me away to college so that I wouldn't become a hairdresser. But when I kept at it, they changed their minds. They came to like the idea that I could give them a very good haircut and it wouldn't cost what they were used to paying.

I've always loved the challenge of making people look good and feel good. It was something I always knew I wanted to do—it was in my heart. Nothing felt more natural to me than to pick up a pair of scissors and transform someone with a beautiful look. But, over time, I wanted more than that. I had this dream to open a day spa, and I went for it.

Learning how to manage and run the daily operations of a day spa was a real challenge for me. Being in a structured environment from day to day, doing payroll and writing manuals—it's been a learning curve. But we started in 1987 with 2,500 square feet and next year we'll be moving to 17,000 square feet on three floors with close to 100 employees, so I can't complain. And if you want to make it in this business, don't complain.

I think the number-one quality that is key to building a loyal clientele is flexibility.

Make yourself available to the client. The other thing that is so important is education. Without continuing education, I do not believe that a business can grow and thrive, and I do not believe that an individual can grow as well. Continuing education is something we insist on, and we have guidelines for in-house training before anyone actually works on a client or even talks to one. Our assistants and apprentices go through programs that can take anywhere from a year to three years, depending on their time and commitment. We take them step-by-step and talk about basic things: introducing yourself to a client, having a consultation, and then, of course, the technical aspects as well. There is so much involved in performing as a team and not being clones of each other, but working in sync.

Selling is vital in our field. You're selling yourself, you're selling your image, you're selling who you are, and you're selling your trade to the public. So many times when students are fresh out of school, they don't consider themselves salespeople because they want to believe that they're artists. Well, yes, we are artists, but the good news is that most hairdressers today do not have to be starving artists! There's no reason why anyone with talent and dedication should not succeed in this field.

Functions of the Skin

The principal functions of the skin are protection, sensation, heat regulation, excretion, secretion, and absorption.

- *Protection.* The skin protects the body from injury and bacterial invasion. The outermost layer of the epidermis is covered with a thin layer of sebum, which renders it waterproof. This outermost layer is resistant to wide variations in temperature, minor injuries, chemically active substances, and many forms of bacteria.
- *Sensation.* By stimulating sensory nerve endings, the skin responds to heat, cold, touch, pressure, and pain. When the nerve endings are stimulated, a message is sent to the brain. You respond by saying "ouch" if you feel pain, by scratching an itch, or by pulling away when you touch something hot. Sensory nerve endings are located near hair follicles (Figure 17–5).
- *Heat regulation.* This means that the skin protects the body from the environment. A healthy body maintains a constant internal temperature of about 98.6° Fahrenheit (37° Celsius). As changes occur in the outside temperature, the blood and sweat glands of the skin make necessary adjustments to allow the body to be cooled by the evaporation of sweat.
- *Excretion.* Perspiration from the sweat glands is excreted through the skin. Water lost through perspiration takes salt and other chemicals with it.
- *Secretion.* Sebum, or oil, is secreted by the sebaceous glands. This oil lubricates the skin, keeping it soft and pliable. Oil also keeps hair soft. Emotional stress can increase the flow of sebum.
- *Absorption.* Absorption is limited, but it does occur. Female hormones, when used as an ingredient of a face cream, can enter the body through the skin and influence it to a minor degree. Fatty materials, such as lanolin creams, are absorbed largely through hair follicles and sebaceous gland openings. 2

17

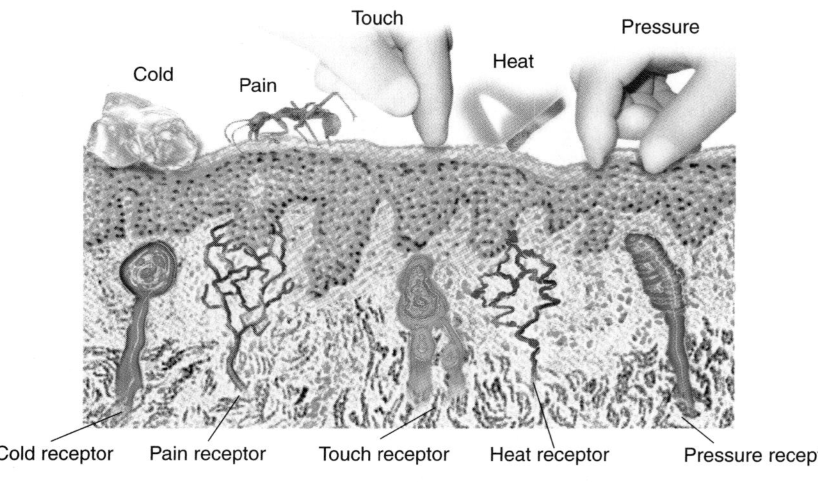

Figure 17–5 Sensory nerve endings in the skin.

Aging of the Skin

Aging of the skin is a process that takes many years and can be influenced by many different factors. One does not necessarily age as one's parents have. Many outside factors like the sun, the environment, health habits, and general lifestyle influence aging to such a great extent that heredity has little to do with the overall process.

The Sun and Its Effects

The sun and its ultraviolet (UV) rays have the greatest impact on how our skin ages. Approximately 80 to 85 percent of our aging is caused by the rays of the sun. As we age, the collagen and elastin fibers of the skin naturally weaken. This weakening happens at a much faster rate when the skin is frequently exposed to ultraviolet rays without proper protection. The UV rays of the sun reach the skin in two different forms, as UVA and UVB rays. Each of the rays influences the skin at a different level.

UVA rays, also called the "aging rays," contribute to 90 to 95 percent of the sun's ultraviolet rays that reach the earth's surface. These rays weaken the collagen and elastin fibers, causing wrinkling and sagging in the tissues.

UVB rays, also referred to as the "burning rays," cause tanning of the skin by affecting the melanocytes, the cells of the epidermis that are responsible for producing melanin, the skin pigment. Melanin is designed to help protect the skin from the sun's UV rays but can be altered or destroyed when large, frequent doses of UV light are allowed to penetrate the skin. Although UVB penetration is not as deep as UVA, these rays are equally damaging to the skin and can damage the eyes as well. On a positive note, UVB rays contribute to the body's synthesis of Vitamin D and other important minerals.

As a consultant to your clients, it is appropriate that you advise them about the necessary precautions to take when they are exposed to the sun:

- Wear a moisturizer or protective lotion with a sunscreen of at least SPF 15 on all areas of potential exposure.
- Avoid exposure to the sun during peak hours, when UV exposure is highest. This is usually between 10AM and 3PM.
- Apply sunscreen liberally after swimming or any activities that result in heavy perspiration. Better yet, sunscreen should be applied periodically throughout the day as a precaution.
- All sunscreen used for protection should be full or broad spectrum to filter out UVA and UVB rays of the sun. Check expiration dates printed on the bottle to make sure that the sunscreen has not expired.
- Avoid exposing children younger than six months of age to the sun.
- If prone to burning frequently and easily, wear a hat and protective clothing when participating in outdoor activities. Redheads are particularly susceptible to sun damage.

In addition to following the above precautions, clients should be advised to regularly see a physician specializing in dermatology for checkups of the skin, especially if any changes in coloration, size, or shape of a mole are detected.

Home self-examinations can also be an effective way to check for signs of potential skin cancer between scheduled doctor visits. When performing a self-care exam, clients should be advised to check for any changes in existing moles and pay attention to any new visible growths on the skin.

Skin Aging and the Environment

While the sun may play the major role in how the skin ages, changes in our environment also greatly influence this aging process. Pollutants in the air from factories, automobile exhaust, and even secondhand smoke can all influence the appearance and overall health of our skin. While these pollutants affect the surface appearance of the skin, they can also change the health of the underlying cells and tissues, thereby speeding up the aging process.

The best defense against these pollutants is the simplest one: follow a good daily skin care routine. Routine washing and exfoliating (removing dead surface skin cells) at night helps to remove the buildup of pollutants that have settled on the skin's surface throughout the day. The application of daily moisturizers, protective lotions, and even foundation products all help to protect the skin from airborne pollutants.

FYI

The American Cancer Society recommends using the ABCD Cancer Checklist to help make potential skin cancer easier to recognize. When checking existing moles, look for changes in any of the following:

A - Asymmetry
B - Border
C - Color
D - Diameter

Changes to any of these should be examined by a physician. For more information, contact the American Cancer Society at www.cancer.org or (800) ACS-2345.

Aging and Lifestyle

Aging of the skin cannot be blamed entirely on the outside influences of the sun and other environmental factors. What we choose to put into our bodies also has a profound effect on the overall aging process. The impact of poor choices can be seen most visibly, however, on the skin. Smoking, drinking, taking drugs, and making poor dietary choices all greatly influence the aging process. It is the responsibility of the cosmetologist to be aware of how these habits affect the skin and to tactfully point out these effects to clients.

Smoking and tobacco use may not only cause cancer, but have also been linked to the premature aging and wrinkling of the skin. Nicotine in tobacco causes contraction and weakening of the blood vessels and small capillaries, which supply blood to the tissues. In turn, this contraction and weakening causes decreased circulation to the tissues. Eventually, the tissues are deprived of essential oxygen, and the effect of this becomes evident on the skin's surface. The skin may appear yellowish or gray in color and can have a dull appearance.

The use of illegal drugs affects the skin as much as smoking does. Some drugs have been shown to interfere with the body's intake of oxygen, thus affecting healthy cell growth. Some drugs can even aggravate serious skin conditions, such as acne. Others can cause dryness and allergic reactions on the skin's surface.

The use of alcohol has an opposite yet equally damaging effect on the skin. Heavy or excessive intake of alcohol overdilates the blood vessels and capillaries. Over time, this constant overdilation and weakening of the fragile capillary walls will cause them to burst. This causes a constant flushed appearance of the skin and red splotches in the whites of the eyes. Alcohol can also dehydrate the skin by drawing essential water out of the tissues, which causes the skin to appear dull and dry.

Both smoking and drinking contribute to the aging process on their own, but the combination of the two can be devastating to the tissues. The constant dilation and contraction that occurs on the tiny capillaries and blood vessels, as well as the constant deprivation of oxygen and water to the tissues, quickly make the skin appear lifeless and dull. It is very difficult for the skin to adjust and repair itself. Usually, the damage done by these lifestyle habits is hard to reverse or diminish. 3

DISORDERS OF THE SKIN

Like any other organ of the body, the skin is susceptible to a variety of diseases, disorders, and ailments. In your work as a cosmetologist you will often see skin and scalp disorders, so you must be prepared to recognize certain common skin conditions and know what you can and cannot do with them. Some skin and scalp disorders can be treated in cooperation with, and under the supervision of, a physician. Medicinal preparations, available only by prescription, must be applied in accordance with the physician's directions. If a client has a skin condition that you do not recognize as a simple disorder, refer the client to a physician.

It is very important that a beauty salon does not serve a client who is suffering from an inflamed skin disorder, infectious or not. The cosmetologist should be able to recognize these conditions and sensitively suggest that proper measures be taken to prevent more serious consequences. Thus, the health of the cosmetologist, as well as the health of other clients, is safeguarded.

Listed below are a number of important terms relating to skin, scalp, and hair disorders that you should be familiar with.

Lesions of the Skin

A **lesion** (LEE-zhun) is an injury or damage that changes the structure of tissues or organs. There are three types of lesions: primary, secondary, and tertiary. The cosmetologist is concerned with primary and secondary lesions only. If you are familiar with the principal skin lesions, you will be able to distinguish between conditions that may or may not be treated in a beauty salon (Figure 17–6).

PRIMARY LESIONS

Bulla (BULL-uh); plural: bullae—A large blister containing a watery fluid; similar to a vesicle but larger (Figure 17–7).

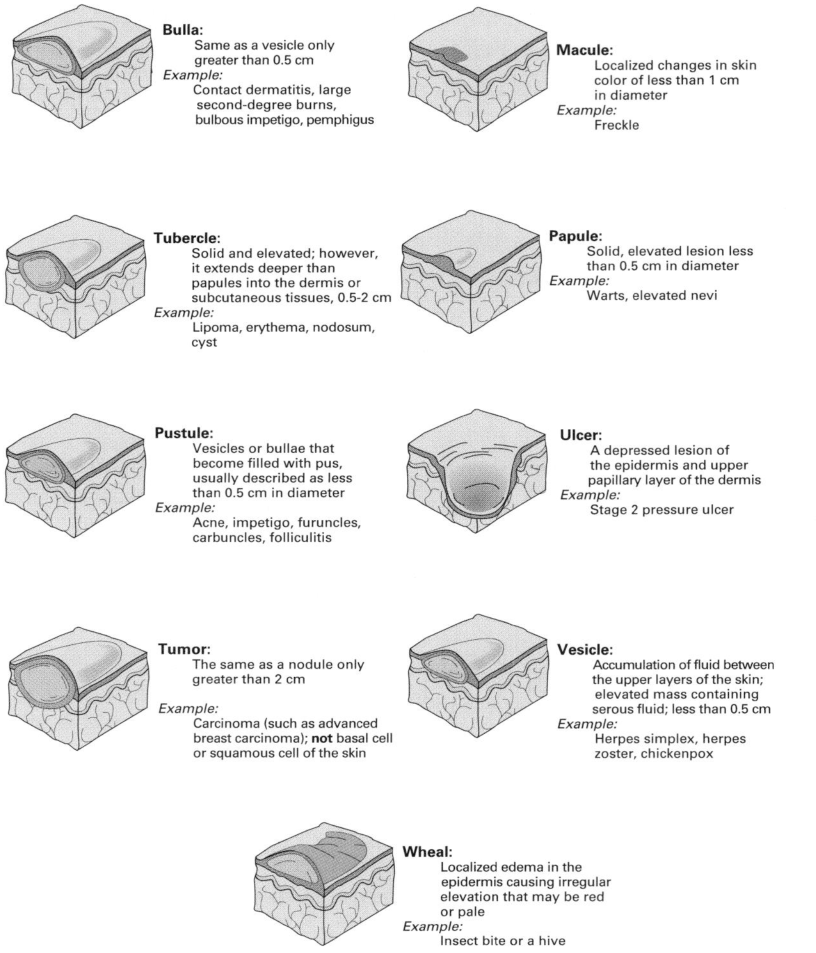

Bulla:
Same as a vesicle only greater than 0.5 cm
Example:
Contact dermatitis, large second-degree burns, bulbous impetigo, pemphigus

Macule:
Localized changes in skin color of less than 1 cm in diameter
Example:
Freckle

Tubercle:
Solid and elevated; however, it extends deeper than papules into the dermis or subcutaneous tissues, 0.5-2 cm
Example:
Lipoma, erythema, nodosum, cyst

Papule:
Solid, elevated lesion less than 0.5 cm in diameter
Example:
Warts, elevated nevi

Pustule:
Vesicles or bullae that become filled with pus, usually described as less than 0.5 cm in diameter
Example:
Acne, impetigo, furuncles, carbuncles, folliculitis

Ulcer:
A depressed lesion of the epidermis and upper papillary layer of the dermis
Example:
Stage 2 pressure ulcer

Tumor:
The same as a nodule only greater than 2 cm
Example:
Carcinoma (such as advanced breast carcinoma); **not** basal cell or squamous cell of the skin

Vesicle:
Accumulation of fluid between the upper layers of the skin; elevated mass containing serous fluid; less than 0.5 cm
Example:
Herpes simplex, herpes zoster, chickenpox

Wheal:
Localized edema in the epidermis causing irregular elevation that may be red or pale
Example:
Insect bite or a hive

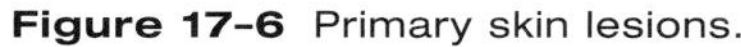

Figure 17-6 Primary skin lesions.

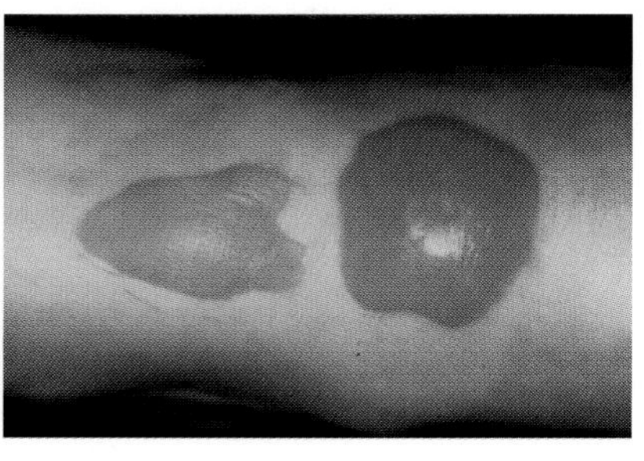

Figure 17-7 Bullae.

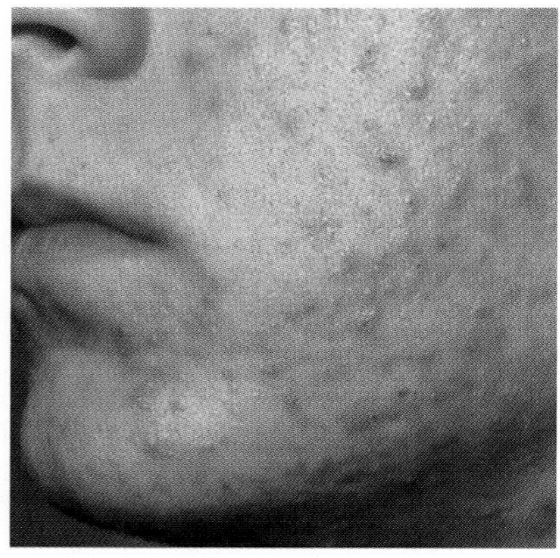

Figure 17-8 Papules and pustules.

Cyst (SIST)—A closed, abnormally developed sac, containing fluid, semifluid, or morbid matter, above or below the skin.

Macule (MAK-yool); plural: maculae (MAK-yuh-ly)—A spot or discoloration on the skin, such as a freckle. Macules are neither raised nor sunken.

Papule (PAP-yool)—A pimple; small circumscribed elevation on the skin that contains no fluid but may develop pus.

Pustule (PUS-chool)—An inflamed pimple containing pus (Figure 17–8).

Tubercle (TOO-bur-kul)—An abnormal rounded, solid lump above, within, or under the skin; larger than a papule.

Tumor (TOO-mur)—A swelling; an abnormal cell mass resulting from excessive multiplication of cells, varying in size, shape, and color. Nodules are also referred to as tumors but are smaller.

Vesicle (VES-ih-kel)—A small blister or sac containing clear fluid, lying within or just beneath the epidermis. Poison ivy and poison oak, for example, produce vesicles (Figure 17–9).

Wheal (WHEEL)—An itchy, swollen lesion that lasts only a few hours; caused by a blow, the bite of an insect, urticaria (skin allergy), or the sting of a nettle. Examples include hives and mosquito bites.

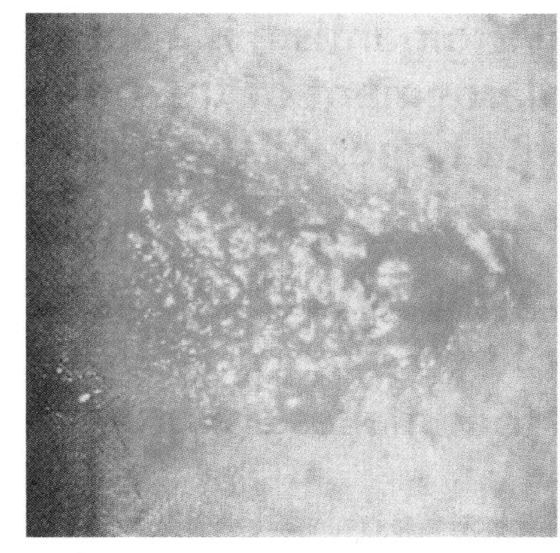

Figure 17-9 Poison oak vesicles.

Secondary Lesions

Secondary skin lesions are those that develop in the later stages of disease (Figure 17–10). These include:

Crust—Dead cells that form over a wound or blemish while it is healing; an accumulation of sebum and pus, sometimes mixed with epidermal material. An example is the scab on a sore.

Excoriation (ek-skor-ee-AY-shun)—A skin sore or abrasion produced by scratching or scraping.

Fissure (FISH-ur)—A crack in the skin that penetrates the dermis. For example, chapped hands or lips.

Keloid (KEE-loyd)—A thick scar resulting from excessive growth of fibrous tissue (Figure 17–11).

Scale—Any thin plate of epidermal flakes, dry or oily. An example is abnormal or excessive dandruff.

Scar or **cicatrix** (SIK-uh-triks)—Light-colored, slightly raised mark on the skin formed after an injury or lesion of the skin has healed.

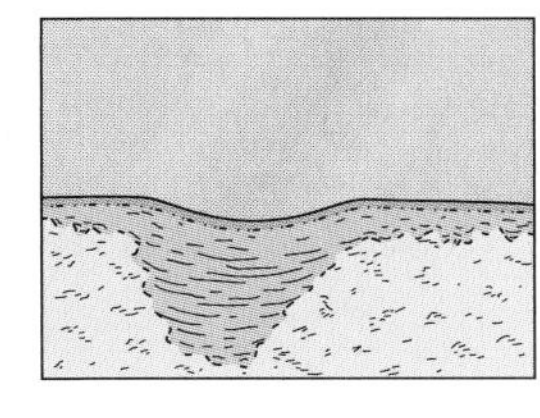

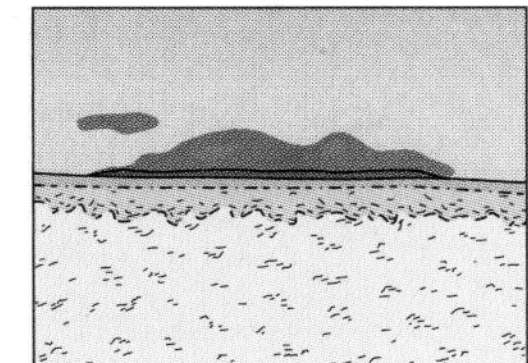

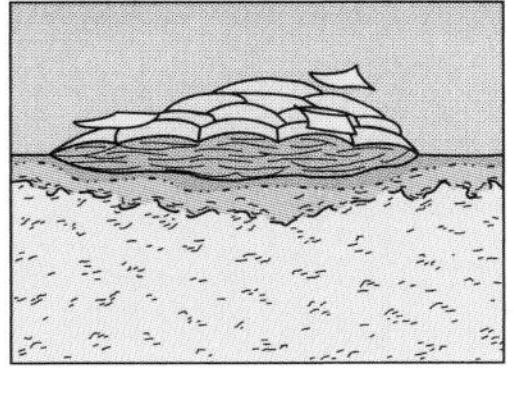

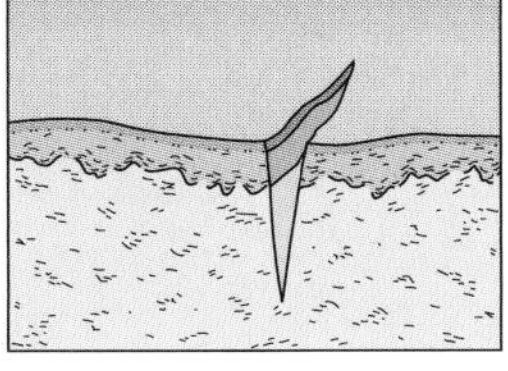

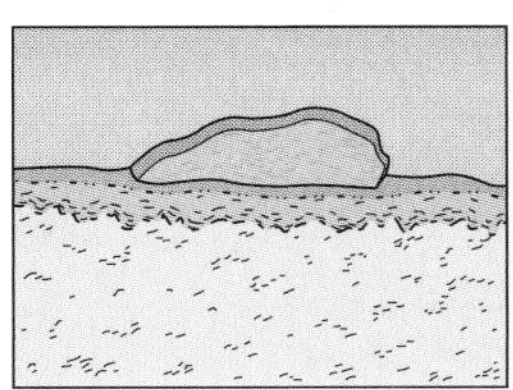

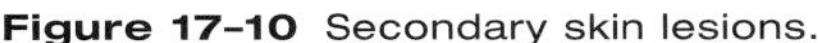

Figure 17-10 Secondary skin lesions.

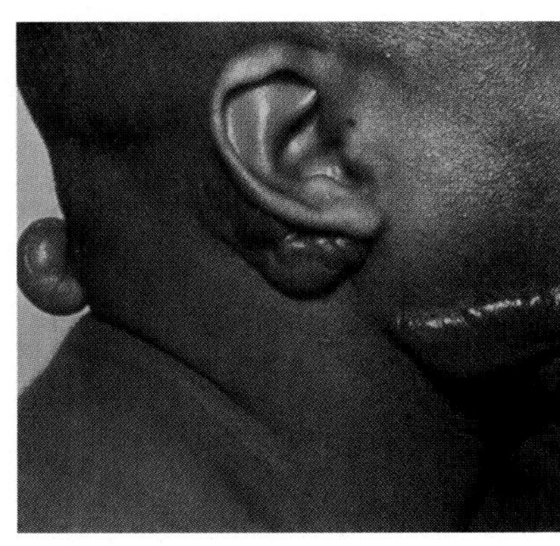

Figure 17-11 Keloids.

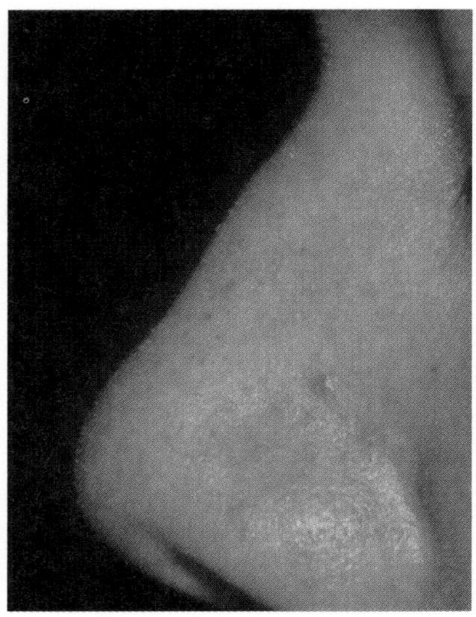

Figure 17–12 Comedones.

Ulcer (UL-sur)—An open lesion on the skin or mucous membrane of the body, accompanied by pus and loss of skin depth.

Disorders of the Sebaceous (Oil) Glands

There are several common disorders of the sebaceous (oil) glands that the cosmetologist should be able to understand and identify.

A **comedone** (KAHM-uh-dohn), or blackhead, is a wormlike mass of hardened sebum in a hair follicle. Comedones appear most frequently on the face, especially on the forehead and nose (Figure 17–12). When the hair follicle is filled with an excess of oil from the sebaceous gland, a blackhead forms and creates a blockage at the mouth of the follicle. Blackheads should be removed under sterile conditions using proper extraction procedures. Should the condition become severe, medical attention is necessary.

Milia (MIL-ee-uh), also called **whiteheads**, are small, whitish, pear-like masses in the epidermis, due to retention of sebum. They can occur on any part of the face, neck, back, chest, and shoulders. Milia are associated with fine-textured, dry types of skin (Figure 17–13).

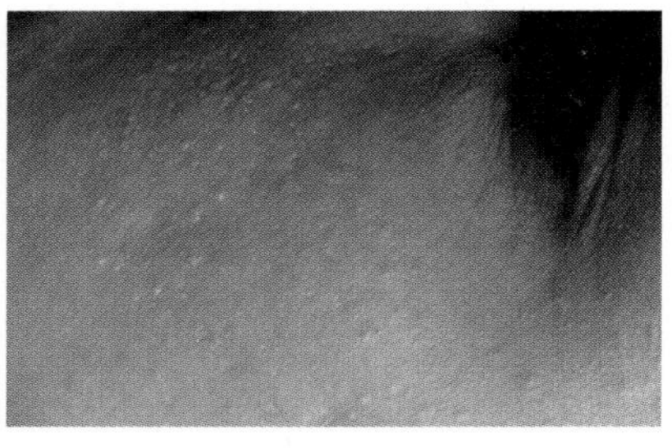

Figure 17–13 Milia.

Acne (AK-nee) is a skin disorder characterized by chronic inflammation of the sebaceous glands from retained secretions. It occurs most frequently on the face, back, and chest. Acne, or common pimples, is also known as acne simplex or acne vulgaris (Figure 17–14).

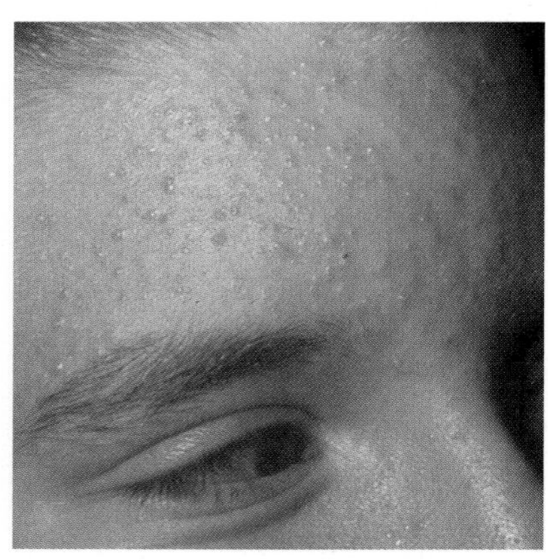

Figure 17–14 Acne.

There are two basic types of acne: simple acne and the more serious acne vulgaris. It is always advisable for the client to have the condition examined and diagnosed by a physician before receiving any service in the salon.

Seborrhea (seb-oh-REE-ah) is a skin condition caused by an abnormal increase of secretion from the sebaceous glands. An oily or shiny condition indicates the presence of seborrhea.

Asteatosis (as-tee-ah-TOH-sis) is a condition of dry, scaly skin due to a deficiency or absence of sebum, caused by old age and by exposure to cold.

Rosacea (roh-ZAY-shee-uh), formerly called acne rosacea, is a chronic congestion appearing primarily on the cheeks and nose, characterized by redness, dilation of the blood vessels, and the formation of papules and pustules. The cause of rosacea is unknown, but certain factors are known to aggravate the condition in some individuals. These include spicy foods, caffeine, alcohol, exposure to extremes of heat and cold or sunlight, and stress (Figure 17–15).

A **steatoma** (stee-ah-TOH-muh) is a sebaceous cyst or fatty tumor. It is filled with sebum and ranges in size from a pea to an orange. It usually appears on the scalp, neck, and back. A steatoma is sometimes called a wen.

Disorders of the Sudoriferous (Sweat) Glands

Anhidrosis (an-hih-DROH-sis)—Deficiency in perspiration, often a result of fever or certain skin diseases. It requires medical treatment.

Bromhidrosis (broh-mih-DROH-sis)—Foul-smelling perspiration, usually noticeable in the armpits or on the feet.

Hyperhidrosis (hy-per-hy-DROH-sis)—Excessive sweating, caused by heat or general body weakness. Medical treatment is required.

Miliaria rubra (mil-ee-AIR-ee-ah ROOB-rah)—Prickly heat; acute inflammatory disorder of the sweat glands, characterized by the eruption of small red vesicles and accompanied by burning, itching skin. It is caused by exposure to excessive heat.

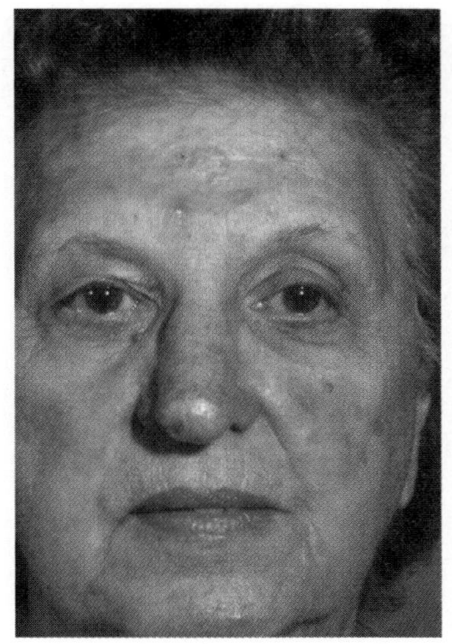

Figure 17–15 Rosacea.

Inflammations of the Skin

Dermatitis (dur-muh-TY-tis)—Inflammatory condition of the skin. The lesions come in various forms, such as vesicles or papules.

Eczema (EG-zuh-muh)—An inflammatory, painful itching disease of the skin, acute or chronic in nature, presenting many forms of dry or moist lesions. All cases of eczema should be referred to a physician for treatment. Its cause is unknown (Figure 17–16).

Herpes simplex (HER-peez SIM-pleks)—Fever blister or cold sore; recurring viral infection. It is characterized by the eruption of a single vesicle or group of vesicles on a red swollen base. The blisters usually appear on the lips, nostrils, or other part of the face, and rarely last more than a week. It is contagious (Figure 17–17).

Psoriasis (suh-RY-uh-sis)—A skin disease chracterized by red patches, covered with white-silver scales usually found on the scalp, elbows, knees, chest, and lower back. It rarely occurs on the face. If irritated, bleeding points occur. It is not contagious (Figure 17–18).

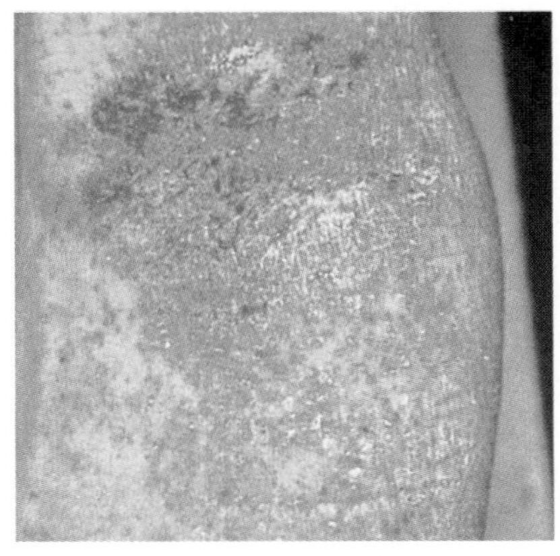

Figure 17–16 Eczema.

Occupational Disorders in Cosmetology

Cosmetologists must be sensitive to skin disorders not only in their clients but in themselves. Frequent contact with chemicals can result in abnormal skin conditions. Some individuals may develop allergies to ingredients in cosmetics, antiseptics, cold waving lotions, and aniline derivative tints. These can cause eruptive skin infections known as **dermatitis venenata** (VEN-uh-nah-tuh). In your work as a cosmetologist, it is important that you employ protective measures, such as the use of rubber gloves or protective creams, whenever possible.

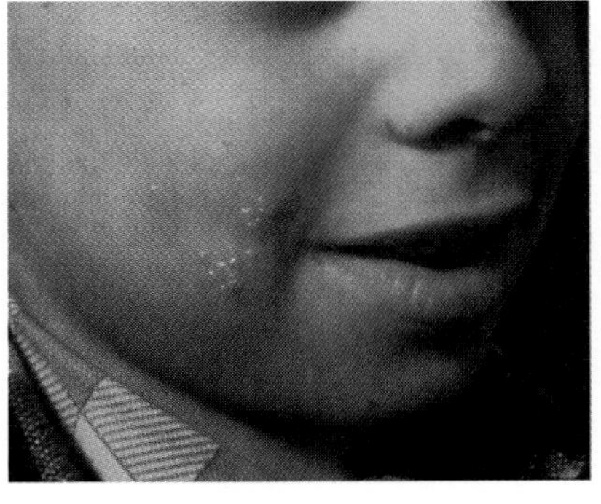

Figure 17–17 Herpes simplex.

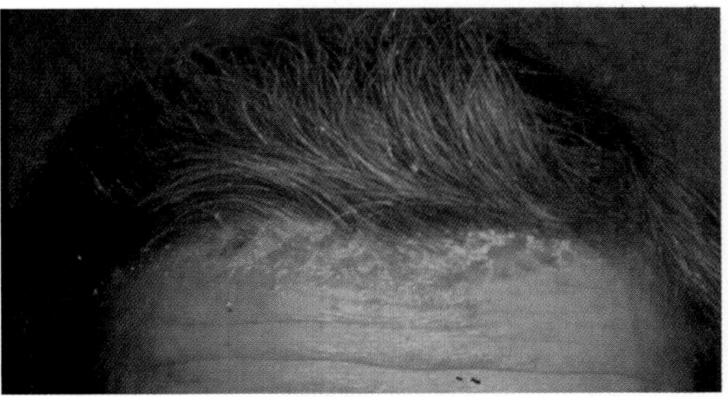

Figure 17–18 Psoriasis.

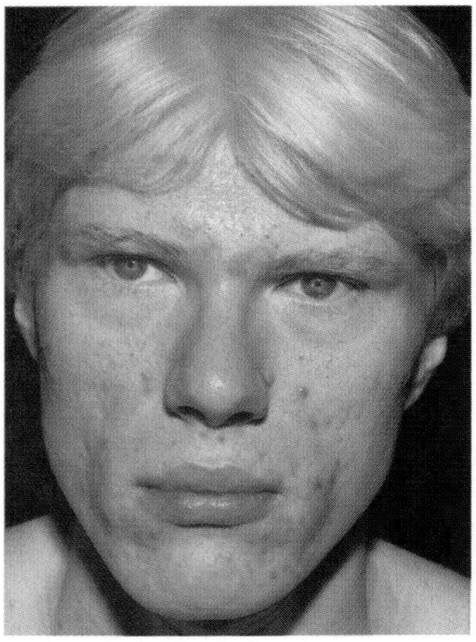

Figure 17-19 Albinism.

Pigmentations of the Skin

Pigment can be affected from inside or outside the body in abnormal conditions, such as prolonged exposure to the sun or other elements. Abnormal coloration also accompanies every skin disorder and many systemic disorders. A change in pigmentation can be observed as well when certain drugs are being taken internally. The following terms relate to changes in the pigmentation of the skin.

Albinism (AL-bi-niz-em)—Congenital leukoderma or absence of melanin pigment of the body, including the skin, hair, and eyes (Figure 17–19). The silky hair is white. The skin is pinkish white and will not tan. Eyes are pink. Skin is sensitive to light and ages early.

Chloasma (kloh-AZ-mah)—Condition characterized by increased pigmentation on the skin, in spots that are not elevated. Chloasma is also called moth patches or liver spots.

Lentigines (len-TIJ-e-neez); singular: lentigo (len-TY-goh)—Technical term for freckles. Small yellow- to brown-colored spots on skin exposed to sunlight and air.

Leukoderma (loo-koh-DUR-muh)—Skin disorder characterized by light abnormal patches; caused by a burn or congenital disease that destroys the pigment-producing cells. It is classified as vitiligo and albinism.

Nevus (NEE-vus)—Small or large malformation of the skin due to abnormal pigmentation or dilated capillaries; commonly known as birthmark.

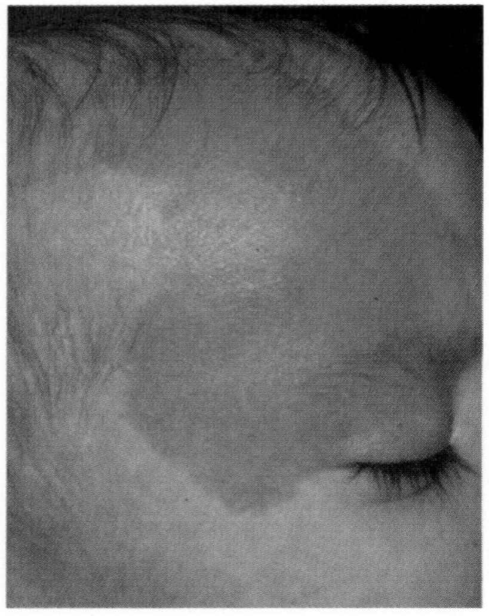

Figure 17-20 Port wine stain.

Stain—Abnormal brown or wine-colored skin discoloration with a circular and irregular shape (Figure 17–20). Its permanent color is due to the presence of darker pigment. Stains occur during aging; after certain diseases; and after the disappearance of moles, freckles, and liver spots. The cause is unknown.

Tan—Change in pigmentation of skin caused by exposure to the sun or ultraviolet rays.

Vitiligo (vih-til-EYE-goh)—Milky-white spots (leukoderma) of the skin; acquired condition (Figure 17–21). Must be protected from overexposure to the sun.

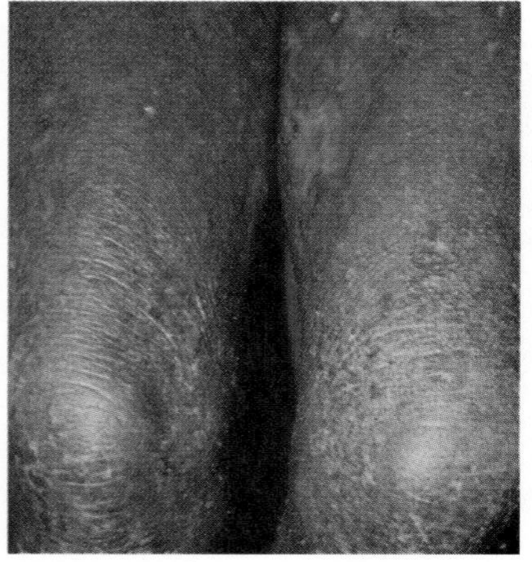

Figure 17-21 Vitiligo.

Hypertrophies of the Skin

A **hypertrophy** (hy-PUR-truh-fee) of the skin is an abnormal growth of the skin. Many hypertrophies are benign, or harmless.

Keratoma (kair-uh-TOH-muh)—An acquired, superficial, thickened patch of epidermis commonly known as callus, caused by pressure or friction on the hands and feet. If the thickening grows inward, it is called a corn.

Mole—A small, brownish spot or blemish on the skin, ranging in color from pale tan to brown or bluish black. Some moles are small and flat, resembling freckles; others are raised and darker in color. Large, dark hairs often occur in moles. Any change in a mole requires medical attention.

Skin tag—Small brown or flesh-colored outgrowth of the skin (Figure 17–22). Skin tags occur most frequently on the neck of an older person.

Verruca (vuh-ROO-kuh)—Technical term for wart; hypertrophy of the papillae and epidermis. It is caused by a virus and is infectious. It can spread from one location to another, particularly along a scratch in the skin.

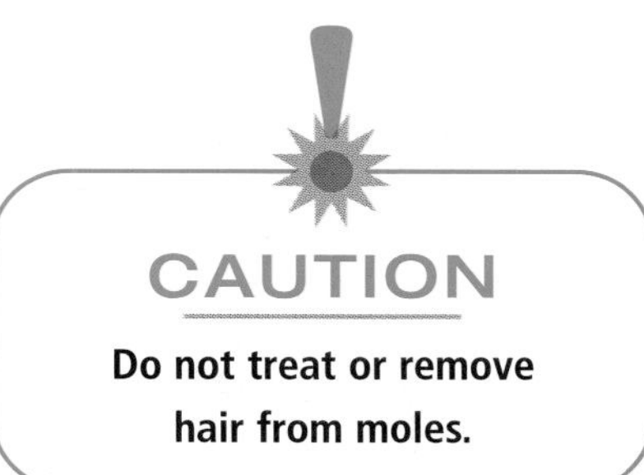

Skin Cancer

Skin cancer from overexposure to the sun comes in three distinct forms, varying in severity. Each is named for the type of cells it affects in the body.

Basal cell carcinoma (BAY-zul SEL kar-sin-OH-muh) is the most common type and the least severe. It is often characterized by light or pearly nodules (Figure 17–23). **Squamous** (SKWAY-mus) **cell carcinoma** is more serious than basal cell carcinoma and often is characterized by scaly red papules or nodules (Figure 17–24). The third and most serious form of skin cancer is **malignant melanoma** (muh-LIG-nent mel-uh-NOH-muh), which is often characterized by black or dark brown patches on the skin that may appear uneven in texture, jagged, or raised (Figure 17–25). Malignant melanomas often appear on individuals who do not receive regular sun exposure and are most commonly located on areas of the body that are not regularly exposed. It is often nicknamed the "city person's cancer." Malignant melanoma is the least common but most dangerous type of skin cancer.

If detected early, anyone with any of these three forms of skin cancer has a good chance for survival. It is important for a cosmetologist to be able to recognize the appearance of serious skin disorders in order to better serve clients. It also important to remember that a cosmetologist should not attempt to diagnose a skin disorder but should sensitively suggest that the client seek the advice of a dermatologist. 4✓ 5✓

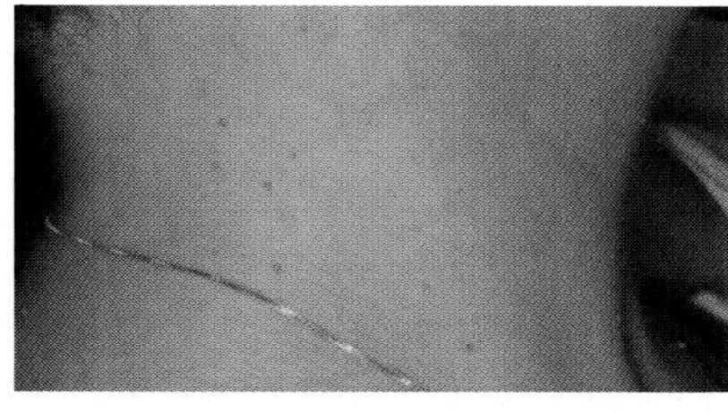

Figure 17-22 Skin tags.

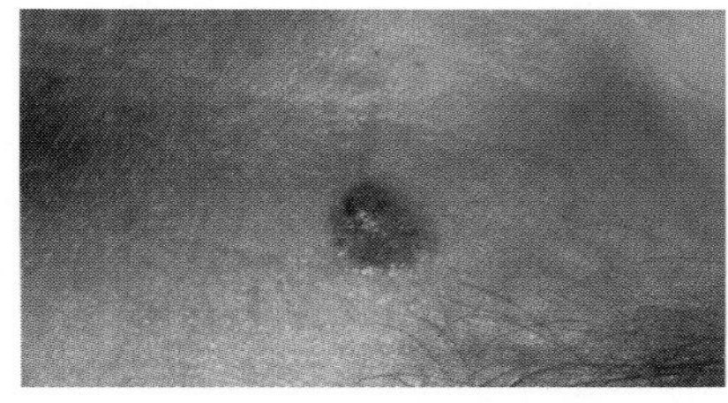

Figure 17-23 Basal cell carcinoma.

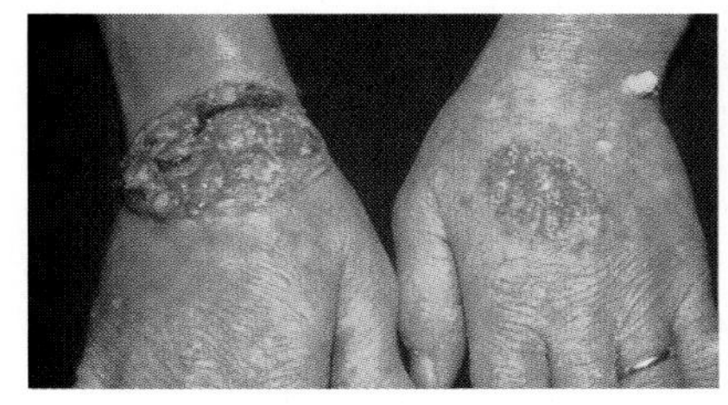

Figure 17-24 Squamous cell carcinoma.

MAINTAINING THE HEALTH OF THE SKIN

For your own benefit as well as the benefit of your clients, you should have a basic understanding of how best to maintain the health of the skin. Let us begin with diet, which is a major factor in maintaining the skin's overall health. In order to keep the skin and the body healthy, the old adage "you are what you eat" still holds true. Proper dietary choices help to regulate hydration (maintaining a healthy level of water in the body), oil production, and overall function of the cells. Eating foods found in all three basic food

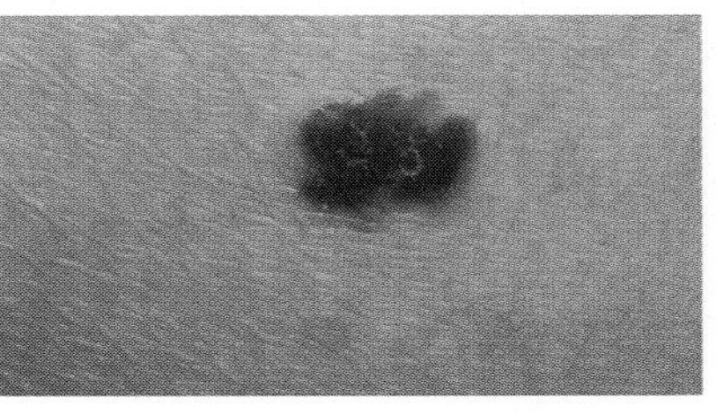

Figure 17-25 Malignant melanoma.

groups—fats, carbohydrates, and proteins—is the best way to support the health of the skin (see Chapter 3 for a discussion of a healthy diet).

Vitamins and Dietary Supplements

Vitamins play an important role in the skin's health, often aiding in healing, softening, and fighting diseases of the skin. Vitamins such as A, C, D, and E have all been shown to have positive effects on the skin's health when taken internally. Although experts agree that taking vitamins internally is still the best way to support the health of the skin, some external applications of vitamins have also been found to be useful in nourishing the skin. The following vitamins relate to the skin in particularly significant ways.

Vitamin A supports the overall health of the skin. This vitamin aids in the health, function, and repair of skin cells. Vitamin A is an antioxidant that can help prevent certain types of cancers, including skin cancer, and has been shown to improve the skin's elasticity and thickness. In its topical acid form as the prescription cream called **retinoic acid** or Retin-A, vitamin A can be used to treat many different types of acne.

Vitamin C, also known as ascorbic acid, is an important element needed for proper repair of the skin and various tissues. This vitamin aids in, and even speeds up, the healing processes of the body. Vitamin C is also vitally important in fighting the aging process and promotes the production of collagen in the skin's dermal tissues, keeping the skin healthy and firm.

Vitamin D promotes the healthy and rapid healing of the skin. The best source of this vitamin is sunlight (in limited amounts). Because vitamin D helps to support the bone structure of the body, it has been made readily available in many fortified foods and dietary supplements.

Vitamin E, or tocopherol, used in conjunction with vitamin A, helps fight against, and protect the skin from, the harmful effects of the sun's rays. Vitamin E also helps to heal damage to the skin's tissues when used both internally and externally. When used externally in topical lotions or creams, vitamin E can help heal structural damage on the skin including severe burns and stretch marks.

Ideally, the nutrients the body needs for proper functioning and survival should come primarily from the foods we eat. If a person's daily food consumption is lacking in nutrients, an effective way to provide them is to take vitamins and mineral supplements (providing the RDA, or recommended daily allowance, is not exceeded).

Water and the Skin

There is one essential nutrient no person can live without, and that is water. In order to function properly, the body and skin both rely heavily on the benefits of water. Water composes 50 to 70 percent of the body's weight. Drinking pure water is essential to the health of the skin and body because it sustains the health of the cells, aids in the elimination of toxins and waste, helps regulate the body's temperature, and aids in proper digestion. All these functions, when performing properly, help keep the skin healthy, vital, and attractive.

The amount of water needed by an individual varies, depending on body weight and level of daily physical activity. The following is an easy formula to help you determine how much water you need every day for maximum physical health: Take your body weight and divide by 2. Divide this number by 8. The resulting number approximates how many 8-ounce glasses of water you should drink every day. For instance, if you weigh 160 pounds, you should drink 10 glasses of water a day. If intense physical activity is performed daily, add two extra glasses of water to the final number. This will help replace extra fluids lost while exercising (Figure 17–26).

Did you know...

It is estimated that 75 percent of Americans are chronically dehydrated. Research suggests that the benefits of water on human health and functioning are many:

- Even mild dehydration will slow metabolism by as much as 3 percent.
- Drinking lots of water can help stop hunger pangs for many dieters.
- Lack of water is the number-one cause of daytime fatigue.
- A 2 percent drop in body water can trigger fuzzy short-term memory and trouble with basic math and can cause difficulty focusing on a computer screen or printed page.

Pass the water, please!

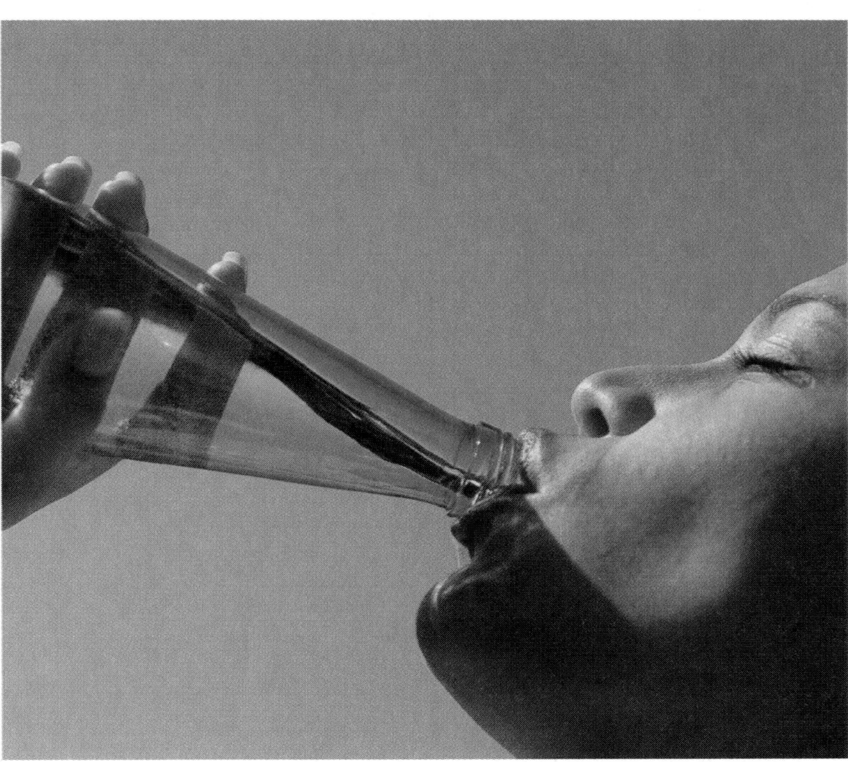

Figure 17-26 Water is essential for healthy skin.

chapter glossary

acne	skin disorder characterized by chronic inflammation of the sebaceous glands from retained secretions
albinism	congenital leukoderma or absence of melanin pigment of the body, including the skin, hair, and eyes
anhidrosis	deficiency in perspiration, often a result of fever or certain skin diseases
asteatosis	condition of dry, scaly skin due to a deficiency or absence of sebum, caused by old age and by exposure to cold
basal cell carcinoma	most common and least severe type of skin cancer; often characterized by light or pearly nodules
bromhidrosis	foul-smelling perspiration, usually noticeable in the armpits or on the feet
bullae (plural: bullae)	large blister containing a watery fluid; similar to a vesicle but larger
chloasma	condition characterized by increased pigmentation on the skin, in spots that are not elevated
collagen	fibrous protein that gives the skin form and strength
comedone	blackhead; worm-like mass of hardened sebum in a hair follicle
crust	dead cells that form over a wound or blemish while it is healing; an accumulation of sebum and pus, sometimes mixed with epidermal material
cyst	closed, abnormally developed sac, containing fluid, semifluid, or morbid matter, above or below the skin
dermatitis	inflammatory condition of the skin
dermatitis venenata	an eruptive skin infection caused by contact with irritating substances such as chemicals or tints
dermatologist	physician engaged in the science of treating the skin, its structures, functions, and diseases
dermatology	medical branch of science that deals with the study of skin and its nature, structure, functions, diseases, and treatment
dermis	underlying or inner layer of the skin; also called the derma, corium, cutis, or true skin
eczema	inflammatory, painful itching disease of the skin, acute or chronic in nature, presenting many forms of dry or moist lesions
elastin	protein base similar to collagen that forms elastic tissue
epidermis	outermost layer of the skin; also called cuticle or scarf skin
esthetician	specialist in the cleansing, preservation of health, and beautification of the skin and body; one who gives therapeutic facial treatments
excoriation	skin sore or abrasion produced by scratching or scraping
fissure	crack in the skin that penetrates the dermis, such as chapped hands or lips
fundus	coiled base of sudoriferous (sweat) gland
herpes simplex	fever blister or cold sore; recurring viral infection

hyperhidrosis	excessive sweating, caused by heat or general body weakness
hypertrophy	abnormal growth of the skin
keloid	thick scar resulting from excessive growth of fibrous tissue
keratin	fiber protein that is the principal component of hair and nails
keratoma	acquired, superficial, thickened patch of epidermis commonly known as callus, caused by pressure or friction on the hands and feet
lentigines	technical term for freckles
lesion	injury or damage that changes the structure of tissues or organs
leukoderma	skin disorder characterized by light abnormal patches; caused by a burn or congenital disease that destroys the pigment-producing cells
macule (plural: maculae)	spot or discoloration on the skin, such as a freckle
malignant melanoma	most serious form of skin cancer; often characterized by black or dark brown patches on the skin that may appear uneven in texture, jagged, or raised
melanin	tiny grains of pigment (coloring matter) deposited in the stratum germinativum of the epidermis and the papillary layers of the dermis
melanocytes	melanin-forming cells
milia	small, whitish, pear-like masses in the epidermis due to retention of sebum; also called whiteheads
miliaria rubra	prickly heat; acute inflammatory disorder of the sweat glands, characterized by the eruption of small red vesicles and accompanied by burning, itching skin
mole	small, brownish spot or blemish on the skin, ranging in color from pale tan to brown or bluish black
nevus	small or large malformation of the skin due to abnormal pigmentation or dilated capillaries; commonly known as birthmark
papillary layer	outer layer of the dermis, directly beneath the epidermis
papule	pimple; small circumscribed elevation on the skin that contains no fluid but may develop pus
psoriasis	skin disease chracterized by red patches, covered with white-silver scales usually found on the scalp, elbows, knees, chest, and lower back, rarely on the face
pustule	inflamed pimple containing pus
reticular layer	deeper layer of the dermis that supplies the skin with oxygen and nutrients; contains cells, vessels, glands, nerve endings, and follicles
retinoic acid	Retin-A; prescription cream for acne

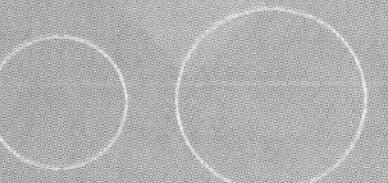

chapter glossary *(continued)*

rosacea	chronic congestion appearing primarily on the cheeks and nose, characterized by redness, dilation of the blood vessels, and the formation of papules and pustules
scale	any thin plate of epidermal flakes, dry or oily, such as abnormal or excessive dandruff
scar or cicatrix	light-colored, slightly raised mark on the skin formed after an injury or lesion of the skin has healed
sebaceous glands	oil glands of the skin, connected to hair follicles
seborrhea	skin condition caused by an abnormal increase of secretion from the sebaceous glands
skin tag	a small brown or flesh-colored outgrowth of the skin
squamous cell carcinoma	type of skin cancer more serious than basal cell carcinoma; often characterized by scaly red papules or nodules
stain	abnormal brown or wine-colored skin discoloration with a circular and irregular shape
steatoma	sebaceous cyst or fatty tumor
stratum corneum	outer layer of the epidermis
stratum germinativum	deepest layer of the epidermis; also known as basal or Malpighian layer
stratum granulosum	granular layer of the epidermis
stratum lucidum	clear, transparent layer of the epidermis under the stratum corneum
subcutaneous tissue	fatty layer found below the dermis that gives smoothness and contour to the body, contains fats for use as energy, and also acts as a protective cushion for the outer skin; also called adipose or subcutis tissue
sudoriferous glands	sweat glands of the skin
tactile corpuscles	small epidermal structures with nerve endings that are sensitive to touch and pressure
tan	change in pigmentation of skin caused by exposure to the sun or ultraviolet rays
tubercle	abnormal rounded, solid lump above, within, or under the skin; larger than a papule
tumor	a swelling; an abnormal cell mass resulting from excessive multiplication of cells, varying in size, shape, and color
ulcer	open lesion on the skin or mucous membrane of the body, accompanied by pus and loss of skin depth
verruca	technical term for wart; hypertrophy of the papillae and epidermis
vesicle	small blister or sac containing clear fluid, lying within or just beneath the epidermis
vitiligo	milky-white spots (leukoderma) of the skin; acquired condition
wheal	itchy, swollen lesion that lasts only a few hours; caused by a blow, the bite of an insect, urticaria, or the sting of a nettle

review questions

1. Briefly describe healthy skin.
2. Name the main divisions of the skin and the layers within each division.
3. How is the skin nourished?
4. List the three types of nerve fibers found in the skin.
5. What is collagen?
6. Name the two types of glands contained within the skin and describe their functions.
7. What are the six important functions of the skin?
8. List the factors that contribute to the aging of the skin.
9. Explain the effect of overexposure to the sun on the skin.
10. Define dermatology.
11. What is a skin lesion?
12. Name and describe at least five disorders of the sebaceous glands.
13. Name and describe at least five changes in skin pigmentation.
14. List at least six skin conditions and disorders that should be referred to a physician.
15. Name and describe the three forms of skin cancer.

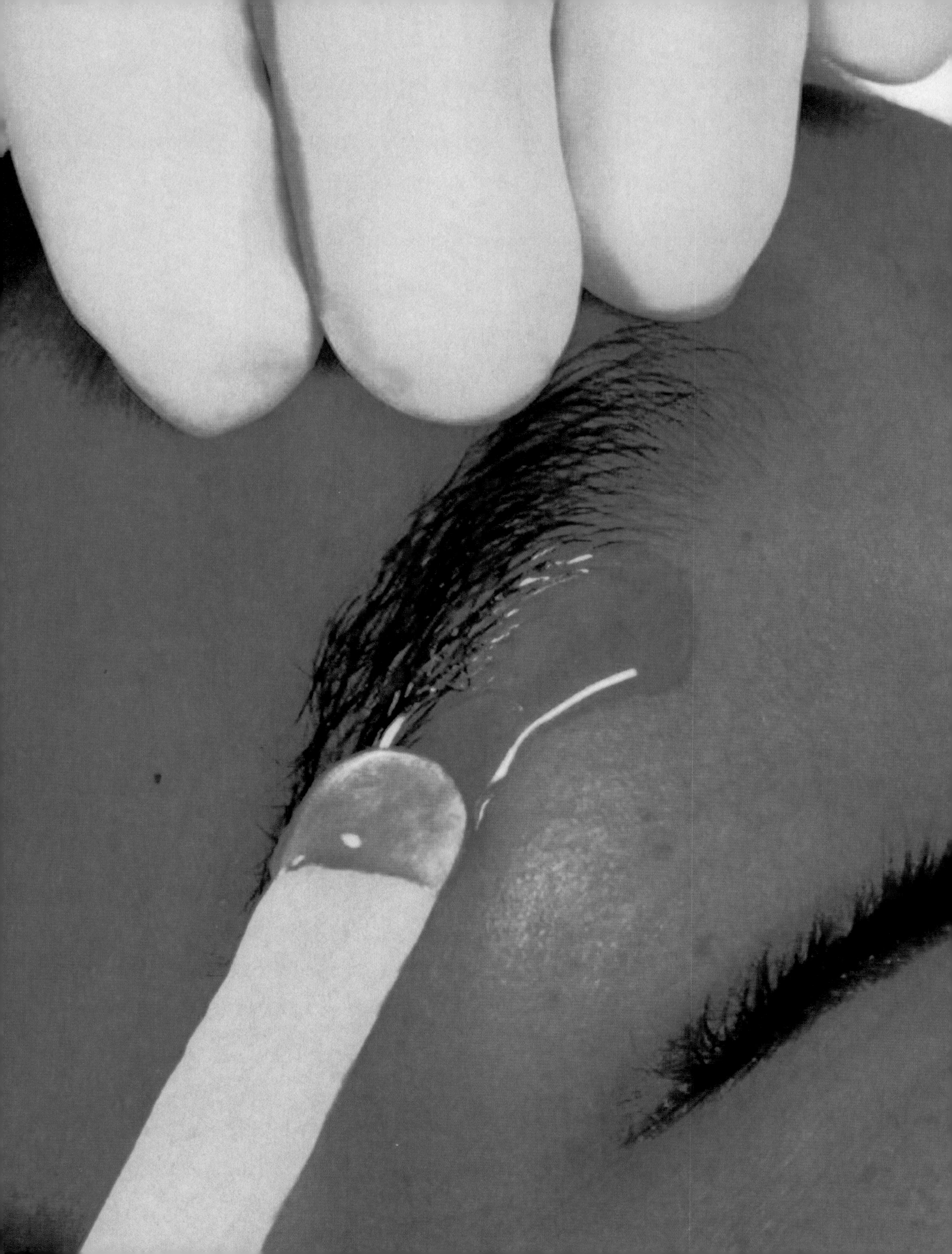

HAIR REMOVAL

Jane Crawford
MEDICAL SPA/DAY SPA CONSULTANT

Chapter Outline

Client Consultation • Permanent Hair Removal
Temporary Methods of Hair Removal

Learning Objectives

After completing this chapter, you should be able to:

1. Describe the elements of a client consultation for hair removal.
2. Name the conditions that contraindicate hair removal in the salon.
3. Identify and describe three methods of permanent hair removal.
4. Demonstrate the techniques involved in temporary hair removal.

National Skill Standards

This chapter provides you with the necessary information to master these National Industry Skill Standards for Entry-Level Cosmetologists.

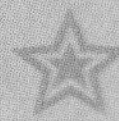
Performing hair removal services.

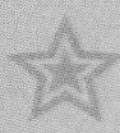
Consulting with clients to determine their needs and preferences.

Conducting services in a safe environment and taking measures to prevent the spread of infectious and contagious diseases.

Key Terms

Page number indicates where in the chapter the term is used.

depilatory pg. 637

electrolysis pg. 636

epilator pg. 642

hirsuties or hypertrichosis pg. 633

laser hair removal pg. 636

photo-epilation pg. 636

sugaring pg. 649

threading pg. 642

Unwanted or overly abundant hair is a common problem that affects both men and women. Fortunately, a variety of hair removal methods are available, ranging from the fairly simple procedures of shaving and tweezing to more complex procedures that require special training.

Hirsuties (hur-SOO-shee-eez) or **hypertrichosis** (hy-pur-trih-KOH-sis) are terms that refer to the growth of an unusual amount of hair on parts of the body normally bearing only downy hair, such as the faces of women or the backs of men.

Unwanted hair has been treated throughout the ages by a variety of methods. Excavations of early Egyptian tombs indicate that abrasive materials, such as pumice stone, were used to rub away hair. Ancient Greek and Roman women were known to remove most of their body hair by similar methods. Native Americans used sharpened stones and seashells to rub off and pluck out hair.

History also records chemical means of removing excess hair. For example, the ancient Turks used *rusma*, a combination of yellow sulfide of arsenic, quicklime, and rose water, as a crude hair removal agent.

Facial and body hair removal has become increasingly popular as evolving technology makes it easier to perform with more effective results. Women comprise the vast majority of hair-removal clients, most often wanting to rid their bodies of hair on the upper lip, cheeks, chin, neck, underarms, navel, bikini line, buttocks, and legs. Hair removal for men is also on the rise. Men may choose to have unsightly hair removed from their backs, shoulders, and chests. If they compete in certain sports like bicycling and swimming, they may want hair removed from their legs and arms to facilitate faster competition times.

Two major types of hair removal are in use today: permanent and temporary. Salon techniques are generally limited to temporary methods.

CLIENT CONSULTATION

Before any hair removal service, a consultation is always necessary. Ask the client to complete a questionnaire that discloses all medications, both topical (applied to the skin) and oral (taken by mouth), along with any known skin disorders or allergies (Figure 18–1). Allergies or sensitivities must be noted and documented. Keep in mind that many changes can occur between client visits. Since the last time you saw them, clients may have been placed on medications such as antidepressants, hormones, cortisone, medicine for blood pressure or diabetes, or such topical prescriptions as Retin-A, Renova, and hydroquinone. A client on any one of these prescriptions may not be a candidate for hair removal. See Figure 18–2 for a sample client assessment form.

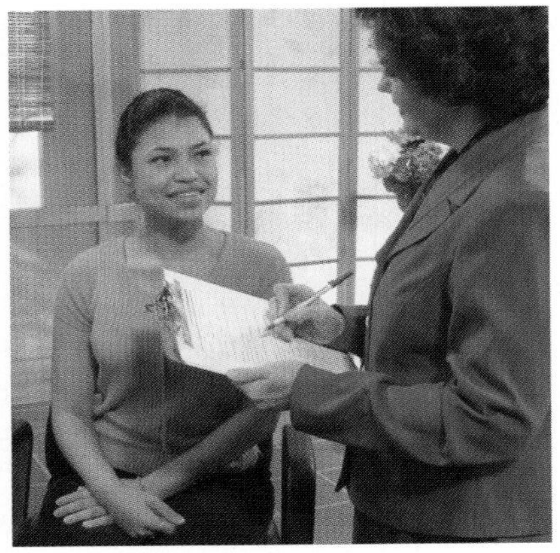

Figure 18–1 Filling out a client questionnaire.

It is imperative that every client fills out a release form for the hair removal service you are going to provide. This should be completed prior to every service. It serves as a reminder to the client to really think about any topical or oral medication they might have started since their last visit. See Figure 18–3 for a sample release form.

Contraindications for Hair Removal

One of the main purposes of the client consultation is to determine the presence of any contraindications for hair removal. Leg waxing should not be performed on clients with varicose veins or phlebitis. Facial waxing or tweezing should not be performed on those clients who have any of the following conditions or treatments:

- rosacea or very sensitive skin
- sunburn
- history of fever blisters or cold sores
- presence of pustules or papules
- recent chemical peel using glycolic, salicylic, or other acid-based product
- recent botox or collagen injections
- cosmetic or reconstructive surgery

Clients using the following medications should also not receive hair removal treatments:

- Retin-A, Renova, hydroquinone, or similar products
- blood-thinning medications
- topical or oral cortisone medication
- Accutane

CLIENT ASSESSMENT FORM

Date ______________

Name ____ Sex __________

Address ____

City ____________________________ State ______________ Zip__________

1. Have you been seen by a dermatologist? Yes _____ No _____If yes, for what reason?
   ____
2. Please list all medications that you take regularly. Include hormones, vitamins, and the like.
   ____
   Are you taking Accutane? Yes ___ No ___ If yes, for how long? ______________
   Do you use Retin-A, Renova, or hydroquinone? Yes ___ No ___
   If yes, for how long? ______________________________________
3. Do you have any allergies? Are you allergic to any medications? Yes ___ No ___
   If yes, please list allergies: ______________________________
4. Are you pregnant or lactating? Yes ___ No ___
5. Have you had any of the following procedures?
   Laser resurfacing Yes___ Date ________ No ___
   Light chemical peel Yes___ Date ________ No ___
   Medium/heavy chemical peel Yes___ Date ________ No ___
6. Do you ever experience tightness or flaking of your skin? Yes ___ No ___
7. Do you frequent tanning booths? Yes ___ No ___
8. Do you have a history of fever blisters or cold sores? Yes ___ No ___

Figure 18–2 Client assessment form.

RELEASE FORM FOR HAIR REMOVAL

I, ______________________________, am _____ am not _____ presently using:

_____ Retin-A

_____ Accutane

_____ any alphahydroxy-based products

_____ any medications such as cortisone, blood thinners, or diabetic medication

_____ I understand that if I begin using any of the above products and do not inform my esthetician/cosmetologist prior to hair removal, I am accepting full responsibility for any skin reactions.

_____ The hair removal process has been thoroughly explained to me, and I have had an opportunity to ask questions and receive satisfactory answers.

Client's Signature ______________________________ Date______________

Technician's Signature____________________________ Date______________

Figure 18–3 Sample release form.

PERMANENT HAIR REMOVAL

Although permanent hair removal services will probably not be offered in your salon, it is useful to know the options that exist. Permanent hair removal methods include electrolysis, photo-epilation (light-based hair removal), and laser hair removal.

Electrolysis

Electrolysis is the removal of hair by means of an electric current that destroys the root of the hair. The current is applied with a very fine, needle-shaped electrode that is inserted into each hair follicle. This technique can be painful, time-consuming, and expensive, and must be performed only by a licensed electrologist.

Photo-Epilation

The U.S. Food and Drug Administration (FDA) has recently approved the use of **photo-epilation** for permanent hair removal. This treatment uses intense light to destroy the hair follicles. This treatment has minimal side effects, requires no needles, and thus eliminates the risk of infection. Clinical studies have shown that photo-epilation can provide 50 percent to 60 percent clearance of hair in twelve weeks. This method can be administered in some salons by cosmetologists and estheticians, depending on state law. Manufacturers of photo-epilation equipment generally provide the special training necessary for administering this procedure.

Laws regarding photo-epilation and laser hair removal services vary in different states and provinces. Be sure to check with your regulatory agency for guidelines.

Laser Hair Removal

Lasers are a new method for the rapid, gentle removal of unwanted hair. In **laser hair removal**, a laser beam is pulsed on the skin, impairing the hair follicles. It is most effective when used on follicles in the growth phase, or anagen.

The laser method was discovered by chance when it was noted that birthmarks treated with certain types of lasers became permanently devoid of hair. Lasers are not for everyone; the absolute requirement is that one's hair must be darker than the surrounding skin. Coarse, dark hair responds best to laser treatment. For some clients, this method brings truly permanent results. The laser can also slow down regrowth.

In certain states and provinces, cosmetologists or estheticians are allowed to perform laser hair removal. This method requires specialized training, most commonly offered by laser equipment manufacturers. 3

TEMPORARY METHODS OF HAIR REMOVAL

The following are temporary methods of hair removal, some of which may be offered in your salon or spa.

Shaving

The most common form of temporary hair removal, particularly of men's facial hair, is shaving. Shaving is usually recommended for women when the unwanted hair covers a large area, such as the underarms and legs. It is most often done by women at home and represents a quick and convenient solution, although it can sometimes result in skin irritation, ingrown hairs, and nicks from the razor blade. A shaving cream or lotion is applied before shaving.

An electric clipper may also be used, particularly to remove unwanted hair at the nape of the neck. The application of a preshaving lotion helps to reduce any irritation.

Tweezing

Tweezing is commonly used to shape the eyebrows and can also be used to remove undesirable hairs from around the mouth and chin. Eyebrow arching is often done as part of a professional makeup service. Correctly shaped eyebrows have a strong, positive impact on the overall attractiveness of the face. The natural arch of the eyebrow follows the orbital bone, or the curved line of the eye socket. Most people have hair growth both above and below the natural line. These hairs should be removed to give a clean and attractive appearance.

Electronic Tweezers

Another method for the removal of superfluous hair used in salons and spas is the electronically charged tweezers. This method transmits radio frequency energy down the hair shaft into the follicle area. The papilla is thus dehydrated and eventually destroyed.

The tweezers are used to grasp a single strand of hair. The energy is then applied, first at a low level to prewarm and then at a higher level for up to two minutes to remove the hair. Most manufacturers suggest that the area be steamed first in order to increase efficiency.

Electronic tweezers are not a method of permanent hair removal. Furthermore, the process of clearing any area of hair by this method is slow.

Depilatories

A **depilatory** is a substance, usually a caustic alkali preparation, used for the temporary removal of superfluous hair by dissolving it at the skin level. It contains detergents to strip the sebum from the hair and adhesives to hold the chemicals to the hair shaft for the five to ten minutes that are necessary to remove the hair. During the application time, the hair expands and the disulfide bonds break. Finally, such chemicals as sodium hydroxide, potassium hydroxide, thioglycolic acid, or calcium thioglycolate destroy the disulfide bonds. These chemicals turn the hair into a soft, jelly-like mass that can be scraped from the skin. Although depilatories are not commonly used in salons, you should be familiar with them in the event that your clients have used them.

If a client requests a chemical depilatory, you should perform a patch test to determine whether the individual is sensitive to the action of the

? Did you know...

Contrary to popular belief, shaving does not cause the hair to grow thicker or stronger. It only seems that way because the razor blunts the hair ends and makes them feel stiff.

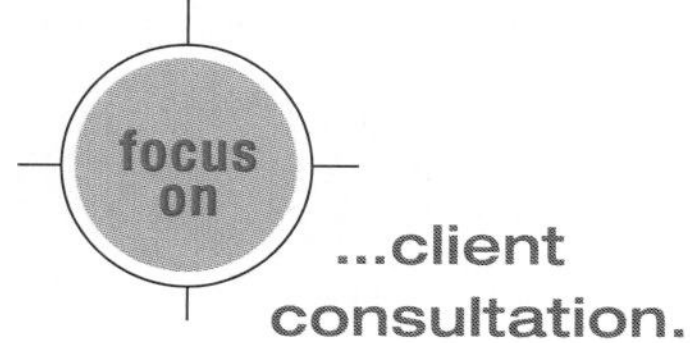

As with any procedure, always perform a client consultation prior to tweezing or waxing the eyebrows. Determine the client's wishes as to final eyebrow shape. If you remove too much hair, it will generally grow back, but the process takes a long time. You will also end up with an unhappy client who is not likely to return for your services. Conducting a thorough consultation beforehand will help you avoid such mistakes.

PROCEDURE 47

SHAVING MEN'S FACIAL HAIR

Shaving a man's face or beard can be performed in a hydraulic salon chair or a barber chair.

Implements and Materials

- towels
- shampoo cape
- shaving lotion or cream
- disposable razor (single- or double-edged)
- after-shaving balm or lotion
- disposable gloves

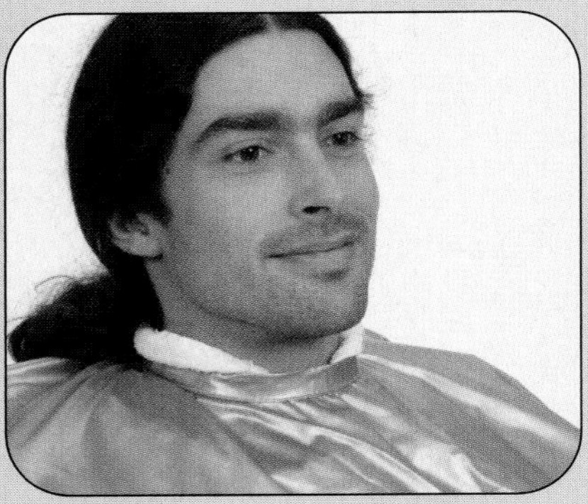

Figure 18–4 Drape the client for shaving.

18

Preparation

1. Seat the client comfortably in the chair.
2. Drape the client. Place a towel around the neck, then place a shampoo cape over the towel and secure in the back. Turn down the towel over the top of the cape (Figure 18–4).
3. Wash and dry your hands and put on disposable gloves.

Procedure

1. Saturate a towel by holding it under hot running water. Wring out the towel until it is fairly dry. It should be comfortably warm, not hot. Use a lukewarm or cool towel on clients with sensitive or rosacea skin.
2. Cleanse the client's face with the towel (Figure 18–5).
3. Dispense shaving cream into a cup or bowl. Apply to the client's face with a disposable brush (Figure 18–6).

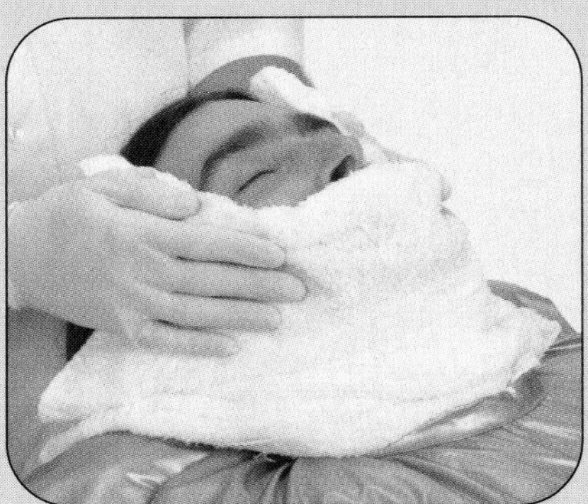

Figure 18–5 Cleanse the client's face.

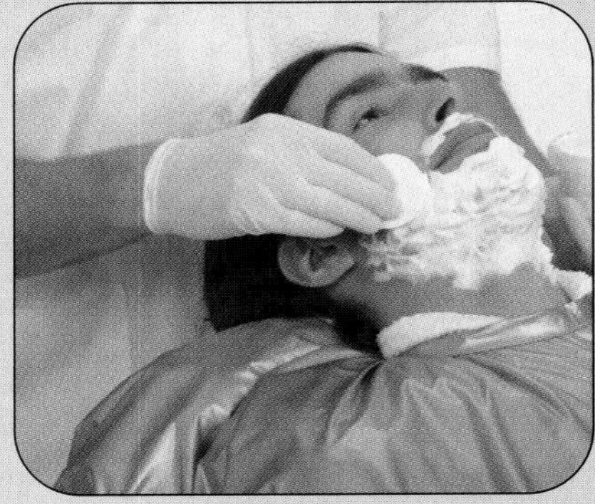

Figure 18–6 Apply shaving cream.

4. Stretching the skin tautly with one hand, use the other to stroke the razor in the direction opposite the hair growth. Start under the jawline on the client's left and shave upward (Figure 18–7). Follow the jawline, moving toward the right side of the face. Then move to the cheekbones and shave downward, moving from the left side to the right (Figure 18–8).
5. Rinse the razor as necessary.
6. When the face has been shaved, cleanse it with another cool or warm, damp towel, depending on the skin type.
7. Apply after-shave lotion or balm (Figure 18–9).

CAUTION

If a client is cut during the shaving procedure, stop the procedure and follow the instructions for blood spill disinfection on page 116.

Cleanup and Sanitation

1. Remove towels and cape from the client and place in a closed hamper.
2. Accompany the client to the reception area.
3. Discard the razor and any other disposable items.
4. Sanitize your workstation, including the hydraulic or barber chair.
5. Wash your hands with soap and warm water.

Some state laws permit only licensed barbers to shave beards. Check with your regulatory agency before performing shaving procedures on male clients.

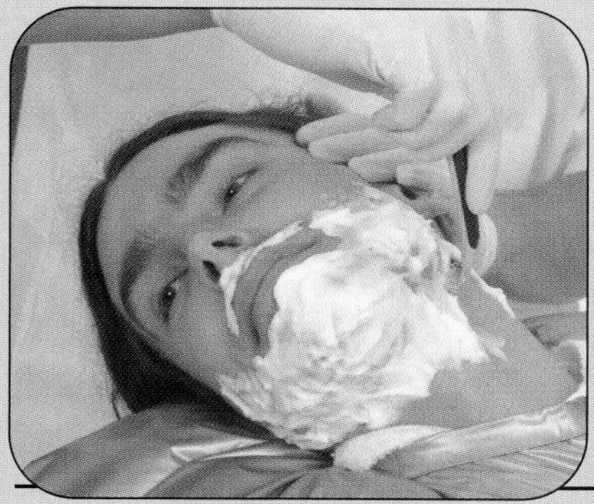

Figure 18–7 Shave upward from under the jaw.

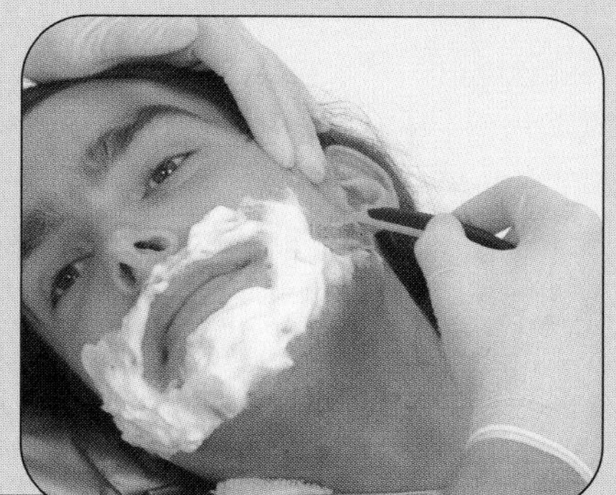

Figure 18–8 Shave downward from the right cheekbone.

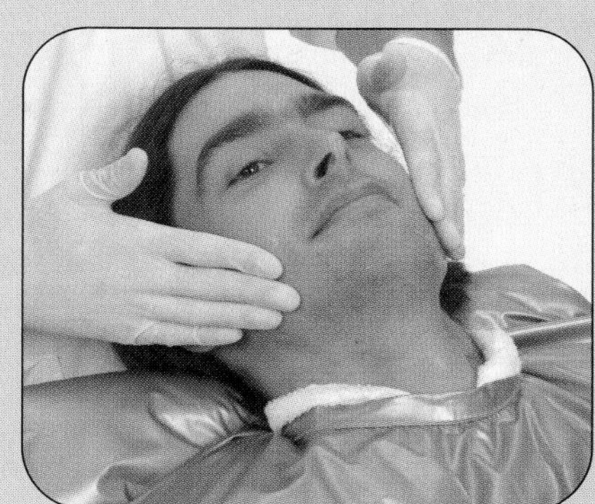

Figure 18–9 Apply after-shave lotion.

18

completed!

PROCEDURE 48

TWEEZING EYEBROWS

Implements and Materials

- towels
- tweezers
- cotton balls
- eyebrow brush
- emollient cream
- antiseptic lotion
- gentle eye makeup remover
- astringent
- disposable gloves

CAUTION

Washing your hands thoroughly with soap and warm water is critical before and after every client procedure you perform. The importance of proper sanitation in these procedures cannot be overemphasized.

Preparation

1. Seat the client in a facial chair in a reclining position, as for a facial massage. Or, if you prefer, seat the client in a half-upright position and work from the side.
2. Discuss with the client the type of eyebrow arch suitable for her facial characteristics.
3. Drape a towel over the client's chest.
4. Wash and dry your hands and put on disposable gloves.

Procedure

1. Cleanse the eyelid area with cotton balls moistened with gentle eye makeup remover.
2. Brush the eyebrows with a small brush to remove any powder or scaliness (Figure 18–10).
3. Soften brows. Saturate two pledgets of cotton or a towel with warm water and place over the brows. Allow them to remain on the brows one to two minutes to soften and relax the eyebrow tissue (Figure 18–11). You may soften the brows and surrounding skin by rubbing emollient cream into them.

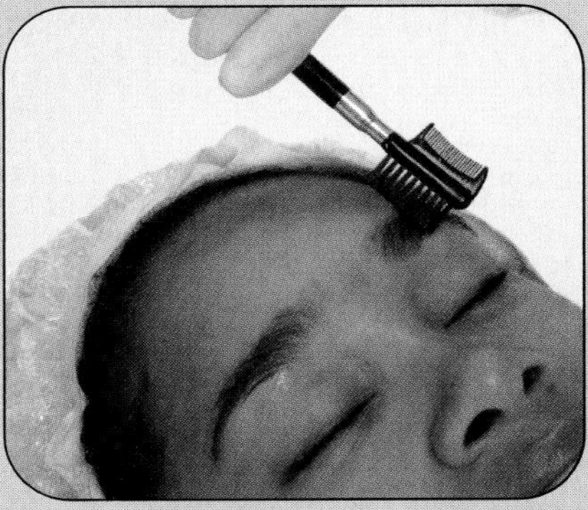

Figure 18–10 Brush the eyebrows with a small brush.

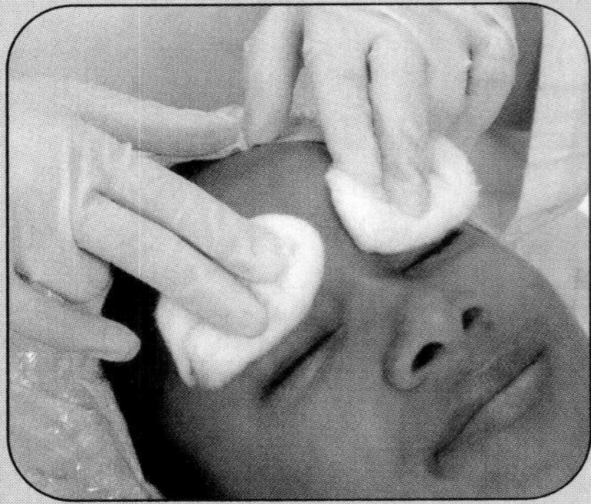

Figure 18–11 Hold a wet cotton pledget over each eyebrow.

4. Use a mild antiseptic on a cotton ball prior to tweezing.
5. Remove the hairs between the brows. When tweezing, stretch the skin taut with the index finger and thumb (or index and middle fingers) of your nondominant hand. Grasp each hair individually with tweezers and pull with a quick motion in the direction of growth (Figure 18–12). Tweeze between the brows and above the brow line first, because the area under the brow line is much more sensitive.
6. Sponge the tweezed area frequently with cotton moistened with an antiseptic lotion to avoid infection.
7. Brush the hair downward. Remove hairs from above the eyebrow line. Shape the upper section of one eyebrow; then shape the other (Figure 18–13). Frequently sponge the area with antiseptic.
8. Brush the hairs upward. Remove hairs from under the eyebrow line. Shape the lower section of one eyebrow; then shape the other. Sponge the area with antiseptic. *Optional:* Apply emollient cream and massage the brows. Remove cream with tissues.
9. After tweezing is completed, sponge the eyebrows and surrounding skin with astringent to contract the skin.
10. Brush the eyebrow hair in its normal position.

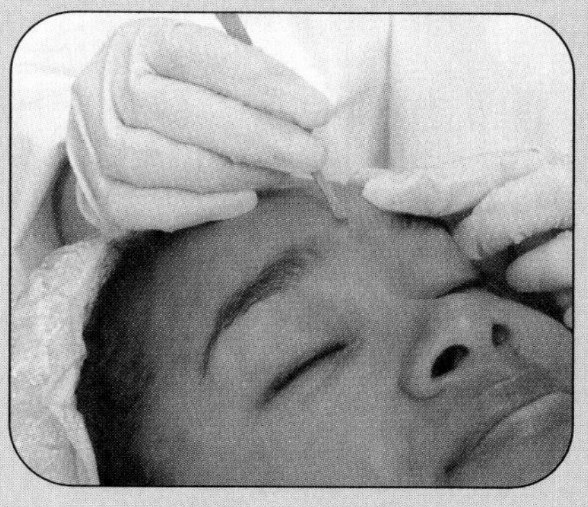

Figure 18-12 Tweeze hair from between eyebrows.

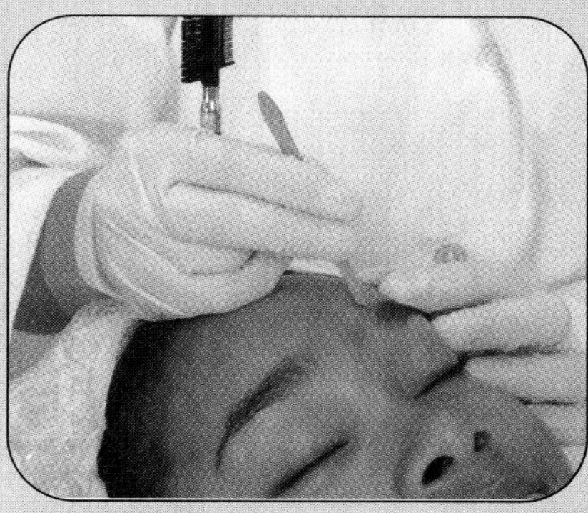

Figure 18-13 Tweeze hair along the upper edge of the eyebrow.

Cleanup and Sanitation

1. If eyebrow tweezing is part of a makeup service, continue the makeup procedure. If not, complete the next steps.
2. Remove the towel from the client and place in a closed hamper.
3. Accompany the client to the reception area and suggest rebooking (the eyebrows should be treated about once a week).
4. Discard disposable materials in a closed receptacle and disinfect implements.
5. Wash your hands with soap and warm water.

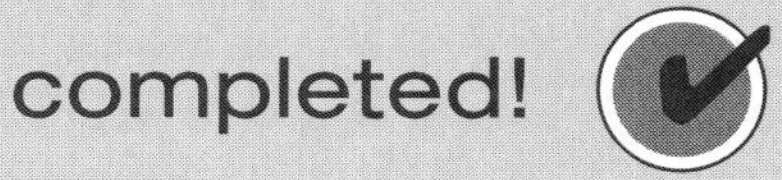

depilatory. Select a hairless part of the arm, apply a small amount according to the manufacturer's directions, and leave it on the skin for seven to ten minutes. If there are no signs of redness, swelling, or rash, the depilatory can probably be used with safety over a larger area of the skin. Follow the manufacturer's directions for application.

Epilators

An **epilator** removes the hair by pulling it out of the follicle. Wax is a commonly used epilator, applied in either hot or cold form as recommended by the manufacturer. Both products are made primarily of resins and beeswax. Cold wax is somewhat thicker and does not require fabric strips for removal. Because waxing removes the hair from the follicle, the hair takes longer to grow back. The time between waxings is generally four to six weeks.

Wax may be applied to various parts of the face and body, such as the eyebrows, cheeks, chin, upper lip, arms, and legs. On male clients, wax may be used to remove hair on the back and nape of the neck. The hair should be at least 1/4 inch (.6 cm) to 1/2 inch (1.25 cm) long for waxing to be effective. Do not remove vellus (lanugo) hair; doing so may cause the skin to lose its softness.

> **CAUTION**
>
> **Beeswax has a relatively high incidence of allergic reaction. Always give a small patch test of the product to be used prior to the service.**

Before beginning a wax treatment, be sure to complete a client consultation card and have the client sign a release form. Wear disposable gloves to prevent contact with any possible bloodborne pathogens.

Safety Precautions

- To prevent burns, always test the temperature of the heated wax before applying to the client's skin.
- Use caution so that the wax does not come in contact with the eyes.
- Do not apply wax over warts, moles, abrasions, or irritated or inflamed skin. Do not remove hair protruding from a mole, as the wax could cause trauma to the mole.
- The skin under the arms is sometimes very sensitive. If so, use cold wax.
- Redness and swelling sometimes occur on sensitive skin. Apply an aloe gel to calm and soothe the skin.

Threading

Threading is a temporary hair removal method that is still practiced in many Eastern cultures today. It involves the manipulation of cotton thread, which is twisted and rolled along the surface of the skin, entwining the hair in the thread and lifting it from the follicle. Threading has become increasingly popular in the United States as an option to other methods. It requires specialized training.

PROCEDURE

HOT WAXING: EYEBROWS

Equipment, Implements, and Materials

- facial chair
- roll of disposable paper
- wax
- single or double wax heater
- wax remover
- small disposable spatula or small wooden applicators
- fabric strips for hair removal
- hair cap or headband
- towels for draping
- disposable gloves
- mild skin cleanser
- emollient or antiseptic lotion

Preparation

1. Melt the wax in the heater. The length of time it takes to melt the wax depends on how full the wax holder is: 15 to 20 minutes if it is full; 10 minutes if it is a quarter to half full. Be sure it is not too hot (Figure 18–14).
2. Complete client consultation.
3. Lay a clean towel over the top of the facial chair, then a layer of disposable paper.
4. Place a hair cap or headband on the client's head to keep hair out of the face.
5. Drape a towel over the client's chest.
6. Wash and dry your hands, and put on disposable gloves.

Figure 18–14 Melt the wax.

Procedure

1. Remove makeup, cleanse the area thoroughly with a mild astringent cleanser, and dry.
2. Test the temperature and consistency of the heated wax by applying a small drop on your wrist. It should be warm but not hot, and it should run smoothly off the spatula (Figure 18–15).

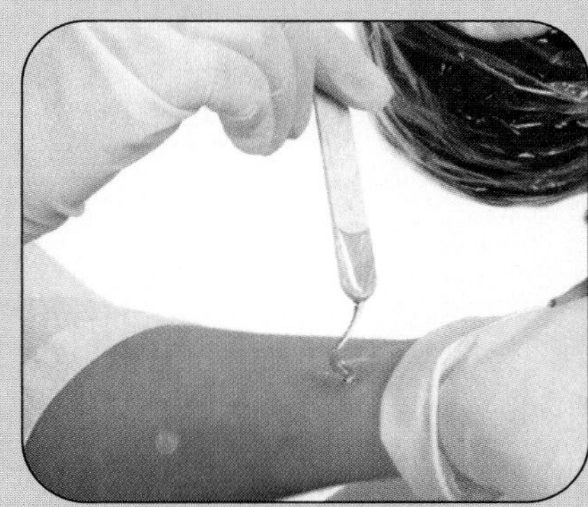

Figure 18–15 Test the temperature of the melted wax.

3. With the spatula or wooden applicator, spread a thin coat of the warm wax evenly over the area to be treated, going in the same direction as the hair growth (Figure 18–16). Be sure not to put the spatula in the wax more than once. Do not double-dip!
4. Apply a sterile fabric strip over the waxed area. Press gently in the direction of hair growth, running your finger over the surface of the fabric three to five times (Figure 18–17).
5. Gently applying pressure to hold the skin taut with one hand, quickly remove the fabric strip and the wax that sticks to it by pulling it in the direction opposite the hair growth. Do not pull straight up on the strip (Figure 18–18).
6. Lightly massage the treated area.
7. Remove any remaining wax residue from the skin with a gentle wax remover.
8. Repeat procedure on the area around the other eyebrow.
9. Cleanse the skin with a mild emollient cleanser and apply an emollient or antiseptic lotion (Figure 18–19).

CAUTION

Be sure not to use an excessive amount of wax, as it will spread when the fabric is pressed and may spread to hair you do not wish to remove.

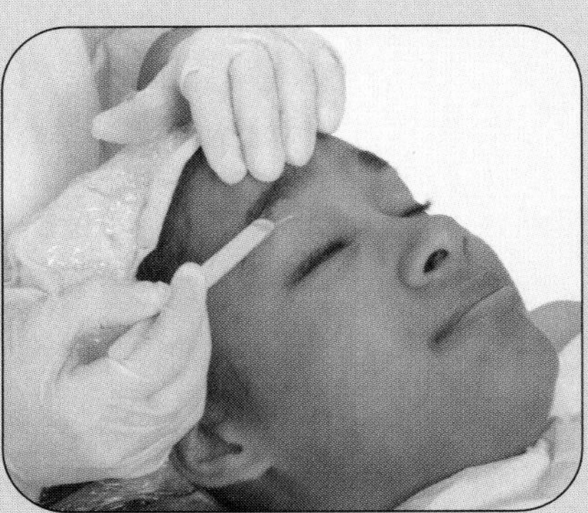

Figure 18–16 Spread warm wax over the eyelid.

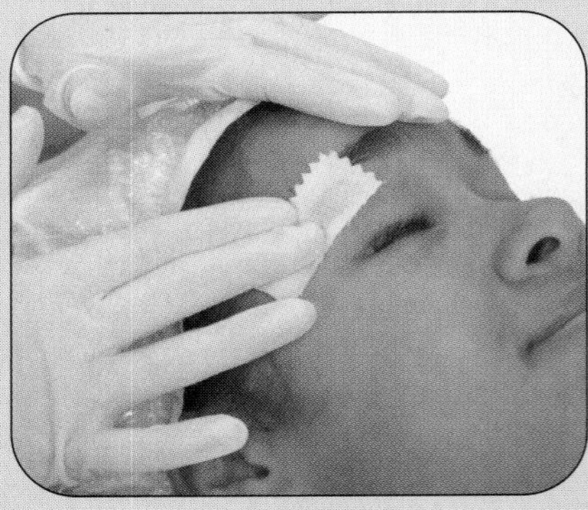

Figure 18–17 Press a fabric strip over the waxed eyelid.

18

Some states or provinces require sanitizing the area prior to tweezing or waxing and applying an antiseptic at the end of the procedure. Always check with your regulatory agency.

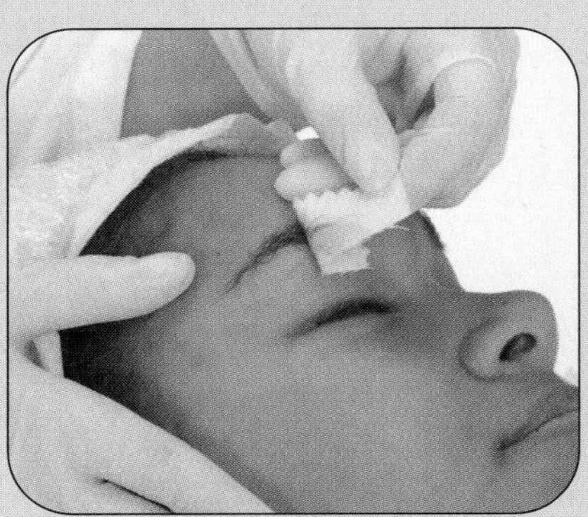

Figure 18–18 Pull off the fabric strip in the direction opposite hair growth.

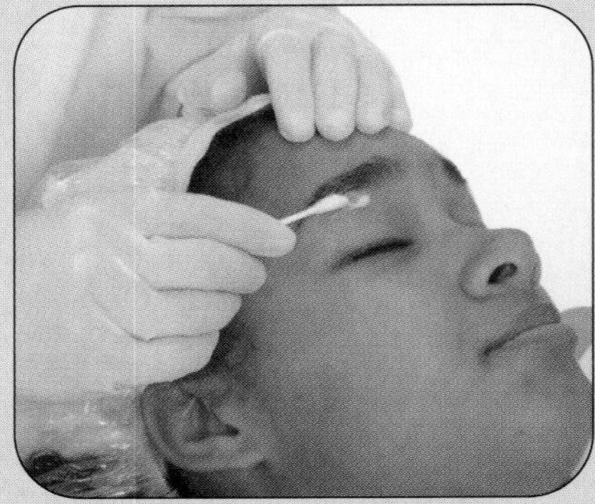

Figure 18–19 Apply emollient or antiseptic lotion to the eyelid.

Cleanup and Sanitation

1. Remove headband and towel drape from the client and place in a closed hamper.
2. Discard all used disposable materials in a closed hazardous waste container. Never reuse wax. Do not lay used spatula, muslin strips, wax, or any other materials used in waxing on the counter.
3. Sanitize the treatment area. This includes counter surfaces, facial chair, wax heater and container, floor, bottle caps, and lids.
4. Wash your hands with soap and warm water.

CAUTION

Never leave the wax heater on overnight, as it is a fire hazard and can damage the wax.

completed!

PROCEDURE

BODY WAXING

Equipment, Implements, and Materials

Use the same equipment as for Procedure 49—eyebrow waxing, with the addition of a metal or disposable wooden spatula. A metal spatula holds the heat longer, but it must not touch the client's skin as you apply the wax. You may find disposable spatulas more convenient.

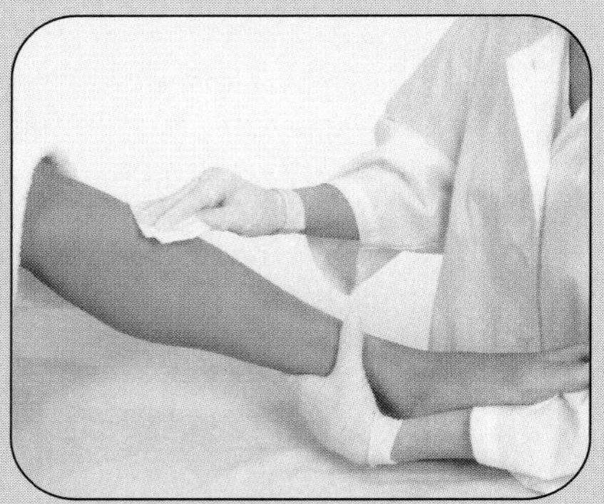

Figure 18-20 Apply a light coating of powder.

Preparation

1. Melt the wax in the heater.
2. Complete your client consultation.
3. Drape the treatment bed with disposable paper or a bed sheet with paper over the top.
4. If bikini waxing, offer the client disposable panties or a small sanitized towel.
5. If waxing the underarms, have the client remove her bra and put on a terry wrap. Offer a terry wrap when waxing the legs as well.
6. Assist the client onto the treatment bed and drape with towels.
7. Wash your hands.

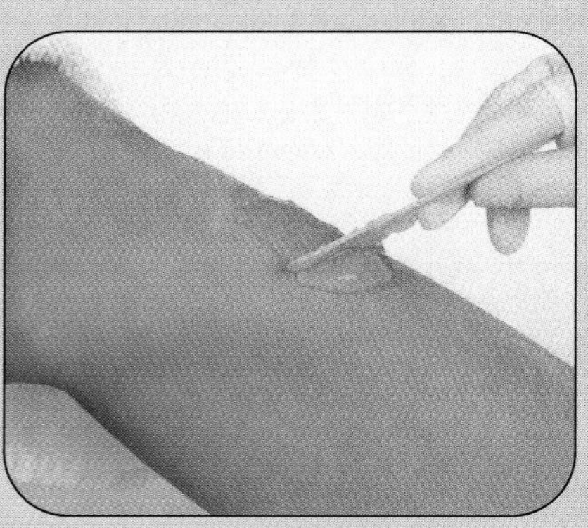

Figure 18-21 Spread warm wax over the top of the leg.

Procedure

1. Thoroughly cleanse the area to be waxed with a mild astringent cleanser and dry.
2. Apply a light covering of powder (Figure 18-20).
3. Test the temperature and consistency of the heated wax by applying a small drop to your wrist.
4. Using a metal or disposable spatula, spread a thin coat of the warm wax evenly over the skin surface in the same direction as the hair growth (Figure 18-21). Be sure not to put the spatula in the wax more than once. If the wax strings and lands in an area you do not wish to treat, remove it with lotion designed to dissolve and remove wax.

5. Apply a sterile fabric strip in the same direction as the hair growth. Press gently, running your hand over the surface of the fabric three to five times (Figure 18–22).
6. Gently apply pressure to hold the skin taut with one hand and quickly remove the adhering wax in the opposite direction of the hair growth (Figure 18–23).
7. Apply gentle pressure and lightly massage the treated area.
8. Repeat, taking a fresh fabric strip as each strip becomes covered with wax.
9. Have the client turn over, and repeat the procedure on the backs of the legs (Figure 18–24).
10. Remove any remaining residue of powder from the skin.
11. Cleanse the area with a mild emollient cleanser and apply an emollient or antiseptic lotion.
12. Undrape the client and escort her to the dressing room.

CAUTION

When waxing sensitive areas such as underarms or bikini lines, be sure the wax is not too hot. Trim the hair with scissors if it is more than ½ inch (1.25 cm) long.

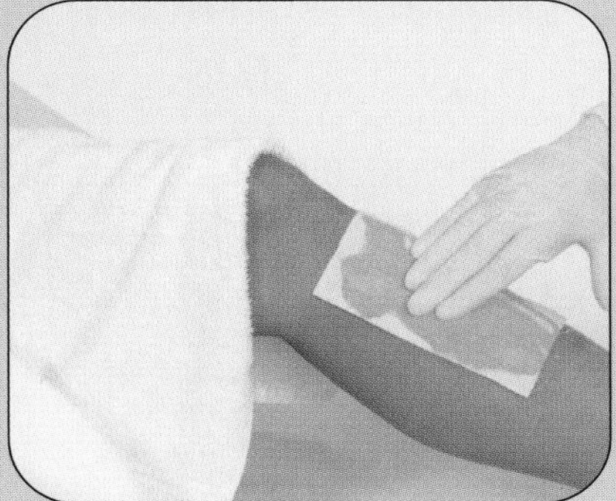

Figure 18–22 Press a fabric strip over the waxed area.

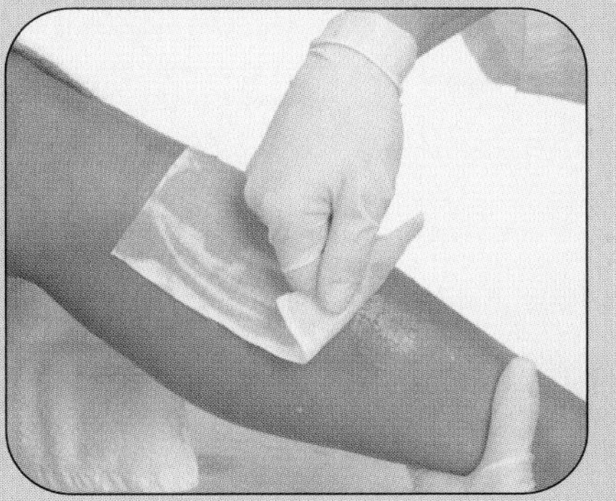

Figure 18–23 Pull off the fabric strip in the direction opposite hair growth.

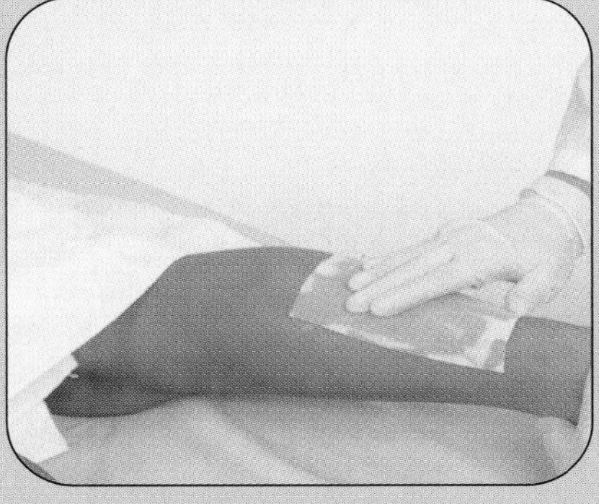

Figure 18–24 Pull the fabric strip from the back of the leg.

18

Cleanup and Sanitation

1. Discard used disposable materials in a closed hazardous waste container.
2. Place linens and robe in a closed hamper.
3. Remove any wax from the metal spatula (if you used one) with wax removal solution. Disinfect the spatula and store in a clean, covered container.
4. Sanitize the treatment bed and counter.
5. Wash your hands with soap and warm water.

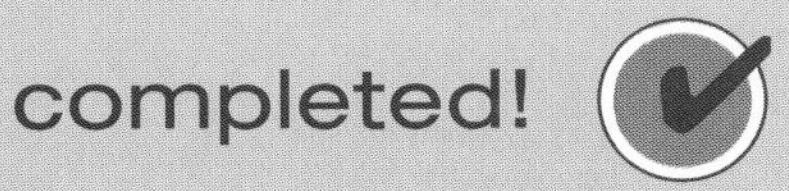

insights

Helen Bickmore

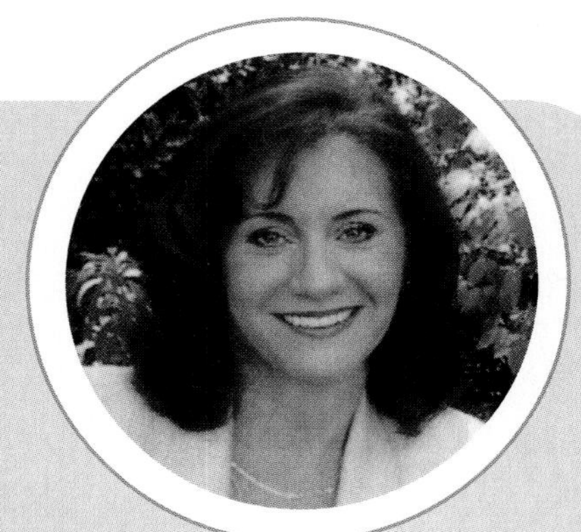

Helen Bickmore, a veteran with 25 years of experience in the industry, is an esthetician in Albany, New York.

As a girl, back in England, I was a carrot-top redhead with white eyelashes and eyebrows. I was educated in a convent and when we wore mascara, the nuns would wash it out with carbolic soap. One day, when I was sixteen, I sneaked off to a beauty salon and had my eyelashes tinted. I got to know that place and I learned to love the environment. The services they provided really made a difference in people's lives.

Providing a hands-on service gives me tremendous satisfaction. That's the thing I most love about my work—providing a service and getting a great response back from the client. I so enjoy the rapport, especially when I've had a client for a long time. It's amazing how you can bond over a bikini wax or electrolysis.

If I were a young stylist looking to get a job in a salon, I would check for cleanliness and professionalism. I'd pay attention to the way people are dressed and how they present themselves. If I walked into a salon and saw a bunch of people standing around looking like they were bored and gossiping because they had nothing better to do, that would be a place I'd run from. The stylists who are not busy should be doing something constructive, whether it's working on each other or discussing a product or dusting shelves.

People skills are so important too. You've got to be able to laugh. You can't be narrow-minded. You have to enjoy people for all their complexities. Sure, you have to be good at selling, but you have to recommend and sell honestly. If you're just looking to get that 3 percent commission, you won't keep that client for long. Most of my clients have been buying from me now for years without my actually having to sell anymore. These relationships are renewing and replenishing. They sustain themselves.

One of the best ways to build a client base is to be honest with your clients. This may mean not performing a service if you don't think it would be a good idea to wax a particular area of the client's face, for instance. It may mean turning someone down because of a contraindication. But you'll win them back in another area; you'll win them back by reputation. So don't sell out your professional ethics for a buck. Be prepared to turn a client away with a contraindication, or recommend another service that would ultimately be best for the client. You'll hang on to that client. You'll get them for something else, or you'll get their sister or their mother.

I would say those two areas are most important: holding yourself to the highest standard of excellence and not selling out your professional ethics.

Body Area	Waxing	Tweezing	Depilatories
Face/upper lips/eyebrows	X	X	
Underarms	X		
Arms	X		X
Bikini line	X	X (after waxing or sugaring)	
Legs	X		X
Top of feet/toes	X		X

Table 18–1 Appropriate Hair Removal Procedures

Sugaring

Sugaring, another epilator treatment, is also becoming more popular and produces the same results as hot or cold wax. It involves the use of a thick, sugar-based paste and is especially appropriate for more sensitive skin types. Removing the residue from the skin is simple, as it dissolves with warm water. (See Table 18–1 for a list of the hair removal procedures described in this chapter and their uses.)

18

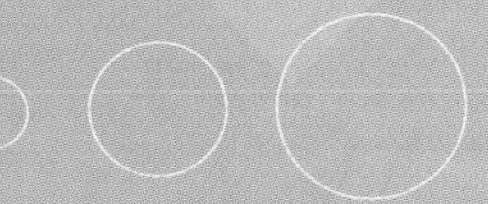

chapter glossary

depilatory	substance, usually a caustic alkali preparation, used for the temporary removal of superfluous hair by dissolving it at the skin level
electrolysis	removal of hair by means of an electric current that destroys the root of the hair
epilator	substance used to remove hair by pulling it out of the follicle
hirsuties or hypertrichosis	growth of an unusual amount of hair on parts of the body normally bearing only downy hair, such as the faces of women or the backs of men
laser hair removal	permanent hair removal treatment in which a laser beam is pulsed on the skin, impairing the hair follicles
photo-epilation	permanent hair removal treatment that uses intense light to destroy the hair follicles
sugaring	temporary hair removal method that involves the use of a thick, sugar-based paste
threading	temporary hair removal method that involves twisting and rolling cotton thread along the surface of the skin, entwining the hair in the thread and lifting it from the follicle

review questions

1. What information should be entered in the client record during the consultation?
2. What conditions, treatments, and medications contraindicate hair removal in the salon?
3. What are the two major types of hair removal? Give examples of each.
4. Define these methods of hair removal: electrolysis, photo-epilation, and laser removal.
5. Which hair removal techniques should not be performed in the salon without special training?
6. What is the difference between a depilatory and an epilator?
7. Why must a patch test be given before waxing?
8. List safety precautions that must be followed for hot and cold waxing.
9. Define threading and sugaring.

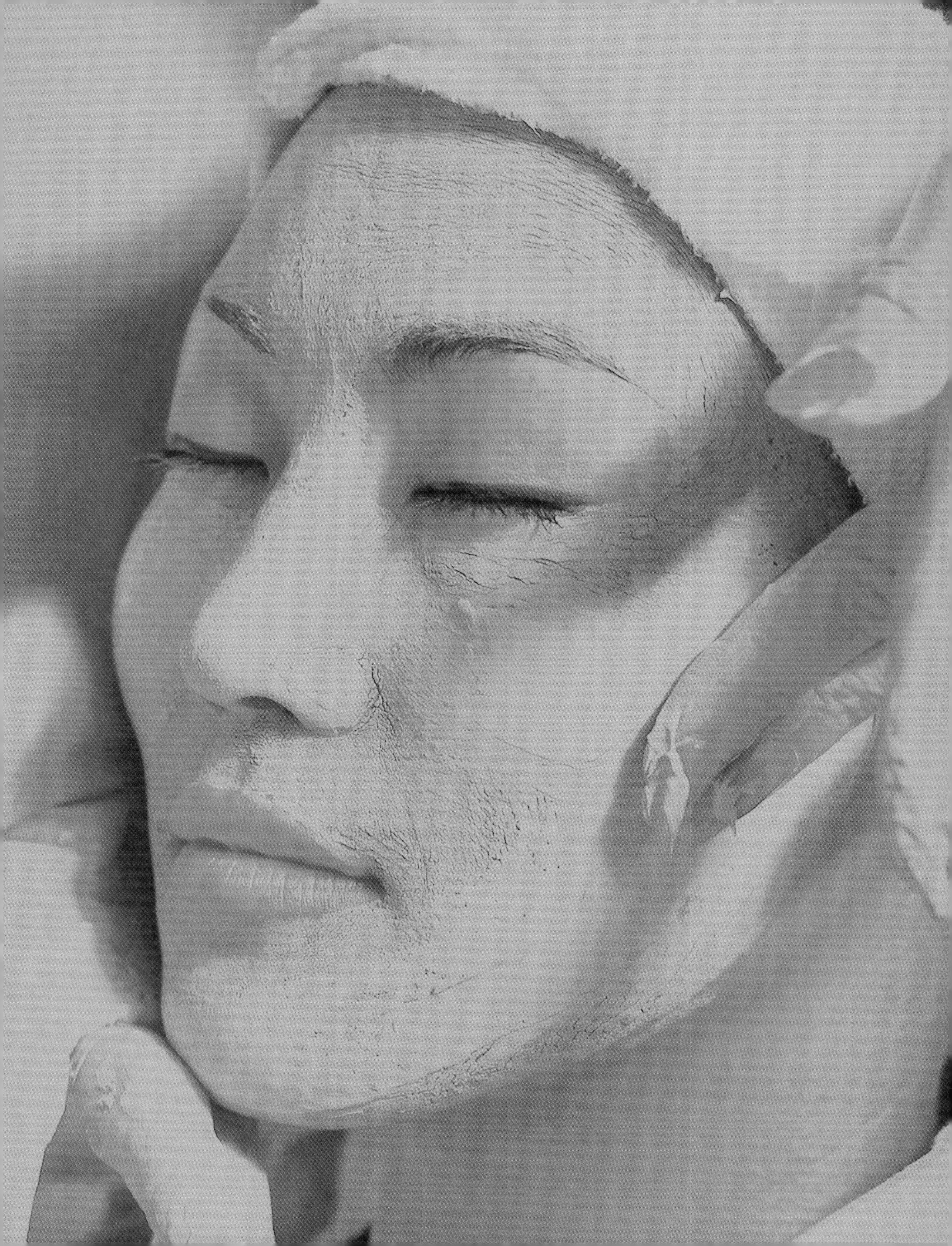

FACIALS

Margrit Altenburg
LICENSED ESTHETICS INSTRUCTOR AND SCHOOL DIRECTOR

Chapter Outline

Learning Objectives

After completing this chapter, you should be able to:

1. List and describe the five main categories of professional skin care products.
2. Explain the different skin types and skin conditions.
3. Identify the various types of massage movements and their physiological effects.
4. List and describe the different types of electrical current used in facial treatments and the safety precautions that must be followed when working with them.
5. Demonstrate the procedure for a basic facial.

National Skill Standards

This chapter provides you with the necessary information to master these National Industry Skill Standards for Entry-Level Cosmetologists.

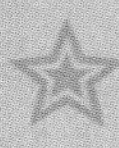
Consulting with clients to determine their needs and preferences.

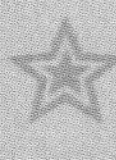
Conducting services in a safe environment, taking measures to prevent the spread of infectious and contagious diseases.

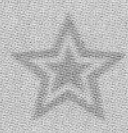
Safely using a variety of salon products while providing client services.

Providing basic skin care services.

Key Terms

Page number indicates where in the chapter the term is used.

alphahydroxy acids Pg. 659
ampules Pg. 662
aromatherapy Pg. 689
astringent Pg. 657
chemical exfoliation Pg. 658
chucking Pg. 667
clay masks Pg. 660
cleansing cream Pg. 656
cleansing lotion Pg. 656
effleurage Pg. 666
electrolyte Pg. 674
electrotherapy Pg. 673
emollients Pg. 656
enzyme peels Pg. 659
exfoliant Pg. 657
exfoliation Pg. 657
face wash Pg. 656
fresheners Pg. 656
friction Pg. 667
fulling Pg. 667
gommage Pg. 659
hacking Pg. 667
keratolytic enzymes Pg. 659
light therapy Pg. 675
mask Pg. 660
massage Pg. 665
massage creams Pg. 660
mechanical exfoliation Pg. 657
microdermabrasion Pg. 658
modelage masks Pg. 660
moisturizers Pg. 660
motor point Pg. 668
packs Pg. 661
paraffin wax masks Pg. 660
petrissage Pg. 666
rolling Pg. 667
sulfur masks Pg. 661
tapotement or percussion Pg. 667
toners Pg. 657
treatment or nourishing creams Pg. 659
vibration Pg. 667
wringing Pg. 667

More and more clients today consider the facial the favorite part of their salon visit. These clients are often juggling the demands of their work, family, and community. If performed correctly and professionally, the facial can serve as an oasis in a busy day, leaving the client feeling refreshed, renewed, and with a desire to return for future services.

As a professional who performs facials, you are working in one of the fastest-growing sectors of the beauty field. Your work can boost a person's self-esteem and confidence and can change the way that person "faces" the world. Your help will be particularly valuable to many of your clients for whom skin problems cause anxiety. Recognize the pleasure that you give and know that the more you develop your expertise at performing facials, the more you will be able to establish yourself as an important member of the salon team (Figure 19–1).

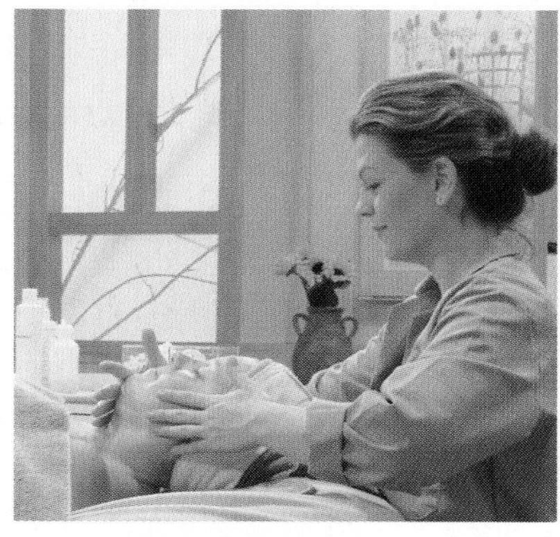

Figure 19–1 A facial is a soothing, pleasurable experience for the client.

BASIC CLASSIFICATION AND CHEMISTRY OF SKIN CARE PRODUCTS

The cosmetic industry is continually turning out a wide array of products designed to improve the condition and appearance of the skin (Figure 19–2). These products can be grouped into five main categories.

1. Cleansing products
2. Exfoliants
3. Treatment and massage creams
4. Moisturizers
5. Intensive care products

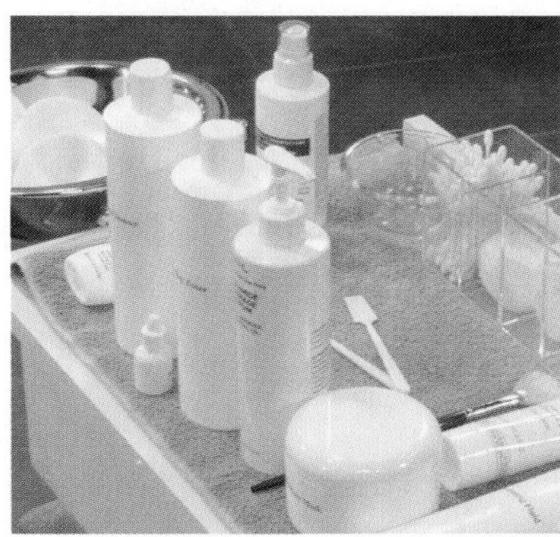

Figure 19–2 There is a wide variety of skin care products for every skin type.

Cleansing Products

All facial cleansing procedures begin with a cleanser and end with the application of a tonic lotion. The quality of your products, joined with the excellence of your skills, will determine the outcome of the facial.

Cleansers

Cleansers are designed for every skin type and skin condition and come in three basic forms: face wash, cleansing lotion, and cleansing cream.

- **Face wash** is a detergent-type foaming cleanser with a neutral or slightly acidic pH. Face washes vary in strength and texture. You should always have face wash available, as many of your clients are used to the foaming action of bar soap and seek that same kind of "squeaky clean" feeling. The consistency of face wash is very much like that of soap. When water is added, it foams moderately. When cleansing is done, it rinses off completely, leaving the skin feeling fresh and clean but often also a little tight. Clients with oily or combination skin (skin that has both dry and oily areas) are especially fond of face wash because it cuts excess amounts of oil. For acne-prone skin, an antimicrobial agent is added to kill bacteria. The danger of face wash is that it can overdry the skin.
- **Cleansing lotion** is formulated to remove makeup and soil. It is a water-based emulsion that can be used twice a day on normal and combination skin. It can also be used on slightly dry skin, although some milk cleansers that contain more oils or **emollients** (agents that soften or smooth the skin surface) may be a better choice. Cleansing lotion can be applied with damp cotton pads or with your hands and should always be removed with a damp soft cloth, cotton, or sponges. Additional ingredients can be added to cleansing lotions to suit certain skin conditions such as sensitivity, dehydration, or capillary problems.
- **Cleansing cream** is a light-textured, oil-based emulsion used primarily to dissolve makeup and soil quickly. It is suitable for basic skin cleansing twice a day on very dry and mature skin. It is considerably heavier than cleansing lotions. Actors and other performers use these products to remove heavy stage makeup. Cleansing cream must only be used with a sponge or a soft cloth; otherwise you run the risk of leaving a residue on the skin. Cleansing creams should be followed by a tonic lotion that is strong enough to remove any residue.

CAUTION

As a cosmetology student, you should always receive hands-on training from your instructor before attempting any of the procedures discussed in this chapter.

19

Tonic Lotions

Fresheners, toners, and astringents are all essentially the same type of product. They perform three specific functions.

1. They remove excess cleanser and residue left behind by face wash cleansers.
2. They have a relatively low pH, helping to restore the skin's natural pH after cleansing.
3. They have a temporary tightening effect on both the skin and the individual follicle openings, helping to temporarily "shrink pores."

Tonic lotions vary in strength and alcohol content.

- **Fresheners**, or skin freshening lotions, have the lowest alcohol content (0 to 4 percent) and are beneficial for dry and mature skin as well as for sensitive skin conditions.

- **Toners** usually have an alcohol content of 4 to 15 percent and are designed for use on normal and combination skin.
- **Astringents** may have an alcohol content of up to 35 percent and are used for oily and acne-prone skin. They remove oil accumulation on the skin.

Tonic lotions can be applied to the face with a cotton pad or can be sprayed directly onto the skin. Always blot the skin dry with a tissue after using tonic lotions so as not to leave the client with a wet feeling on her face.

CAUTION

It is important to note that the cosmetologist's domain is the hair and the superficial epidermis. The cosmetologist must not perform treatments that involve the live layers of the skin.

Exfoliants

The term **exfoliation** refers to the peeling and shredding of the horny (outer) layer of the skin. An **exfoliant** is an ingredient that assists in this process. Many different types of peeling and exfoliation treatments are available, ranging from brushing treatments and light enzyme peels to strong surgical peels that can be administered only by dermatologists and plastic surgeons.

Removing cell layers from the surface of the skin can be used to treat a variety of both cosmetic and medical problems. There are two basic types of exfoliation treatments: mechanical and chemical.

Mechanical Exfoliants

During the process of **mechanical exfoliation**, some method of physical contact is used to literally scrape or bump cells off the skin. Examples of mechanical peeling treatments include granular scrubs, such as those made with almond meal or jojoba beads, or treatments that use a brushing machine. When the granules of these scrubs or the bristles of a brushing machine come into contact with the surface corneum cells, the movement of the granules or the bristles literally "bump off" cells from the surface of the corneum (Figure 19–3 and Figure 19–4).

The removal of dry, dead surface cells can help the skin in the following ways:

- it can make the skin appear much smoother.
- it makes the extraction of clogged pores easier.

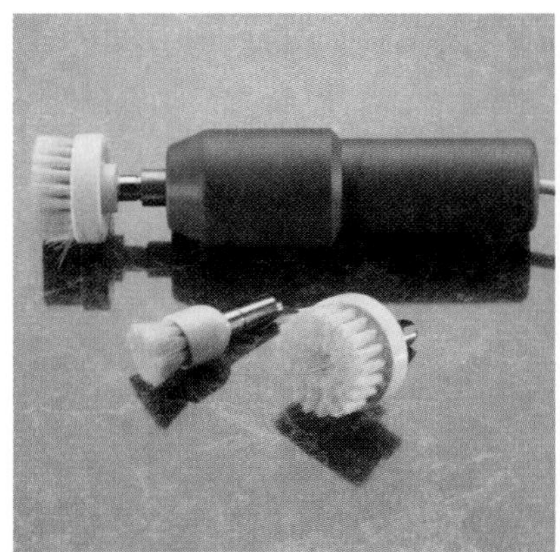

Figure 19-3 A skin brushing machine.

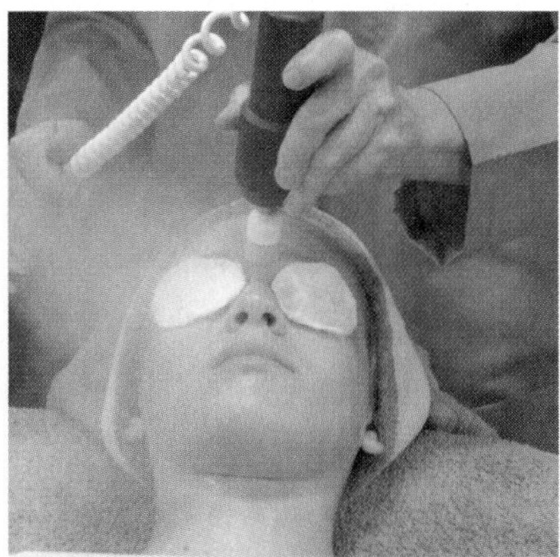

Figure 19-4 Using a skin brushing machine on a client's face.

CAUTION

Do not use brushing machines, scrubs, or any harsh mechanical peeling techniques on these skin types and conditions:

- **skin with many visible capillaries.**
- **thin skin that reddens easily.**
- **older skin that is thin and bruises easily.**
- **skin being medically treated with tretinoin (retinoic acid or Retin-A), Accutane, azelaic acid, adapalene (Differin), alphahydroxy acid (AHA), or salicylic acid (found in many common skin products).**
- **acne-prone skin with inflamed papules and pustules.**

- it brings lower-level cells to the surface more quickly and improves the skin's moisture content.
- it allows for deeper delivery of moisturizers and other treatments into the epidermis.
- it makes it easier to apply makeup more evenly.
- the mechanical treatment used in exfoliation stimulates blood flow to the surface of the skin.

Granular scrubs for normal to dry skin are usually recommended two to three times per week.

One of the most recent advances in mechanical exfoliation is known as **microdermabrasion**. If you have ever watched an old building being cleaned by sandblasting, you'll understand the basic concept of microdermabrasion. A microdermabrasion machine uses aluminum chloride, corundum, or sodium chloride crystals to sandblast dead cells off the surface of the skin. These crystals, directed at the skin through a vacuum or air pulsating wand, abrade the stratum corneum (Figure 19–5). At the same time, dead skin cells are picked up along with the crystal residue. Depending on the skin and the quantity of dead cells, it may be necessary to pass the wand over the skin several times.

Microdermabrasion has been used in Europe for many years and was first introduced in the United States during the mid-1990s. The procedure respects the integrity of the skin, promotes even healing, and complements most treatment programs.

Microdermabrasion has been used to treat:

- aging and sun-damaged skin
- some types of acne scarring and acne
- altered pigmentation
- stretch marks
- fine lines and wrinkles

Results may include:

- improved skin tone
- even skin color
- refined skin pores
- fewer breakouts
- healthy glow
- renewed elasticity
- diminished appearance of scars

Microdermabrasion should be performed only after extensive training.

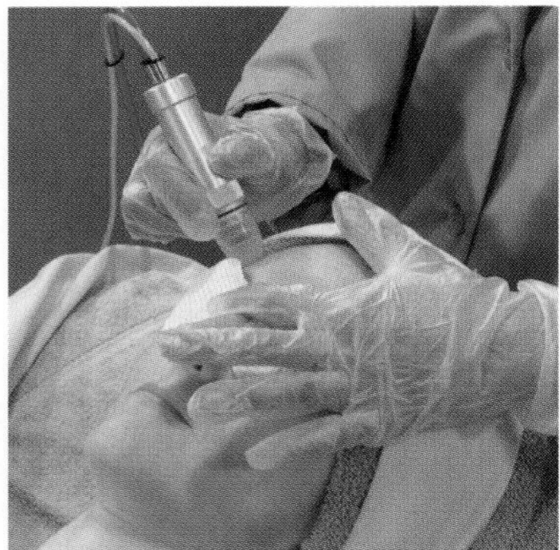

Figure 19-5 Microdermabrasion.

Chemical Exfoliants

In **chemical exfoliation**, dead skin cells or the intercellular "glue" that holds them together is dissolved by chemical agents such as alphahydroxy acids and enzymes. Superficial chemical exfoliants are very gentle. You might consider using them when mechanical exfoliation is not appropriate. These exfoliating procedures, called **enzyme peels**, involve the use of substances called **keratolytic enzymes** (kair-uh-tuh-LIT-ik), which help speed up the breakdown of keratin, the protein in skin.

One enzyme often used in keratolytic enzyme peels is papain (puh-PAY-in), which is derived from juice of the papaya fruit. Another frequently used enzyme is pancreatin (pan-KREE-uh-tin), which is derived from beef by-products.

There are two basic types of keratolytic enzyme peels. In one, a cream is applied to the skin before steaming. This cream may contain paraffin or oatmeal, which dries in about seven minutes to form a hardened crust. The crust is then massaged or "rolled" off the skin. Products of this type are often called "vegetal peelings" or **gommage** (gom-AHZH). This treatment is actually a combination of an enzyme and a mechanical peeling (Figure 19–6).

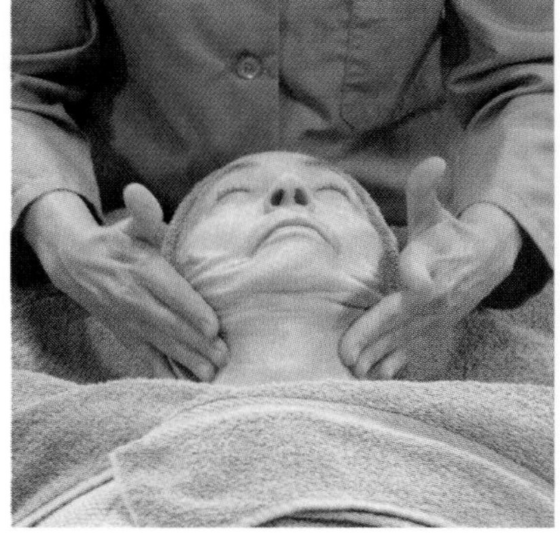

Figure 19-6 Rolling a gommage mask off the face.

The second, and perhaps more popular, type of enzyme peel uses a powdered form of enzyme. Mixed with warm water immediately before application, this product stays soft during application and does not dry to a crust. This type of enzyme treatment generally produces a more even peeling of the cell buildup and helps to slightly dilate the follicle openings. Enzyme peelings are suitable for the following conditions:

- oily, clogged skin with blackheads and whiteheads and minor acne breakouts.
- dry or dehydrated skin with cell buildup, flaking, and a tight dry surface.
- dull, lifeless-looking skin. This skin condition actually has a tremendous buildup of dead cells that produces a slight gray color on the surface.
- clients who desire a smoother skin appearance and a more even surface for makeup application.

Another group of chemical exfoliants are those that use **alphahydroxy acids**. These acids are derived from plants, mostly fruit. On oily or acne-prone skin, they loosen clogged pores to treat and prevent the excessive buildup of dead cells that can cause acne lesions. Alphahydroxy acid exfoliation should only be performed when the client has first been using a 5 to 10 percent concentration gel, lotion, or cream at home for at least two weeks. If a client does not do this first, the alphahydroxy acid exfoliation may cause discomfort and more redness and irritation afterward.

Treatment and Massage Creams

Treatment creams, also referred to as **nourishing creams**, are designed to hydrate and condition the skin during the night, when normal tissue repair is taking place. Treatment creams are often heavier in consistency and texture than moisturizers and contain more emollient and active ingredients. The amount of emollient added to the treatment cream depends on the type of skin it is designed for. More emollient content means that the product is designed for dry and mature skin types. Less emollient content means that

?

Did you know...

A valuable ingredient in moisturizers is sunscreen; its presence is particularly important in day creams. Not only does sunscreen guard against premature aging of the skin, but, when used consistently, it is one of the best ways to help prevent skin cancer.

the product is designed for normal or combination skin types. Treatment creams for oily skin usually have very little or no emollient.

Massage creams are lubricants with very few or no active ingredients. They are designed to give the practitioner a good slip (slippery quality) during massage, so that the skin is not stretched. These products must be removed from the skin after massage and before mask application, to allow the active ingredients in the mask a chance to penetrate.

Moisturizers

Moisturizers are products formulated to add moisture to the skin. They are water-based emulsions, which are absorbed quickly without leaving any residue on the surface of the skin. They are applied at the end of the facial and are ideal for daily use as a day cream or makeup base. Moisturizers are available for various skin types, from acne-prone to extremely mature skin.

Moisturizers usually contain an ingredient that helps retain water within the surface layers of the skin. They may also contain emollients or other active ingredients depending on which skin type they are intended for.

Intensive Care Products

Intensive care products include masks, packs, and ampules.

Masks and Packs

Masks and packs are special cosmetic preparations applied to the face to benefit and beautify the skin. They require a short application time and allow a practitioner to treat different skin conditions on the same face at the same time (Figure 19–7).

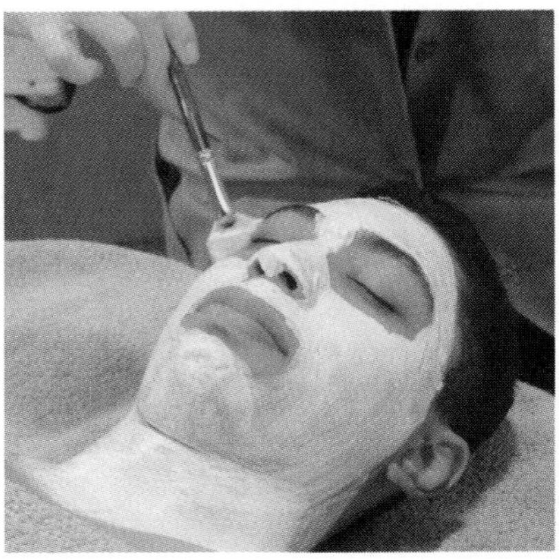

Figure 19–7 Applying a mask to a male client.

19

A **mask** is usually a setting product, which means that it dries after application and provides a complete closure to the environment on top of the skin. Ingredients such as alginate, paraffin wax, and gypsum (a kind of plaster) generally account for this effect. Masks may also use such special ingredients as clay, kaolin, and silica for their tightening and sebum-absorbing effects.

- **Clay masks** are clay preparations used to stimulate circulation and temporarily contract the pores of the skin. They are ready-to-use products with ingredients simiilar to those in treatment creams, but they also contain clay, kaolin, or silica. They absorb sebum and are used on oily and combination skin. Clay masks are applied with a mask brush and are allowed to set for about 10 minutes.
- **Paraffin wax masks** are specially prepared facial masks containing paraffin and other beneficial ingredients. They are melted at a little more than body temperature before application. The paraffin quickly cools to a lukewarm temperature and hardens to a candle-like consistency. Paraffin masks are used with a treatment cream because the paraffin, which has no treatment properties of its own, allows for deeper penetration of the cream's ingredients into the skin. Eye pads and gauze are also used in a paraffin mask application, as facial hair could stick to the wax if not covered and the mask would be difficult and painful to remove.
- **Modelage masks** (MAHD-lahzh) contain special crystals of gypsum, a plaster-like ingredient (Figure 19–8). As with paraffin masks, modelage

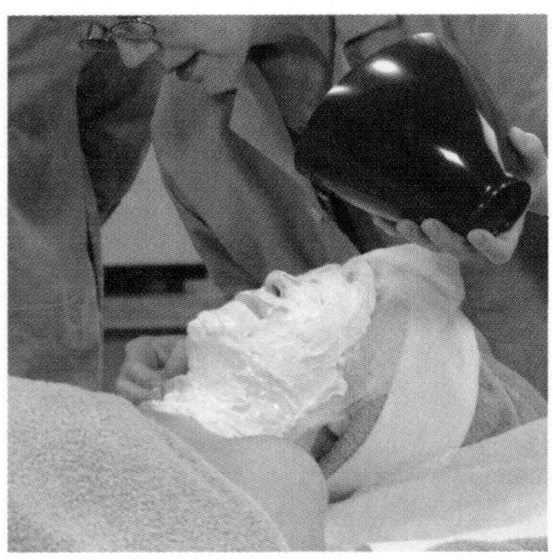

Figure 19–8 A modelage mask.

masks are used with a treatment cream. When mixed with cold water immediately before application and applied about ¼ inch (.6 cm) thick, the modelage mask hardens. The chemical reaction that occurs when the plaster and the crystals mix with water produces a gradually increasing temperature that reaches approximately 105°F. As the mask is left on the skin, the temperature gradually cools until it has cooled down completely. The setting time for modelage masks is approximately 20 minutes.

The heat increases blood circulation and is very beneficial for dry, mature skin or skin that is dull and lifeless-looking. This type of mask is not recommended for use on sensitive skin, skin with capillary problems, oily skin, or skin with blemishes. Massage is not recommended prior to or after modelage mask application because blood circulation will already be increased by the mask itself. Modelage masks can become quite heavy on the face and should not be applied to the lower neck or to clients who suffer from claustrophobia, a fear of being closed in or confined.

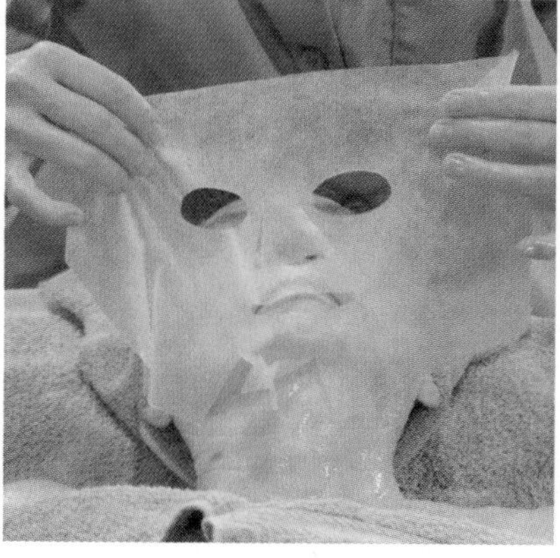

Figure 19–9 Placing gauze on the client's face.

- **Sulfur masks** contain sulfur, a common chemical, as their most important ingredient. Sulfur has been found to have a beneficial effect in reducing the production of sebum.
- You will usually use prepared masks, such as clay and paraffin masks, but sometimes a client may prefer a custom-designed mask made from fresh fruits, vegetables, milk, yogurt, or eggs. Some ingredients such as honey and almond meal or oatmeal can be mixed into a paste with milk for use as a mask. These masks are generally beneficial unless the client is allergic to a particular substance. Be sure to ask the client about any allergies before applying a mask. Custom-designed masks are generally left on the face for 10 to 15 minutes during a one-hour treatment.

Packs, also referred to as cream masks or gel masks, are very similar in composition to treatment creams. They remain soft and creamy throughout their entire setting time. Packs are highly beneficial when used to condition sensitive skin and have excellent hydrating properties. They are applied with a mask brush and are allowed to set for about 10 minutes.

The Use of Gauze for Mask Application

Gauze is a thin, open-meshed fabric of loosely woven cotton. It can be used to hold in place certain mask ingredients that tend to run, such as sliced or crushed fruits or vegetables. Cheesecloth is sometimes used as well. These ingredients can be applied over a layer of gauze. The gauze holds the mask on the face but allows the ingredients to seep through to benefit the skin. In some cases, it is necessary to apply a second layer of gauze over the mask to keep the ingredients from sliding off. Gauze is also used to keep paraffin and gypsum/plaster masks from sticking to the skin and the tiny hairs on the skin.

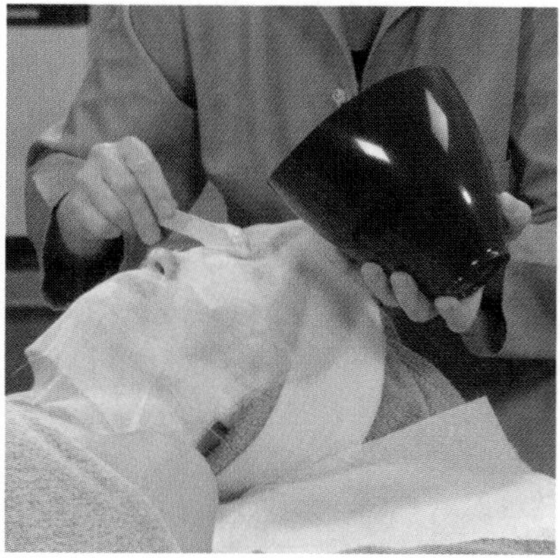

Figure 19–10 Applying a mask over the gauze.

To prepare gauze, cut a piece large enough to cover the entire face and neck. Cut out spaces for the eyes, nose, and mouth. Although the client is able to breathe through the gauze, the cut-out spaces will make it more comfortable (Figure 19–9 and Figure 19–10).

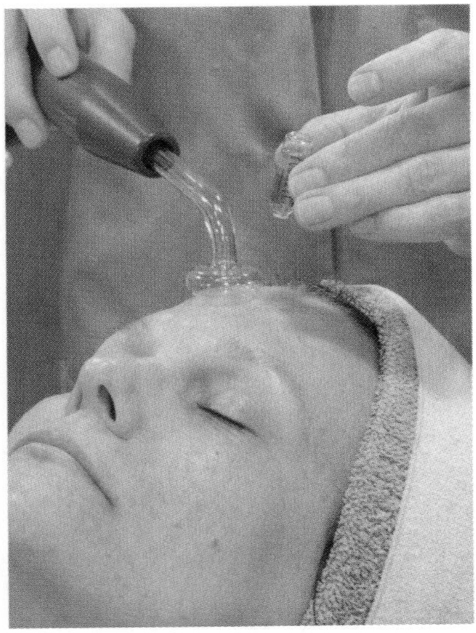

Figure 19–11 Skin treatment in an ampule.

AMPULES

Ampules (AM-pyools) are small, sealed glass vials containing a single application of a highly concentrated extract in a water or oil base. These extracts are applied under a night cream or fluid or a massage cream. They are available for a wide variety of skin types and problems. Some are used in a series once a month or several times a year. Others are designed to be used nightly. The advantage of ampules is that they deliver highly concentrated active ingredients in a premeasured amount (Figure 19–11).

After cleansing and exfoliation, the extract is applied to the client's face with light massage movements until it has been completely absorbed. 1

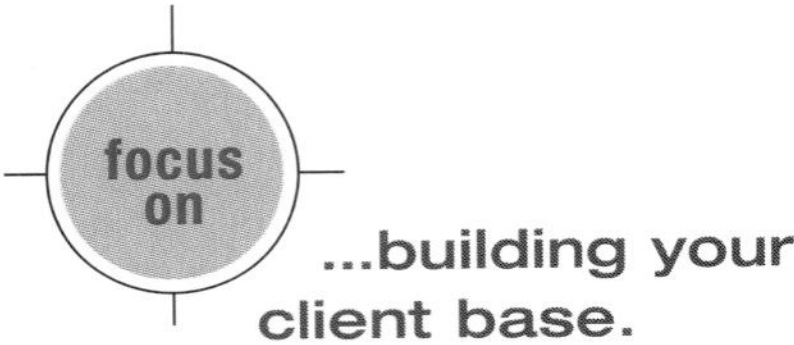

...building your client base.

It is useful to note on the consultation card how the client was referred to the salon. This helps you determine what kind of advertising draws your clients. If the referral has come from another salon client, you will want to make a point of thanking that client. This small courtesy can well lead to other valuable referrals.

CLIENT CONSULTATION

The salon should designate a quiet area for facial treatments. Not only does the relaxing nature of a facial call for a quiet spot, but the area also needs to be quiet enough that you can conduct a thorough consultation with your client. All facial treatments should begin with such a consultation.

Record-Keeping

During the consultation, keep client record cards at hand so that you can write down all necessary information (Figure 19–12). The record card should contain the following information:

- the client's name, home address, and home telephone number.
- the client's occupation and date of birth (this is useful so that you can determine if any signs of aging are, in fact, premature).
- the client's medical history and whether the client is presently taking or using any kind of medication. It should also be noted if the client is under the care of a physician or dermatologist.
- any contraindications—a pacemaker, metal implants, pregnancy, diabetes, epilepsy, allergies, high blood pressure—that call for alternative methods of treatments.
- information as to whether the client has had facials before and what kind of treatments were used.
- information on any skin care products the client is currently using.
- a notation of how the client was referred to the salon.
- observations on the client's skin type, skin condition, and any abnormalities of the skin.

Use the back of the consultation card to record the date and type of service and/or treatment being performed, the products that are being used, and products purchased by the client for home care. Often, a client will want to purchase a product that he has used before but has lost or discarded the container and cannot remember the name of the product (Figure 19–13).

CONSULTATION CARD				
Name				Date of Consultation
Address				D.O.B.
City	State	Zip		Occupation
Tel. (Home)	(Business)			Ref. by
				Contraindications
Medical History				
Current Medication				
Previous treatments				
Home Care Products used				
SKIN TYPE	Oily	Normal	Dry	Combination
SKIN CONDITION	Clogged pores	Sensitive	Dehydrated	Mature
Skin Abnormalities				
Remarks				

Figure 19–12 Client consultation card (front).

FACIAL RECORD			
Date	Type of treatment	By	Products purchased
2/14	Cleansing, Peel - Relaxing Massage	Mary	Moisturizer with sunscreen
3/16	Cleansing, Peel Modelage Mask	Mary	Cleanser, Toner
4/5	Cleansing, Peel High Frequency indirect	Mary	Moisturizer, Foundation # 7
4/26 5/13	Cleansing, Peel Massage Alginate Mask Cleansing, Peel Iontophoresis Paraffin Mask Skin is showing marked improvement.	John Mary	 Night cream for dry skin Lipstick # 43
6/1	Cleansing, Peel Relaxing Massage	Mary	Eye contour mask

Figure 19–13 Client consultation card (back).

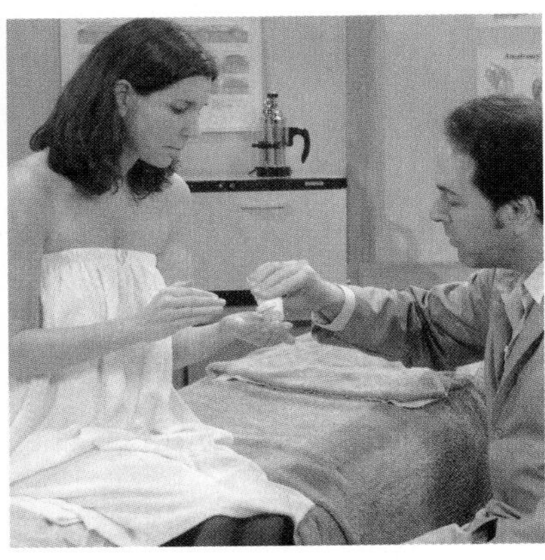

Figure 19–14 Recommend skin care products to the client.

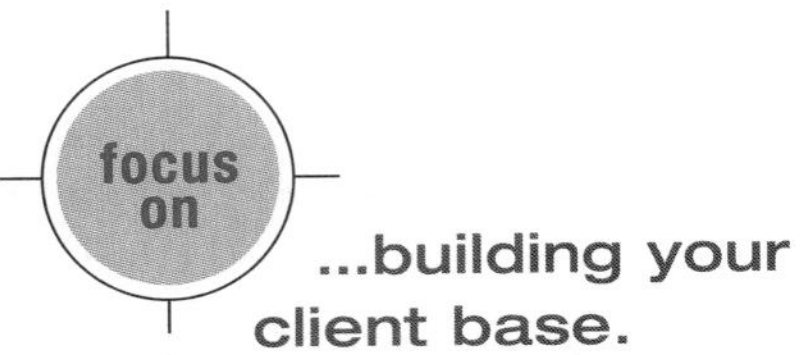

...building your client base.

Send your client a birthday card for his or her birthday. This way of advertising is not expensive and is always greatly appreciated.

Ask for your clients' e-mail addresses for this purpose and for other kinds of communications. E-mail is the preferred mode of communicating now for many people, who may also like to book their appointments this way.

As part of the consultation, do not hesitate to recommend services and products that will be beneficial to the client (Figure 19–14). Since the client has taken the initiative to come into the salon, she will feel disappointed if you neglect to discuss treatments and products as well as proper home care for the skin. Also, if you do not recommend professional products, your client may go elsewhere for advice, such as a department store or drugstore. She might not get the kind of product you would have advised, and you and the salon will not get the retail income.

Make it clear to your client that if she wishes to achieve the best results from a treatment, she must follow a proven routine of skin care at home with products that reinforce the salon treatments. Be careful, however, not to make the client feel that the sole purpose of the consultation is to sell products. Review appropriate and discreet retailing techniques with your instructor to make sure you achieve the right tone with your client.

Classification of Skin Types

During the first consultation and before every subsequent facial treatment, it is important to perform a thorough analysis of the client's skin prior to cleansing. If the skin is oily, it will often look shiny or greasy. If the skin is dry, it may look flaky. Table 19–1 lists brief descriptions of basic skin types.

Skin Type	Description
Oily Skin	Has overabundance of sebum; may or may not be blemished. Treatments will help to clear blemishes and normalize production of sebum.
Normal Skin	Usually in good condition; has adequate supply of sebum and moisture. Usually free of blemishes but can benefit from maintenance treatments to keep it healthy and attractive.
Dry Skin	Lacking in oil; often dehydrated. Treatments can stimulate sebaceous glands to produce natural oils needed to keep skin lubricated.
Combination Skin	May have either oily and normal areas or normal and dry areas. Treatments help normalize functioning of sebaceous glands and improve health and appearance of skin.

Table 19–1 Skin Types

Skin Conditions

While specific skin types can contribute to specific skin conditions, there are a number of conditions that can affect any type of skin. Some of the more common conditions include the following:

- If oily skin is not cleansed properly, sebum and dead cells can clog pores and lead to comedones (blackheads). These are breeding grounds for infectious bacteria and, if not given proper attention, can develop into pimples. An occasional pimple may develop into acne.
- Sensitivity can occur in all skin types as a reaction to such enemies of the skin as air pollution, chemicals present in water, and preservatives in food. Today, it is more important than ever to treat the skin with proper daily care.
- Dehydration can occur in every skin type, regardless of how oily the skin is. A client's skin may have a sufficient amount of oil but can still feel dry and flaky because of an insufficient amount of water in the body. This is known as dehydration. Insufficient fluid intake, too much sun, or the use of drying cosmetics are just some of the factors that can cause dehydration. The application of moisturizers in the morning and evening, along with regular facial treatments, can help the skin maintain the proper moisture content.
- Mature or aging skin is usually loose, wrinkled, and/or lined. Treatments may be effective in slowing down the aging process and can help diminish surface lines.

CAUTION

The cosmetologist does not treat skin diseases or disorders. However, as a professional, you must be able to recognize the presence of various skin ailments in order to suggest that the client seek medical advice from a physician.

Skin Abnormalities

Among the notes on your consultation card will be any skin abnormalities that you observe on your client (see Chapter 17). These can include:

- abnormalities of the sebaceous gland and hair follicle (comedones, papules, pustules, ingrown hair)
- abnormalities of the capillaries (dilated capillaries [not broken], rosacea)
- abnormalities of pigmentation (freckles, liver spots, moles, vitiligo)
- abnormalities of the corneum layer (psoriasis)
- abnormalities of the connective tissue (skin tags, scars, keloids)
- other abnormalities (warts, cold sores, or herpes simplex)

FACIAL MASSAGE

Massage is the manual or mechanical manipulation of the body by rubbing, pinching, kneading, tapping, and other movements to increase metabolism and circulation, promote absorption, and relieve pain. Cosmetologists massage their clients to help them keep their facial skin healthy and their muscles firm.

FYI

As a cosmetologist, your services are limited to certain areas of the body: scalp, face, neck, and shoulders; the upper chest and back; the hands and arms; and the feet and lower legs. Therapeutic massage, such as deep muscle and tissue massage and lymph drainage, should only be performed by therapists specialized in working on the different kind of tissues. Therapeutic massage requires special training and, in most cases, licensure.

To master massage techniques, you must have a basic knowledge of anatomy and physiology as well as considerable practice in performing the various movements. It is important that you use a firm, sure touch when giving a massage. To do this, you must develop flexible hands, a quiet temperament, and self-control.

Keep your hands soft by using creams, oils, and lotions. File and shape your nails to avoid scratching your client's skin. Your wrists and fingers should be flexible, your palms firm and warm. Cream or oil should be applied to your hands to permit smoother and gentler hand movements and to prevent drag or damage to the client's skin.

Basic Massage Manipulations

All massage treatments combine one or more basic movements or manipulations. Each manipulation is applied to the superficial muscles in a certain way to achieve a certain end. The impact of a massage treatment depends on the amount of pressure, the direction of movement, and the duration of each type of manipulation involved.

The direction of movement is always from the insertion of the muscle toward its origin. The insertion is the portion of the muscle at the more movable attachment (where it is attached to another muscle or to a movable bone or joint). The origin is the portion of the muscle at the fixed attachment (to an immovable section of the skeleton). Massaging a muscle in the wrong direction could result in a loss of resiliency and sagging of the skin and muscles.

Effleurage

Effleurage (EF-loo-rahzh) is a light, continuous stroking movement applied with the fingers (digital) or the palms (palmar) in a slow, rhythmic manner. No pressure is used. The palms work the large surfaces, while the cushions of the fingertips work the small surfaces, such as those around the eyes (Figure 19–15). Effleurage is frequently used on the forehead, face, scalp, back, shoulder, neck, chest, arms, and hands for its soothing and relaxing effects. Every massage should begin and end with effleurage.

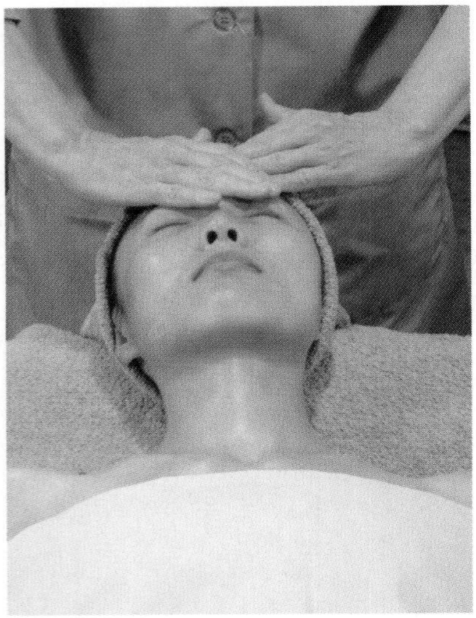

Figure 19–15 Palmar stroking of the face.

When performing effleurage, hold your whole hand loosely and keep your wrist and fingers flexible. Curve your fingers slightly to conform to the shape of the area being massaged, with just the cushions of the fingertips touching the skin. Do not use the ends of the fingertips. They are pointier than the cushions and will cause the effleurage to be less smooth. Also, the free edges of your fingernails may scratch the client's skin.

Petrissage

Petrissage (PEH-treh-sahzh) is a kneading movement performed by lifting, squeezing, and pressing the tissue with a light, firm pressure. Petrissage offers deeper stimulation to the muscles, nerves, and skin glands, and improves the circulation. These kneading movements are usually limited to the back, the shoulders, and the arms.

Although usually used on larger surface areas such as the arms and shoulders, digital kneading can also be used on the cheeks with light pinching movements (Figure 19–16). The pressure should be light but firm. When grasping and releasing the fleshy parts, the movements must be rhythmic, never jerky.

Fulling is a form of petrissage in which the tissue is grasped, gently lifted, and spread out, used mainly for massaging the arms. With the fingers of both hands grasping the arm, apply a kneading movement across the flesh, with light pressure on the underside of the client's forearm and between the shoulder and elbow.

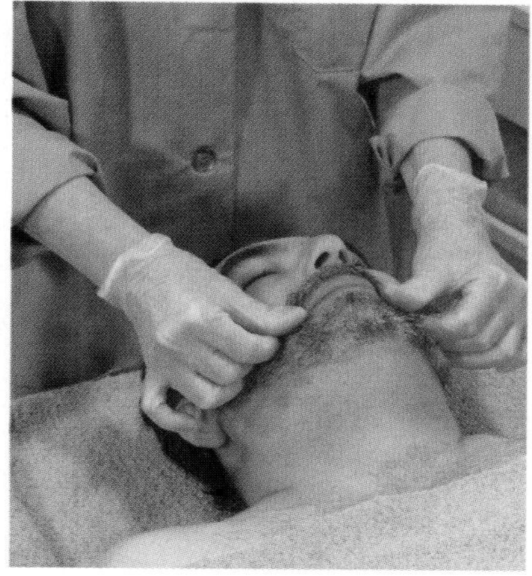

Figure 19-16 Digital kneading of the cheeks.

Friction

Friction (FRIK-shun) is a deep rubbing movement in which you apply pressure on the skin with your fingers or palm while moving it over an underlying structure. Friction has been known to have a significant benefit on the circulation and glandular activity of the skin. Circular friction movements are usually used on the scalp, arms, and hands. Light circular friction is used on the face and neck (Figure 19–17).

Chucking, rolling, and wringing are variations of friction and are used mainly to massage the arms and legs, as follows:

- **Chucking**. Grasping the flesh firmly in one hand and moving the hand up and down along the bone while the other hand keeps the arm or leg in a steady position.
- **Rolling**. Pressing and twisting the tissues with a fast back-and-forth movement.
- **Wringing**. Vigorous movement in which the hands, placed a little distance apart on both sides of the client's arm or leg and working downward, apply a twisting motion against the bones in the opposite direction.

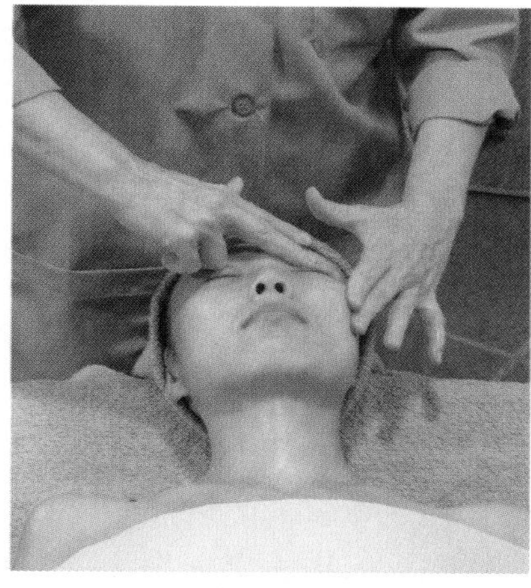

Figure 19-17 Circular friction on the face.

Tapotement

Tapotement (tah-POHT-mant), or **percussion** (per-KUSH-un), consists of short, quick tapping, slapping, and hacking movements. This form of massage is the most stimulating and should be applied with care and discretion. Tapotement movements tone the muscles and impart a healthy glow to the area being massaged.

In facial massage, use only light digital tapping. Bring the fingertips down against the skin in rapid succession. Your fingers must be flexible enough to create an even force over the area being massaged (Figure 19–18).

In slapping movements, keeping your wrists flexible allows your palms to come in contact with the skin in light, firm, and rapid slapping movements. One hand follows the other. With each slapping stroke, lift the flesh slightly.

Hacking is a chopping movement performed with the edges of the hands. Both the wrists and hands move alternately in fast, light, firm, and flexible motions against the skin. Hacking and slapping movements are used only to massage the back, shoulders, and arms.

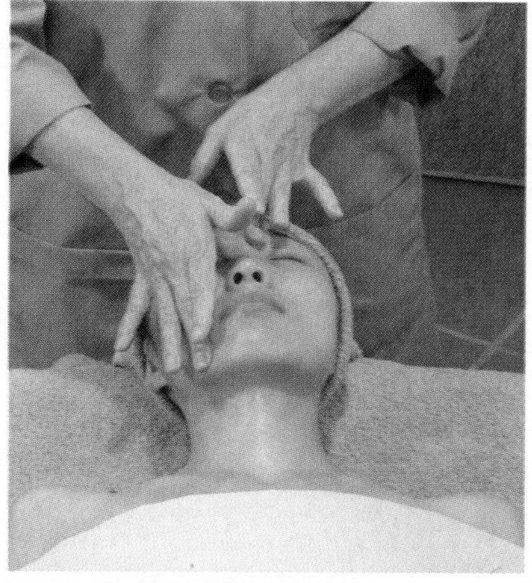

Figure 19-18 Digital tapping on the face.

Vibration

Vibration (vy-BRAY-shun) is a rapid shaking of the body part while the balls of the fingertips are pressed firmly on the point of application. The

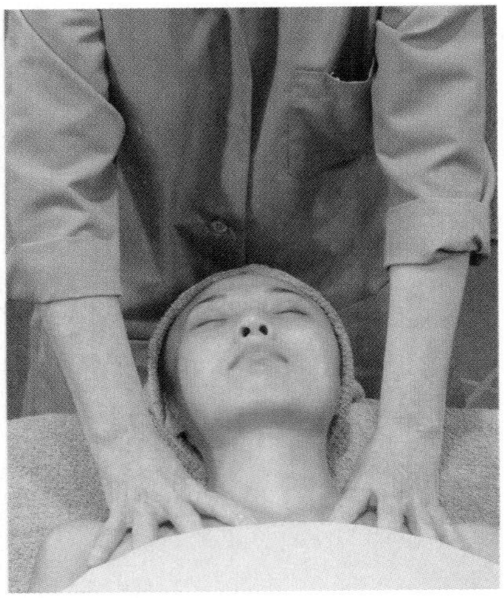

Figure 19-19 Vibration on the shoulders.

movement is accomplished by rapid muscular contractions in your arms. It is a highly relaxing movement, and should be applied at the end of the massage (Figure 19–19). Deep vibration in combination with other classical massage movements can also be produced by the use of a mechanical vibrator to stimulate blood circulation and increase muscle tone in muscles of the body.

Physiological Effects of Massage

To obtain proper results from a scalp or facial massage, you must have a thorough knowledge of all the structures involved: muscles, nerves, connective tissues, and blood vessels. Every muscle has a **motor point**, which is a point on the skin over the muscle where pressure or stimulation will cause contraction of that muscle. Some examples are illustrated here (Figure 19–20 and Figure 19–21). In order to obtain the maximum benefits from a facial massage, you must consider the motor points that affect the underlying muscles of the face and neck. The location of motor points varies among individuals due to differences in body structure. However, a few manipulations on the proper motor points will relax the client early in the massage treatment.

Relaxation is achieved through light but firm, slow, rhythmic movements, or very slow, light hand vibrations over the motor points for a short time. Another technique is to pause briefly over the motor points, using light pressure.

Skillfully applied massage directly or indirectly influences the structures and functions of the body. The immediate effects of massage are first noticed on the skin. The area being massaged shows increased circulation, secretion, nutrition, and excretion. The following benefits may be obtained by proper facial and scalp massage:

- the skin and all its structures are nourished
- the skin becomes softer and more pliable
- the circulation of the blood is increased

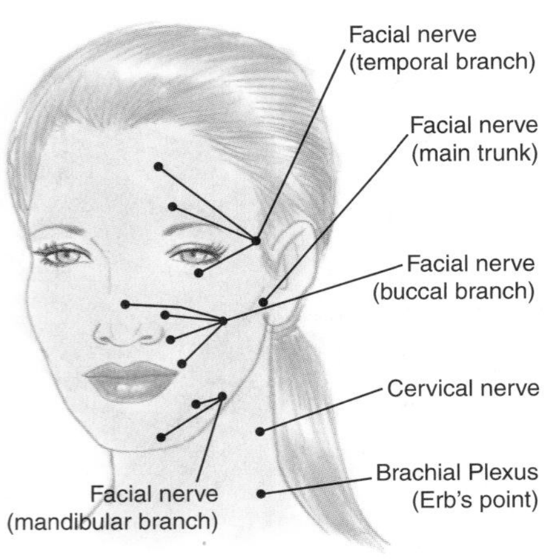

Figure 19-20 Motor nerve points of the face.

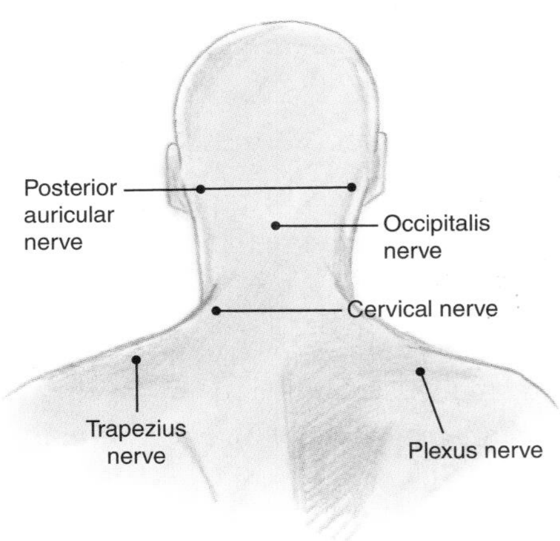

Figure 19-21 Motor nerve points of the neck.

- the activity of the skin glands is stimulated
- the muscle fibers are stimulated and strengthened
- the nerves are soothed and rested
- pain is sometimes relieved

The frequency of facial or scalp massage depends on the condition of the skin or scalp, the age of the client, and the condition being treated. As a general rule, normal skin or scalp can be kept in excellent condition with the help of a weekly massage, accompanied by proper home care.

CAUTION

Do not massage a client who has high blood pressure, a heart condition, or has had a stroke. Massage increases circulation and may be harmful to such a client. Have the client consult a physician first. If a client has arthritis, be very careful to avoid vigorous massage of the joints. Communicate with your client throughout the massage and adjust your touch according to the needs that she expresses.

Facial Manipulations

Now that we have had an overview of basic massage/manipulation techniques and guidelines, let us examine in more depth how best to use manipulations on the face. When performing facial manipulations, keep in mind that an even tempo, or rhythm, brings on relaxation. Do not remove your hands from the client's face once you have started the manipulations. Should it become necessary to remove your hands, feather them off, then gently replace them with feather-like movements. Remember that massage movements are generally directed from the insertion toward the origin of a muscle, in order to avoid damage to muscular tissues.

The following illustrations show the different movements that may be used on the various parts of the face, chest, and back. Each instructor may have developed her own routine, however. For example, some instructors and estheticians prefer to start massage manipulations at the chin, while others prefer to start at the forehead. Both are correct. Be guided by your instructor.

- *Chin movement.* Lift the chin, using a slight pressure (Figure 19–22).
- *Lower cheeks.* Using a circular movement, rotate from chin to ears (Figure 19–23).
- *For mouth, nose, and cheek movements,* follow the diagram (Figure 19–24).
- *Linear movement over the forehead.* Slide fingers to the temples and then stroke up to hairline, gradually moving your hands across the forehead to the right eyebrow (Figure 19–25).

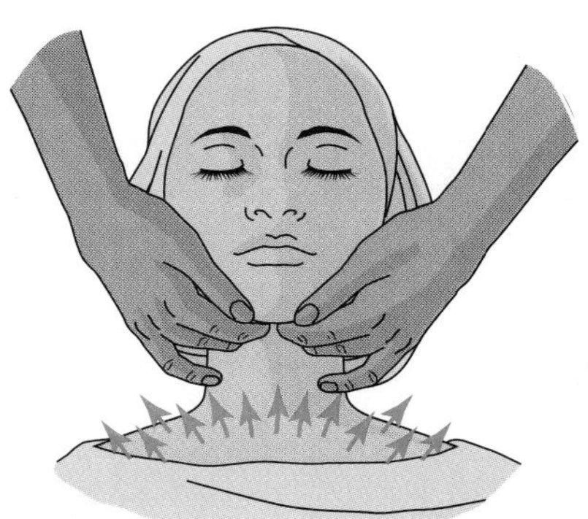

Figure 19-22 Chin movement.

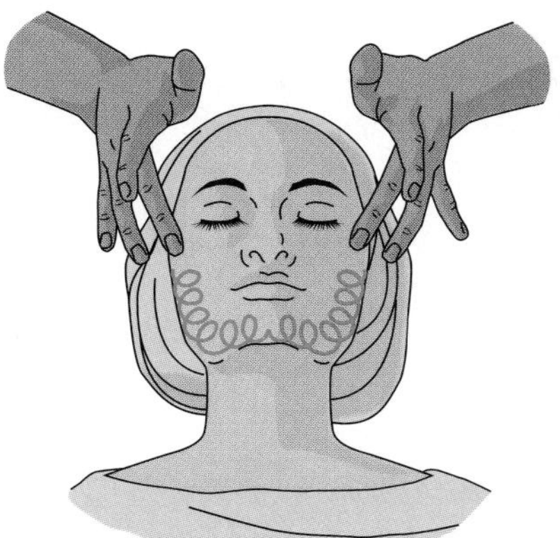

Figure 19-23 Circular movement of lower cheeks.

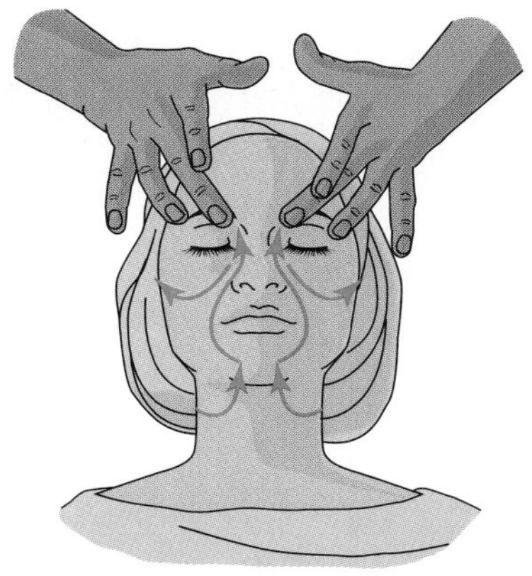

Figure 19-24 Mouth, nose, and cheek movements.

- *Circular movement over the forehead.* Starting at the eyebrow line, work across the middle of the forehead and then toward the hairline (Figure 19–26).
- *Crisscross movement.* Start at one side of forehead and work back (Figure 19–27).
- *Stroking (headache) movement.* Slide your fingers toward the center of the forehead and then draw your fingers, with slight pressure, toward the temples and rotate (Figure 19–28).
- *Brow and eye movement.* Place your middle fingers at the inner corners of the eyes and your index fingers over the brows. Slide them toward the outer corners of the eyes, under the eyes, and then back to the inner corners (Figure 19–29).
- *Nose and upper cheek movement.* Slide your fingers down the nose. Apply a rotary movement across the cheeks to the temples and rotate gently. Slide your fingers under the eyes and then back to the bridge of the nose (Figure 19–30).

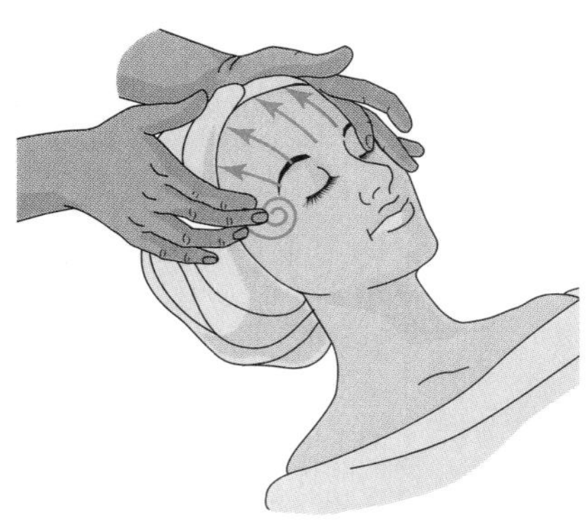

Figure 19-25 Linear movement over forehead.

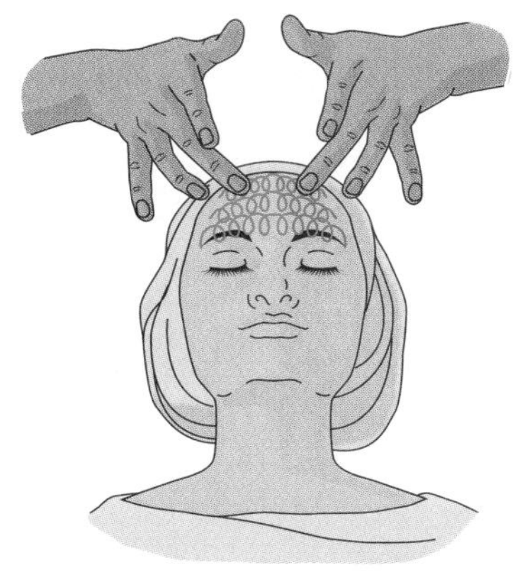

Figure 19-26 Circular movement over forehead.

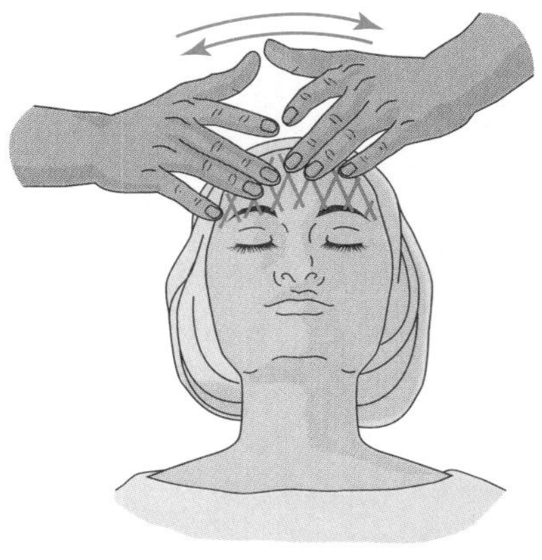

Figure 19-27 Crisscross movement.

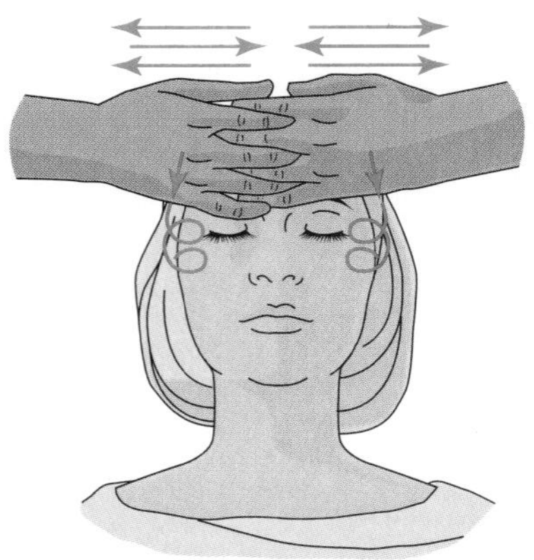

Figure 19-28 Stroking (headache) movement.

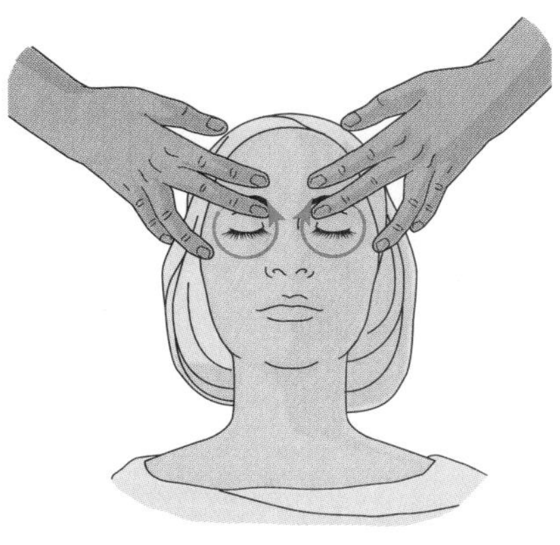

Figure 19-29 Brow and eye movement.

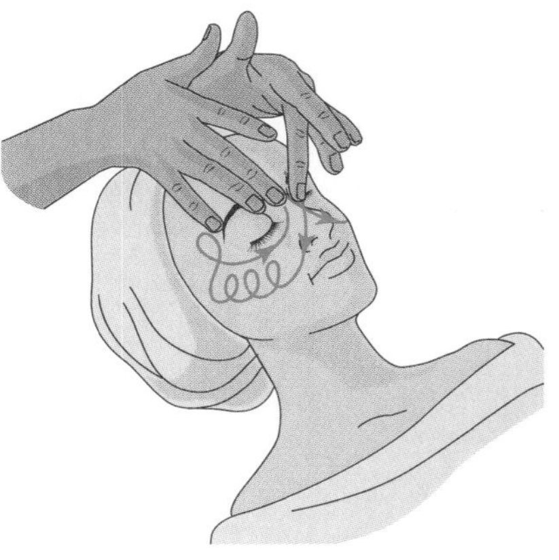

Figure 19-30 Nose and upper cheek movement.

- *Mouth and nose movement.* Apply a circular movement from the corners of the mouth up to the sides of the nose. Slide your fingers over the brows and then down to the corners of the mouth up to the sides of nose. Follow by sliding your fingers over the brows and down to the corners of the mouth again (Figure 19–31).
- *Lip and chin movement.* From the center of the upper lip, draw your fingers around the mouth, going under the lower lip and chin (Figure 19–32).
- *Optional movement.* Hold the head with your left hand and draw the fingers of your right hand from under the lower lip and around mouth, moving to the center of the upper lip (Figure 19–33).
- *Lifting movement of the cheeks.* Proceed from the mouth to the ears, and then from the nose to the top part of the ears (Figure 19–34).
- *Rotary movement of the cheeks.* Massage from the chin to the ear lobes, from the mouth to the middle of the ears, and from the nose to the top of the ears (Figure 19–35).

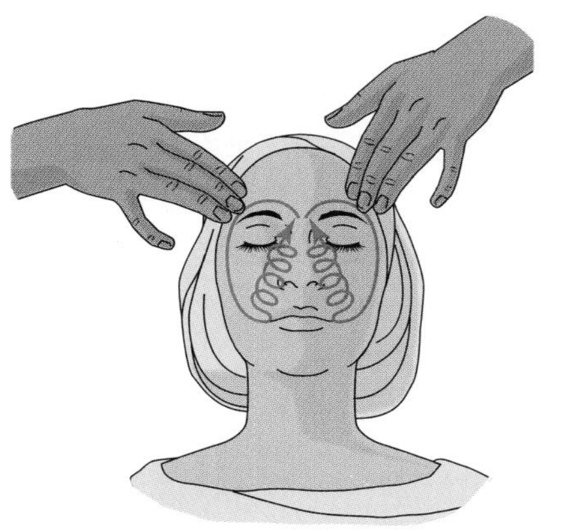

Figure 19-31 Mouth and nose movement.

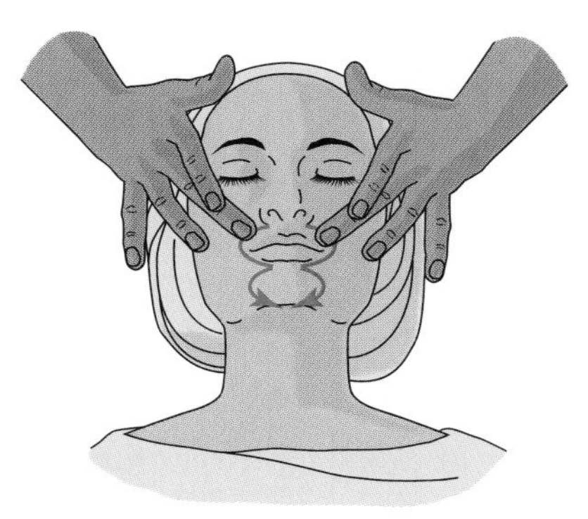

Figure 19-32 Lip and chin movement.

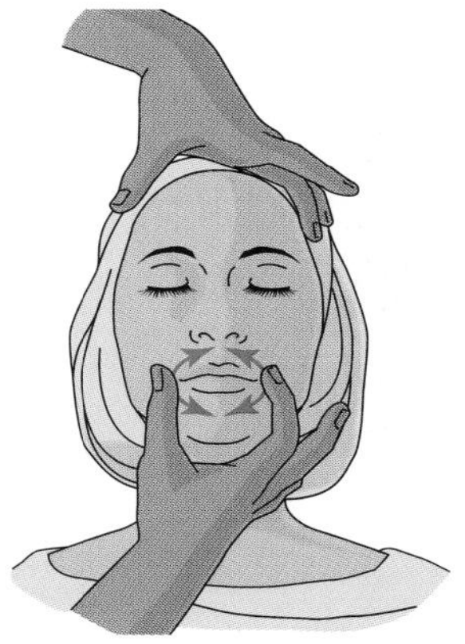

Figure 19-33 Optional movement.

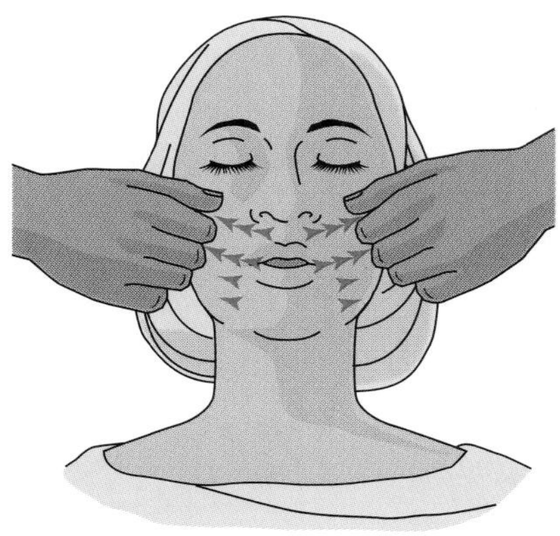

Figure 19-34 Lifting movement of cheeks.

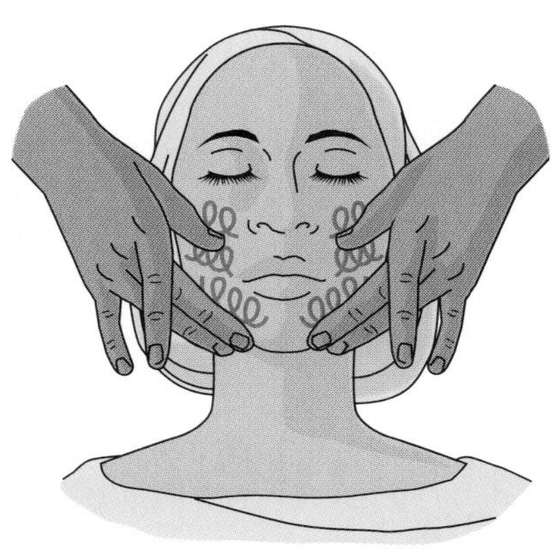

Figure 19-35 Rotary movement of cheeks.

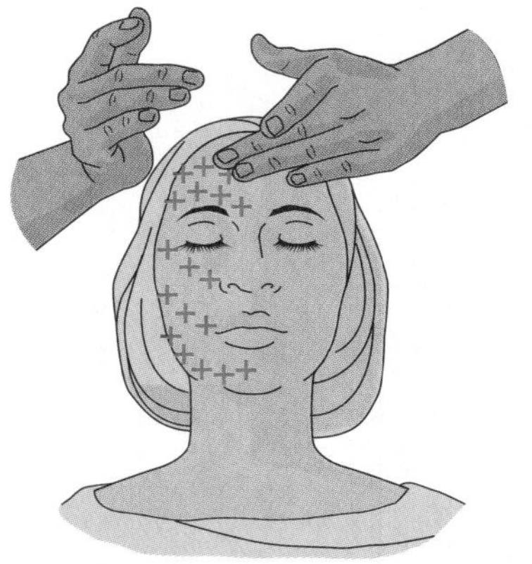

Figure 19–36 Light tapping movement.

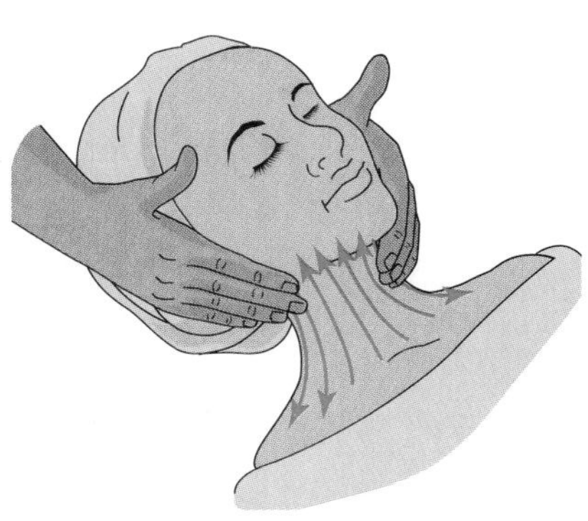

Figure 19–37 Stroking movement of neck.

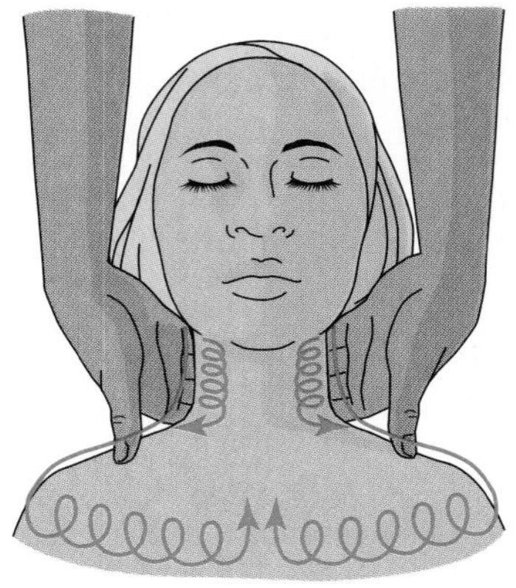

Figure 19–38 Circular movement over neck and chest.

- *Light tapping movement.* Work from the chin to the earlobe, from the mouth to the ear, from the nose to the top of the ear, and then across the forehead. Repeat on the other side (Figure 19–36).
- *Stroking movement of the neck.* Apply light upward strokes over the front of the neck. Use heavier pressure on the sides of neck in downward strokes (Figure 19–37).
- *Circular movement over the neck and chest.* Starting at the back of the ears, apply a circular movement down the side of the neck, over the shoulders, and across the chest (Figure 19–38).

Chest, Back, and Neck Manipulations (Optional)

Some instructors prefer to treat these areas first before starting the regular facial. Apply cleanser, then remove with a tissue or a warm moist towel. Then apply massage cream and perform the following manipulations:

- *Chest and back movement.* Use a rotary movement across the chest and shoulders, then down to the spine. Slide your fingers to the base of the neck. Rotate three times.
- *Shoulders and back movement.* Rotate the shoulders three times. Glide your fingers to the spine and then to the base of the neck. Apply circular movement up to the back of the ear, and then slide your fingers to the front of the earlobe. Rotate three times.
- *Back massage.* To stimulate and relax the client, use your thumbs and bent index fingers to grasp the tissue at the back of the neck. Rotate six times. Repeat over the shoulders and back to the spine.

Remove cream with tissues or a warm, moist towel. Dust the back lightly with talcum powder and smooth.

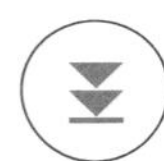

Here's a tip:

Male skin is not all that different from female skin. However, it needs more attention in the areas of the face where there is hair growth. For your male clients, use downward movements in the area of beard growth. It feels very uncomfortable if you massage against hair growth. Pressure point massage in the beard area is much appreciated by your male clients.

ELECTROTHERAPY AND LIGHT THERAPY

Electric facial machines are special appliances and equipment that are used to enhance the effectiveness of facial treatments. Electrical facial treatments are called **electrotherapy**. The currents used in electrical facial and scalp treatments are referred to as modalities. Each produces a different effect on the skin. There are many types of modalities, but cosmetologists are concerned with only the galvanic, faradic, sinusoidal, and high-frequency currents. Some devices have all four currents, and some have only one or two. (For a review of these modalities, refer to Chapter 7.)

An electrode is an applicator for directing the electric current from the machine to the client's skin (Figure 19–39). Except for the high-frequency modality, each of these modalities requires two electrodes, one negative and one positive, to conduct the flow of electricity through the body. A negative electrode is called a cathode, has a black plug and cord, and is marked with an "N" or a minus (–) sign. A positive electrode is called an anode, has a red plug and cord, and is marked with a "P" or a plus (+) sign (Figure 19–40).

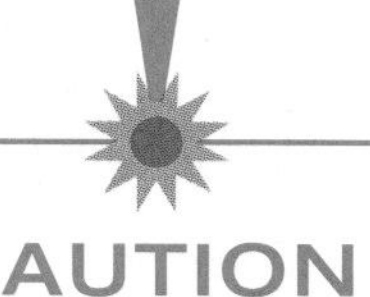

CAUTION

Do not use the galvanic current on the following clients:

- **with metal implants, a pacemaker, or any heart insufficiency.**
- **with epilepsy.**
- **who are pregnant.**
- **with high blood pressure, fever, or any infection.**
- **with insufficient nerve sensibility.**
- **with open or broken skin (wounds, new scars) or a pustular acne condition**
- **who are afraid of electrical current.**

Galvanic Current

The most commonly used device is the galvanic current machine (Figure 19–41). Significant chemical changes are produced when this current is used. Depending on which electrode is used on the area treated—negative or positive—galvanic current will produce two different chemical reactions.

Your client will experience the effects of the galvanic current as the current passes through the body from one electrode to the other and completes a circuit. Both the positive and negative poles must be functioning to complete the circuit. All electrodes must be firmly wrapped with a moistened cotton pledget.

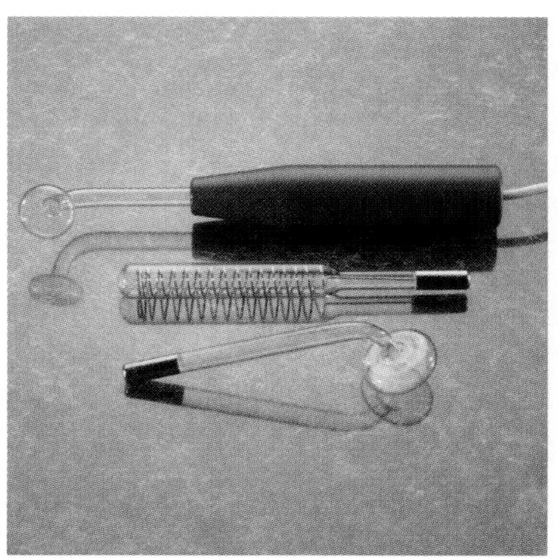

Figure 19-39 A variety of electrodes.

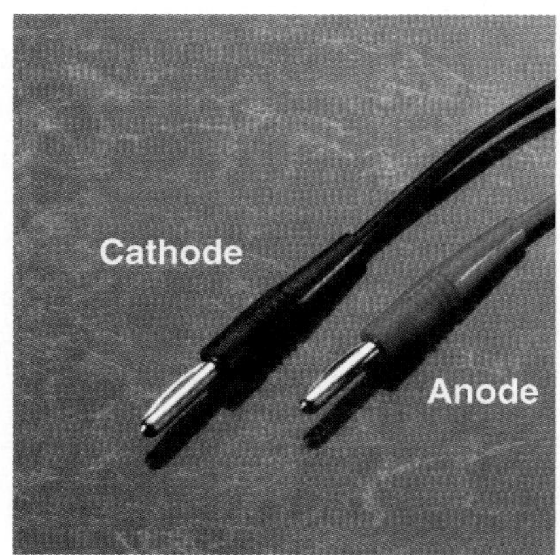

Figure 19-40 Cathodes.

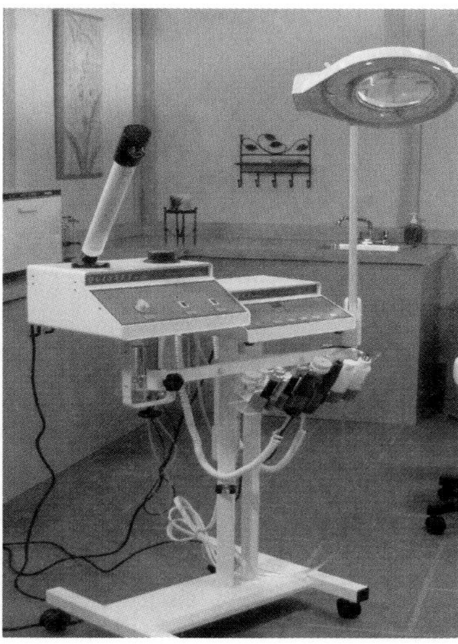

Figure 19-41 "Five-in-one" machine, including galvanic electrodes.

Figure 19–42 Applying galvanic current.

Application of Galvanic Current

The active electrode is the electrode used on the area to be treated. The negative pole is the active electrode when negative reactions are desired on the face, such as forcing negative ions into the skin, opening follicles, or liquefying sebum. Plug the black cord into the metal roller or flathead stick (mushroom-shaped) electrode. This is the electrode you use on the client's face and is also referred to as a desincrustator, although it is not used for desincrustation only (Figure 19–42).

The passive electrode actually is not passive at all but is called passive because it is not used on the client's face. Either your client can hold the metal stick or cylinder, wrapped in a moistened cotton pledget, or you can place the wet pad on the client's right upper arm or under the right shoulder.

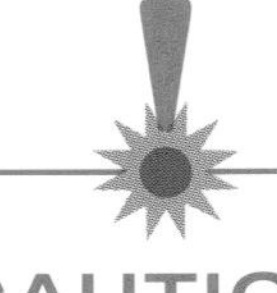

CAUTION

Place the passive electrode on the right side of the client's body only (never on the left side), to avoid current flow through the heart.

Desincrustation

Desincrustation (or disincrustation) is the process of softening and emulsifying grease deposits and blackheads in the follicles for easier extraction. The active electrode is wrapped with a cotton pledget saturated with an **electrolyte** (any compound that conducts a current of electricity). Salt water serves this purpose perfectly.

The passive electrode is wrapped in cotton moistened with water. The client holds the passive electrode in her right hand, or the wet pad is placed on a comfortable spot on the right side of the body. The active electrode (negative polarity) is placed on the client's face and moved slowly over the oily areas of the face for three to five minutes (Figure 19–43). After the procedure, all the liquefied sebum is removed from the skin before the facial continues.

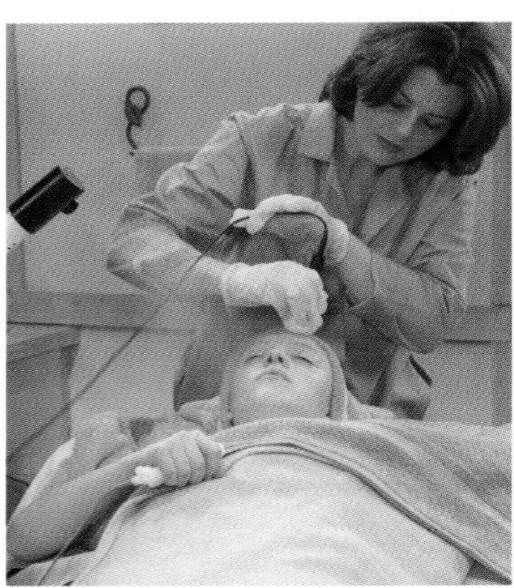

Figure 19–43 Client holding passive electrode.

Iontophoresis

The word *iontophoresis* comes from the Greek and means "moving ions." This process is used to force water-soluble products that contain ions deeper into the skin with the help of electric current such as galvanic current. The negative pole (cathode) forces negatively charged ions (anions) into the skin, in a process called anaphoresis. With the positive pole (the anode), positively charged ions (cations) are forced into the skin in a process called cataphoresis (see Chapter 7).

Faradic and Sinusoidal Currents

Faradic and sinusoidal currents produce impulses on the muscles and force them to contract. They are used during a facial to tone the facial muscles.

Application of Faradic and Sinusoidal Current

Two electrodes (one negative and one positive) are required to complete the faradic or sinusoidal circuit. The cathode is placed on the insertion of the muscle and the anode on the origin of the muscle. Let each muscle contract five to ten times and then move on to the next muscle.

To perform muscle stimulation treatments using faradic or sinusoidal current, you must know exactly where the facial muscles are and how to locate their insertions and origins. An in-depth study and thorough hands-on training is absolutely necessary.

High-Frequency Current

High-frequency (HF) current, discovered by Nikolas Tesla, has a germicidal effect, which makes it very beneficial for acne-prone skin. After treatment with a high-frequency machine, the skin is well stimulated and has increased blood supply. Any products applied after a high-frequency treatment penetrate more deeply.

The electrodes for high-frequency current are made of glass, and you need only one electrode to perform a service. The facial electrode for direct HF is mushroom-shaped and comes in a variety of sizes. The long electrode for indirect HF has a metal coil inside. As the air around the glass electrode vibrates, tiny violet sparks are emitted. Some units have neon gas in the tube, which produces an orange glow. All units produce the same effects.

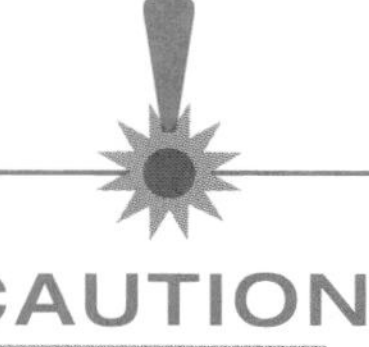

CAUTION

Do not use faradic current if it causes pain or discomfort. The same contraindications that apply to galvanic current apply as well to faradic and sinusoidal current.

Application of High-Frequency (Tesla) Current

All treatments given with high-frequency current should start with a mild intensity and gradually increase to the required strength. The length of the treatment depends on the condition being treated. Allow about five minutes for a general facial HF treatment. For proper use, always follow the manufacturers' instructions.

There are two methods for using high-frequency current.

1. *Direct surface application.* Do not apply any product to the client's face. If the glass electrode is hard to move on the skin, use some gauze over it. The cosmetologist holds the handpiece, where the glass electrode is inserted, and applies it directly to the client's skin, moving it slowly over the entire face for stimulation. When you apply and remove the electrode from the skin, you must hold your finger on the glass electrode to prevent sparking. Remove your finger once the electrode has been placed on the skin. Dab the electrode on a spot to cause sparking for stronger germicidal effect.
2. *Indirect application.* The client holds the tube electrode (with the metal coil inside) while you massage the face with your hands (Figure 19–44). At no time do you hold the electrode. To prevent shock, turn on the current only after the client has firmly grasped the electrode. Turn the current off before you remove the electrode from the client's hand. The indirect application of high-frequency current stimulates all cell functions without the irritation that could occur with direct application. This treatment is highly beneficial for sensitive, dehydrated skin. 4

In some states it is illegal to cause visible muscle contractions with faradic or sinusoidal currents. Always check with your regulatory agency.

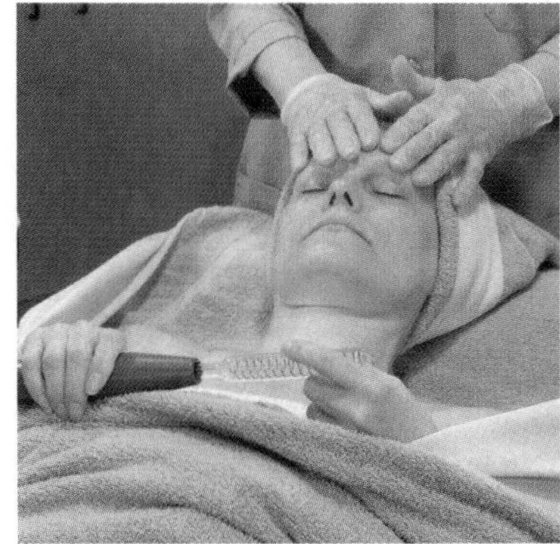

Figure 19–44 Client holding electrode as stylist massages the face.

Light Therapy

Light therapy refers to the application of light rays to the skin for the treatment of disorders. (Refer to Chapter 7 for a detailed discussion of light rays.) Light therapy makes use of infrared and ultraviolet rays as well as the white, blue, and red lights of the visible spectrum of light. Each of these produces a different effect on the skin. Refer to Table 19–2 for the effects of the various kinds of light therapy.

Artificial light rays are produced by an electrical apparatus called a therapeutic (ther-ah-PYOO-tic) lamp. The lamp has a dome-shaped

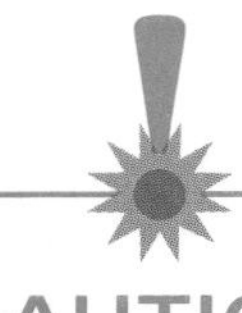

CAUTION

For high-frequency current, either direct or indirect, the same contraindications apply as for galvanic current. In addition, the client should avoid any contact with metal, such as chair arms, stools, jewelry, and metal bobby pins during the treatment. A burn may occur if such contact is made.

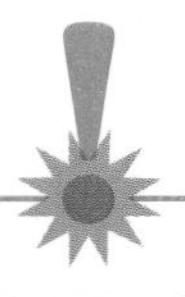

CAUTION

The client's eyes always should be protected during any light ray treatment. Use cotton pads saturated with alcohol-free freshener or distilled water. The eye pads protect the eyes from the glare of the reflecting rays.

Type of Light	Beneficial Effects
Ultraviolet	Increases the elimination of waste products Improves the flow of blood and lymph Has a germicidal and antibacterial effect Produces vitamin D in the skin Can be used to treat rickets, psoriasis, and acne Produces a tan
Infrared	Heats and relaxes the skin Dilates blood vessels and increases circulation Produces chemical changes Increases metabolism Increases production of perspiration and oil Deep penetration relieves pain in sore muscles Soothes nerves
White Light	Relieves pain in the back of the neck and shoulders Produces some chemical and germicidal effects Relaxes muscles
Blue Light	Soothes nerves Improves skin tone Provides some chemical and germicidal effects Used for mild cases of skin eruptions Produces little heat
Red Light	Improves dry, scaly wrinkled skin Relaxes muscles Penetrates the deepest Produces the most heat

Table 19-2 Effects of Light Therapy

reflector mounted on a pedestal with a flexible neck. The dome usually has a highly polished metal lining capable of reflecting the rays from the different types of light.

FACIAL TREATMENTS

A professional facial is one of the most enjoyable and relaxing services available to the salon client. Clients who have experienced this very restful yet stimulating experience do not hesitate to return for more. When

insights

Renée Poignard

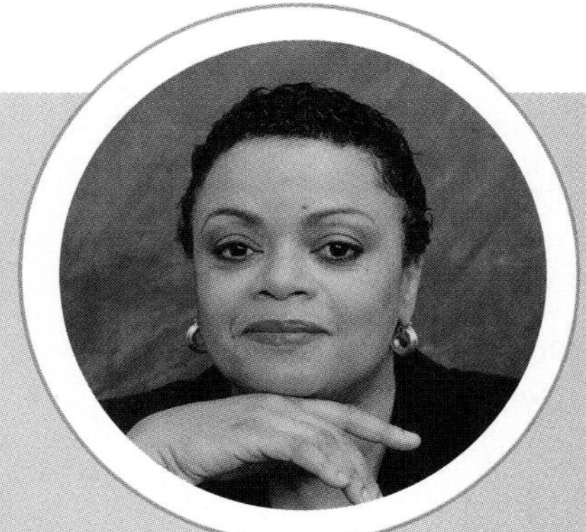

Renée Poignard, an esthetician in Atlanta, holds a Cidesco Diplomate, the highest certification an esthetician can achieve and one that demonstrates an understanding of both the American and European techniques of esthetics.

Back in 1977, I was a divorced mother and had to find a job. Since a lot of people always complimented me on my makeup, I decided to try that route. I applied for a position and when they asked me what my best quality was, I immediately said, "Honesty." Well, it was the right answer, because this salon had recently had a problem with employees pilfering products.

I knew from the beginning that this was the perfect job for me. It allowed me to use my creative side, but, even more than that, I realized that I had a love for people. I enjoyed the people I met, I enjoyed servicing them, and I liked learning about all the new things my clients told me about. Understanding what a person could achieve by working very, very hard was a thrill for me.

Now, after more than 25 years in the industry, I have to say that the aspect of my career I love the most is being an esthetics teacher and educating people in how to improve their physical appearance, their wellness, and their mental state. I think educating the client as to what is going on with their skin is an essential factor in building up a loyal client base. To keep your clients loyal, you have to educate them, satisfy their needs, stand behind your word, and make sure that you do everything you say you're going to do.

Patience is also a critical quality in a cosmetologist. If you have these qualities, then the retailing follows very naturally. For me, the key factor in retailing is keeping accurate records of my clients' visits and services—not only their basic health history, but also what they have purchased and what services they have and have not received. You need to be able to look at your records and know what products you sold your client three months ago and what she might need now. Every night, I examine the records of the clients I expect to see the next day. When I demonstrate my awareness of my client's history, she feels, "Wow. This is personal. She remembers this. She knows my products."

I teach a class on how to make more money in this industry, and that is the winner right there: to always preplan your day with your clients' service cards. Even when I teach to licensed professionals who have been in the business for five or six years, they're amazed. I give examples of the way little things can add up to as much as $500 or even $1000 per week extra for you. Isn't it exciting to think about going into a field where you can make that kind of "extra" money?

CAUTION

For sanitary reasons, never remove products from containers with your fingers. Always use a spatula.

focus on ...sharpening your personal skills.

If a client seems dissatisfied with a facial treatment, check to see if you have been guilty of any of the following:

- offensive breath or body odor.
- rough, cold hands or ragged nails that may have scratched the client's skin.
- allowing cream or other substances to get into the client's eyes, mouth, nostrils, or hairline.
- towels that were too hot or too cold.
- talking too much.
- manipulating the skin roughly or in the wrong direction.
- being disorganized and interrupting the facial to get supplies.

received on a regular basis, facials result in a noticeable improvement in the client's skin tone, texture, and appearance.

Facial treatments fall into two categories.

1. *Preservative*. Maintain the health of the facial skin by cleansing correctly, increasing circulation, relaxing the nerves, and activating the skin glands and metabolism through massage.
2. *Corrective*. Correct some facial skin conditions, such as dryness, oiliness, comedones, aging lines, and minor conditions of acne.

As with other forms of massage, facial treatments help to increase circulation, activate glandular activity, relax the nerves, maintain muscle tone, and strengthen weak muscle tissues.

Guidelines for Facial Treatments

Your facial treatments are bound to be successful and to inspire return visits if you follow some simple guidelines:

- Help the client to relax by speaking in a quiet and professional manner. Explain the benefits of the products and service, and answer any questions the client may have.
- Provide a quiet atmosphere, and work quietly and efficiently.
- Maintain neat, clean, sanitary conditions in the facial work area with an orderly arrangement of supplies.
- Follow systematic procedures.
- If your hands are cold, warm them before touching the client's face.
- Keep your nails smooth and short so as not to scratch the client's skin.

Another guideline you must always be sure to follow is to perform an analysis of your client's skin. After the client is draped and seated in the facial bed, you should inspect the skin to see if it is dry, normal, or oily; if fine lines or creases exist; if blackheads or acne are present; if dilated capillaries are visible; if the skin texture is smooth or rough; and if the skin color is even. The results of your analysis will determine what products to use for the massage, what areas of the face need special attention, how much pressure to use when massaging, and what equipment should be used.

Basic Facial

The steps for performing a basic facial are listed in Procedure 54. Some procedures may vary, however, so be guided by your instructor.

A note on the implements and materials you will need: the following list includes items for a basic facial. You can add other items if you wish. There are several types of head coverings on the market. Some are a turban design; others are designed with elastic, like a shower cap. They are generally made of either cloth or paper towels. For the paper towel procedure, be guided by your instructor.

Special Problems

There are a number of special problems that must be considered when you are performing a facial. These include dry skin, oily skin and blackheads, and acne.

Dry skin is caused by an insufficient flow of sebum (oil) from the sebaceous glands. The facial for dry skin helps correct this condition.

PROCEDURE

BASIC FACIAL

Equipment, Implements, and Materials

- facial bed or chair
- facial steamer
- garbage can
- magnifying lamp
- makeup tray
- trolley for products and implements

Implements and Materials

- clean sheet or other covering (blanket if necessary)
- cotton (roll)
- cotton pads
- cotton swabs and pledgets
- gauze
- headband or head covering
- salon gown
- towels
- plastic bobby pins/safety pins
- spatulas
- sponges
- tissues

Products

- antiseptic lotion
- astringent
- cleansers and makeup removers
- hand sanitizer
- massage cream or lubricating oil
- masks
- moisturizers
- sun protection products
- tonic lotions

Optional

- specialty or intensive care products
- infrared lamp
- other electrical equipment

Preparation

1. Wash your hands with soap and warm water before each client.
2. Greet the client in a friendly and professional way. This helps to put the client at ease.
3. Ask the client to remove any jewelry such as a necklace or earrings, and store it in a safe place. Clients may wish to keep their handbags nearby during the facial.

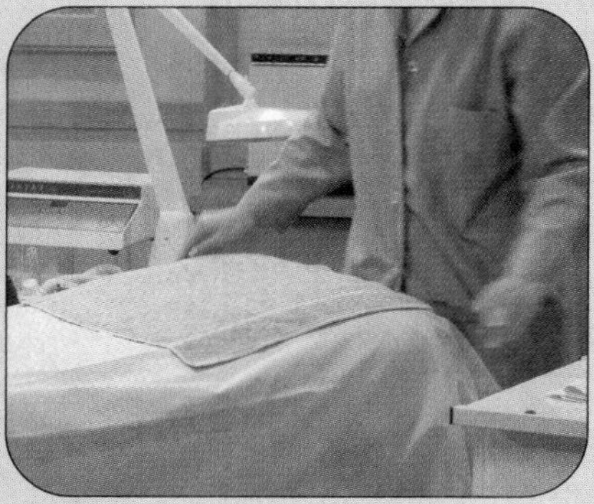

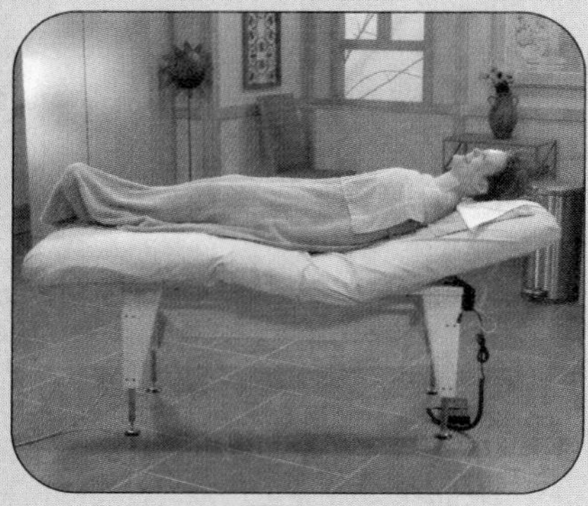

Figure 19-45 Place a towel across the back of the facial bed.

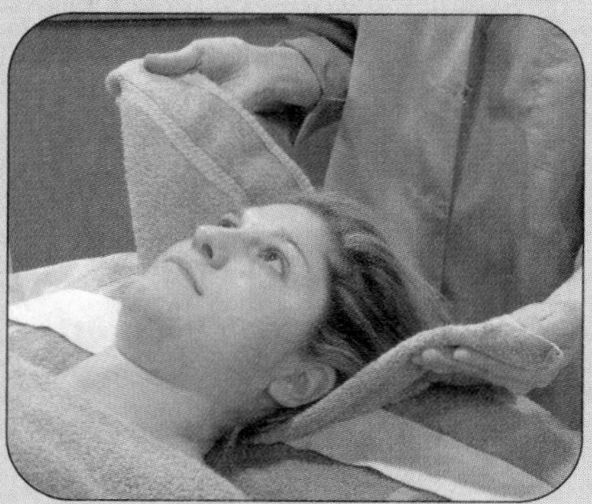

Figure 19-46 Client in facial bed.

4. Show the client to the dressing room and offer assistance if needed.
5. Place a clean towel across the back of the facial bed to prevent the client's bare shoulders from coming into contact with the bed (Figure 19–45).
6. Assist the client onto the facial bed (offer assistance if needed) and place a towel across the client's chest. Next, place a coverlet or sheet over the client's body and fold the top edge of the towel over it. Remove the client's shoes and tuck the coverlet around the feet (Figure 19–46). Some salons provide disposable slippers that can be worn to and from the dressing room.
7. Fasten a headband lined with tissue, a towel, or other head covering around the client's head to protect the hair. To drape the head with a towel, follow these steps:
   a. Fold the towel lengthwise from one of the top corners to the opposite lower corner, and place it over the headrest with the fold facing down. Place the towel on the headrest before the client enters the facial area.
   b. When the client is in a reclined position, the back of the head should rest on the towel, so that the sides of the towel can be brought up to the center of the forehead to cover the hairline (Figure 19–47 and Figure 19–48).
   c. Use a headband with a Velcro closure or a T-pin to hold the towel in place (Figure 19–49). Make sure that all stands of hair are tucked under the towel, that the earlobes are not bent, and that the towel is not wrapped too tightly (Figure 19–50).
8. Remove lingerie straps from a female client's shoulders. *Alternative method*: If client is given a strapless gown to wear, tuck the straps into the top of the gown.

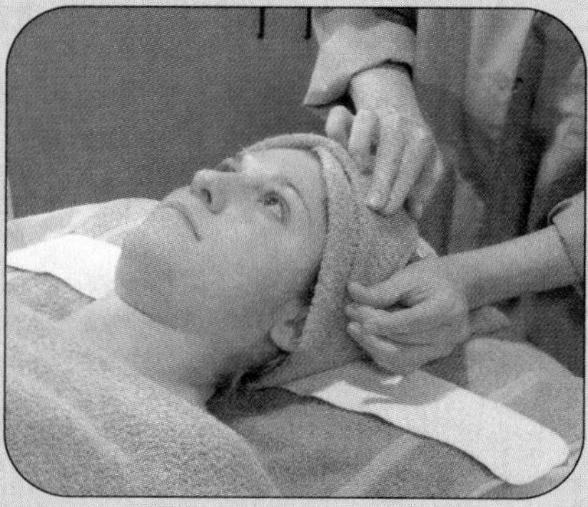

Figure 19-47 Bring the sides of the towel around the client's head.

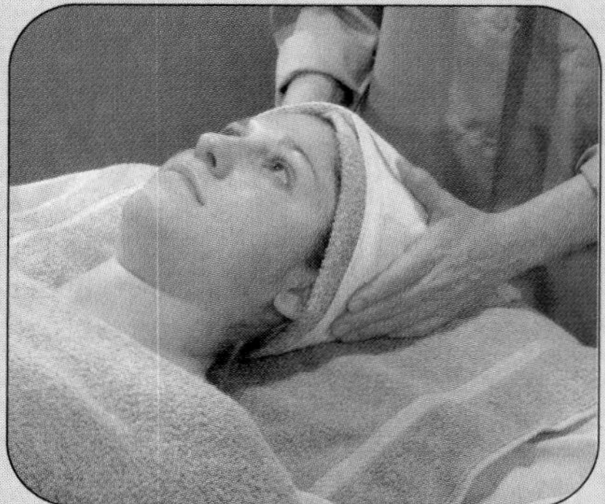

Figure 19-48 Bring one side of the towel over the other.

Figure 19-49 Secure the towel with a terrycloth headband.

9. Wash your hands with soap and warm water.
10. Perform a client consultation.

Procedure

1. If your client wears makeup, use the following steps to remove it. If your client has no makeup, skip this part and proceed to Step 2.
   a. Apply a pea-sized amount of eye makeup remover to each of two damp cotton pads and place them on the client's closed eyes. Leave them in place for one minute (Figure 19–51).
   b. Meanwhile, apply another pea-sized amount of eye makeup remover to a damp cotton pad and gently remove the client's lipstick with even strokes from the corners of the lips toward the center. Repeat the procedure until the lips are clean.
   c. Now, remove the eye makeup in the same way, gently stroking down and outward with the cotton pad. Do one eye first, then the other. Repeat the procedure until the eyelids and lashes are clean (Figure 19–52).
   d. Ask the client to look up, then remove any makeup underneath the eyes. Always be gentle around the eyes; never rub or stretch the skin, as it is very delicate and thin.
2. Apply cleanser
   a. Remove about a teaspoon of cleanser from the container with a clean spatula. Blend with your fingers to soften it.

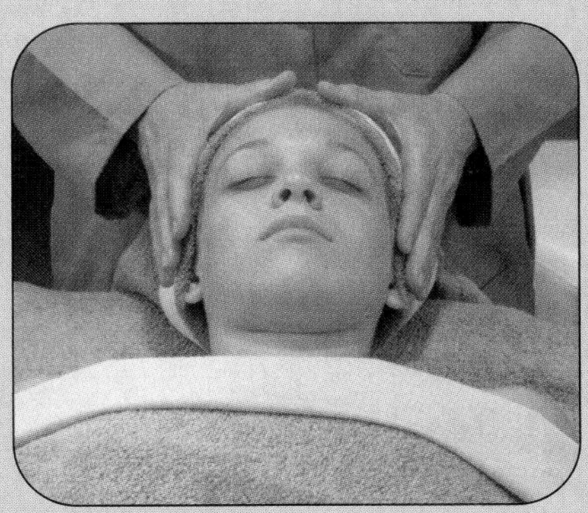

Figure 19-50 The client is prepared for the facial.

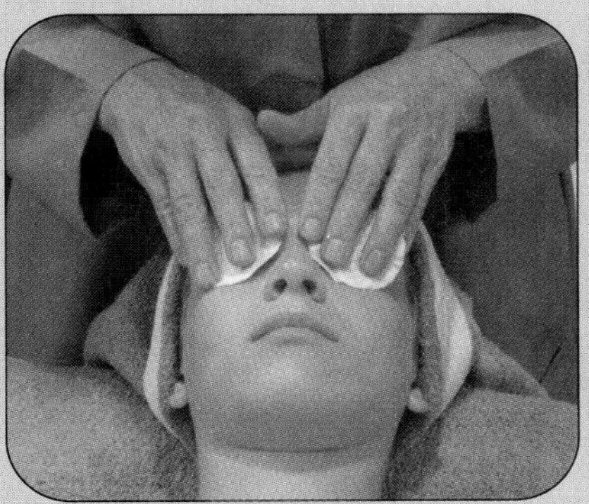

Figure 19-51 Leave cotton pads on the client's eyes.

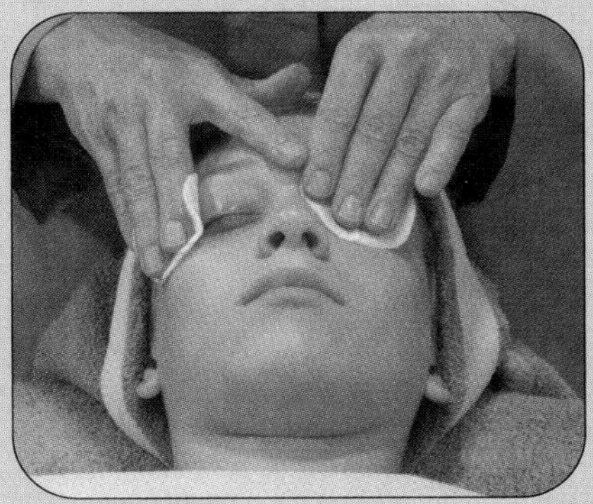

Figure 19-52 Stroke down and outward with the pads.

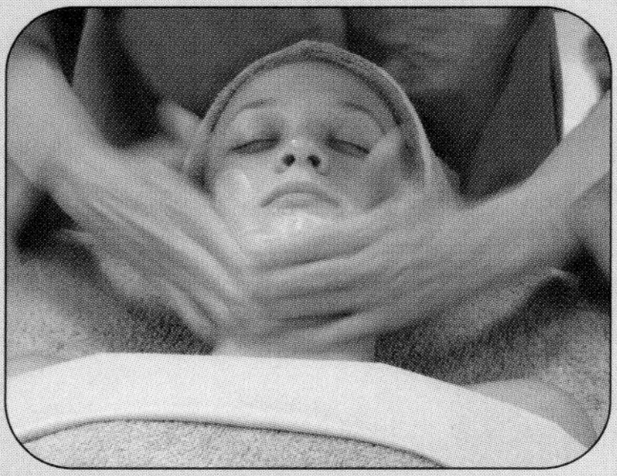

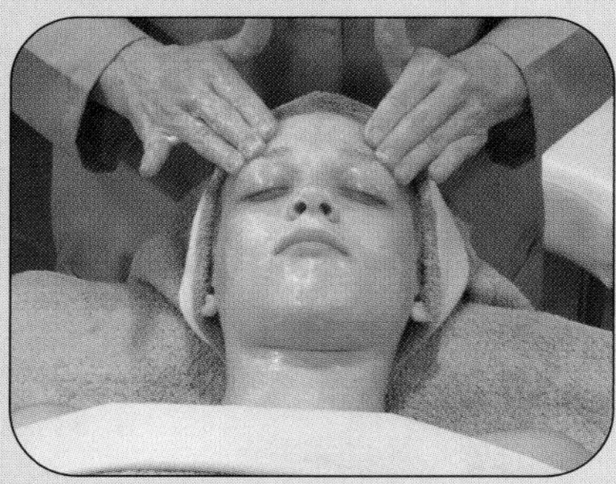

Figure 19-53 Spread cleanser over the neck.

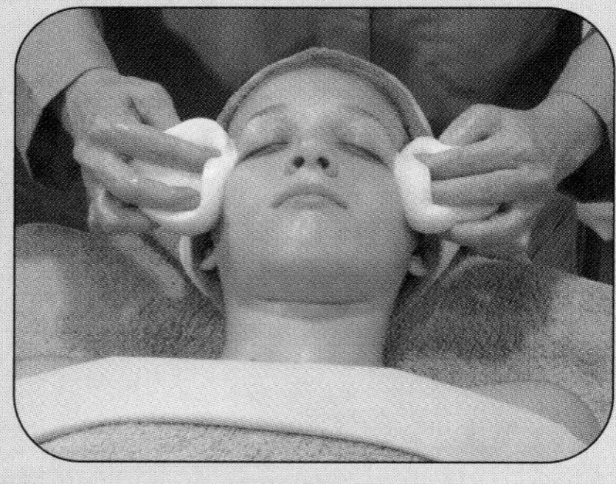

Figure 19-54 Spread cleanser over the forehead.

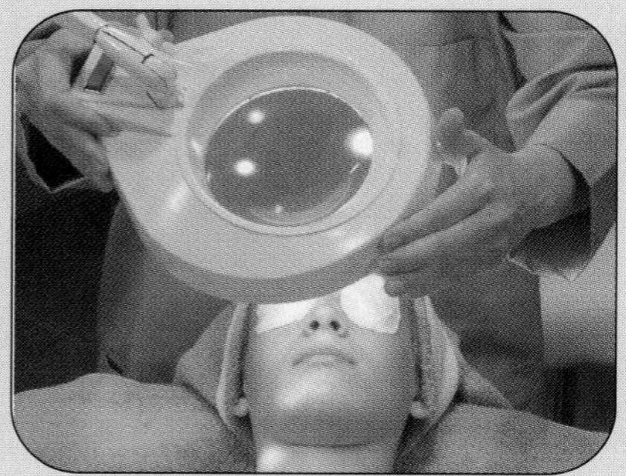

Figure 19-55 Remove cleanser with facial sponges.

b. Starting at the neck with a sweeping movement, use both hands to spread the cleanser upward on the chin, jaws, cheeks, and the base of the nose to the temples and along the sides and the bridge of the nose (Figure 19–53). Make small circular movements with your fingertips around the nostrils and sides of the nose. Continue the upward sweeping movements between the brows and across the forehead to the temples.

c. Take additional cleanser from the container with a clean spatula, and blend. Smooth down the neck, chest, and back with long, even strokes.

d. Starting at the center of the forehead, move your fingertips lightly in a circle around the eyes to the temples and then back to the center of the forehead (Figure 19–54).

e. Slide your fingers down the nose to the upper lip, from the temples through the forehead, lightly down to the chin, then firmly up the jawline back toward the temples and forehead.

3. Remove the cleanser with facial sponges, tissues, moist cotton pads, or warm, moist towels. Start at the forehead and follow the contours of the face. Remove all the cleanser from one area of the face before proceeding to the next. Finish with the neck, chest, and back (Figure 19–55).
4. Analyze the skin to determine the products and procedures to be used, as described on page 662-665 (Figure 19–56). *Optional:* If exfoliation or eyebrow arching is to be done, it should be done at this time.
5. Steam the face mildly with warm, moist towels or with a facial steamer to open the pores so they can be cleansed of oil and comedones. If you use a steamer, cover the client's eyes with cotton pads moistened with distilled water or alcohol-free freshener. Steam helps to soften superficial lines and increases blood circulation to the surface of the skin (Figure 19–57 and Figure 19–58).
6. Select a massage cream appropriate to the client's skin type. Using the same procedure as for the cleanser, apply the massage cream to the

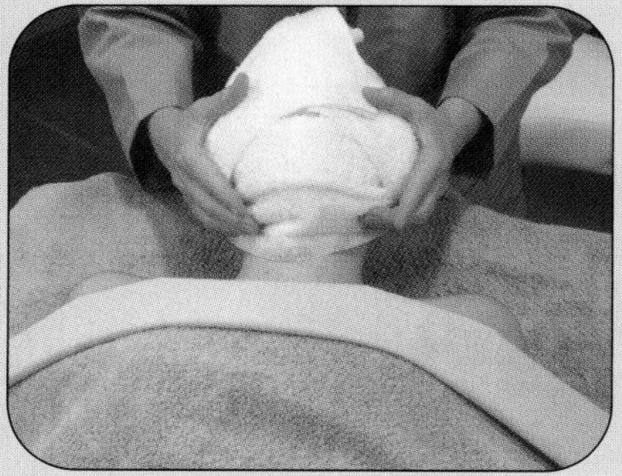

Figure 19-56 Analyze the skin.

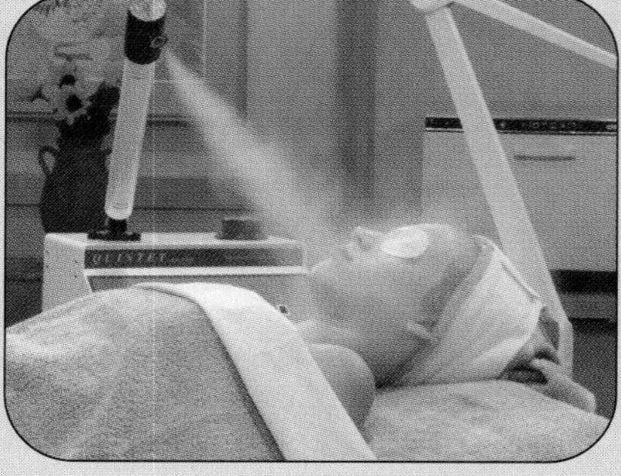

Figure 19-57 Steam the face with warm, moist towels.

Figure 19-58 You may also use a steamer to steam the face.

face, neck, shoulders, chest, and back (Figure 19–59). If needed, apply lubrication oil or cream around the eyes and on the neck. An optional step is exposing the face to infrared light. Place the lamp about 30 inches (76 cm) from the face. Cover the client's eyes with eye pads, and expose the face to infrared rays for no more than three to five minutes.

7. Massage the face, using the facial manipulations described on pages 669–672.
8. Remove massage cream with tissues, warm, moist towels, moist cleansing pads, or sponges. Follow the same procedure as for removing cleanser.
9. Sponge the face with cotton pledgets moistened with toner or freshener (Figure 19–60).
10. Apply a treatment mask formulated for the client's skin condition.
    a. Remove the mask from its container with a clean spatula and place it in a little cup.
    b. Apply the mask with a natural bristle brush, starting at the neck. Use long slow strokes from the center outward.
    c. Proceed to the jawline and apply the mask on the face from the center outward on one-half of the face, then the other (Figure 19–61).
    d. Allow it to remain on the face for seven to ten minutes.
11. Remove the mask with wet cotton pledgets, sponges, or towels (Figure 19–62).
12. Apply toner, astringent, or freshener.
13. Apply a moisturizer or sunscreen.

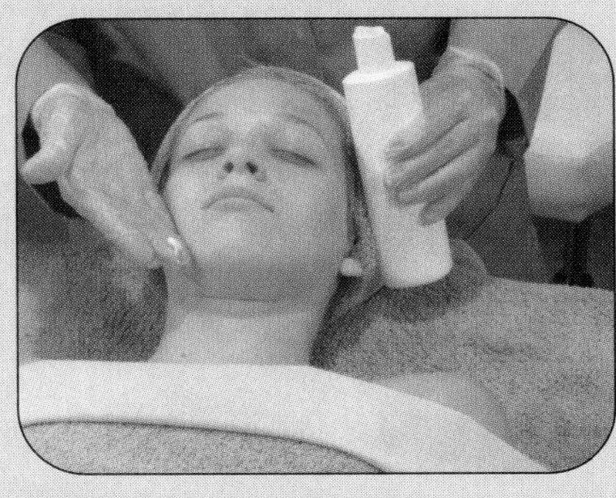

Figure 19-59 Apply massage cream.

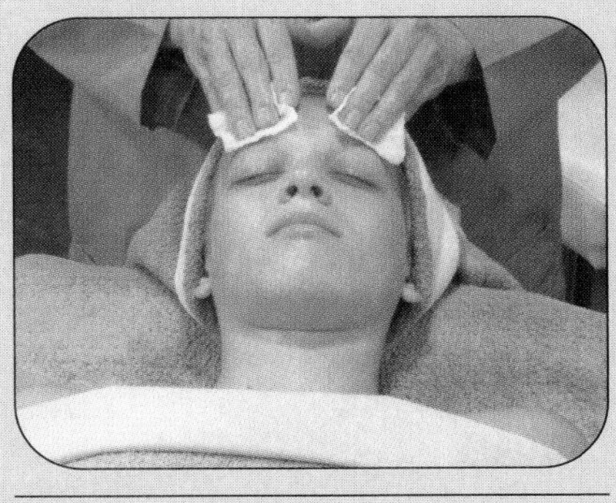

Figure 19-60 Apply tonic lotion or freshener.

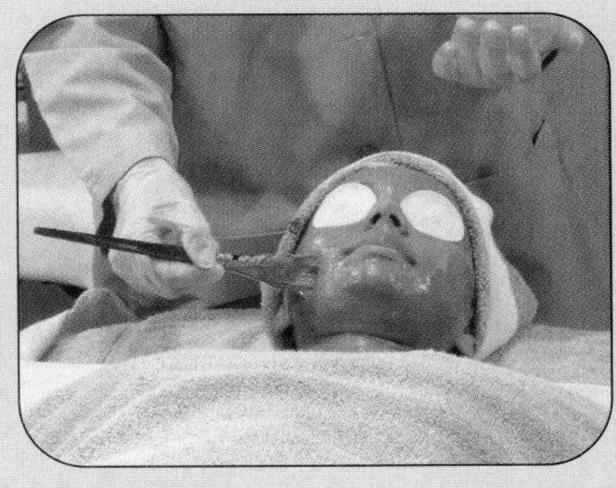

Figure 19-61 Apply a mask, starting at the neck.

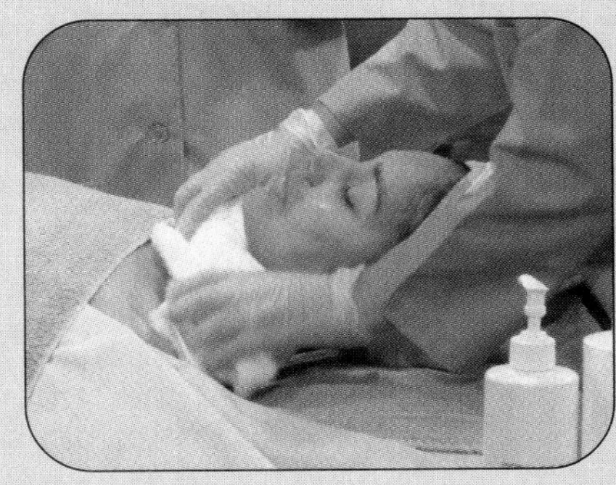

Figure 19-62 Remove the mask.

Cleanup and Sanitation

1. Remove the head covering and show the client to the dressing room, offering assistance if needed.
2. Discard all disposable supplies and materials.
3. Close product containers tightly, clean them, and put them away in their proper places. Return unused cosmetics and other items to the dispensary.
4. Place used towels, coverlets, head covers, and other linens in hamper.
5. Sanitize your workstation, including the facial bed.
6. Wash your hands with soap and warm water.

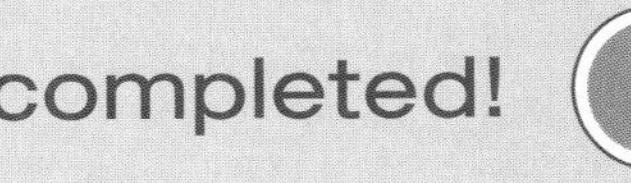

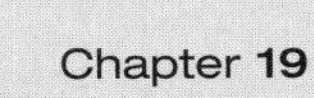
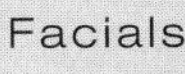

PROCEDURE

FACIAL FOR DRY SKIN

Electrotherapy in a dry skin facial can be performed using infrared rays, galvanic current, or high-frequency current.

Equipment, Implements, and Materials

These materials are in addition to those listed for Procedure 51— basic facial.

- infrared lamp, galvanic machine, or high-frequency machine, depending on treatment
- tonic lotion for dry skin
- nonalcohol freshener
- eye cream

Preparation

Prepare the client as for Procedure 51— basic facial.

19

CAUTION

For dry skin, avoid using lotions that contain a high percentage of alcohol. Read the manufacturers' directions.

Procedure with Infrared Rays

1. Apply cleanser, then remove with tissues or a warm, moist towel.
2. Sponge the face with tonic lotion.
3. Apply massage cream.
4. Apply eye cream over and under the eyes.
5. Apply lubricating oil over the neck.
6. Cover the client's eyes with cotton pads moistened with a nonalcohol freshener.
7. Expose the face and neck to infrared rays for not more than five minutes.
8. Perform manipulations, three to five times each movement.
9. Remove massage cream and oil with tissues or with a warm, moist towel.
10. Apply a tonic lotion suitable for dry skin. Blot the face with tissues.
11. Apply a moisturizer or base foundation suitable for the client's skin.
12. Complete and clean up as for a plain facial.

Procedure with Galvanic Current

1. Follow Steps 1 to 3 of the procedure for infrared rays.
2. Apply a thick layer of ionized, oil-free gel to the face and neck.
3. Apply negative galvanic current for five to seven minutes (Figure 19–63).
4. Reapply ionized, oil-free gel to the face and neck.
5. Apply positive galvanic current for four to six minutes.
6. Follow Steps 3 to 5 of the procedure with infrared rays.
7. Follow Steps 8 to 12 of the procedure with infrared rays.

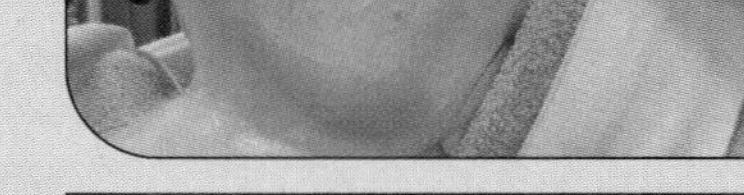

Figure 19–63 Apply galvanic current.

Procedure with Indirect High-Frequency Current

1. Follow Steps 1 through 5 of the procedure for infrared rays.
2. Have the client hold the electrode in his or her right hand.
3. Give manipulations, using the indirect method of applying high-frequency current, for seven to ten minutes (Figure 19–64). Do not use tapping movements. Do not lift your hands from the client's skin.
4. Apply two or three cold towels to the face and neck.
5. Follow Steps 9 to 12 of the procedure for a facial with infrared rays.

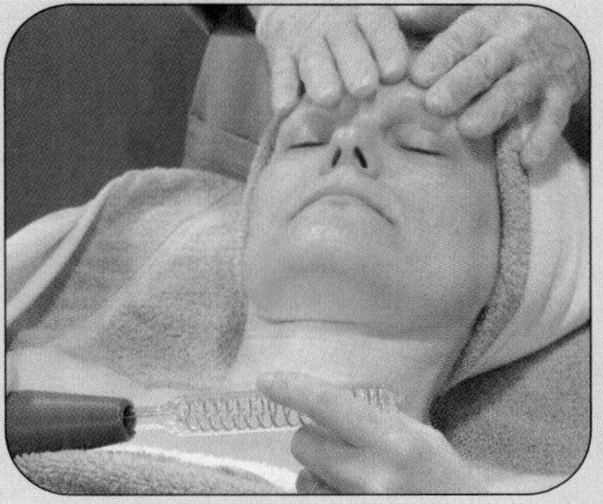

Figure 19–64 Apply indirect high-frequency current.

completed!

PROCEDURE 53

FACIAL FOR OILY SKIN AND BLACKHEADS

Equipment, Implements, and Materials

These materials are in addition to those listed for Procedure 51— basic facial.

- nonalcoholic freshener
- astringent lotion for oily skin
- gloves
- blue light (optional)

Preparation

Prepare the client as for Procedure 51—basic facial.

CAUTION

Some people are allergic to latex or rubber. Check with your client to determine whether a latex allergy exists, and, if so, make a note of this on the client card. Then proceed, using vinyl gloves.

Procedure

1. Apply cleanser and remove it with a warm, moist towel, moist cotton pads, or facial sponges.
2. Place moistened eye pads on the client's eyes and analyze the skin under a magnifying lamp.
3. Steam the face with moist, warm towels three or four times or a facial steamer to open the pores (Figure 19–65).
4. Wear latex gloves and, covering your fingertips with cotton, gently press out comedones. Place your middle fingers on either side of the comedone, stretching the skin first. Push your fingers down to reach underneath the follicle, and then squeeze gently, "massaging" out the comedone. Do not press so hard as to bruise the skin, and make sure you are not squeezing with bare fingers or fingernails (Figure 19–66).

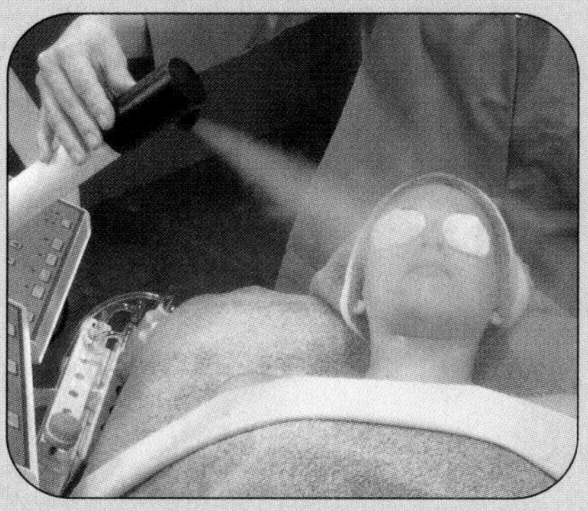

Figure 19-65 Steam the face.

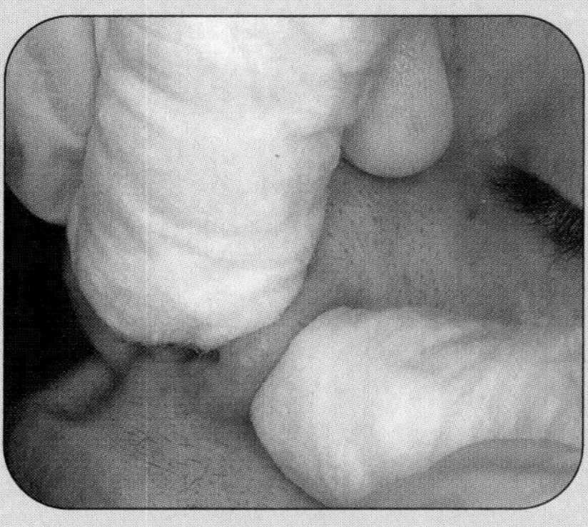

Figure 19-66 Press out comedones.

5. Sponge the face with astringent.
6. *Optional*: Cover the client's eyes with pads moistened with a nonalcohol freshener. Apply blue light over the skin for three to five minutes.
7. Apply a massage cream that is suitable for the skin condition. Perform facial manipulations.
8. Remove the massage cream with a warm, moist towel, cotton pads, or facial sponges.
9. Moisten a cotton pad with an astringent lotion. Apply it to the face and neck with upward and outward movements to constrict the pores. When treating a male client, use downward and outward movements in the direction of the beard hair growth.
10. Blot the skin dry with tissues.
11. Apply moisturizer or a protective lotion according to the skin type.
12. Complete and clean up as for Procedure 51—basic facial.

completed!

PROCEDURE

FACIAL FOR ACNE

Equipment, Implements, and Materials

These materials are in addition to those listed for a basic facial.

- acne cream or lotion
- astringent lotion for oily skin
- appropriate mask
- gloves
- high-frequency machine (optional)

Preparation

Prepare the client as for Procedure 51—basic facial.

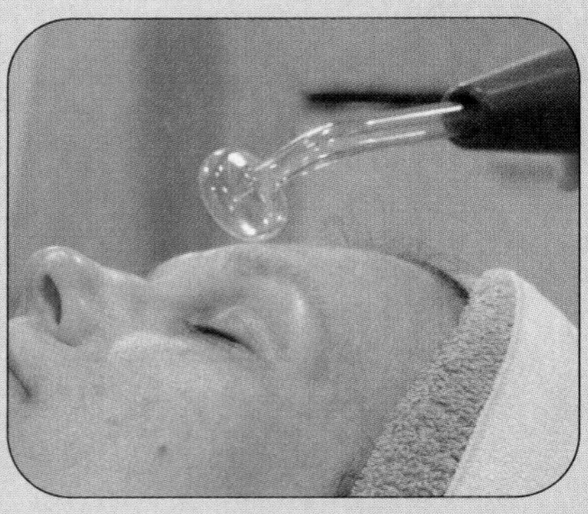

Figure 19-67 Apply high-frequency current with a facial electrode.

19

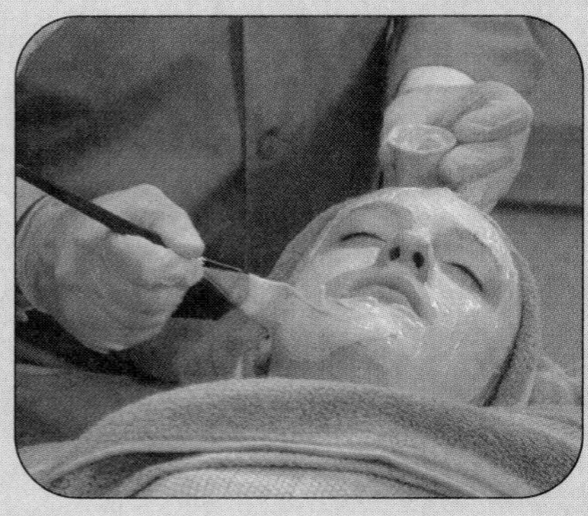

Figure 19-68 Apply a facial mask for acne skin.

Procedure

1. Cleanse the client's face as in Procedure 51—basic facial.
2. Place cotton eye pads over the client's eyes and analyze the skin under the magnifying lamp.
3. Apply warm, moist towels to the face to open the pores for deep cleansing.
4. Extract comedones as in previous procedure.
5. Cleanse the face with a wet cotton pad that has been sprinkled with astringent.
6. *Optional*: Apply high-frequency current with direct application (facial electrode) over the affected area for not more than five minutes (Figure 19–67). Be guided by your instructor.
7. Leave the eye pads on and apply a treatment mask that is suitable for acne skin. Allow it to remain on the face for about eight to ten minutes (Figure 19–68).
8. Remove the mask with moist cotton pads.
9. Apply astringent to the face with a wet cotton pad.
10. Apply special acne lotion or protective fluid.
11. Complete cleanup and sanitation procedures as for Procedure 51— basic facial.

completed!

Although it can be given with or without an electrical current, the use of electrical current provides better results.

Oily skin is often characterized by blackheads, or open comedones, which are caused by hardened masses of sebum formed in the ducts of the sebaceous glands. Oily skin can benefit from the facial procedure described below.

Acne is a disorder of the sebaceous glands that requires thorough and sometimes ongoing medical attention. If the client is under medical care, the role of the cosmetologist is to work closely with the client's physician, following the physician's instructions for the kind and frequency of facial treatments. Generally, medical direction limits the cosmetologist to the following measures in the treatment of acne:

- cleansing the skin
- reducing the oiliness of the skin by local applications
- removing blackheads, using proper procedures
- using special medicated preparations

Because acne skin contains infectious matter, you must wear protective gloves and use disposable materials such as cotton cleansing pads.

CAUTION

Aromatherapy is a healing method that should not be used on clients without proper training. It requires in-depth study of plants, essential oils, and the chemistry of those oils, as well as sound knowledge of human anatomy and physiology. A cosmetologist must not attempt to perform healing treatments with aromatherapy.

AROMATHERAPY

The therapeutic use of essential oils, which we now call **aromatherapy**, dates back to 2000 B.C. The ancient Egyptians, Greeks, and Romans all used oils derived from plants for many purposes, including healing, perfumes, hypnosis, and meditation.

Today, the skilled use of essential oils can enhance a person's physical, emotional, mental, and spiritual well-being. Using various oils and oil blends for specific benefits can create positive effects on the body, mind, and spirit (Figure 19–69).

Essential oils can be used in a variety of ways. Lighting a cinnamon candle in the winter can give the salon a cozy feeling and cheer up both clients and service givers. You can use a spray bottle to spray well-diluted essential oils on yourself, the treatment room, or the sheets. For a more balanced massage, you can create your own aromatherapy massage oil by adding a few drops of essential oil into basic massage oil, cream, or lotion. Always be careful to use essential oils lightly, however, as they sometimes have a tendency to be overpowering.

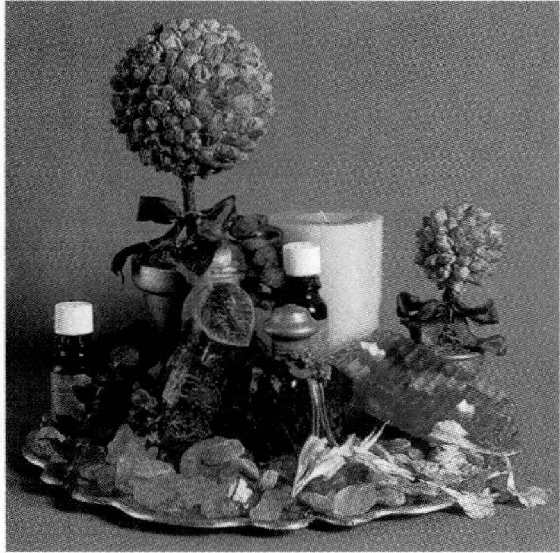

Figure 19–69 Some ingredients for aromatherapy.

focus on ...sharpening your personal skills.

The importance of following proper hygiene and sanitation guidelines when giving facials cannot be overemphasized. As much as possible, perform your sanitation procedures in the presence of your clients. When they see you doing this, they will feel more confidence in you as a professional.

FACE VALUE

You can see from the chapter you have just studied that the range of options open to the professional who performs facials is extensive and exciting. There is a lot to learn, with new advances coming every year. It is important to stay on top of your craft, to continue to learn as much as you can, and to be open to people. Your sensitivity to your clients will carry you far. If you do your job well, you will find yourself in great demand. It is very rewarding to make people feel good during a facial service and confident about how they look when they go out into the world.

chapter glossary

alphahydroxy acids	acids derived from plants, mostly fruit, and used in chemical exfoliants
ampules	sealed glass vials containing highly concentrated extract in a water or oil base
aromatherapy	therapeutic use of essential oils
astringents	tonic lotions with an alcohol content of up to 35 percent; used to remove oil accumulation on oily and acne-prone skin
chemical exfoliation	exfoliation in which dead skin cells or the intercellular "glue" that holds them together is dissolved by chemical agent such as alphahydroxy acids and enzymes.
chucking	massage movement accomplished by grasping the flesh firmly in one hand and moving the hand up and down along the bone while the other hand keeps the arm or leg in a steady position
clay masks	clay preparations used to stimulate circulation and temporarily contract the pores of the skin
cleansing cream	light-textured, oil-based emulsion used primarily to dissolve makeup and soil quickly
cleansing lotion	lotion formulated to remove makeup and soil
effleurage	light, continuous stroking movement applied with the fingers (digital) or the palms (palmar) in a slow, rhythmic manner
electrolyte	any compound that conducts a current of electricity
electrotherapy	electrical facial treatments
emollients	agents that soften or smooth the surface of the skin
enzyme peels	chemical exfoliants that involve the use of enzymes that help speed up the breakdown of keratin, the protein in skin
exfoliant	ingredient that assists in the process of exfoliation
exfoliation	peeling and shredding of the horny (outer) layer of the skin
face wash	detergent-type foaming cleanser with a neutral or slightly acidic pH
fresheners	tonic lotions with the lowest alcohol content (0 percent to 4 percent); beneficial for dry and mature skin and sensitive skin conditions
friction	deep rubbing movement requiring pressure on the skin with the fingers or palm while moving it over an underlying structure
fulling	form of petrissage in which the tissue is grasped, gently lifted, and spread out; used mainly for massaging the arms
gommage	enzyme peels in which a cream is applied to the skin before steaming and forms a hardened crust that is then massaged or "rolled" off the skin; also called "vegetal peeling"
hacking	chopping movement performed with the edges of the hands in massage
keratolytic enzymes	substances that help speed up the breakdown of keratin, the protein in skin

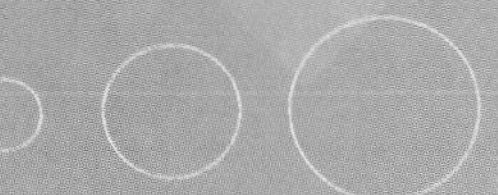

chapter glossary *(continued)*

light therapy	the application of light rays to the skin for the treatment of disorders
mask	special cosmetic preparation applied to the face to benefit and beautify the skin; usually a setting product
massage	manual or mechanical manipulation of the body by rubbing, pinching, kneading, tapping, and other movements to increase metabolism and circulation, promote absorption, and relieve pain
massage creams	lubricants designed to give the practitioner a good slip (slippery quality) during massage
mechanical exfoliation	exfoliation in which some method of physical contact is used to scrape or bump cells off the skin
microdermabrasion	mechanical exfoliation that involves "shooting" aluminum oxide or other crystals at the skin with a hand-held device that exfoliates dead cells
modelage masks	facial masks containing special crystals of gypsum, a plaster-like ingredient
moisturizers	products formulated to add moisture to the skin
motor point	point on the skin over the muscle where pressure or stimulation will cause contraction of that muscle
packs	special cosmetic preparations applied to the face to benefit and beautify the skin; condition sensitive skin and have excellent hydrating properties
paraffin wax masks	specially prepared facial masks containing paraffin and other beneficial ingredients; usually used with treatment cream
petrissage	kneading movement performed by lifting, squeezing, and pressing the tissue with a light, firm pressure
rolling	massage movement in which the tissues are pressed and twisted using a fast back-and-forth movement
sulfur masks	facial masks containing sulfur, which helps to reduce the production of sebum
tapotement or percussion	most stimulating massage movement, consisting of short, quick tapping, slapping, and hacking movements
toners	skin lotions with an alcohol content of 4 to 15 percent, designed for use on normal and combination skin
treatment or nourishing creams	creams designed to hydrate and condition the skin during the night; heavier in consistency and texture than moisturizers
vibration	in massage, the rapid shaking of the body part while the balls of the fingertips are pressed firmly on the point of application
wringing	vigorous movement in which the hands, placed a little distance apart on both sides of the client's arm or leg and working downward, apply a twisting motion against the bones in the opposite direction

review questions

1. What are the five main categories of professional skin care products?
2. On what skin types should you not use a mechanical exfoliant?
3. What is the difference between treatment creams and massage creams?
4. How are paraffin and modelage masks used?
5. Explain the importance of the client consultation with regard to facials.
6. What information should be written on the record card?
7. Why is it important to give home care advice?
8. Briefly describe the four basic skin types.
9. Explain the purpose of massage.
10. Name and briefly describe the five categories of massage manipulations.
11. Name the different kinds of electrical current used in facials.
12. Name and define the two basic categories of facial treatments.
13. List the steps involved in giving a basic facial.

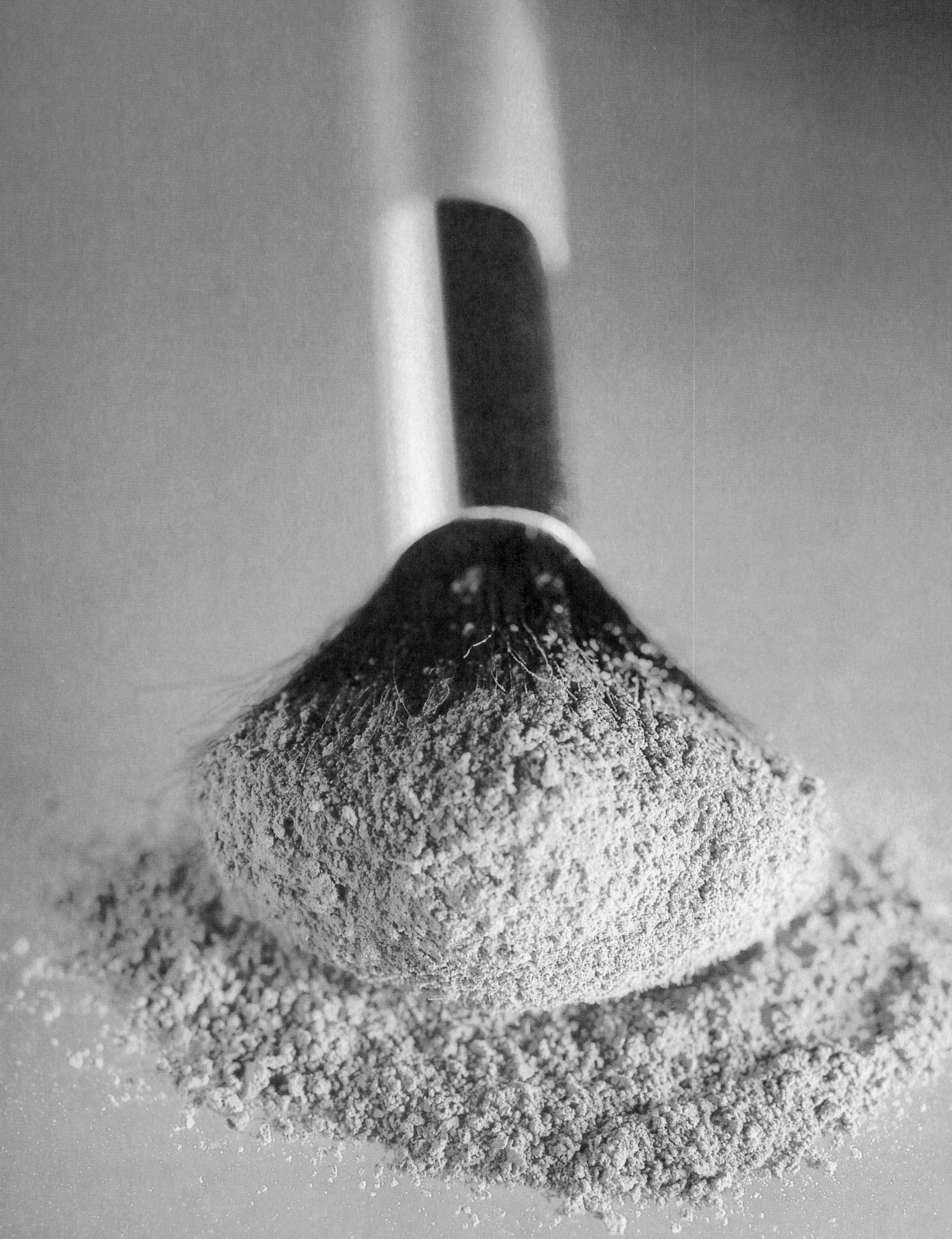

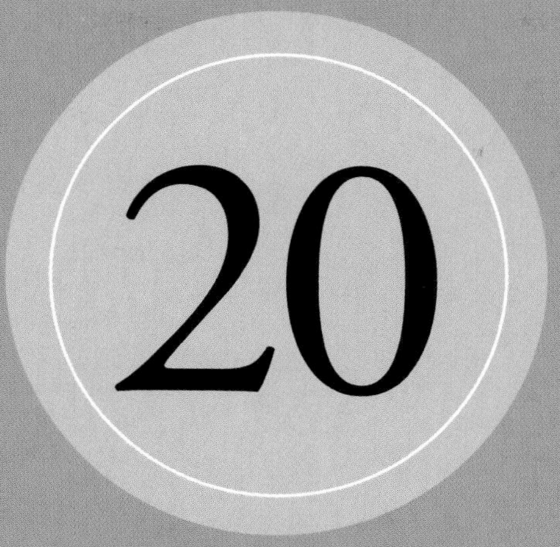

FACIAL MAKEUP

Teresa Sammarco
FREELANCE MAKEUP ARTIST AND EDUCATOR

Chapter Outline

Cosmetics for Facial Makeup • Makeup Color Theory
Client Consultation • Corrective Makeup
Artificial Eyelashes • Safety Precautions

Learning Objectives

After completing this chapter, you should be able to:

1. Describe the different types of cosmetics and their uses.
2. Demonstrate an understanding of cosmetic color theory.
3. Demonstrate a basic makeup procedure for any occasion.
4. Identify different facial types and demonstrate procedures for basic corrective makeup.
5. Demonstrate the application and removal of artificial lashes.
6. List safety measures to be followed during makeup application.

National Skill Standards

This chapter provides you with the necessary information to master these National Industry Skill Standards for Entry-Level Cosmetologists.

Consulting with clients to determine their needs and preferences.

Applying appropriate cosmetics to enhance a client's appearance.

Conducting services in a safe environment and taking measures to prevent the spread of infectious and contagious diseases.

Effectively marketing professional salon products.

Key Terms

Page number indicates where in the chapter the term is used.

band lashes
pg. 728

cake (pancake) makeup
pg. 704

cheek color
pg. 700

concealers
pg. 699

cool colors
pg. 708

eyebrow pencils
pg. 703

eyelash adhesive
pg. 728

eyeliner
pg. 703

eye makeup removers
pg. 704

eye shadows
pg. 702

eye tabbing
pg. 732

face powder
pg. 699

foundation
pg. 698

greasepaint
pg. 704

lip color
pg. 701

lip liner
pg. 701

mascara
pg. 704

matte
pg. 698

warm colors
pg. 708

Makeup has a magical quality that speaks to both the cosmetologist and the client. It brings to mind weddings, proms, and glamorous events and is often the secret ingredient in film and theater. Each year brings increased sophistication to the art and science of makeup. In the 21st century, the magic of makeup is more powerful than ever, thanks to technological advances and the intensive training of cosmetologists such as yourself.

For most clients, makeup application should be subtle. The main objective is to emphasize the client's most attractive facial features while minimizing those features that are less attractive. There is no fixed pattern for applying facial makeup; application will vary from client to client, based on your analysis of each client's face and her individual needs. When applying makeup, you must take into consideration the structure of the face; the color of the eyes, skin, and hair; how the client wants to look; and the results you can realistically achieve (Figure 20–1).

You will be better equipped to make use of cosmetics in your professional services when you have learned the chemical composition and preparation of cosmetics. Once you know these basics, you can use makeup to create optical illusions with shadowing, highlighting, and color. The client's natural beauty can be enhanced by a blend of facial makeup, hairstyle, and clothing colors.

Figure 20–1 Enhancing a client's natural beauty.

COSMETICS FOR FACIAL MAKEUP

The cosmetics industry offers a wide range of products designed to improve the skin's appearance as well as its condition. The cosmetics available today meet the needs of every skin type (Figure 20–2).

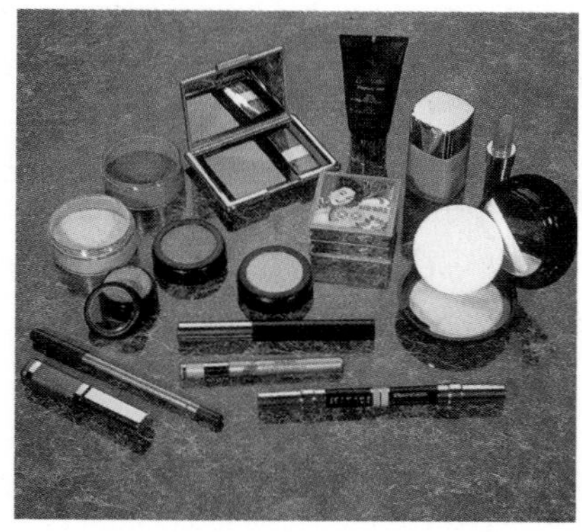

Figure 20–2 A wide variety of cosmetics is available to you and your client.

focus on ...retailing.

Retailing cosmetics is a great way to increase your income. Most salons will pay you 5 to 10 percent of every product you retail. If you focus on retailing to every client, this amount will add up quickly. It is not unusual for a cosmetologist who is retailing makeup on a daily basis to pay for a vacation or even make car payments using these rewards. And you will be helping your client out by giving her professional advice and allowing her to shop for makeup while she is receiving other salon services. So take advantage of this terrific opportunity. If you don't, the department store down the street surely will!

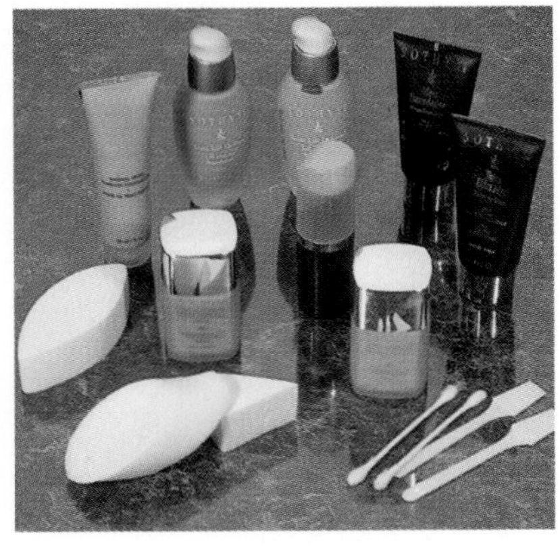

Figure 20-3 Foundations.

Here's a tip:

The label "oil-free" on a foundation only means that it is free of mineral oil. Most foundations contain some amount of oil, which provides consistency in binding properties. Oil levels vary, so ask if a product is safe for oily or acne skin.

Foundation

Foundation is a cosmetic, usually tinted, that is used as a base or as a protective film applied before makeup and/or powder. Foundation evens skin tone and color, conceals minor imperfections of the skin, and protects the skin from climate, dirt, and debris.

Liquid foundation, stick foundation, cream-to-powder foundation, and tinted moisturizer are the most widely used types and give a natural coverage with a slight sheen. They usually contain mineral oil or essential oil and are referred to as oil-based. These products are a good choice for normal to dry skin. Oil-free products are referred to as water-based, water being the main ingredient. Water-based liquid foundation, cream-to-powder foundation, or powder foundations generally give a more **matte** (dull, nonshiny) finish and help conceal minor blemishes and discolorations. These foundations are particularly effective for oily skin as they will not add more oil to the skin (Figure 20–3).

Foundation Chemistry

Cream foundations are predominantly water, mineral oil, stearic acid, cetyl alcohol, propylene glycol, triethanolamine, lanolin derivatives, borax, and insoluble pigments. Foundations may also contain surfactants (detergents), emulsifiers, humectants, perfume, and preservatives such as paraben. The formulation of these products is generally suited for dry to normal skin and gives medium to full coverage.

Liquid foundations are suspensions of organic and inorganic pigments in alcohol and water-based solutions. Most liquid foundations must be shaken before use, but bentonite is added to help keep the products blended. The formulation of this product is generally suited for clients with oily to normal skin conditions who desire sheer to medium coverage.

Powder foundations consist of a powder base mixed with a coloring agent (pigment) and perfume, and are especially effective for oily skin. Cream-to-powder foundations are moist on application but dry to a powdery finish.

Many foundations contain barrier agents, such as sunscreen and silicone, to protect the complexion from environmental damage.

Using Foundation

The success of the entire makeup application depends on the correct color selection and application of the foundation. When correctly matched and applied, foundation creates an even canvas for the rest of the makeup application.

Skin tone determines the selection of foundation color. Skin tones are generally classified as warm, cool, or neutral. Warm tones are generally classified as yellow, orange, or red-orange. Cool tones are generally referred to as blue, blue-green (olive), or blue-red (pink). Neutral skin has equal amounts of warm and cool tones (see "Makeup Color Theory" later in this chapter).

Foundation should always be matched as closely as possible to the actual skin tone. If foundation color is too light, it will have a chalky or gray appearance and will "sit" on top of the skin, exaggerating imperfections. If the color is too dark, it will look dirty or muddy on the skin. The best way to determine the correct foundation color for your client is to apply a stripe of color to clean skin on the jawline. Blend slightly, then repeat with two or three colors. The color that "disappears" on the skin is the correct tone. Avoid creating a contrast between the color of the face and the color of the neck. Makeup should be matched in color and blended smoothly with no visible line of demarcation.

Liquid foundation, tinted moisturizer, and tube foundation are taken from the container with a spatula, then applied to the face with the fingertips or a facial sponge. Powder and cream-to-powder foundation may be applied with a moist or dry facial sponge.

Concealers

Concealers are used to cover blemishes and discolorations and may be applied before or after foundation. They are available in pots, pencils, wands, and tubes or sticks in a range of colors to coordinate with or match natural skin tones. Any form of concealer may contain moisture or control oil, depending on the brand. Some specifically treat acne and oiliness, while others provide anti-aging ingredients and moisturizing benefits.

Generally, pot concealer is the heaviest and provides the most coverage. Pencil concealer gives sheer to medium coverage and may contain some moisture. Wand concealer is usually sponge- or brush-tipped and in fluid consistency. Tube or stick concealer is usually medium to sheer and may double as a foundation.

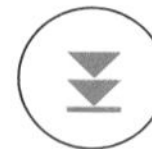

Here's a tip:

Concealer may be worn alone, without foundation, if chosen and blended correctly. Be sure to use it sparingly and soften the edges so that the complexion looks like clear, even skin rather than a heavy makeup application.

Concealer Chemistry

The chemical composition of concealers is similar to that of cream foundation.

Using Concealer

Concealer is removed from the container with a spatula and may be applied with a concealer brush or sponge. Place it sparingly over blemishes or areas of discoloration and blend it into the surrounding skin with a facial sponge. It is important to match concealer color to skin as closely as possible. Concealer that is noticeably lighter than skin can appear "raccoon-like," and can actually draw attention to a problem area such as dark circles. If covering a blemish, match skin very closely so as not to highlight the blemish. The principles that apply to choosing foundation colors also apply to concealer colors.

20

Face Powders

Face powder is a fine cosmetic powder, sometimes tinted and scented, that is used to add a matte or dull finish to the face. It improves the overall attractiveness of the skin by enhancing the skin's natural color, helping to conceal minor blemishes and discolorations, and toning down excessive color and shine. Face powder is also used to set the foundation (Figure 20–4).

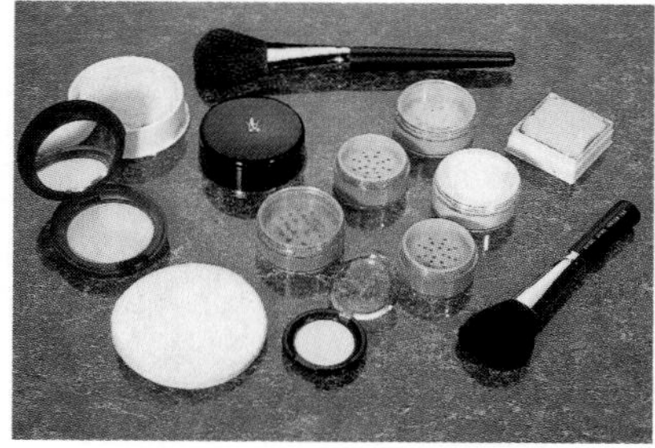

Figure 20-4 Commonly used forms of powder.

Face Powder Chemistry

Two forms of face powder are widely used in the salon: loose powder and pressed powder. Both types have the same basic composition; pressed powders are simply compressed and held together with binders so they will not crumble.

Face powder consists of a powder base mixed with a coloring agent (pigment) and perfume. Ingredients in most powders include talc, zinc oxide, titanium dioxide, kaolin, chalk, zinc stearate, and magnesium stearate. Bactericides are also added to inhibit the growth of bacteria and preserve the product.

Using Face Powder

Face powders are available in a variety of tints and shades and in different weights. Light and medium weights are generally best for dry to normal skin, while a heavier weight is effective on skin that is normal to oily. Face powder should match the natural skin tone and work well with the foundation. It should never appear caked, spotted, or streaked on the face. Translucent powder (colorless and sheer) blends with all foundations and will not change color when applied.

Apply face powder after foundation using a fresh cotton puff. Press the powder over the face in the desired areas, then use a powder brush or another puff to remove the excess.

When suggesting products to a client, recommend both loose and pressed powders. Pressed powder is compact and easy to carry for quick touch-ups during the day. Loose powder is best used at home.

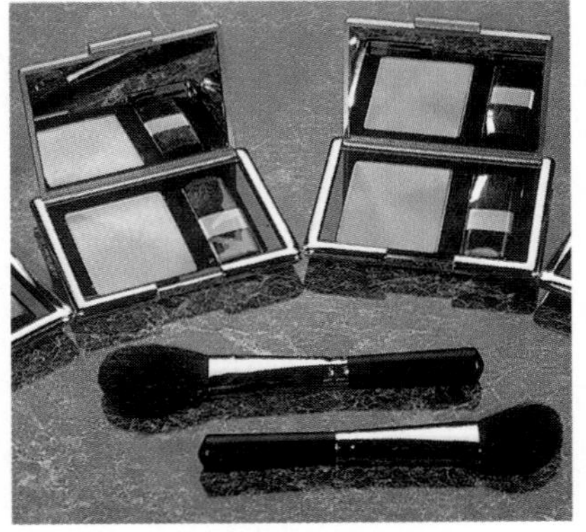

Figure 20–5 Cheek colors.

Cheek Color

Cheek color (also called blush, blusher, or rouge) is a cream, liquid, dry (pressed), or loose powder cosmetic used to color the cheeks and the skin beneath the cheekbones. It gives a natural-looking glow to the face and also helps to create more attractive facial contours (Figure 20–5).

Cheek Color Chemistry

Powder cheek color is simply pressed or loose powder with coloring added. Cream and liquid cheek colors fall into two categories: oil-based and emulsions. The oil-based formulations are combinations of pigments in an oil or fat base. Blends of waxes (carnauba wax and ozokerite) and oily liquids (isopropyl myristate and hexadecyl stearate) create a water-resistant product. In addition, cream cheek colors contain water, thickeners, and a variety of surfactants or detergents that enable particles to penetrate the hair follicles and cracks in the skin.

Using Cheek Color

Cheek colors are applied over foundation.

- Cream or gel cheek colors resemble cream foundation and are generally preferred for dry and normal skin. These colors are applied with a facial sponge.
- Liquid cheek color blends well and is suitable for all skin types. It is applied with a facial sponge.
- Dry (pressed) cheek color imparts a matte finish and is the most widely used. It is applied with a brush or cotton puff.

- Loose powder cheek color comes in a variety of shades. It is applied with a brush or cotton puff.

Cheek color accents the part of the face where it is applied. The following are general rules for application:

- Apply cheek color where natural color would normally appear in the cheeks. Do not apply the color in toward the nose beyond the center of the eye.
- Do not extend color above the outer corner of the eye.
- Do not apply color in a bright, round circle. Blend the color so that it fades softly into the foundation.

Lip Color

Lip color (also called lipstick or gloss) is a cosmetic in paste form, usually in a metal or plastic tube, manufactured in a variety of colors. It is used to color the lips and to enhance or correct the shape of the lips. Some lip colors contain sunscreen to protect the lips from the harmful effects of the sun. Others contain moisturizers to keep lips from becoming dry or chapped (Figure 20–6).

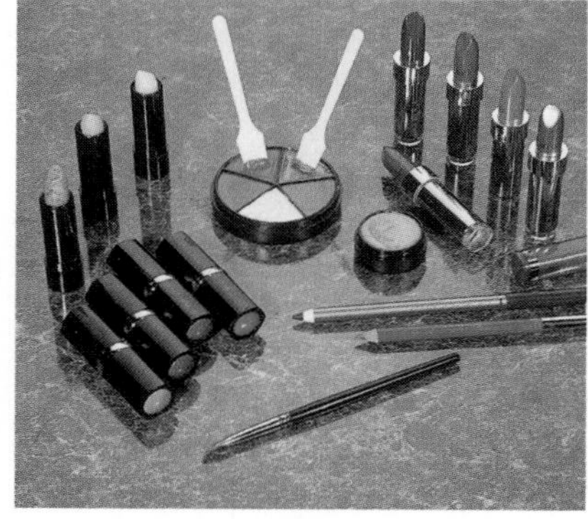

Figure 20–6 Lip colors.

Lip Color Chemistry

Lip color is available in a variety of forms: creams, glosses, pencils, gels, and sticks. All are formulas of oils, waxes, and dyes. Castor oil is the primary ingredient in lipsticks; other oils used are olive, mineral, sesame, cocoa butter, petroleum, lecithin, and hydrogenated vegetable oils. Waxes commonly included in the ingredients are paraffin, beeswax, carnauba, and candelilla wax. Bromic acid, D&C Red No. 27, D&C Orange No. 17 Lake, and related tints are examples of common coloring agents. Iron oxides, mica, and annatto are natural colorants sometimes used in lip colors.

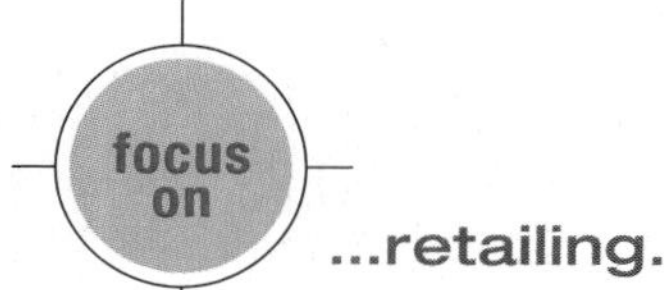

Lip colors create a huge opportunity for retail. Think of how many lipsticks you own. Most women own several lipsticks, glosses, and pencils. Some carry more than five at a time in their purses. Suggest a few colors to a client in a variety of finishes. Lip color is a simple way to change a look, and it provides a great way for your client to give herself a treat and brighten her day.

Using Lip Color

Artistry and a keen sense of fashion are essential when it comes to selecting the appropriate lip color shade or tint. The current fashion trend might call for a certain look, lighter or darker colors, or a certain style of application, such as heavily lined or glossy, lightly stained or matte. Consider the client's preferences, eye color, skin tone, and lip shape before selecting and applying lip color.

Lip color must not be applied directly from the container unless it belongs to the client. Use a spatula to remove the lip color from the container, then take it from the spatula with a disposable lip brush. Use the tip of the brush to line the lips, beginning at the outer corner of the upper lip and working toward the middle. Repeat on the opposite side. Connect the center peaks using rounded strokes, following the natural lip line. Repeat on the bottom lip, working from the outer corners in and connecting in the middle. Aim for symmetry and balance.

Lip Liner

Lip liner is a colored pencil used to outline the lips. It also helps to keep lip color from feathering. It is often used when doing corrective makeup. Lip

focus on ...retailing.

One of the biggest challenges women face when purchasing cosmetics is finding the correct colors and finishes. When you start to use specific and "colorful" language, you will see a great improvement in your selling technique. Consider persuasive phrases such as these:

- "This cocoa shadow will really make your green eyes look beautiful."
- "You have a great smile. This new peach lipstick will show it off."
- "What a great dress. This silver eyeliner would look great with it."

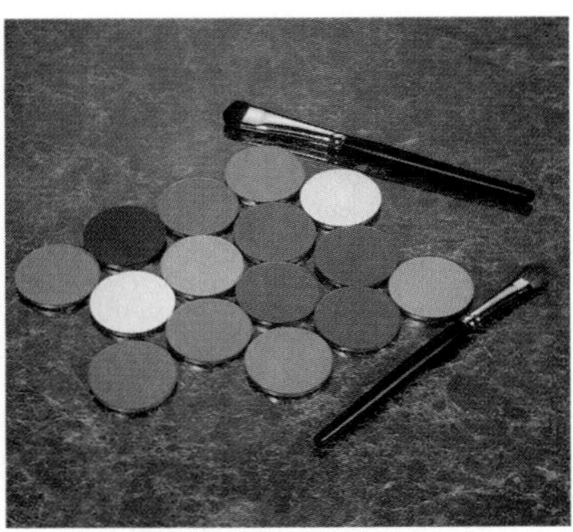

Figure 20–7 Eye shadows.

20

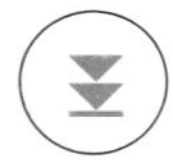

Here's a tip:

Eye shadow in pressed powder form may be applied to the eyes with an eyeliner brush to create a softer lined effect. Whether using shadow or pencil liner, it may be helpful to pull the skin taut, from right below the eyebrow up, to ensure smooth application.

liner comes in thin or thick pencil form and is available in a variety of finishes. Some lip liners double as lipstick for ease of application.

Lip liner is usually applied before lip color to ensure proper shape and definition of the lips. Choose a lip liner that coordinates with the chosen lip color. The liner color should not be dramatically darker or brighter than the lip shade. If a darker liner is desired, fill in most of the lip with the liner and blend the lip color and lip liner to avoid harsh lines.

Sharpen the lip liner pencil and wipe with a clean tissue before each use. Also, remember to sanitize the sharpener before every use.

Line the lips, beginning at the outer corner of the upper lip and working toward the middle. Repeat on the opposite side. Connect the center peaks with rounded strokes, following the natural line of the lip. Outline the lower lip from the outer corners in, and then apply liner on the lips, staying within the outline.

Eye Shadow

Eye shadows are cosmetics applied on the eyelids to accentuate or contour them. They are available in almost every color of the rainbow, from warm to cool, neutral to bright, and light to dark. Some powder eye shadows are designed to be used wet or dry. They also come in a variety of finishes, including metallic, matte, frost, shimmer, or dewy.

Eye Shadow Chemistry

Eye shadow is available in stick, cream, pressed, and dry powder form, and usually comes with an applicator (Figure 20–7). Stick and cream shadows are water-based with oil, petrolatum, thickener, wax, perfume, preservatives, and color added. Water-resistant shadows have a solvent base, such as mineral spirits. Pressed and dry powder shadows are composed much the same as pressed face powder and powdered cheek color.

Using Eye Shadow

When applied to the lids, eye color or shadow makes the eyes appear brighter and more expressive. Matching eye shadow to eye color creates a flat field of color and should generally be avoided. Using color other than the actual eye color (that is, a contrasting or complementary color) can enhance the eyes. Using light and dark can also bring attention to the eyes.

Generally, a darker shade of eye color makes the natural color of the iris appear lighter, while a lighter shade makes the iris appear deeper. However, the only set rules for selection of eye makeup colors are that they should enhance the client's eyes and that color choices should be more subtle for daytime. If desired, eye makeup color may match or coordinate with the client's clothing color.

Eye shadow colors are generally referred to as highlight, base, and contour colors.

- A highlight color is lighter than the client's skin tone and may have any finish. Popular choices include matte or iridescent (shiny). As the name suggests, these colors highlight a specific area, such as the brow bone.

Remember that a lighter color will make an area appear larger.

- A base color is generally a medium tone that is close to the client's skin tone. It is available in a variety of finishes. This color is generally used to even skin tone on the eye. It is often applied all over the lid and brow bone, from lash to brow, before other colors are applied, thus providing a smooth surface for the blending of other colors. If used this way, a matte finish is generally preferred.
- A contour color is a color, in any finish, that is deeper and darker than the client's skin tone. It is applied to minimize a specific area, to create contour in a crease, or to define the eyelash line.

To apply eye shadow, remove the product from its container with a spatula, then use a fresh applicator or clean brush. Unless you are doing corrective makeup, apply the eye color close to the lashes on the upper eyelid, sweeping the color slightly upward and outward. Blend to achieve the desired effect. More than one color may be used if a particular effect is desired.

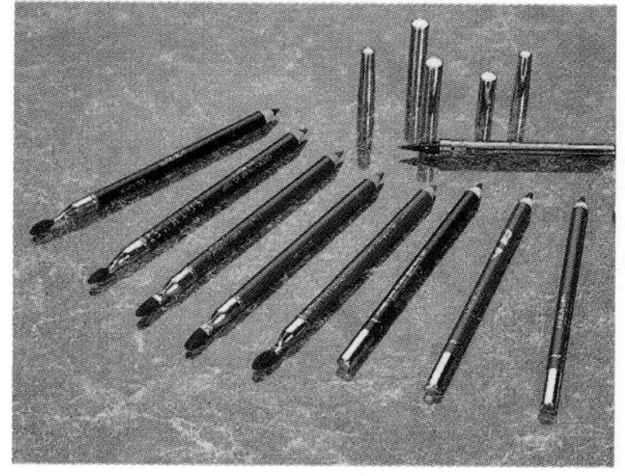

Figure 20–8 Eyeliners.

Eyeliners

Eyeliner is a cosmetic used to outline and emphasize the eyes. It is available in a variety of colors, in pencil, liquid, pressed (cake), or felt tip pen form. With eyeliner you can create a line on the eyelid close to the lashes to make the eyes appear larger and the lashes fuller (Figure 20–8).

Eyeliner Chemistry

Eyeliner pencils consist of a wax (paraffin) or hardened oil base (petrolatum) with a variety of additives to create color. They are available in both soft and hard form for use on the eyebrow as well as the upper and lower eyelid.

Liquid and cake eyeliners contain alkanolamine (a fatty alcohol), cellulose, ether, polyvinylpyrrolidone, methylparaben, antioxidants, perfumes, and titanium dioxide.

CAUTION

According to the American Medical Association, eye pencils should not be used to color the inner rim of the eyes, because this can lead to infection of the tear duct, causing tearing, blurring of vision, and permanent pigmentation of the mucous membrane lining the inside of the eye.

Using Eyeliners

Most clients prefer eyeliner that is the same color as the lashes or mascara for a more natural look. More dramatic colors may be chosen depending on seasonal color trends.

Be extremely cautious when applying eyeliner. You must have a steady hand and be sure that your client remains still. Sharpen the eyeliner pencil and wipe with a clean tissue before each use. Also, remember to sanitize the sharpener before each use. Apply to the desired area with short strokes and gentle pressure; the most common placement is close to the lash line. For powder shadow liner application, scrape a small amount onto a tissue and apply to the eyes with a disposable applicator or clean brush. If desired, wet the brush before the application for a more dramatic look.

Eyebrow Color

Eyebrow pencils or shadows are used to add color and shape to the eyebrows, usually after tweezing or waxing. They can be used to darken the eyebrows, correct their shape, or fill in sparse areas.

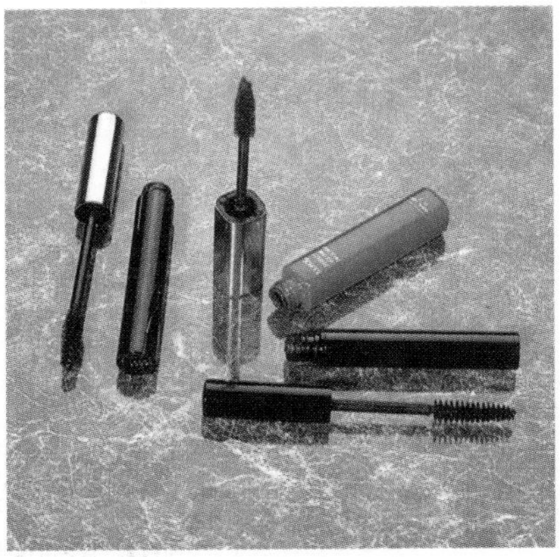

Figure 20-9 Mascara products.

Eyebrow Color Chemistry

The chemistry of eyebrow pencils is similar to that of eyeliner pencil. The chemical ingredients in eyebrow shadows are also similar to those in eye shadows.

Using Eyebrow Color

Sharpen the eyebrow pencil and wipe with clean tissue before each use. Sanitize the sharpener before each use. For powder shadow application, scrape a small amount onto a tissue and use a disposable applicator or clean brush to apply shadow to brows. Avoid harsh contrasts between hair and eyebrow color, such as pale blonde or silver hair with black eyebrows.

Mascara

Mascara is a cosmetic preparation used to darken, define, and thicken the eyelashes. It is available in liquid, cake, and cream form and in a variety of shades and tints (Figure 20–9). Mascara brushes can be straight or curved, with fine or thick bristles. The most popular mascara colors are shades of brown and black, which enhance the natural lashes, making them appear thicker and longer. Mascara and eyebrow pencils should generally coordinate so there is no harsh contrast.

Mascara Chemistry

Mascara is available in tube and wand applicators. Both are polymer products that include water, wax, thickeners, film-formers, and preservatives in their formulation. The pigments in mascara must be inert (unable to combine with other elements) and usually are carbon black, carmine, ultramarine, chromium oxide, and iron oxides. Some wand mascaras contain rayon or nylon fibers to lengthen and thicken the hair fibers.

Here's a tip:

If you are using an eyelash curler, you must curl the lashes before applying mascara. If lashes are curled after mascara, eyelashes may be broken or pulled out. Use extreme caution whenever using an eyelash curler. It is easiest to learn how to use this tool by first observing its use. Ask your instructor to demonstrate before attempting to use an eyelash curler on someone else.

Using Mascara

Mascara may be used on all the lashes, from the inner to outer corners. Using a disposable wand, dip into a clean tube of mascara and apply from close to the base of the lashes out toward the tips, making sure your client is comfortable throughout the application. Dispose of the wand. Never double-dip.

Apply mascara carefully. The most common injury with mascara application is poking the eye with the applicator. Practice applying mascara repeatedly until you feel confident enough to apply it on clients.

Other Cosmetics

Eye makeup removers do just that: remove eye makeup. Most eye makeup products are water-resistant, so plain soap and water is less effective for removal. Eye makeup removers are either oil-based or water-based. Oil-based removers are generally mineral oil with a small amount of fragrance added. Water-based removers are a water solution to which acetone, boric acid, oils, lanolin or lanolin derivatives, and other solvents have been added.

Greasepaint is a heavy makeup used for theatrical purposes. **Cake (pancake) makeup** is a shaped, solid mass applied to the face with a moistened cosmetic sponge. It gives good coverage and is generally used to cover scars and pigmentation defects.

Makeup Brushes and Other Tools

Makeup brushes come in a variety of shapes and sizes (Figure 20–10). They may be made of synthetic or animal hair with wooden or metal handles. Commonly used makeup brushes and implements include the following items.

- *Powder brush.* Large, soft brush used to apply powder or blush and for blending edges of color.
- *Blush brush.* Smaller, more tapered version of the powder brush, excellent for applying powder cheek color.
- *Concealer brush.* Usually narrow and firm with a flat edge, used to apply concealer around the eyes or over blemishes.
- *Lip brush.* Similar to the concealer brush, with a more tapered edge; may be used to apply concealer or lip color.
- *Eye shadow brushes.* Available in a variety of sizes, from small to large, and in finishes from soft to firm. The softer and larger the brush, the more diffused and blended the shadow will be. A firm brush is better for depositing dense color than for blending it.
- *Eyeliner brush.* Fine, tapered, firm bristles; used to apply liquid liner or shadow to the eyes.
- *Angle brush.* Firm, thin bristle; angled for ease of application of shadow to the eyebrows or shadow liner to the eyes.
- *Lash and brow brush.* Comb-like brush used to remove excess mascara on lashes or to comb brows into place.
- *Tweezers.* Available in metal or plastic; used to remove excess facial hair.
- *Eyelash curler.* Metal or plastic device used to give lift and upward curl to the upper lashes.

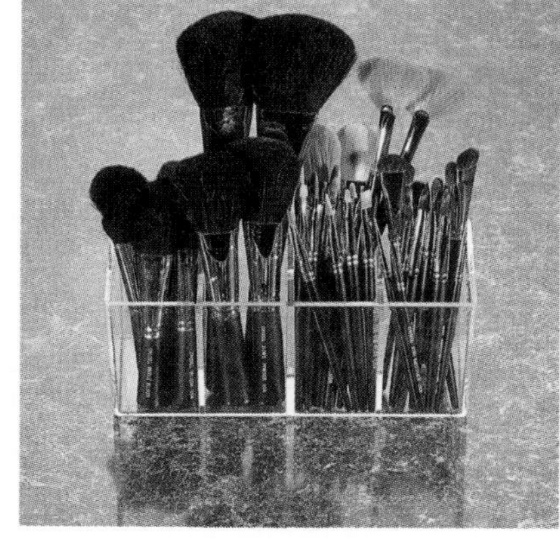

Figure 20–10 Makeup brushes.

Caring for Makeup Brushes

If you invest in high-quality makeup brushes, you will have them for years. Take good care of your brushes by cleaning them gently.

A commercial sanitizer can be used for quick cleaning, although spray-on instant sanitizers contain a high level of alcohol and will dry brushes over time. A gentle shampoo or brush solvent should be used to truly clean the brushes. These products will not hurt brushes and may actually help them last longer. One caution: the brush should always be put into running or still water with the ferrule (the metal ring that keeps bristles and handle together) pointing downward. If the brush is pointed up, the water may remove the glue that keeps the bristles in place. Rinse brushes thoroughly after cleansing. Because they will dry in the shape they are left in, reshape the wet bristles and lay the brushes flat to dry.

Guidelines for cleaning and sanitizing brushes vary from state to state, so check with your regulatory agency.

Disposable Implements

Disposable implements include the following items.

- *Sponges.* Come in a variety of sizes and shapes, including wedges and circles, and work well to apply and blend foundation, cream or powder blush, powder, or concealer.
- *Powder or cotton puffs.* May be made of velour or cotton and are used to apply and blend powder, powder foundation, or powder blush.
- *Mascara wands.* Usually plastic; used to apply mascara on a client; generally disposable, so as to ensure proper hygiene.

- *Spatulas.* Wooden or plastic, with a wide, flat base; used to remove makeup such as lipstick, foundation, concealer, powder, blush, and shadow from their containers.
- *Disposable lip brushes.* May be plastic or another synthetic; used to hygienically apply lip color to a client.
- *Sponge-tipped shadow applicators.* Used to apply shadow and lip color or to blend eyeliner; may be used to remove unwanted makeup from eyes or lips
- *Cotton swabs.* May be used to apply shadow, blend eyeliner, or remove unwanted makeup from the eyes or lips.
- *Cotton pads or puffs.* May be used with astringents or makeup removers; also used to apply powder products.
- *Pencil sharpener.* Used before each application of eye or lip liner pencil to ensure hygienic application.

MAKEUP COLOR THEORY

A strong understanding of how color works is vital to effective makeup application. Everyone sees color a little differently, and it may take a while to learn to see color naturally and easily. Let us review how to identify primary, secondary, and tertiary colors, as well as warm, cool, and complementary colors. Once you understand these basics of color theory, you can use your creative instincts to invent any color palette you desire.

Primary colors are fundamental colors that cannot be obtained from a mixture. The primary colors are yellow, red, and blue (Figure 20–11).

Secondary colors are obtained by mixing equal parts of two primary colors. Yellow mixed with red makes orange. Red mixed with blue makes violet. Yellow mixed with blue makes green (Figure 20–12).

Tertiary colors are formed by mixing equal amounts of a secondary color and its neighboring primary color on the color wheel. These colors are named by primary color first, secondary color second. For example, when we mix blue (a primary) with violet (a neighboring secondary), we call the resulting color blue-violet (Figure 20–13).

A primary and secondary color directly opposite each other on the color wheel are called complementary colors. When mixed, these colors cancel each other out to create a neutral brown or gray color. When complementary colors are placed next to each other, each color makes the other look brighter, resulting in greater contrast. For example, if you place blue next to orange, the blue seems bluer, the orange brighter. Try this with magic markers or colored paper to compare. The concept of complementary colors is useful when determining color choice. For example, the use of complementary colors will emphasize eye color, making the eyes appear brighter (Figure 20–14).

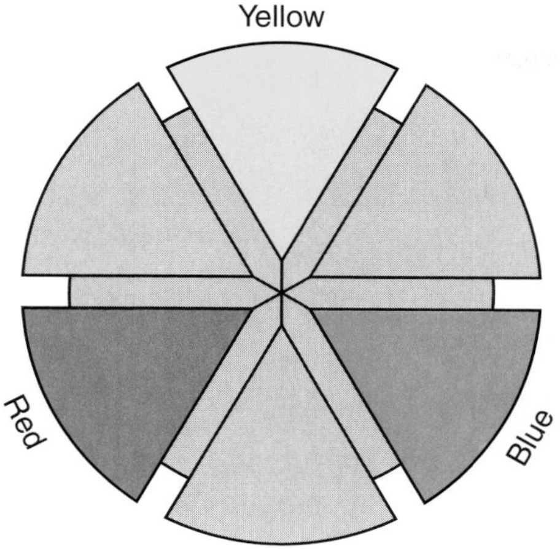

Figure 20-11 Primary colors.

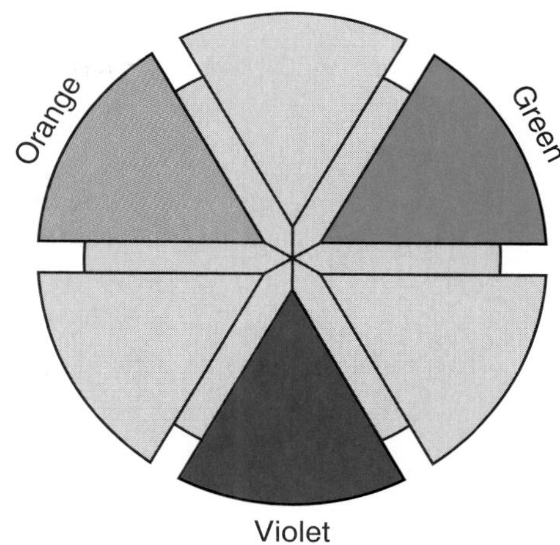

Figure 20-12 Secondary colors.

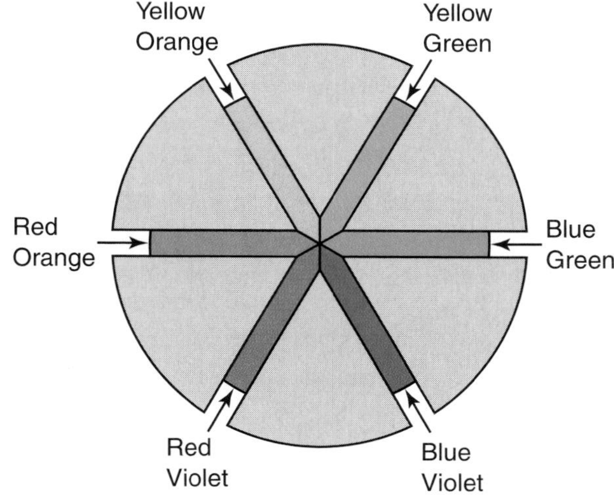

Figure 20-13 Tertiary colors.

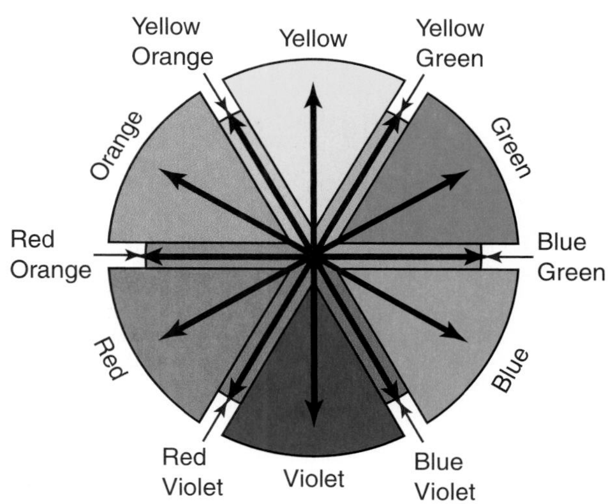

Figure 20-14 Complementary colors.

Warm and Cool Colors

Learning the difference between warm and cool colors is essential to your success as a makeup artist. This is the basis of all color selection, and understanding the difference will enable you to properly enhance your client's coloring.

20

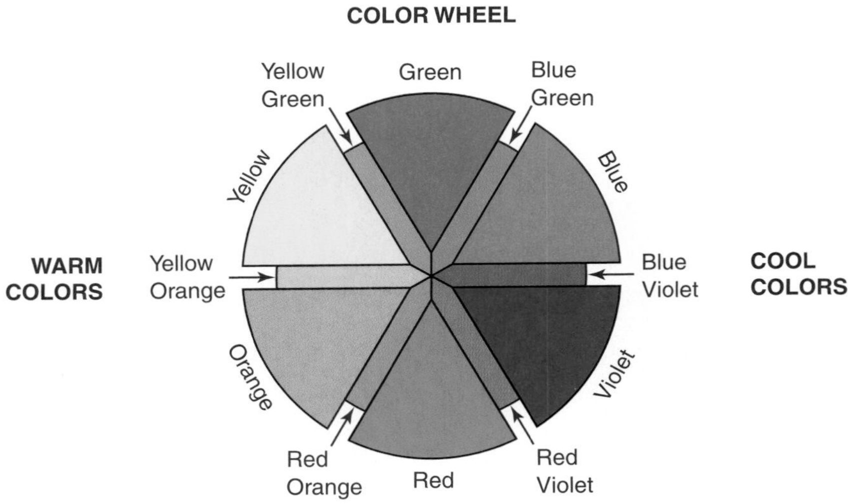

COLOR WHEEL

Yellow Green
Green
Blue Green
Yellow
Blue
WARM COLORS
Yellow Orange
Blue Violet
COOL COLORS
Orange
Violet
Red Orange
Red
Red Violet

Figure 20–15 Warm and cool colors.

Warm colors are the range of colors from yellow and gold through the oranges, red-oranges, most reds, and even some yellow-greens. **Cool colors** suggest coolness and are dominated by blues, greens, violets, and blue-reds (Figure 20–15). You will notice that reds can be both warm and cool. If the red is orange-based, it is warm. If it is blue-based, it is cool. Green is similar: if a green contains more gold, it is warm; if it contains more blue, it is cool.

You may hear people refer to a color as having a lot of blue in it. For example: "This lipstick has a blue base" or "That blush is very blue." This does not mean that the color is truly blue. Rather, it means that when the pigments were mixed to create that cosmetic, more blue color was added. What you are seeing might look primarily violet or magenta.

Selecting Makeup Colors

Now that we have determined warms and cools, it is time to learn a system that will help you feel more comfortable when choosing colors for your clients. Keep in mind this is simply one way of choosing colors. The art of makeup application allows for more than one way to achieve the result you are looking for. However, once you learn the rules of a basic color selection system, you can then go on to break them if you so desire.

As you look at the color wheel, think of it as a tool in determining color choice. There are three main factors to consider when choosing colors for a client: skin color, eye color, and hair color.

Determining Skin Color

When determining skin color, you must first decide if the skin is light, medium, or dark in level. Then determine whether the tone of the skin is warm or cool (use Table 20–1 as a guide). You may not see skin colors truly in the beginning. Give yourself time and practice to develop your eye.

Skin Colors	Warm	Cool
Light skin	yellow, gold, pale peach	pink or slightly ruddy (reddish); florid undertones
Medium skin	yellow, yellow-orange, red	olive (yellow-green)
Dark skin	red, orange-brown, red-brown	dark olive, blue, blue-black, ebony

Table 20–1 Skin Colors and Tones

A neutral skin tone contains equal elements of warm and cool, no matter how light or dark the skin is. Remember to always match your foundation color to the color of the skin, or use the corrective techniques discussed later in this chapter.

Once you have determined if the skin is light, medium, or dark, you may choose eye, cheek, and lip colors to match the skin color in level, or try contrast for more impact. Most skin tones and levels can wear a surprisingly wide range of eye, cheek, and lip colors.

- If skin color is light, you may use light colors for a soft, natural look. Medium to dark colors will create a more dramatic look.
- If skin color is medium, medium tones will create an understated look. Light or dark tones will provide more contrast and will appear bolder.
- If skin color is dark, dark tones will be most subtle. Medium to medium-light or bright tones will be striking and vivid (Figure 20–16).

Be cautious when choosing tones lighter than the skin. If the color is too light, it will turn gray or chalky on the skin. Look for translucent, shimmery colors if you are choosing these tones.

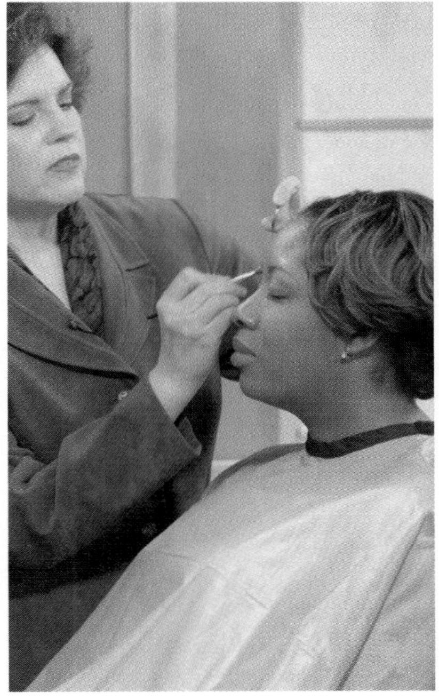

Figure 20–16 Choose cosmetics to enhance your client's skin and hair color.

Complementary Colors for Eyes

As you begin recommending eye, cheek, and lip colors, neutrals will always be your safest choice. They contain elements of warm and cool and work well on any skin tone, eye color, or hair color. They come in variations of brown or gray. For instance, they may have a warm or cool base with brown tones. Or you might choose a plum-brown, which would be considered a cool neutral. An orange-brown would be considered a warm neutral. Charcoal gray is a cool neutral, as is blue-gray.

Contrary to popular belief, matching eye color with shadow color is not the best way to enhance it; it only creates a flat region of color. By contrasting eye color with complementary colors, you emphasize the color most effectively.

The following is a guideline for eye color selection. You may refer back to the color wheel for additional help in determining complementary colors.

- *Complementary colors for blue eyes.* Orange is the complementary color to blue. Because orange contains yellow and red, shadows with any of these colors in them will make your eyes look bluer. Common choices include gold, warm orange-browns like peach and copper, red-browns like mauves and plum, and neutrals like taupe or camel.
- *Complementary colors for green eyes.* Red is the complementary color to green. Because red shadows tend to make the eyes look tired or bloodshot, pure red tones are not recommended. Instead, use brown-based reds or other color options next to red on the color wheel. These include red-orange, red-violet, and violet. Popular choices are coppers, rusts, pinks, plums, mauves, and purples.
- *Complementary colors for brown eyes.* Brown eyes are neutral and can wear any color. Recommended choices include such contrasting colors as greens, blues, grays, and silvers.

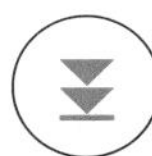

Here's a tip:

It is not recommended to mix warms and cools on a face. They will compete with each other and will result in an "off" appearance. Staying within the color ranges you have chosen will ensure a balanced, beautiful look.

Adding Cheek and Lip Color

After you have chosen eye makeup, use the color wheel to determine whether your choices are warm or cool and then coordinate cheek and lip makeup in the same color family as the eye makeup. For example, if your client has green eyes, you recommended plums for her, which are cool. Now you should stay with cool colors for the cheeks and lips in order to coordinate with the eye makeup. You may also choose neutrals, as these contain both warm and cool elements and coordinate with any makeup colors.

Hair Color and Eye Color

Hair color needs to be taken into account when determining eye makeup color. For example, if a woman has blue eyes, your instinct might be to select orange-based eye makeup as the complementary choice. But if she has cool blue-black hair, the orange will not be flattering. In this case, you would choose cool colors to coordinate with the hair color. Red-violets (plums) would be a more flattering choice. Look at orange on the color wheel: it is warm. Go around the wheel toward the cool end. Red-violets are the closest to orange on the color wheel while still remaining cool. As stated earlier, there is a range of colors to choose from for any client. Use Table 20–2 as a general guide.

Reviewing Color Selection Steps

1. Determine skin level: light, medium, or dark.
2. Determine skin undertone: warm, cool, or neutral.
3. Determine eye color: blue, green, brown, and so forth.
4. Determine complementary colors.
5. Determine hair color: warm or cool.
6. Choose eye makeup colors based on complementary or contrasting colors.
7. Coordinate cheek and lip colors within the same color family: warm, cool, or neutral.
8. Apply makeup.

The best thing about choosing colors is the unlimited number of choices you have. Try one or all methods of choosing color. You may choose colors

Hair Color	Warm	Cool
Blonde hair	yellow, orange	white-blonde, ash
Red hair	gold, copper, orange, red	red-violet, violet
Brown hair	yellow, gold, orange	ash
Dark brown/black hair	copper, red	violet, blue

Table 20-2 Determining Hair Color Tones

based only on skin tone, or you might find that working with complementary colors makes you feel more comfortable. Bring out hair color by matching or contrasting with it, or by blending all three areas as discussed here.

CLIENT CONSULTATION

The first step in the makeup process, as with all other services that take place in the salon, is the client consultation. This is where you ask the client the questions that will bring out her wishes and concerns. Listen closely and try not to impose your own opinions too much. Your role is to hear your client's wishes and concerns and to make recommendations based on your knowledge. If she chooses not to act on your recommendations, do not take it personally. In time, perhaps she will.

Consultation Area

The area that you use for consultations must be clean and tidy. No one wants to see a messy makeup unit or dirty brushes lying about. Clean your brushes after each use and tidy your makeup area daily. Also, keep a portfolio in the consultation area that includes photographs of your own work or pictures from magazines. The client can go through your portfolio to find styles and colors that appeal to her.

activity

Apply makeup to a partner, using color theory to choose and coordinate makeup colors. Have fun and experiment. Keep track of which colors enhance her appearance and coordinate with her wardrobe, and which ones don't. And remember, while a haircut or haircolor may represent a big commitment, makeup does not. If you don't like it, you can simply wash it off and try again!

Lighting

Adequate and flattering lighting is essential for both the consultation and application parts of the makeup process. Be sure your client's face is evenly lit and without dark shadows. Natural light is the best choice, but if it is necessary to use artificial light, it should be a combination of incandescent light (warm bulb light) and fluorescent light (cool industrial tube light). If you must choose between the two, incandescent light will be more flattering.

Make sure that the light always shines directly and evenly on the face. And remember, good lighting makes a client look good, and clients who look good are more likely to purchase the products you recommend. When this happens, everyone comes out a winner.

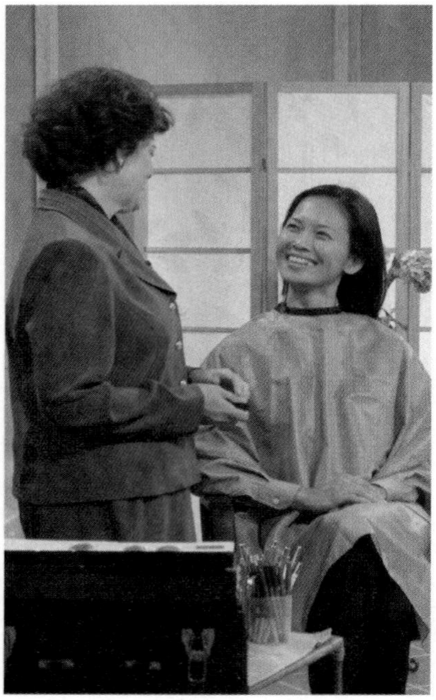

Figure 20-17 Client consultation.

Makeup Consultation

A makeup service should always begin with a warm introduction to your client. Visually assess her to understand her personal style. This will give you cues as you continue your consultation (Figure 20–17).

Engaging the client in conversation will help you determine her needs. Gather whatever information you can on her skin condition, how much or how little makeup she wears, daily versus special occasion makeup, the amount of time she spends applying makeup, colors she likes or dislikes, and any makeup areas she's having trouble with.

Record this information on a client consultation card. Also, write down your recommendations so that you may refer back to them at the end of the makeup application. Reviewing and restating your written advice with the client at the end of the service will also help you sell the retail products you hope she will purchase (Figure 20–18). Escort your client to the reception area where you can assist her in gathering the products that you have recommended. Ask her if she has any other questions and, if so, give clear answers. If possible, set up a time for her next appointment. Then give her a business card with your name on it and shake her hand as you turn her over to the receptionist who will check her out.

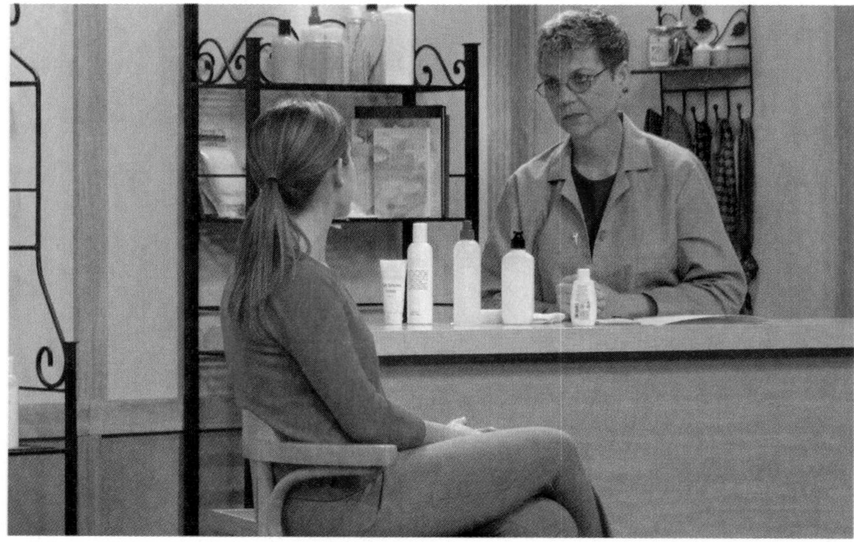

Figure 20-18 Retailing cosmetic products.

PROCEDURE

PROFESSIONAL MAKEUP APPLICATION

Equipment, Implements, and Materials

Skin care:

- cleansers
- astringent and skin-freshening lotion
- moisturizers

Makeup:

- foundations
- concealers
- face powders
- cheek colors
- lip colors
- lip liners
- eye shadows
- eyeliner pencils
- mascara

Accessories:

- towels and draping sheets, if desired
- makeup cape
- headband or hair clip
- eyelash curler
- assorted makeup brushes (for eye shadow, eyeliner, lip color, concealer, blush, powder, and flat or slanted brush for brows or eyeliner)
- small makeup palette

Disposables:

- mascara wands
- shadow applicators
- sponge wedges
- tissues
- pencil sharpener
- disposable lip brushes
- cotton swabs
- spatulas
- cotton pads or puffs

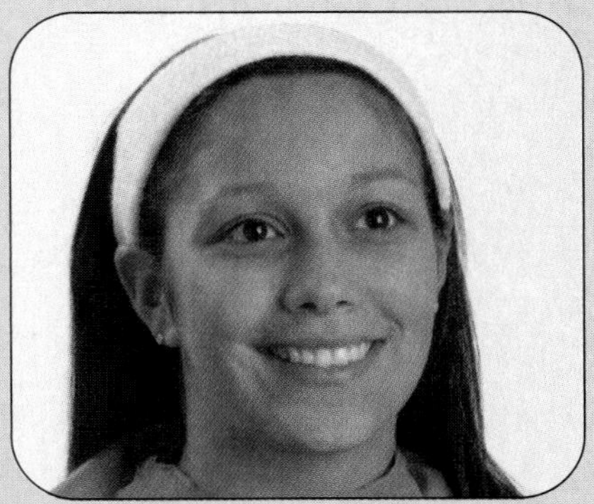

Figure 20-19 Use a headband to keep the client's hair off her face.

Preparation

1. Client consultation. Determine the client's needs and choose products and colors accordingly.
2. Wash your hands.
3. Drape the client and use a headband or hair clip to keep the hair out of the face (Figure 20–19).

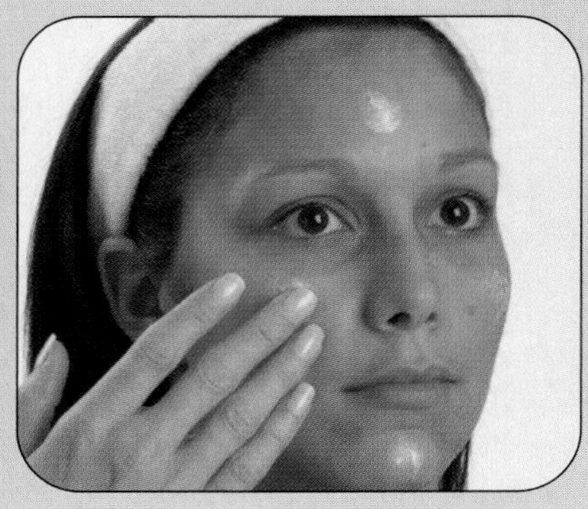

Figure 20-20 Apply cleansing cream or lotion.

4. Apply cleansing cream or lotion. Remove a small quantity of cleanser from the container with a spatula and place it in the palm of the left hand, or apply a dab of lotion to an applicator. With the fingertips of the right hand, place dabs of cleanser on the forehead, nose, cheeks, chin, and neck. Spread the cleanser over the face and neck with light upward and outward circular movements (Figure 20–20).
5. Remove the cleanser with tissue mitts or moistened cotton pads, using an upward and outward motion (Figure 20–21). Be especially gentle around the eyes. If makeup or color is particularly heavy on the eyes and lips, apply the cleanser a second time, as needed.
6. Apply astringent lotion or toner. For oily skin, apply astringent lotion; for dry skin, apply a skin toner. Moisten a cotton pad with the lotion and pat it lightly over the entire face and under the chin and neck. Blot off excess moisture with tissues or a cotton pad (Figure 20–22).
7. When necessary, as in the case of dry and delicate skin, apply a moisturizing lotion. Dab a small amount of the moisturizer on the forehead, cheeks, and chin. Blend upward over the face. Remove excess with a tissue, cotton pad, or facial sponge.
8. Groom the eyebrows. Eyebrow arching (tweezing) is a complete service in itself (see Chapter 18). You may, however, choose to remove a few stray hairs before a facial makeup by tweezing the hair in the same direction in which it grows.

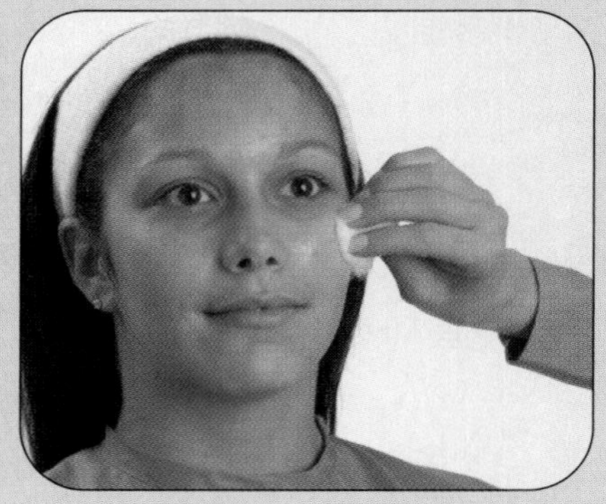

Figure 20-21 Remove the cleanser.

Procedure

1. Apply foundation. Test the color by blending the foundation on the client's jawline. When you are satisfied with your choice, place a small amount of the foundation on a palette, in the palm, or on the back of

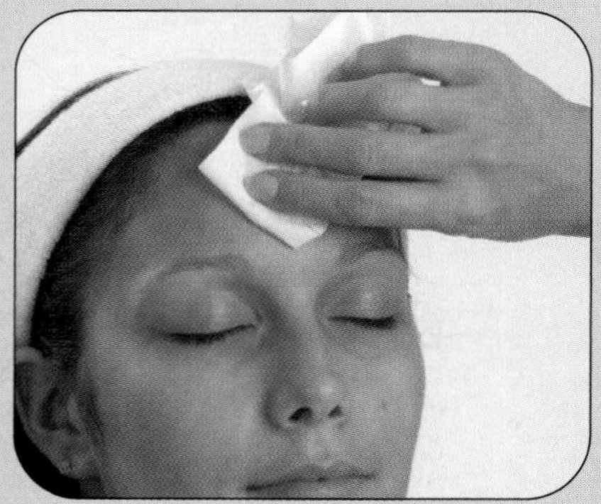

Figure 20-22 Blot excess moisture.

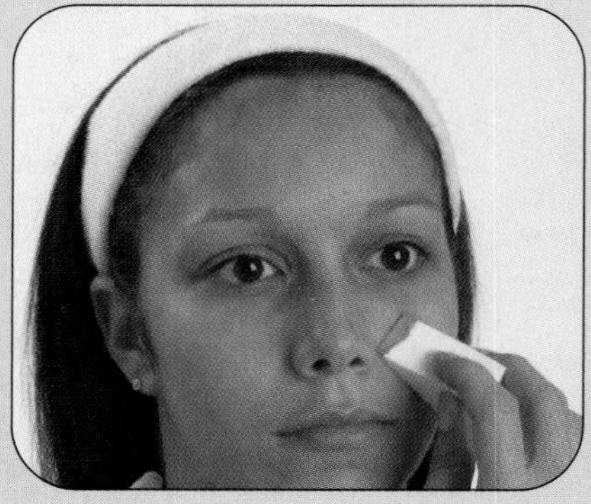

Figure 20-23 Apply foundation.

your hand and, using the tips of your fingers or a cosmetic sponge, apply sparingly and evenly over the entire face and around the neckline. Starting at the center of the face, blend with outward and downward motions (Figure 20–23). Blend near the hairline, and remove excess foundation with a cosmetic sponge or cotton pledget.

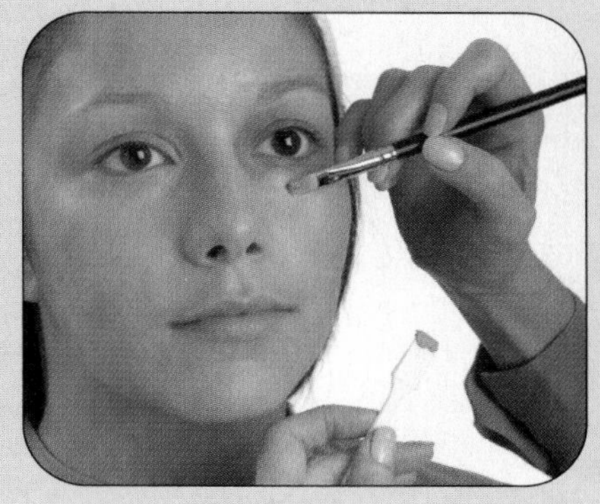

Figure 20-24 Apply concealer.

2. Apply concealer. Select the appropriate type and color of concealer and then scrape a small amount onto a spatula. Using a brush or fingertips, apply the concealer lightly where needed (under the eyes, over blemishes, to cover redness). Blend in with a patting motion. If a powder foundation is being used, the concealer must be applied before the foundation (Figure 20–24). Your instructor may prefer a different method that may be equally correct.
3. Apply powder. Apply the powder with a sanitary puff or cosmetic sponge, pressing it over the face and whisking off the excess with a puff or powder brush (Figure 20–25). A moistened cosmetic sponge may be pressed over the finished makeup to give the face a matte look.
4. Apply eye color. Select a complementary color in a medium tone and then, beginning at the lash line or crease, apply lightly and blend outward with a brush or disposable applicator (Figure 20–26).
5. Apply eyeliner. Select pencil, pressed, or liquid liner in a color to harmonize with the mascara you will be applying. Pull the eyelid taut as the client looks down, and draw a very fine line along the entire lid (Figure 20–27). You may apply to the top lash line and/or bottom lash line. If eyeliner pencil is used, the point should be fine and care should be taken to avoid injury or discomfort. Be sure to trim the pencil before each use.

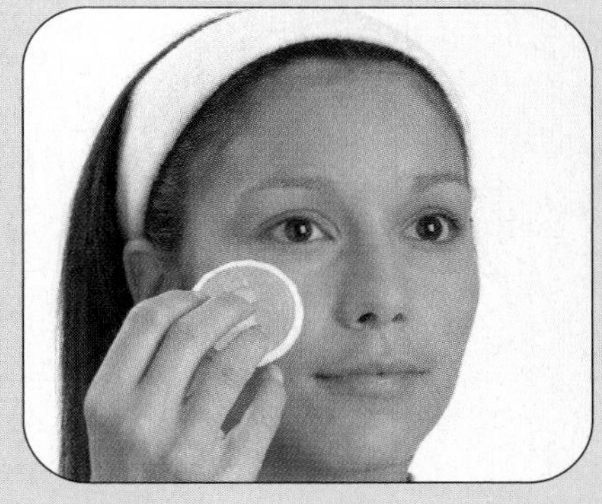

Figure 20-25 Apply powder.

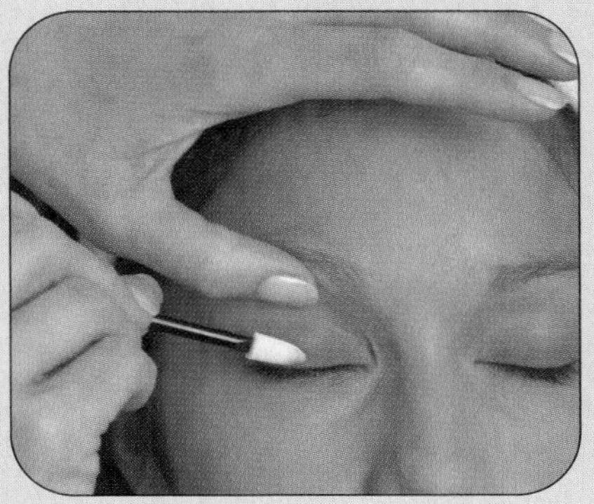

Figure 20-26 Apply eye color.

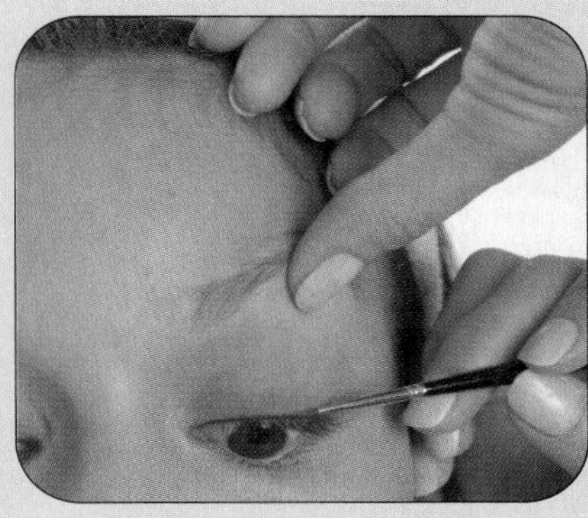

Figure 20-27 Apply eyeliner.

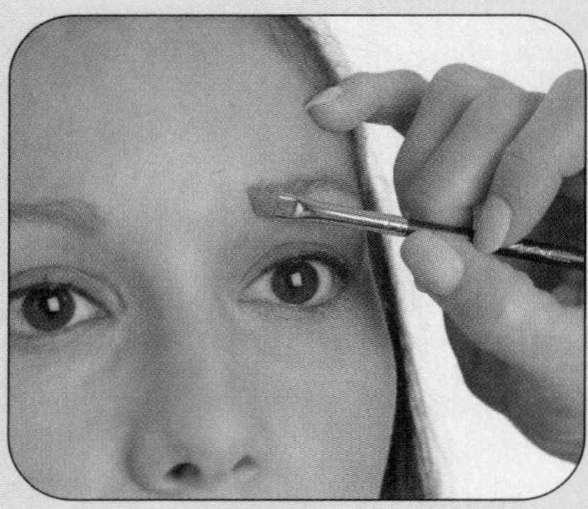

Figure 20-28 Apply eyebrow color.

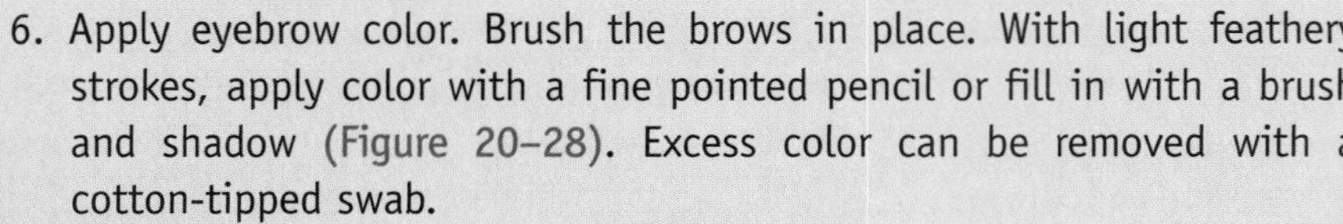

6. Apply eyebrow color. Brush the brows in place. With light feathery strokes, apply color with a fine pointed pencil or fill in with a brush and shadow (Figure 20–28). Excess color can be removed with a cotton-tipped swab.
7. Apply mascara to the top and underside of the upper lashes with careful, gentle strokes until the desired effect is achieved (Figure 20–29). Use a fresh brush or applicator to separate the lashes. Mascara may be applied to lower lashes if desired, but the effect should be subtle.
8. Apply cheek color. Have the client smile, to raise the cheeks, and then apply powder cheek color, blending outward and upward toward the temples (Figure 20–30). Liquid or cream cheek color is applied with a sanitized applicator before powder, and sometimes on bare skin.
9. Apply lip color. Use a freshly sharpened pencil to line the lips, beginning at the outer corner of the upper lip and working toward the middle (Figure 20–31a). Repeat on the opposite side. Connect the center peaks using rounded strokes, following the natural line of the lip. Outline the lower lip from the outer corners in, and then apply liner on the lips, staying within the outline. For sanitary reasons, lip color must not be applied directly from the container unless it belongs to the client. Use a spatula to remove the lip color from the container, then take it from the spatula with a lip brush. Rest your ring finger on the client's chin to steady your hand. Ask the client to relax her lips and

CAUTION

Remember, when applying mascara, use a disposable mascara wand and dip into a clean tube of mascara. Then dispose of the wand. Never "double dip."

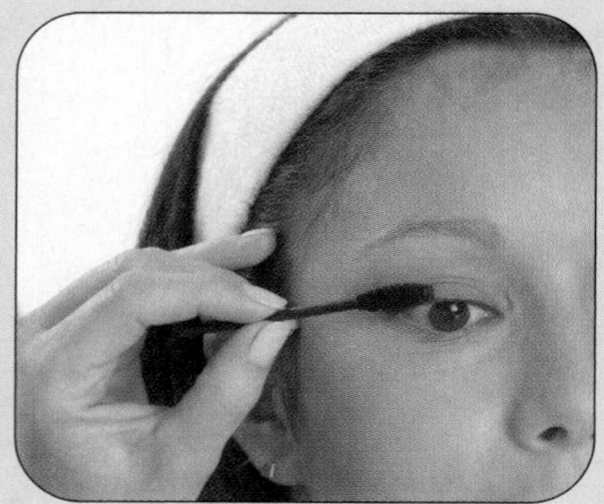

Figure 20-29 Apply mascara.

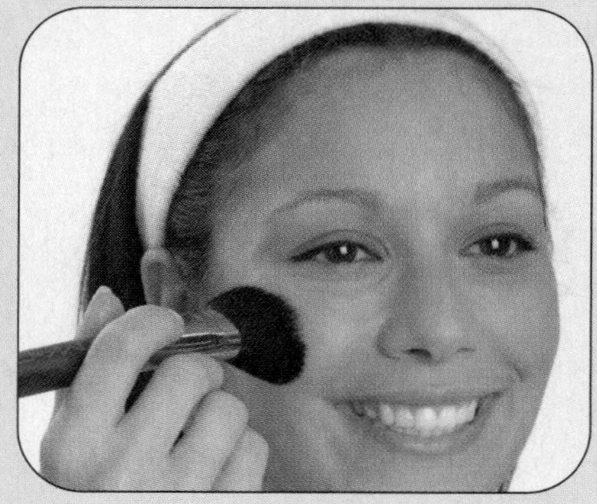

Figure 20-30 Apply cheek color.

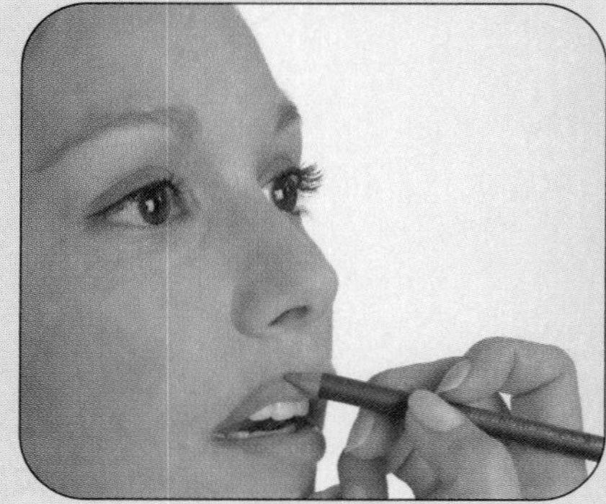

Figure 20-31a Outline the lips with lip liner.

part them slightly. Brush on the lip color (Figure 20–31b). Then ask the client to smile slightly so that you can smooth the lip color into any small crevices. Blot the lips with tissue to remove excess product and set the lip color. Powdering is not recommended, as a moist look is more desirable for lips (Figure 20–32).

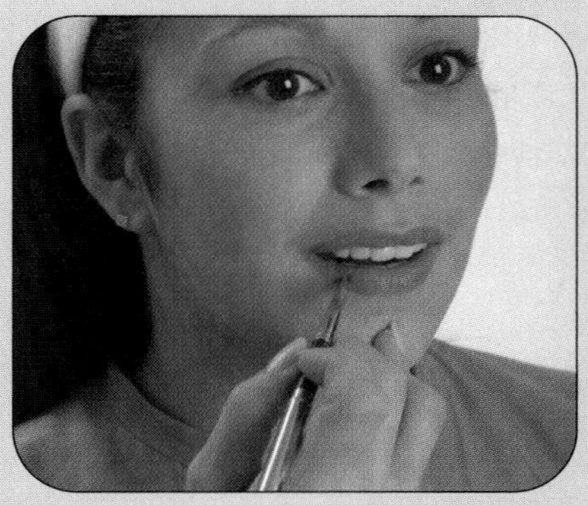

Figure 20–31b Apply lip color.

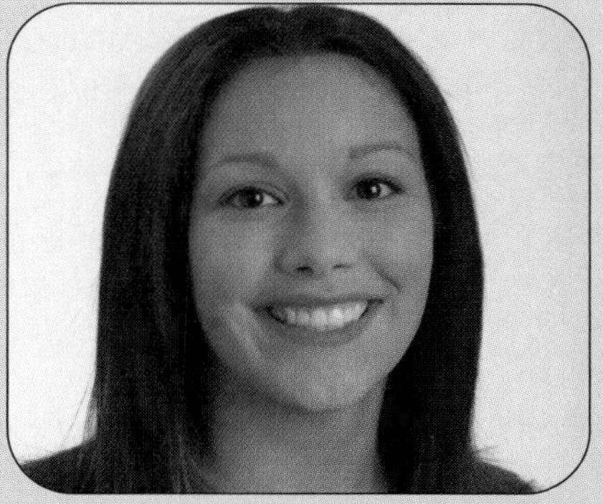

Figure 20–32 Finished makeup application.

Cleanup and Sanitation

1. Discard all disposable items, such as sponges, pads, spatulas, and applicators, after each use.
2. Disinfect implements such as eyelash curlers.
3. Clean and sanitize brushes using a commercial brush sanitizer.
4. Place towels, linens, makeup cape, and other washable items in a hamper.
5. Sanitize your workstation.
6. Wash your hands with soap and warm water.

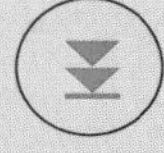

Here's a tip:

Skin varies in color and tone from person to person, regardless of ethnic background. When applying makeup, always remember to analyze the skin and choose makeup that will enhance the client's skin, eyes, and hair color, as well as her features.

completed!

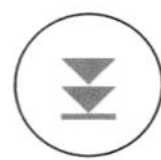

Here's a tip:

It is not recommended that you intensify every feature, as this will tend to look overdone and garish. For example, you can intensify the eyes and lips, or the cheeks and lips, but not the eyes, cheeks, and lips.

Special-Occasion Makeup

When a client asks for makeup for a special occasion, that is the time for you to work your magic. Special occasions often come with special conditions. For instance, many are evening events, when lighting is subdued. That means that more definition is required for the eyes, cheeks, and lips. You may also add drama by applying false lashes and using shimmery colors on the eyes, lips, cheeks, or complexion. If the special occasion is a wedding, however, where photography is an issue, matte colors are recommended, since shimmer may reflect light too much. Follow the basic makeup procedure above but consider the following pointers.

Special Occasion Makeup for Eyes

Option 1: *Striking Contour Eyes*

1. Apply the base color from the lashes to the brow with a shadow brush or applicator.
2. Apply medium tone on the lid, blending from lash line to crease with the shadow brush or applicator.
3. Apply medium to deep color in the crease, blending up toward the eyebrow, but ending below it.
4. Apply highlight shadow under the brow bone with the shadow brush or applicator.
5. Apply eyeliner on the upper lash line from the outside corner in, tapering as you reach the inner corner. Blend with the small brush or applicator.
6. Apply shadow in the same color as the liner, directly over the liner. This will give longevity and intensity to the liner. Repeat on the bottom lash line, if desired.
7. Apply mascara with a disposable wand (Figure 20–33).

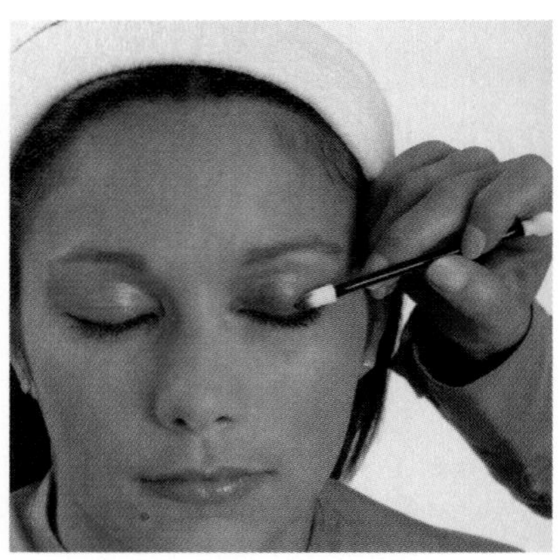

Figure 20-33 Striking contour eyes.

Option 2: *Dramatic Smoky Eyes*

1. Encircle the eye with dark gray, dark brown, or black eyeliner.
2. Smudge with a small shadow brush or disposable applicator.
3. Using the shadow brush or applicator, apply dark shadow from the upper lash line to the crease, softening and blending as you approach the crease. The shadow should be dark from outer to inner corner. You may choose shimmering or matte finish eye shadows.

20

activity

Using a model (or yourself) and two different color applications, divide the face in half. Try different foundations, colors, and intensity on each side. This will give you a visual example of how makeup will work on a face. Actually applying makeup is the best way to learn how to use it.

4. Repeat on the lower lash line, carefully blending any hard edges.
5. If desired, add a highlight color in a shimmering or matte finish to the upper brow area with the shadow brush or applicator.
6. Apply mascara with a disposable wand (Figure 20–34).
7. Add individual or band lashes if desired.

Special-Occasion Makeup for Cheeks

Refer to the next section on corrective makeup for techniques you can use to remedy less attractive aspects of the cheeks. You can also try either of these two steps.

1. Use a darker blush color under the cheekbones to add definition. Apply with a blush brush or applicator and blend carefully. Add a brighter, lighter cheek color to the apples of the cheeks and blend.
2. Use a cheek color with shimmer or glitter over the cheekbones for highlight. You may use cream or powder colors.

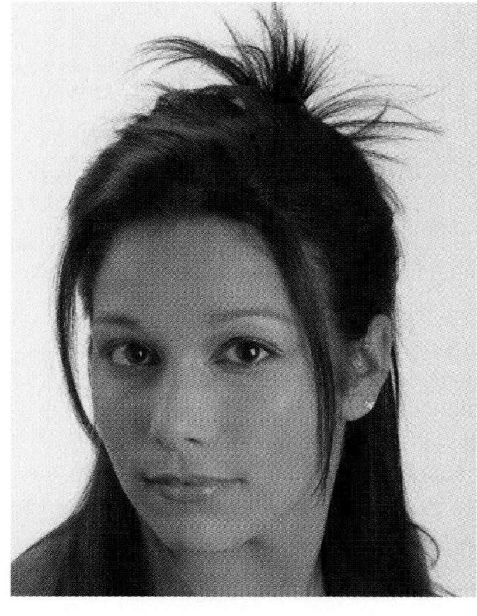

Figure 20-34 Dramatic smoky eyes.

Special-Occasion Makeup for Lips

Most clients prefer brighter or darker colors for special occasions. You may use shimmer colors or matte colors, if desired.

1. Apply liner color to the lips. Fill in the lip line with pencil and blot.
2. Add similar color in lipstick over the entire mouth with a lip brush or applicator.
3. Apply gloss to the center of the lips with a lip brush or applicator.

CORRECTIVE MAKEUP

All faces are interesting in their own special ways, but few are perfect. When you analyze a client's face, you might see that the nose, cheeks, lips, or jawline are not the same on both sides, or that one eye might be larger than the other, or that the eyebrows might not match. In fact, these tiny imperfections can make the face more interesting if treated artfully. In any case, facial makeup can create the illusion of better balance and proportion when so desired.

Facial features can be accented with proper highlighting, subdued with correct shadowing or shading, and balanced with the proper hairstyle. A basic rule for the application of makeup is that highlighting emphasizes a feature, while shadowing minimizes it. A highlight is produced when a cosmetic, usually foundation that is lighter than the original foundation is used on a particular part of the face. A shadow is formed when the

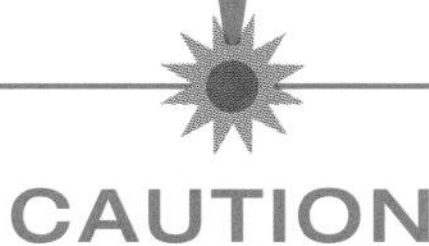

CAUTION

Corrective makeup can be very effective if applied properly. However, a less experienced cosmetologist should proceed with caution, as improper application, insufficient blending, or the wrong choice of colors can make the face look dirty and artificial.

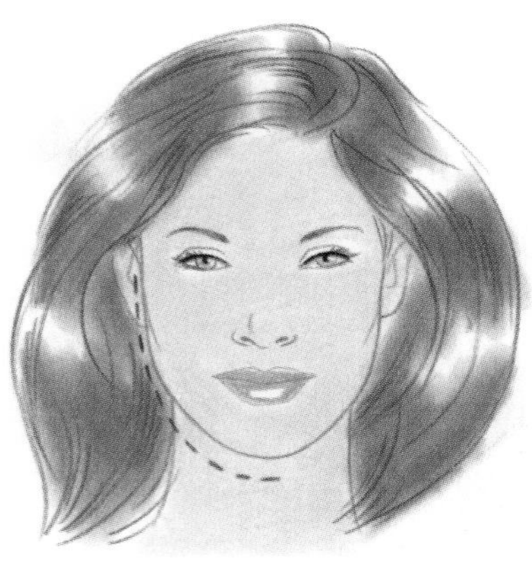

Figure 20–35 Oval face.

foundation is darker than the original color. The use of shadows (dark colors and shades) minimizes prominent features so that they are less noticeable.

Before you undertake any kind of corrective makeup application, you should have a clear sense of how to analyze the shape of the faces you will be working with.

Analyzing Features and Face Shape

The basic rule of makeup application is to emphasize the client's attractive features while minimizing features that are less appealing. Learning to see the face and its features as a whole and determining the best makeup for an individual takes practice. While the oval face with well-proportioned features has long been considered the ideal, other face shapes are just as attractive in their own way. The goal of effective makeup application is to enhance the client's individuality, not to "remake" her image according to some ideal standard.

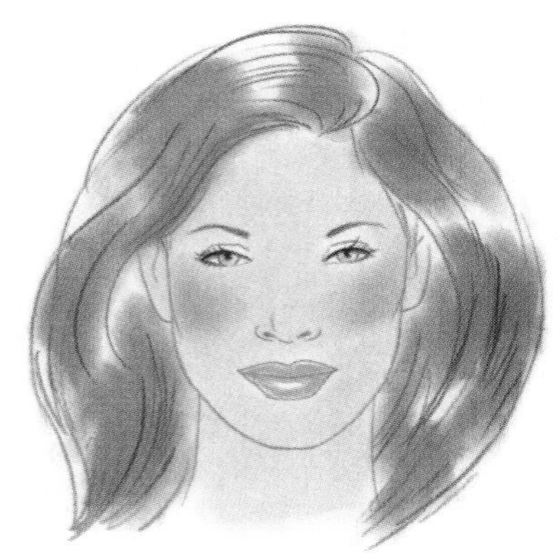

Figure 20–36 Oval face with makeup.

Oval-Shaped Face

The artistically ideal proportions and features of the oval face are the standard to which you will refer when learning the techniques of corrective makeup application. The face is divided into three equal horizontal sections. The first third is measured from the hairline to the top of the eyebrows. The second third is measured from the top of the eyebrows to the end of the nose. The last third is measured from the end of the nose to the bottom of the chin.

The ideal oval face is approximately three-fourths as wide as it is long. The distance between the eyes is the width of one eye (Figure 20–35 and Figure 20–36).

Round Face

The round face is usually broader in proportion to its length than the oval face. It has a rounded chin and hairline. Corrective makeup can be applied to slenderize and lengthen the face (Figure 20–37 and Figure 20–38).

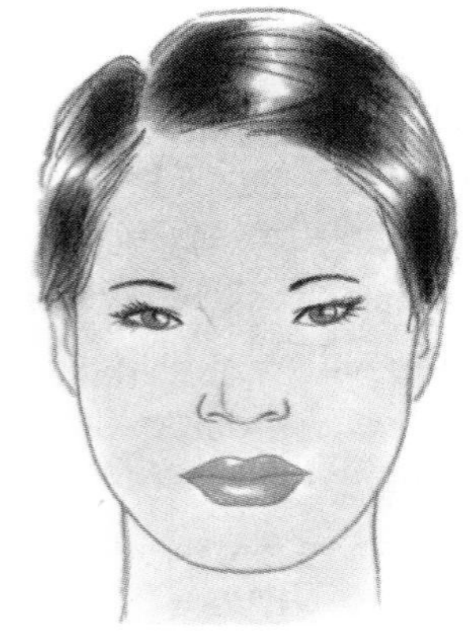

Figure 20–37 Round face.

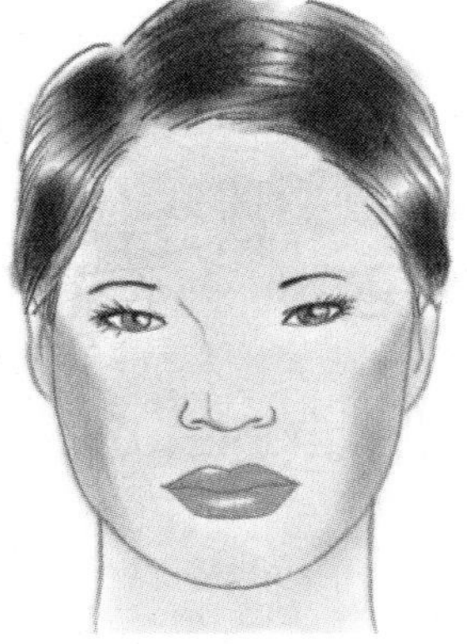

Figure 20–38 Round face with corrective makeup.

insights

Kimberly Woodall

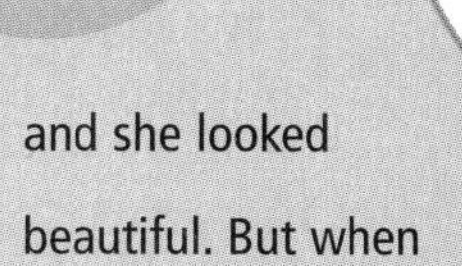

After eight years as a hairstylist and five years doing makeup, Kimberly Woodall, a freelancer, has gotten a good overview of what you need to know to survive—and thrive—in this business.

I started out doing styling for friends and family and little photo shoots just for fun. With the compliments I was getting, I worked up the courage to do what I'm doing now, which is styling clients and doing shots for magazines and fashion shows here in New York City. I'm basically an independent contractor. I'll go wherever the work is, whether it's a photo shoot, a wedding, or whatever.

The biggest challenge for me is keeping up with my craft and knowing all the current styles. Selling yourself is also a challenge. If you don't package yourself or present yourself in a proper way, you're not going to get the response you're looking for. You can learn how to do that from someone you admire.

I think the key to building up a loyal client base is staying professional. You have to be punctual; you have to show courtesy. You also have to make time for continuing education. My schedule is busy, but I make time because the trends are constantly changing and it's crucial to keep up with them.

My worst professional mishap was the first wedding I had to do, which was also my first professional freelance job. I did the bride's makeup in her house, and she looked beautiful. But when we got the pictures back, her face from the chin up was pale white and the rest of her skin looked tanned. What I learned from that is that when you apply makeup and foundation you have to be under good lighting to see how it's blending in with that person's natural skin tones, especially for an outdoor wedding. It definitely opened my eyes. I thought I could just put it on, it's easy. But that wasn't the case, and that's where advanced training comes in.

Before I do a shoot, I do a lot of planning. I try to take some test shots with a particular model if I have access to that model. You might even have to do things you never thought you'd have to do. For instance, I was having a hard time finding a professional photographer, so I decided to do the photography myself. I took some classes and it's worked out pretty well.

Each client is different, and that keeps it interesting and challenging for me because what may look good on one person does not look good on another. I like that. What I love most about my work is the satisfaction I get from my clients—the look on their faces when they see how much they can improve how they look. And that gives them encouragement, helps them feel better about themselves.

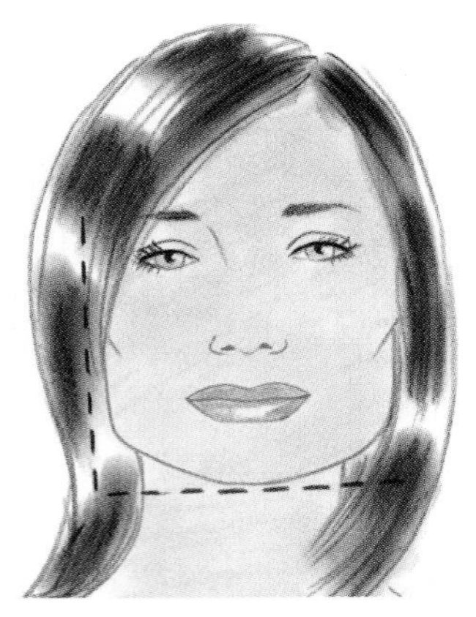

Figure 20-39 Square face.

Square-Shaped Face

The square face is composed of comparatively straight lines with a wide forehead and square jawline. Corrective makeup can be applied to offset the squareness and soften the hard lines around the face (Figure 20–39 and Figure 20–40).

Triangular (Pear-Shaped) Face

A jaw that is wider than the forehead characterizes the pear-shaped face. Corrective makeup can be applied to create width at the forehead, slenderize the jawline, and add length to the face (Figure 20–41 and Figure 20–42).

Inverted Triangle (Heart-Shaped) Face

The inverted triangle or heart-shaped face has a wide forehead and narrow, pointed chin. Corrective makeup can be applied to minimize the width of the forehead and to increase the width of the jawline (Figure 20–43 and Figure 20–44).

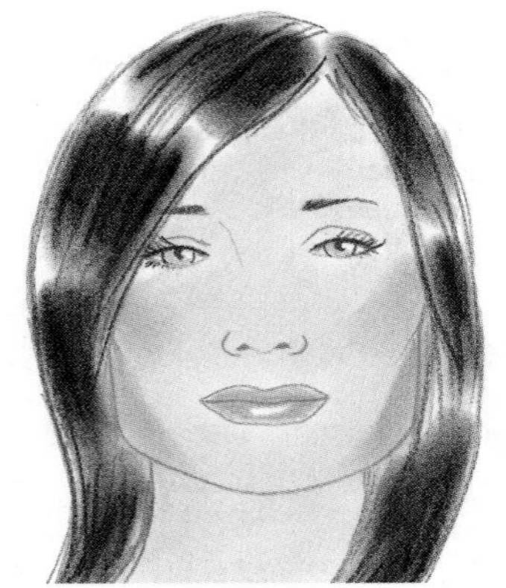

Figure 20-40 Square face with corrective makeup.

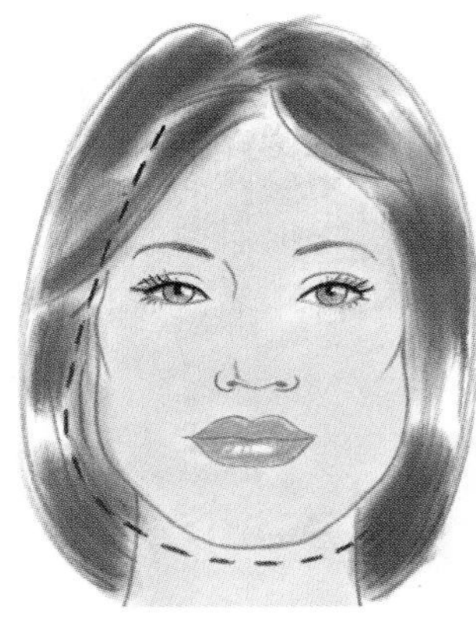

Figure 20-41 Triangular face.

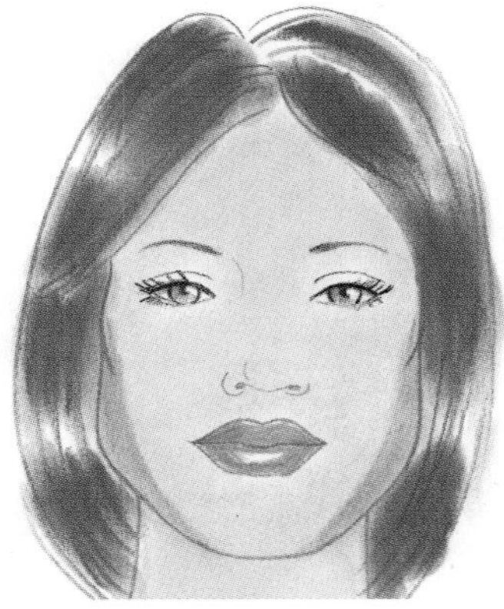

Figure 20-42 Triangular face with corrective makeup.

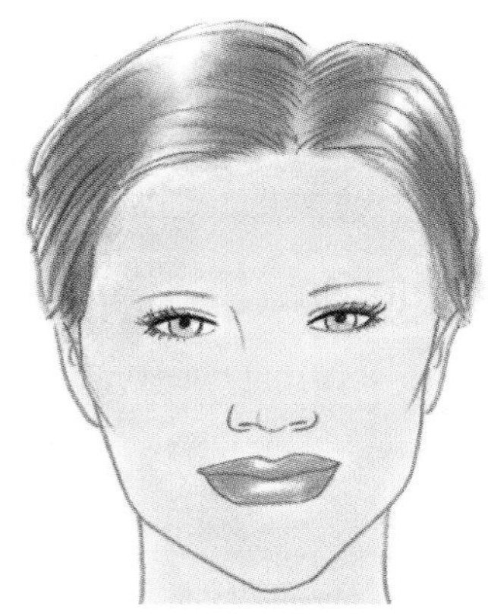

Figure 20-43 Inverted triangle-shaped face.

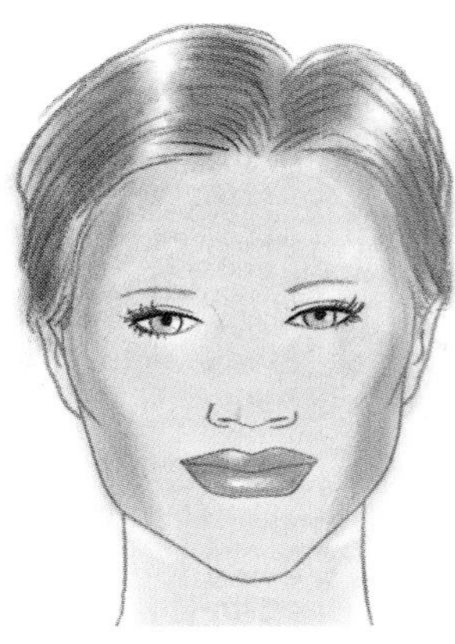

Figure 20-44 Inverted triangle-shaped face with corrective makeup.

Diamond-Shaped Face

This face has a narrow forehead. The greatest width is across the cheekbones. Corrective makeup can be applied to reduce the width across the cheekbone line (Figure 20–45 and Figure 20–46).

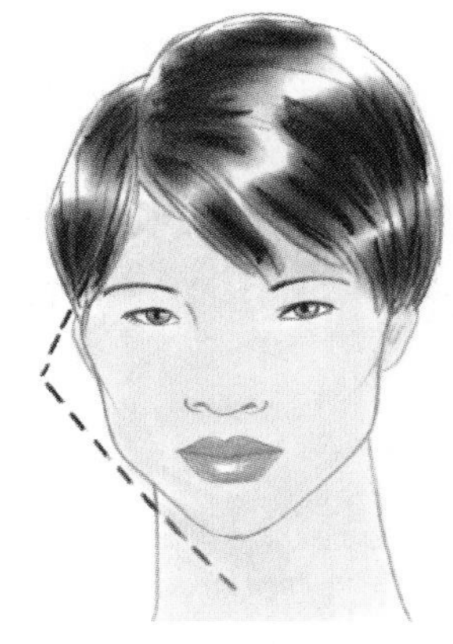

Figure 20-45 Diamond-shaped face.

Oblong Face

This face has greater length in proportion to its width than the square or round face. It is long and narrow. Corrective makeup can be applied to create the illusion of width across the cheekbone line, making the face appear shorter (Figure 20–47 and Figure 20–48).

Forehead Area

For a low forehead, the application of a lighter foundation lends a broader appearance between the brows and hairline. For a protruding forehead, applying a darker foundation over the prominent area gives an illusion of fullness to the rest of the face and minimizes the bulging forehead. A suitable hairstyle also goes a long way toward drawing attention away from the forehead (Figure 20–49).

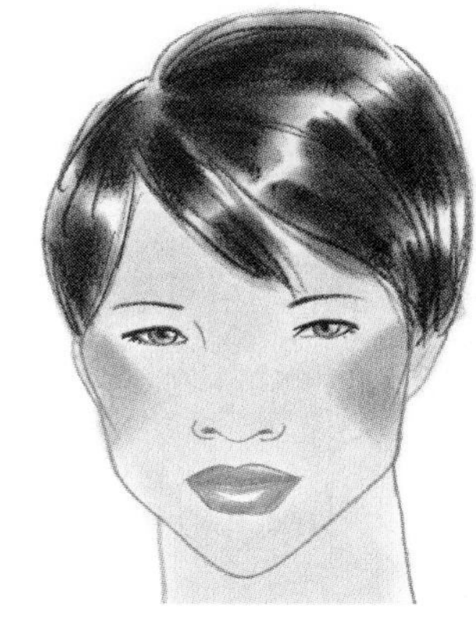

Figure 20-46 Diamond-shaped face with corrective makeup.

Nose and Chin Areas

For a large or protruding nose, apply a darker foundation on the nose and a lighter foundation on the cheeks at the sides of the nose. This will create fullness in the cheeks and will make the nose appear smaller. Avoid placing cheek color close to the nose.

For a short and flat nose, apply a lighter foundation down the center of the nose, ending at the tip. This will make the nose appear longer and larger.

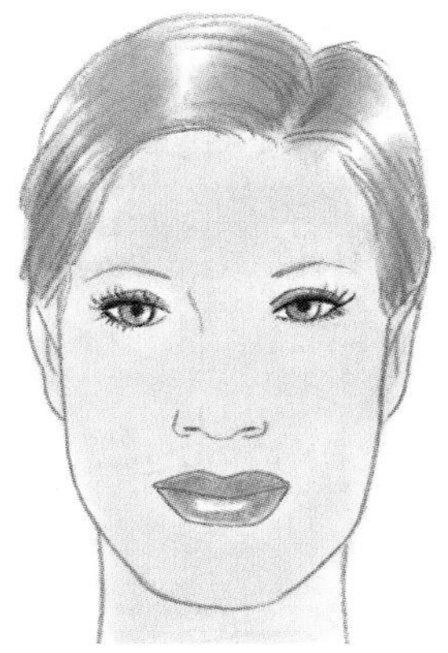

Figure 20-47 Oblong face.

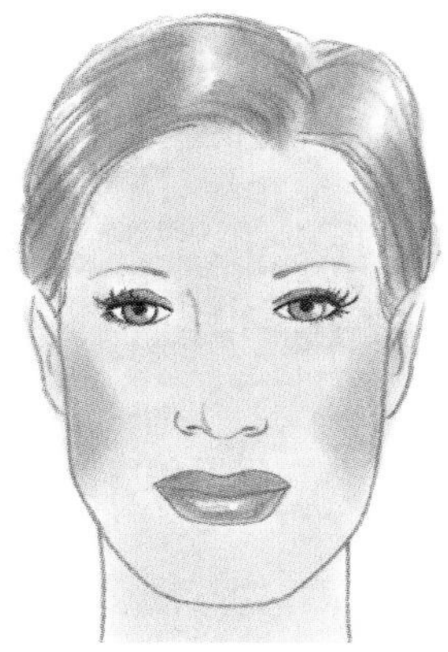

Figure 20-48 Oblong face with corrective makeup.

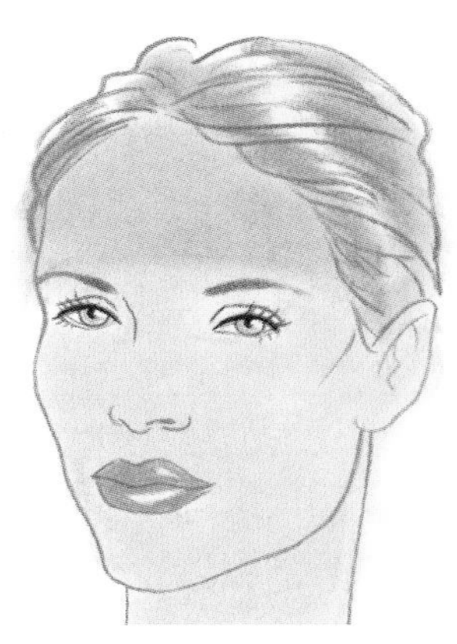

Figure 20-49 Protruding forehead with corrective makeup.

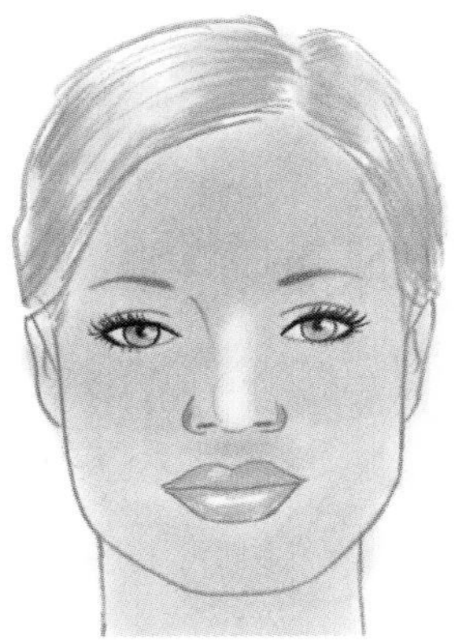

Figure 20-50 Short flat nose with corrective makeup.

If the nostrils are wide, apply a darker foundation to both sides of the nostrils (Figure 20–50).

For a broad nose, use a darker foundation on the sides of the nose and nostrils. Avoid carrying this dark tone into the laugh lines because it will accentuate them. The foundation must be carefully blended to avoid visible lines (Figure 20–51).

For a protruding chin and receding nose, shadow the chin with a darker foundation and highlight the nose with a lighter foundation. For a receding chin, highlight the chin by using a lighter foundation than the one used on the face.

For a sagging double chin, use a darker foundation on the sagging portion, and use a natural skin tone foundation on the face (Figure 20–52).

Jawline and Neck Area

The neck and jaw are just as important as the eyes, cheeks, and lips. When applying makeup, blend the foundation onto the neck so that the client's color is consistent from face to neck. Always set with a translucent powder to avoid transfer onto the client's clothing.

To correct a broad jawline, apply a darker shade of foundation over the heavy area of the jaw, starting at the temples. This will minimize the lower part of the face and create an illusion of width in the upper part of the face (Figure 20–53).

To correct a narrow jawline, highlight by using a lighter foundation shade (Figure 20–54).

For a round, square, or triangular face, apply a darker shade of foundation over the prominent part of the jawline. By creating a shadow over this area, the prominent part of the jaw will appear softer and more oval.

For a small face and a short, thick neck, use a darker foundation on the neck than the one used on the face. This will make the neck appear thinner.

For a long, thin neck, apply a lighter shade of foundation on the neck than the one used on the face. This will create fullness and counteract the long, thin appearance of the neck (Figure 20–55).

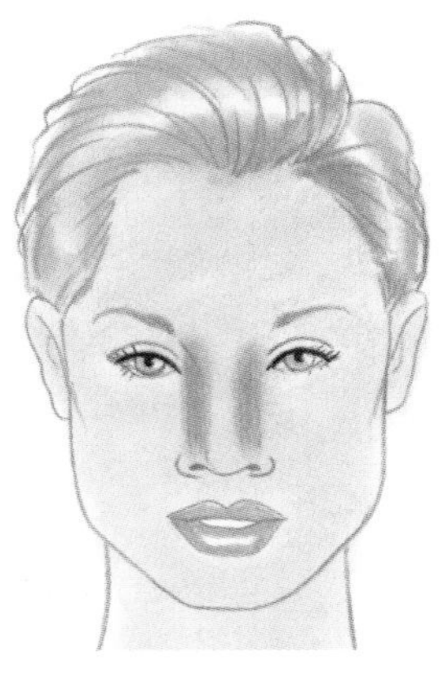

Figure 20-51 Broad nose with corrective makeup.

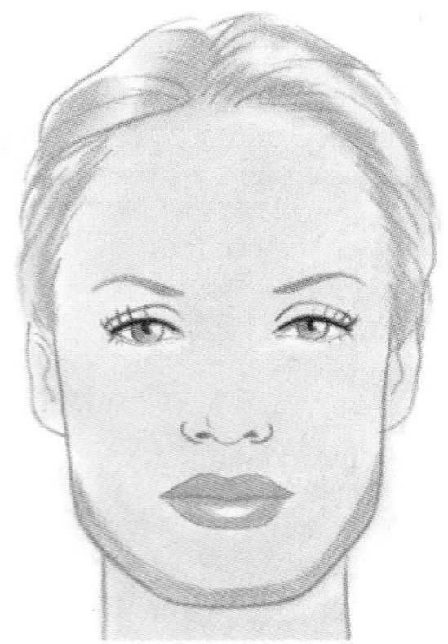

Figure 20-52 Double chin with corrective makeup.

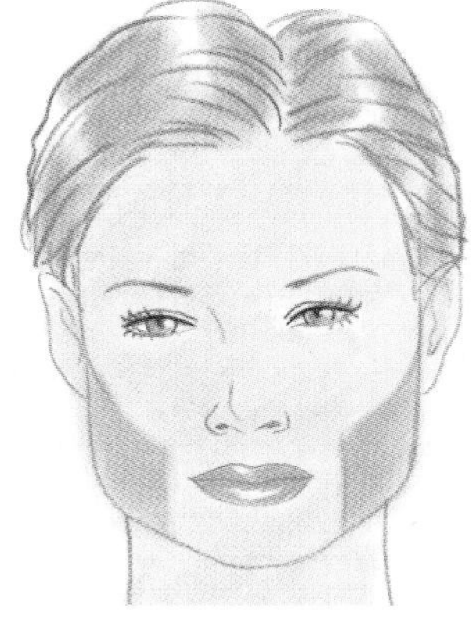

Figure 20-53 Broad jawline with corrective makeup.

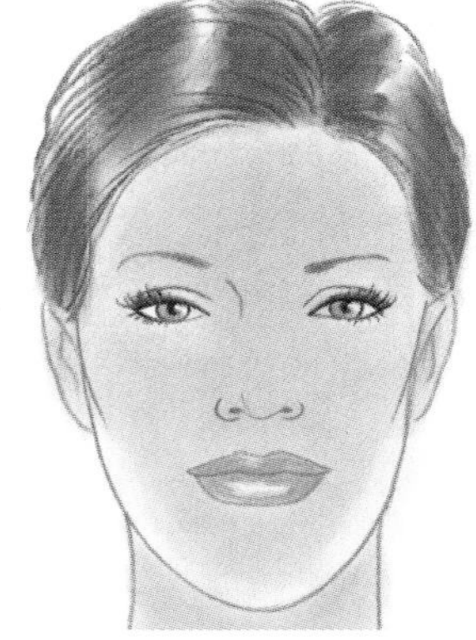

Figure 20-54 Narrow jawline with corrective makeup.

Corrective Makeup for the Eyes

The eyes are very important when it comes to balancing facial features. The proper application of eye colors and shadow can create the illusion of the eyes being larger or smaller, and will enhance the overall attractiveness of the face.

Round eyes can be lengthened by extending the shadow beyond the outer corner of the eyes (Figure 20–56 and Figure 20–57).

Close-set eyes are closer together than the length of one eye. For eyes that are too close together, lightly apply shadow up from the outer edge of the eyes (Figure 20–58 and Figure 20–59).

Protruding or bulging eyes can be minimized by blending the shadow carefully over the prominent part of the upper lid, carrying it lightly toward the eyebrow. Use a medium to deep shadow color (Figure 20–60 and Figure 20–61).

Heavy-lidded eyes. Shadow evenly and lightly across the lid from the edge of the eyelash line to the small crease in the eye socket (Figure 20–62 and Figure 20–63).

Small eyes. To make small eyes appear larger, extend the shadow slightly above, beyond, and below the eyes.

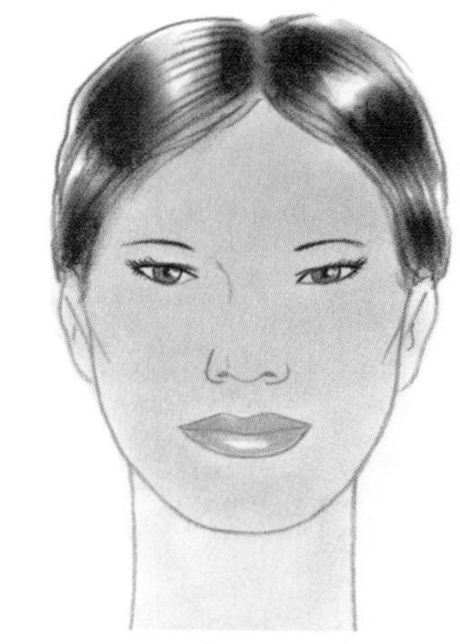

Figure 20-55 Long, thin neck with corrective makeup.

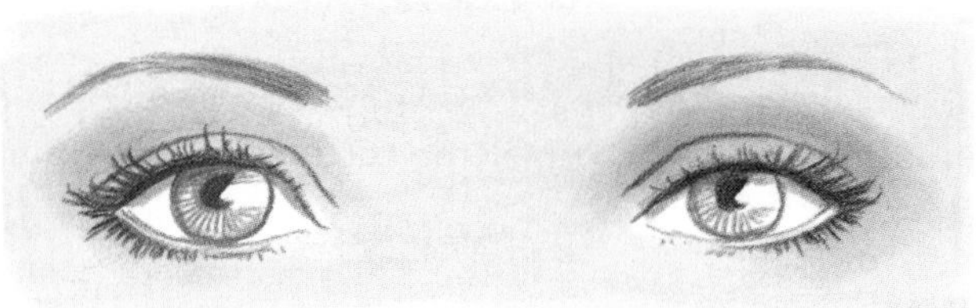

Figure 20-56 Round eyes.

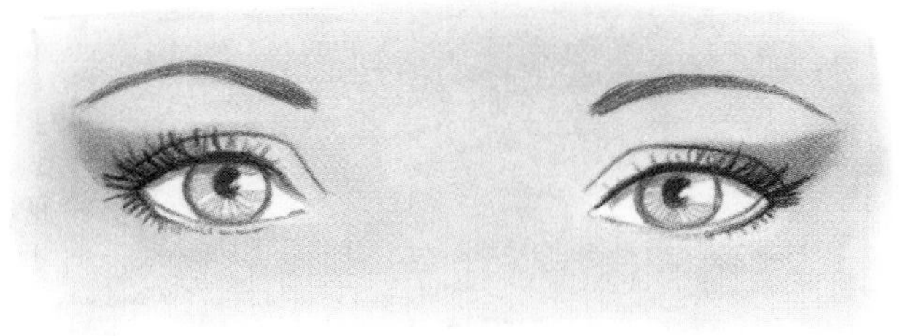

Figure 20-57 Round eyes with corrective makeup.

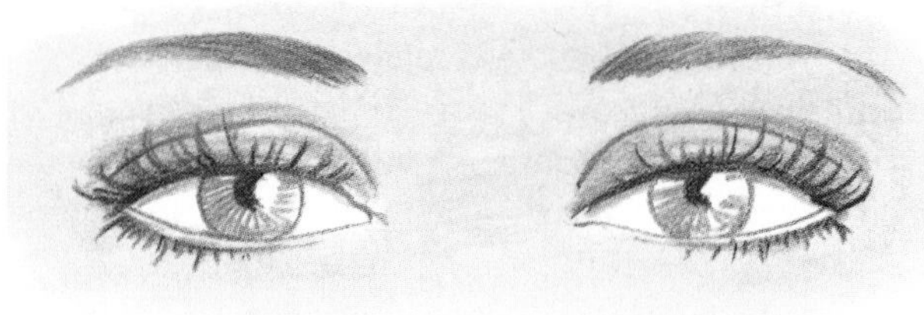

Figure 20-58 Close-set eyes.

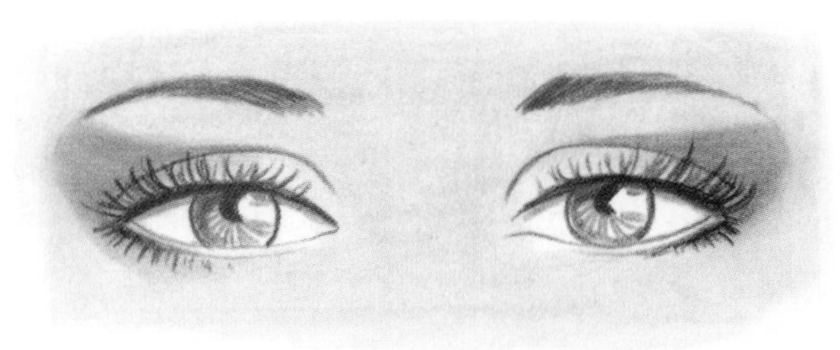

Figure 20-59 Close-set eyes with corrective makeup.

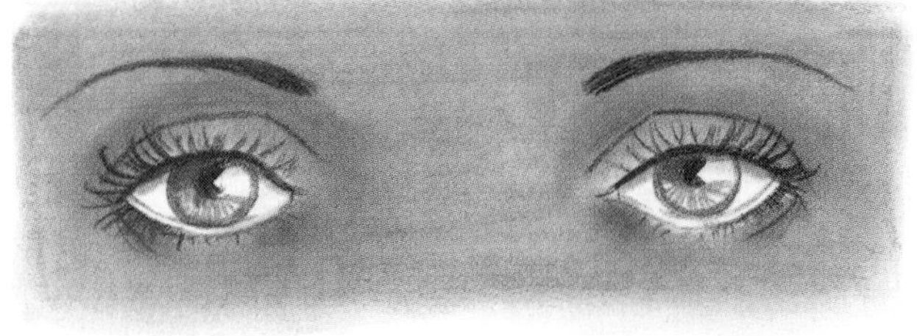

Figure 20-60 Protruding eyes.

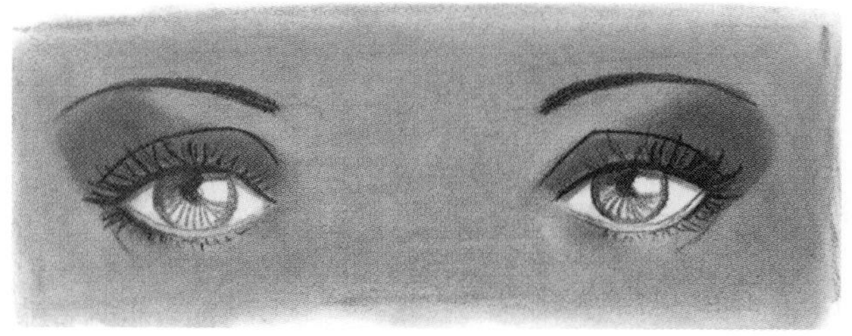

Figure 20-61 Protruding eyes with corrective makeup.

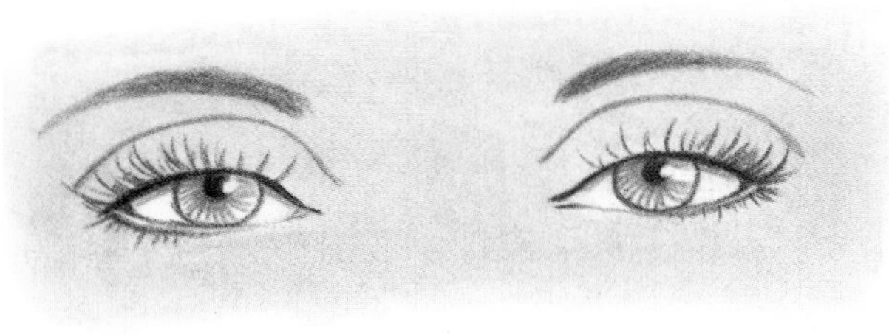

Figure 20-62 Heavy-lidded eyes.

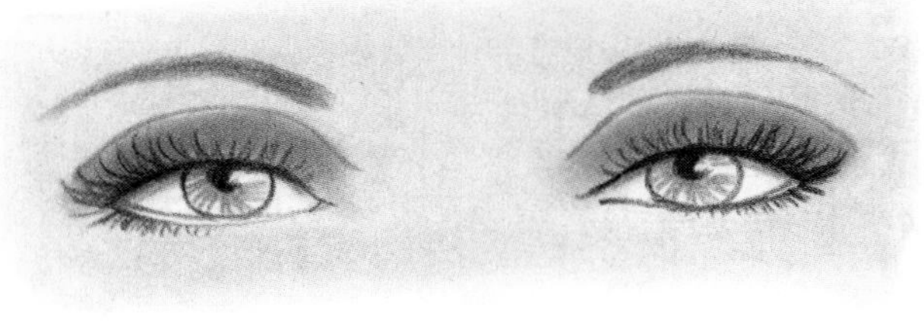

Figure 20-63 Heavy-lidded eyes with corrective makeup.

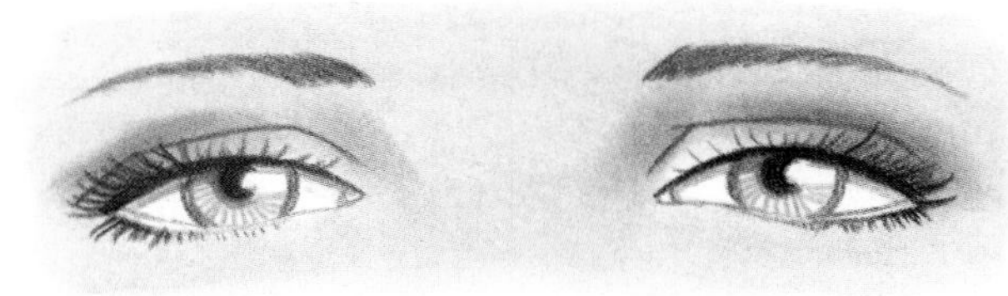

Figure 20-64 Deep-set eyes.

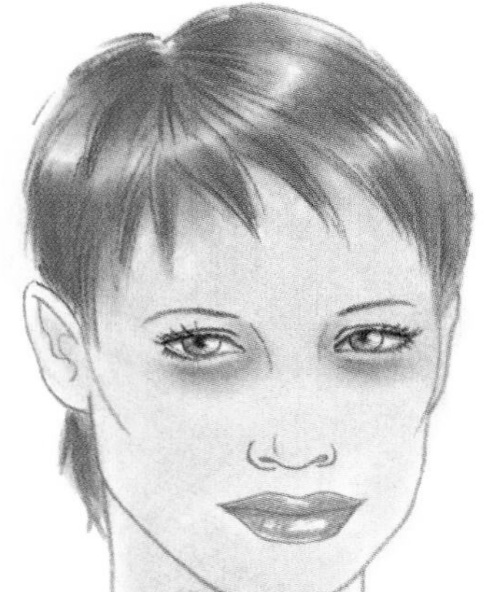

Figure 20-65 Dark circles under eyes.

Wide-set eyes. Apply the shadow on the upper inner side of the eyelid, toward the nose, and blend carefully.

Deep-set eyes. Use bright, light, reflective colors. Use the lightest color in the crease, and a light to medium color sparingly on the lid and brow bone (Figure 20–64).

Dark circles under eyes. Apply concealer over the dark area, blending and smoothing it into the surrounding area. Set lightly with translucent powder (Figure 20–65).

Eyebrows

Reshaping and defining eyebrows can be an art unto itself. Well-groomed eyebrows are part of a complete and effective makeup application. The eyebrow is the frame for the eye. Overgrown eyebrows can cast a shadow on the brow bone or between the two eyebrows. Overtweezed eyebrows can make the face look puffy or protruding, or may give the eyes a surprised look.

When a client wants to correct eyebrow shape, begin by removing all unnecessary hairs and then demonstrate how to use the eyebrow pencil or shadow to fill in until the natural hairs have grown in again. When there are spaces in the eyebrow hair, they can be filled in with hairlike strokes of an eyebrow pencil or shadow, applied with an angled brush. Use an eyebrow brush to soften the pencil or shadow marks.

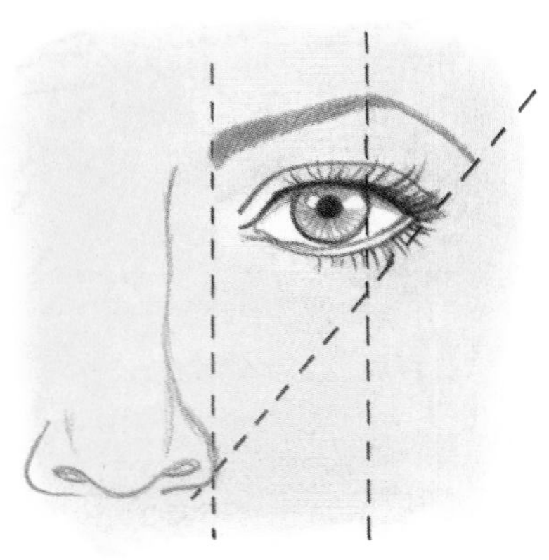

Figure 20-66 Ideal eyebrow shape.

The ideal eyebrow shape can be drawn in three lines (Figure 20–66). The first line is vertical, from the inner corner of the eye upward. This is where the eyebrow should begin. The second line is drawn at an angle from the outer corner of the nose to the outer corner of the eye. This is where the eyebrow should end. The third line is vertical, from the outer circle of the iris of the eye upward. The client should be looking straight ahead as you determine this line. This is where the highest part of the arch would ideally be. Of course, not everyone's eyebrows fit exactly within these measurements, so use them only as guidelines.

When the arch is too high, remove the superfluous hair from the top of the brow and fill in the lower part with eyebrow pencil or shadow. Build up the shape by layering color lightly until the desired effect is achieved.

Adjustments to eyebrow shape can also be used to correct other facial shortcomings.

- *Low forehead.* A low arch gives more height to a very low forehead.
- *Wide-set eyes.* The eyes can be made to appear closer together by extending the eyebrow lines to the inside corners of the eyes. However, care must be taken to avoid giving the client a frowning look.
- *Close-set eyes.* To make the eyes appear farther apart, widen the distance between the eyebrows and slightly extend them outward.
- *Round face.* Arch the brows high to make the face appear narrower. Start on a line directly above the inside corner of the eye and extend to the end of the cheekbone.
- *Long face.* Making the eyebrows almost straight can create the illusion of a shorter face. Do not extend the eyebrow lines farther than the outside corners of the eyes.
- *Square face.* The face will appear more oval if there is a high arch on the ends of the eyebrows. Begin the lines directly above the corners of the eyes and extend them outward.

The Lips

Lips are usually proportioned so that the curves or peaks of the upper lip fall directly in line with the nostrils. In some cases, one side of the lips may differ from the other. Lips can be very full, very thin, or uneven. The illustrations on this page and the next show various lip lines and how lip color can be used to create the illusion of better proportions (Figure 20–67, Figure 20–68, Figure 20–69, Figure 20–70, Figure 20–71, Figure 20–72, Figure 20–73, Figure 20–74 and Figure 20–75).

Skin Tones

For whatever reason, some clients may wish to alter their skin tone. In terms of corrective makeup, you will be dealing with two basic skin tones.

- *For ruddy skin* (skin that is red, wind-burned, or affected by rosacea), apply a yellow or green foundation to affected areas, blending carefully.

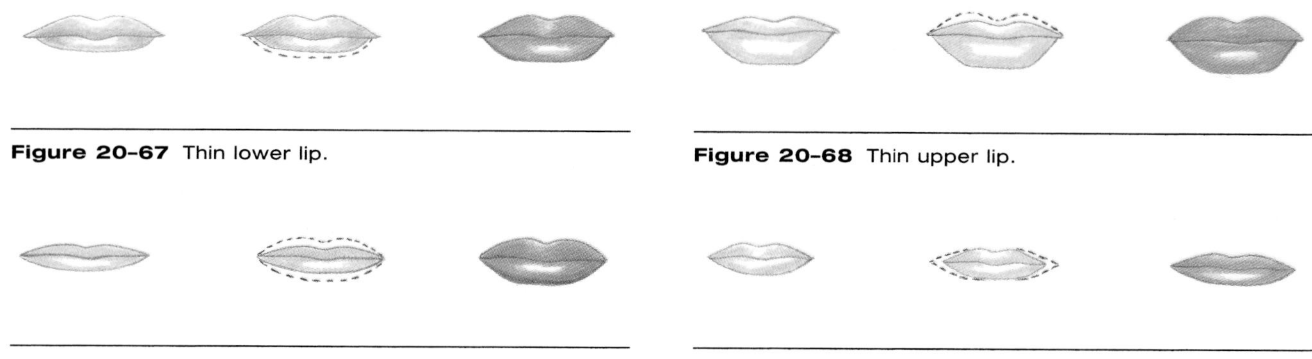

Figure 20-67 Thin lower lip.

Figure 20-68 Thin upper lip.

Figure 20-69 Thin lips.

Figure 20-70 Small mouth.

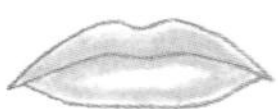 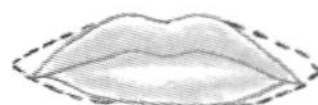 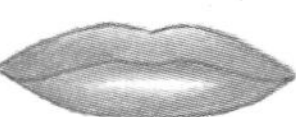

Figure 20-71 Drooping corners.

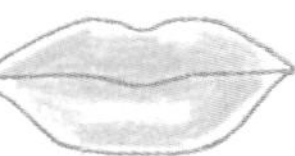 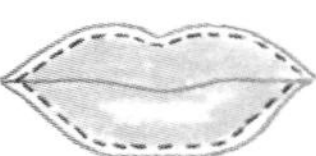 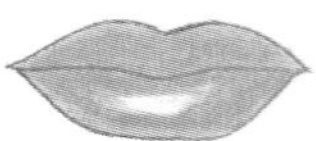

Figure 20-72 Large, full lips.

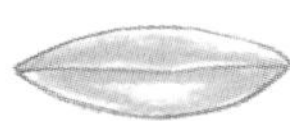 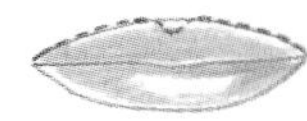 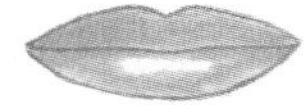

Figure 20-73 Oval lips.

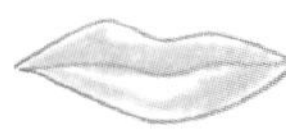 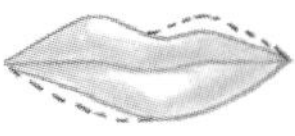 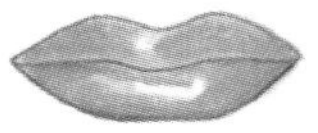

Figure 20-74 Sharp peaks.

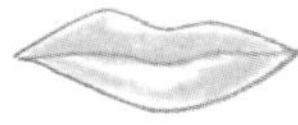 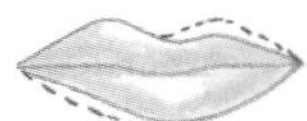 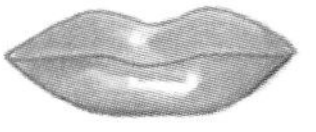

Figure 20-75 Uneven lips.

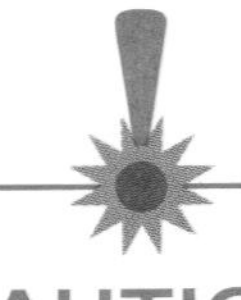

CAUTION

Some clients may be allergic to adhesive. When in doubt, give the client an allergy test before applying the lashes. This test may be done in one of two ways:

1. **Put a drop of the adhesive behind one ear.**
2. **Attach a single individual eyelash to each eyelid.**

In either case, if there is no reaction within 24 hours, it is probably safe to proceed with the application.

You may then apply a light layer of foundation with a yellow base over the entire complexion. Set it with translucent or yellow-based powder. Avoid red or pink blushes.

- *For sallow skin* (skin that has a yellowish hue), apply a pink-based foundation on the affected areas and blend carefully into the jaw and neck. Set with translucent powder. Avoid yellow-based colors for eyes, cheeks, and lips.

Wrinkles

Age lines and wrinkles due to dry skin can be minimized with a foundation. Apply the foundation sparingly and evenly, in a light, outward, circular motion over the entire surface of the face. Care should be taken to remove any foundation that collects in lines and wrinkles of the face.

20

ARTIFICIAL EYELASHES

The use of artificial eyelashes has grown enormously for a number of reasons: the technology has improved dramatically, and fashion has become more reliant on these accessories. Clients with sparse lashes and clients who want to enhance their eyes for special occasions are most likely to request this service. The objective is to make the client's own lashes look fuller, longer, and more attractive without appearing unnatural.

Two types of artificial eyelashes are commonly used. **Band lashes** (also called strip lashes) are eyelash hairs on a strip that are applied with adhesive to the natural lash line. Individual lashes are separate artificial eyelashes that are applied to the eyelids one at a time. **Eyelash adhesive** is the product used to make artificial eyelashes adhere, or stick, to the natural lash line.

PROCEDURE 56

APPLYING BAND LASHES

Implements and Materials

- wet sanitizer for metal implements
- headband or hair clip
- tweezers
- cotton swabs
- eyelash brushes
- eyelash curler
- hand mirror
- manicure scissors
- adjustable light (gooseneck lamp)
- makeup chair
- lash adhesive
- adhesive tray
- eyelid and eyelash cleanser
- eyelash remover
- cotton pads
- eye makeup remover
- makeup cape
- trays of artificial eyelashes
- pencil sharpener

Preparation

1. Client consultation. Discuss with the client the desired length of the lashes and the effect she hopes to achieve.
2. Wash your hands.
3. Place the client in the makeup chair with her head at a comfortable working height. The client's face should be well and evenly lit, but avoid shining the light directly into the eyes. Work from behind or to the side of the client. Avoid working directly in front of the client whenever possible.
4. Properly drape the client to protect her clothing and have her use a hairline strip, headband, or turban during the procedure.
5. If the client wears contact lenses, they must be removed before starting the procedure.
6. If the client has not already done so, remove all eye makeup so that the lash adhesive will adhere properly. Work carefully and gently. Follow the manufacturers' instructions carefully.

Procedure

1. Brush the client's eyelashes to make sure they are clean and free of foreign matter, such as mascara particles. If the client's lashes are straight, they can be curled with an eyelash curler before you apply the artificial lashes.
2. Carefully remove the eyelash band from the package.
3. Start with the upper lash. If it is too long to fit the curve of the upper eyelid, trim the outside edge. Use your fingers to bend the lash into a horseshoe shape to make it more flexible so it fits the contour of the eyelid.

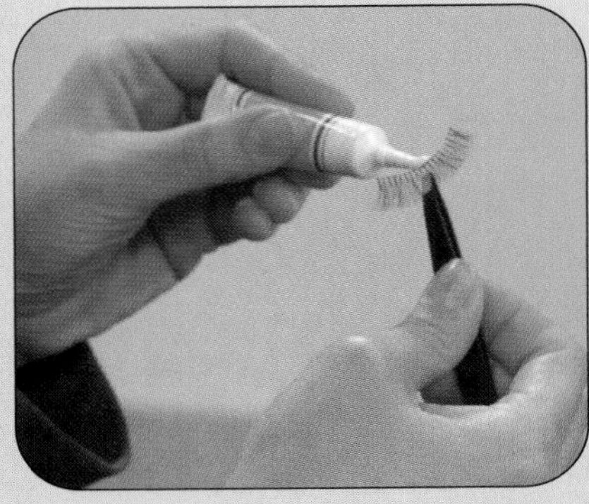
Figure 20-76 Feather the band lashes.

4. Feather the lash by nipping into it with the points of your scissors. This creates a more natural look (Figure 20–76).
5. Apply a thin strip of lash adhesive to the base of the lash and allow a few seconds for it to set (Figure 20–77).
6. Apply the lash. Start with the shorter part of the lash and place it on the inner corner of the eye, toward the nose. Position the rest of the artificial lash as close to the client's own lash as possible. Use the rounded end of a lash liner brush or tweezers to press the lash on (Figure 20–78). Be very careful and gentle when applying the lashes. If eyeliner is to be used, the line is usually drawn on the eyelid before the lash is applied and retouched when the artificial lash is in place (Figure 20–79).
7. Apply the lower lash, if desired. Lower lash application is optional, as it tends to look more unnatural. Trim the lash as necessary and apply adhesive in the same way you did for the upper lash. Place the lash on top of the client's lower lash. Place the shorter lash toward the center of the eye and the longer lash toward the outer part of the lid (Figure 20–80).

Figure 20-77 Apply lash adhesive to the band lashes.

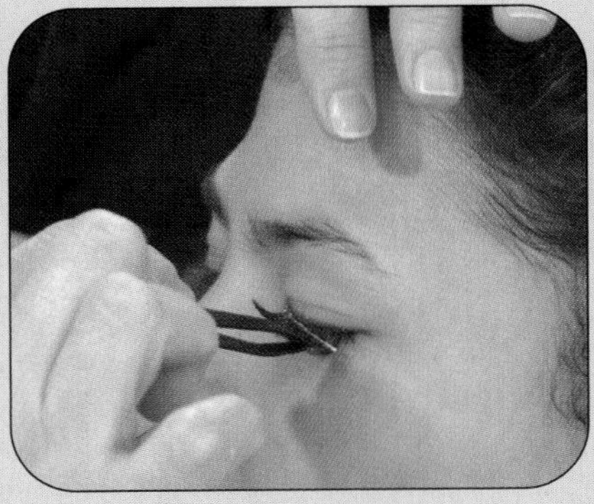
Figure 20-78 Apply the band lashes to the eyelid.

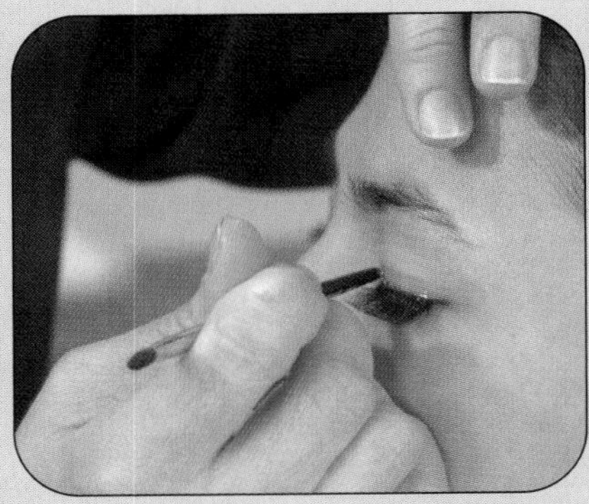
Figure 20-79 Retouch the lash line with eyeliner.

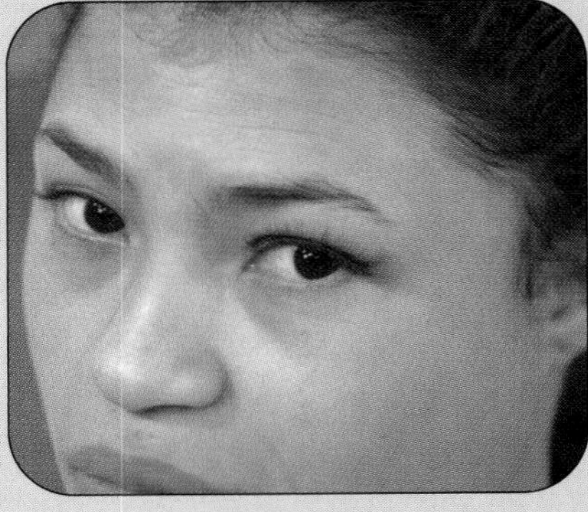
Figure 20-80 Finished band eyelash application.

Cleanup/Sanitation

1. Discard all disposable items, such as sponges, pads, spatulas, and applicators.
2. Disinfect implements, such as the eyelash curler.
3. Clean and sanitize brushes using a commercial brush sanitizer.
4. Place all towels, linens, and makeup cape in a hamper.
5. Sanitize your workstation.
6. Wash your hands with soap and warm water.

CAUTION

Remind the client to take special care with artificial lashes when swimming, bathing, or cleansing the face. Water or cleansing products will loosen artificial lashes.

completed!

Applying Band Lashes

Band lashes (sometimes referred to as strip lashes) are available in a variety of sizes, textures, and colors. They can be made from human hair, certain animal hair such as mink, or synthetic fibers. Synthetic fiber eyelashes are made with a permanent curl and do not react to changes in weather conditions. Artificial eyelashes are available in natural colors ranging from light to dark brown and black or light to dark auburn, as well as bright, trendy colors. Black and dark brown are the most popular choices.

Removing Band Eyelashes

You may use commercial preparations, such as pads saturated with special lotions, to remove band eyelashes. The lash base may also be softened by applying a face cloth or cotton pad saturated with warm water and a gentle facial cleanser. Hold the cloth over the eyes for a few seconds to soften the adhesive. Starting from the outer corner, remove the lashes carefully to avoid pulling out the client's own lashes. Use cotton tips to remove any makeup and adhesive remaining on the eyelid.

Individual Lashes

Individual eyelashes are synthetic and attach directly to a client's own lashes at their base. This procedure is sometimes referred to as **eye tabbing**. Follow the manufacturers' instructions for attaching individual lashes.

SAFETY PRECAUTIONS

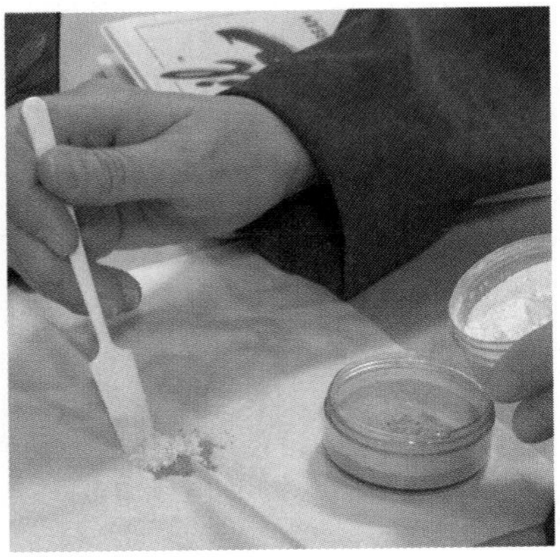

Figure 20–81 Remove cosmetics from containers with a spatula.

- Wash your hands thoroughly with soap and warm water before and after every makeup application.
- Properly drape the client to protect her clothing and have her use a headband or hair clip during the makeup procedure.
- Protect the client's hair and skin from direct contact with the facial chair.
- Keep your fingernails smooth to avoid scratching the client's skin.
- Use only sanitized brushes and implements.
- Use a shaker-type container for loose powder.
- Pour all lotions from bottle containers.
- Always use a clean spatula or cosmetic applicator to remove cosmetics from their containers (Figure 20–81).
- Never apply lip color directly from the container to the client's lips. Use a spatula or disposable applicator to remove the product from the container, then use a brush to apply.
- Use an antiseptic on tweezed areas of the eyebrow to avoid infection.
- Discard all disposable items, such as sponges, pads, spatulas, and applicators, after use.
- Place all towels, linens, makeup capes, and other items that can be washed and sanitized in the proper containers.
- Keep your workstation sanitary, neat, and well organized.

chapter glossary

band lashes	eyelash hairs on a strip that are applied with adhesive to the natural lash line
cake (pancake) makeup	shaped, solid mass applied to the face with a moistened cosmetic sponge; gives good coverage
cheek color	cream or powder cosmetic used to color the cheeks and the skin beneath the cheekbones; also called blush, blusher, or rouge
concealers	cosmetics used to cover blemishes and discolorations; may be applied before or after foundation
cool colors	colors that suggest coolness and are dominated by blues, greens, violets, and blue-reds
eyebrow pencils	pencils used to add color and shape to the eyebrows
eyelash adhesive	product used to make artificial eyelashes adhere, or stick, to the natural lash line
eyeliner	cosmetic used to outline and emphasize the eyes
eye makeup removers	cosmetic preparations for removing eye makeup
eye shadows	cosmetics applied on the eyelids, eyebrows, or lash line to accentuate or contour
eye tabbing	procedure in which individual synthetic eyelashes are attached directly to a client's own lashes at their base
face powder	fine cosmetic powder, sometimes tinted and scented, that is used to add a matte or dull finish to the face
foundation	cosmetic, usually tinted, that is used as a base or as a protective film applied before makeup and/or powder
greasepaint	heavy makeup used for theatrical purposes
lip color	cosmetic in paste form, usually in a metal or plastic tube, manufactured in a variety of colors and used to color the lips; also called lipstick or gloss
lip liner	colored pencil or brush used to outline the lips and to help keep lip color from feathering
mascara	cosmetic preparation used to darken, define, and thicken the eyelashes
matte	dull, nonshiny
warm colors	the range of colors from yellow and gold through oranges, red-oranges, most reds, and even some yellow-greens

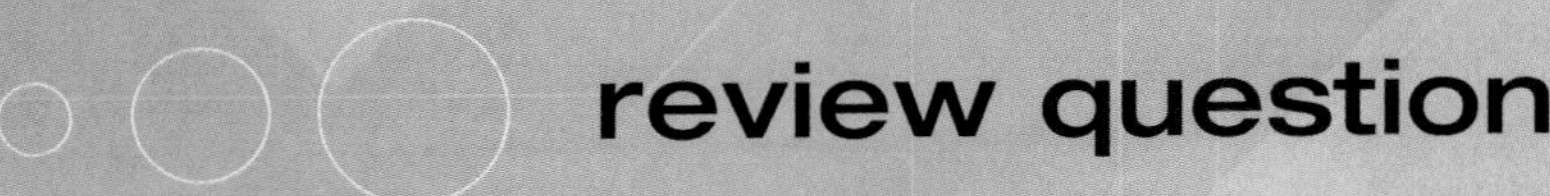

review questions

1. What is the main objective of makeup application?
2. List eight types of facial cosmetics and how they are used.
3. Name the different types and uses of foundation.
4. Name four types of cheek color.
5. Name the three different types of eye shadow and how they are used.
6. List the primary and secondary colors.
7. Name the colors in the warm range and the cool range.
8. What are complementary colors?
9. List the cosmetics used in a basic makeup procedure, in the order in which they are applied.
10. What are the seven facial types?
11. Name and describe the two types of artificial eyelashes.
12. List at least ten safety measures that should be followed when applying makeup.

part 5

NAIL CARE

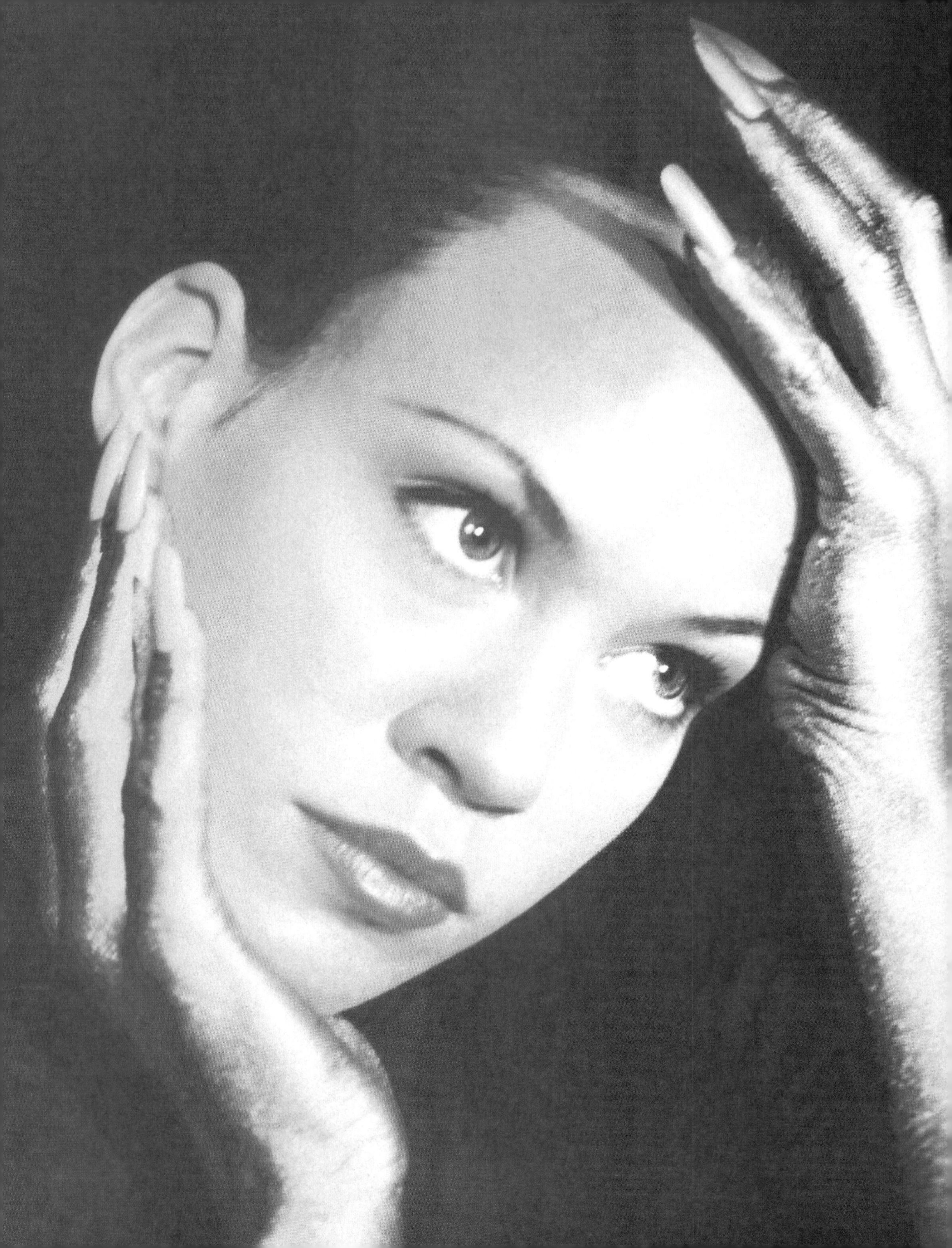

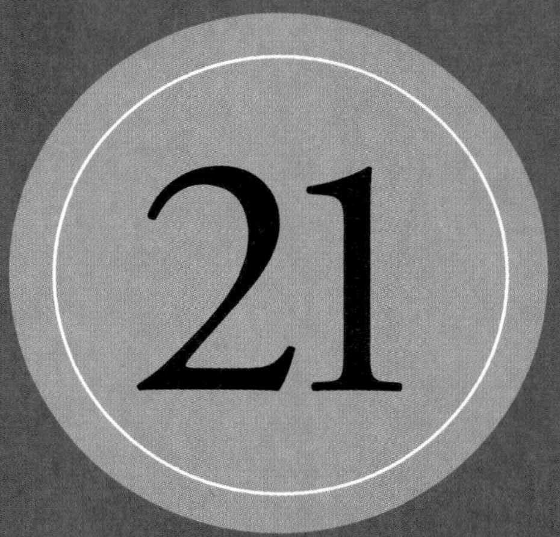

NAIL STRUCTURE AND GROWTH

Sue Ellen Schultes
INTERNATIONAL NAIL JUDGE AND CEO,
NOTORIOUS NAILS SEMINARS

Chapter Outline

Learning Objectives

After completing this chapter, you should be able to:

1. **Describe the structure and composition of nails.**

2. **Discuss how nails grow.**

3. **List and describe the various disorders and irregularities of nails.**

4. **Recognize diseases of the nails that should not be treated in the salon.**

National Skill Standards

This chapter provides you with the necessary information to master this National Industry Skill Standard for Entry-Level Cosmetologists.

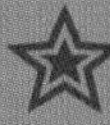

Conducting services in a safe environment and taking measures to prevent the spread of infectious and contagious diseases.

Key Terms

Page number indicates where in the chapter the term is used.

bed epithelium pg. 740

blue nails pg. 742

bruised nails pg. 742

corrugations pg. 742

cuticle pg. 740

eggshell nails pg. 742

eponychium pg. 740

free edge pg. 740

furrows pg. 743

hangnail or agnail pg. 743

hyponychium pg. 740

leukonychia pg. 743

ligament pg. 741

lunula or half moon pg. 740

mantle pg. 741

matrix bed or nail root pg. 740

melanonychia pg. 743

nail pg. 739

nail bed pg. 740

nail disorder pg. 742

nail folds pg. 741

nail grooves pg. 741

nail plate or nail body pg. 740

onychatrophia pg. 744

onychauxis or hypertrophy pg. 744

onychia pg. 748

onychocryptosis pg. 748

onychogryposis or onychogryphosis pg. 748

onycholysis pg. 750

onychomadesis pg. 750

onychophagy pg. 744

onychophosis pg. 750

onychoptosis pg. 750

onychorrhexis pg. 744

onychosis pg. 748

onyx pg. 739

paronychia pg. 750

plicatured nail pg. 744

Pseudomonas aeruginosa pg. 747

pterygium pg. 745

pyogenic granuloma pg. 751

tile-shaped nails pg. 745

tinea or ringworm pg. 751

tinea pedis pg. 751

tinea unguium or onychomycosis pg. 751

trumpet or pincer nail pg. 745

The **nail** is the horny protective plate located at the end of the finger or toe. It is an appendage of the skin and is, therefore, part of the integumentary system. The nails protect the tips of the fingers and toes and reflect the general health of the body.

A normal, healthy nail is firm and flexible and should be shiny and slightly pink in color. Its surface should be smooth and unspotted, without any hollows or wavy ridges. Systemic problems in the body can show up in the nails as nail disorders or poor nail growth. To provide professional service and care to your clients, you must educate yourself about the nail's structure and function.

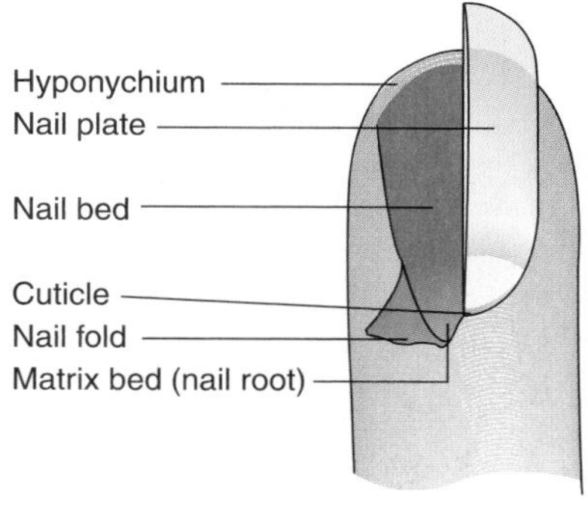

Figure 21–1 The structure of the nail.

THE NAIL

The **nail**, which is technically referred to as **onyx** (AHN-iks), is composed mainly of keratin, the same protein found in skin and hair. The keratin in nails is harder than the keratin in hair or skin. A healthy nail should be whitish and translucent in appearance, with the pinkish color of the nail bed below showing through. The horny nail plate contains no nerves or blood vessels.

The nail is quite porous; water will pass through it much more easily than it will pass through normal skin. The water content of the nail is related to the relative humidity of the surrounding environment. The nail may look like a dry hard plate, but it actually has between 10 and 30 percent water content. The water content directly affects the nail's flexibility. The lower the water content, the more brittle the nail becomes. Using an ointment-based nail conditioner or nail enamel on the nail will reduce the loss of water.

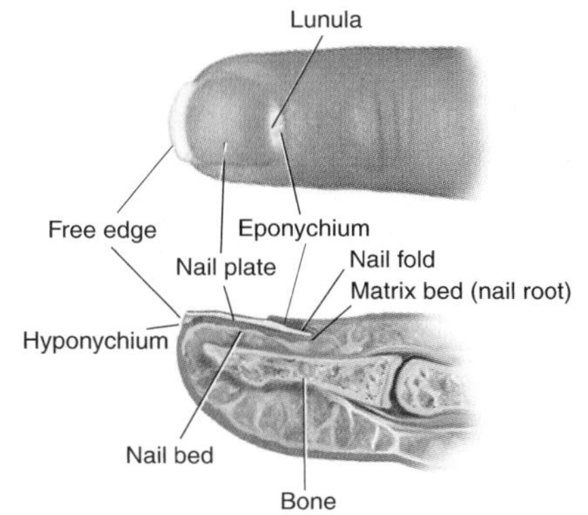

Figure 21–2 Cross section of the nail.

Nail Anatomy

The nail unit consists of six basic parts (Figure 21–1 and Figure 21–2).

- Nail bed
- Matrix bed (nail root)
- Nail plate (nail body)
- Cuticular system (cuticle, eponychium, hyponychium)

21

- Specialized ligaments
- Nail folds

The nail anatomy is the same in both fingernails and toenails.

Nail Bed

The **nail bed** is the portion of the skin on which the nail plate rests. Because it is richly supplied with blood vessels, it is seen, under the nail plate, as a pinkish area extending from the lunula (half moon) to the area just before the free edge of the nail. The nail bed is supplied with many nerves and is attached to the nail plate by a thin layer of tissue called the **bed epithelium** (ep-ih-THEE-lee-um). The bed epithelium forces the plate to grow toward the end of the digit (finger or toe) instead of growing straight up off the matrix bed.

Matrix Bed

The **matrix bed** (**nail root**) is where the nail is formed. The matrix bed is composed of matrix cells that produce the nail plate. It contains nerves, lymph, and blood vessels to nourish the nail. The matrix will continue to grow as long as it receives nutrition and is kept in healthy condition. It extends from under the nail fold at the base of the nail plate, where it can be seen as a whitish half-moon shape. This visible portion of the matrix bed is called the **lunula** or **half moon** (LOO-nuh-luh). The light color of the lunula is caused by the reflection of light where the matrix and the connective tissue of the nail bed join.

The matrix bed may be roughly divided into three parts: the proximal matrix, the intermediate or middle matrix, and the distal matrix. The nail plate grows from all three. Growth of the nails can be affected if an individual is in poor health, if a nail disorder or disease is present, or if there has been an injury to the nail matrix.

Nail Plate

21

The horny **nail plate,** or **nail body**, rests on and is attached to the nail bed. It is formed by the matrix cells and is the most visible and functional part of the nail unit. The nail plate seems to be one piece, but is actually constructed in layers. This structure can be readily seen, in both length and thickness, when a nail splits. The **free edge** is the part of the nail plate that extends over the tip of the finger or toe.

Cuticular System

The **cuticle** (KYOO-tih-kul) is the crescent of toughened skin around the base of the fingernails and toenails. A normal cuticle should be loose and flexible. It seals the area against foreign material and microorganisms, thus helping to prevent injury and infection. The **eponychium** (ep-oh-NIK-ee-um) is the extension of the cuticle at the base of the nail body that partly overlaps the lunula. The perion ychium is the portion of the epidermis surrounding the entire nail border.

The **hyponychium** (hy-poh-NIK-eeum) is the thickened stratum corneum of the epidermis that lies underneath the free edge of the nail. It seals the free edge of the nail to the normal skin, thus preventing external moisture, bacteria, or fungi from getting under the nail.

Specialized Ligaments

A **ligament** is a tough band of fibrous tissue that connects bones or holds an organ in place. Specialized ligaments attach the nail bed and matrix bed to the underlying bone. They are located at the base of the matrix and around the edges of the nail bed.

Nail Folds

The **nail folds** are folds of normal skin that surround the nail plate. These folds form the **nail grooves**, the slits or furrows on the sides of the nail on which it moves as it grows. The **mantle** (MAN-tul) is the deep fold of skin in which the matrix bed (nail root) is lodged. 1

NAIL GROWTH

The growth of the nail is affected by nutrition and a person's general health. A normal nail grows forward, starting at the matrix and extending over the tip of the finger. Normal, healthy nails can grow in a variety of shapes, depending on the individual (Figure 21–3). The shape of the matrix bed, its length, and the speed with which it produces the nail plate are all factors that determine the thickness of the nail. A longer matrix bed will produce more nail to make a thicker nail plate.

The average rate of nail growth in the normal adult is about ⅛ inch (.3 cm) per month. Nails grow faster in the summer than they do in the winter. Children's nails grow more rapidly, whereas those of elderly persons grow at a slower rate. The nail of the middle finger grows fastest and the thumbnail grows the most slowly. Although toenails grow more slowly than fingernails, they are thicker and harder.

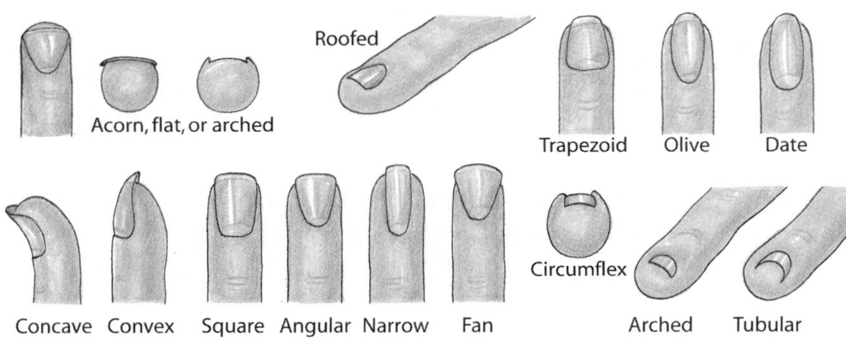

Figure 21-3 Various shapes of nails.

Nail Malformation

If disease, injury, or infection occurs in the matrix, the shape or thickness of the nail plate can change. A normal nail will be replaced as long as the matrix remains in good condition. If the nail plate is separated from the nail bed through injury, it becomes distorted or discolored. Should the nail bed be injured after the loss of a nail, the new nail will be badly formed. Ordinarily, replacement of the nail takes about four to six months. It should be noted that nails are not shed automatically or periodically, as is the case with hair. 2

Nail Disorders

A **nail disorder** is a condition caused by injury to the nail or some disease or imbalance in the body. Most, if not all, of your clients have experienced some type of common nail disorder at some time in their lives. The technician should recognize normal and abnormal nail conditions and understand why they occur. You may be able to help your clients with nail disorders in one of two ways.

- You can tell clients that they may have a disorder and refer them to a physician.
- You can cosmetically improve the disorder if the nail irregularities and blemishes fall within the province of cosmetology.

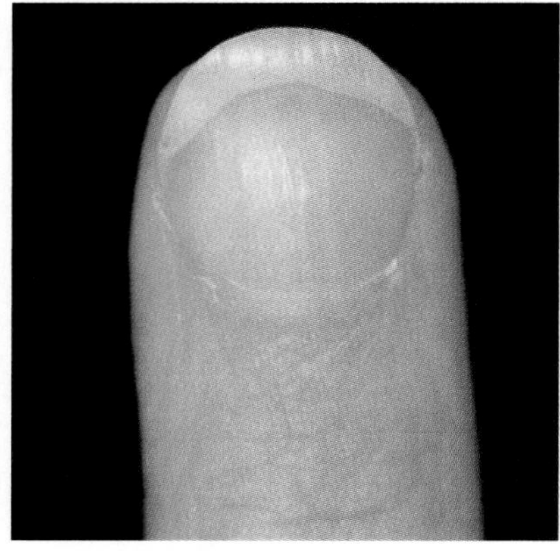

Figure 21-4a Eggshell nail, front view.

It is your responsibility to know which option to choose. The rule is, if the nail or skin to be worked on is infected, inflamed, broken, or swollen, you should not service the client. Instead, the client should be referred to a physician.

Blue nails or discolored nails is a condition caused by poor blood circulation, a heart disorder, or topical and oral medications. The nails turn a variety of colors, not only blue but blue-gray, green, yellow, red, or purple. This condition may indicate the presence of a systemic disorder. A client with this condition can benefit from a regular manicure with polish, artificial tips, or wraps.

21

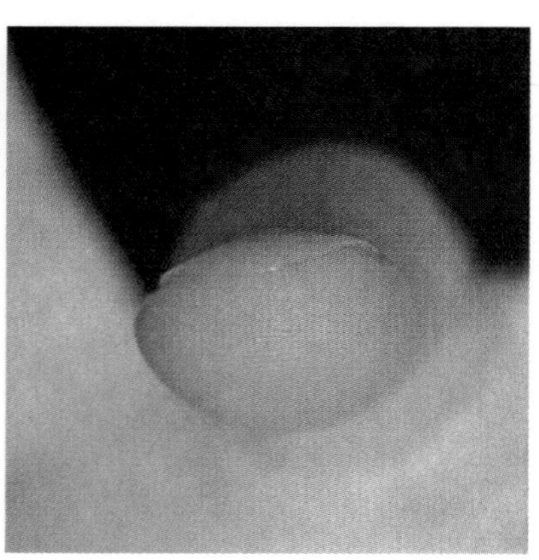

Figure 21-4b Eggshell nail, end view.

Bruised nails is a condition in which a blood clot forms under the nail plate, forming a dark purplish spot, usually due to injury. The dried blood attaches itself to the nail and grows out with it. Treat this injured nail gently. Avoid pressure.

Corrugations, or wavy ridges, are caused by uneven growth of the nails, usually the result of illness or injury. When manicuring a client with this condition, carefully buff the nails. This helps to remove or minimize the ridges. Ridge filler used with colored polish can give a smooth look to the nail.

Eggshell nails have a noticeably thin, white nail plate and are more flexible than normal. The nail plate separates from the nail bed and curves at the free edge (Figure 21–4a and Figure 21–4b). The condition is caused by improper diet, internal disease, medication, or nervous disorders. Be very careful when manicuring these nails because they are fragile and can break easily. Use the fine side of an emery board to file them gently and do not use pressure with a metal pusher at the base of the nail.

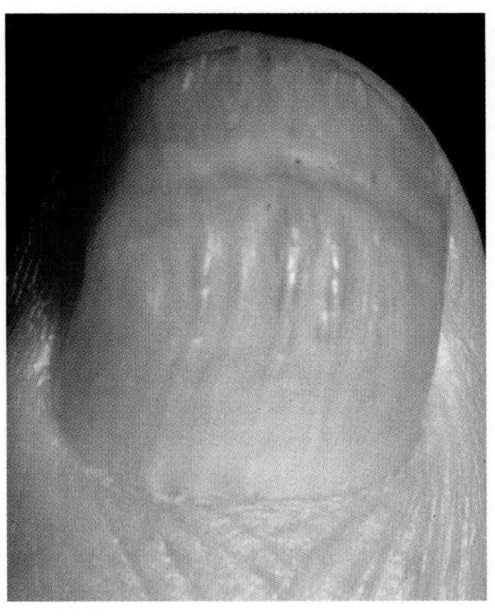

Figure 21-5 Furrows.

Furrows (depressions) in the nails can run either lengthwise or across the nail (Figure 21–5). These usually result from illness or from an injury to the nail cells in or near the matrix. They can also be caused by pregnancy or stress. Some lengthwise ridges are normal in adult nails and then increase with age. Lengthwise ridges can also be caused by conditions such as psoriasis, poor circulation, and frostbite. Since these nails are exceedingly fragile, great care must be exercised when giving a manicure. Avoid the use of the metal pusher; instead, use a disinfected plastic pusher or a new cotton-tipped orangewood stick around the cuticle.

Hangnail or **agnail** (AG-nayl) is a condition in which the cuticle splits around the nail (Figure 21–6). Dryness of the cuticle, cutting off too much cuticle, or carelessly removing cuticle tissue can result in hangnails. Advise the client that proper nail care, such as hot oil manicures, will aid in correcting such a condition. If not properly cared for, a hangnail can become infected.

Infected finger. In the case of an infected finger, the client should be referred to a physician. Signs of infection are redness, pain, swelling, or pus.

Leukonychia (loo-koh-NIK-ee-ah), or white spots, are a whitish discoloration of the nails, usually caused by injury to the base of the nail (Figure 21–7). They appear frequently in the nails but do not indicate disease. As the nail continues to grow, these white spots eventually disappear.

Melanonychia (mel-uh-nuh-NIK-ee-uh) is darkening of the fingernails or toenails. It may be seen as a black band under or within the nail plate, extending from the base to the free edge. In some cases, it may affect the entire nail plate. A localized area of increased pigment cells (melanocytes), usually within the matrix bed, is responsible for this condition. As matrix

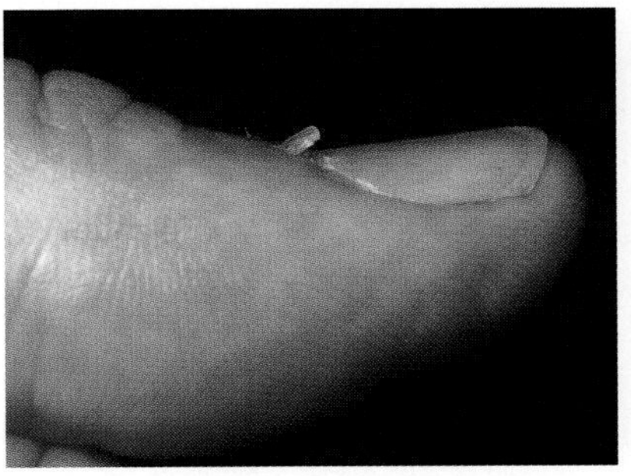

Figure 21-6 Hangnail.

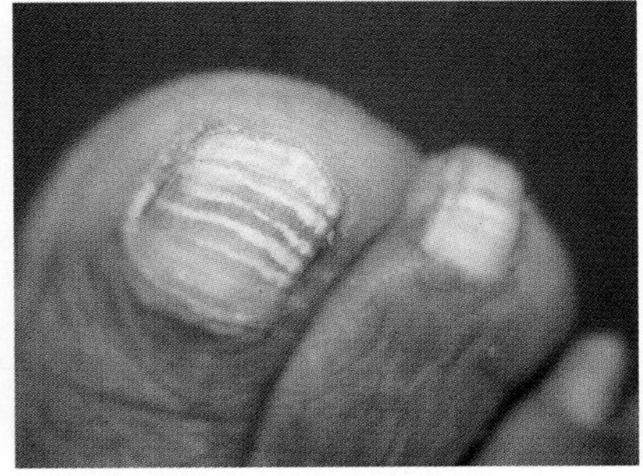

Figure 21-7 Leukonychia.

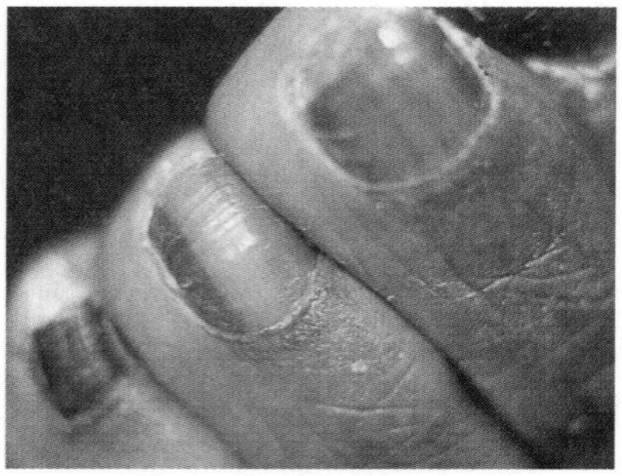

Figure 21-8 Melanonychia.

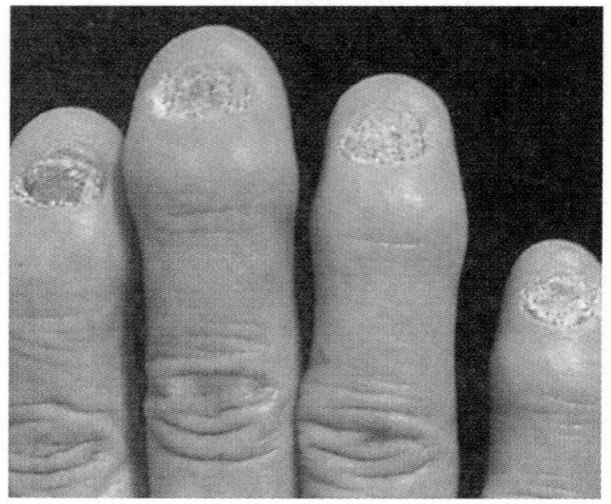

Figure 21-9 Onychatrophia.

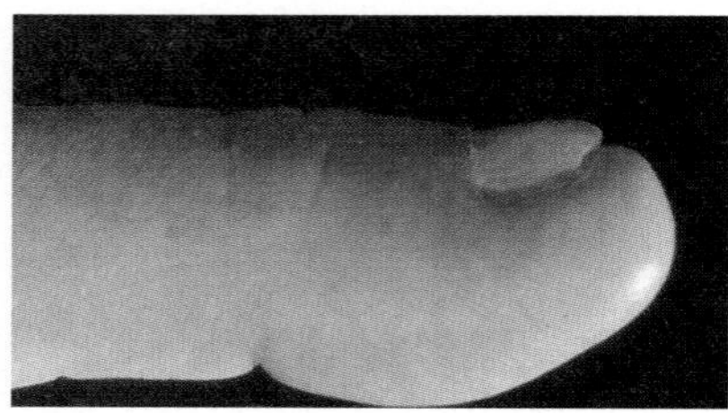

Figure 21-10a Onychauxis, side view.

cells form the nail plate, melanin is laid down within the plate by the melanocytes (Figure 21–8).

Onychatrophia (ahn-ih-kuh-TROH-fee-uh) is the atrophy or wasting away of the nail (Figure 21–9). The nail loses its luster, becomes smaller, and sometimes is shed entirely. Injury or disease might account for this nail irregularity. File the nail smooth with the fine side of the emery board and do not use a metal pusher. Advise the client to protect the nail from further injury and from exposure to strong soaps and detergents.

Onychauxis (ahn-ih-KAHK-sis), or **hypertrophy** (hy-PUR-truh-fee), is an overgrowth of the nail, usually in thickness rather than length (Figure 21–10a and Figure 21–10b). It is usually caused by a local infection or an internal imbalance but can also be hereditary. If infection is present, the nail should not be manicured. If infection is not present, you may file the nail smooth and buff.

Onychophagy (ahn-ih-koh-FAY-jee), or bitten nails, is the result of an acquired nervous habit that prompts the individual to chew the nail or the hardened cuticle (Figure 21–11). Advise the client that frequent manicures and care of the hardened cuticle often help to overcome this habit. Sometimes, the application of nail enhancements can beautify deformed nails and discourage the client from biting the nails.

Onychorrhexis (ahn-ih-koh-REK-sis) is abnormal brittleness with striation (lines) of the nail plate (Figure 21–12). Among the causes of brittle or split nails are injury to the finger, careless filing of the nails, vitamin deficiencies, illness, frequent exposure to strong soap and water, and excessive use of cuticle solvents and nail polish removers. You may want to suggest oil manicures to deal with this problem.

Plicatured nail (plik-a-CHOORD) literally means "folded nail" (Figure 21–13). The surface of the nail is generally flat while one or both of the edges of the plate are folded at an angle of 90 degrees or more down into the soft-tissue nail margins. This disorder may result from an injury that

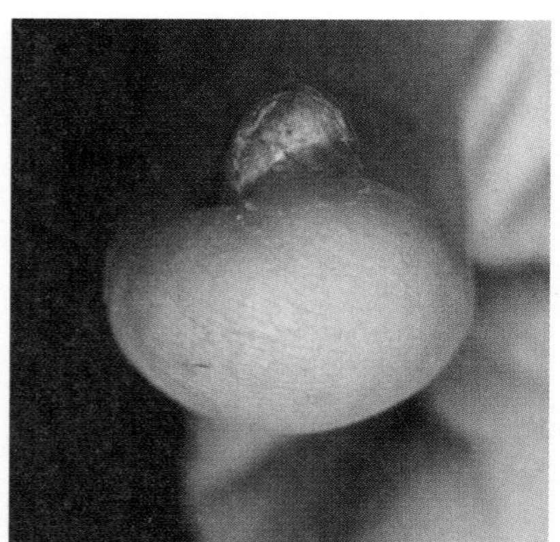

Figure 21-10b Onychauxis, end view.

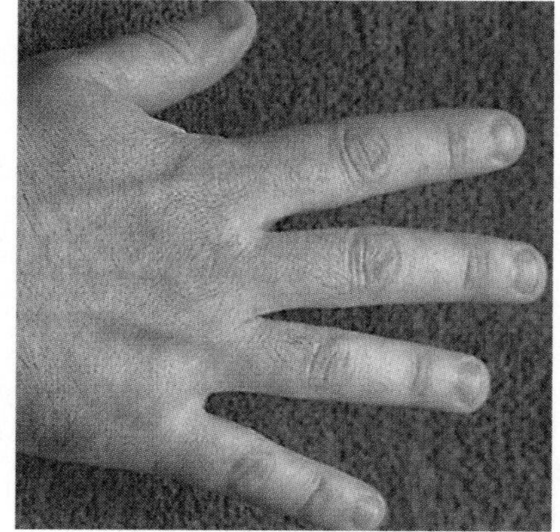

Figure 21-11 Onychophagy.

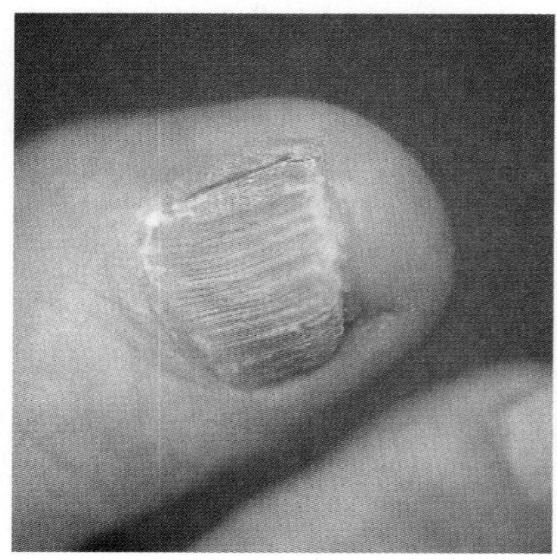

Figure 21-12 Onychorrhexis.

deforms the matrix bed. Plicatured nails are not the same as ingrown nails but could develop into them.

Pterygium (teh-RIJ-ee-um) is the forward growth of the eponychium (cuticle), with adherence to the surface of the nail (Figure 21–14). Do not treat pterygium by pushing the extension of skin back with an instrument. Doing so will cause more injury to the tissues and will make the condition worse. The gentle massage of cuticle creams and conditioners into the affected area may be beneficial. However, once the disorder has occurred, it is usually not reversible. Oil manicures may be helpful.

Tile-shaped nails have an increased crosswise curvature throughout the nail plate caused by an increased curvature of the matrix bed itself. The borders of the nail are parallel to each other. This nail type usually does not cause discomfort to the individual (Figure 21–15).

Trumpet or **pincer nail** is a disorder in which the edges of the nail plate curl around to form the shape of a trumpet or cone at the free edge. The nail bed becomes constricted and may be painful. In most instances, you may carefully trim the margins of the nail to make the client comfortable (Figure 21–16).

A brief summary of nail disorders is found in Table 21–1. 3

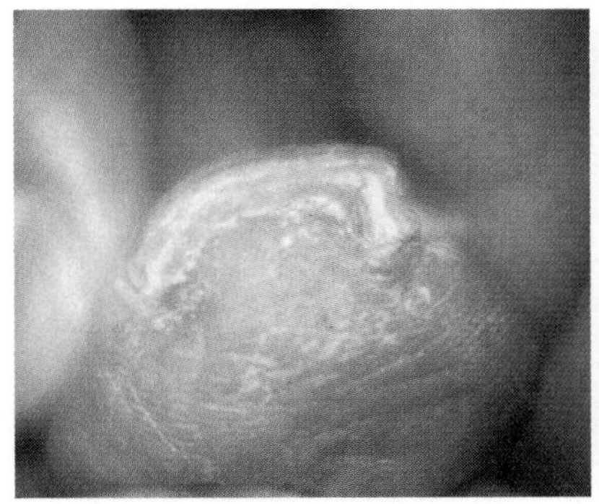

Figure 21-13 Plicatured nail.

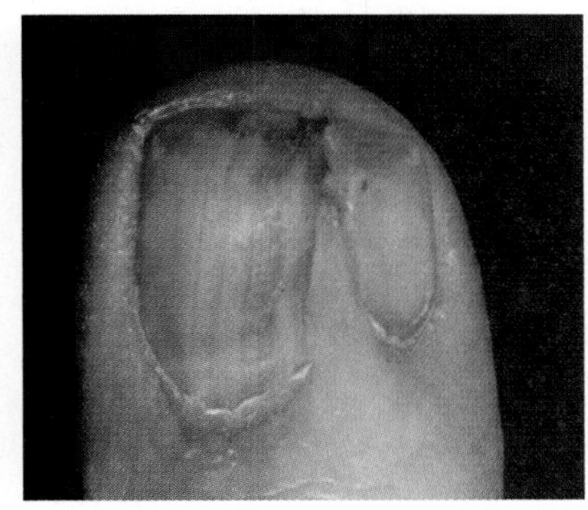

Figure 21-14 Pterygium.

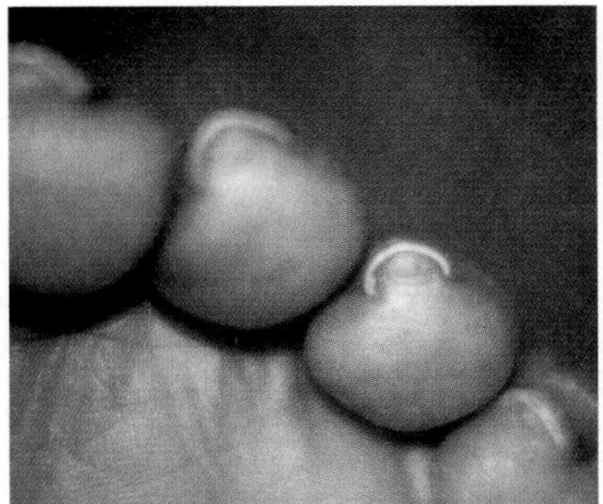

Figure 21-15 Tile-shaped nails.

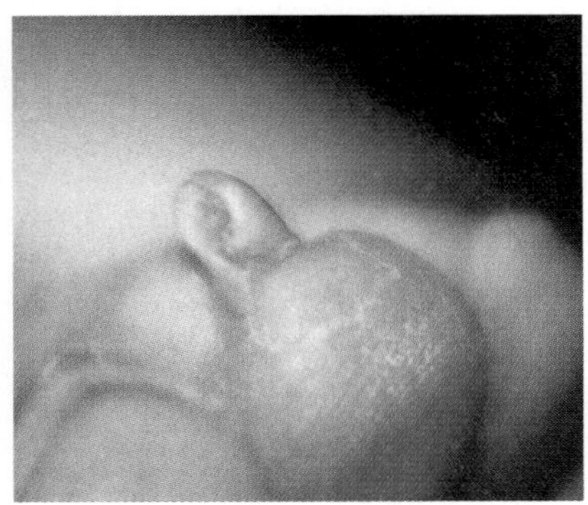

Figure 21-16 Trumpet nail.

Disorder	Signs or Symptoms
Blue nails (discolored nails)	Nails turn variety of colors; may indicate systemic disorder
Bruised nails	Dark purplish spots; usually due to injury
Corrugations	Wavy ridges caused by uneven nail growth; usually result of illness or injury
Eggshell nails	Noticeably thin white nail plate that is more flexible than normal; may be caused by diet, illness, or medication
Furrows	Depressions in the nail that run either lengthwise or across the nail; result from illness or injury, stress, or pregnancy
Hangnail (Agnail)	The cuticle splits around the nail
Infected finger	Redness, pain, swelling, or pus; refer to physician
Leukonychia (white spots)	Whitish discoloration of the nails; usually caused by injury to the base of the nail
Melanonychia	Darkening of the fingernails or toenails
Onychatrophia	Atrophy or wasting away of the nail; caused by injury or disease
Onychauxis (hypertrophy)	Overgrowth in thickness of the nail; caused by local infection, internal imbalance, or may be hereditary.
Onychophagy	Bitten nails
Onychorrhexis	Abnormal brittleness with striation (lines) of the nail plate
Plicatured nails	Folded nails
Pterygium	Forward growth of the cuticle
Tile-shaped nails	Increased crosswise curvature throughout the nail plate
Trumpet nails (pincer nails)	Edges of the nail plate curl around to form the shape of a trumpet or cone around the free edge

Table 21-1: Overview of Nail Disorders

NAIL FUNGUS

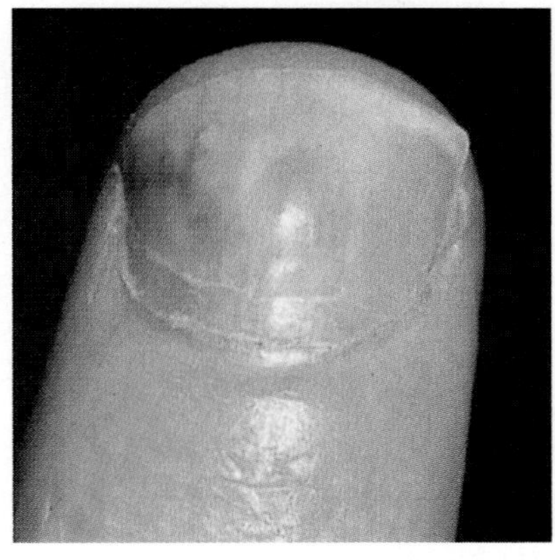

Figure 21–17 *Pseudomonas aeruginosa.*

Fungi (FUN-jy) (singular fungus, FUNG-gus) are vegetable parasites, including all types of fungus and mold (see Chapter 5). Nail fungi are of concern to the salon because they are contagious and can be transmitted from one client to the other through unsanitary implements and work conditions. Fungi can spread from nail to nail on the client's hands and from the client to the nail technician. With proper disinfection and sanitation practices, however, fungi can be avoided.

Nail fungi usually appear under the nails of the hands and feet as a cheesy, sticky residue that progresses to a dry and crusty texture under the nail plate. Clients with suspected nail fungus must be referred to a physician.

"Nail Mold" Is Not Mold

Formerly, discolorations between the nail plate and artificial enhancements were referred to as "molds." The discoloration is actually a bacterial infection caused by a bacteria called ***Pseudomonas aeruginosa***. This naturally occurring bacteria on our skin can grow out of control and cause an infection under certain conditions (Figure 21–17).

Infection can be caused by the use of implements that are contaminated with bacteria. An infection can also result from moisture that is trapped between an unsanitized natural nail and such artificial nail products as tips, wraps, gels, or acrylics. This produces the anaerobic (no oxygen) conditions loved by *Pseudomonas aeruginosa*. The infection can be identified in the early stages as a yellow-green spot that becomes darker in its advanced stages. The color usually changes from yellow to green to brown to black. If the nail has been infected for a period of time, the nail may begin to soften and smell bad, and the nail plate becomes sensitive to the touch. If these conditions continue, the nail will probably fall off, but usually the client will return to the salon for removal of the artificial product from the sore nail plate before it reaches such a point.

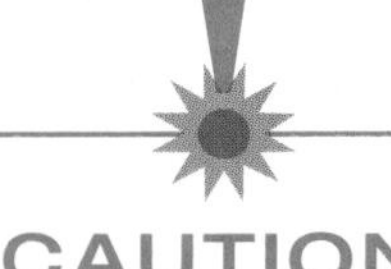

CAUTION

Infection by *Pseudomonas aeruginosa* and fungus may be avoided by strict sanitary precautions. Do not take shortcuts or omit any of the sanitation steps when performing an artificial nail service. Do not perform nail services for clients who are suspected of having fungus on their nails. If you repeatedly encounter fungus or *Pseudomonas aeruginosa* infections on your clients' nails, you should reexamine your sanitation and application techniques.

Exposing the Natural Nail

You should not provide nail services for a client who has a nail fungus or bacterial infection, but the client may want you to remove any artificial nail covering to expose the natural nail. Once the natural nail is exposed, the client should see a physician. *Pseudomonas aeruginosa* is easily killed by exposure to air. Remember, it is anaerobic bacteria, meaning that it cannot live in the presence of oxygen.

Removal can be as simple as filing off the artificial product in the area of and around the stain and exposing the infected surface to the air, or soaking off the nail. Alcohol is applied to remove and dry the contaminated moisture from the surface of the nail. The remaining stain, however, cannot be removed and must be allowed to grow out. The client should be assured that the remaining color is stain, not live bacteria, and that it will grow out with the nail.

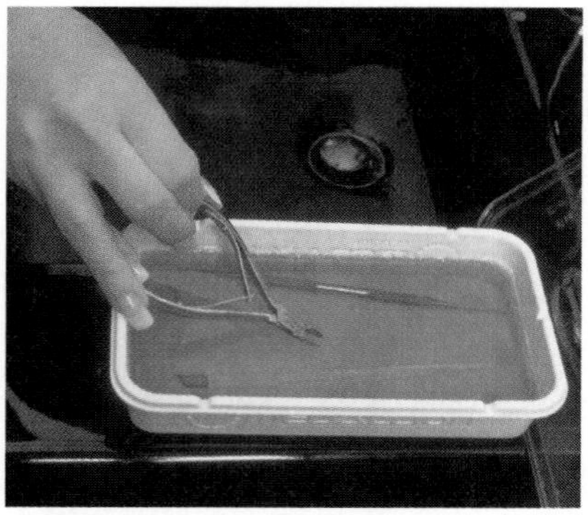

You should always wear gloves during the removal of artificial nails. Make sure to follow the manufacturers' directions for removal. When the artificial nail has been removed, discard orangewood sticks, abrasives, and any other porous product you use that cannot be disinfected. Completely disinfect all other metal and reusable implements, wash linens or replace with disposable towels, and sanitize the table surface before and after the procedure (Figure 21–18).

Figure 21–18 Always practice strict sanitation when working with the nails.

NAIL DISEASES

There are several nail diseases that you may come across. Any nail disease that shows signs of infection or inflammation (redness, pain, swelling, or pus) should not be treated in the salon. Medical treatment is required for all nail diseases.

A person's occupation can cause a variety of nail infections. For instance, infections develop more readily in people who regularly place their hands in alkaline solutions. Natural oils are removed from the skin by frequent exposure to soaps, solvents, and other substances. The cosmetologist's hands are exposed daily to chemical materials. Many of these materials are harmless, but some are potentially dangerous. Always protect your hands and nails when working with chemicals.

Onychosis (ahn-ih-KOH-sis) is the technical term applied to any deformity or disease of the nails.

Onychia (uh-NIK-ee-uh) is an inflammation of the matrix of the nail with formation of pus and shedding of the nail. Any opening of the skin allows the entry of bacteria, fungi, or foreign materials, which may result in onychia. Be careful not to cause an abrasion or opening in the tissues around the nail plate while performing a nail service. Improperly disinfected nail implements and bacterial infection can cause this disease.

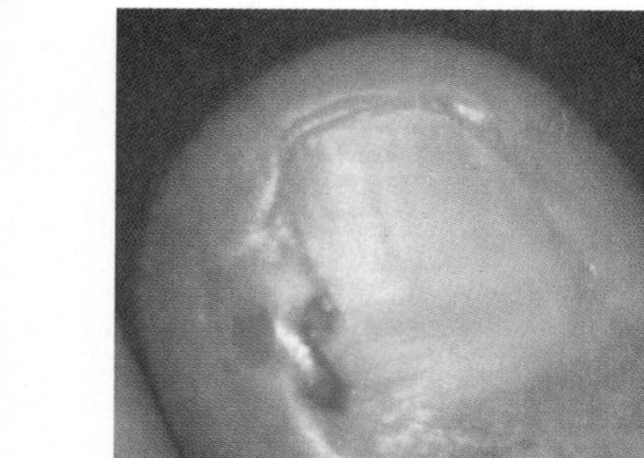

Figure 21–19 Onychocryptosis.

Onychocryptosis (ahn-ih-koh-krip-TOH-sis), or ingrown nails, can affect either the fingers or toes (Figure 21–19). In this condition, the nail grows into the sides of the tissue around the nail. The movements of walking can press the soft tissues up against the nail margin, contributing to the problem. If the tissue around the nail is not infected or if the nail is not too deeply imbedded in the flesh, you can trim the corner of the nail in a curved shape to relieve the pressure on the nail groove. You may not work on an infected ingrown nail. Refer the client to a physician.

Onychogryposis (ahn-ih-koh-gry-POH-sis), also known as **onychogryphosis** (ahn-ih-koh-gry-FOH-sis), is the thickening and increased curvature of the nail. It is also called "ram's horn nail" and is usually the result of injury to the matrix. It may be hereditary and can also occur as the result of long-term neglect. It is most commonly seen in the great toe but may be seen in other toes as well as in fingernails. The nail

insights

Nancy King

Nail technician Nancy King, with over 23 years in the industry, is committed to standards. This has led her to her current position as director of Electric File Manufacturers.

How did I get into this field? Well, back in 1980 I had someone do my nails, and she was ferocious. She used a hand file and hurt me badly. I had her do my right hand only, and I did my left hand myself. She said I was better than a lot of people out of school, and she suggested that I get my license. I got into school and then worked part-time with a few clients. But, as a single mom, I couldn't afford to lose clients. I needed to know that I would always have clients, so I went to work for a salon.

My philosophy has always been that you have to pay your dues and do your homework. Open your mind and learn. If you know everything there is to know about an industry or a job, it's time to move on to another career. But you can't know everything. It all changes so much. I learn something every day. That's why I like getting up in the morning. Bad things happen, but that doesn't make it a bad day. As long as I learn something, it's a good day.

I love making people happy by doing a good job for them. But I also love doing the work I've done with state boards and improving the level of safety. I got four new laws passed in Maryland and was appointed to the Maryland Board of Cosmetologists. I started a new organization devoted to educating state boards.

As a client, the number one thing I would be looking for in a salon is cleanliness. I want to see licenses. As a cosmetologist, I believe that if you want to be successful, you need to listen to what people want. You need to learn to ask the right questions. Never gossip. Make a point of always being on time. Regard yourself as a professional, just as a doctor or lawyer would. You need to follow your state guidelines, and read and truly understand your state regulation book. And you must value and show your appreciation for your clients.

This year, I thought I'd have a party for all my clients. I have a neighbor who owns a French restaurant and he gave me a great price. I had 340 people to dinner, just before the holidays. These people are worth $1,000 a year to me, so I can spring for a $30 dinner for them. Basically, the gift amounted to a free service. It was a way of saying "thank you" to valued customers for their dedication and loyalty.

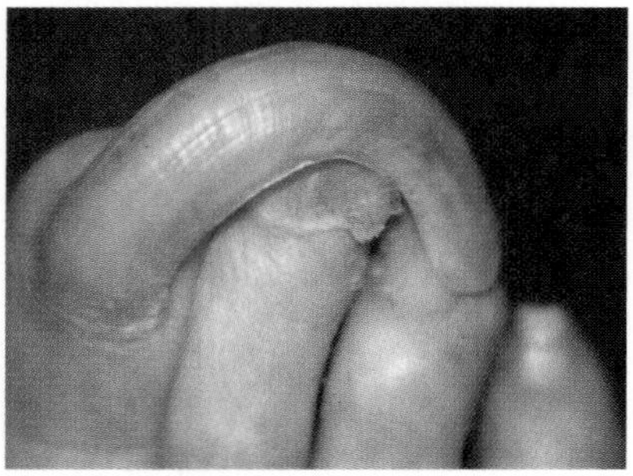

Figure 21-20 Onychogryposis.

usually has many crosswise grooves and ridges, is brownish in color, and one side of the nail grows faster than the other, curving the nail plate and giving it its typical "ram's horn" configuration (Figure 21–20). The thick curved nail is hard to cut so the nail remains untrimmed, adding to the severity of the problem. If no infection is present, you can trim the nail with the proper nail nipper and a file. Each of the grooves is a weak area of the nail plate. Trim the nail across the plate at a groove, taking only small bites, and the nail will break off when it has been trimmed about halfway across.

Onycholysis (ahn-ih-KAHL-ih-sis) is the loosening of the nail without shedding, usually beginning at the free edge and continuing to the lunula (Figure 21–21). It is frequently associated with an internal disorder, trauma (Figure 21–22), infection, nail fungi, and allergy to nail enhancement products, or may result from certain drug treatments.

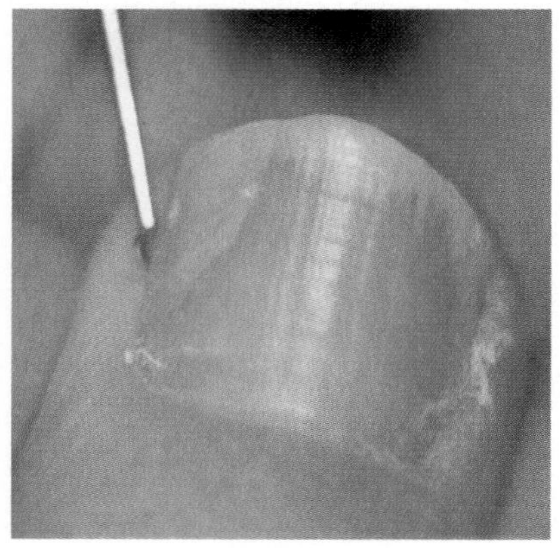

Figure 21-21 Onycholysis.

Onychomadesis (ahn-ih-koh-muh-DEE-sis), is the separation and falling off of a nail from the nail bed. It can occur on fingernails and toenails (Figure 21–23). In most cases, the cause can be traced to a localized infection, minor injuries to the matrix bed, or a severe systemic illness. Some chemotherapy treatments or X-ray treatments for cancer may also cause it. When the cause is removed, a new nail plate will form. If onychomadesis is present, do not apply enhancements to the nail. If there is no active infection present, a basic manicure or pedicure service may be given.

Onychophosis (ahn-ih-kahf-OH-sis) refers to a growth of horny epithelium in the nail bed.

Onychoptosis (ahn-ih-kahp-TOH-sis) is the periodic shedding of one or more nails, in whole or in part. This condition might follow certain diseases such as syphilis, or can result from fever, trauma, system upsets, or a reaction to prescription drugs.

Paronychia (payr-uh-NIK-ee-uh), or felon (FEL-un), is a bacterial inflammation of the tissues surrounding the nail (Figure 21–24). Pus is usually present, along with a gradual thickening and brownish discoloration of the nail plate. Paronychia around the entire nail is sometimes referred to as "runaround paronychia" (Figure 21–25). Chronic paronychia is most

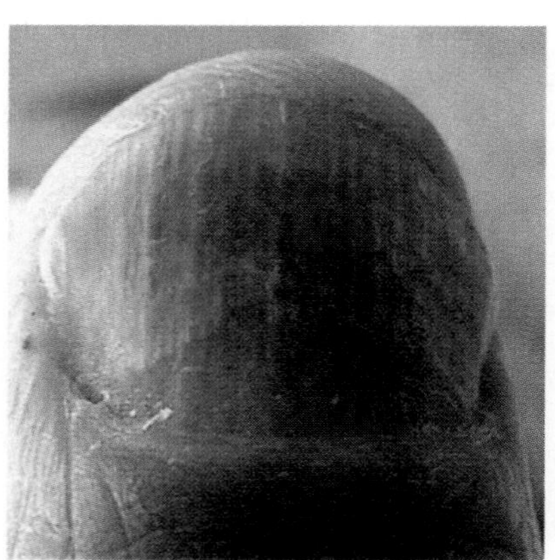

Figure 21-22 Onycholysis caused by trauma.

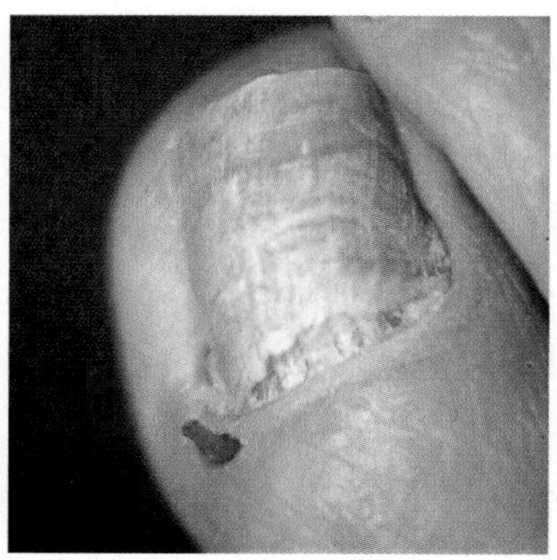

Figure 21-23 Onychomadesis of a toenail.

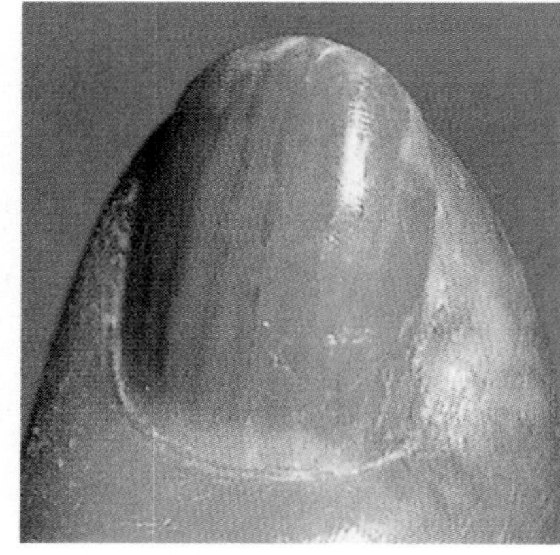

Figure 21-24 Paronychia.

often caused by a yeast infection of the soft tissues around the nail but can also be traced to a bacterial infection (Figure 21–26). Individuals who work with their hands in water, such as dishwashers and bartenders, or who must wash their hands continually, such as health care workers and food processors, are quite prone to this type of infection. Toenails, because of perspiration and footgear, may often exhibit chronic paronychia infections. Do not aggressively push back the cuticle in the presence of paronychia. There are products available that will safely remove and soften excess cuticle formations.

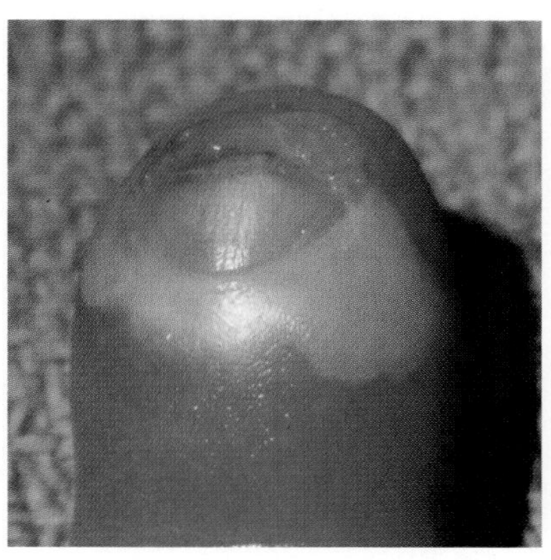

Figure 21-25 Runaround paronychia.

Pyogenic granuloma (py-oh-JEN-ik gran-yoo-LOH-muh) is a severe inflammation of the nail in which a lump of red tissue grows up from the nail bed to the nail plate (Figure 21–27).

Tinea (ringworm) is a highly contagious skin disease caused by a vegetable parasite or fungus. It is characterized by itching, scales, and, sometimes, painful circular lesions. Most cases of dermatitis of the hands resemble tinea but are actually a contact dermatitis plus a staphylococcic infection. Only a physician can determine this condition.

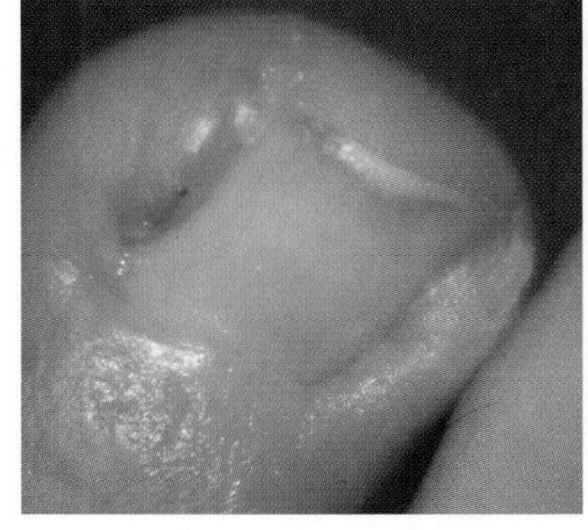

Figure 21-26 Chronic paronychia.

Tinea pedis is the medical term for athlete's foot or ringworm of the foot. In acute conditions, deep, itchy, colorless vesicles (blisters) appear (Figure 21–28). These appear as isolated blisters or in groups, and sometimes on only one foot. They spread over the sole and between the toes, perhaps involving the nail fold and infecting the nail. When the vesicles rupture, the skin becomes red and oozes. The lesions dry as they heal. Fungus infection of the feet is likely to become chronic.

Tinea unguium (TIN-ee-uh UN-gwee-um) or **onychomycosis** (ahn-ih-koh-my-KOH-sis) is ringworm of the nails (Figure 21–29). A common form is whitish patches that can be scraped off the surface of the nail. A second form is long, yellowish streaks within the nail substance. The disease invades the free edge and spreads toward the root. The infected portion is thick and discolored. In a third form, the deeper layers of the nail are invaded, causing the superficial layers to appear irregularly thin. These infected layers peel off and expose the diseased parts of the nail bed.

21

Refer to Table 21–2 on the following page for a brief summary of nail diseases.

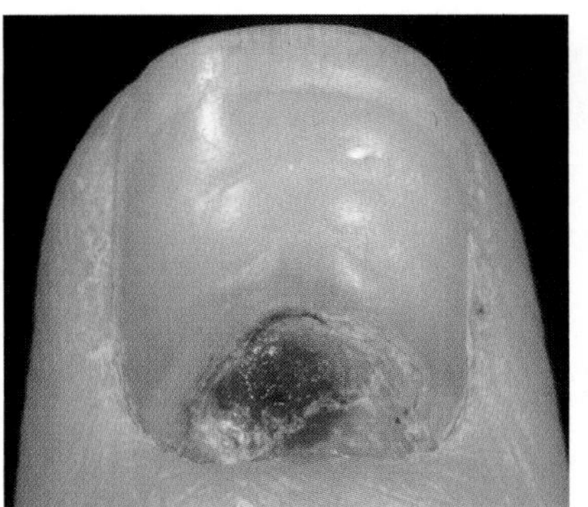

Figure 21-27 Pyogenic granuloma.

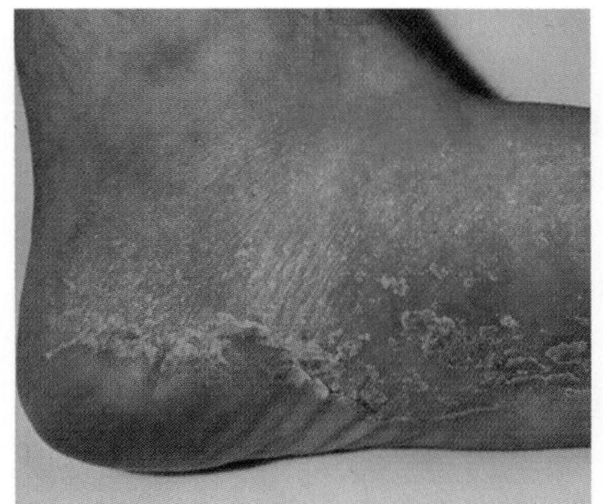

Figure 21-28 Tinea pedis.

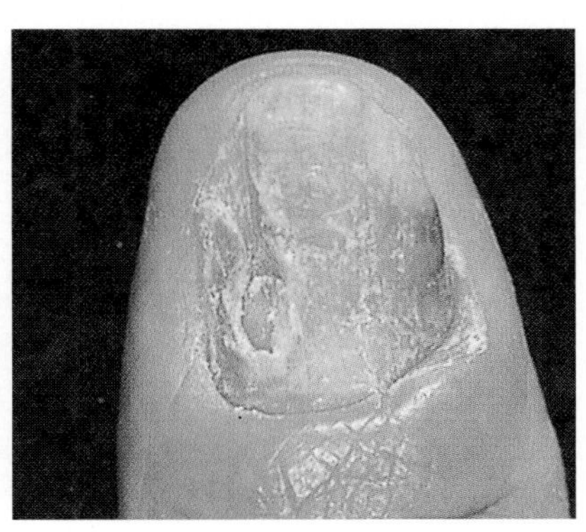

Figure 21-29 Tinea unguium (onychomycosis).

Disease	Signs or Symptoms
Onychia	Inflammation of the matrix with pus and shedding of the nail
Onychocryptosis	Ingrown nails
Onychogryposis	Thickening and increased curvature of the nail
Onycholysis	Loosening of the nail without shedding
Onychomadesis	Separation and falling off of a nail from the nail bed
Onychophosis	Growth of horny ephithelium in the nail bed
Onychoptosis	Periodic shedding of one or more nail
Paronychia (felon)	Bacterial inflammation of the tissues around the nail; pus, thickening, and brownish discoloration of the nail plate
Pyogenic granuloma	Severe inflammation of the nail in which a lump of red tissue grows up from the nail bed to the nail plate
Tinea (ringworm)	Reddened patches of small blisters; slight or severe itching
Tinea pedis (ringworm of the foot or athlete's foot)	Deep, itchy, colorless blisters
Tinea unguium (onychomycosis or ringworm of the nails)	Whitish patches on the nail that can be scraped off or long yellowish streaks within the nail substance

Table 21-2: Overview of Nail Diseases

KNOW YOUR NAILS

Many cosmetology professionals are interested in nails because of the creative opportunities that can be explored there. As with every other area of cosmetology, the creativity must be grounded in a full awareness of the structure and physiology of the body part with which you are working. Working on good, strong, healthy nails can be a pleasure. Working on unhealthy nails can be a danger, both to your clients and to yourself. Begin with the knowledge and grow from there.

chapter glossary

bed epithelium	thin layer of tissue between the nail plate and the nail bed
blue nails	condition caused by poor blood circulation, a heart disorder, or topical and oral medications
bruised nails	condition in which a blood clot forms under the nail plate, forming a dark purplish spot, usually due to injury
corrugations	wavy ridges; caused by uneven growth of the nails, usually the result of illness or injury
cuticle	crescent of toughened skin around the base of the fingernails and toenails
eggshell nails	nails with a noticeably thin, white nail plate that are more flexible than normal
eponychium	extension of the cuticle at the base of the nail body that partly overlaps the lunula
free edge	part of the nail plate that extends over the tip of the finger or toe
furrows	depressions in the nails can run either lengthwise or across the nail
hangnail or agnail	condition in which the cuticle splits around the nail
hyponychium	thickened stratum corneum of the epidermis that lies underneath the free edge of the nail
leukonychia	whitish discoloration of the nails, usually caused by injury to the base of the nail; white spots
ligament	a tough band of fibrous tissue that connects bones or holds an organ in place
lunula or half moon	whitish, half-moon shape at the base of the nail plate, caused by the reflection of light where the matrix bed and connective tissue of the nail bed join
mantle	deep fold of skin in which the matrix bed (nail root) is lodged
matrix bed or nail root	where the nail is formed; composed of matrix cells that produce the nail plate
melanonychia	darkening of the fingernails or toenails; may be seen as a black band under or within the nail plate, extending from the base to the free edge
nail	horny protective plate located at the end of the finger or toe
nail bed	portion of the skin on which the nail plate rests
nail disorder	condition caused by injury to the nail or some disease or imbalance in the body
nail folds	folds of normal skin that surround the nail plate
nail grooves	slits or furrows on the sides of the nail on which the nail moves as it grows
nail plate or nail body	horny plate resting on and attached to the nail bed
onychatrophia	atrophy or wasting away of the nail
onychauxis or hypertrophy	an overgrowth of the nail, usually in thickness rather than length
onychia	inflammation of the matrix of the nail with formation of pus and shedding of the nail
onychocryptosis	ingrown nails; nail grows into the sides of the tissue around the nail

chapter glossary *(continued)*

onychogryposis or onychogryphosis	the thickening and increased curvature of the nail; also called "ram's horn nail"; usually the result of injury to the matrix
onycholysis	the loosening of the nail without shedding, usually beginning at the free edge and continuing to the lunula
onychomadesis	the separation and falling off of a nail from the nail bed; can occur on fingernails and toenails
onychophagy	bitten nails; the result of an acquired nervous habit that prompts the individual to chew the nail or the hardened cuticle
onychophosis	growth of horny epithelium in the nail bed
onychoptosis	periodic shedding of one or more nails, in whole or in part
onychorrhexis	abnormal brittleness with striation (lines) of the nail plate
onychosis	technical term applied to any deformity or disease of the nails
onyx	nail of the fingers or toes
paronychia	bacterial inflammation of the tissues surrounding the nail; pus is usually present, also a gradual thickening and brownish discoloration of the nail plate
plicatured nail	"folded nail"; disorder in which the surface of the nail is generally flat while one or both of the edges of the plate are folded at a 90-degree (or more) angle down into the soft-tissue nail margins
Pseudomonas aeruginosa	naturally occurring bacteria that can cause nail infection when nail services are performed in unsanitary conditions
pterygium	forward growth of the eponychium (cuticle), with adherence to the surface of the nail
pyogenic granuloma	severe inflammation of the nail in which a lump of red tissue grows up from the nail bed to the nail plate
tile-shaped nails	increased crosswise curvature throughout the nail plate caused by an increased curvature of the matrix bed itself
tinea or ringworm	highly contagious skin disease caused by a vegetable parasite, or fungus; characterized by itching, scales, and sometimes painful circular lesions
tinea pedis	medical term for athlete's foot or ringworm of the foot
tinea unguium or onychomycosis	ringworm of the nails that invades from the free edge and spreads toward the root
trumpet or pincer nail	disorder in which the edges of the nail plate curl around to form the shape of a trumpet or cone at the free edge

review questions

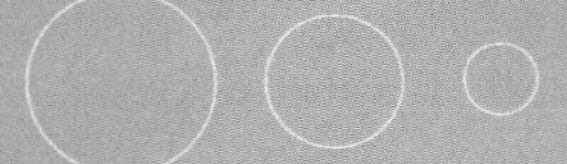

1. Describe a normal healthy nail.
2. What is the technical term for nail?
3. What is the nail composed of?
4. Name the six basic parts of the nail.
5. What part of the nail contains the nerve and blood supply?
6. Explain how the nail grows.
7. How does the nail become malformed?
8. In what situation should a nail service not be performed?
9. What is *Pseudomonas aeruginosa*? Why is it important to learn about it?
10. Name at least eight nail disorders that can be treated in the salon.
11. What is the most effective way to avoid fungal or bacterial infections among your clients?

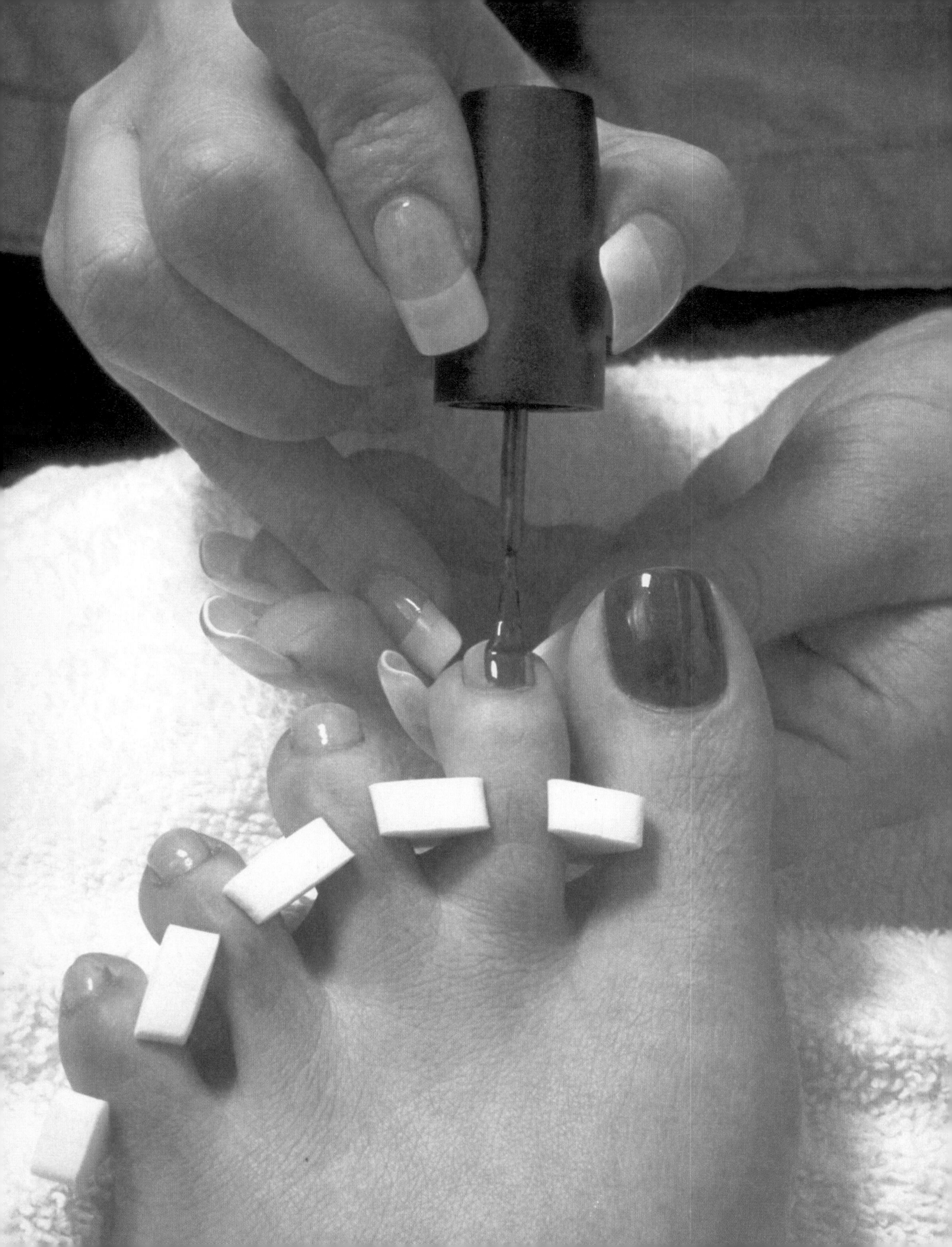

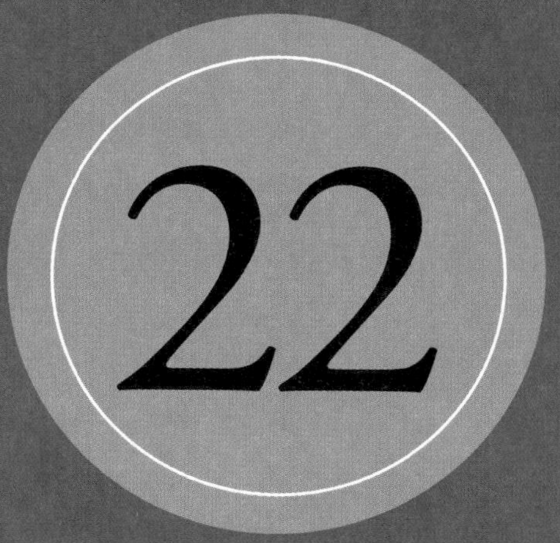

MANICURING AND PEDICURING

Sue Ellen Schultes

INTERNATIONAL NAIL JUDGE AND CEO, NOTORIOUS NAILS SEMINARS

Chapter Outline

Nail Care Tools • The Manicure Table • Client Consultation
The Plain Manicure • Other Types of Manicures • Pedicures
Safety Rules in Manicuring and Pedicuring • A Valuable Service

Learning Objectives

After completing this chapter, you should be able to:

1. List the abilities that make a good nail technician.
2. Demonstrate the proper use of implements, cosmetics, and materials used in manicuring and pedicuring.
3. Identify the five basic nail shapes.
4. Demonstrate massage techniques used when giving a) a manicure or b) a pedicure.
5. Demonstrate a plain manicure.
6. Demonstrate a plain pedicure.
7. List the sanitary and safety precautions that should be observed when performing a manicure or a pedicure.

National Skills Standards

This chapter provides you with the necessary information to master these National Industry Skill Standards for Entry-Level Cosmetologists.

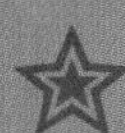

Providing basic manicure and pedicure.

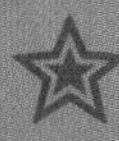

Conducting services in a safe environment, taking measures to prevent the spread of infectious and contagious diseases.

Key Terms

Page number indicates where in the chapter the term is used.

The ancients regarded long, polished, and tinted fingernails as a mark of distinction between aristocrats and common laborers. The care of the hands and feet, once considered a luxury for the few, are now services used by many. Manicures and pedicures make up one of the biggest growth areas in salon services today. A client pleased with a professional manicure or pedicure is likely to return regularly for these services, as well as for other beauty services.

The word **manicure** (MAN-i-kyoor) is derived from the Latin *manus* (hand) and *cura* (care), and means the artful treatment and care of the hands and nails. The word **pedicure** has its root in the Latin *ped*, for foot, and means the care of the feet and toenails. The purpose of manicures and pedicures is to improve the appearance of the hands, the feet, and their nails. Once you have gained the basic knowledge and mastered the fundamental techniques in this chapter, you will be able to provide a service that is in great demand (Figure 22–1).

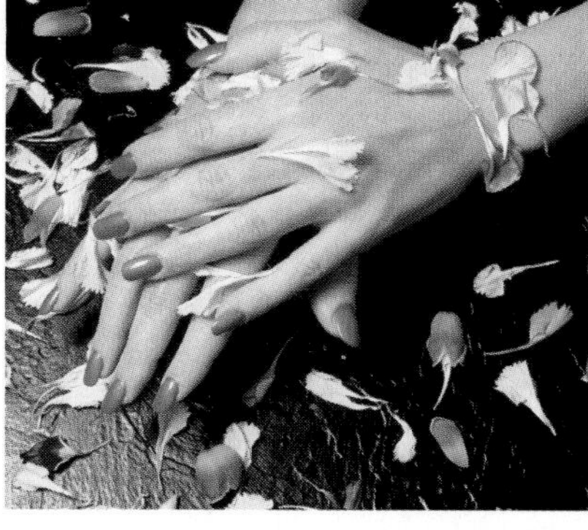

Figure 22–1 Manicures are a popular service.

A professional nail technician should have:

- knowledge of the structure of the nail.
- knowledge of the composition of the cosmetics used in manicuring.
- the ability to give a manicure and pedicure efficiently and effectively.
- the ability to care for the client's manicuring problems or concerns.
- the knowledge to be able to distinguish between disorders that may be treated in the salon and those that must be treated by a physician.
- a thorough awareness of the procedures involved in sanitation and disinfection. 1

NAIL CARE TOOLS

As a professional, it is imperative that you develop competence in working with the tools that are required for nail care. These tools can be grouped into four basic categories: equipment, implements, nail cosmetics, and materials. Let us look more closely at each.

Equipment

Equipment consists of the permanent tools you will be using to perform nail services. They do not require replacement unless they are no longer in good repair. They include the following items.

- *Manicure table with adjustable lamp.* Most standard tables include a drawer for storing implements and cosmetics (Figure 22–2). Some tables come with an attached, adjustable lamp with a 40-watt bulb. The heat from a higher wattage might interfere with the manicure or other advanced nail procedures, while a lower wattage will not adequately warm a client's nails if the room is cool.
- *Nail technician's chair and client's chair.* These should be selected for ergonomic value, comfort, durability, and ease of sanitation.
- *Client's cushion.* This cushion, with a standard size of eight inches by twelve inches, is especially made for manicuring purposes. It should be covered with a clean and/or disposable towel before each appointment.
- *Supply tray.* Used for holding cosmetics such as polishes, polish remover, and creams, it should be durable, balanced, and easy to clean and sanitize.
- *Finger bowl.* Designed for soaking the client's fingers in warm water with a liquid soap added, it is generally made of plastic, china, or glass so it can be easily sanitized.

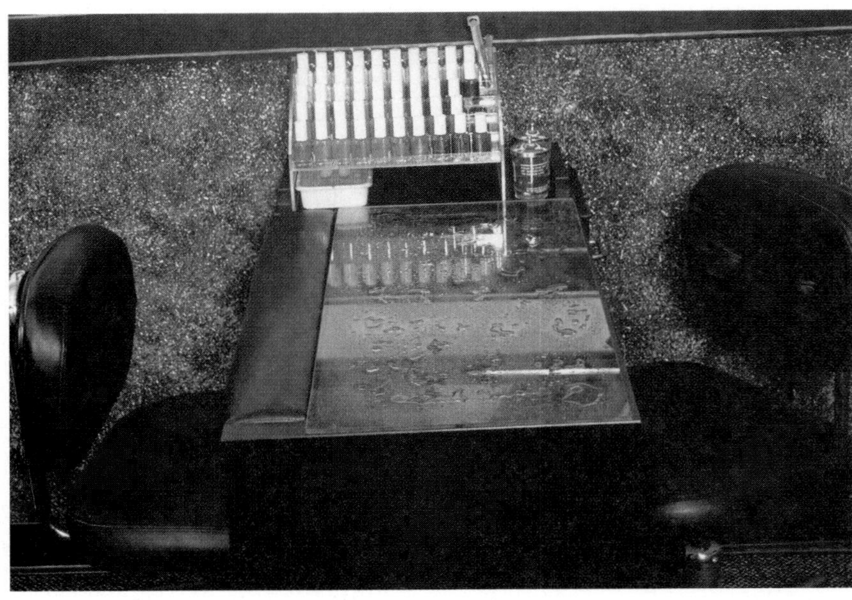

Figure 22–2 Manicure table.

- *Container*. For holding clean absorbent cotton.
- *Electric heater*. For heating oil when giving a hot oil manicure.
- *Disinfectant container*. This is a particularly important piece of equipment. It should be large enough to hold a disinfectant solution in which all implements requiring sanitization can be completely immersed. Disinfectant containers come in a variety of shapes, sizes, and materials (Figure 22–3). They should have a lid, which is used to keep the solution from becoming contaminated when not in use. Some containers have a lift tray that allows the implements to be removed from the solution automatically. After lifting implements from the disinfectant container, spray them thoroughly with water or alcohol. If your container does not have a lift tray, remove the implements with tongs or tweezers. Never allow your fingers to come in contact with the solution, as this can cause contamination. Never return used implements to the disinfectant container until they have been properly cleaned.

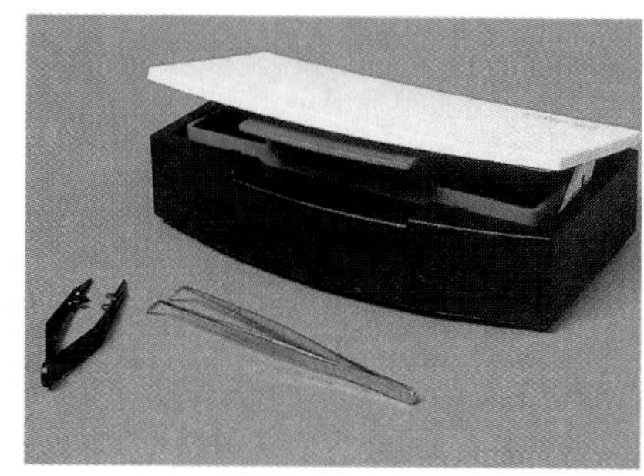

Figure 22-3 Disinfectant container.

Implements

Implements are instruments or tools that must be disinfected, sanitized, or disposed of after use with each client. They are small enough to fit in the disfectant container. The following is a list (in alphabetical order) of the implements you will need for most services.

- **Cuticle nipper.** Small cutting tool used to nip or cut excess cuticle at the base of the nail (Figure 22–4). Reusable.
- **Cuticle pusher**. Implement used to loosen and push back the cuticle around the fingernails or toenails. It is shaped to conform to the shape of the nails (Figure 22–5). Reusable.
- **Emery board**. Disposable manicuring instrument with rough cutting ridges, used for shaping the nails with the coarse side, and for smoothing them with the finer side (Figure 22–6). To bevel, hold the emery board at a 45-degree angle and, using light pressure, file on the top or underside of the nail. The board cannot be sanitized, so either give it to the client or break it in half and discard after use. Do not keep an emery board in a plastic bag for individual clients from one visit to the next. Bacteria can grow on the unsanitized implement in between appointments.
- **Nail brush**. Small brush used to clean under and around the nails, with the aid of warm water and soap. Reusable.

In some states or provinces it is a violation of sanitary codes to have metal implements on your table when not in use. Keep them in a closed container or cabinet sanitizer instead. Check with your regulatory agency.

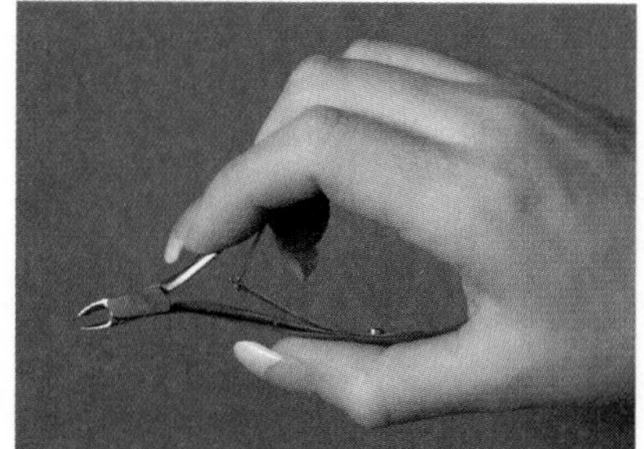

Figure 22-4 Cuticle nipper.

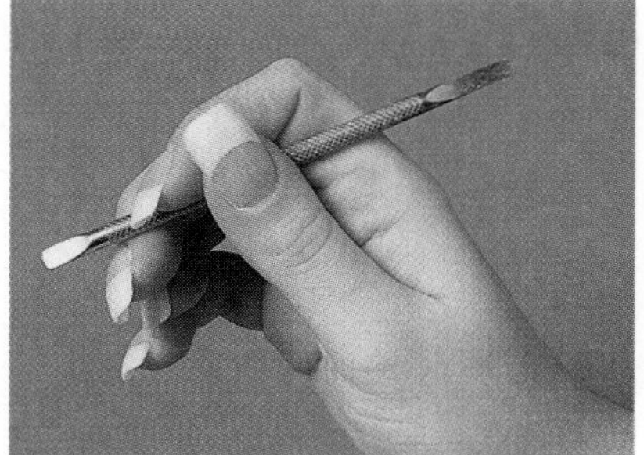

Figure 22-5 Cuticle pusher.

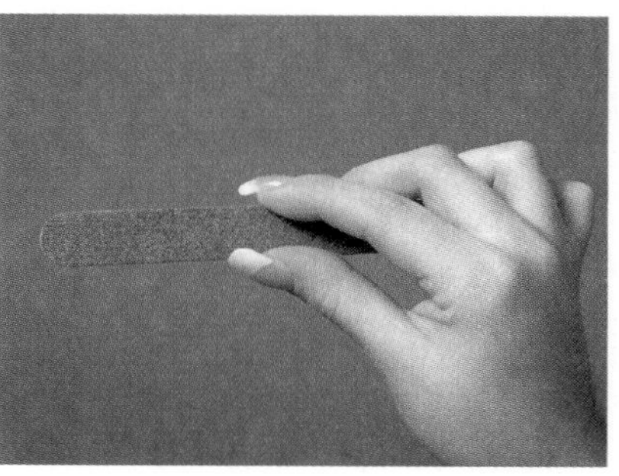

Figure 22-6 Emery board.

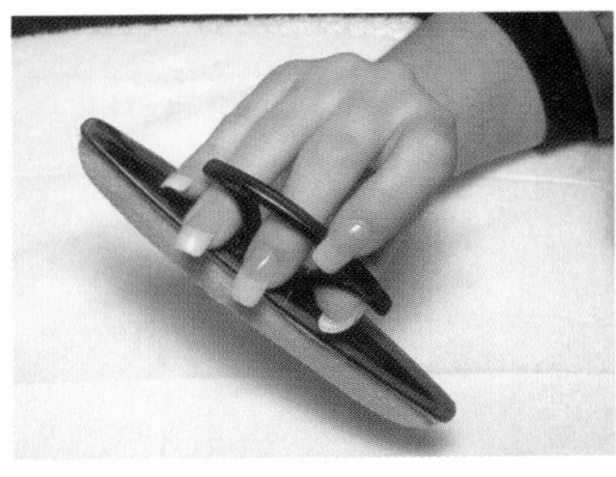

Figure 22-7 Nail buffer.

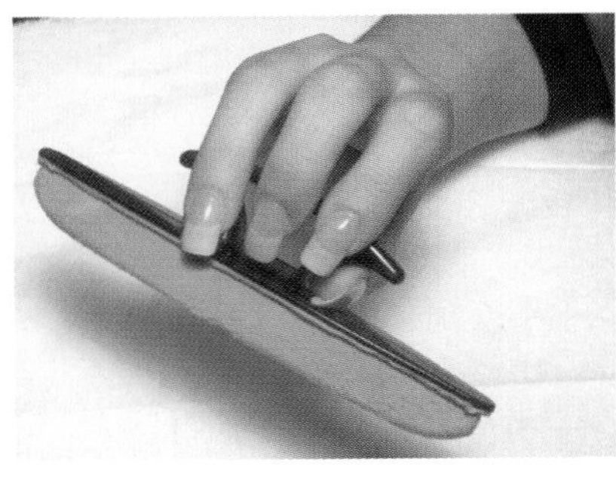

Figure 22-8 Alternate way to hold nail buffer.

- **Nail buffer**. Instrument made of leather or chamois; used with a polishing powder to polish the nails to a high luster. Chamois buffers are designed with a removable frame so that the chamois cover can be changed for each client. Let your instructor guide you on how to hold the chamois buffer (Figure 22–7 and Figure 22–8). Some states and provinces do not permit the use of a chamois buffer and recommend a disposable buffer that should be discarded after each use.
- **Nail clippers**. Implement used to shorten nails. If your client's nails are very long, clipping will reduce filing time. Reusable.
- **Nail file**. Metal instrument with a specially prepared surface used to file and shape the nails (Figure 22–9). Most professional nail technicians use a 7-inch or 8-inch file as some states and provinces do not allow the use of shorter files. Reusable; strict sanitation guidelines must be followed before using metal files for any nail service.
- **Orangewood stick**. Stick made from the wood of the orange tree, used to loosen the cuticle around the base of the nail or to clean under the free edge. An orangewood stick cannot be sanitized, so you may give it to your client or break it in half and discard it after use (Figure 22–10).
- **Tweezers**. Implement used to lift small bits of cuticle from the nail. Reusable.

Table 22–1 lists disposable and reusable implements.

Sanitation for Implements

It is a good idea to have two complete sets of metal implements so you will always have a completely disinfected set ready for each client, with no waiting time between appointments. If you have only one set of implements, remember that it takes approximately 10 to 20 minutes to sanitize implements after each use. Follow these steps for proper sanitation.

1. Wash all implements thoroughly with soap and warm water and rinse off all traces of soap with plain water (Figure 22–11). Dry thoroughly with a clean and/or disposable towel.
2. Metal implements should be completely immersed in a container filled with an approved disinfectant (Figure 22–12). Follow

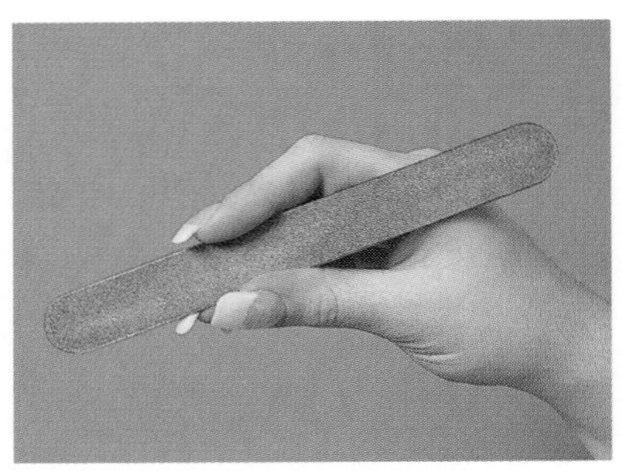

Figure 22-9 Metal nail file.

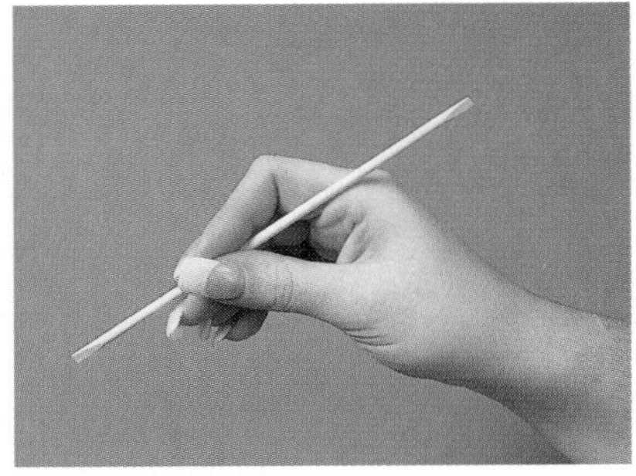

Figure 22-10 Orangewood stick.

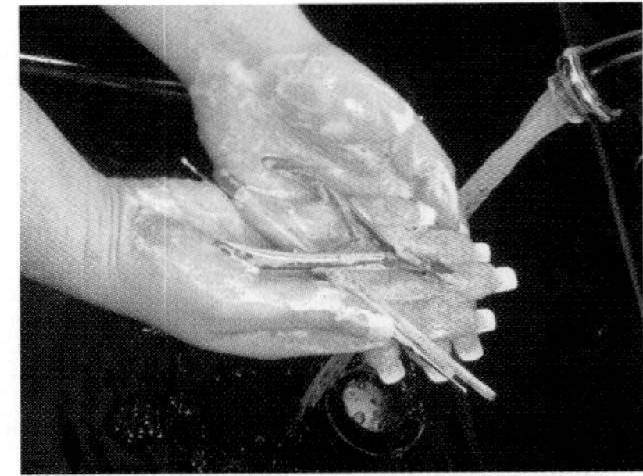

Figure 22-11 Wash implements first.

Disposable (must be discarded after each client)	Reusable (must be disinfected after each client)
orangewood sticks	fingernail clippers
emery boards	tweezers
chamois cover on buffer (depending on state and/or province regulations)	nail brush
	cuticle nipper metal cuticle pusher metal nail file

Table 22–1: Disposable and Reusable Implements.

manufacturers' instructions for the required disinfection time. Rinse implements after disinfecting to prevent overexposure to the disinfectant, which can irritate your skin as well as the client's. Dry the implements with a clean and/or disposable towel when you remove them from the disinfection container.

3. Follow your state or province regulations for storage of sanitized manicuring implements. The regulations will tell you whether to store them in sealed containers, sealed plastic bags, or in a cabinet sanitizer until they are ready for use.

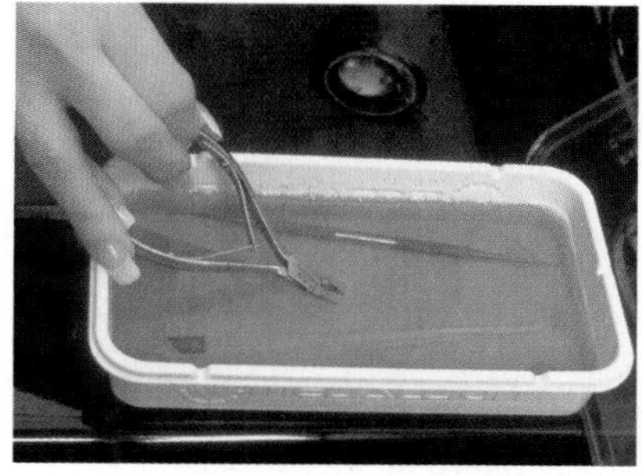

Figure 22–12 Place implements in disinfectant.

Nail Cosmetics

As a professional, you must develop a strong working knowledge of nail cosmetics and what ingredients they contain. You need to know how to apply each cosmetic and when to avoid using a product because of a client's allergies or sensitivities. Nail and hand cosmetics vary in their composition and usage depending on the purpose for which they are designed. Here are some of the most important nail cosmetics, in alphabetical order (Figure 22–13).

- *Antiseptic.* Used to prevent infection when there are minor injuries to tissues surrounding the nails.
- **Base coat**. Colorless liquid applied to the natural nail before the application of colored polish. Allows the nail polish to adhere readily to the nail surface; forms a hard gloss, which prevents the color in the nail polish from staining the nail plate.
- **Cuticle creams**. Special creams that usually have a base of lanolin, petroleum, or beeswax. Designed to prevent or correct brittle nails and dry cuticles and are suitable for use on a daily basis.

22

Figure 22-13 Nail cosmetics.

There should be a Material Safety Data Sheet, or MSDS, on all the products you use in your nail services. They should be kept for easy reference in a file or a notebook. The company from which you order supplies can provide you with the MSDS. Be guided by your instructor concerning the information and importance of the MSDS.

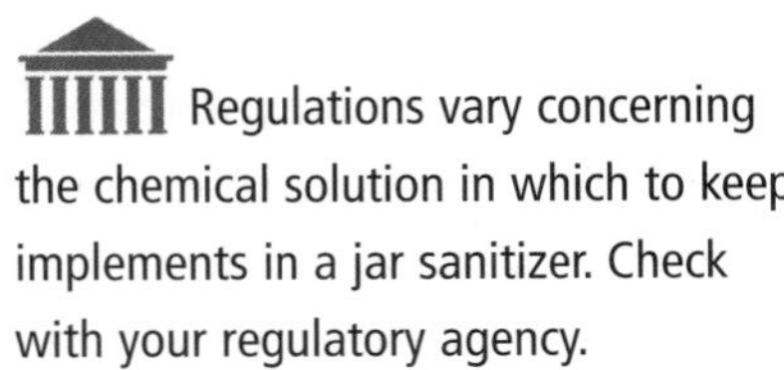

Regulations vary concerning the chemical solution in which to keep implements in a jar sanitizer. Check with your regulatory agency.

- **Cuticle oil**. Special oil used to soften and lubricate the cuticle around the fingernails and toenails.
- **Cuticle remover** or solvent. Solution of alkali, glycerin, and water used to soften and remove dead cuticle from around the nail.
- **Dry nail polish**. Powder or paste used with chamois buffer to add shine to the nails.
- **Hand creams** and **hand lotions**. Recommended for dry, chapped, or irritated skin. Hand creams are made up of emollients and humectants and add a finishing touch to a manicure. Hand lotions are similar in composition to hand creams but have a thinner consistency due to a higher oil content. Hand cream or lotion can be used as oil in a hot oil manicure.
- **Liquid nail polish** or **lacquer**. Thick liquid used to color or gloss the nail. It is a solution of nitrocellulose in such volatile solvents as amyl acetate, mixed with a plasticizer such as castor oil to prevent too rapid drying. Resin and color are also present. In addition to the finished nail appearance, the purpose of the polish application is to build layers allowing for adhesion and staying power. Always keep the polish thin enough to flow freely. If the polish is thick, add a little polish solvent and shake well.
- **Nail bleach**. Product used to remove stains and whiten the nails.
- **Nail conditioner**. Product that contains moisturizing ingredients to combat dryness and brittleness. Used independently of a manicure, usually overnight, on clean, dry nails.
- **Nail dryer**. Solution that protects the nail polish against stickiness and dulling. Can be used either as a spray or brush-on and is applied over the top coat or directly on the nail polish.

- **Nail hardener** or strengthener. Product designed to prevent nails from splitting or peeling. Applied before the base coat to nails that must be thoroughly clean, free of oils or creams, and dry. There are three types of hardeners: protein, formaldehyde, and nylon fiber.
- **Formaldehyde hardeners** utilize keratin fibers to strengthen the nail and contain no more than 5 percent formaldehyde, because more than that could cause damage to the nail.
- **Nylon fiber hardeners** are a combination of clear polish and nylon fibers, applied first vertically, then horizontally, on the nail plate.
- **Protein hardeners** are a combination of clear polish and a protein such as collagen.
- **Polish remover**. An organic solvent used to dissolve and remove nail polish. To offset the drying action of the solvent, oil is frequently present in nail polish remover. Use nonacetone polish remover for clients who have artificial nails, because acetone will weaken or dissolve tips, wrap glues, and sculptured nail compound.
- **Polish thinner**. Product used to thin out nail polish where it has thickened; contains acetone or some other solvent.
- **Top coat** or **sealer**. Liquid, colorless nail enamel applied over polish to protect the polish, prevent chipping, and impart a high gloss.

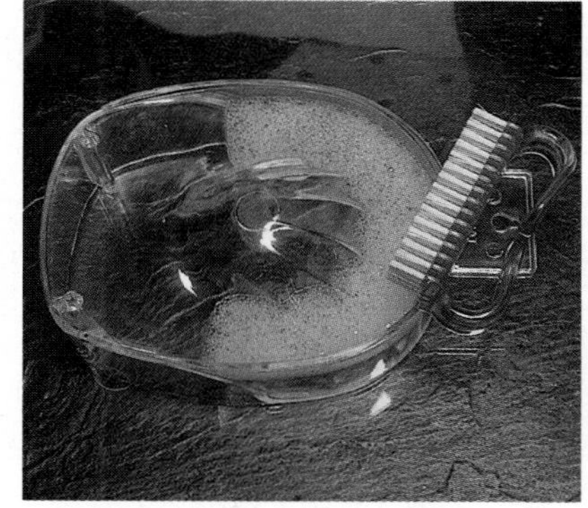

Figure 22–14 Finger bath with soapy water.

Materials

Materials are those supplies used during a service that must be replaced for each client. Materials include the following.

- *Absorbent cotton, cotton balls, or cotton pledgets.* For application of cosmetics to the nails.
- *Approved solution for jar sanitizer.* This is where implements are kept during a manicure.
- *Chamois.* For replacing soiled chamois on buffer (if allowed in your state or province).
- *Cleanser for finger baths* (liquid or other form) (Figure 22–14).
- *Cleansing tissue.* For use whenever necessary.
- *Plastic bag.* Tape or clip a bag to the side of the manicuring table to hold the used materials you discard during a service. The bag should be replaced after each client.
- *Plastic cups.* For use in oil manicure heater.
- *Plastic spatula.* For removing creams from jars.
- *Powdered alum or alum solution.* Aluminum salt used as a **styptic** (agent used to stop bleeding).
- *Terry cloth towel.* Fresh for each client.
- *Trash container.* Should have a lid that can be operated by a foot pedal. Should be lined and kept closed when not in use. Empty it at the end of each day. 2

CAUTION

Styptic pencils are not permitted for use in most states and provinces because they are unsanitary. Use powdered alum or other styptic instead.

22

THE MANICURE TABLE

A messy manicure table creates a bad impression. Seeing a neat table will help your client feel confident about your abilities. Everything—containers, bowls, instruments, and materials—must be in perfect order. Everything you will need during a service should be at your fingertips (Figure 22–15).

When giving a professional manicure, all the rules of sanitation and disinfection must be followed. Disinfect manicuring implements after each use. Do not ask the client to sit at the table with the remains of the previous manicure in sight. Always clear the table immediately after the completion of one manicure so that it will be ready for the next. This will make the manicure more pleasant for the client, and will put her in a more receptive mood for your advice and suggestions. The actual placement of supplies on the table is a suggestion. Since regulations regarding table setup vary from state to state and province to province, be guided by your instructor.

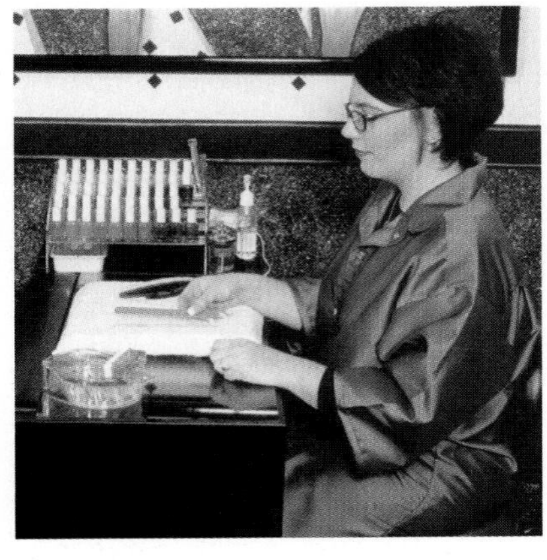

Figure 22-15 Basic manicure table setup.

Preparing the Manicure Table

1. Sanitize the manicure table and drawer with approved disinfectant.
2. Place a clean or disposable towel over the client's cushion.
3. Place a bowl of warm, soapy water to the left of the client. If you are giving a hot oil manicure, replace the fingerbowl and brush with an electric hot oil heater.
4. Place disinfected metal implements and a new orangewood stick on a clean or disposable towel.
5. Arrange cream or lotion bottles and nail polishes in the order to be used and place them to the left of the manicurist.
6. Place the disinfected abrasive and fresh emery boards to the right of the manicurist.
7. Attach a small plastic bag to the table with adhesive tape, on either the right or left side, for waste materials.
8. Prepare a fresh disinfectant solution for your implements on a daily basis.

The manicuring table drawer always should be clean and neat. Do not use it to store money, pencils, or waste materials. Use the plastic bag for wastes.

CLIENT CONSULTATION

Before you perform a service on a client, you should take some time to talk with the client, and complete a client health record and a service and product record. During this consultation, you will discuss the client's general health, the health of his nails and skin, the client's lifestyle and needs, and the nail services you can offer. You will use your knowledge of skin, nails, and nail services to help your client select the most appropriate service. If the client has a nail or skin disorder that prevents you from performing a service, you should refer that client to his physician and offer to perform a service as soon as the disorder has been treated.

A consultation has two parts: the analysis and the recommendations. For best results, you should perform them separately and distinctly.

1. *Analysis.* This is the information-gathering part of the consultation. Ask questions, looking closely at the client's skin and nails. Touch the skin and nails, pointing out their texture, moisture content, coloration, and condition to the client. Ask relevant questions concerning the client's lifestyle and at-home care. Ask what goals the client has in mind for the nail service (Figure 22–16).
2. *Recommendations.* These are offered only after the information above has been gathered. When you know the client's goals, you can then make recommendations for the appropriate service. Explain the benefits and results of the service and recommend home-care products with instructions on how and when they are to be used.

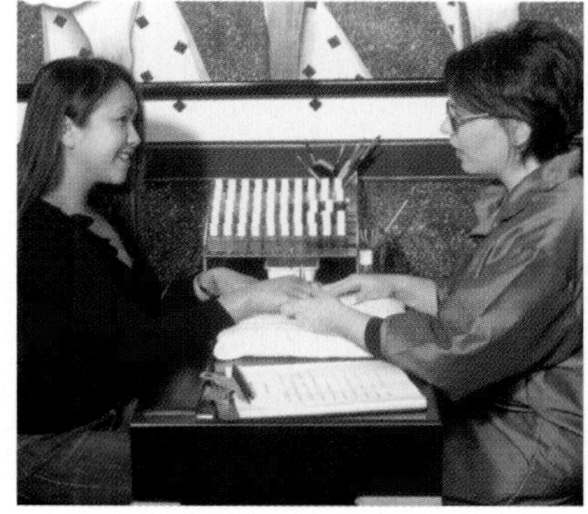

Figure 22–16 Client consultation.

The consultation is your first opportunity to portray yourself as a professional to your client. It should be performed in a straightforward and confident manner. You will need to:

- focus on the client.
- look at the client directly while speaking in a tone that demonstrates integrity and confidence.
- support your recommendations with facts and information.
- be friendly and helpful.

A well-handled consultation will help establish you in the eyes of a client. It demonstrates the difference between being a professional and just "performing a service."

Discussing the Client's General Health

To safeguard your client, you should ask relevant questions concerning her general health. Always read the completed health record so that you will be alert to precautions you must take during services. For example, be particularly careful while filing the nails or pushing back the pterygium (forward growth of the cuticle) of a diabetic client, and *never* nip the cuticles. Diabetics heal slowly and easily get infections that will not heal quickly, sometimes not at all. The damage can be deadly if the skin is cut or scraped. Clients with arthritis should have their hands held gently during the service, while clients who have a circulatory disease, such as varicose veins, should be massaged very carefully, if at all. It is the responsibility of the technician to seek out information that will ensure the health of all clients (Figure 22–17).

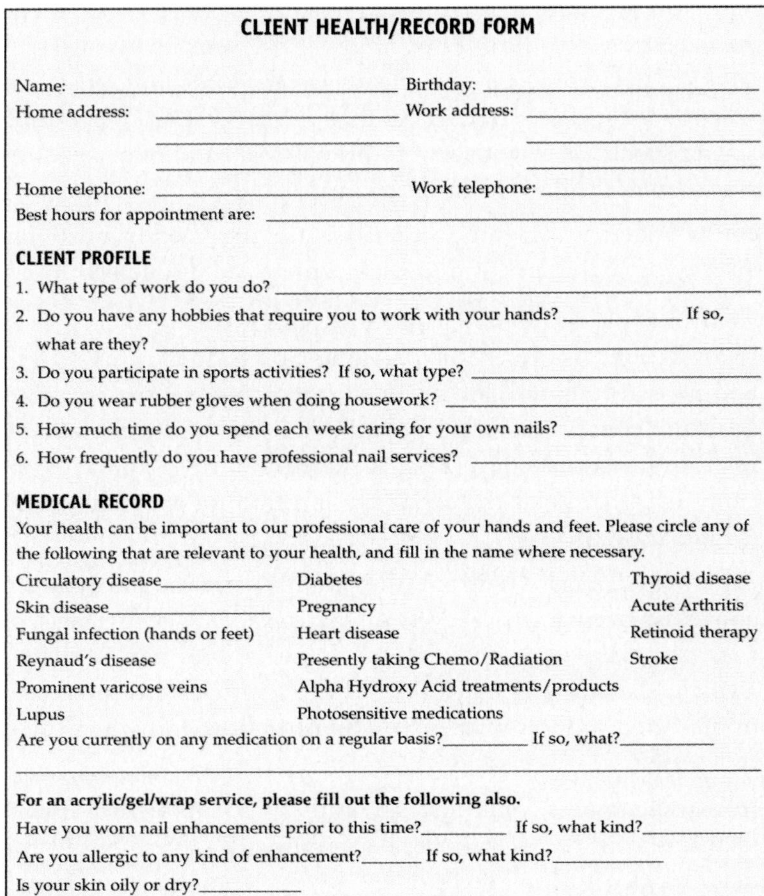

CLIENT HEALTH/RECORD FORM

Name: ______________________ Birthday: ______________________
Home address: ______________________ Work address: ______________________
______________________ ______________________
______________________ ______________________
Home telephone: ______________________ Work telephone: ______________________
Best hours for appointment are: ______________________

CLIENT PROFILE

1. What type of work do you do? ______________________
2. Do you have any hobbies that require you to work with your hands? __________ If so, what are they? ______________________
3. Do you participate in sports activities? If so, what type? ______________________
4. Do you wear rubber gloves when doing housework? ______________________
5. How much time do you spend each week caring for your own nails? ______________________
6. How frequently do you have professional nail services? ______________________

MEDICAL RECORD

Your health can be important to our professional care of your hands and feet. Please circle any of the following that are relevant to your health, and fill in the name where necessary.

Circulatory disease__________	Diabetes	Thyroid disease
Skin disease__________	Pregnancy	Acute Arthritis
Fungal infection (hands or feet)	Heart disease	Retinoid therapy
Reynaud's disease	Presently taking Chemo/Radiation	Stroke
Prominent varicose veins	Alpha Hydroxy Acid treatments/products	
Lupus	Photosensitive medications	

Are you currently on any medication on a regular basis?________ If so, what?__________
____

For an acrylic/gel/wrap service, please fill out the following also.

Have you worn nail enhancements prior to this time?________ If so, what kind?__________
Are you allergic to any kind of enhancement?______ If so, what kind?__________
Is your skin oily or dry?__________
Comments: ______________________
____

Figure 22-17 Client health record.

Choosing a Nail Shape

Before you begin to work on a client's nails, both you and the client should agree on which nail shape is desired. Nails naturally vary greatly in shape, but are usually classified into five general shapes: square, squoval (square with rounded edges), round, oval, and pointed (Figure 22–18). Keep in mind the following considerations when deciding which shape to go with:

- the shape of the client's hands
- the length of the fingers
- the shape of the cuticles
- the type of work the client does

It is generally felt that the nails should be shaped to mirror the shape of the cuticles. Only an attractive hand can afford to direct attention to itself by exaggerated shape and color. People who perform work with their hands usually require shorter nails in order to avoid nail breakage and injury.

The square nail is completely straight across the free edge with no rounding at the edges. The length depends on the client's preference.

Squoval Round
Oval Pointed Square

Figure 22-18 Nail shapes.

insights

Natalie Wilkson

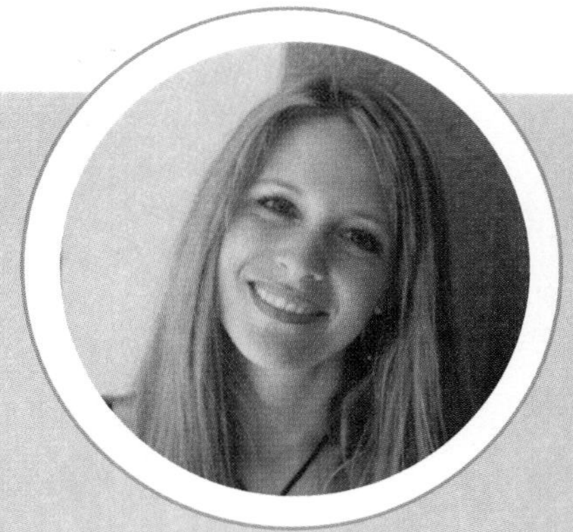

Natalie Wilkson, a nail technician and makeup artist in St. Petersburg, Florida, rates her job satisfaction a perfect 10.

I was a stay-at-home mother for many years, but I have always had an interest in cosmetology. My sister-in-law is a nail technician, and she is a big part of why I went into the industry. She really enjoys her job and has been in the industry for more than 10 years. I thought cosmetology would be perfect for me because I'm able to schedule my own hours. Also, I really missed speaking with people—at least, *adult* people—having been at home with a four-year-old and a 10-year-old all day.

I work about 35 to 36 hours a week as a nail technician and also doing makeup (I'm not certified to do makeup, but in the state of Florida you don't need a license to do makeup). I think this field is perfect for single mothers as well as moms like me who want to go back to work. You can make your own hours, the money is good, and you can be at home. If you're able to schedule your own hours, you can even arrange to be at home with your children in the afternoon.

I really enjoy the one-on-one contact that you have with other women. At the resort where I work, there are so many different types of people who come in, and you hear so many stories. I met several people from New York after the 9/11 tragedy and it really helped me to have a better understanding of what those poor people went through. I think it's important for a cosmetologist to be able to listen and have a good conversation with people. People come in and they want to relax and enjoy themselves. Personality is key in this industry.

When I go into a salon, I pay attention to how I'm greeted. I take into account the personality of the salon. I also look for cleanliness, of course. For me, right now, the biggest challenge is selling retail. Retail is a huge part of the industry. I don't like to be pushy with my clients, but I feel I should try to get good at selling.

The field is full of challenges. Recently, I had a gentleman come in who worked in construction. His nails were worn down with indentations and black spots where he had dropped equipment on them. He wanted acrylic overlays to cover the damage, and that was hard. But I like a good challenge!

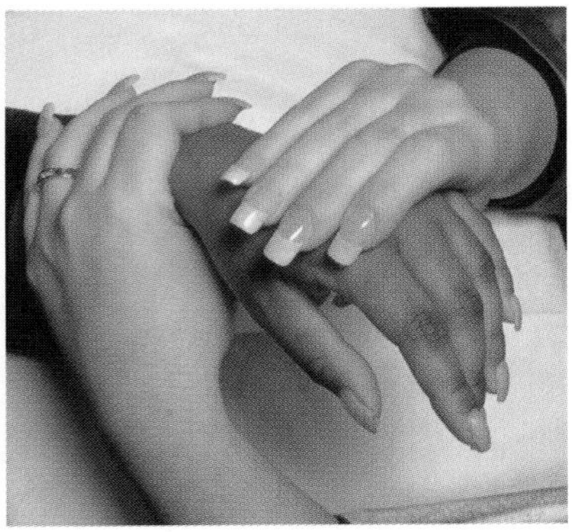

Figure 22-19 Movement to limber the wrist.

The round nail should extend only slightly past the tip of the finger with the nail tip rounded off. The entire nail may be polished with a slight half moon left at the base and a white margin left at the sides of the nail.

The oval nail is the ideal nail shape and can be styled by either covering the entire nail with polish, leaving the free edge white, or leaving the half moon at the base of the nail white.

The pointed nail is well suited for the thin, delicate hand. The nail should be tapered somewhat longer than usual to enhance the slender appearance of the hand. The nail can be completely polished, or a half moon can be left at the base.

The **squoval** nail is a square nail with the ends rounded or taken off. As the name suggests, the shape is a combination of square and oval.

Hand Massage

A hand massage is a very appealing option to offer with each manicure. It keeps the hands flexible, well groomed, and smooth. A typical manicure sequence is as follows.

1. Holding the client's hand, place a dab of hand lotion on the back of the client's hand and spread it out to the fingers and wrist.
2. Hold the client's hand firmly. Bend the hand slowly with a forward and backward movement to limber the wrist. Repeat three times (Figure 22–19).
3. Grasp each finger, one at a time, and gently bend it to limber the top of the hand and finger joints. As the fingers and thumb are bent, slide your thumb down toward the fingertips (Figure 22–20).
4. With the client's elbow resting on the table, hold the hand upright. Massage the palm of the hand with the cushions of your thumbs, using a circular movement in alternating directions. This movement will completely relax the client's hand (Figure 22–21).

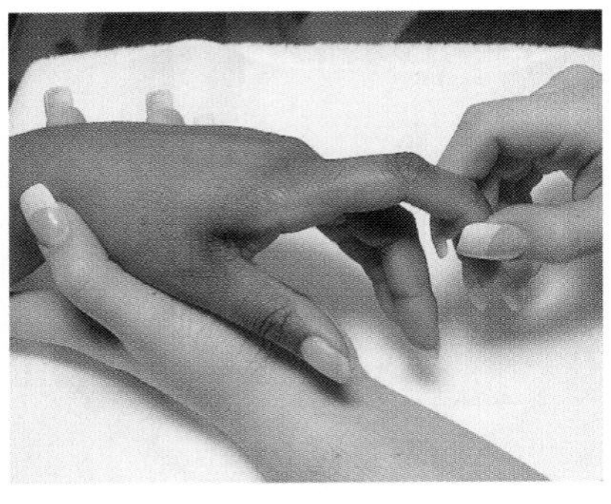

Figure 22-20 Limber top of hand and finger joints.

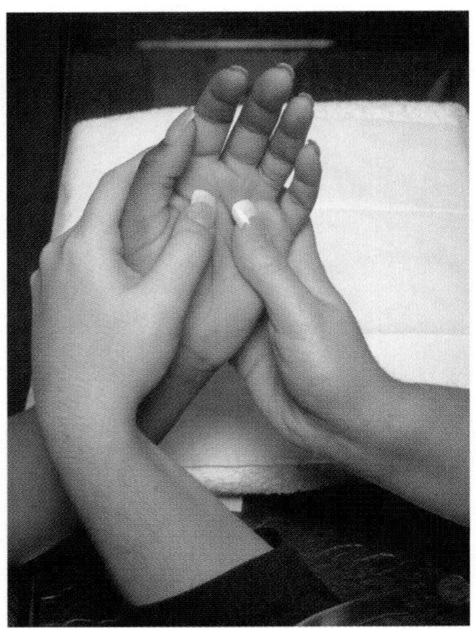

Figure 22-21 Movement to relax the hand.

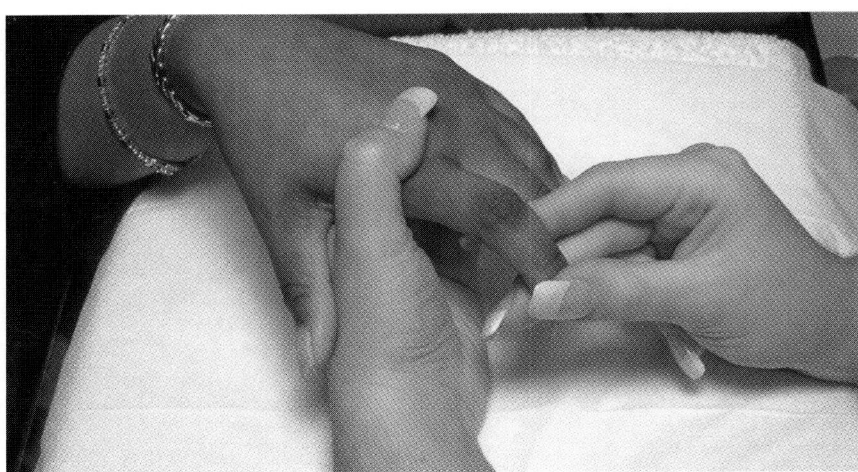

Figure 22-22 Grasp each finger and rotate.

5. Rest the client's arm on the table. Grasp each finger and rotate it gently in large circles, ending with a gentle squeeze of the fingertips. Repeat three times (Figure 22–22).
6. Hold the client's hand. Massage the wrist, then the top of the hand with a circular movement. Slide back and with both hands, wring the wrist in the opposite direction three times. Repeat the whole action three times (Figure 22–23).
7. Finish the massage by tapering each finger. Beginning at the base of the finger, rotate, pause, and then squeeze with gentle pressure. Pull lightly with some pressure until the tip is reached. Repeat three times (Figure 22–24).
8. Repeat Steps 1 through 7 on the other hand.

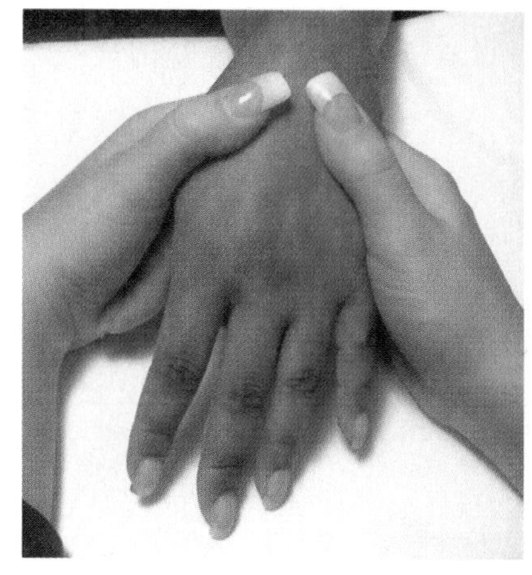

Figure 22-23 Massage wrist and top of hand.

Hand and Arm Massage

This procedure is a special service that may be offered in addition to the plain manicure. It is very similar to the hand massage, except that all applications are extended to the forearm, including the elbow.

1. Complete the hand massage as described above.
2. Place the client's arm on the table, with the palm turned downward. Massage the arm from the wrist to the elbow, using a slow, circular motion in alternate directions. Repeat three times. Turn the client's palm upward and repeat the same movements three times (Figure 22–25).
3. Firmly massage the underside of the arm to the elbow, using the fingers of both your hands in alternate crosswise directions. Repeat three times (Figure 22–26).
4. Massage the top of the arm from the wrist to the elbow. Apply your thumbs in opposite directions with a squeezing motion. Repeat three times (Figure 22–27).

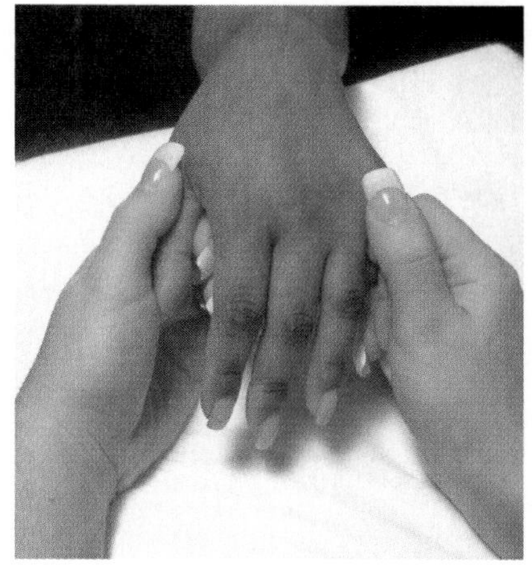

Figure 22-24 Taper each finger.

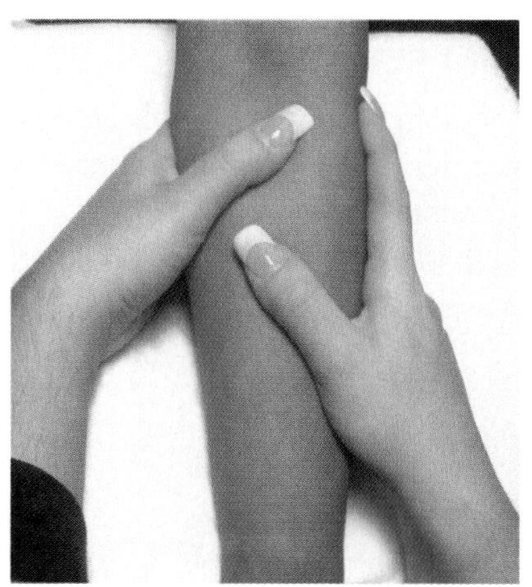

Figure 22-25 Massage arm from wrist to elbow.

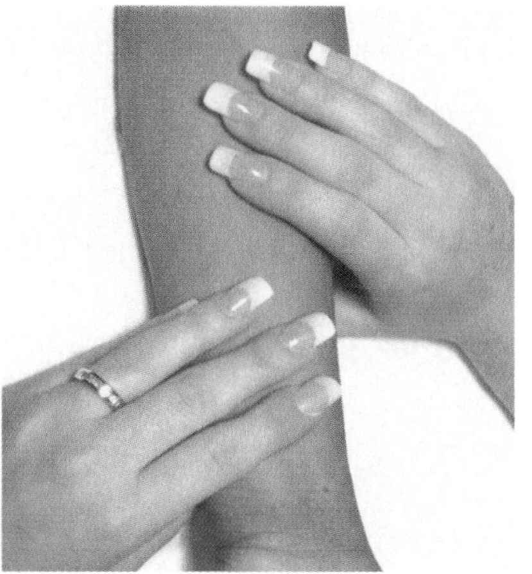

Figure 22-26 Massage underpart of arm to elbow.

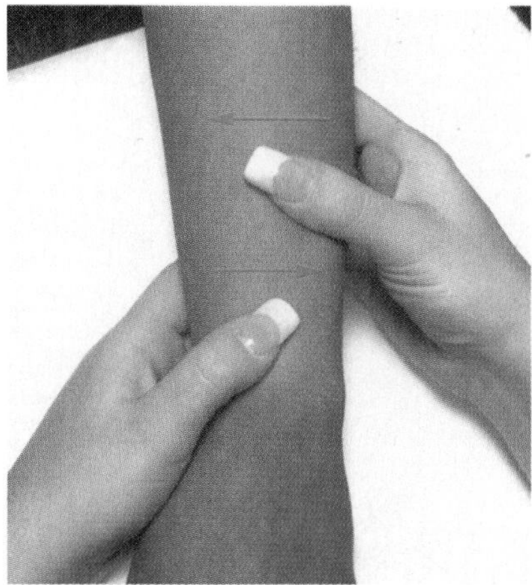

Figure 22-27 Massage top of arm from wrist to elbow.

5. Cup the elbow joint in your hand. Massage the elbow with a circular motion. Repeat three times (Figure 22–28).
6. Stroke the arm firmly in opposite directions, from the elbow to wrist (Figure 22–29). Finally, stroke each finger, ending with a gentle squeeze of the fingertips.
7. Repeat Steps 1 through 6 on the other arm.

Figure 22-28 Massage elbow.

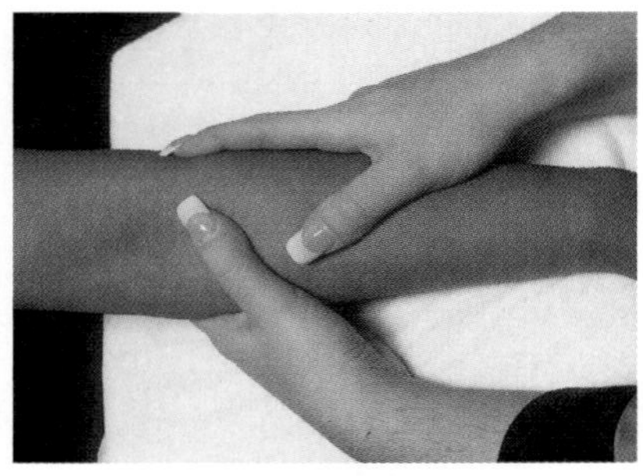

Figure 22-29 Stroke arm in opposite directions.

THE PLAIN MANICURE

The routine outlined below is just one of several correct ways to provide a plain manicure. Whatever routine your instructor outlines for you will be equally correct.

As a professional nail technician, you will follow a three-part procedure for all services you perform. This sequence includes a preservice function, the actual procedure, and a postservice function.

During the actual manicure procedure, discuss with your client the products you are using and suggest that those products be purchased in order to maintain the nails and skin in between appointments. Before applying polish, ask your client to replace jewelry, locate keys, pay for the service as well as any retail products, and put on any outer clothing such as sweaters or jackets. Having your client do these things ahead of the polish application decreases the chances of smudging the polish once the application has been completed.

Nail Problems

Here are a few common problems you may encounter during a manicure.

- A fringe of loose skin left around the nail after a manicure can be caused by trimming the cuticle closer than necessary and then rolling back the epidermis. To prevent this, trim the cuticle only enough to allow a tiny margin to remain.
- Callus growth at the fingertips can be softened by the application of creams and lotions. Gentle rubbing with pumice powder or an abrasive is also a good way to begin the process of removal.
- Stains on fingernails may be bleached with prepared nail bleach or peroxide. You may also remove stains by slightly dampening pumice powder and using it to buff the nails.

PROCEDURE

PLAIN MANICURE

Implements and Materials

The setup for a plain manicure includes all the items listed under "Nail Care Tools" described on pages 760-762.

Preservice (Preparation)

1. Sanitize the table.
2. Sanitize all additional equipment, tools, and implements.
3. Set up the standard table.
4. Wash your hands with soap and warm water.
5. Cordially greet your client.
6. Have your client remove all jewelry and place the items in a safe, secure place.
7. Have your client wash her hands with soap and warm water and dry them thoroughly with a clean and/or disposable towel.
8. Perform a client consultation.

NOTE: Begin working with the hand that is not the client's favored hand. The favored hand will need to soak longer, because it is used more often. If the client is left-handed, begin with the right hand, and if the client is right-handed, begin with the left hand. This procedure is written for a left-handed client.

Procedure

1. Remove old polish, starting with the little finger of the right hand. Moisten cotton with nail polish remover and press over the nail for a few moments to soften the polish. With a firm movement, bring the cotton from the base of the nail to the tip. Do not smear the old polish into the cuticle or surrounding tissues (Figure 22–30). An alternate method of removing nail polish is to moisten small pledgets of cotton with nail polish remover and place them over the old polish on each nail. Then moisten another pledget of cotton with nail polish remover and use it to remove the small pledgets on the nails. The pressed-on pledget acts as a blotter and does not leave a polish smear on the cuticle.

Figure 22–30 Remove polish.

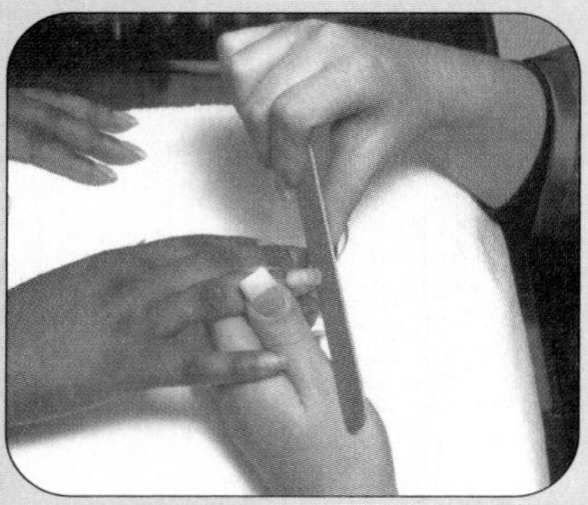

Figure 22-31 Shape the nails.

2. Shape the nails. Having decided on the nail shape during the client consultation, proceed with that in mind. File the nails of the right hand, starting with the little finger and working toward the thumb, in the following manner.
   a. Hold the client's finger between the thumb and first two fingers of your left hand.
   b. Hold the file or emery board in your right hand and tilt it slightly so that filing is confined mainly to the underside of the free edge.
   c. File each nail from corner to center, going from right to left and then from left to right (Figure 22-31). File nails according to the way they grow avoids splitting. If the nails need shortening, they can be cut with fingernail clippers. This will save time during the filing process. Avoid filing deep into the corners of the nails. They will look longer and be stronger if permitted to grow out at the sides.
3. Soften the cuticle. After filing the nails of the right hand, file two nails of the left hand. Then immerse the right hand into the finger bowl (soap bath) to soften of the cuticle (Figure 22-32). Finish filing the nails of the left hand. Remove the right hand from the finger bowl. Clean the nails by brushing them with a sanitized brush. Use downward strokes, starting at the first knuckle and brushing toward the free edge.

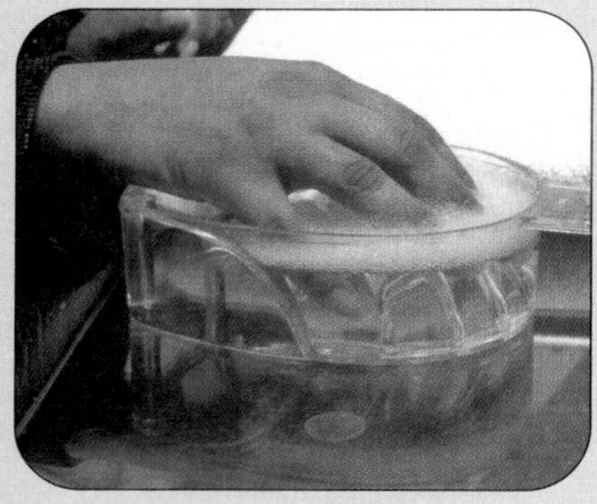

Figure 22-32 Soak hand in finger bowl.

4. Dry the fingertips. Holding a towel with both hands, carefully dry the right hand, including the area between the fingers. With the towel, gently loosen and push back the cuticle on each nail (Figure 22-33).
5. Wind a thin layer of cotton around the blunt edge of a new orangewood stick for use as an applicator. Apply cuticle remover around the cuticle of the right hand (Figure 22-34).
6. Use the spoon end of the cuticle pusher to gently loosen the cuticle. Keep the cuticle moist while working. Use the cuticle pusher, in a safe position, to remove dead cuticle adhering to the nail without scratching the nail plate (Figure 22-35). Use a circular movement to help lift cuticles that cling to the nail plate. The cuticle remover will probably

22

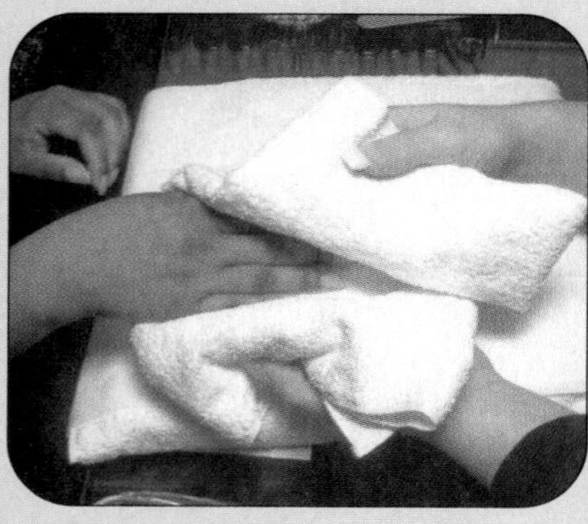

Figure 22-33 Dry the fingertips.

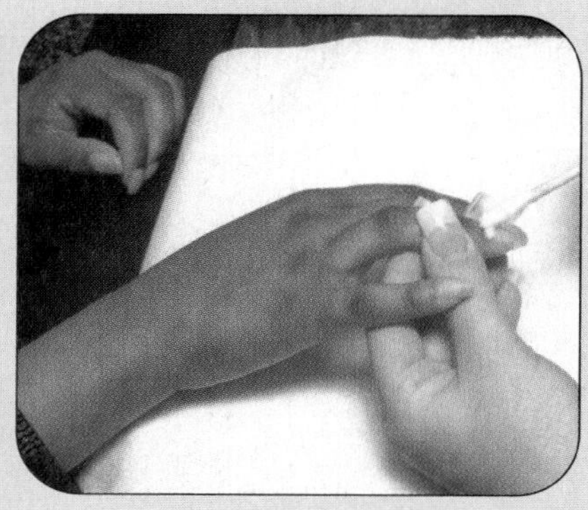

Figure 22-34 Apply cuticle solvent.

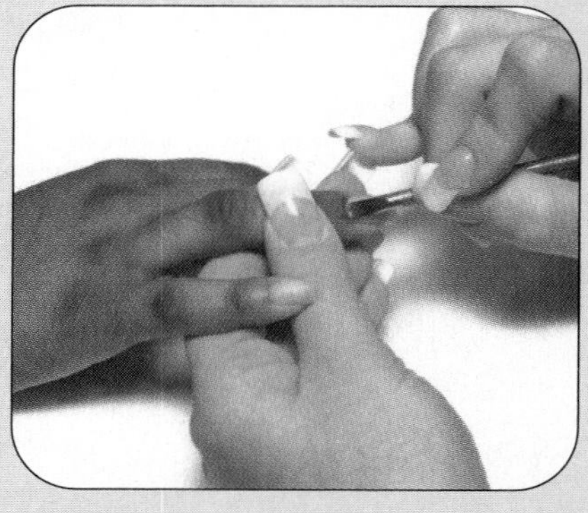

Figure 22-35 Loosen dead cuticle.

remove enough cuticle so that you won't need to clip any. Light pressure should be used to avoid damaging the area at the root of the nail and the nail plate.

7. Use a cotton-tipped orangewood stick, dipped in soapy water, to clean under the free edge, working from the center toward each side with gentle pressure (Figure 22–36).
8. If necessary, use cuticle nippers to remove dead cuticle, uneven cuticle, or hangnails. When cutting the cuticle, be careful to remove it as a single segment (Figure 22–37).
9. When cutting the cuticle of the middle finger of the right hand, immerse fingers of the left hand into finger bowl, while continuing to manicure the right hand.
10. An optional step here is to bleach under the free edge. With a cotton-tipped orangewood stick, apply hydrogen peroxide or other bleaching preparation under the free edge of each nail.
11. Apply cuticle oil or cream around the sides and base of the nail and massage with the thumb in a rotary movement.
12. Remove the left hand from the finger bowl. Manicure the nails and cuticles of the left hand as described in Steps 4 through 11.
13. Brush the nails over the finger bowl, using a downward movement, to clean the nails of both hands. Dry the hands and nails thoroughly.
14. Reexamine the nails and cuticles for any defects. Use the fine side of an emery board to give the nails a smooth beveled edge and remove any remaining pieces of cuticle.
15. If required, repair split or broken nails (see Chapter 23).
16. As an added service, a hand or hand and arm massage may be given at this time. Use an emollient hand cream when performing the massage.
17. Apply the base coat, beginning with the right hand. Use long strokes, starting with the little finger and working toward the thumb (Figure 22–38). Allow the base coat to dry until "slick to a light touch." If using a nail strengthener and/or hardener, apply it under the base coat.

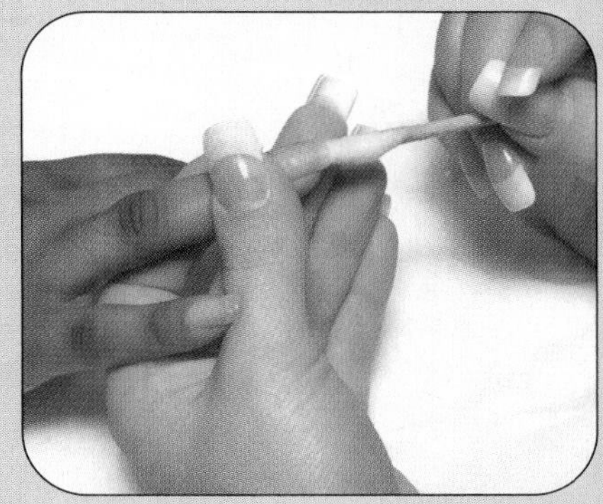

Figure 22-36 Clean under free edge.

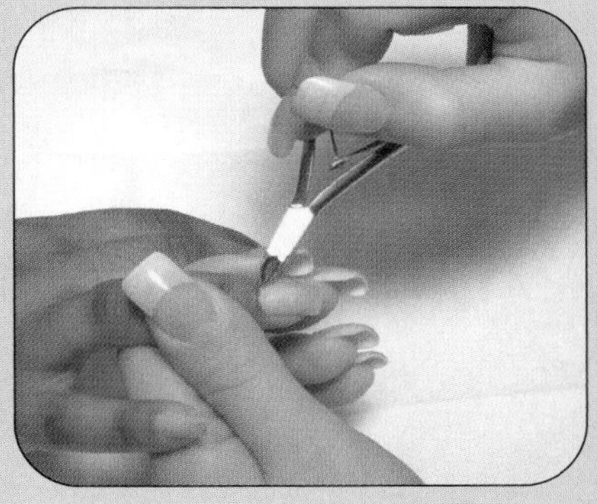

Figure 22-37 Trim cuticle with nippers.

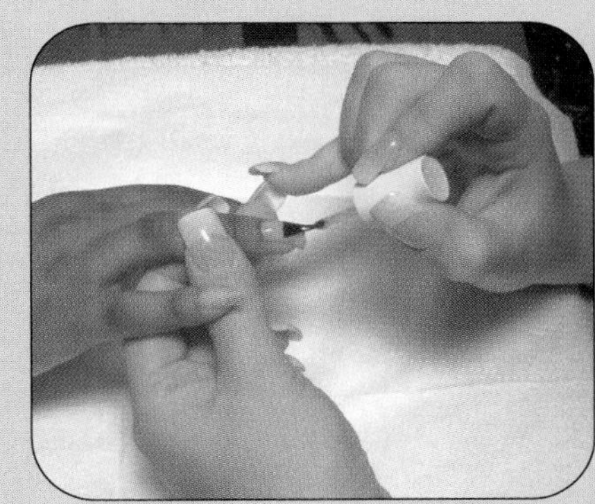

Figure 22-38 Apply base coat.

Some states or provinces do not permit nail technicians to nip cuticles or hangnails. Be guided by your instructor or check with your regulatory agency.

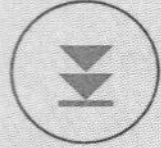

Here's a tip:

Never shake polish bottles. Shaking will cause air bubbles to form and will make the polish application appear rough and irregular. Gently roll the polish bottle between your palms to mix.

18. Choose a color of liquid polish and apply. Remove the brush from the bottle and wipe the side away from you on the neck of the bottle. You should have a bead of polish on the end of the brush, enough to complete the polish application in three strokes without having to dip the brush back into the bottle (Figure 22–39).
19. Hold the brush at approximately a 30-degree angle. Starting in the center of the nail, place the brush 1/16 inch (.2 cm) away from the cuticle. Brush toward the free edge (Figure 22–40). If you go back and dab at any spots you missed, the polish will not appear smooth on the nail. The more strokes you use, the more lines and lumps will appear on the polished nails. If you miss a small area on the nail, you can cover this area when you apply the second coat. Practice covering the entire nail each time, especially near the cuticle, so as not to create a shadow of polish. Wait until the polish settles before continuing, as bubbles could cause a problem.
20. Remove excess polish. Dip a cotton-tipped orangewood stick into nail polish remover. Apply it carefully around the cuticles and nail edges to remove excess polish (Figure 22–41).
21. Using long strokes, apply top or seal coat first to the right hand, then to the left hand. Brush around and under the tips of the nails for added support and protection. A UV top coat can be used instead of an air-dry top coat. Place both the client's hands under a UV lamp dryer (Figure 22–42).
22. Instant nail dry is optional; if used, apply it at this time. Apply it to each nail to prevent smudging, dulling, and to decrease drying time. The basic manicure is now complete (Figure 22–43).

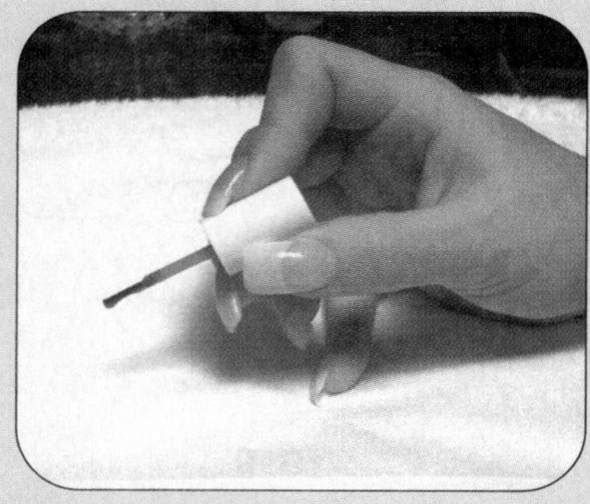

Figure 22–39 Bead of polish on brush.

22

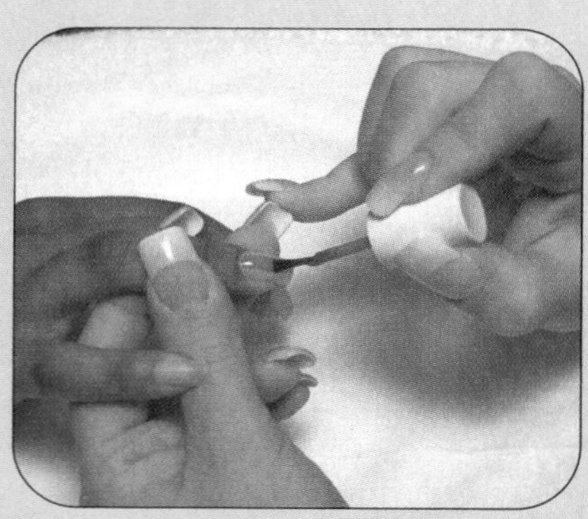

Figure 22–40 Apply polish.

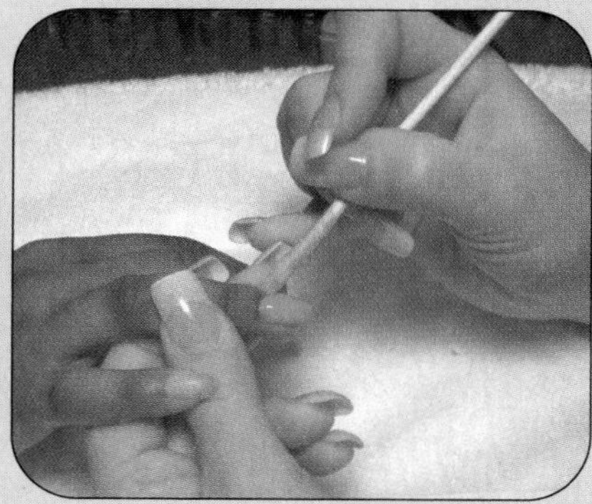

Figure 22–41 Remove excess polish.

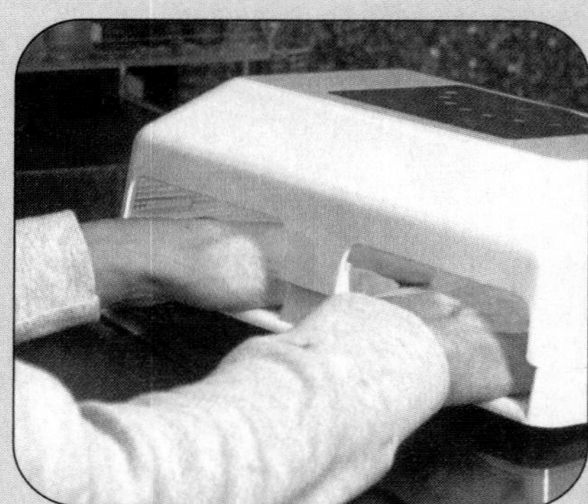

Figure 22–42 Place client's hands under UV lamp dryer.

Postservice (Cleanup and Sanitation)

1. Schedule your client's next appointment. Set up the date and time and determine which services will be performed.
2. Write down the information for the client on your business or appointment card.
3. Clean up your work area and properly dispose of all used materials and nonsantitizable implements.
4. Sanitize your table and additional equipment, tools, and implements.
5. Record the service information on your client's health and/or record card.

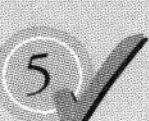

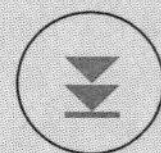

Here's a tip:

A flat nylon bristle brush, size 6 or 8, can also be used to remove polish. Dip it into acetone, touch it to the towel to release excess acetone, and clean around the perimeter of the nail. Never let the brush sit in the acetone, as it will loosen the bristles from the ferrule. This brush can be sanitized.

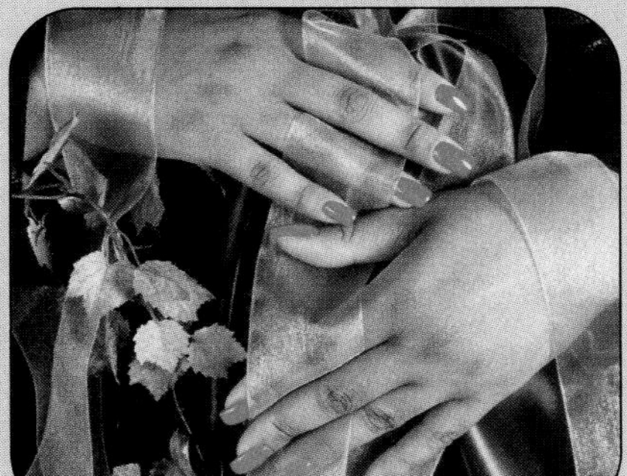

Figure 22-43 Finished basic manicure.

22

completed!

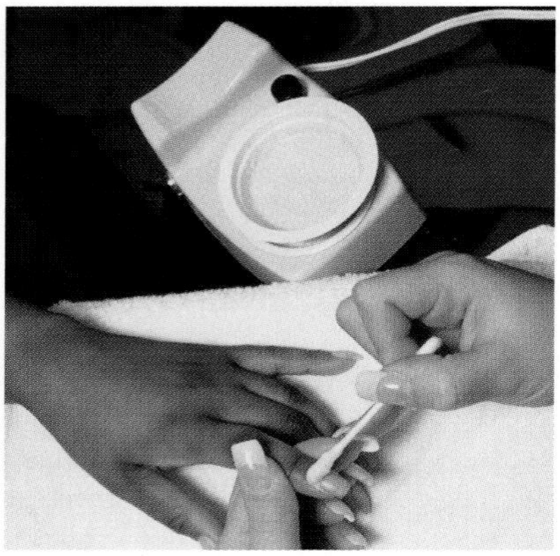

Figure 22-44 Oil heater.

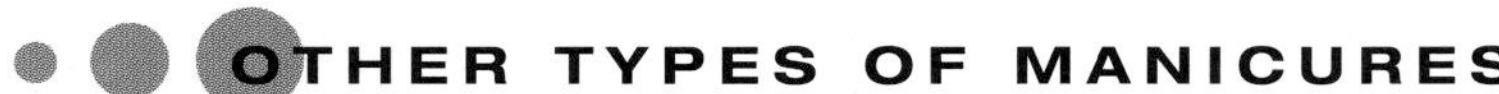

OTHER TYPES OF MANICURES

There are a number of other manicures you should learn in addition to the plain manicure described above.

Hot Oil Manicure

A **hot oil manicure** is one in which a heated oil, cream, or lotion is applied to the cuticles to soften them before pushing them back. It is beneficial for ridged and brittle nails and dry cuticles. You may use vegetable oil (olive oil is good) or a commercial product such as a hand cream or lotion. It is suggested that a reconditioning hot oil manicure be performed once a week, as it will add moisture to the skin and nails. Hot oil manicures are also beneficial for people who bite their nails because it helps keep rough cuticles soft.

A hot oil manicure calls for the same table setup as the plain manicure, plus an oil heater and the cream, lotion, or oil of your choice (Figure 22–44). Preheat the oil for 15 minutes. Perform a plain manicure to the point at which you would place the client's hand in the finger bowl. Instead, have the client place her fingers in the heated oil or apply the oil to each finger using a cotton-tipped swab. Push the cuticles back carefully (cuticle remover or cuticle oil is not needed). Massage the hands and wrists with the oil. Wipe each nail carefully with polish remover to remove all traces of the oil before applying the base coat. Then complete as you would a plain manicure.

French Manicure

A **French manicure** is one in which the free edge of the nail is polished, tipped, or sculpted in an opaque color while the nail plate is polished or left a more translucent color. It is a popular service in the salon. This technique creates nails that appear clean and natural and offers a good base for designs with flat nail art, airbrushing, rhinestones, pearls, or striping tape. A French manicure usually uses a more dramatic white on the free edge of the nail, whereas the American manicure calls for a more subtle white.

Men's Manicure

Men usually prefer a conservative manicure. File the nails either round or square, but remember to ask if your client has a preference. You can apply a dry polish instead of a liquid polish.

Implements and materials are the same as those used for a plain manicure. Follow the same procedure for a plain manicure up to the application of a base coat.

Buff nails with a chamois buffer (where permitted). Apply a small dab of paste polish over the buffer. Then buff the nails with downward strokes, from the base to the free edge of each nail, until a smooth, clear gloss has been obtained (Figure 22–45). To prevent a hot or burning sensation, lift the buffer from the nail after each stroke. Buffing the nails increases the circulation of the blood to the fingertips, smooths the nails, and gives them a natural gloss or sheen. Another option is a three-way buffer, which you can discard after use or give to the client.

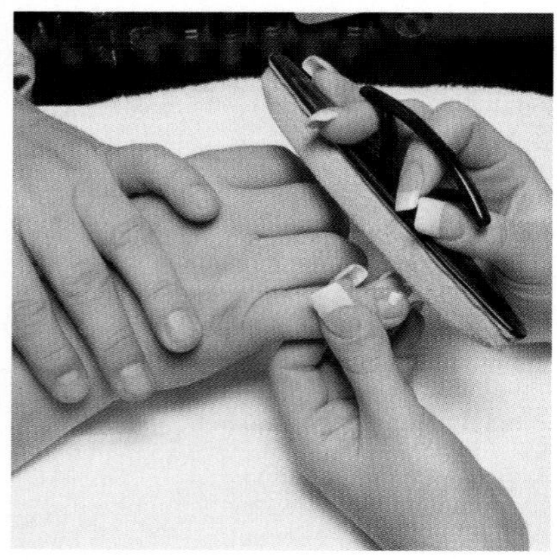

Figure 22-45 Buff the nails.

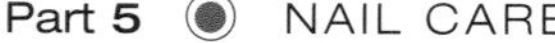

PROCEDURE

FRENCH MANICURE

Implements and Materials

Same table setup as for Procedure 57—plain manicure.

Preparation

Perform preservice procedure in Procedure 57—plain manicure.

Procedure

1. Perform the procedure for the plain manicure up to polish application.
2. If the nail has pitting, lines, or ridges, use a ridge-filling base coat. It will help the nail to appear smooth after the translucent polish is applied (Figure 22–46).
3. Apply opaque white polish. Start at one side of the free edge (usually the left side of the nail) and sweep across toward the center of the free edge on a diagonal line (Figure 22–47). Repeat this on the right side of the nail (Figure 22–48). This will form a V-shape. Some clients like this look, called a "chevron French." If not, fill in the open top of the V so that you have an even line across the free edge (Figure 22–49). Allow the white polish to dry.

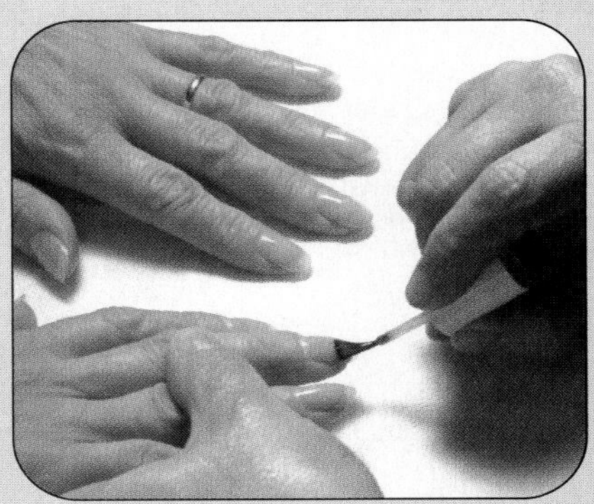

Figure 22–46 Apply base coat.

22

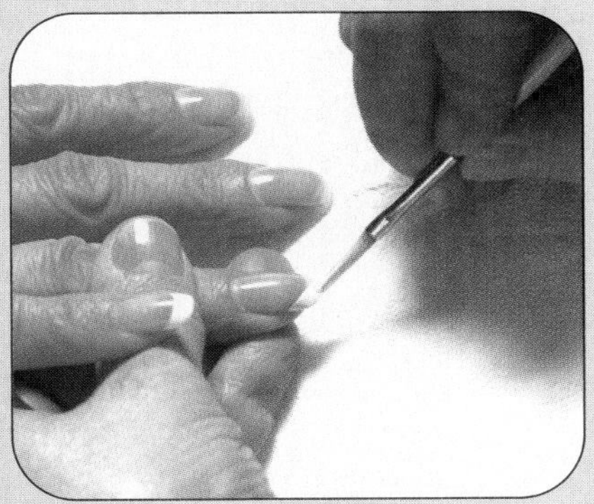

Figure 22–47 Apply white polish to center of nail.

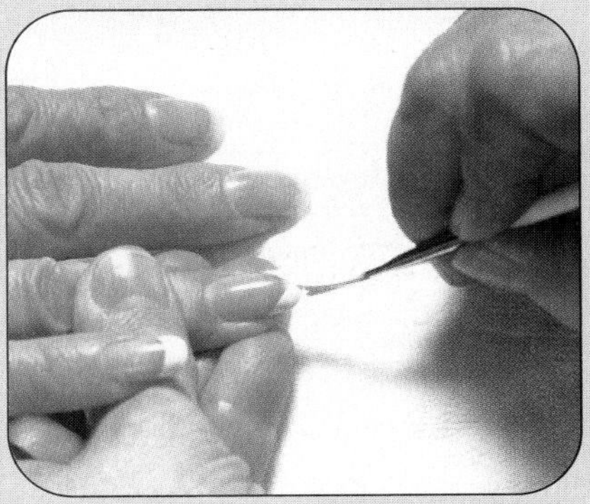

Figure 22–48 Repeat on the other side.

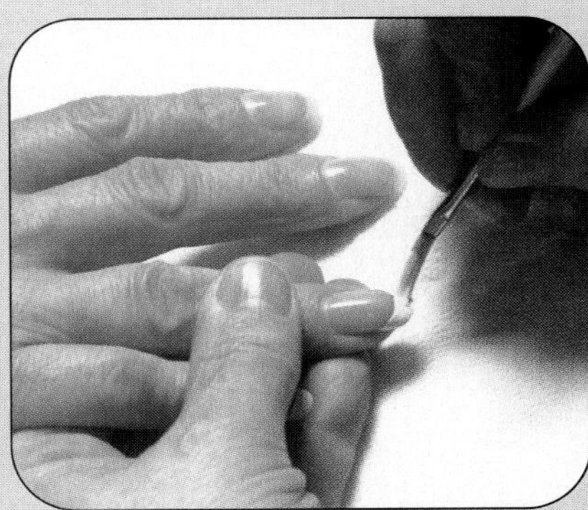

Figure 22–49 Fill in the top of the V.

4. Apply a translucent white, pink, natural, or peach color polish from the base to the free edge. Be careful not to get any on the cuticle (Figure 22-50).
5. Apply a top coat over the entire nail plate and around the free edge to seal and protect the white (Figure 22-51).
6. Perform postservice procedure in Procedure 57—plain manicure.

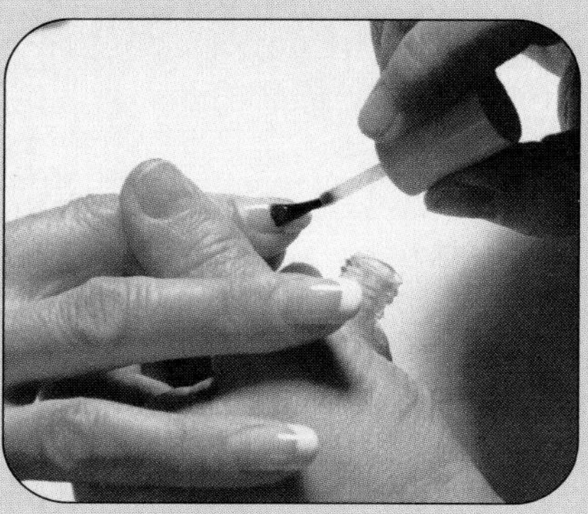

Figure 22-50 Apply translucent polish.

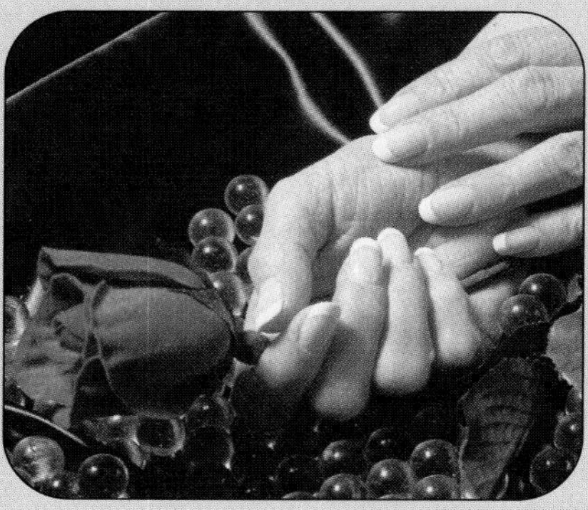

Figure 22-51 Finished French manicure.

completed!

Remove all residue from the nails by washing and drying the fingertips. If a clear liquid polish is used, buffing is not required. If polish application is requested, apply a base coat and a clear top coat, followed by instant nail dry. A satin or matte polish is available if your client prefers. Apply polish in the same manner as for a plain manicure.

A citrus or musk-scented hand cream, rather than a flowery one, is recommended for a man's hand massage.

Booth Manicure

A **booth manicure** is a manicure that is given in the booth and not at the manicuring table. It is usually given while the client is receiving another service, such as a pedicure or a haircut.

Electric Manicure

The electric manicure is given with a portable device operated by a small motor. It uses a variety of attachments, including an emery wheel, cuticle pusher, callus attachment, and chamois buffer. Videos and instructional classes are offered by manufacturers of electric files. Should you need training, be sure to seek out these opportunities.

Before using an electric file, read the manufacturers' instructions carefully. State regulations regarding this procedure may vary, so be guided by your instructor. All drill bits must be properly disinfected after each client use.

PEDICURES

Pedicuring has become an important salon service because of popular shoe styles that expose the heels and toes. During the warmer months, we are particularly aware of rough, harsh heels and unattractive toenails. Foot care not only improves personal appearance but also adds to the comfort of the feet. It is particularly important for clients who are on their feet much of the day, such as dancers, nurses, sales clerks, and cosmetologists.

When making a pedicure appointment, suggest that the client wear open-toed shoes or sandals so that the polish will not smear. Another alternative would be to offer pedicure thongs along with open-toed socks to keep those the feet in colder weather.

Not all clients will want or need a full pedicure service. Some only need a professional nail trimming. You can help your client decide what is most suitable.

Equipment, Implements, and Materials

The equipment, implements, and materials required for pedicuring are the same as those for manicuring, with the following additions:

- *Client's chair with armrests.*
- *Low stool for cosmetologist or pedicurist.*

CAUTION

Your role as a provider of pedicures does not qualify you to treat any medical disorders you may encounter. Abnormal foot conditions, such as corns and infected ingrown nails, are best treated by a podiatrist (a physician who treats diseases of the feet). Never perform a pedicure on feet with a contagious disease such as ringworm (athlete's foot), which can be spread from one person to another. For an in-depth explanation of nail diseases, see Chapter 21.

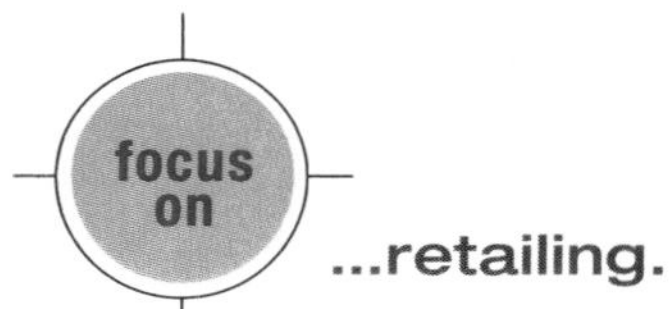

...retailing.

During the actual pedicure procedure, talk with your client about the products that are needed to maintain the service between salon visits. You might suggest polish, top coat, foot cream, and a foot file.

22

- *Ottoman on which to rest the client's foot.*
- *Basin* large enough to hold warm, soapy water in which to soak the client's feet.
- *Waterproof apron,* or an extra towel, to place over the lap to protect the uniform.
- *Two towels* for drying the client's feet.
- *Liquid soap*
- *Antiseptic foot spray.* Contains an antifungal agent as well as a mild antiseptic.
- *Toe separators.* Foam rubber toe separators or cotton used to keep toes apart during the pedicure.
- *Cuticle nippers.*
- *Toenail clippers.* Two types of toenail clippers are available; both are acceptable for a professional pedicure.
- *Cotton pledgets.*
- *Witch hazel or other astringent.*
- *Foot lotion or cream.* Used during the foot massage.
- *Foot powder.* Contains an antifungal agent for keeping feet dry after pedicuring.
- *Pedicure slippers.* Disposable paper or foam slippers for clients who have not worn open-toed shoes.
- *Toenail nippers.* Use only the professional nippers made specifically for cutting toenails. They come with either curved or straight jaws. They allow you to trim the corner of a toenail properly; trimming improperly can cause an ingrown toenail.
- **Curette** (optional). This small spoon-shaped implement, if carefully used, is the ideal tool for cleaning the debris from the nail margins. In most clients, you will only have to use it along the margins of the great toenails. Only occasionally is it necessary to clean along the lesser toenail margins. Most curettes are quite sharp on their edges.
- **Nail rasp** (optional). This tool is constructed so that it only cuts or files in one direction. It is used to smooth off the edges of the nail in the nail groove and reduce the possibility of the nail cutting into the skin. To use the file, gently place it in the nail groove against the free edge of the nail plate and pull it along the edge of the nail toward the end of the toe. This process may be repeated to make sure there are no rough edges remaining along the nail margin. Like the curette, this file is used mainly along the nail margins of the great toenail. The lesser toenails do not usually require filing along their margins. As you become proficient in the use of this file, you will find it an invaluable and time-saving tool.
- **Diamond nail file** (optional). This implement files the free edge of the toenails and in some cases, thins them. It is metal with diamond dust embedded in the metal. It comes in coarse, medium, and fine grits. The

coarse grit is usually best for toenails. The file is thin and flexible and can be used in the same manner as other nail files. Its major advantage is that it is easily sanitized and can be kept in disinfectant solutions. Therefore, it can be used safely on many different clients. This file is not easily worn out, making the initial expense extremely cost-effective.

- **Foot file or paddle** (optional). This implement is used to remove dry flaky skin and smooth calluses on the foot. It comes in many different grits and shapes. The main disadvantage is that most are not easily disinfected. You should pick a file that is advertised as "sanitizable" and can be immersed in disinfection solution many times without falling apart.

Some states or provinces do not allow the use of implements such as curettes and nail rasps in the salon. Be guided by your instructor or check with your regulatory agency.

Foot Massage

Performing a good, thorough foot massage is an excellent way to build client loyalty. Be gentle but firm when handling the foot. Too light a touch or hold will produce a tickling sensation, which is not relaxing for most clients. Massage movements are described more fully in Chapter 19.

Here are some techniques and illustrations for the massage of the left foot; make the necessary adjustments for massaging the right foot.

1. *Relaxer movement to the joints of the foot.* Rest the client's foot on the footrest. Grasp the leg just above the ankle with your left hand. This will brace the client's leg and foot. Use your right hand to hold the left foot just beneath the toes and rotate the foot in a circular motion (Figure 22–52).
2. *Effleurage (light or hard stroking movements) on top of the foot.* Place both thumbs on top of the foot at the instep. Move your thumbs, using circular movements in opposite directions, down the center of the top of the foot. Continue this movement to the toes. Keeping one hand in contact with the foot or leg, firmly slide one hand at a time back to the instep and rotate back down to the toes. This is a relaxing movement. Repeat three to five times (Figure 22–53).

CAUTION

Callus is there for a reason: it protects the underlying skin from irritation. Remove only enough callus to make the client comfortable. Calluses should be softened and smoothed, not removed.

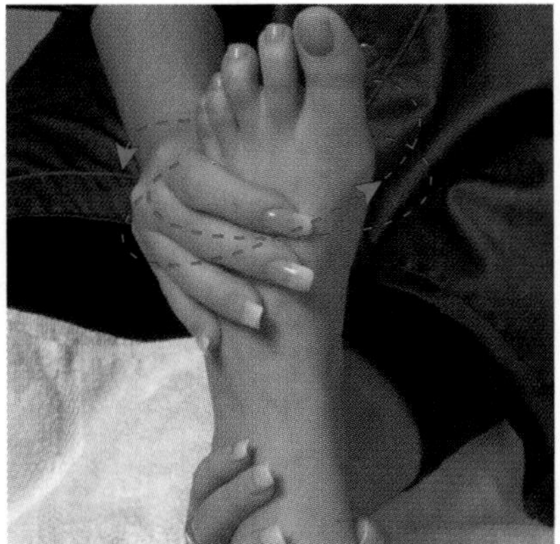

Figure 22-52 Relaxer movement to the joints of the foot.

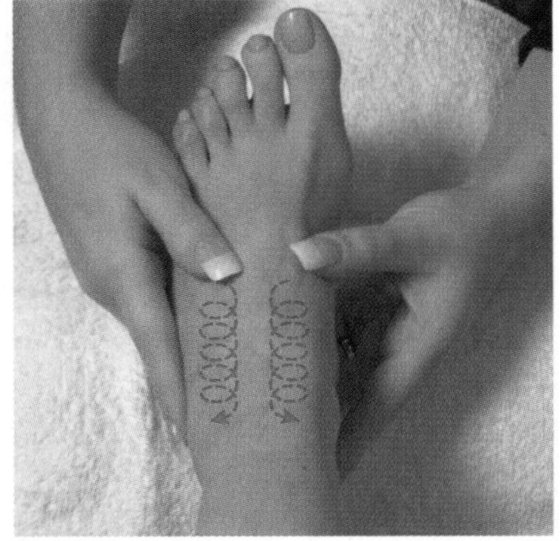

Figure 22-53 Effleurage movement on top of foot.

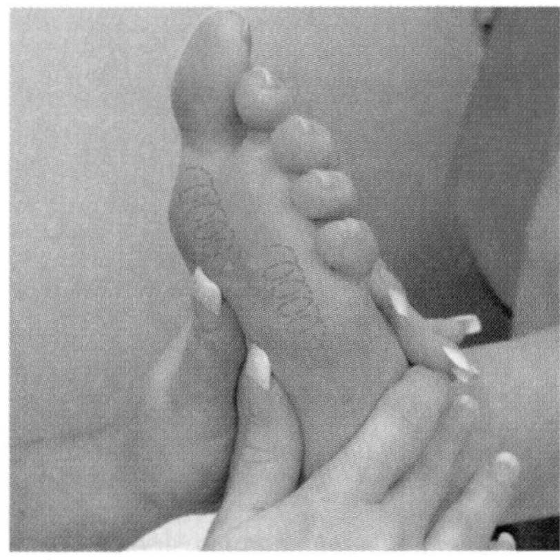

Figure 22-54 Effluerage movement on bottom of foot.

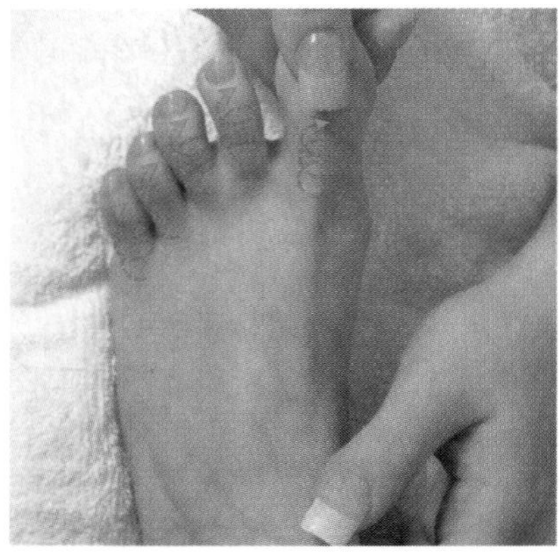

Figure 22-55 Effleurage on toes.

3. *Effleurage on the heel (bottom of foot).* Use the same thumb movement that you used on top of the foot. Start at the base of the toes and move from the ball of the foot to the heel, rotating your thumbs in opposite directions. Slide your hand back to the top of the foot. This is a relaxing movement. Repeat three to five times (Figure 22–54).
4. *Effleurage movement on toes.* Starting with the little toe, place your thumb on the tip and your index finger on the bottom of the foot. Hold each toe and rotate with your thumb. Start at the base of the toe and work toward the end of the toes. This is relaxing and soothing. Repeat three to five times (Figure 22–55).
5. *Joint movement for toes.* Start with the little toe and make a figure eight with each toe. Repeat three to five times (Figure 22–56).
6. *Thumb compression (friction movement).* Make a fist with your fingers, keeping your thumb out. Apply firm pressure with your thumb and move your fist up the heel toward the ball of the foot. Work from the left side of the foot and back down the right side toward the heel. As you massage over the bottom of the foot, check for any nodules or bumps. If you find one, be very gentle because the area may be tender (Figure 22–57).
7. *Metatarsal scissors.* Place your fingers on top of the foot along the metatarsal bones with your thumb underneath the foot. Knead up and down along each bone by raising your thumb and lowering your fingers to apply pressure. This is a petrissage or kneading movement that promotes flexibility and stimulates blood flow. Repeat three to five times (Figure 22–58).
8. *Fist twist compression.* Place your left hand on top of the foot and make a fist with your right hand. Your left hand will apply

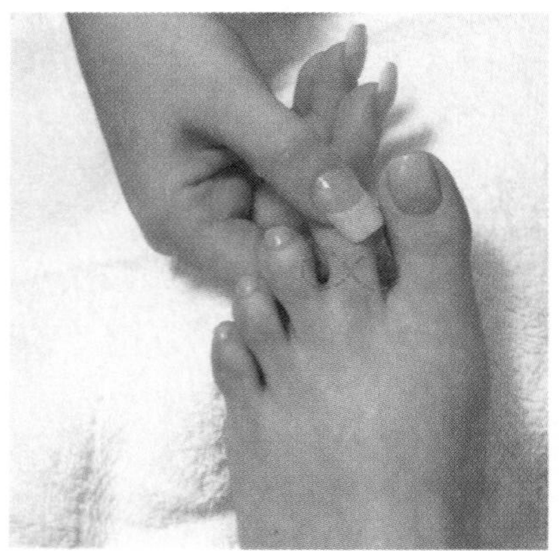

Figure 22-56 Joint movement for toes.

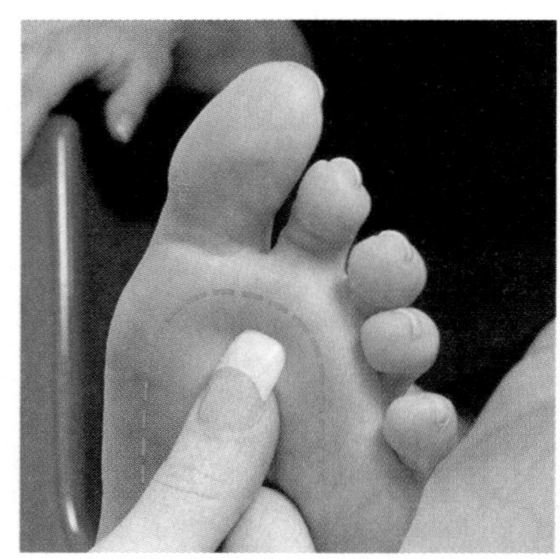

Figure 22-57 Thumb compression.

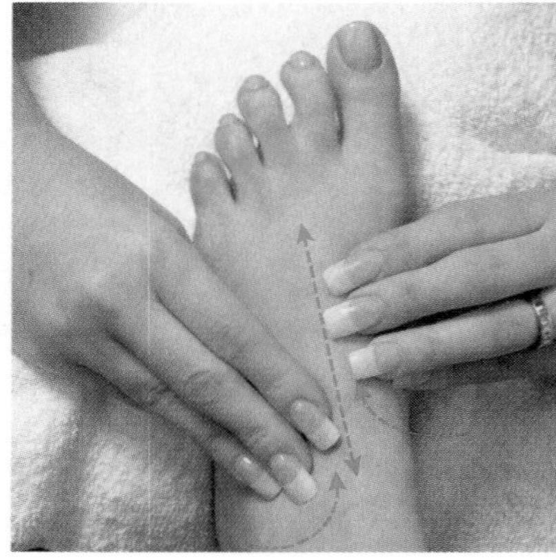

Figure 22-58 Metatarsal scissors.

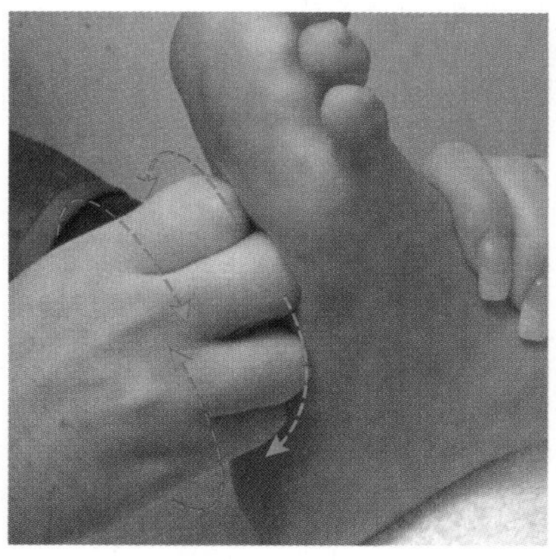

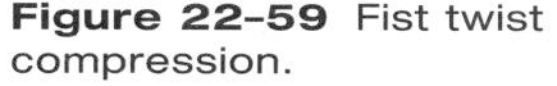

Figure 22-59 Fist twist compression.

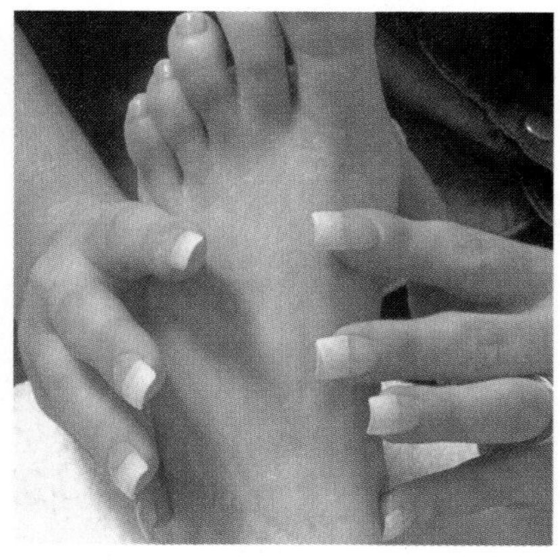

Figure 22-60 Tapotement movements on foot.

Do not massage a client who has high blood pressure, a heart condition, or has had a stroke. Massage increases circulation and may be harmful to such a client. Have your client consult a physician before receiving a massage, then request a doctor's release. Also, if the client has had any form of foot surgery, inquire as to whether or not massage is appropriate.

pressure while your right hand twists around the bottom of the foot. This helps stimulate blood flow. Repeat three to five times up and around foot (Figure 22–59).

9. *Percussion or tapotement movement.* Use your fingertips to perform tapotement movements, lightly tapping over the entire foot to reduce blood circulation as you complete the massage (Figure 22–60).

Leg Massage

The foot massage may be extended up to the knee. Do not massage over the shinbone or above the knee. Limit the pressure to the muscular tissue on either side of the shinbone. On the calf area of the leg, you may use kneading movements up to the backside of the knee. 4

SAFETY RULES IN MANICURING AND PEDICURING

"Safety first" is the rule you need to follow when manicuring. Your goal is to prevent accidents and injury to the client and to yourself. The following safety rules will guide you in your work.

- Keep all containers covered and labeled.
- Make sure your hands are dry when holding or moving containers.
- Handle sharp or pointed implements carefully and avoid dropping them.
- Dull very sharp cutting edges with an emery board.
- Bevel a sharp nail edge with an emery board.
- Do not file too deeply into nail corners.
- Do not use a sharp, pointed implement to clean under the nail.
- Avoid excessive friction in nail buffing.
- Immediately apply an antiseptic if the skin is accidentally cut.

PROCEDURE

PLAIN PEDICURE

Equipment, Implements, and Materials

Basic pedicure setup described on pages 781-783.

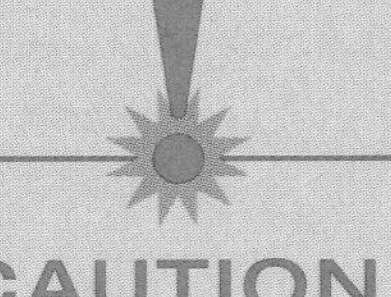

CAUTION

Be sure the floor around the pedicure area is dry, because wet floors are slippery. You or your client might fall. When water is spilled, wipe it up immediately.

Preservice (Preparation)

1. Arrange required equipment, implements, and materials.
2. Greet the client cordially.
3. Seat the client in the chair and have her remove her shoes and stockings.
4. Place the client's feet on a clean or disposable towel on the footrest.
5. Wash your hands with soap and warm water.
6. Fill the basin with enough warm water to cover the ankles.
7. Add antiseptic or liquid soap to the basin. Spray the feet with foot spray or wipe them with antiseptic.
8. Place both feet in the bath for five to ten minutes to wash and sanitize the feet before you begin the pedicure.
9. Remove the client's feet from the basin and wipe them dry. Place them on a clean terry cloth towel.

Procedure

1. Remove old polish from the nails of both feet (Figure 22–61).
2. Clip the toenails of the left foot first, taking care that they are even with the end of the toe. In some cases, a small corner of the nail should be trimmed out. Trimming the corner of a toenail, if done properly, does not cause an ingrown toenail (Figure 22–62).

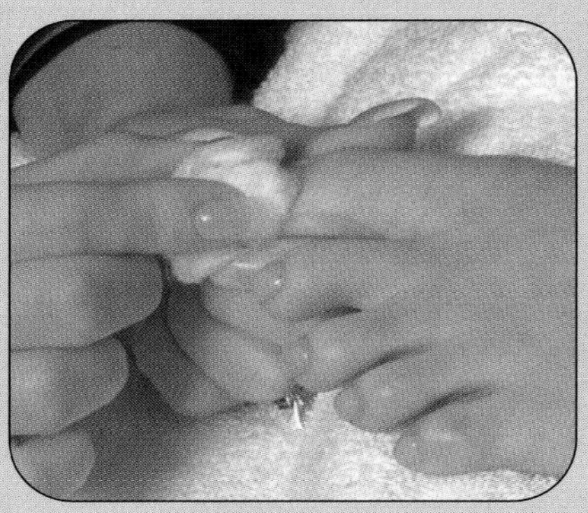

Figure 22-61 Remove old polish.

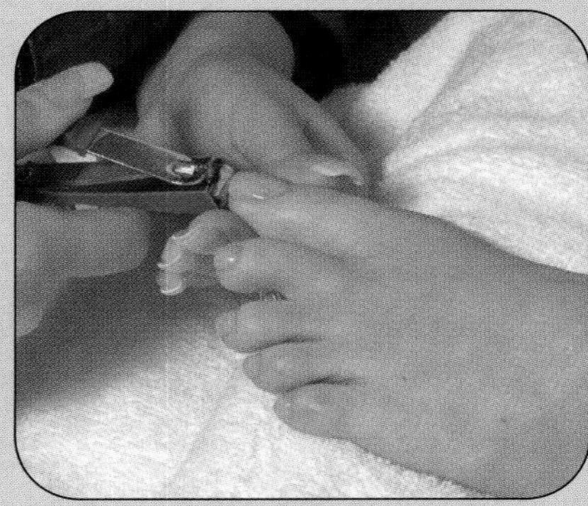

Figure 22-62 Trim toenails.

3. Using both hands, carefully insert toe separators between the toes of the left foot (Figure 22–63).
4. File toenails of the left foot with a new emery board, having already softened the edges. File the toenails straight across, rounding them slightly at the corners to conform to the shape of the toes. Smooth any rough edges with the fine side of the emery board (Figure 22–64).
5. Use a foot file on the ball and heel of the left foot to remove dry skin and smooth down callus growths (Figure 22–65). Do not file too much, because it can cause irritation and bleeding.
6. Remove toe separators and place the left foot in warm, soapy water.
7. Repeat Steps 2 through 6 on the right foot, through soaking (Figure 22–66).
8. Remove the left foot from the foot bath and brush the nails with a nail brush. Rinse the foot in the rinse bath and dry thoroughly (Figure 22–67). Insert toe separators between toes.
9. With a new cotton-tipped orangewood stick, apply cuticle solvent to the cuticle and under the free edge of each toenail of the left foot.
10. Loosen the cuticle gently with the cotton-tipped orangewood stick. Keep the cuticle moist with additional lotion or water. Do not use excessive pressure (Figure 22–68).

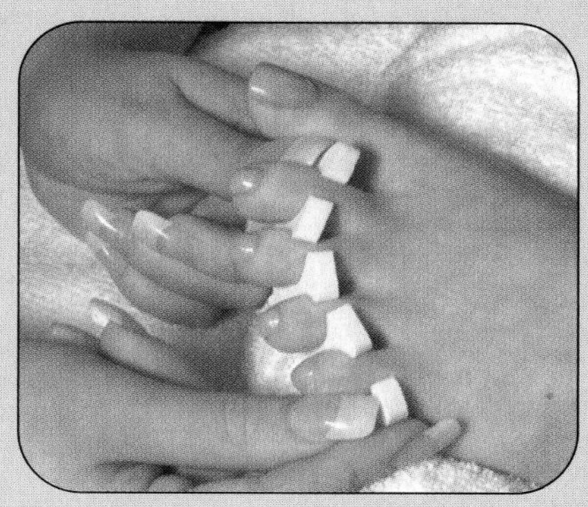

Figure 22-63 Insert toe separators.

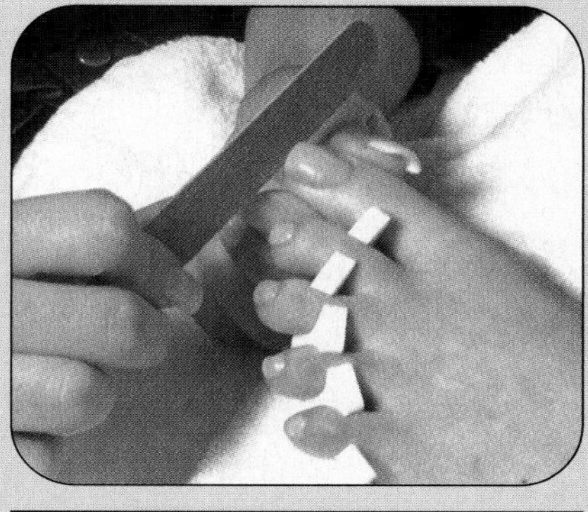

Figure 22-64 File toenails.

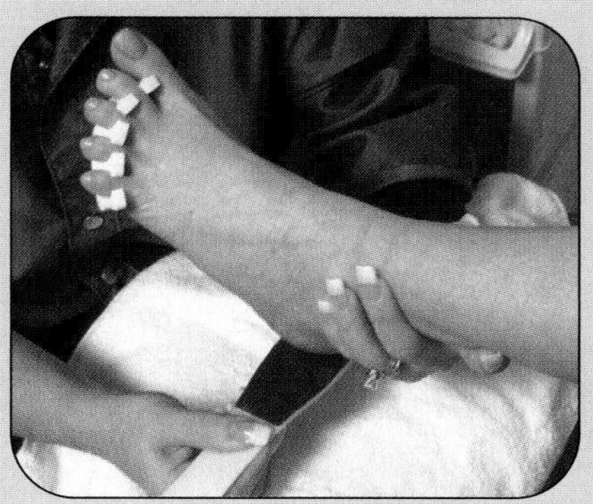

Figure 22-65 Use foot file.

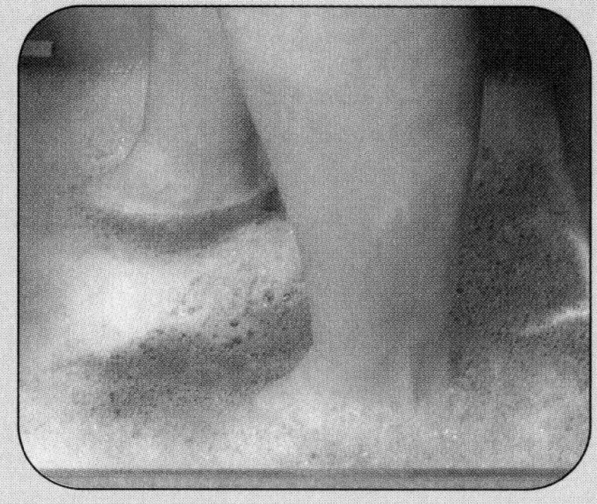

Figure 22-66 Soak the feet.

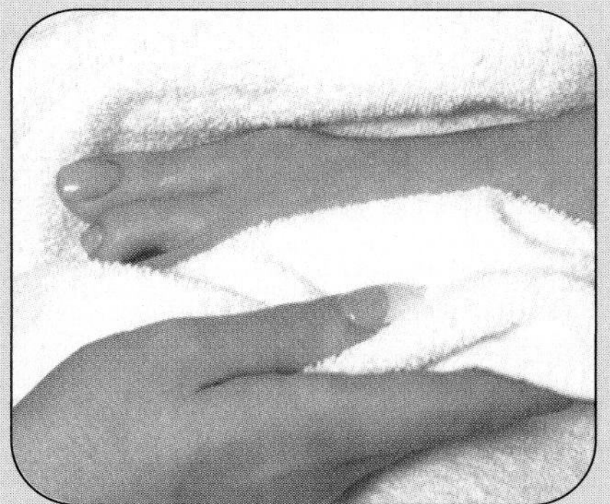

Figure 22-67 Dry the foot.

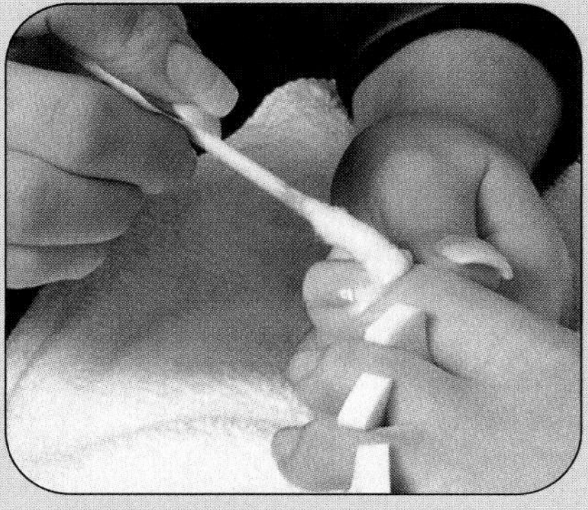

Figure 22-68 Loosen cuticle.

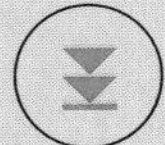

Here's a tip:

Focus on your client. There should be no distractions for you or the client during the pedicure. Make the client feel you have nothing more to do than take care of her every wish. Develop your procedures so there are no wasted motions.

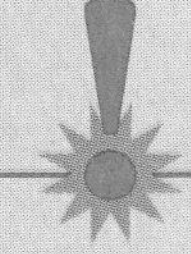

CAUTION

Failure to follow proper disinfection procedures with foot spas and basins can lead to the spread of infections among your clients such as that caused by *Mycobacterium fortuitum furunculosis* (see Chapter 5). Do not take shortcuts or neglect any of the steps in disinfection procedures. Not only are your clients' health and safety at stake, but the salon may be served with fines and lawsuits as well. Practicing correct, complete disinfection procedures is part of your professional responsibility.

11. Do not cut the cuticle. Nip only large, ragged hangnails.
12. Rinse the left foot and dry it.
13. Apply cream or lotion.
14. Massage the left foot and place it on a clean towel on the floor.
15. Repeat Steps 8 through 14 on right foot.
16. Remove traces of lotion or cream from the toenails. Place feet in disposable paper or foam pedicure slippers for those clients who have not worn open-toed shoes. Apply base coat, two coats of color, and top coat to the toenails (Figure 22–69). Spray with instant nail dry. Place the feet on a towel to dry (Figure 22–70).

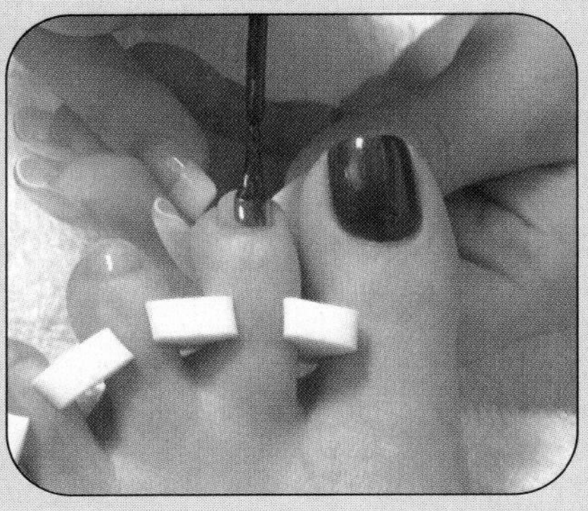

Figure 22-69 Apply polish to toenails.

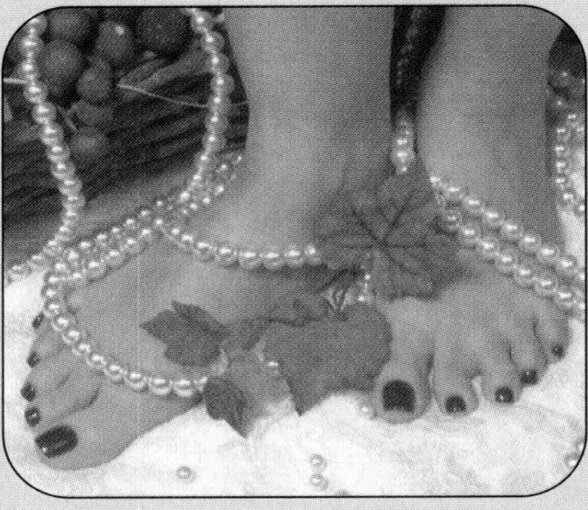

Figure 22-70 Finished pedicure.

Postservice (Cleanup and Sanitation)

1. Schedule another pedicure appointment for your client.
2. Advise your client about proper foot care. Remind her that wearing tight shoes and very high heels can cause problems with the feet.
3. Suggest that the client purchase the retail products you have discussed during the pedicure.
4. Clean the pedicure work area. Empty the basin and wipe it down with a hospital-grade disinfectant. Dry the basin and put it away. Wipe the chair and footrest with hospital-grade disinfectant. For disinfection procedures for foot spas, refer to page 115 in Chapter 5.
5. Discard used materials in the plastic bag at the side of the table. Discard it in a closed pail and attach a new bag to the table.
6. Sanitize all implements. Return the pedicure area to its basic setup.

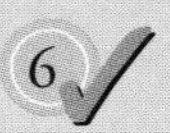

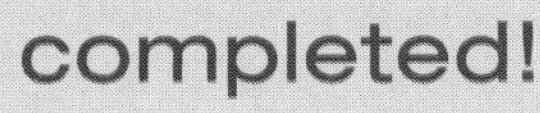

- Apply alum powder or solution to stop the bleeding from a small cut. Never use a styptic pencil.
- Avoid pushing the cuticle back too far.
- Avoid too much pressure at the base of the nail.
- Do not work on a nail when the surrounding skin is inflamed or infected.
- Any disposable sharp objects, such as files, or materials, such as cotton that come in contact with blood or body fluids must be disposed of in a sealed plastic bag.
- If bleeding occurs during a procedure, stop the service and follow the procedure for handling blood spills. Clean and disinfect the implement, or use another implement. Do not risk cutting yourself with a sharp tool that has blood on it.

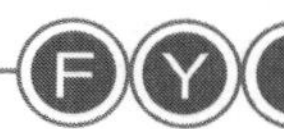

The elderly need care and maintenance for their feet on a year-round basis. A large number of elderly people cannot reach their feet and need help. Many who can reach their feet suffer from arthritis and cannot squeeze the nail implements. These clients need the proper foot care that a good pedicurist can provide. The technician who offers pedicures for this segment of the population will be doing these individuals a tremendous favor.

Procedure for Handling Blood Spills

At times during a manicure, bleeding may occur as a result of too much filing or some other reason. The safety and sanitation factors involved in an incident of this nature are of the utmost importance for both you and your client. If bleeding should occur, follow this procedure.

1. Immediately put on gloves and inform your client of what has happened. Apologize and proceed.
2. Apply slight pressure to the bleeding site with cotton and an antiseptic.
3. Apply powdered alum or other styptic (liquid or spray), using the end of a cotton-wrapped orangewood stick. Do not contaminate the container. Never place the orangewood stick back into the container once it has been applied to an opened area on the skin. Do not use a styptic pencil.
4. Apply a bandage to the cut, if necessary.
5. Discard any blood-contaminated disposable implements and materials (such as cotton or towels) by double-bagging (place the waste in a plastic bag and then in a trash bag). Use a biohazard sticker (red or orange) or a container for contaminated waste. Deposit sharp disposables in a sharps box.
6. Once you have removed your gloves, wash your hands with soap and warm water.
7. Complete the service as called for.
8. Properly and thoroughly disinfect all implements that have come in contact with blood or body fluid in an EPA-registered, hospital-grade, tuberculocidal disinfecting solution. 7 ✓

22

A VALUABLE SERVICE

Many people have come to recognize the good hygiene and wellness that are associated with regular hand and foot care. Those who have not yet discovered these benefits should be educated. As a technician, you should feel confident that the manicures and pedicures you provide can make all the difference in a person's mobility, comfort, and appearance. Do good work and enjoy the good you do!

chapter glossary

alum	aluminum salt used as a styptic (agent used to stop bleeding) in powder form or solution
base coat	colorless liquid applied to the natural nail before the application of colored polish
booth manicure	manicure that is given in the booth and not at the manicuring table
curette	small spoon-shaped implement used for cleaning the debris from the nail margins
cuticle creams	special creams that usually have a base of lanolin, petroleum, or beeswax; designed to prevent or correct brittle nails and dry cuticles
cuticle nipper	small cutting tool used to nip or cut excess cuticle at the base of the nail
cuticle oil	special oil used to soften and lubricate the cuticle around the fingernails and toenails
cuticle pusher	implement used to loosen and push back the cuticle around the fingernails or toenails; shaped to conform to the shape of the nails
cuticle remover	solution of alkali, glycerin, and water used to soften and remove dead cuticle from around the nail
diamond nail file	metal implement with diamond dust embedded in the metal; files the free edge of the toenails and in some cases thins them
dry nail polish	powder or paste used with chamois buffer to add shine to the nails
emery board	disposable manicuring instrument with rough cutting ridges, used for shaping the nails with the coarse side and smoothing them with the finer side
foot file or paddle	implement used to remove dry flaky skin and smooth calluses on the foot
formaldehyde hardeners	nail hardeners that utilize keratin fibers to strengthen the nail and contain no more than 5 percent formaldehyde
French manicure	manicure in which the free edge of the nail is polished, tipped, or sculpted in an opaque color while the nail plate is polished or left a more translucent color
hand creams	creams made up of emollients and humectants, recommended for dry, chapped, or irritated skin
hand lotions	lotions similar in composition to hand creams but with a thinner consistency due to a higher oil content
hot oil manicure	manicure in which a heated oil, cream, or lotion is applied to the cuticles to soften them before pushing them back
liquid nail polish or lacquer	thick liquid used to color or gloss the nail
manicure	the artful treatment and care of the hands and nails
nail bleach	product used to remove stains and whiten the nails
nail brush	small brush used to clean under and around the nails, with warm water and soap
nail buffer	instrument made of leather or chamois; used with a polishing powder to polish the nails to a high luster
nail clippers	implement used to shorten nails

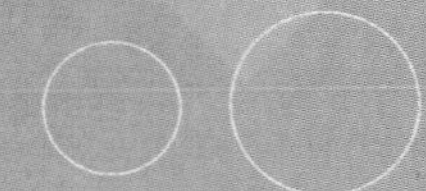

chapter glossary *(continued)*

nail conditioner	product containing moisturizing ingredients to combat nail dryness and brittleness
nail dryer	solution that protects the nail polish against stickiness and dulling
nail file	metal instrument with a specially prepared surface used to file and shape the nails
nail hardener	product designed to prevent nails from splitting or peeling
nail rasp	tool that cuts or files in only one direction; used to smooth off the edges of the nail in the nail groove and reduce the possibility of the nail cutting into the skin
nylon fiber hardeners	nail hardeners that are a combination of clear polish and nylon fibers, applied first vertically, then horizontally, on the nail plate
orangewood stick	stick made from the wood of the orange tree, used to loosen the cuticle around the base of the nail or to clean under the free edge
pedicure	the care of the feet and toenails
polish remover	organic solvent used to dissolve and remove nail polish
polish thinner	product used to thin out nail polish where it has thickened; contains acetone or some other solvent
protein hardeners	nail hardeners that are a combination of clear polish and a protein such as collagen
squoval	term describing a square nail with the ends rounded or taken off
styptic	agent used to stop bleeding
top coat or sealer	liquid, colorless nail enamel applied over polish to protect the polish, prevent chipping, and impart a high gloss
tweezers	Implement used to lift small bits of cuticle from the nail

review questions

1. What are the Latin root words for manicure and pedicure?
2. What are the six areas of knowledge that every nail technician should master?
3. What are the four basic categories of nail care tools?
4. What is the most important difference between equipment and implements?
5. List the implements used in a plain manicure. Which ones are disposable?
6. Describe the three types of nail hardeners.
7. What are the five basic nail shapes?
8. List the eight steps of a manicure preservice procedure.
9. What is the proper way to file fingernails? Toenails?
10. Explain the value of a hot-oil manicure.
11. Define French manicure.
12. Why is pedicuring an important salon service?
13. Why is it critical that proper disinfection procedures be followed after a pedicure service?
14. List at least 10 safety rules that should be followed when manicuring.

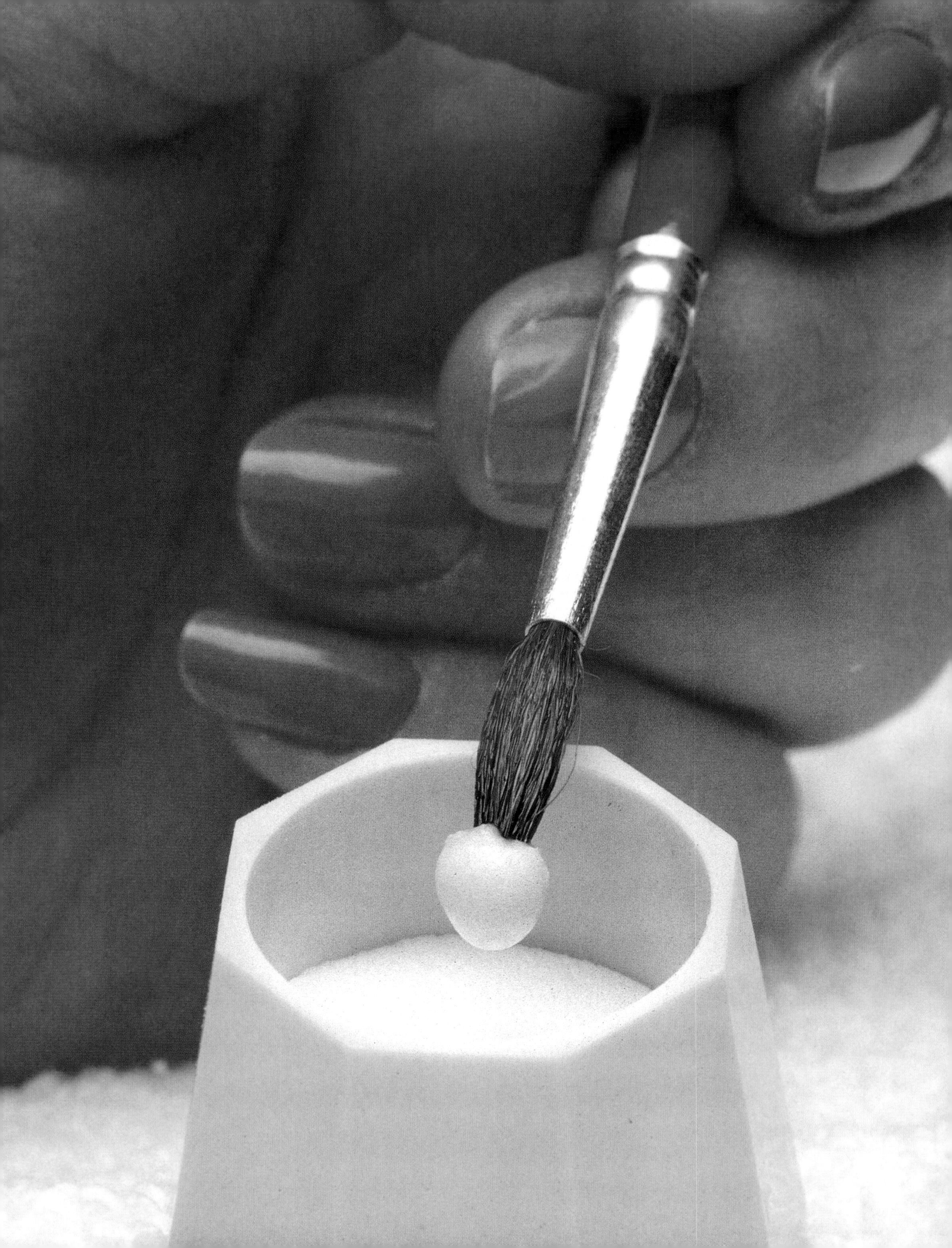

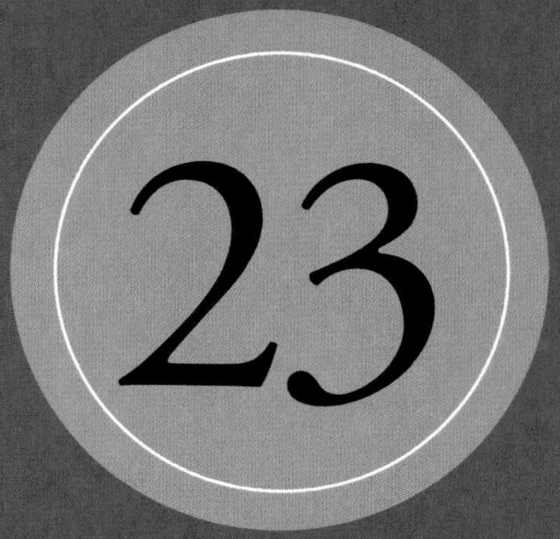

ADVANCED NAIL TECHNIQUES

Sue Ellen Schultes

INTERNATIONAL NAIL JUDGE AND CEO, NOTORIOUS NAILS SEMINARS

Chapter Outline

Learning Objectives

After completing this chapter, you should be able to:

1. List the preservice and postservice steps of an artificial nail procedure.
2. Demonstrate the basic procedures for applying: a) tips, b) wraps, c) acrylic nails, and d) gels.
3. Explain the chemistry of acrylic nails.
4. List the safety precautions that must be followed when applying artificial nails.

National Skill Standards

This chapter provides you with the necessary information to master these National Industry Skill Standards for Entry-Level Cosmetologists

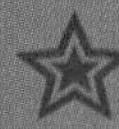

Consulting with clients to determine their needs and preferences.

Using a variety of salon products while performing client services.

Conducting services in a safe environment and taking measures to prevent the spread of infectious and contagious diseases.

Key Terms

Page number indicates where in the chapter the term is used.

acrylic nails pg. 808

acrylic overlays pg. 809

catalyst pg. 809

curing pg. 809

dipped nails pg. 820

fill pg. 809

gels pg. 816

light-cured gels pg. 816

liquid nail wrap pg. 808

monomer pg. 808

nail tips pg. 799

nail wrapping pg. 803

no-light gels pg. 820

overlay pg. 799

polymer pg. 808

position stop pg. 799

primer pg. 809

rebalancing pg. 816

When you meet someone new, chances are your eyes go first to the face and then to the hands, particularly the fingernails. Chipped, cracked, bitten, or dirty nails and cuticles are unattractive and embarrassing. Fortunately, there are many ways to help clients who want their nails to look better.

If a client has a problem growing natural nails to the length and strength desired, the solution may be advanced nail techniques, which include nail tips, nail wraps, acrylics, gels, and dipped nails. When applied properly, these techniques yield artificial nails that are durable, attractive, and natural-looking (Figure 23–1).

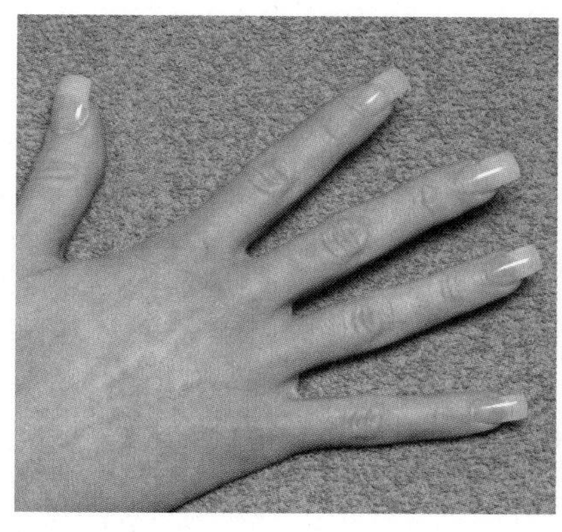

Figure 23–1 Nail enhancements add length and beauty to natural nails.

Artificial nails may be used for the following purposes:

- to mend or conceal broken or damaged nails
- to improve the appearance of very short or badly shaped nails
- to help overcome the habit of nail-biting
- to protect a nail or nails against splitting or breakage

If you recognize any of these problems in a client, explain the merits of artificial nails and what they can do for a person's image and self-esteem.

PRESERVICE AND POSTSERVICE PROCEDURES

As with other procedures, the artificial nail service begins with the client consultation. During this session, you will be asking questions that will help both you and your client determine the type of nail service best suited to her lifestyle. The format of the consultation for artificial nail procedures is the same as the format for other nail service consultations described. Let us focus on the preservice and postservice procedures you should always follow. They are designed to ensure that the service you provide will be efficient, effective, safe, and sanitary.

The preservice procedure consists of the following steps.

1. Rinse all implements with cool running water and then wash them with soap and warm water. Make sure to brush all grooved items and any open hinges (Figure 23–2).

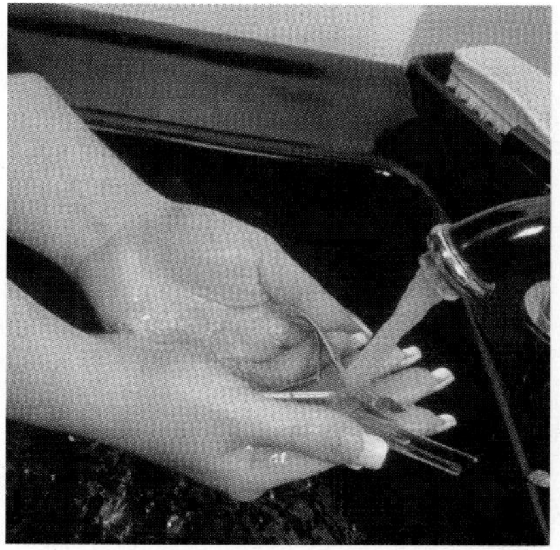

Figure 23–2 Wash nail implements with soap and water.

2. Rinse the implements in plain warm water, taking care to wash away all traces of soap, which can interact with disinfectants and cause them to become inactive. Dry thoroughly with a clean and/or disposable towel.
3. Completely immerse all implements in an EPA-registered, hospital-level disinfectant for the required time (usually 10 minutes) (Figure 23–3). Use tongs or rubber gloves to avoid skin contact with the disinfectant.
4. Wash your hands with liquid soap and warm water. Rinse well and dry with a clean and/or disposable towel.
5. Remove the implements from the disinfectant solution with tongs or while wearing rubber gloves, and rinse them well in water (Figure 23–4). Wipe them dry with a clean and/or disposable towel to prevent rusting.
6. When storing sanitized manicuring implements, follow your state or province regulations. Generally, sanitized implements are stored in sealed containers or kept in a closed cabinet sanitizer until ready to be used.
7. Sanitize the manicure table by wiping with disinfectant or sanitizing solution (Figure 23–5).
8. Disinfect all working surfaces. Spray the surfaces with an EPA-registered disinfectant that is approved by your state or province. Allow surfaces to remain wet for 10 minutes and then wipe dry. Spray again and allow the surfaces to air-dry.
9. Wrap the manicuring cushion with a clean and/or disposable towel. Be sure to use a fresh towel for each client.
10. Refill all disposable materials—abrasive (file), orangewood stick, cotton balls, and other such materials—on the manicuring table. These materials are discarded after they have been used.

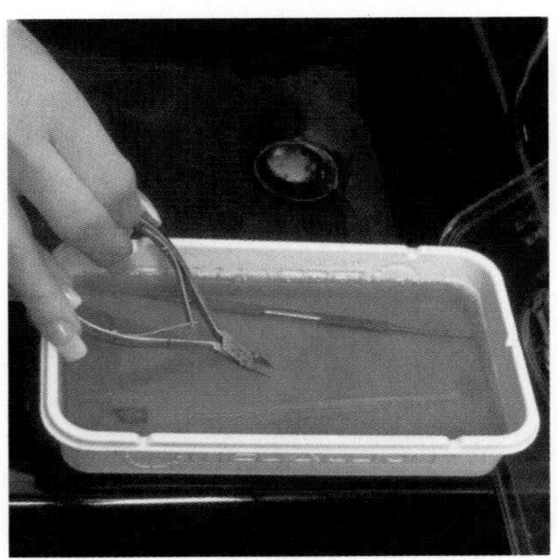

Figure 23-3 Immerse implements in disinfectant.

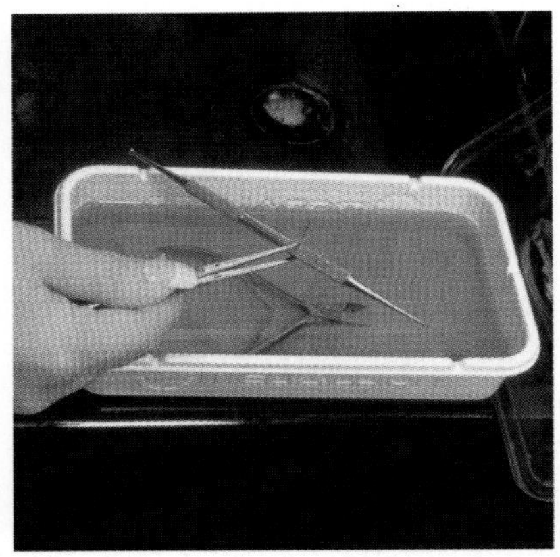

Figure 23-4 Remove implements with tongs.

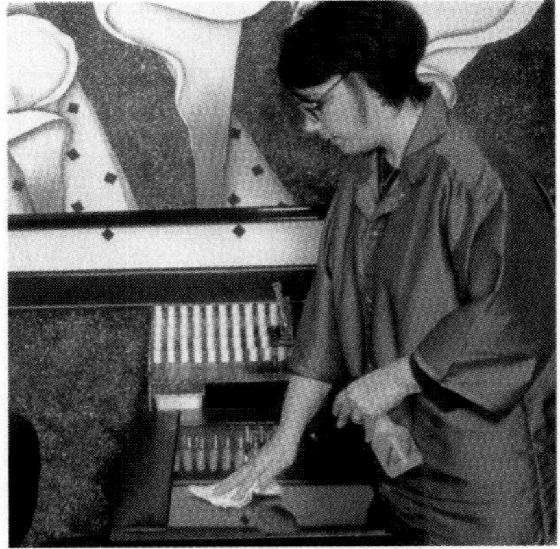

Figure 23-5 Sanitize the manicure table.

11. Set up the standard manicuring table, adding the items you need for the advanced nail service you are performing.
12. Greet your client (Figure 23–6). Ask the client to wash her hands with a soap and warm water. Wash your hands as well, using a waterless hand sanitizer gel or wipe. Dry hands and nails thoroughly with a clean and/or disposable towel.
13. Perform a client consultation. Record your observations and the client's responses on a client card. Determine if the client's nails and hands are healthy enough for you to perform the service. If the client has a nail or skin disorder and should not receive a service, explain why and refer the client to a physician. If you determine that it is safe to proceed with the service, you can then discuss your client's needs and wants.

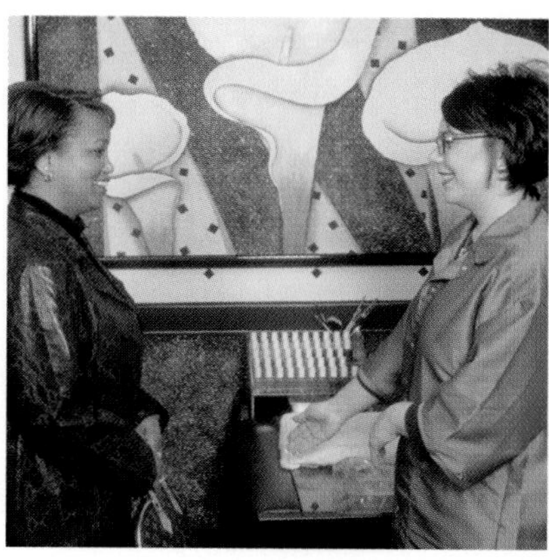

Figure 23-6 Welcome your client.

The postservice procedure consists of the following steps:

1. Book another appointment with your client in order to maintain her nails according to the prescribed maintenance schedule.
2. Offer retail products that will help your client take care of the nails between appointments. Polish, lotion, and top coat are just a few of the valuable aids you can offer (Figure 23–7).
3. Clean your table and the surrounding area. Allow enough time to restore the basic setup.
4. Discard all used materials in a closed pail.
5. Sanitize your table and disinfect your implements. Perform the complete preservice sanitation procedure described above. 1

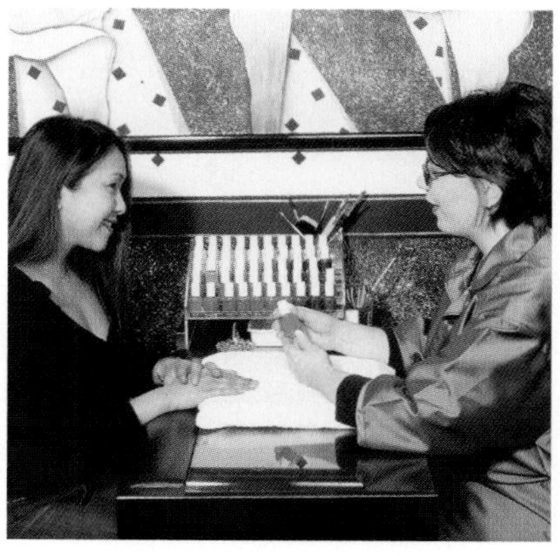

Figure 23-7 Retailing is an important part of every nail service.

NAIL TIPS

One of the most popular advanced nail techniques is **nail tips**, which are preformed artificial nails applied to the tips of the natural fingernails. Nail tips are commonly made of plastic, nylon, or acetate and are used to add extra length. Usually, tips are combined with another artificial nail service, such as wraps, acrylic, or gel. A tip worn with no **overlay** (any wrap, acrylic, or gel applied over the entire natural nail plate) is very weak and is considered a temporary service.

Nail tips are secured to the natural nails with glue or bonding agents. These agents come in either a tube with a pointed applicator tip, a one-drop applicator, or as a brush-on.

All nail tips have a well that serves as the point of contact with the nail plate. The **position stop** is the point where the nail plate meets the tip before it is glued to the nail. Tips are designed with either a partial or full well (Figure 23–8). The tip should never cover more than half of the natural

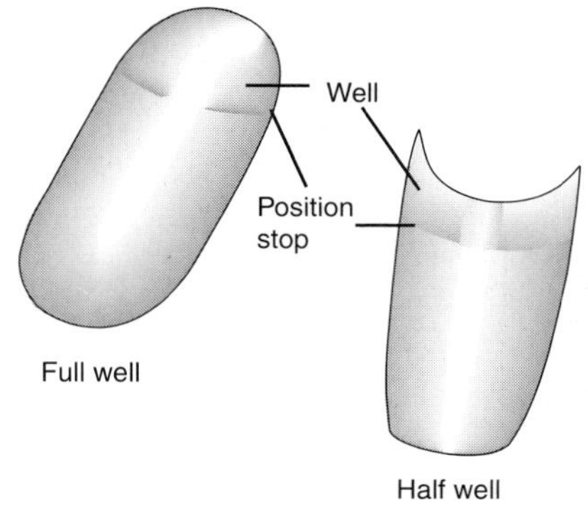

Figure 23-8 Tip with half well and tip with full well.

23

PROCEDURE

APPLYING NAIL TIPS

Implements and Materials

In addition to the materials on your basic manicuring table, you will need the following:

- polish remover
- medium fine file
- adhesive
- tip clipper or large nail clippers
- buffer block
- nail tips

Preparation

Complete the preservice procedure listed on pages 797-799.

CAUTION

Nail polish remover containing acetone will damage plastic artificial nails. Use only polish remover that has an oily base and is nonacetone.

23

Procedure

1. Remove any old polish from the client's nails, working from little finger to thumb.
2. Push back the cuticle.
3. Buff the nails to remove shine and any natural oils (Figure 23–9). Remove the dust.
4. Select the proper size tip. Make sure it completely covers the nail plate from sidewall to sidewall but never covers more than half the length of the nail (Figure 23–10). Trim the tip to the right size if the well covers too much of the nail.
5. Apply nail antiseptic to remove the remaining natural oil and to dehydrate the nail for better adhesion. Again, begin with the little

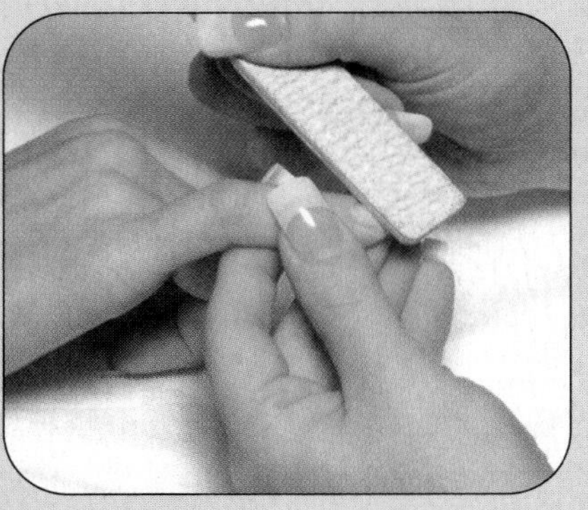

Figure 23-9 Buff the nails.

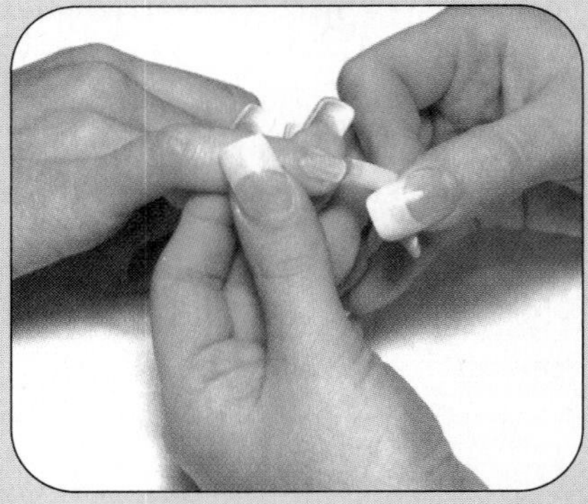

Figure 23-10 Select the proper size tip.

finger (Figure 23–11). If you accidentally touch the nails after you apply antiseptic, you must clean them again and reapply antiseptic.

6. Apply adhesive on the nail plate to cover the area where the tip will be placed. Do not let adhesive run onto the skin. Apply adhesive from the middle of the nail plate to the free edge (Figure 23–12). An alternate method is to apply adhesive to the well of the tip. This may ensure that fewer air bubbles are trapped in the adhesive.
7. Slide on the tip. Use a stop, rock, and hold procedure:

   Stop: find the stop against the free edge at a 45-degree angle (Figure 23–13).

   Rock: rock the tip on slowly.

   Hold: hold in place for 5 to 10 seconds until dry.
8. Apply a bead of adhesive to the seam between the natural nail plate and the tip to strengthen the stress point (Figure 23–14).

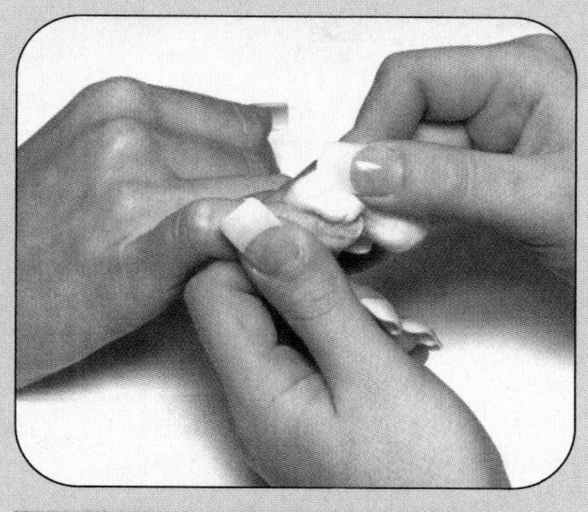

Figure 23-11 Apply nail antiseptic.

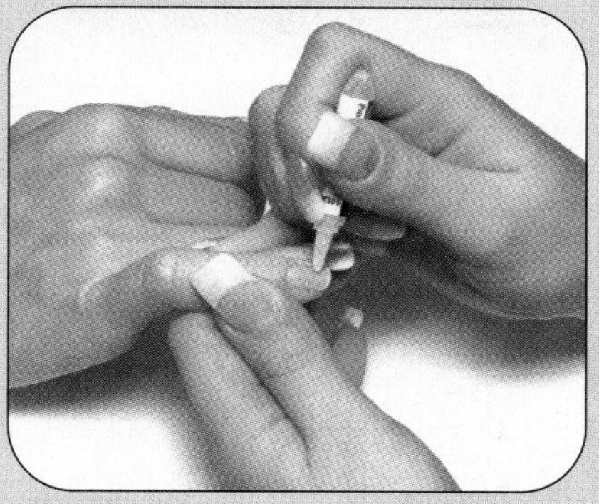

Figure 23-12 Apply adhesive.

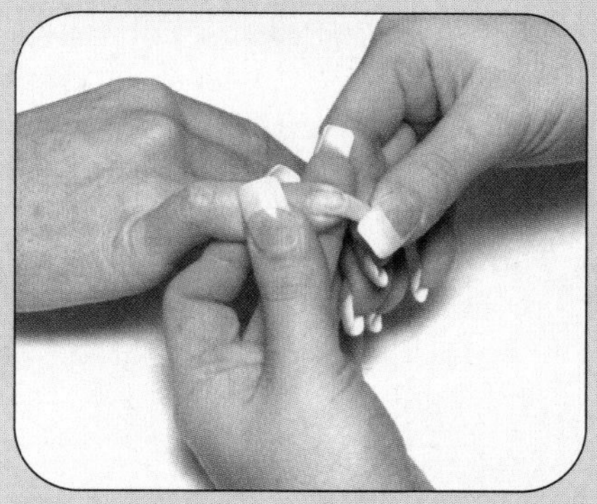

Figure 23-13 Find the stop at a 45 degree angle.

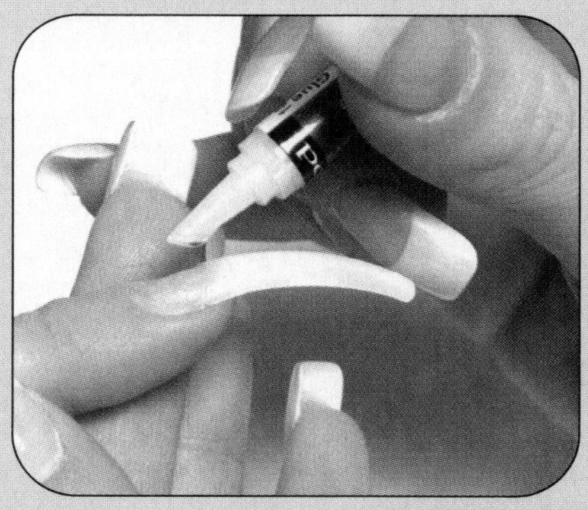

Figure 23-14 Apply adhesive bead to seam.

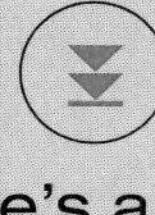

Here's a tip:

Before you apply the tips, spray the nails, one hand at a time, with a glue activator, also called an accelerator, booster, or catalyst. You will have an immediate bond and will not have to hold the tip in place as the glue dries.

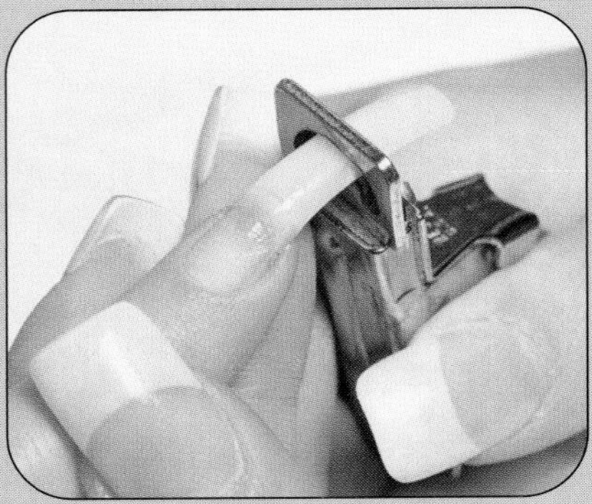

Figure 23-15 Trim the nail tip.

9. Trim the nail tip to the desired length, using a tip clipper or large nail clippers. Cut from one side, then the other, if you are using the nail clippers. Cutting the tip straight across weakens the plastic (Figure 23–15).
10. Blend the tip into the natural nail. File the shine off the tip, keeping the file flat on the nail at all times. Never hold the file at an angle, because doing so can form a groove in the nail plate (Figure 23–16).
11. Buff the tip for a perfect blend between the natural nail plate and the tip extension. There should be no visible line or cloudiness between the two (Figure 23–17).
12. Shape the nail (Figure 23–18).
13. Proceed with any other service that may be desired. Tips are seldom worn without an additional service such as wraps, acrylics, or gels. If your client is only wearing tips as a temporary service, add a drop of cuticle oil to each nail and then buff (Figure 23–19).
14. Perform postservice procedure on page 799.

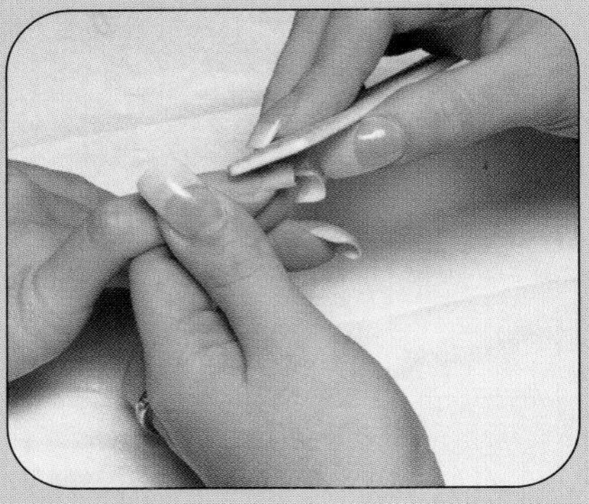

Figure 23-16 Blend tip into natural nail.

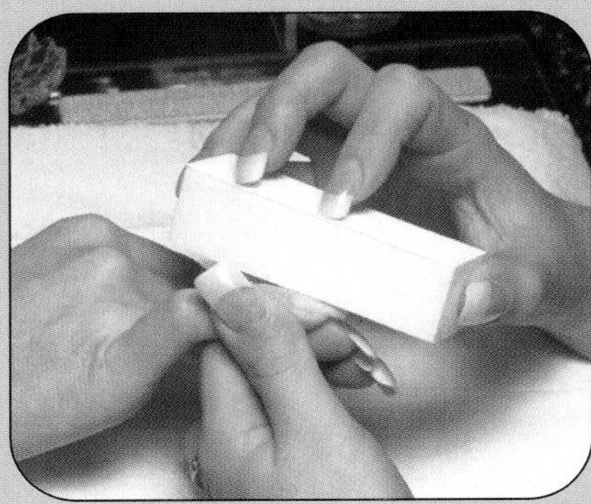

Figure 23-17 Buff the tip.

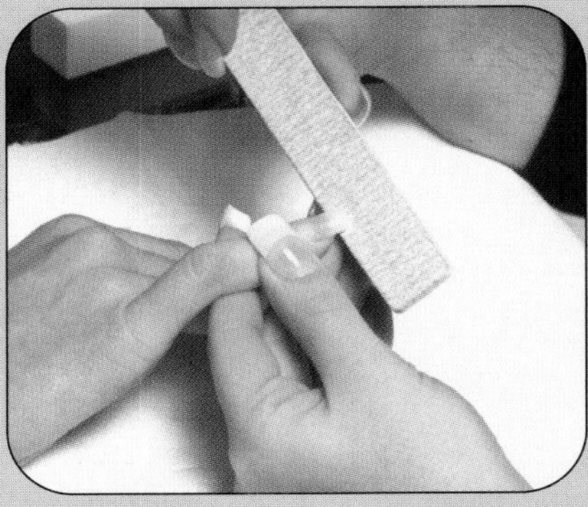

Figure 23-18 Shape the tip.

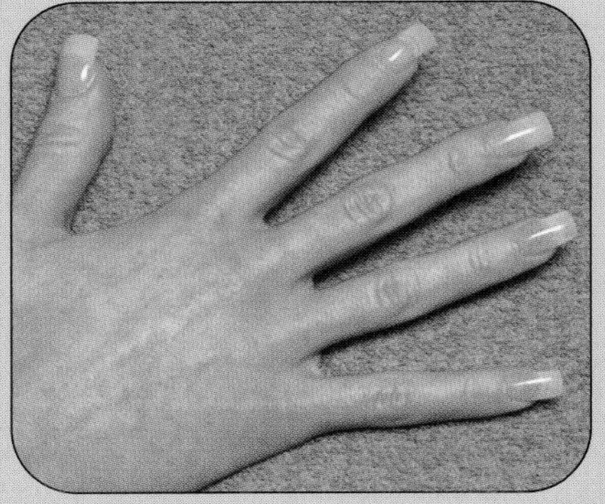

Figure 23-19 Finished tip application.

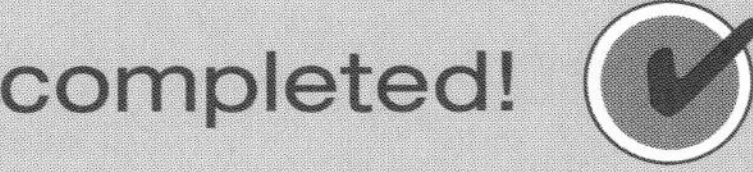

nail plate. Nail tips should also be prebeveled along the edge closest to the cuticle to thin out the plastic. Tips that are prebeveled require less filing on the natural nail after application. This cuts down the potential for damage to the natural nail.

Tips come in an assortment of sizes, shapes, and colors. With such a wide assortment, it is easier to fit each client with the precise size and shape tip for her needs.

CAUTION

Even the smallest amount of glue in the eyes can be highly dangerous. Always wear safety glasses when performing this nail procedure and offer them to your client as well.

Tip Maintenance

Clients wearing tips will need weekly or biweekly manicures to allow for regluing and rebuffing. With temporary tips, reglue at the seam between the natural nail and the tip. Most tips will require nonacetone polish remover, as acetone removers will dissolve the tips. If the client has an overlay on her tips, follow the recommended maintenance procedure for that product.

Tip Removal

When removing tips, begin by removing any and all polish. Place the client's fingertips in a bowl with enough acetone to cover the nails and soak them for the amount of time recommended by the manufacturer. Use a fresh orangewood stick or a metal pusher to slide off the softened tips (Figure 23–20). Do not pry them off, as this can be damaging to the nail bed and mantle.

Buff the nails with a block buffer to remove any glue residue. Have the client wash her hands with soap and warm water. Condition the cuticle and surrounding skin with cuticle cream or oil. Suggest a reconditioning hot oil manicure.

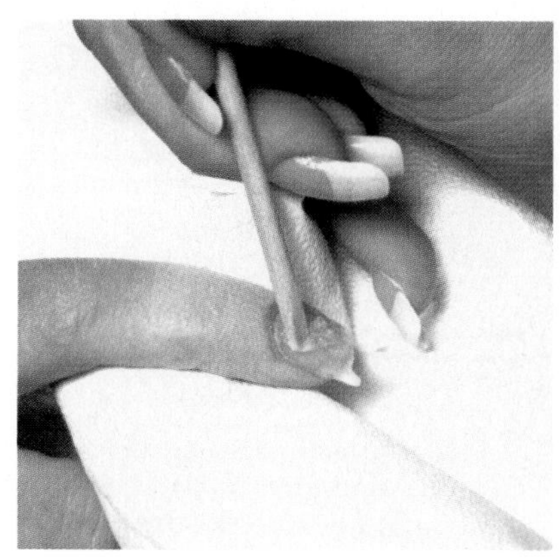

Figure 23–20 Slide the tip off.

NAIL WRAPS

Nail wrapping is a corrective treatment that forms a protective coating for a damaged or fragile nail. Nail wraps can be applied over the natural nail or over a set of tips. Silk, linen, fiberglass, and paper are among the materials commonly used in this procedure.

- *Silk* nail wraps give a smooth, even appearance to the nail. They become almost transparent when adhesive is applied.
- *Fiberglass* is a very thin synthetic mesh with a loose weave that makes it easy for adhesive to penetrate. It is strong and durable.
- *Linen* provides a durable wrap, but the coarse material requires a colored polish to cover the completed nail. It is much thicker than silk or fiberglass and remains opaque even after adhesive is applied.
- *Paper* wraps are made of very thin paper and dissolve in both acetone and nonacetone remover. For this reason, paper wraps are temporary, rarely used, and must be reapplied when polish is removed. They are glued both on top and under the free edge of the nail.

PROCEDURE 61

NAIL WRAPPING

Implements and Materials

In addition to the materials on your basic manicuring table, you will need the following:

- nail wrap fabric
- small, sharp scissors for cutting fabric
- nail adhesive
- adhesive dryer
- small piece of plastic
- medium fine file
- buffer block

Preparation

Complete the preservice procedure listed on pages 797-799.

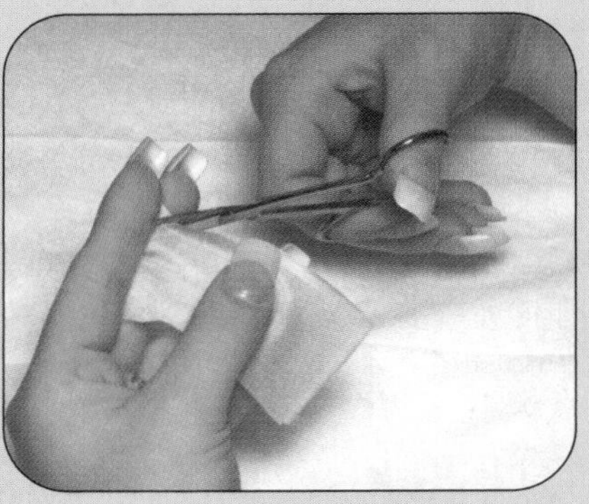

Figure 23-21 Cut fabric.

Procedure

1. Remove all old polish, working from little finger to thumb.
2. Push back the cuticle.
3. Use the abrasive to remove the oil and shine from the natural nail.
4. Spray or wipe on nail antiseptic to remove the remaining natural oil and to dehydrate the nail for better adhesion. Apply nail tips if they are to be used and shape them as needed.
5. Cut the wrapping material to fit the nail (Figure 23-21).
6. Place a line of adhesive down the center of the nail (Figure 23-22). Alternatively, coat the entire nail plate and under the free edge with adhesive.

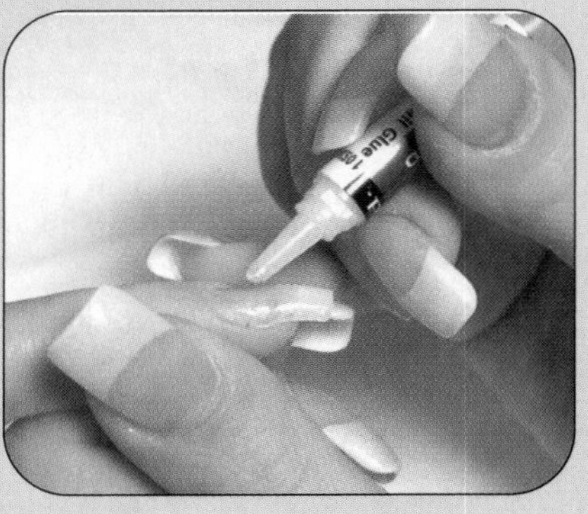

Figure 23-22 Apply adhesive.

7. Using two fingers, place the wrapping material over the nail and press it down until it adheres (Figure 23–23). Starting at the middle of the nail, use a fresh orangewood stick to push the material in all directions, toward the edges and tip of the nail. Continually dip the orangewood stick into the polish remover and pat the material until it is smooth.
8. Trim away any excess material that extends past the free edge and the sides of the nails (Figure 23–24).
9. Apply adhesive to the entire nail to strengthen and seal the wrap. Do not touch the cuticle (Figure 23–25).
10. Use adhesive dryer to hasten drying.
11. Lightly file the entire nail (top, sides, and free edge) until all is smooth (Figure 23–26).

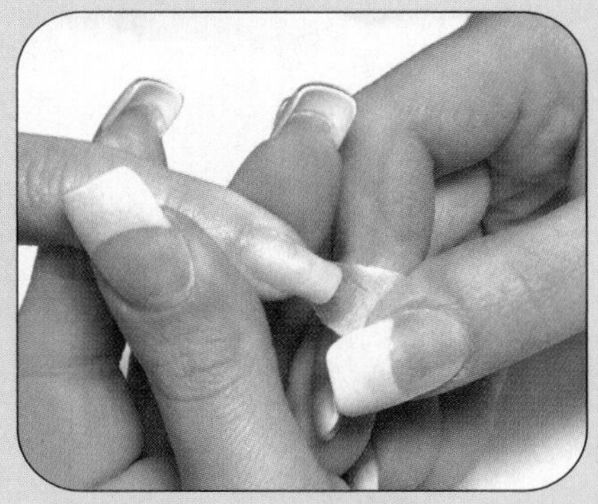

Figure 23-23 Apply fabric.

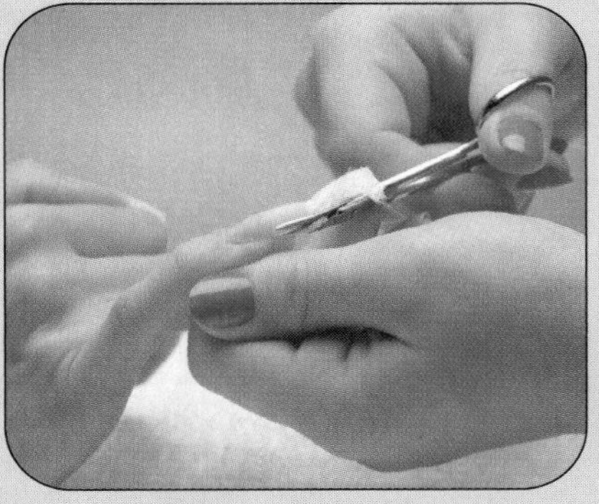

Figure 23-24 Trim fabric.

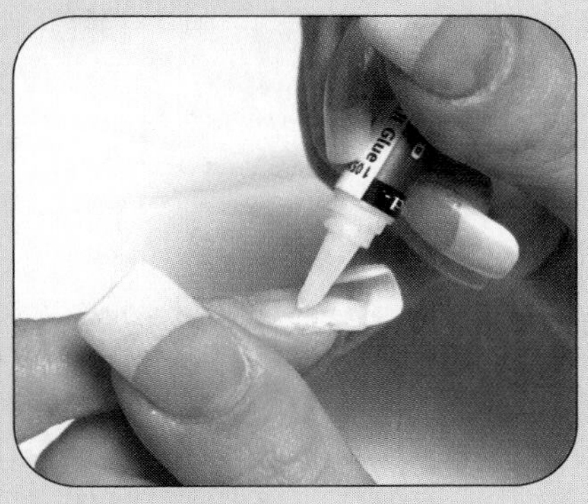

Figure 23-25 Apply adhesive.

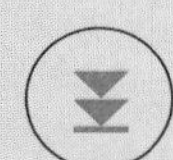

Here's a tip:

Using a 6 x 4 inch piece of plastic wrap to press fabric onto the nail will prevent the transfer of dust and oil from you to your client. Use a fresh area of the plastic for each finger.

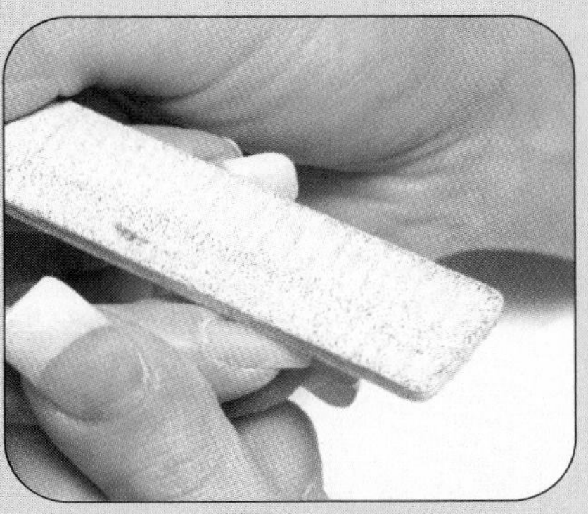

Figure 23-26 File entire nail surface smooth.

CAUTION

Never use the same orangewood stick on more than one client, as this implement cannot be sanitized.

12. Apply one or two more coats of adhesive to the top and sides of the free edge of the nail. Buff between coats with a buffing block.
13. Apply a protective base coat to the top and underside of the free edge of the nail, and allow it to dry. Apply nail enamel and top coat or sealer, as in a basic manicure (Figure 23–27).
14. Complete postservice procedure on page 799. Store unused fabric in a sealable plastic bag to protect it from oil and dust.

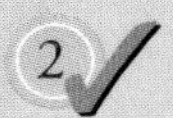

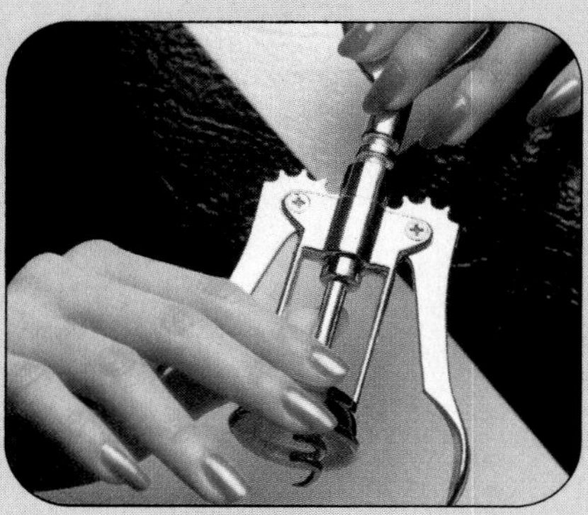

Figure 23–27 Finished fabric wraps.

Small swatches of the mending material of your choice, cut to fit the nail size and shape, are available. You may choose instead to use a precut wrap with an adhesive backing. The nail adhesive is a glue or bonding agent used to secure the nail tip or fabric to the natural nail. You may also want to use an adhesive dryer, which is a brush-on spray that allows for quick drying of the nail adhesive. Remember, when working with adhesives, be sure to protect your eyes with goggles and offer them to your clients as well.

Removing Nail Wraps

The process for the removal of nail wraps is relatively simple. First, have your client soak her fingertips in a small bowl of acetone for a few minutes to remove all polish. The acetone should be approximately 1 inch (2.5 cm) above the nails. Gently remove the loosened wrap with an orangewood stick or a metal pusher, and proceed with a basic manicure or a hot oil version. Buff the client's nails gently with a fine block buffer. Condition the cuticles and surrounding skin with cuticle oil or lotion.

Fabric Wrap Maintenance and Repairs

It is critical that fabric wraps be regularly maintained in order to keep them looking fresh. This means that glue "fills" will be required after two weeks and glue and fabric fills will be necessary after four weeks. Cutting corners can lead to problems.

Two-Week Maintenance

1. Complete the nail wrap preservice.
2. Remove all old polish.
3. Clean the nails and push back the cuticles.
4. File the nails to remove any shine. Make sure the line between the new growth and the existing wrap is smooth. The bottom of the previous wrap near the cuticle should not be visible.
5. Apply a nail antiseptic.
6. Apply adhesive to the new nail growth area, taking care not to touch the skin. Hasten drying with an adhesive dryer.
7. Apply adhesive to the entire nail. Follow with the adhesive dryer.
8. Shape and refine the nails.
9. Buff the nails. Remove dust and all traces of oil.
10. Apply polish.
11. Complete the nail wrap postservice.

Four-Week Maintenance

After four weeks, new fabric must be applied to the area of new growth on the nail. Follow the procedure for the two-week maintenance up to and including Step 5, then continue with these additional steps.

1. Cut a piece of fabric large enough to cover the new growth area and slightly overlap the old wrap.
2. Apply adhesive to the regrowth area.

3. Apply fabric to the area and smooth it down.
4. Apply adhesive a second time.
5. Spray, brush, or drop on adhesive dryer to dry the adhesive more quickly.
6. Apply adhesive again.
7. Apply a second coat of adhesive dryer and finish as you would a two-week maintenance visit.

Repairs with Fabric Wraps

Small pieces of fabric can be used to strengthen a weak point or repair a break in the nail. A stress strip is a strip of fabric cut to 1/8 inch and applied to the weak point of the nail using the four-week maintenance procedure. A repair patch is a piece of fabric that is cut to completely cover the crack or break in the nail. Use the four-week maintenance procedure for this procedure as well.

Liquid Nail Wrap

Liquid nail wrap is a polish made with tiny fibers designed to strengthen and preserve the natural nail as it grows. It is brushed on the nail in several directions to create a network that, when hardened, protects the nail. It is similar to nail hardener, though it is of a thicker consistency and contains more fiber.

ACRYLIC NAILS

23

Acrylic (uh-KRIL-ik) **nails**, often referred to as sculptured nails, are artificial nails that are created by combining a liquid acrylic product with a powdered product. When joined, the two products form a soft ball that can easily be molded into a nail shape. Acrylic nails can be applied directly onto a natural nail or over a tip, or they can be sculpted onto a paper or metal nail form. These nails are sometimes referred to as "built." Acrylics can be used to strengthen or extend the nail or to repair weak, bitten, or torn nails.

The Science of Acrylic Nails

There are three basic ingredients in the acrylic nail process.

- A **monomer** (MON-oh-mer) is a substance made up of many small molecules that are not attached to one another. Liquid acrylic is a type of monomer.
- A **polymer** (PAHL-uh-mur) is a hard substance formed by combining many small molecules (monomers), usually in a long chain-like structure. Polymers and monomers are developed from the same chemistry except that one remains in liquid form (monomer) while the other is powdered (polymer).

- A **catalyst** (KAT-ul-est) is any substance having the power to increase the velocity (speed) of a chemical reaction. Powdered acrylic is a combination of ground-up polymer and a catalyst. The process begins when the liquid from the brush (the monomer) picks up the powder from the jar (the polymer). The catalyst "explodes" when it comes in contact with the monomer, causing heat. The heat starts a chain reaction from one polymer bead to the other. This transfer continues until the last polymer bead receives heat. This hardening process is also referred to as **curing**. 3

CAUTION

When performing an acrylic service, it is critical that your work area be well ventilated. Consider wearing a safety mask as well to prevent the inhalation of dust.

Acrylic Nails over Forms

Nail forms are versatile, easy-to-apply artificial nails made of adhesive-backed coated paper or mylar. They also come in preshaped plastic or aluminum; these nail forms must always be sanitized. Acrylic nails can be colored with a variety of acrylic powders, including many shades of pink, white, clear, and natural. For more artistic or ambitious nail extension projects involving patterns and florals, there is a range of other acrylic colors from which you can choose. Acrylics can be created either by using one-color powder for the entire nail or by using pink powder on the nail plate and white powder for the free edge to produce a French manicure look.

Before you learn how to apply acrylic nails, you should understand the role that primers play in the process. A **primer** is a substance that improves adhesion, or attachment, and prepares the nail surface for bonding with the acrylic material. Acid primer is widely used to help bind the acrylic to the natural nail. Nonacid primer is noninvasive to the natural nail and not corrosive on the skin but may not be as effective as acid primer.

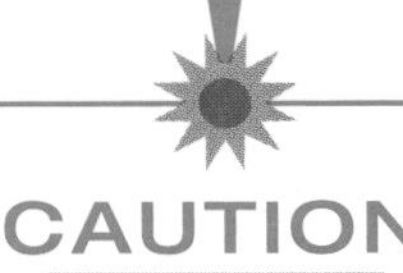

CAUTION

Primers are very effective but can cause serious, sometimes irreversible, damage to the skin and eyes. Be sure to read the label and follow the manufacturers' instructions when using primer and always wear gloves and safety glasses.

Most primer bottles have self-contained brushes. These brushes hold too much primer and can cause primer burn. Use a separate brush to apply a dot of primer on the natural nail surface. The primer will spread evenly without your having to move the brush over the entire nail surface. Make sure that you do not overuse primer. Overly primed nails can become too slick and can cause the acrylic to lift. Allow the primer to dry naturally to a chalky white.

Acrylic Overlays on Tips or Natural Nails

Acrylic overlays are artificial nails that use the same acrylic material as sculptured nails but are applied directly to the natural nail surface instead of being extended. These overlays are useful for strengthening weak nails or repairing damaged ones.

The procedure for applying acrylic on the natural nail or on a tip is similar to sculpting, but somewhat simpler. Follow the procedure for applying tips, then apply the acrylic as you would on a nail form. The natural nail may be shorter than a tip or sculptured nail, so you might need to use only two balls of acrylic.

Fills for Acrylic Nails

As the natural nail grows, the acrylic nails are pushed farther up the nail plate (Figure 23–28). A **fill** is the application of acrylic product to the new

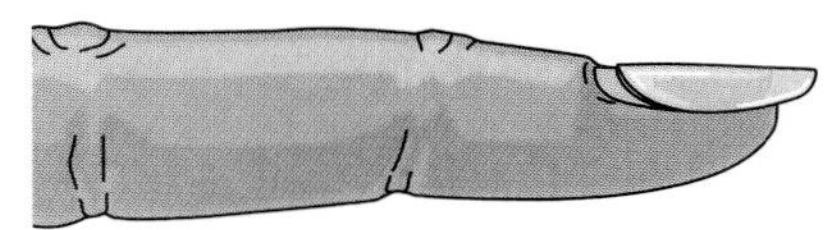

Figure 23-28 Acrylic nail needing fill.

PROCEDURE

APPLYING ACRYLIC NAILS OVER FORMS

Implements and Materials

In addition to the materials on your basic manicuring table, you will need the following:

- acrylic liquid
- acrylic powder
- dehydrator
- primer
- dappen dishes (small cups for liquid and powdered acrylic)
- nail forms
- brush
- plastic gloves
- safety glasses and safety mask (recommended)

Preparation

Complete the preservice procedure on pages 797-799.

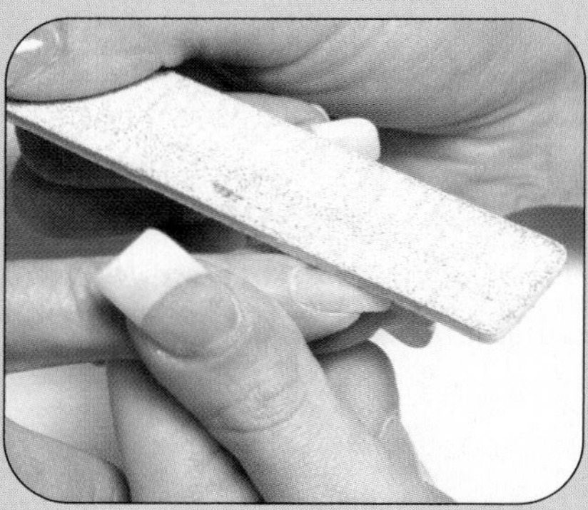

Figure 23-29 Buff nails to remove shine.

Procedure

1. Remove all polish.
2. Push back the cuticle.
3. Remove any shine from the natural nail surface. Buff lightly over the nail plate with an abrasive to remove the natural oil. Remove dust (Figure 23–29).
4. If using a dehydrator, liberally apply it to the natural plate only, to cleanse and remove surface moisture on the nail plate prior to acrylic application.
5. Apply nail antiseptic with cotton or spray (Figure 23–30).

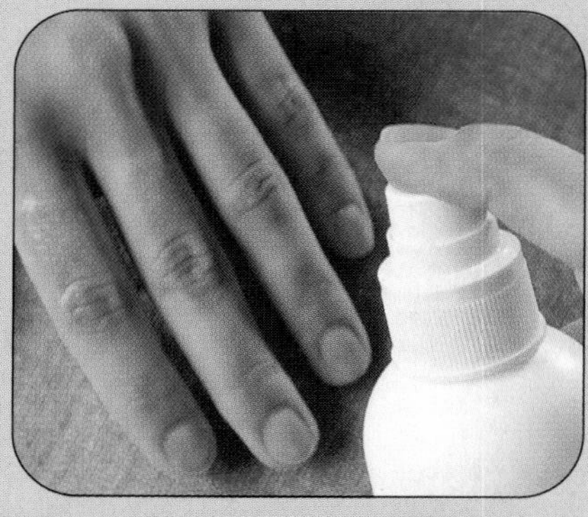

Figure 23-30 Apply nail antiseptic.

6. Position the nail forms. If you are using disposable forms, peel the nail form from its paper backing and, using the thumb and index finger of both hands, bend the form into an arch to fit the client's natural nail shape. Slide the form onto your client's finger and press the adhesive backing to the sides of the finger. Make sure the form is snug under the free edge and level with the natural nail (Figure 23–31).
7. If you are using reusable nail forms, slide the form onto the client's finger, making sure the free edge is over the form and that it fits snugly. Be careful not to cut into the part of the skin under the free edge. Tighten the form around the finger by squeezing lightly.
8. Apply primer (Figure 23–32). Remember to put on plastic gloves and safety glasses and offer a pair to your client as well.
9. Dip the brush into the liquid mixture, wipe any excess material on the side of the bowl, and then immediately dip the tip of the brush into the powder, rotating it slightly as you draw it toward yourself to form a smooth ball of acrylic (Figure 23–33 and Figure 23–34). If you are using the two-color acrylic method, use the white powder at this point.
10. Place the ball of acrylic on the nail form at the point where the free edge joins the nail form (Figure 23–35).

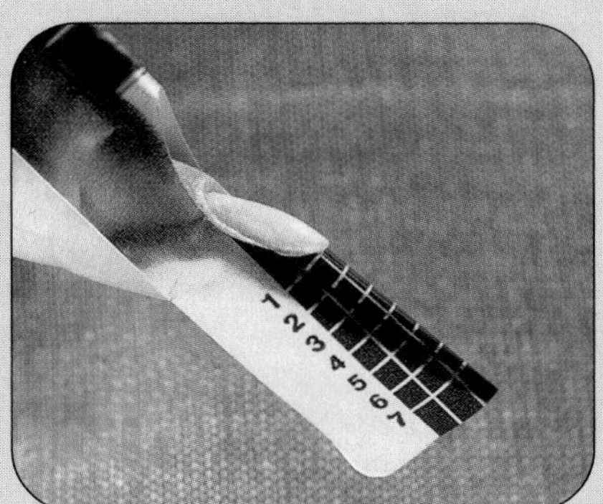

Figure 23-31 Position the nail form.

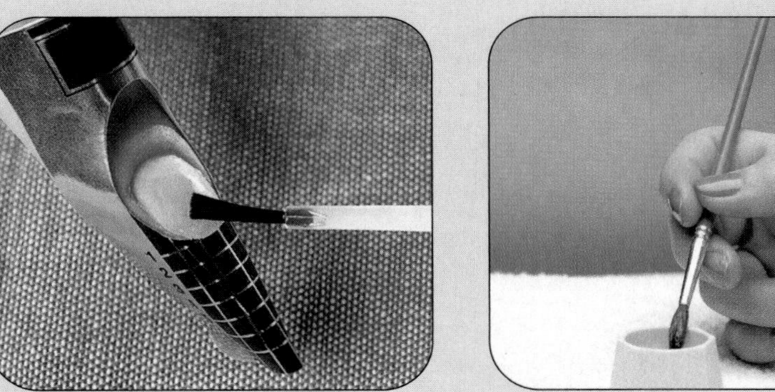

Figure 23-32 Apply primer.

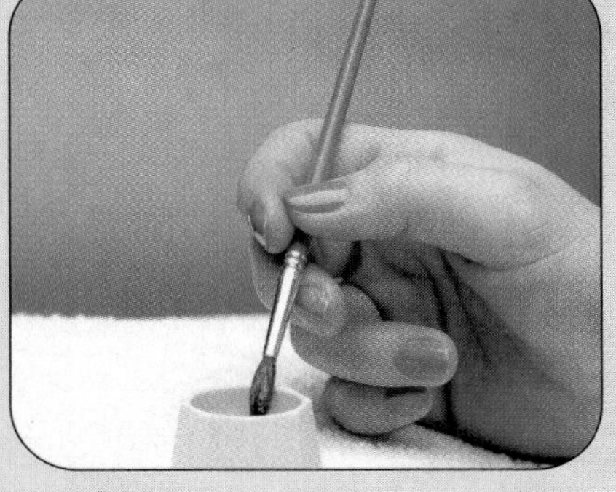

Figure 23-33 Dip brush into acrylic liquid.

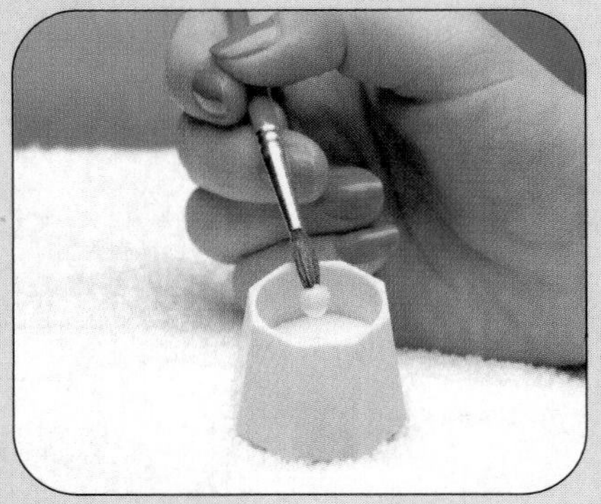

Figure 23-34 Form ball of acrylic.

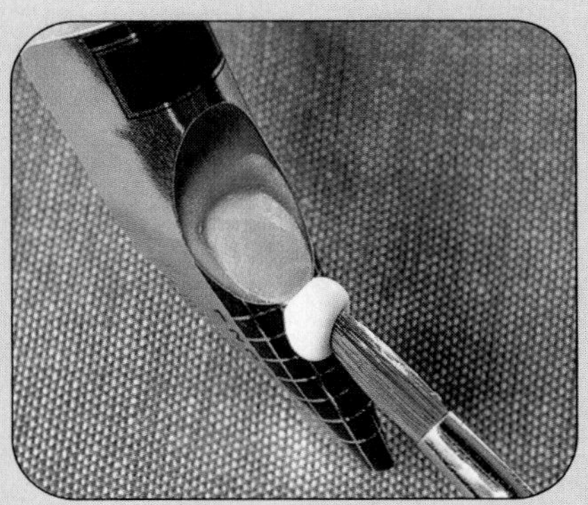

Figure 23-35 Place ball of acrylic on nail form.

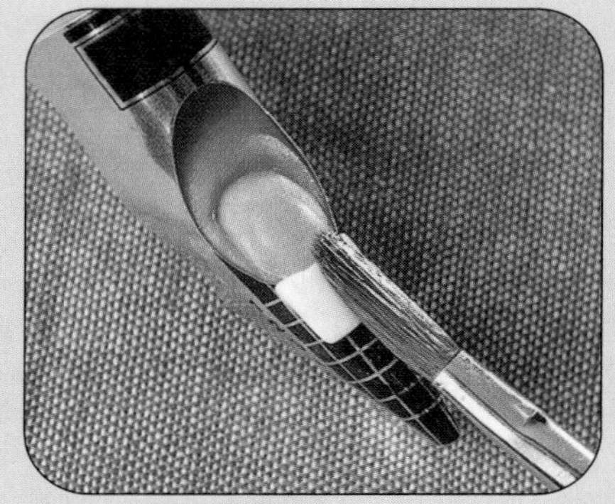

Figure 23-36 Dab and press acrylic with the middle portion of brush.

11. Shape the free edge. Use the middle portion of your sable brush to dab and press the acrylic to form an extension. Do not "paint" the acrylic onto the nail. Dabbing and pressing the acrylic produces a more natural-looking nail than you will get by "painting" (Figure 23–36). Keep the sidewall lines parallel and shape the acrylic continuously along the free edge line. If you are using the two-color acrylic method, make sure you follow the natural free edge line with the white powder to produce the French manicure look (Figure 23–37).
12. Form a second ball of acrylic of medium consistency and place it on the natural nail next to the free edge line in the center of the nail (Figure 23–38). Dab and press the product to the sidewalls, making sure that the product is very thin around all the edges (Figure 23–39). If you are using a two-color acrylic product, use the pink powder for this step.
13. Make an extremely wet acrylic mixture, using very little powder, and place it at the center of the lower half of the nail. Spread the mixture to the sides of the nail, being careful not to touch the cuticle (Figure 23–40). The application near the cuticle, the sidewall, and the free edge should be kept extremely thin in order to achieve a natural-looking nail.

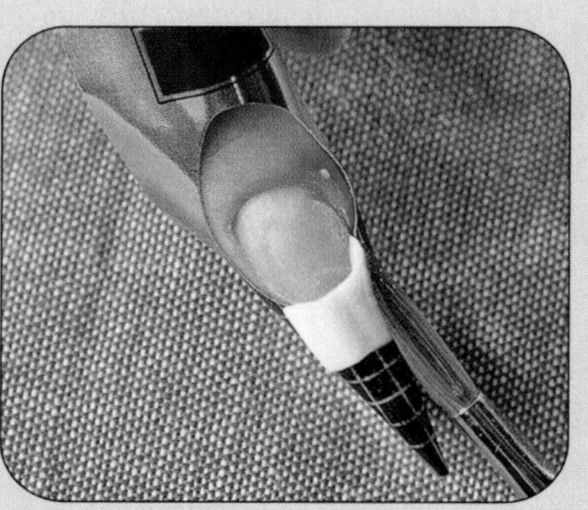

Figure 23-37 Shape free edge.

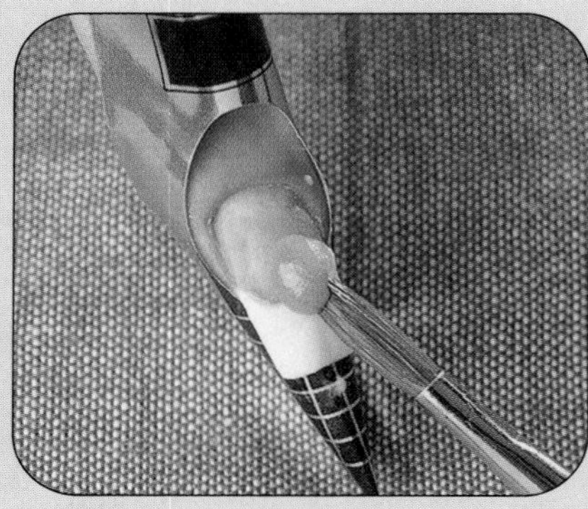

Figure 23-38 Place second ball on natural nail.

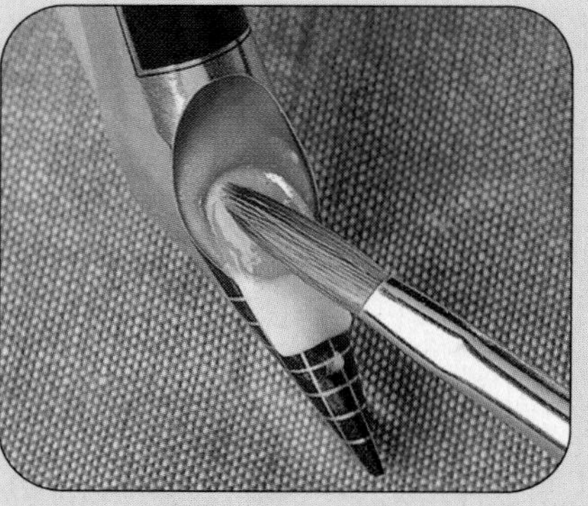

Figure 23-39 Shape second ball of acrylic.

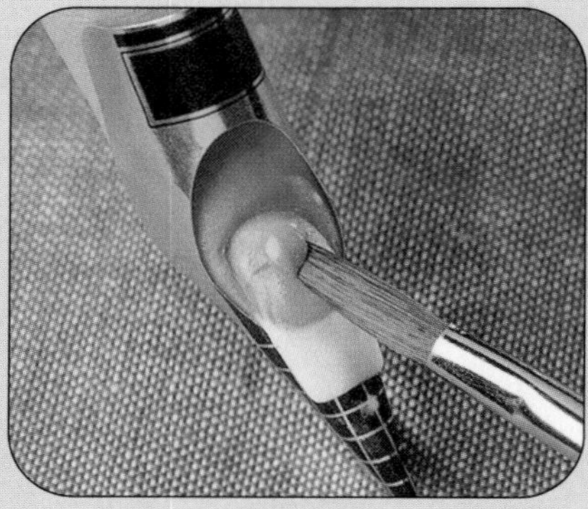

Figure 23-40 Apply acrylic to the sides of the nail.

14. Apply the acrylic to the remaining nails.
15. Allow the nails to dry and then remove the nail forms. The nails are dry when they make a clicking sound if lightly tapped.
16. File the new nails to the desired shape and then buff the nails until the entire surface is smooth.
17. Wash the nails thoroughly. Allow them to dry.
18. Apply a base coat, polish, and top coat sealer (Figure 23–41).
19. Complete the postservice procedure on page 799. Clean the brush by dipping it into polish remover and wiping it clean. Clean dappen dishes by lifting hardened content out with the pusher. 2

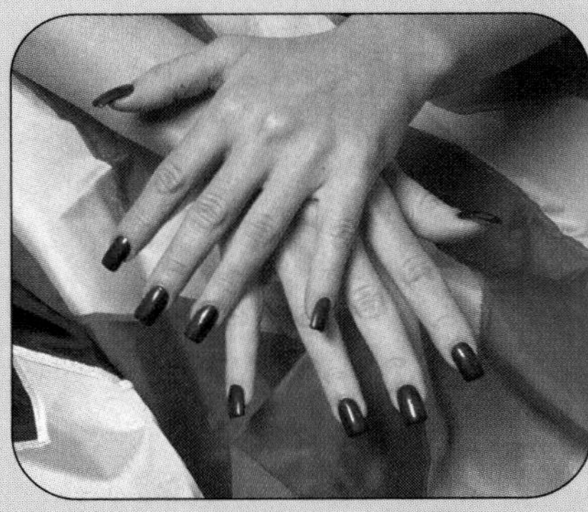

Figure 23–41 Finished acrylic nails.

completed!

insights

Sue Ellen Schultes

The greatest moment in Sue Schultes's career was the day a set of nails she painted was entered into the permanent collection at the Smithsonian Museum in Washington, DC.

I was an artist before I got into any of this. I didn't have a degree, but I studied with many different artists. Then I stayed home with my son, and after about 14 years I decided to go back into the workforce. My sister, who's a cosmetologist, bugged me to go into nail art. I have no nails myself, and I'm allergic to nail polish and acrylics and gels. But my sister kept insisting, so I started painting her nails. Then I did her friends, and everyone thought my work was wonderful, so I wound up getting a job and I loved it. I loved the people and the process and the excitement. Most of all, I loved the pleasure I gave. I got thanked twenty or thirty times a day.

I had my own nail salon for several years, and it was a challenge. You have to change your hat so many times a day. You're the boss; you're a mentor, a technician, an artist, and a salesperson. People think that because we're nail technicians we have no pressure, that we sit and talk all day. But you have time constraints. As an owner you have to make that money, and as a technician you want to do a good job. So you're always trying to get everything done within a certain time period, along with all the interruptions. It's like a comedy on TV sometimes. Each day has its own culture; each group of people has its own discussions.

One of the things I like best about being a nail technician is that you're facing your client and holding her hand, and you get a lot and give a lot. It's much more personal than doing hair. And if you make a mistake, it's much more easily remedied.

The key to building a loyal client base is professionalism. You're there for the client, and everything else comes second. If I had to name three people skills that contribute to success as a manicurist, they would be listening, service, and a sense of humor.

Having a set of nails in the Smithsonian is a great thrill. A client of mine attended the senior President Bush's inaugural ball in Washington, and as she was signing a book a photographer said, "Oh my God, what do you have on your nails?" So she showed him, and he said, "Do they come off?" And she lied and said yes. Then she called me up and told me to paint another set right away. So I did. It was the bald eagle, the flag, the Capitol, and the Washington Monument. The nails are in the museum's archives now. Because of the work I did for a client, I got into the Smithsonian—it's marvelous!

PROCEDURE

APPLYING ACRYLIC NAIL FILLS

Implements and Materials

See Procedure 62—applying acrylic nails over forms.

Preparation

Perform the preservice procedure on pages 797-799.

Procedure

1. Remove all old polish.
2. With a medium abrasive, smooth the ledge between the new growth and the acrylic nail.
3. Place your client's hand in a fingerbowl filled with warm water and liquid soap and use a nail brush to gently wash the nails. Do not soak the nails.
4. Use a fresh cotton-tipped orangewood stick to gently push back the cuticle.
5. Buff lightly over the nail plate with a medium/fine abrasive to remove the natural oil. Brush off filings.
6. Apply nail antiseptic to the nails.
7. Brush the exposed area with primer, following the manufacturers' instructions. Use safety glasses and gloves when working with primer.
8. Dip the tip of your brush first into the liquid acrylic and then into the powder acrylic to form a small ball.
9. Place the ball on the exposed area, pressing and shaping it with the base of the brush until it blends into the existing sculptured nail. Let the area dry and then reshape the nail with abrasive, buffing for a smooth appearance.
10. Apply polish.
11. Complete the postservice procedure on page 799.

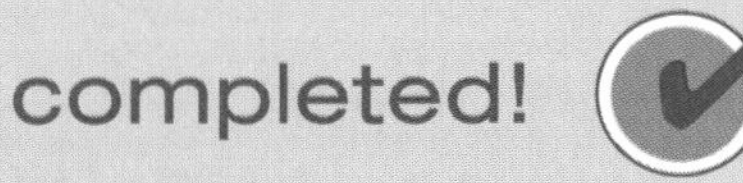

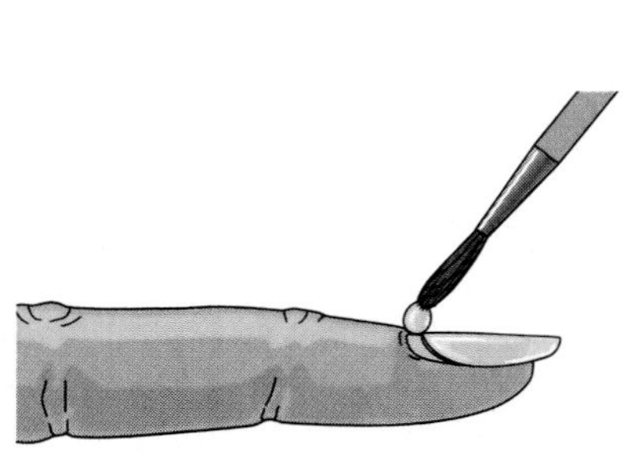

Figure 23-42 Apply the acrylic fill.

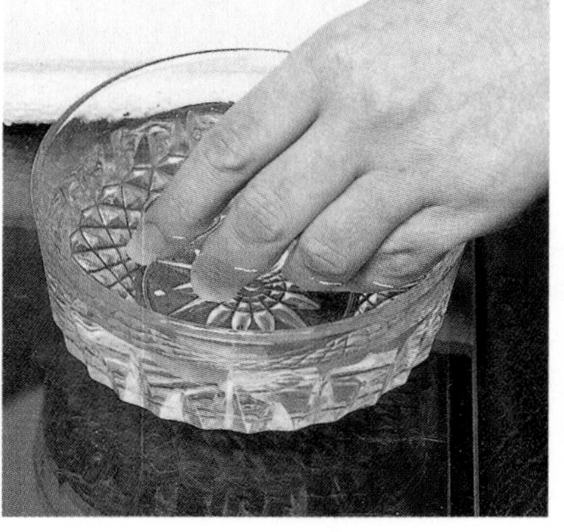

Figure 23-43 Soak fingertips in solvent.

growth (Figure 22–42). Acrylic nails should be filled in every two to three weeks, depending on how fast the nail grows. During the course of a fill, the shape of the nail should be defined again. This is called **rebalancing**. Without rebalancing, the nail will begin to look unnatural and uneven as it grows longer, and the new growth area will be noticeable.

Crack Repair

If an acrylic nail is badly chipped or cracked, your choice is to file a V shape into the crack or to file flush to remove the crack. If necessary, a new nail form can be attached and acrylic material added to the free edge of the nail. If any area of the natural nail is involved, be sure to prime the area. Then form a new tip and blend it with whatever old material is still adhering to the nail.

Removing Acrylic Nails

To remove an acrylic nail, begin by soaking the nail in a solvent specified by the manufacturer or your instructor (Figure 23–43). Use a fresh orangewood stick or a metal pusher to gently push off the softened acrylic nail. Repeat until all acrylic has been removed. Never try to pry off the acrylic with nippers, as this will damage the natural nail plate.

CAUTION

When sculptured nails lift, crack, or grow out and are not maintained in a responsible manner, moisture and dirt may become trapped under the nail, creating an environment in which bacteria can grow. A change in the color of the natural nail indicates that bacteria may be present under the acrylic. If left unattended, this can lead to nail injury or loss. Most primers have ingredients that sterilize the nail before acrylic is applied, thus preventing infection. To help ensure that contamination does not occur, do not touch the nail after the primer has been applied.

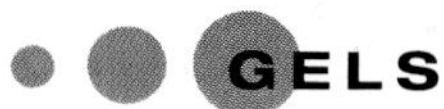

GELS

Gels are strong, durable artificial nails that are brushed onto the nail plate. They have a chemical consistency very similar to that of acrylic nails, but they require a separate catalyst to ensure hardening.

There are two types of gels.

1. **Light-cured gels** harden when they are exposed to a special light source, either ultraviolet or halogen.

PROCEDURE

LIGHT-CURED GEL ON TIPS OR NATURAL NAILS

Implements and Materials

In addition to the materials on your basic manicuring table, you will need the following:

- nail antiseptic
- light-cured gel
- curing light
- brush
- primer (if recommended by manufacturer)
- nail tips
- nail prep
- adhesive

Preparation

Perform the preservice procedure on pages 797-799.

Procedure

1. Remove all old polish.
2. Push back the cuticles.
3. Buff the nails to remove shine. Apply nail antiseptic.
4. Apply tips if desired.
5. Apply nail prep or primer as recommended by the manufacturer.
6. Apply gel #1 or base coat gel from the pinky finger to the index finger (Figure 23–44). Firmly brush the gel onto the entire nail surface, including the rim of the free edge. Keep the gel from touching the cuticle or sidewalls. If necessary, remove excess gel with a fresh orangewood stick.

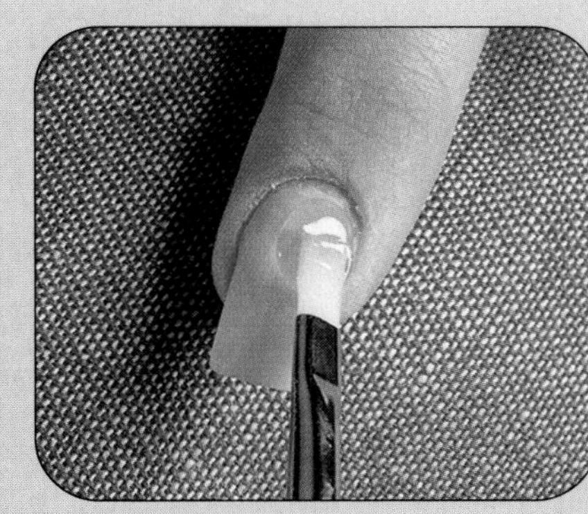

Figure 23–44 Apply gel to entire nail.

completed!

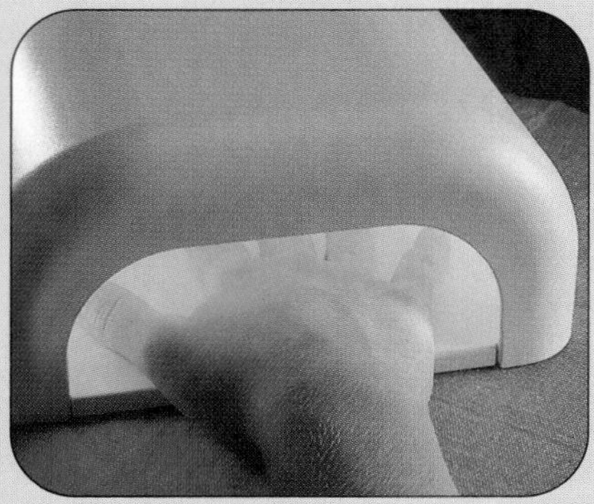

Figure 23-45 Cure gel.

7. Place the client's hand under a curing lamp for the manufacturer's suggested cure time (Figure 23-45).
8. Repeat Steps 6 and 7 on the other hand. Repeat the same steps for both thumbs.
9. Apply gel #2 or building gel to the first hand. Dispense a generous amount of gel down the center from the cuticle to the free edge over the cured sticky first layer (Figure 23-46). As you drag the gel across the first layer, the tacky surface will pull the gel off the brush or from the tube. Apply this line of gel on all four nails from pinky to index finger.
10. Place the client's hand under the lamp for 20 seconds. This will "freeze" the gel in place yet leave it ready for additional, thinner layers.
11. Repeat Steps 9 and 10 on the other hand, then on both thumbs.
12. Dispense a slightly smaller amount of gel. Starting from the cuticle, stroke down one side of the gel line and repeat down the other side toward the free edge using a light polishing stroke. Wrap the gel around the entire free edge to seal and protect the free edge of the natural nail or tip. Apply to all four nails from pinky to index finger.
13. Cure the gel. Check the manufacturers' cure time.
14. Repeat Steps 12 and 13 on the other hand, then on both thumbs.
15. Remove any tacky residue. Wipe all nail surfaces with cleanser, following the manufacturer's directions (Figure 23-47). The cleanser is usually acetone-based or alcohol.
16. Check nail contours. Using 180 grit abrasive, refine the surface contour (gels are easily filed) (Figure 23-48).

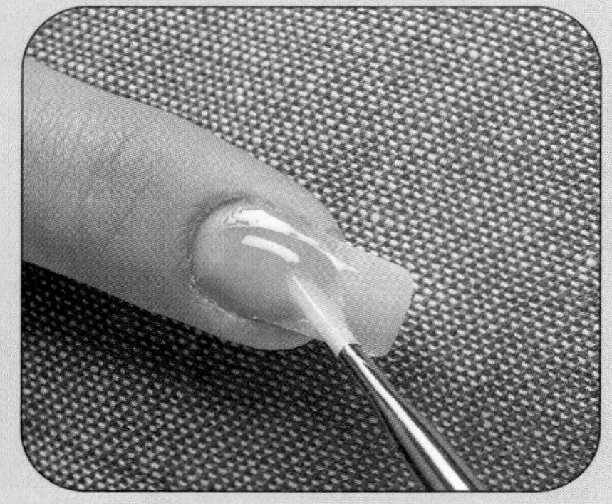

Figure 23-46 Apply gel #2 or building gel.

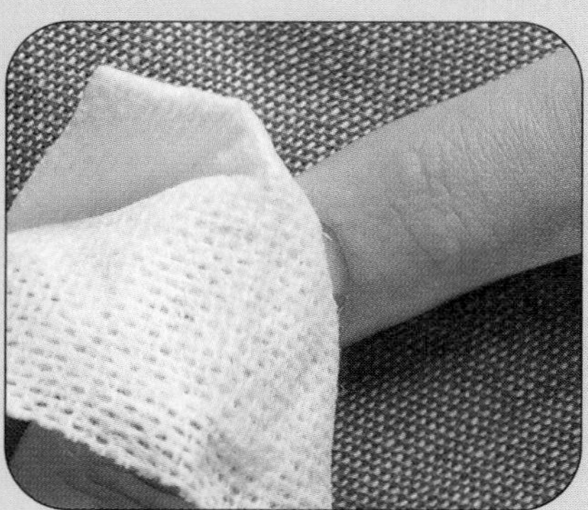

Figure 23-47 Wipe nails with cleanser.

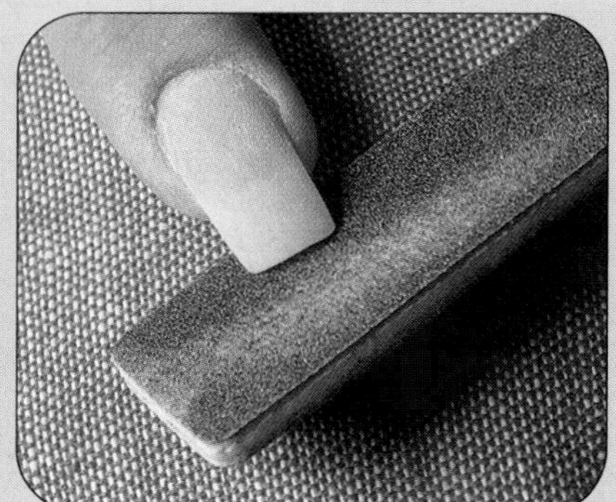

Figure 23-48 Refine the entire nail surface.

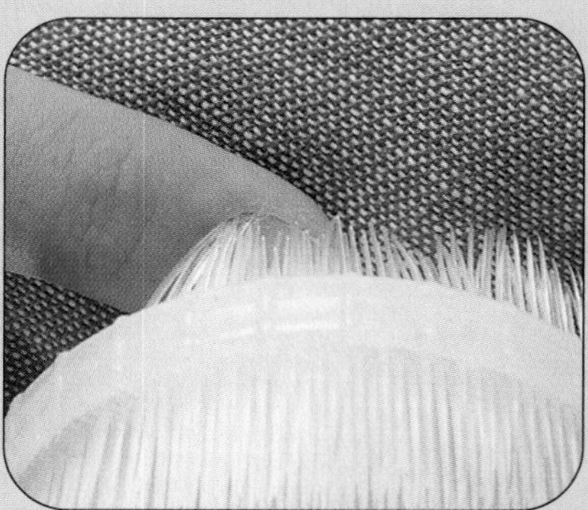

Figure 23-49 Remove dust filings.

17. Vigorously buff the entire nail to a smooth finish. Remove dust filings with a manicure brush (Figure 23–49).
18. Apply a top coat gel.
19. Repeat Steps 15 to 18.
20. Rub cuticle oil into the surrounding skin and nail surface if you are leaving the nails free of polish. Otherwise, clean the nails and proceed to polish (Figure 23–50).
21. Complete the postservice procedure on page 799. 2

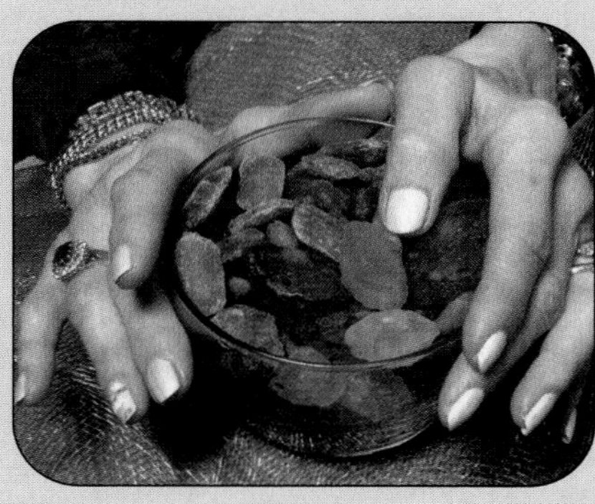

Figure 23-50 Finished gel nails.

completed!

2. **No-light gels** harden when an activator or accelerator is sprayed or brushed on, or when they are soaked in water. They are thicker glues that can be applied either by themselves or over a silk or fiberglass wrap. Follow manufacturer's instructions for application of no-light gels.

Gel Maintenance

Both light-cured and nonlight-cured gels should be maintained every two to three weeks, depending on how fast the client's nails grow. Use a medium abrasive file and buff the entire nail to remove any shine. If you find that a regrowth ledge has developed, you can eliminate it by gliding a file or an abrasive over the ledge area. Hold the file flat at the ledge, not at an angle, because this can make a groove and might damage the natural nail plate. Continue buffing until there is no line between the hardened gel and the natural nail. Be careful not to damage the natural nail plate by buffing too roughly. When the nail is smooth, follow the procedure for the application of gel on natural nails.

Gel Removal

UV gels must be buffed off layer by layer and will not soak off in acetone. No-light gels, on the other hand, can be soaked off. Soak the client's nails in a small bowl filled with acetone for 15 to 25 minutes without lifting the hands from the bowl. Always be sure to read and follow manufacturers' instructions. Using a metal pusher, scrape gently from the cuticle to the free edge to slide off the softened product. Follow with a gentle buffing of the natural nail using a fine block buffer. This will remove the glue residue. Complete the service with a manicure.

DIPPED NAILS

Dipped nails are created by dipping the nails into acrylic powder (the powder may also be sprinkled on). Most dipped nails do not rely on an acrylic monomer but use instead a cyanoacrylate (si-ah-no-ah-KRILL-ate), a very fast-setting glue which comes in different viscosities and can be applied in several ways.

Begin the procedure by applying a thick brush-on glue to the nail surface with or without a tip extension. Dip the nail into the powder or sprinkle the powder on. Reapply the glue, dip again, and glue again. The glue hardens as it absorbs the powder. Some systems require an activator to complete the hardening process. Once dry, the overlay is filed and shaped to a finished nail and polished. Follow normal pre- and postservice procedures.

SAFETY PRECAUTIONS

- Use a new orangewood stick with each client.
- Keep all products from touching the skin. They may cause sensitivities.
- Keep alcohol nearby in case the acrylic gets hot from the chemical action of the product. Because it evaporates quickly, alcohol has a cooling effect.
- Soften the edges on your abrasive. A new file can etch a groove in the nail during filing.
- If you accidentally touch the nails after you apply antiseptic, you must clean them again and reapply.
- When working with primer, put on safety gloves and safety glasses. Offer safety glasses to your client.
- Check primer for clarity on a regular basis to make sure it is not contaminated with bacteria. If bacteria is present, the primer will appear cloudy.
- Use primer sparingly. It can cause irritation or primer burn if it touches the skin.
- If you accidentally spill primer on your clothing, remove the soiled garment immediately.
- Acrylic applied too thickly near the cuticle or touching the cuticle will lift.
- Do not use a nipper to clip away loose acrylic. Nipping may make the lifting problem worse and can damage the nail plate. If lifting is excessive, soak off the acrylic and start fresh with a new nail application
- Make sure bottles are tightly capped when not in use.
- Do not store acrylic products near heat or use near an open flame.
- Do not apply acrylic to injured or inflamed skin.
- Make sure that your work area is well ventilated.

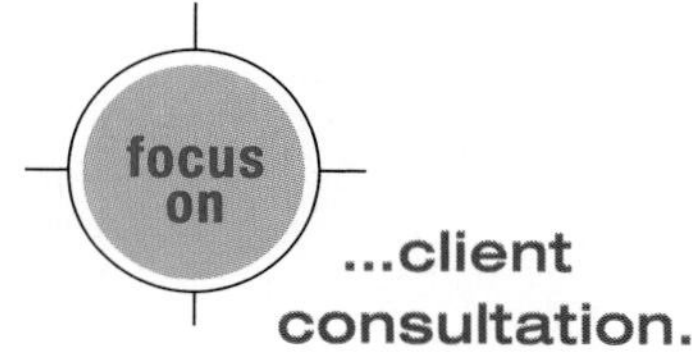

...client consultation.

As part of your client consultation, remind your client to follow common-sense measures with her new nails. Suggest that she always wear gloves when gardening, for instance, or doing household work. She should protect her nails from contact with cleaning products and other chemicals and from extended soaking in water. Remember, these simple measures to protect the nails will also protect the hands.

NAIL ART

Nail art offers endless creative opportunities and is favored by many clients who see it as a way to express their unique personalities. Advanced technology allows for exciting custom designs, which has made nail art one of the most popular add-on services salons can offer.

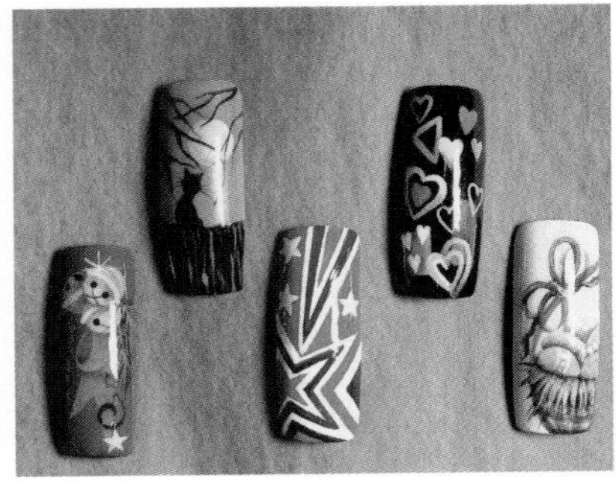

Figure 23-51 Examples of nail art.

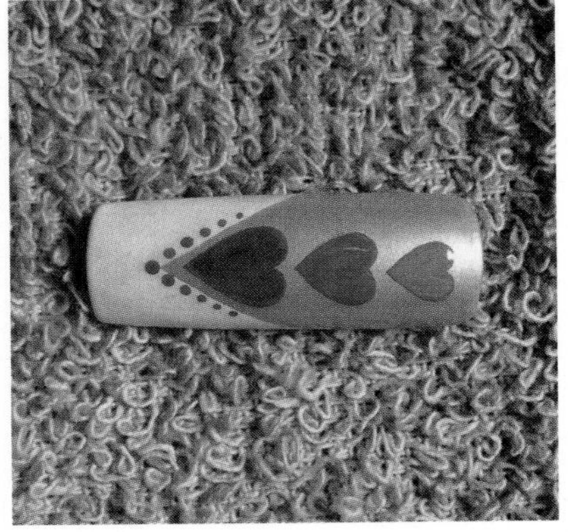

Figure 23-52 Freehand nail art.

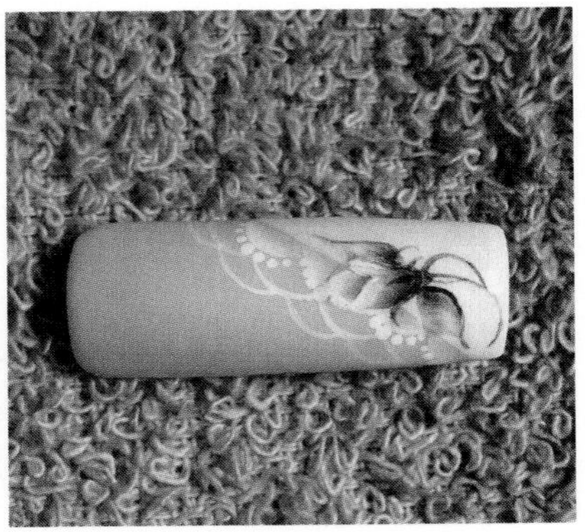

Figure 23-53 Freehand nail art.

Nail art can be conservative and appropriate to an office environment or it can utilize flamboyant holiday designs and expressive specialty art forms (Figure 23–51). Consider the following nail art innovations.

- *Gems.* Tiny rhinestones in different sizes, colors, and shapes are used for the design itself or as sparkling accents.
- *Striping tape.* This tacky-backed tape helps you create more linear or graphic designs. It comes in many widths, colors, and metallic finishes.
- *Foil.* Colored foils are pressed onto the entire nail or part of the nail.
- *Gold leaf or nuggets.* Gold leaf, which comes in very fragile sheets, is applied to the nail in large pieces or in tiny pieces that resemble nuggets.
- *Airbrushing.* An airbrush and a compressor combine air and paint to form an atomized spray for painting. Stencils are sometimes used to create scenes, graphics, or fades.
- *Freehand.* A paintbrush and an endless palette of colors will allow you to customize your client's nails to match any outfit (Figure 23–52 and Figure 23–53).

Manufacturers and distributors of nail art tools and supplies offer instructional classes and videos to help you hone your skills. Seek them out at trade shows, in trade magazines, and on the Internet. Try any one of these specialty services alone or in combination with other nail techniques.

NEW HORIZONS

Until fairly recently, many of the advanced nail techniques we have described did not even exist. The world of nail technology is exploding from year to year and has made this area one of the most lucrative in the salon profession. Enjoy your work and never stop learning. The more training you have in this area, the better your end results will be. And the better your results, the faster your client base will grow.

chapter glossary

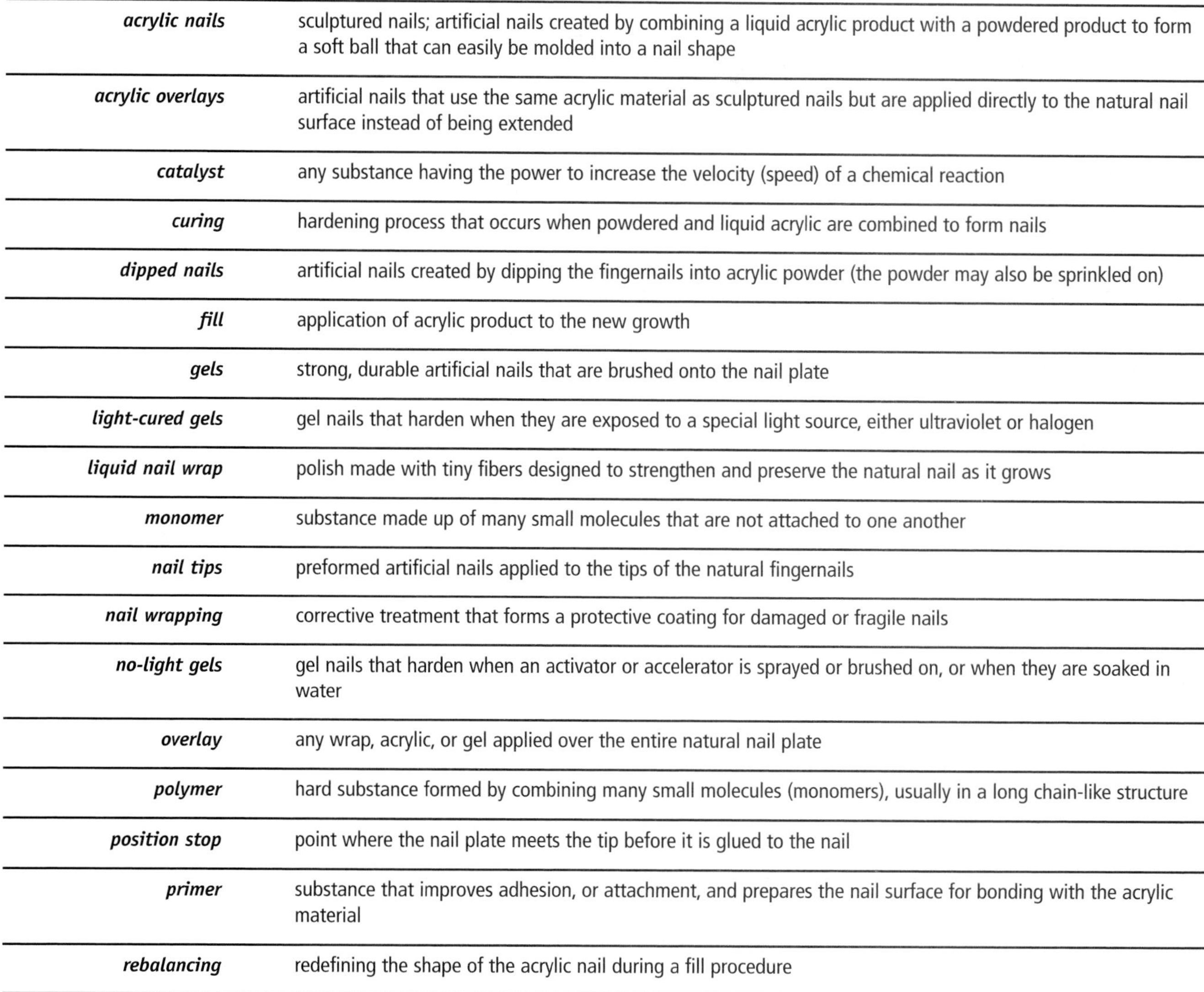

acrylic nails	sculptured nails; artificial nails created by combining a liquid acrylic product with a powdered product to form a soft ball that can easily be molded into a nail shape
acrylic overlays	artificial nails that use the same acrylic material as sculptured nails but are applied directly to the natural nail surface instead of being extended
catalyst	any substance having the power to increase the velocity (speed) of a chemical reaction
curing	hardening process that occurs when powdered and liquid acrylic are combined to form nails
dipped nails	artificial nails created by dipping the fingernails into acrylic powder (the powder may also be sprinkled on)
fill	application of acrylic product to the new growth
gels	strong, durable artificial nails that are brushed onto the nail plate
light-cured gels	gel nails that harden when they are exposed to a special light source, either ultraviolet or halogen
liquid nail wrap	polish made with tiny fibers designed to strengthen and preserve the natural nail as it grows
monomer	substance made up of many small molecules that are not attached to one another
nail tips	preformed artificial nails applied to the tips of the natural fingernails
nail wrapping	corrective treatment that forms a protective coating for damaged or fragile nails
no-light gels	gel nails that harden when an activator or accelerator is sprayed or brushed on, or when they are soaked in water
overlay	any wrap, acrylic, or gel applied over the entire natural nail plate
polymer	hard substance formed by combining many small molecules (monomers), usually in a long chain-like structure
position stop	point where the nail plate meets the tip before it is glued to the nail
primer	substance that improves adhesion, or attachment, and prepares the nail surface for bonding with the acrylic material
rebalancing	redefining the shape of the acrylic nail during a fill procedure

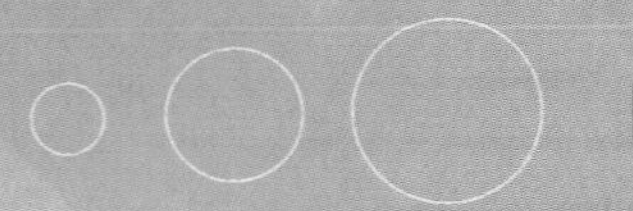

review questions

1. List the four uses of artificial nails.
2. List the steps of the preservice procedure.
3. List the steps of the postservice procedure.
4. Define nail tips, nail wraps, acrylic nails, and gels.
5. Explain briefly how nail tips are applied. How are they removed?
6. Describe the four kinds of nail wraps.
7. Describe briefly how nail wraps are applied. How are they removed?
8. Explain the chemistry of acrylic nails.
9. Explain briefly how acrylic nails are applied using forms. How are they applied over tips or the natural nail?
10. What are the two types of gels?
11. List at least 10 safety precautions you should always follow when performing artificial nail services.

part 6

THE BUSINESS OF COSMETOLOGY

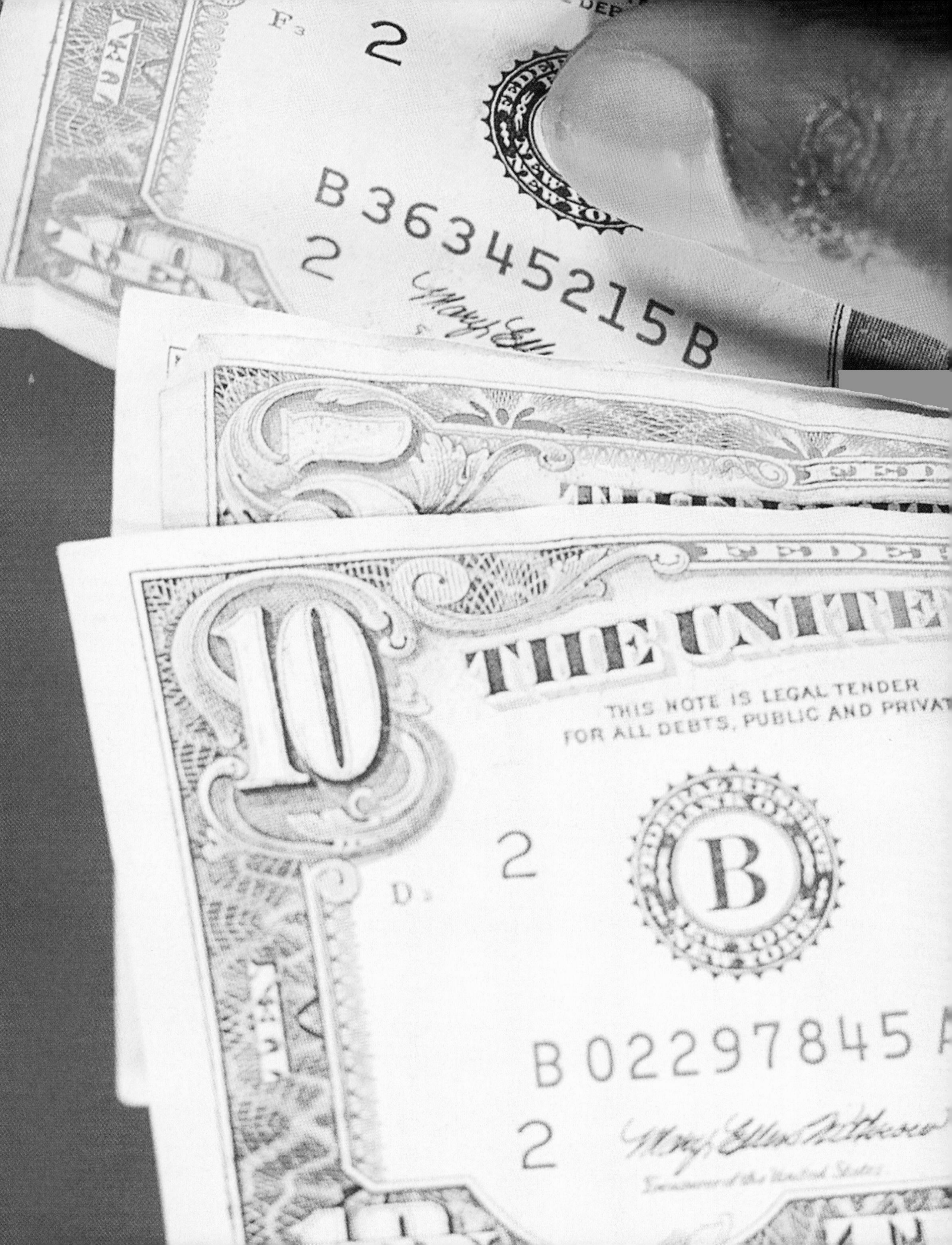
B36345215B
10
THE UNITE
THIS NOTE IS LEGAL TENDER
FOR ALL DEBTS, PUBLIC AND PRIVAT
B
B02297845

THE SALON BUSINESS

Catherine Frangie
BEAUTY INDUSTRY CONSULTANT

Chapter Outline

Learning Objectives

After completing this chapter, you should be able to:

1. List the two ways in which you may go into business for yourself.
2. List the factors to consider when opening a salon.
3. Name and describe the types of ownership under which a salon may operate.
4. Explain the importance of keeping accurate business records.
5. Discuss the importance of the reception area to a salon's success.
6. Demonstrate good salon telephone techniques.
7. List the most effective forms of salon advertising.

National Skill Standards

This chapter provides you with the necessary information to master these National Industry Skill Standards for Entry-Level Cosmetologists.

 Consulting with clients to determine their needs and preferences.

 Interacting effectively with coworkers as part of a team.

 Managing time to provide efficient client service.

 Taking necessary steps to develop and retain clients.

 Marketing professional salon products.

 Maintaining business records on client development, income, and expenses.

 Managing product supply for salon use and retail sales.

 Participating in lifelong learning to stay current with trends, technology, and techniques pertaining to the cosmetology industry.

Key Terms

Page number indicates where in the chapter the term is used.

booth rental
pg. 829

business plan
pg. 833

capital
pg. 836

consumption supplies
pg. 839

corporation
pg. 834

demographics
pg. 832

partnership
pg. 834

personnel
pg. 842

proprietor
pg. 834

retail supplies
pg. 839

As you become more and more proficient in your craft and in your ability to manage yourself and others, you may decide to reach for one of the many exciting opportunities that exist in the field of cosmetology. Perhaps you will decide that it is time to become a salon owner yourself, or the manager of a salon. Having worked for someone else first and having honed your artistic, technical, and managerial skills, the time might seem right for such a venture. The information in this chapter can get you started on the road to realizing your ambitions.

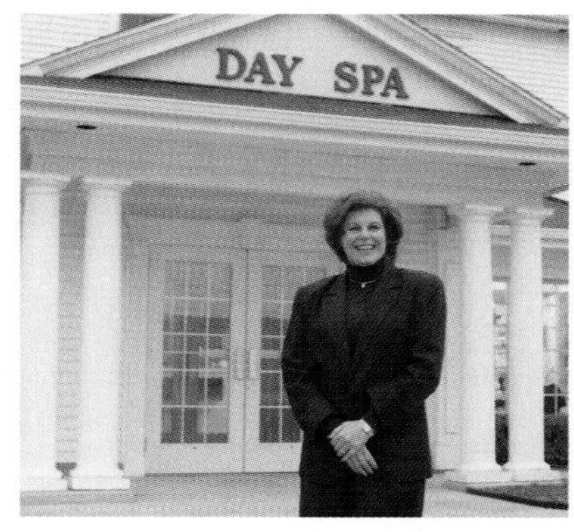

Figure 24-1 Opening your own salon or spa is a big step.

Starting your own business is an enormous responsibility and is not a step to be taken lightly. Much serious planning is necessary. You will need a thorough knowledge of business principles, bookkeeping, business laws, insurance, salesmanship, and psychology before you can take on the role of salon owner and/or manager. This chapter covers some of the basics, but it is only a beginning. Think of it as a useful overview of what you will need to research in more depth before opening your own business. Remember, the more information you have, the better prepared you will be. And the better prepared you are, the greater your chances of success (Figure 24-1).

24

GOING INTO BUSINESS FOR YOURSELF

If you come to a point in your life when you feel you are ready to become your own boss, you will have two main options to consider: opening a salon of your own or renting a booth in an existing salon. Both options have their pros and cons. 1

Booth Rental

Many people see **booth rental**, or renting a booth in a salon (also known as chair rental), as a more desirable alternative to owning a salon, and it has grown in popularity in recent years. In a booth rental arrangement, a stylist

Some state boards of cosmetology require a license for booth rental. Check with your regulatory agency before setting up this arrangement.

generally rents a station in a salon from either a salon owner or a landlord, and is solely responsible for his own clientele, supplies, record-keeping, and accounting. The only obligation to the salon owner is weekly rent for the use of the booth, along with whatever utilities fees are agreed on.

The advantages are that you can become your own boss for a very small amount of money. Your initial investment is not as large as it would be if you were to open your own business. Another advantage is that your expenses are fairly low, limited to your supplies and your rent. For many booth renters, this low overhead balances nicely with the income generated right at the beginning, even if the clientele is small. Booth rental is ideal for someone who is interested in working part time or is supplementing another income. But before becoming a booth renter, you must be sure that you have a large enough clientele to cover your costs.

Although it may sound like a good option, booth renting has its share of obligations, some of which may feel burdensome to some individuals. For one thing, you will need to keep your own records for income tax purposes and other legal reasons. You will need to carry your own malpractice insurance and health insurance, as well as inventory, purchasing, and advertising expenses. You will not enjoy the same benefits as an employee of a salon would, such as paid days off or vacation time. Remember, if you are not there to do the work, you do not get paid. In many ways, you will be on your own and will need to be prepared for that.

Opening Your Own Salon

Opening a salon is a kind of Mount Everest for many stylists; it is the dream they wish to attain. But climbing Mount Everest is a huge undertaking, and opening your own salon can be a huge undertaking as well. Entire books have been written on each of the topics we will touch on in this chapter, so be prepared to read and research your business idea extensively before you make any final decisions. Regardless of the type of salon you hope to open, there are some basic factors you should consider carefully, such as location, written agreements, business regulations, laws, insurance, salon operation, record-keeping, and salon policies.

Location

A good location is one of the most important factors in predicting the success of a business. How can you determine what makes a location good? Essentially, a good location has the visibility and accessibility to attract a volume of customers. It is always best for the salon to be located near other active businesses, such as supermarkets, restaurants, department stores, specialized clothing stores, shoe stores, and other fashion-related shops. That way, the salon can become part of the "one-stop" shopping that is so important to busy people today. Unless you can afford to do a lot of advertising, it is difficult to operate a successful salon in a low-traffic area.

In general, the location you select should reflect your target market. If you are targeting high-income clients, head for a high-income area. If you plan to open a high-volume operation, you will need a high-traffic area with convenient access to public transportation.

insights

Pearl Bailey-Anderson

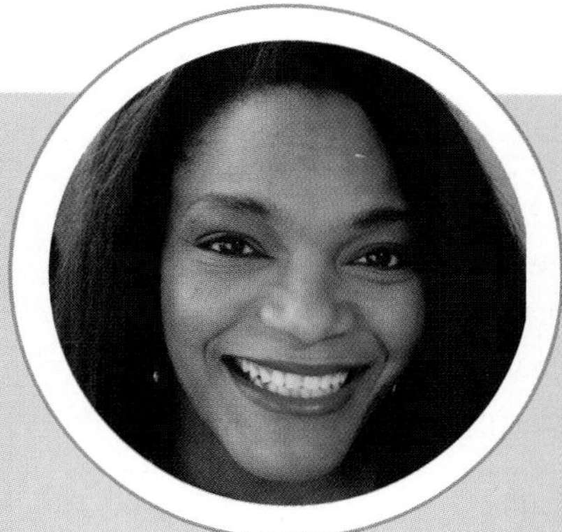

Something of a genius at braiding, Pearl Bailey-Anderson owns a salon and day spa in Philadelphia.

I started out after the last of my four children was five and ready for school. I wore my hair braided, and one day I couldn't get an appointment for a redo, so I redid my hair myself. That's how I found out I could braid hair. The first person I tried braids on was my sister. She lived one block from me. Between the time she left my house and got back to hers, I had three other clients. I became the braid queen.

Then I went to school and did very well, but it was a challenge, juggling the kids and all. When I got out, I worked in a few different salons until my dad gave me the money to start my own business.

Now that I own my own salon, I realize how important it is for the stylist and the salon to be well matched. The first thing I'd do, if I was a young stylist starting out, is to go to the salon and have my hair done as if I were just a client. That way, I'd get to see how they handle people. I would probably be a client for a little while without telling them.

Now, on the other side, what I'm looking for when I hire a stylist is someone who speaks well, who can handle sales, and who is going to be with me for a long time. I'm not looking for someone to come in here and learn what there is to learn and then go across the street and open up her own salon.

In my salon, we call everyone Mr. and Ms. I don't call my clients by their first names, and they don't call me by mine. When I start calling them by their first names, they start asking me for favors. The best thing I can do for my clients, and the reason they stay loyal to me, is I have the products they need when they come in. I never bombard my clients with products they don't need. You have to know each client's personality, too. If you don't know their personality, you don't know when to shut up, you don't know when to talk, you don't know the things you need to know. You have to find out more about your clients. You have to ask them about their lifestyles. Do they work out? What's their hair goal? Where does their daughter go to school? You have to get to know them as people, and when you do, the relationship just grows and grows.

Study the Area

Determine the area's **demographics**, information about the size, average income, and buying habits of the population. The best way to do this is to talk to other business owners who are located near the site in which you are interested. Ask them if they think a salon with the clientele you envision would do well in the area. Many people, when considering starting their own business, actually spend hours or days sitting in a car or a coffee shop, counting the number of people who walk by at any given hour.

Be Visible

No matter what the location, a salon should be clearly visible and sufficiently eye-catching to attract the attention of people walking or driving by (Figure 24–2). Be sure that all signs are easy to see and, whenever possible, have the salon's name on a billboard along with the names of other businesses if you are in a strip mall. Try not to select a name that is difficult to spell or pronounce. Remember that people may want to look you up in the phone book, and if the name of your salon is an alternate spelling of some other name—Kristofer's, for instance—that might present a problem.

Parking Facilities

When selecting a site for a new business, or when planning to take over an established business, consider the parking facilities. People hesitate to patronize a business that is inconvenient to reach, particularly in bad weather. Ample and convenient parking is a must. Also, if the salon is near a parking lot that requires payment or has meters, be sure to inform your clients about this when they call to schedule an appointment. Since most salons remain open even after nightfall, it is also very important that the parking area be well lit, for your safety and that of your clients.

Competition

Competition is a fact of life. In fact, competition can be a positive and motivating force. For most new businesses, however, too much direct

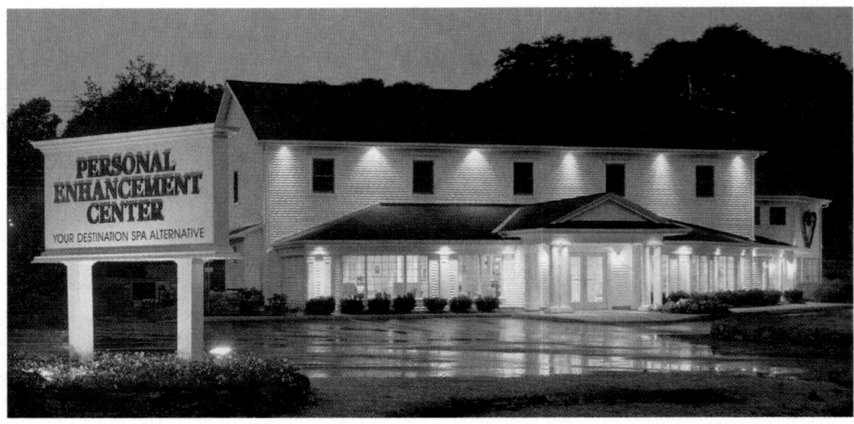

Figure 24–2 A salon should be visible and attractive.

competition in the immediate area can raise the stakes too high. It is better to be located in an area where yours is the only salon of its type. Salons can be located near each other provided that each is trying to attract a different clientele. An upscale salon can operate close to a budget salon and both may be successful because they are focusing on different markets. This can be tricky to determine, so do your homework. Visit all the salons in the neighborhood to determine how closely they will be competing with yours. 2

Business Plan

Before you open a salon, you must develop a **business plan**, a written description of your business as you see it today and as you foresee it in the future. A business plan is like a blueprint; it will always point you in the right direction if you become confused or if you wander away from your original focus. If you are considering obtaining financing, it is essential that you have a business plan in place first. The plan should include a general description of the business and the services it will provide; a statement of the number of personnel to be hired; salaries and other benefits; an operations plan that includes price structure and expenses such as equipment, supplies, repairs, advertising, taxes, and insurance; and a financial plan that includes a profit and loss statement.

Your business plan will tell the world just how serious you are about committing to the success of your new venture. There are lots of books on the market that can help you understand what goes into a business plan. There is also computer software for writing the business plan. You may choose to consult a professional, such as an accountant or a small-business consultant. If you are not sure where to find these professionals, ask other business owners for recommendations, or call your city's chamber of commerce or Small Business Alliance.

In this crucial early stage, make sure you ask for enough working capital to open your salon and to keep you afloat long enough to build the business. You may think that when you leave your current situation you will be able to take all your clients with you, thereby ensuring enough of a cash flow to pay your bills. It is more likely, however, that not all your current clients will make the transition, so you will need to allow time to rebuild your clientele. In addition, you are now solely responsible for all expenses, so you will need a cushion of funds to protect you if you are caught off guard by any unplanned business expenses. One or two surprises can kill a new business.

Regulations, Business Laws, and Insurance

When you decide to open your salon or to rent a booth, you are responsible for complying with local, state, and federal regulations and laws. Since the laws vary from state to state, it is important that you contact your local authorities regarding business licenses and other regulations. In general, you must contact your local (city) officials regarding any building renovations and business codes. Sales taxes, licenses, and employee compensation are covered by state laws. Federal laws cover the payment of Social Security, unemployment compensation or insurance, and cosmetics and luxury tax payments.

When you open your business, you will need to purchase insurance. Insurance covers malpractice, premises liability, fire, burglary and theft, and business interruption. You will need to have disability policies as well. Make sure your policies cover you for all the monetary demands you will have to meet on your lease.

Finally, you must know and comply with all federal OSHA guidelines, including those that require the ingredients of cosmetic preparations (including permanent wave solutions and hair tints) be displayed prominently for clients. OSHA distributes MSDS sheets for this purpose. Refer to Chapter 5 for a more complete discussion of MSDS sheets.

Types of Salon Ownership

A salon can be owned and operated by an individual, a partnership, or a corporation. Before deciding which type of ownership is most desirable, research each thoroughly. There are excellent reference tools available, and you can also consult an attorney for advice.

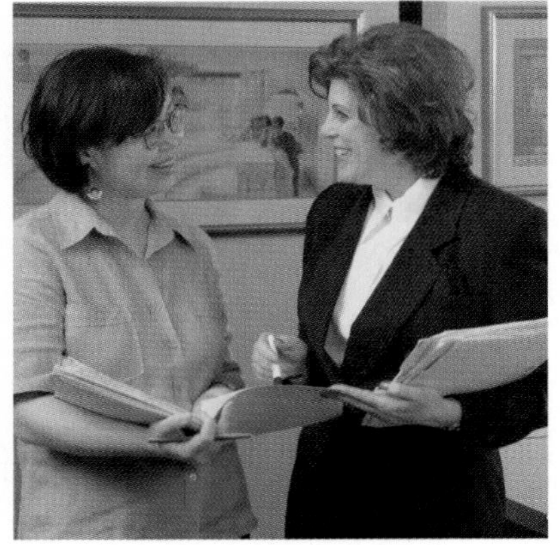

Figure 24-3 Partners share the work and the responsibilities.

Individual Ownership

- The **proprietor** is the owner and manager.
- The proprietor determines policies and has the last say in decision-making.
- The proprietor assumes expenses, receives profits, and bears all losses.

If you like to make your own rules and are responsible enough to meet all the duties and obligations of running a business, individual ownership may be the best arrangement for you.

Partnership

- Two or more people share ownership in a **partnership**, although not necessarily equally. One reason for going into a partnership arrangement is to have more capital for investment.
- Two or more people pool their skills and talents, making it easier to share work, responsibilities, and decision-making (Figure 24–3).
- Each partner assumes the other's unlimited liability for debts.

Partnerships may mean more opportunity for increased investment and growth. They can be magical if the right chemistry is struck, or they can be disastrous if you find yourself linked with someone you wish you had known better in the first place.

Corporation

- Ownership is shared by three or more people called stockholders.
- A charter, required by the state, identifies each individual in the new entity called the **corporation**.
- A corporation is subject to taxation and regulation by the state.

- Management is in the hands of a board of directors who determine policies and make decisions in accordance with the corporation's charter.
- The division of profits is proportionate to the number of shares owned by each stockholder.
- The stockholders cannot lose more than their original investment in the corporation.

There are many corporately owned salons in the beauty business today. They generally employ large numbers of stylists and can offer excellent benefits and opportunities. 3

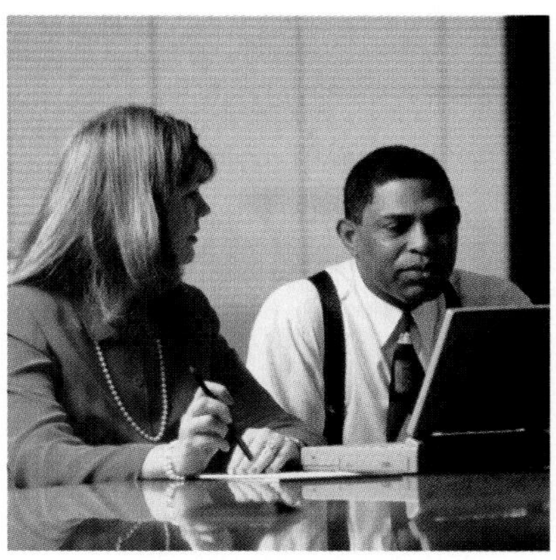

Figure 24–4 A lawyer is a good source of professional advice.

Purchasing an Established Salon

Purchasing an existing salon could be an excellent opportunity, but, as with anything else, you have to look at all sides of the picture. For instance, you may think you are buying an established clientele, but you may, in fact, lose some customers who will see this as an opportunity to try a new salon. You will also probably be buying used fixtures, which could save you a lot of money; on the other hand, you cannot be completely sure of what you are buying. You could, however, work out warranty arrangements with the seller to offer you some protection.

If you choose to buy an established salon, seek professional assistance from an accountant and a lawyer (Figure 24–4). In general, any agreement to buy an established salon should include the following:

- A written purchase and sale agreement to avoid any misunderstandings between the contracting parties.
- A complete and signed statement of inventory (goods, fixtures, and the like) indicating the value of each article.
- If there is a transfer of a note, mortgage, lease, and bill of sale, the buyer should initiate an investigation to determine if there is any default in the payment of debts.
- Identity of owner.
- Use of the salon's name and reputation for a definite period of time.
- Disclosure of any and all information regarding the salon's clientele and its purchasing and service habits.
- A statement regarding competition stating that the seller will not compete with the new owner within a specified distance from the present location.

Drawing Up a Lease

In many cases, owning your own business does not mean that you own the building that houses your business. When renting or leasing space, you must have an agreement between yourself and the building's owner that has been well thought out and well written. The lease should specify clearly who owns what and who is responsible for which repairs and expenses. You should also secure the following:

- An exemption of fixtures or appliances that might be attached to the salon so that they can be removed without violating the lease.

- An agreement about necessary renovations and repairs, such as painting, plumbing, fixtures, and electrical installation.
- An option from the landlord that allows you to assign the lease to another person. In this way, the obligations for the payment of rent are kept separate from the responsibilities of operating the business should you need to bring in another person or owner.

Protection Against Fire, Theft, and Lawsuits

- Keep the premises securely locked.
- Purchase liability, fire, malpractice, and burglary insurance, and do not allow these policies to lapse while you intend to remain in business.
- Do not violate the medical practice laws of your state by attempting to diagnose, treat, or cure a disease or illness. Always refer your client to a physician for diagnosis and treatment.
- Become thoroughly familiar with all laws governing cosmetology and with the sanitary codes of your city and state.
- Keep accurate records of the number of employees, their salaries, lengths of employment, and Social Security numbers as required by various state and federal laws that monitor the social welfare of workers.

Ignorance of the law is no excuse for violating it. Always check with your regulatory agency if you have any questions about a law or regulation.

Business Operation

Whether you are an owner or a manager, there are certain skills you must develop in order to successfully run a salon. To run a people-oriented business, you need excellent business sense, knowledge of sound business principles, ability, good judgment, and diplomacy. It takes time to develop these skills. As a new business owner, the best thing you can do is establish a circle of contacts—business owners, if not specifically salon owners—on whose experience you can draw. Consider joining a local entrepreneur group or your city's chamber of commerce to extend the reach of your networking.

Smooth business management depends on the following factors:

- *Sufficient investment capital.* Before you open your business, determine how much money, or **capital**, you will need to run it for at least the first two years. Many small businesses fail because their plans and their capital funds are not well matched.
- *Efficiency of management.* How many times have you been delighted to see a business open up nearby, thinking it was just what the neighborhood needed, only to see it close after a few months? Even the best business ideas cannot withstand poor management decisions or business operations. Managers must make informed business decisions. If they do not have the experience or expertise, they should consult other sources before it is too late.
- *Good business procedures.* Nothing can erode a client base faster than a business that does not follow specific procedures for the services it offers or one that does not monitor quality control. Following good business procedures includes everything from complying with local, state, and federal laws to managing cash flow and buying inventory responsibly. Quality control means that when clients come to the salon, they can

reasonably expect services to be performed to the same high standards every time.

- *Cooperation between management and employees.* No business can remain in existence very long if employees and managers do not show respect for one another and a true desire to work together harmoniously. If you are having difficulties with employees, do not expect these difficulties to resolve themselves. Do your best to address the problems and resolve them quickly, thoroughly, and diplomatically. Your business success depends on your ability to do this, even if it means finding and training new employees.
- *Trained and experienced salon personnel.* In order to provide excellent service that will keep clients coming back to your salon, all your employees should be trained to the same high level (Figure 24–5). As the salon owner, you should be an example to your employees when it comes to learning and bettering your technical, business, and interpersonal skills.
- *Pricing of services.* Cost of services is generally established according to the location of the salon and the type of clientele you expect to serve. Keep a price list posted where it can be seen by all clients, usually at the reception desk. The salon's pricing strategy should meet the level and quality of service provided. Be sure to monitor what your competition is charging for comparable services and goods and remain competitive in your pricing (Figure 24–6).

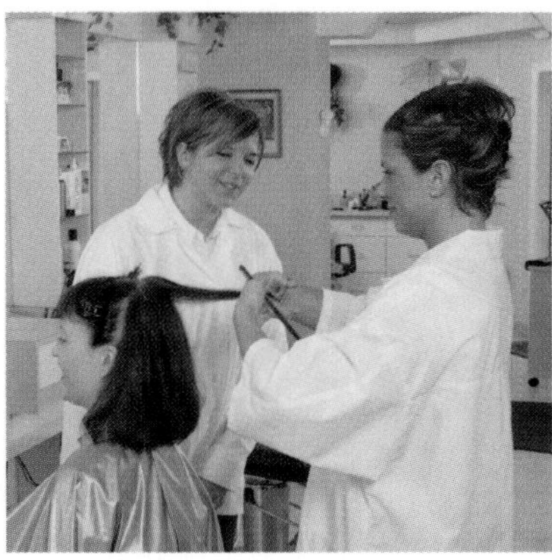

Figure 24-5 Teaching a new stylist how to cross-check a haircut.

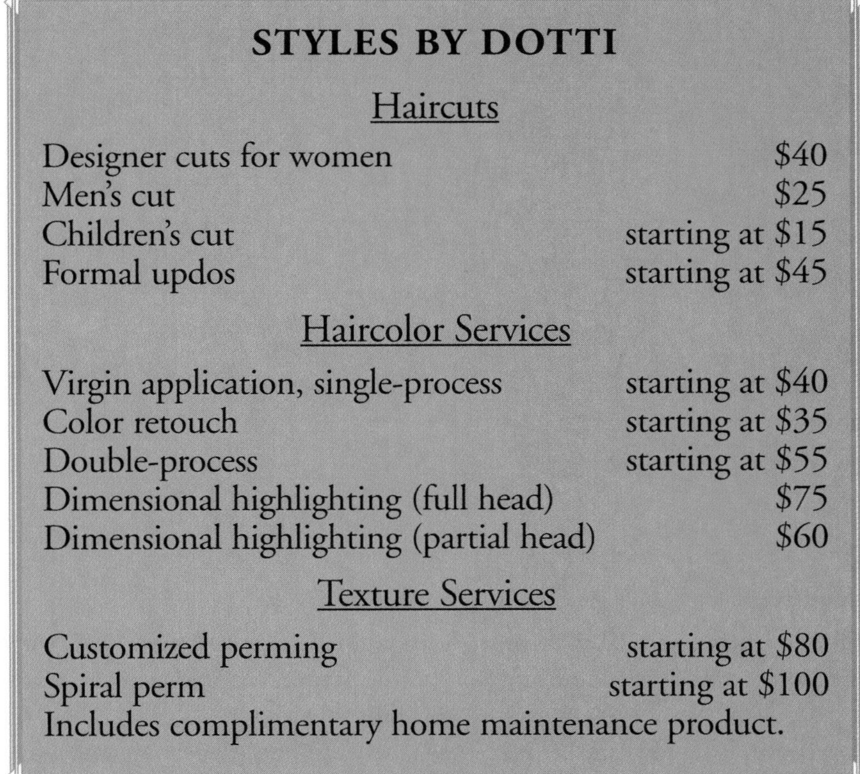

STYLES BY DOTTI

Haircuts

Designer cuts for women	$40
Men's cut	$25
Children's cut	starting at $15
Formal updos	starting at $45

Haircolor Services

Virgin application, single-process	starting at $40
Color retouch	starting at $35
Double-process	starting at $55
Dimensional highlighting (full head)	$75
Dimensional highlighting (partial head)	$60

Texture Services

Customized perming	starting at $80
Spiral perm	starting at $100

Includes complimentary home maintenance product.

Figure 24-6 A typical salon price list.

Expenses	Percent of Total Gross Income
Salaries and commissions (including payroll taxes)	53.5
Rent	13.0
Supplies	5.0
Advertising	3.0
Depreciation	3.0
Laundry	1.0
Cleaning	1.0
Light and power	1.0
Repairs	1.5
Insurance	.75
Telephone	.75
Miscellaneous	1.5
Total expenses	85.0
Net profit	15.0
Total	100.0

Table 24–1 Average Expenses for Salons in the United States

24

Allocation of Money

As a business operator, you must always know where your money is being spent. A good accountant and accounting system are indispensable. The figures in Table 24–1 serve as a guideline but may vary depending on locality. In large towns, and cities, items such as rent might run higher, while in small towns, rents might be lower but utilities and telephone rates could be higher.

The Importance of Record-Keeping

Good business operation requires a simple and efficient record system. Proper business records are necessary to meet the requirements of local, state, and federal laws regarding taxes and employees. Records are of value only if they are correct, concise, and complete. Proper bookkeeping methods include keeping an accurate record of all income and expenses. Income is usually classified as receipts from services and retail sales. Expenses include rent, utilities, insurance, salaries, advertising, equipment, and repairs. Retain check stubs, canceled checks, receipts, and invoices. A professional accountant is recommended to help keep records accurate.

You must record all business transactions in order to:

- determine income, expenses, profit, or loss.
- assess the value of the salon for prospective buyers.
- arrange a bank loan or financing.
- provide necessary data on income tax, Social Security, unemployment and disability insurance, accidents, and for percentage payments of gross income required in some leases.

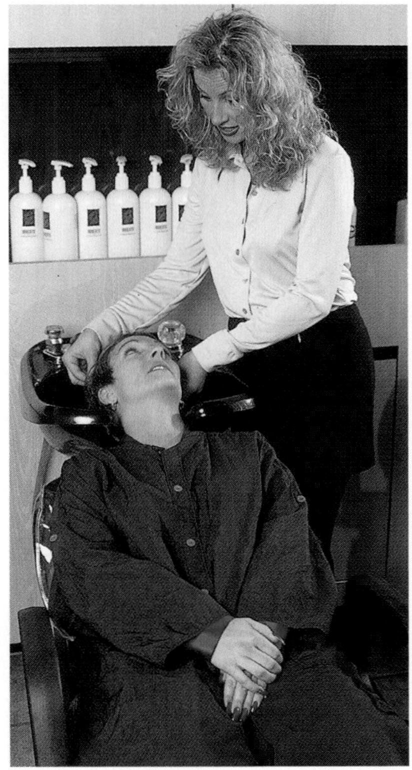

Figure 24–7 Consumption supplies at the shampoo station.

Weekly and Monthly Records

Certain financial records are best kept on a weekly or monthly basis, so that you can:

- make comparisons with other years.
- detect any changes in demands for services.
- check on the use of materials according to the type of service rendered.
- control expenses and waste.

Daily Records

Keeping daily records enables the owner or manager to know just how well the business is functioning. Each expense item affects the total gross income. Accurate records show the cost of operation in relation to income. Keep daily sales slips, appointment book, and a petty cash book for reference when completing your income tax reports. Your accountant will tell you how long to keep these documents. Payroll book, canceled checks, and monthly and yearly records are usually held for at least seven years. Service and inventory records are also important to keep.

Purchase and Inventory Records

An area that should be closely monitored is the purchase of inventory and supplies. Purchase records help maintain a perpetual inventory, which prevents overstock or shortage of needed supplies, and also alert you to any incidents of pilfering (petty theft by employees). These records also help establish the net worth of the business at the end of the year.

Keep a running inventory of all supplies and classify them according to their use and retail value. Those to be used in the daily business operation are **consumption supplies** (Figure 24–7). Those to be sold to clients are **retail supplies**.

Inventory records can tell you which merchandise sells most quickly and which does not. You can then judge how much of each product to order so that it can be used or sold within a reasonable period of time. It is better to have slightly more than "just enough" supplies. Try to plan major purchases around those times when distributors or supply stores offer special prices and other incentives.

Service Records

Always keep service records or client cards that describe treatments given and merchandise sold to each client. Either a card file system or memorandum book kept in a central location will serve this purpose. All service records should include the name and address of the client, the date of each purchase or service, the amount charged, products used, and results obtained. Clients' preferences and tastes should also be noted. For more information on filling out these cards and for examples of a client record card, refer to Chapter 4. 4

OPERATING A SUCCESSFUL SALON

There is only one way to guarantee that you will stay in business and have a prosperous salon, and that is to take excellent care of your clients. Clients visiting your salon should feel they are being well taken care of and look forward to their next visit. To accomplish this, your salon should be physically attractive, well organized, smoothly run, and, above all, sparkling clean.

Planning the Salon's Layout

One of the most exciting opportunities ahead of you is planning and constructing the best physical layout for the type of salon you envision. Maximum efficiency should be the primary concern. For example, if you are opening a low-budget salon offering quick service, you will need several stations for operators to work at and a small- to medium-sized reception area since clients will be moving in and out of the salon fairly quickly. Your retail area may also be on the small side, since your clients may not have a lot of disposable income to spend on retail products (**Figure 24–8**).

However, if you are opening a more luxurious day spa, where clients expect the quality of the service to be matched by the environment, you will want to plan for more room in the waiting areas. You may, in fact, choose to have several areas in which clients can lounge between services with beverages or light snacks. Some upscale salons feature small coffee bars that lend an air of sophistication to the environment. Others offer quiet, private areas where clients can pursue business activities such as phone work or laptop activities between services. This type of salon also requires several private treatment rooms and a comfortable changing area. The retail area should be spacious, inviting, and well lit.

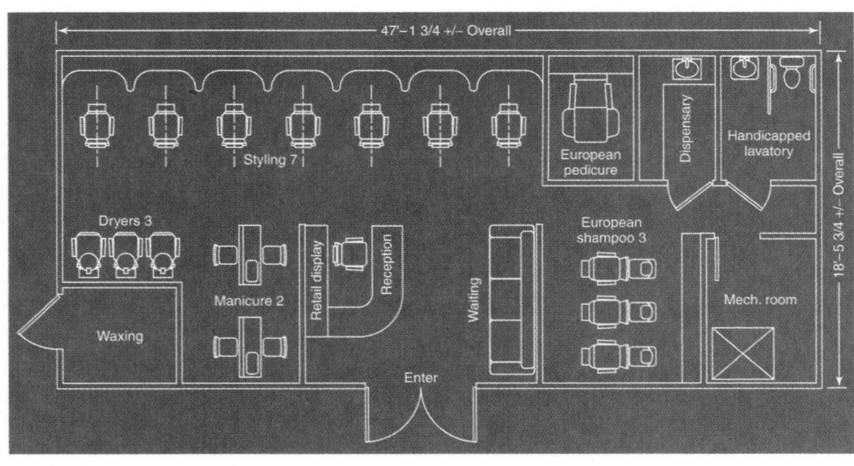

Figure 24-8 A layout for a typical salon.

As you can see, layout is crucial to the smooth operation of a salon. Once you have decided the type of salon you wish to run, seek the advice of an architect. For minor renovations, a professional equipment and furniture supplier might be able to help you.

Regardless of the type of salon you plan to open, the goal is maximum efficiency. A few things to keep in mind when planning layout are:

- flow and volume of operational services to and from the reception area.
- adequate aisle space.
- adequate space for equipment, such as hair dryers and heat lamps.
- furniture, fixtures, and equipment chosen on the basis of cost, durability, utility, and appearance.
- a color scheme that is restful, flattering, and expressive of the mood and purpose of the salon you envision.
- adequate and appropriate lighting to help achieve the most flattering look when performing haircolor and makeup applications and other services.
- a dispensary or "back room" (Figure 24–9).
- storage space for products and additional equipment or furniture that may not be needed at all times.
- a restroom for clients and employees.
- good plumbing and lighting to ensure satisfactory services.
- good ventilation, air conditioning, and heating, especially if you plan to offer manicure and nail extension services.
- adequate closets and changing areas for clients.

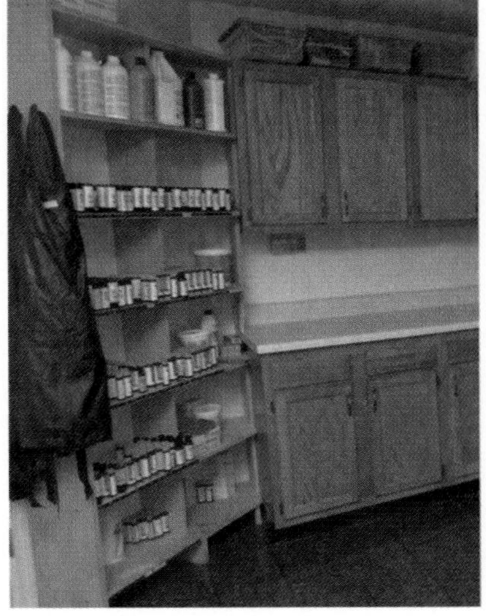

Figure 24-9 A salon dispensary.

Personnel

The size of your salon will determine the size of your staff. Large salons and day spas require receptionists, hairstylists, manicurists, shampoo persons, colorists, massage therapists, facials specialists, and hair removal specialists.

Smaller salons have some combination of these **personnel** who perform more than one service. For example, the stylist might also be the colorist and texture specialist.

The success of a salon depends on the quality of the work done by the staff. When interviewing potential employees, consider the following:

- level of skill
- personal grooming
- image as it relates to the salon (are they too progressive or too conservative for your environment?)
- overall attitude (do they seem more negative than positive in their responses to your questions?)
- communication skills (are they able to understand your questions and can you understand their responses?)
- the clients they will bring with them

Making good hiring decisions is crucial; undoing bad hiring decisions is painful to all involved and can be more complicated than you might expect.

Payroll and Employee Benefits

In order to have a successful business, one in which everyone feels appreciated and is happy to work hard and service clients, you must be willing to share your success with your staff whenever it is financially feasible to do so. You can do this in a number of ways.

- Make it your top priority to meet your payroll obligations. In the allotment of funds, this comes first.
- Whenever possible, offer hardworking and loyal employees as many benefits as possible and cover the cost of these benefits. If your financial situation does not allow you to cover the entire cost of these benefits, at least make them available to employees and allow them to decide if they can cover the cost themselves. Although employees may

24

activity

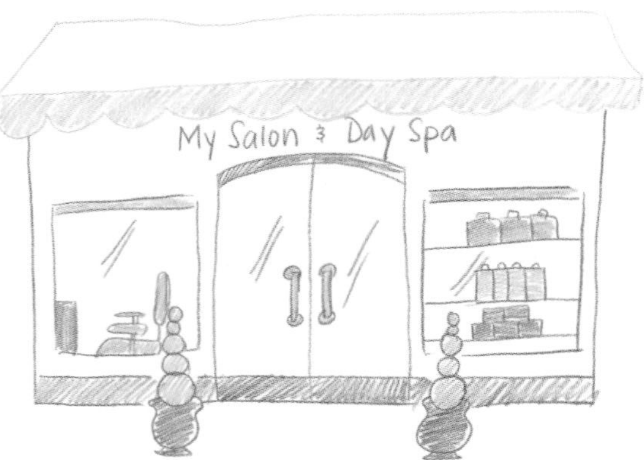

Figure 24-10 What does your dream salon look like?

What would your "dream salon" look like? Try your hand at designing a salon that would attract the kinds of clients you want, offer the services you would like to specialize in, and provide an efficient, comfortable working environment for cosmetologists. Draw pictures, use word pictures, or try a combination of both. Pay attention to practical requirements, but feel free to dream a little, too. Skylights? Fountains? An employee exercise room? You name it. It's your dream! (Figure 24–10)

have to pay their own way, group policies, especially for health insurance, are generally less expensive than individual policies.

- Provide staff members with a schedule of employee evaluations. Make it clear what is expected of them if they are to receive pay increases.
- Create and stay with a tipping policy. It is a good idea both for your employees and your clients to know exactly what is expected.
- If offering a commission system instead of a salary, be sure to put it into writing, with a copy to each employee should questions arise.
- Create incentives by giving your staff opportunities to earn more money, prizes, or tickets to educational events and trade shows.
- Create salon policies and stick to them. Everyone in the salon should be governed by the same rules, and that includes you!

Managing Personnel

As a new salon owner, one of your most difficult tasks will be to manage personnel (your employees or staff). But this can also be very rewarding. If you are good at managing others, you can make a positive impact on the lives of your employees and their ability to earn a living. If managing people does not come naturally to you, do not despair. People can learn how to manage, just as they learn how to drive a car or overcome fears. Keep in mind that managing others is a serious job, and whether it comes naturally to you or not, it takes time to become comfortable with the role. Here are some tips for becoming an effective manager.

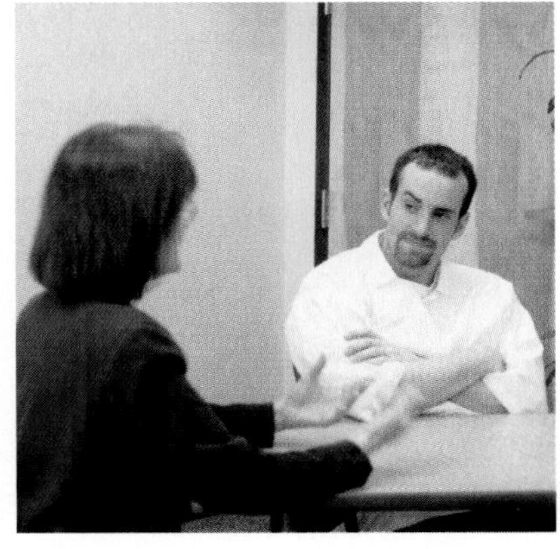

Figure 24–11 Providing feedback to employees is part of managing a salon.

- *Always be honest with employees.* Tell them immediately what you are thinking, whether it is positive or negative. Unless clients are present, it is not a good idea to wait before providing feedback, as the impact of your thoughts and words may diminish as time goes by (Figure 24–11).
- *Expect the best.* Always give your employees the benefit of the doubt and expect the best intentions from them. Never jump automatically to a negative conclusion. Most times, you will find that employees really are trying to be helpful, even if they do not quite know how to go about accomplishing it. Also, make it your practice to recognize your employees' efforts and to thank them for their good work. "You did a great cut on Mrs. Lim" or "I really appreciate your staying late today" will be welcome words to your employees' ears.
- *Be a mentor.* When you hire employees, you will be viewed as an experienced veteran, so it is your responsibility to help, guide, and mentor them whenever possible. The benefits are not only increased harmony and loyalty, but should these employees move on, you and they can share the experience of being in a growing network of professional colleagues in your area.
- *Share information.* There is no better way to help employees feel they are part of the process than to share information with them regarding important salon decisions that need to be made. Share only appropriate information with the staff. Too much information, if it is not the correct kind, can cause unnecessary concern and worry.

- *Follow the rules.* Just as you will expect your employees to follow the rules you set for them and for the salon, so too must you follow the rules and provide a good example. If you find your own rules too burdensome, imagine how your employees feel.
- *Be reliable.* Never make a promise you cannot deliver. Your employees need to believe you are reliable. They need to know you will come through for them.
- *Teach them what you know.* When you find yourself in the position to make management decisions that are of significance to the entire salon, explain your thinking behind these decisions, and include your employees in the decision-making process when appropriate. This way, your employees will learn how many factors must enter every decision. Their respect will go far in strengthening your relationship.

The Front Desk

Most salon owners believe that the quality and pricing of the services are the most important elements of running a successful salon. Certainly these are crucial, but too often the front desk—the "operations center"—is overlooked. The best salons employ professional receptionists to handle the job of scheduling appointments and greeting clients.

The Reception Area

First impressions count, and since the reception area is the first thing clients see, it needs to be attractive, appealing, and comfortable. Here is where your receptionist will sit, where your retail merchandise will be on display, where your dressing area may be located, and where your phone system is centered. In other words, the reception area is the salon's nerve center. Make sure the reception area is stocked with business cards and a prominently displayed price list that shows at a glance what your clients should expect to pay for various services. 5

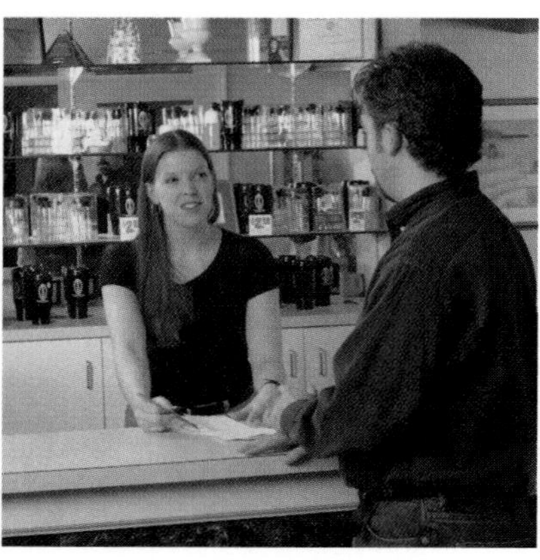

Figure 24–12 A good receptionist is key to a salon's success.

24

The Receptionist

Second only in importance to your stylists is your receptionist. A well-trained receptionist is the "quarterback" of the salon and will be the first person the client will see on arrival. The receptionist should be pleasant, greeting each client with a smile and addressing her by name. Efficient service fosters good will, confidence, and satisfaction.

In addition to filling the crucial role of greeter, the receptionist handles other important functions, including answering the phone, booking appointments, informing the stylist that a client has arrived, preparing the daily appointment information for the staff, and recommending other services to the client. The receptionist should have a thorough knowledge of all of the retail products the salon carries, so that she can also serve as a salesperson and information source for clients (Figure 24–12).

During slow periods, it is customary for the receptionist to perform certain other duties and activities, such as straightening up the reception area and maintaining inventory and daily reports. The receptionist should also reserve these slow times for making any necessary personal calls or otherwise being away from the front desk.

Booking Appointments

One of the most important duties the receptionist has is booking appointments. This must be done with care, as services are sold in terms of time on the appointment page. Appointments must be scheduled to make the most efficient use of everyone's time. Under ideal circumstances, a client should not have to wait for a service, and a stylist should not have to wait for the next client.

Booking appointments may be the main job of the receptionist, but when she is not available, the salon owner or manager, or any of the stylists, can help with scheduling. Therefore, it is important for each person in the salon to understand how to book an appointment and how much time is needed for each service.

Regardless of who actually makes the appointment, anyone who answers the phone or deals with clients must have a pleasing voice and personality. In addition, the receptionist must have the following qualities.

- *An attractive appearance.* Since the salon will, to some degree, be judged by the way the employees look, the receptionist's hairstyle and makeup should be contemporary and flattering, reflecting the work of the salon.
- *Knowledge of the various services offered.* The receptionist should have a thorough knowledge of all the services the salon offers, their cost, and how much time they take.
- *Unlimited patience with both clients and salon personnel.* The receptionist will be busy, often very busy, at the front desk. Even so, she must be able to work with clients who may need extra time or cannot make decisions about the services retail products they want. The receptionist may also need to help staff members with telephone calls or other issues that may tax her time. Patience and graciousness are crucial to making this position work.

Appointment Book

The appointment book helps stylists arrange time to suit their clients' needs. It should accurately reflect what is taking place in the salon at any given time. In most salons, the receptionist prepares the appointment schedule for staff members; in smaller salons, each person may prepare his own schedule (Figure 24–13).

The appointment book may be an actual book that sits atop the reception desk or it may be a computerized appointment book that is easily accessed through the salon's computer system.

Use of the Telephone in the Salon

An important part of the salon business is handled over the telephone. Good telephone habits and techniques make it possible for the salon owner and stylists to increase business and improve relationships with clients and

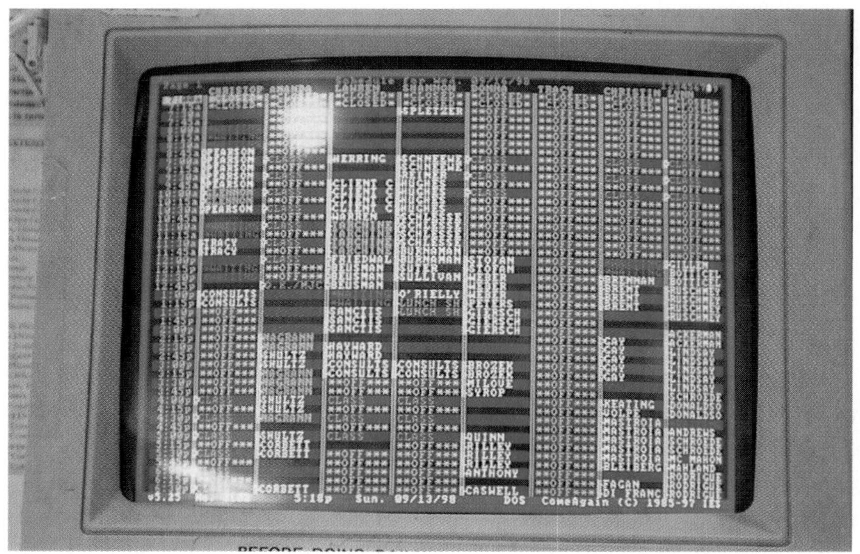

Figure 24-13 A computerized appointment book.

suppliers. With each call, a gracious, appropriate response will help build the salon's reputation.

The telephone is used to:

- make or change appointments.
- seek new business.
- try to determine why you have lost a client.
- remind clients of their appointments.
- answer questions and provide friendly service.
- handle complaints to the client's satisfaction.
- receive messages.
- order equipment and supplies.

Good Planning

The telephone is usually located at the reception desk. Because it can be noisy, business calls to clients and suppliers should be made at a quiet time of the day or from a telephone placed in a quieter area of the salon.

When using the telephone, you should:

- have a pleasant telephone voice, speak clearly, and use correct grammar. A "smile" in your voice counts for a lot.
- show interest and concern when talking with a client or a supplier.
- be polite, respectful, and courteous to all, even though some people may test the limits of your patience.
- be tactful. Do not say anything to irritate the person on the other end of the line.
- plan what is to be said during the call. Make a list of the main points you want to discuss. Knowing what you want to say in advance will help you

project an image of confidence and efficiency. It is also useful to jot down key points of the other person's responses or questions. That can help you address the speaker's concerns.

Incoming Telephone Calls

Incoming phone calls are the lifeline of a salon. Clients usually call ahead for appointments with a preferred stylist, or they might call to cancel or reschedule an appointment. The person answering the phone should develop the necessary telephone skills to handle these calls.

In addition, here are some guidelines for answering the telephone.

- When you answer the phone, say, "Good morning (afternoon or evening), Milady Salon. May I help you?" or "Thank you for calling Milady Salon. This is Jane speaking. How may I help you?" Some salons require that you give your name to the caller. The first words you say tell the caller something about your personality. Let callers know that you are glad to hear from them.
- Answer the phone promptly. On a system with more than one line, if a call comes in while you are talking on another line, ask to put the person on hold, answer the second call, and ask that person to hold while you complete the first call. Take calls in the order in which they came.
- If you do not have the information requested by a caller, either put the caller on hold and get the information, or offer to call the person back with the information as soon as you have it.
- Do not talk with a client standing nearby while you are speaking with someone on the phone. You are doing a disservice to both clients.

Booking Appointments by Phone

When booking appointments, take down the client's first and last name, phone number, and service booked. Many salons call the client to confirm the appointment one or two days before it is scheduled.

You should be familiar with all the services and products available in the salon and their costs, as well as which cosmetologists perform specific services such as color correction. Be fair when making assignments. Try not to schedule six appointments for one stylist and only two for another. However, if someone calls to ask for an appointment with a particular cosmetologist on a particular day and time, every effort should be made to accommodate the client's request. If the stylist is not available when the client requests, there are several ways to handle the situation:

- suggest other times that the stylist is available
- if the client cannot come in at any of those times, suggest another stylist
- if the client is unwilling to try another stylist, offer to call the client if there is a cancellation at the desired time

Handling Complaints by Telephone

Handling complaints, particularly over the phone, is a difficult task. The caller is probably upset and short-tempered. Respond with self-control, tact, and courtesy, no matter how trying the circumstances. Only then will the caller be made to feel that she has been fairly treated.

The tone of your voice must be sympathetic and reassuring. Your manner of speaking should convince the caller that you are really concerned about the complaint. Do not interrupt the caller. After hearing the complaint in full, try to resolve the situation quickly and effectively. The following are suggestions for dealing with some kinds of problems.

- Tell the unhappy client that you are sorry for what happened and explain the reason for the difficulty. Assure the client that the problem will not happen again.
- Sympathize by saying that you understand and that you regret the inconvenience suffered. Express appreciation that the person has called this matter to your attention.
- Ask the client how the salon can remedy the situation. If the request is fair and reasonable, check with the owner or manager for approval.
- If the client is dissatisfied with the results of a service, suggest another visit to the salon to see what can be done to remedy the problem.
- If a client is dissatisfied with the behavior of a stylist, call the owner or manager to the phone.

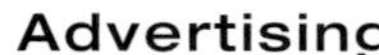

Advertising

A new salon owner will want to get business up and running as soon as possible to start earning some revenue and begin to pay off debts. One of the first things the new salon owner should consider is how to advertise the salon. It is important to understand the many aspects of advertising.

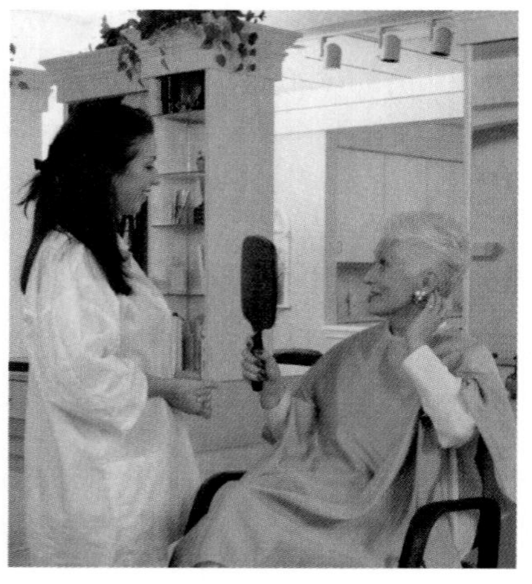

Figure 24–14 Customer satisfaction is your best advertising.

- Advertising includes all activities that promote the salon favorably from a newspaper ad to radio spots to a charity event, such as a fashion show that the salon participates in.
- Advertising must attract and hold the attention of readers, listeners, or viewers so as to create a desire for a service or product. In general, the best form of paid advertising for the salon business remains newspaper and local radio ads.
- A satisfied client is the very best form of advertising, because she will refer your salon to friends and family. So make your customers happy! (Figure 24–14)
- If you have some experience developing ads, you may decide to do your own advertising. If, however, you need help, you can hire a small local agency or ask a local newspaper or radio station to help you produce the ad.
- As a general rule, an advertising budget should not exceed 3 percent of your gross income. Try to concentrate your advertising on those slow periods that inevitably occur.
- Plan well in advance for holidays and special yearly events such as proms, New Year's Eve, or the wedding season.

Here are some advertising venues that may prove fruitful for you.

- *Newspapers.* This is generally the most cost-effective way to advertise. If you use a coupon in your ad, you can track how many new or returning clients your advertising has attracted (Figure 24–15).
- *Direct mail.* This is a great way to target those potential clients for whom your salon has been conceived. Mailing lists are available through local direct marketers and chambers of commerce. Also make sure you have the name, address, and phone number of every client who walks into the salon to add to your mailing list. The quality of your direct mail pieces should reflect the kind of client you wish to attract. If you are planning a budget operation, for instance, your mailing can look simple, with no frills, without detracting from its value. If you are opening a high-end salon, however, your direct mailing piece needs to be beautifully designed and produced.
- *Classified advertising.* A listing in the yellow pages of the local telephone book is a wonderful and relatively inexpensive way to reach lots of

Spring Specials
at
The Manor Day Spa

Celebrate the coming of spring!
Let us pamper you with one of our new deluxe packages

The Getaway:	Swedish massage, facial, manicure, pedicure, makeup, haircut and styling (includes complimentary lunch)	$200
The Refresher:	deep cleansing facial, makeup, haircut and styling	$100
Body Sensations:	aromatherapy massage, facial, makeup	$75
Tips and Toes:	spa manicure, hot stones pedicure	$55

Feb. 15 through May 15 only

Deep conditioning treatment with every haircolor service!

Call now to reserve an hour, two hours, or a whole day of relaxation and pampering at the Manor.

Bring in this ad to receive a 5% discount on any service.

The Manor Day Spa, 123 Main Street, Hometown, USA 12345
(300-555-1111)

Open Tuesday - Friday 10-6,
Saturday 10-4

Figure 24-15 A newspaper advertisement for services at a salon.

potential customers. Larger-size ads may be worth the additional expense as well.

- *Giveaway promotional items*. A salon that produces combs, emery boards, key chains, refrigerator magnets, calendars, or other giveaway promotional items is using its advertising budget wisely. These items often are carried around in a customer's purse or pocket and serve as daily reminders of the salon's existence.
- *Window display*. Making use of your salon's window is a great way to attract attention and to inform passersby of what is happening at the salon. Set up scenes with your retail products, use signs, or simply put a menu of service specials in the window.
- *Radio*. The radio is another terrific way to reach potential clients, since most people listen to the radio in their cars and at their offices. Radio advertising is more expensive than newspaper advertising and is not as easy to track, but it can be very effective.
- *Television*. TV is a high-impact but expensive way to advertise and probably will not be right for your salon for several years at least. You would use TV advertising only after you have established a solid client base and can really afford to be on TV consistently.
- *Community outreach*. Getting out to community events is an excellent means of advertising, especially through personal public appearances at women's and men's clubs, church functions, political gatherings, charitable affairs, and on TV and radio talk shows. Letting your market see that you and your business are involved in the community will make people feel they know you and may inspire them to patronize the salon. Volunteering your services at local bridal and fashion shows and speaking at high school career days are other effective ways of getting yourself in the public eye.
- *Client referrals*. Your current clients can help you get new clients if you ask them to help and give them small incentives for doing so, such as a 10 percent discount on services and retail purchases for each client they refer to the salon.
- *Contacting clients*. Your goal is to get and keep new clients. When you notice that a client has not been in the salon for a while, you may want to phone and invite him back in for a service. This can be a very effective practice. You should also consider seasonal greeting cards, giveaway calendars, and other ways to stay in touch with your clientele.
- *Telemarketing*. Using the telephone can be an effective way to tell your customers about products and services, so long as you are careful not to disturb clients at inopportune times. Keep in mind that many people react in a negative way to telemarketing, so it should be used wisely, if at all.
- *Videos*. You may receive videos or taped promotions from various distributors or product manufacturers. To promote your salon and its goods, why not show them in your reception area? Many clients enjoy watching them while waiting for their appointments. 7

SELLING IN THE SALON

An important aspect of the salon's financial success revolves around the sale of additional salon services and take-home or maintenance products. Whether you own or manage a large salon with several employees or you are a booth renter with only yourself to worry about, adding services or retail sales to your service ticket means additional dollars in your pocket and benefits everyone in the salon.

Hairstyling professionals, in general, seem to feel uncomfortable about having to make sales of products or additional services, and sometimes decide that they "just can't sell." It is important to work at overcoming this feeling. When stylists are reluctant to sell, it is often because they carry a negative stereotype of salespeople—pushy or aggressive—and they do not want to be seen this way themselves. While certainly there are salespeople like that, remember that there are also very helpful and knowledgeable sales professionals who make customer concern and care their top priority. These people play a major role in the lives of their customers and are very valuable to them because they offer good advice.

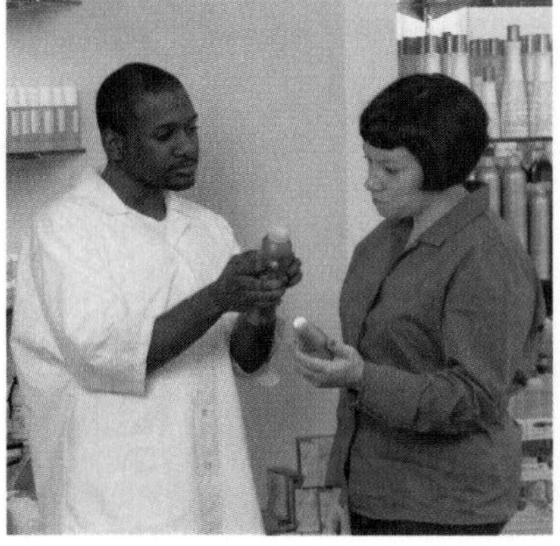

Figure 24-16 Selling retail products benefits everyone.

Work with your employees to develop their confidence at retailing. Suggest that they approach each client with sincere concern and recommend only what is truly in the client's best interest, even if such products may not be the most profitable for the salon at first (Figure 24–16). Once the client's trust and loyalty has been won, the salon—and the stylist—will undoubtedly gain financially as well, for the present and the future (see Chapter 26 for tips on retailing).

There is a tremendous opportunity to make sales in the salon today, especially as more and more products are added to salon operations. The person who is equally proficient as cosmetologist and salesperson is the one most likely to succeed in this business. As owner or manager of the salon, it is in your best interest to train and encourage your employees in the fine points of selling, thereby enhancing their morale, confidence, and self-esteem, and ensuring the salon's success.

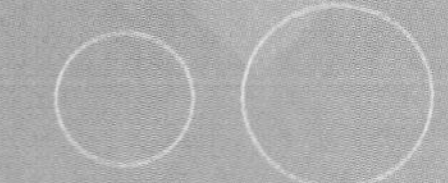

chapter glossary

booth rental	renting a booth or station in a salon (also known as chair rental)
business plan	a written plan of a business, as it is seen in the present and envisioned in the future
capital	the money needed to start a business
consumption supplies	supplies used in daily business operations
corporation	a business whose ownership is shared by three or more people called stockholders
demographics	information about the size, average income, and buying habits of the population
partnership	a business structure in which two or more people share ownership, although not necessarily equally
personnel	employees; staff
proprietor	the owner and manager of a business
retail supplies	supplies sold to clients

review questions

1. What are the two ways in which you may go into business for yourself?
2. List five factors to consider when opening a beauty salon.
3. Name three types of ownership under which a business may operate.
4. What purpose do accurate records serve?
5. What two types of supplies make up a beauty salon's inventory?
6. Why is the reception area of a salon important?
7. Why is the receptionist called the "quarterback" of the salon?
8. Explain the elements of good telephone technique.
9. List six different kinds of advertising.
10. What is the best form of advertising? Why?

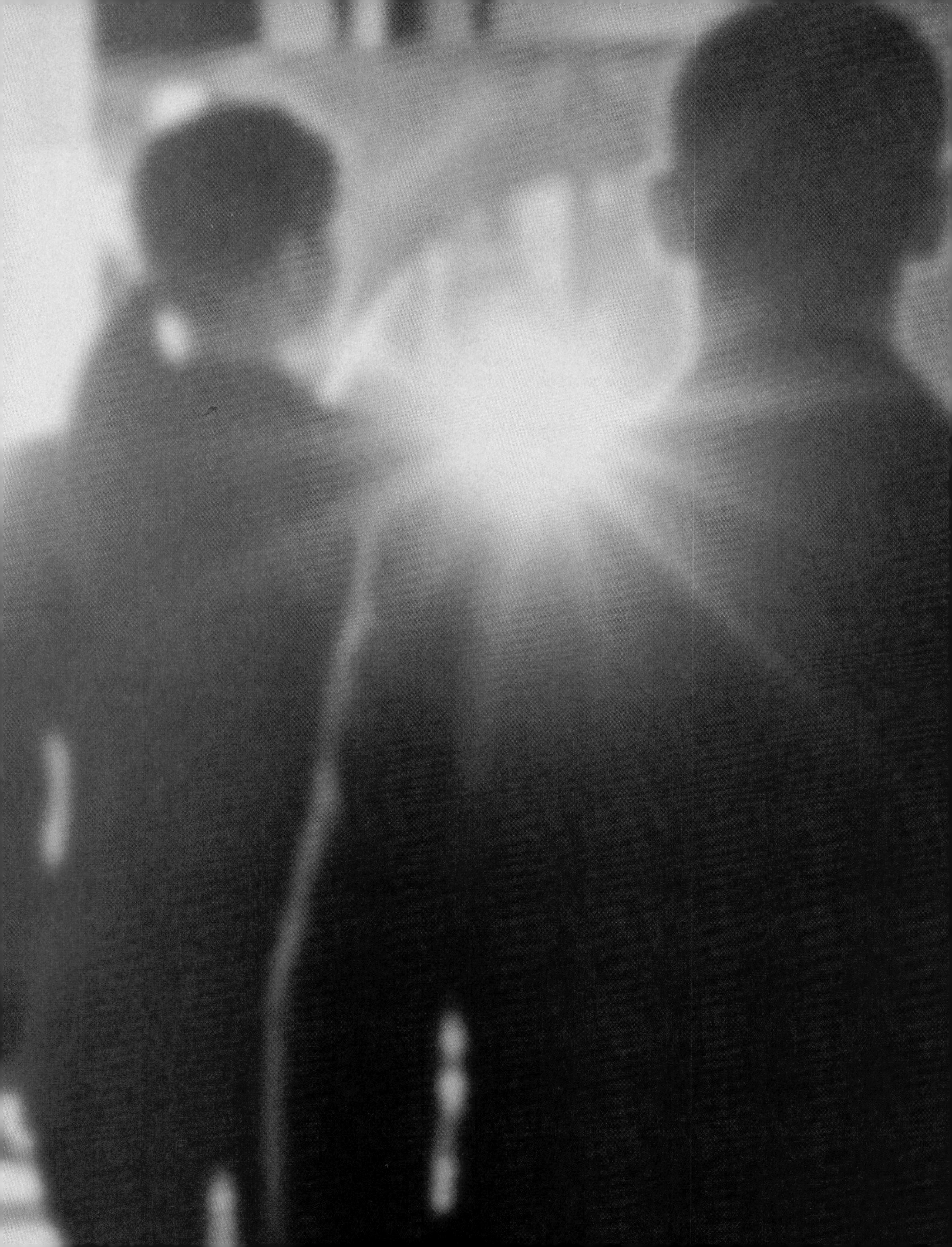

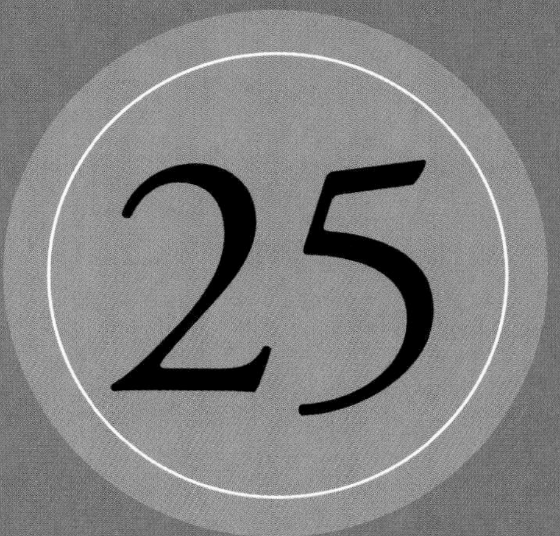

SEEKING EMPLOYMENT

Letha Barnes
COSMETOLOGY EDUCATOR AND DIRECTOR OF THE CAREER INSTITUTE

Chapter Outline

Preparing for Licensure • Preparing for Employment
You Are on Your Way • Doing It Right

Learning Objectives

After completing this chapter, you should be able to:

1. Discuss the essentials of becoming test-wise.
2. Explain the steps involved in preparing for employment.
3. List and describe the different types of salon businesses.
4. Write an achievement-oriented resume and prepare an employment portfolio.
5. Explain how to explore the job market and research potential employers.
6. Be prepared to complete an effective employment interview.

National Skill Standards

This chapter provides you with the necessary information to master this National Industry Skill Standard for Entry-Level Cosmetologists.

Participating in lifelong learning to stay current with trends, technology, and techniques pertaining to the cosmetology industry.

Key Terms

Page number indicates where in the chapter the term is used.

deductive reasoning
pg. 859

employment portfolio
pg. 872

resume
pg. 867

test-wise
pg. 858

transferable skills
pg. 870

work ethic
pg. 865

There is so much about cosmetology that works for you: the creative outlet, the community of stimulating people, the opportunity to make your clients look their best, the self-esteem that comes with knowing that you can do something well. There is only one piece still missing from this picture: the job.

The good news is that there are plenty of great jobs out there for energetic, hardworking, talented people. If you look at the top professionals in the field, you will find that they were not born successful; they achieved success with their motivation, energy, and persistence. Like you, these stylists first began by enrolling in cosmetology school, and they stuck with it. They were the ones who used their time wisely, planned for the future, went the extra mile, and drew on a reservoir of self-confidence to meet any challenge. They owe their success to no one but themselves, because they created it.

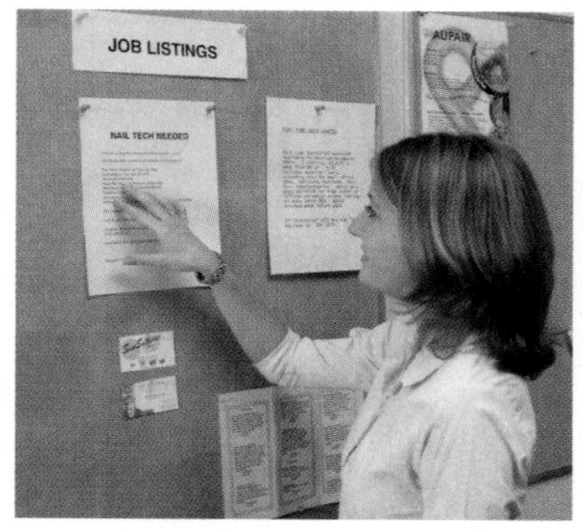

Figure 25–1 Job listings are often posted on the school bulletin board.

If you want to enjoy the same success as these top industry professionals, you need to be prepared for the opportunities that await you. That is why you are putting in your time in school and learning the basics of your craft. And look how much you already know! What you have learned will go a long way as you search out the "right" salon or establishment for you.

No matter what changes occur in the economy, there are often more jobs available for entry-level cosmetologists than there are people to fill them. This is a tremendous advantage for you. It does not mean, however, that you do not have to do thorough research before you take that giant first step and commit to your first job. If you choose the right first job, your career will be launched on the road to success. If you make the wrong choice, it will not be a tragedy, but it will be an unnecessary delay.
So let us discuss how to go about choosing the right first job (Figure 25–1).

PREPARING FOR LICENSURE

Before you can obtain the career position you are hoping for, you must first pass your state licensing examination and secure the required credentials. Many factors will affect how well you perform during that licensing examination and on tests in general. They include your physical and psychological state, your memory, time management, and the skills you have developed in reading, note-taking, writing, test-taking, and general learning.

Of all the factors that will affect your test performance, the most important is your mastery of course content. Even if you have truly learned the material, however, it will still benefit you greatly to have strong test-taking skills to draw on. Being test-wise means having a complete and thorough knowledge of your subject matter and understanding the strategies for taking tests successfully.

Preparing for the Test

A **test-wise** student begins to prepare for test-taking by practicing the daily habits and time management that are such an important part of effective studying. These habits include:

- having a planned, realistic study schedule.
- reading content carefully and becoming an active studier.
- keeping a well-organized notebook.
- developing a detailed vocabulary list.
- taking effective notes during class.
- organizing and reviewing handouts.
- reviewing past quizzes and tests.
- listening carefully in class for cues and clues about what can be expected on the test.

In addition, there are other, more holistic (having to do with "the whole you") hints to keep in mind. These include:

- making yourself mentally ready and developing a positive attitude toward taking the test.
- following a healthy diet to ensure that your body and mind are clear and ready.
- exercising regularly during the weeks prior to the test.
- getting plenty of rest the night before the test.
- dressing comfortably (if unsure of the weather or temperature, dress in layers so that you can adjust if necessary).
- anticipating some anxiety (feeling concerned about the test results may actually help you do better).
- avoiding cramming the night before an examination.

On Test Day

After you have taken all the necessary steps to prepare for your test, there are a number of strategies you can adopt on the day of the actual exam that may be helpful (Figure 25–2).

1. Relax and try to slow down physically. Take slow, deep breaths to calm yourself.
2. If possible, review the material lightly the day of the exam.
3. Arrive early with a self-confident attitude; be alert, calm, and ready for the challenge.
4. Read all written directions and listen carefully to all verbal directions before beginning.
5. Ask the test examiner questions if there is anything you do not understand.
6. Skim the entire test before beginning.
7. Budget your time to ensure that you have plenty of opportunity to complete the test; do not spend too much time on any one question.
8. Wear a watch so you can monitor the time.
9. Begin work as soon as possible and mark the answers in the test booklet carefully but quickly.
10. Answer the easiest questions first in order to save time for the more difficult ones. Quickly scanning all the questions first may clue you in to the more difficult questions.
11. Mark the questions you skip so you can find them again later.
12. Read each question carefully to make sure you know exactly what the question is asking and that you understand all the parts of the question.
13. Answer as many questions as possible; for questions you are unsure of, guess or estimate.
14. Look over the test when you are done to be sure you have read all questions correctly and have answered as many as possible.
15. Make changes to answers only if there is a good reason to do so.
16. Check the test booklet carefully before turning it in (for instance, you might have forgotten to put your name on it!).

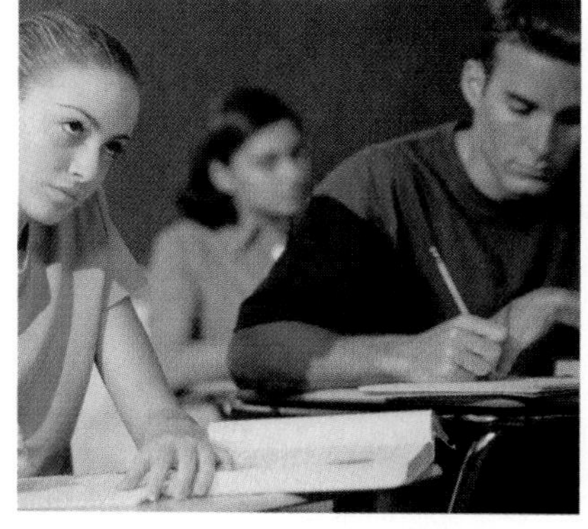

Figure 25–2 Candidates taking the licensing examination.

25

Deductive Reasoning

Another technique that students should learn to use for better test results is called **deductive reasoning**. Deductive reasoning is the process of reaching logical conclusions by employing logical reasoning.

Some strategies associated with deductive reasoning include:

- *Eliminating options known to be incorrect.* The more answers you can eliminate as incorrect, the better your chances of identifying the correct one.

- *Watching for "key" words or terms.* Look for any qualifying conditions or statements. Keep an eye out for such words and phrases as: *usually, commonly, in most instances, never, always,* and the like.
- *Studying the stem* (the basic question or problem). It will often provide a clue to the correct answer. Look for a match between the stem and one of the choices.
- *Watching for grammatical clues.* For instance, if the last word in a stem is "an," the answer must begin with a vowel rather than a consonant.
- *Looking at similar or related questions.* They may provide clues.
- In answering essay questions, watch for words such as *compare, contrast, discuss, evaluate, analyze, define,* or *describe* and develop your answer accordingly.
- In reading-type tests that contain long paragraphs followed by several questions, read the questions first. This will help identify the important elements in the paragraph.

Understanding Test Formats

There are a few additional tips that all test-wise learners should know, especially with respect to the state licensing examination. Keep in mind, of course, that the most important strategy of test-taking is to *know your material.* With that said, however, consider the following tips on the different kinds of question formats.

True/False

- Watch for qualifying words (*all, most, some, none, always, usually, sometimes, never, little, no, equal, less, good, bad*). Absolutes (*all, none, always, never*) are generally *not* true.
- For a statement to be true, the *entire* statement must be true.
- Long statements are more likely to be true than short statements. It takes more detail to provide truthful, factual information.

Multiple Choice

- Read the entire question carefully, including all the choices.
- Look for the best answer; more than one choice may be true.
- Eliminate incorrect answers by crossing them out (if taking the test on the test form).
- When two choices are close or similar, one of them is probably right.
- When two choices are identical, both must be wrong.
- When two choices are opposites, one is probably wrong and one is probably correct, depending on the number of other choices.
- "All of the above" types of responses are often the correct response.
- Pay special attention to words like *not, except, but.*
- Guess if you do not know the answer (providing there is no penalty).
- The answer to one question may be in the stem of another (Figure 25–3).

FINAL EXAM

1. The study of the hair is called:
   a) hairology — c) trichology
   b) dermatology — d) biology
2. Hair is not found on the palms of the hands, soles of the feet, lips, and:
   a) neck — c) ankles
   b) eyelids — d) wrists
3. The technical term for eyelash hair is:
   a) cilia — c) capilli
   b) barba — d) supercilia
4. Hair is composed chiefly of:
   a) oxygen — c) melanin
   b) keratin — d) sulfur
5. The two main divisions of the hair are the hair root and:
   a) hair shaft — c) papilla
   b) follicle — d) bulb
6. The hair root is located:
   a) above the skin surface — c) under the cuticle
   b) below the skin surface — d) within the cortex
7. The hair root is encased by a tubelike depression in the skin known as the:
   a) bulb — c) papilla
   b) arrector pili — d) follicle
8. The club-shaped structure that forms the lower part of the hair root is the:
   a) arrector pili — c) papilla
   b) bulb — d) hair shaft

Figure 25-3 Sample of a multiple-choice test.

Matching

- Read all items in each list before beginning.
- Check off items from the brief response list to eliminate choices.

Essays

- Organize your answer according to the cue words in the question.
- Think carefully and outline your answer before you begin writing.
- Make sure that what you write is complete, accurate, relevant to the question, well organized, and clear.

Remember that even though you may understand test formats and effective test-taking strategies, this does not take the place of having a complete understanding of the material on which you are being tested. In order to be successful at test-taking, you must follow the rules of effective studying and be thoroughly knowledgeable of the exam content for both the written and the practical examination.

In order to be better prepared for the practical portion of the examination, the new graduate should follow these tips.

- Practice the correct skills required in the test as often as you can.
- Participate in "mock" licensing examinations, including the timing of applicable examination criteria.
- Familiarize yourself with the content contained in the examination bulletins sent by the licensing agency.
- Make certain that all equipment and implements are clean, sanitary, and in good working order prior to the exam.
- If allowed by the regulatory or licensing agency, observe other practical examinations prior to taking yours.
- Locate the examination site the day before the exam to ensure that you are on time for the actual exam.
- As with any exam, listen carefully to the examiner's instructions and follow them explicitly.
- Focus on your own knowledge and do not allow yourself to be concerned with what other test candidates are doing.
- Follow all sanitation and safety procedures throughout the entire examination.

PREPARING FOR EMPLOYMENT

When you chose to enter the field of cosmetology, your primary goal was to find a good job after being licensed. Now you need to reaffirm that goal by reviewing a number of important questions. What do you really want out of a career in cosmetology? On what particular areas within the beauty industry do you wish to concentrate? What are your strongest practical skills and in what ways do you wish to use them? What personal qualities will help you have a successful career? One way you can answer these questions is to make a copy of, then complete the Personal Inventory of Characteristics and Skills (Figure 25–4).

After you have completed this inventory and have identified the areas that need further attention, you can then determine where to focus the remainder of your training. In addition, you should have a better idea of what type of establishment would best suit you for your eventual employment. During your training, you may have the opportunity to network with various industry professionals who are invited to be guest speakers. Be prepared to ask them questions about what they like least and most in their current positions. Ask them for any tips they might have that will assist you in your search for the right establishment. In addition, be sure to take advantage of your institution's in-house placement assistance program when you begin your employment search (Figure 25–5).

Your willingness to work hard is a key ingredient to your success. The commitment you make now in terms of time and effort will pay off later in

INVENTORY OF PERSONAL CHARACTERISTICS

PERSONAL CHARACTERISTIC	Exc.	Good	Avg.	Poor	Plan for Improvement
Posture, Deportment, Poise					
Grooming, Personal Hygiene					
Manners, Courtesy					
Communications Skills					
Attitude					
Self-Motivation					
Personal Habits					
Responsibility					
Self-esteem, Self Confidence					
Honesty, Integrity					
Dependability					

INVENTORY OF TECHNICAL SKILLS

TECHNICAL SKILLS	Exc.	Good	Avg.	Poor	Plan for Improvement
Hair shaping/cutting					
Hairstyling					
Hair Coloring					
Texture Services, Perming					
Texture Services, Relaxing					
Manicuring, Pedicuring					
Artificial Nail Extensions					
Skin Care, Facials					
Facial Makeup					
Other					

After analyzing the above responses, would you hire yourself as an employee in your firm? Why or why not?
State your short-term goals that you hope to accomplish in 6 to 12 months:
State your long-term goals that you hope to accomplish in 1 to 5 years:

Ask yourself: Do you want to work in a big city or small town? Are you compatible with a sophisticated, exclusive salon or a trendy salon? Which clientele are you able to communicate with more effectively? Do you want to start out slowly and carefully or do you want to jump in and throw everything into your career from the starting gate? Will you be in this industry throughout your working career or is this just a stopover? Will you only work a 30 or 40 hour week or will you go the extra mile when opportunities are available? How ambitious are you and how many risks are you willing to take?

Figure 25–4 Inventory of Personal Characteristics and Skills.

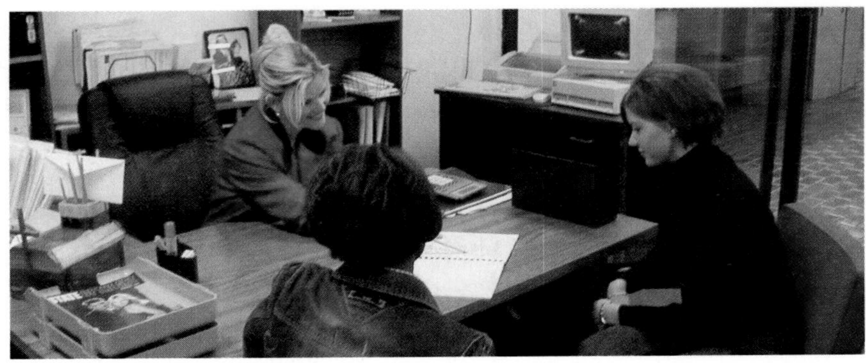

Figure 25-5 Your school counselor can help you find employment.

the workplace, where your energy will be appreciated and rewarded. Having an enthusiasm for getting the job done can be contagious, and when everyone works hard, everyone benefits. You can begin to develop that enthusiasm by establishing good work habits as a student.

How to Get the Job You Want

There are several key personal characteristics that will not only help you get the position you want but will help you keep it. These characteristics include the following points.

- *Motivation.* This means having the drive to take the necessary action to achieve a goal. Although motivation can come from external sources—parental or peer pressure, for instance—the best kind of motivation is internal.
- *Integrity.* When you have integrity, you are committed to a strong code of moral and artistic values. Integrity is the compass that keeps you on course over the long haul of your career.
- *Good technical and communication skills.* It has been determined that about 80 percent of your success will depend on your "people" skills, and the remaining 20 percent will be based on your technical skills. You must develop both to reach the level of success you desire.

activity

For one week, keep a daily record of your performance in the following areas and ask a few of your fellow students to provide feedback as well.

- positive attitude
- professional appearance
- punctuality
- regular class and clinic attendance
- diligent practice of newly learned techniques
- interpersonal skills
- teamwork
- helping others

- *Strong work ethic.* Success comes when you have developed a solid **work ethic**; that is, when you believe that work is good and you are committed to delivering worthy service for the value received from your employer.
- *Enthusiasm.* Try never to lose your eagerness to learn, grow, and expand your skills and knowledge.

A Salon Survey

In the United States alone, the professional salon business numbers over 250,000 establishments. These salons employ more than one million active cosmetologists. This year, like every year, thousands of cosmetology school graduates will find their first position in one of the types of salons described below.

Small Independent Salons

Owned by an individual or two or more partners, this kind of operation makes up the majority of professional salons. The average independent salon has one to three styling chairs. Usually, the owner or owners are hairstylists who maintain their own clientele while managing the business end and the hiring and training of other stylists. There are nearly as many different kinds of independent salons as there are owners. Their image, decor, services, prices, and clientele all reflect the owner's experience and taste. Depending on the owner's willingness to help a newcomer learn and grow, a beginning stylist can learn a great deal in an independent salon and earn a good living.

Independent Salon Chains

These are usually chains of 10 or fewer salons owned by one individual or two or more partners. Independents, both single and chain, range from basic hair salons to full-service salons to day spas, from low-priced to very high-priced. In the larger of these (10 or more styling stations and a minimum of 10 full-time staff), stylists can advance to specialized positions in color, nail care, skin care, or other chemical services. Some larger salons also employ education directors and styles directors, and stylists are often hired to manage the different locations.

Large National Salon Chains

These companies operate salons throughout the country and even internationally. They can be budget or value-priced, haircut-only or full-service, mid-price or high-end. Some salon chains operate within department store chains. Management and marketing professionals at the corporate headquarters make all the decisions for each salon, such as size, decor, hours, services, prices, advertising, and profit targets. Many newly licensed cosmetologists seek their first jobs in national chain salons because of the secure pay and benefits, additional paid training, management opportunities, and corporate advertising. Because the chains are large and widespread, employees have the added advantage of being able to transfer from one location to another.

Franchise Salons

This is another form of chain salon organization, one with a national name and consistent image and business formula throughout the chain.

Franchises are owned by individuals who pay a fee to use the name; these individuals then receive a business plan and can take advantage of national marketing campaigns. Such decisions as size, location, decor, and prices are determined in advance by the parent company. Franchises are generally not owned by stylists but by investors who seek a return on their investment. Franchise salons often offer employees the same benefits as corporate-owned chain salons.

Basic Value-Priced Operations

Often located in busy, low-rent strip shopping centers that are anchored by a nearby supermarket or other large business, these outlets depend on a high volume of walk-in traffic. They hire recent cosmetology graduates and generally pay them by the hour, sometimes adding commission-style bonuses if individual sales pass a certain level. Haircuts are usually priced around $10, sometimes even less, and stylists are trained to work fast, with no frills. Shampoo and conditioning services are available, usually for an additional charge. Texture or color services, if offered at all, are limited. These salons may have their own "private label" retail products, which are also sold at budget prices. Men and children tend to be the typical clients. This type of salon may be a good starting place for the recent graduate. It provides exposure to a variety of clients and allows the new licensee the chance to practice many types of haircuts which increases self-confidence and speed. If you enjoy a busy schedule with an in-and-out flow of customers and can handle the challenge of giving a good haircut in 15 to 20 minutes, you might consider this kind of operation as an option.

Mid-priced Full-Service Salons

These salons cater to men, women, and children with a complete menu of hair, nail, and skin services and retail products. Successful mid-priced salons promote their most profitable services and often offer "service and retail packages" to entice haircut-only clients. They also run strong marketing programs to encourage client returns and referrals. These salons train their professional styling team to be as productive and profitable as possible. If you are inclined to give more time to each client during the consultation, you may like working in a full-service salon. Here you will have the opportunity to build a relationship with clients that may extend over time.

High-End "Image" Salons or Day Spas

At the other end of the salon spectrum from the value-priced operation is the salon where clients not only have their hair styled by a well-known stylist but can also be pampered with luxurious, higher priced services and treatments if they choose. Most high-end salons are located in trendy, upscale sections of large cities; others may be located in elegant mansions, high-rent office and retail towers, or luxury hotels and resorts. Clients expect a high level of personal service, and such salons hire proven stylists whose technical expertise, personal appearance, and communication skills meet their high standards. If you have a flair for fashion and style and are skilled at the demanding, more time-consuming hair, skin, or nail services offered by a high-end salon, this may be an interesting direction for you (Figure 25–6).

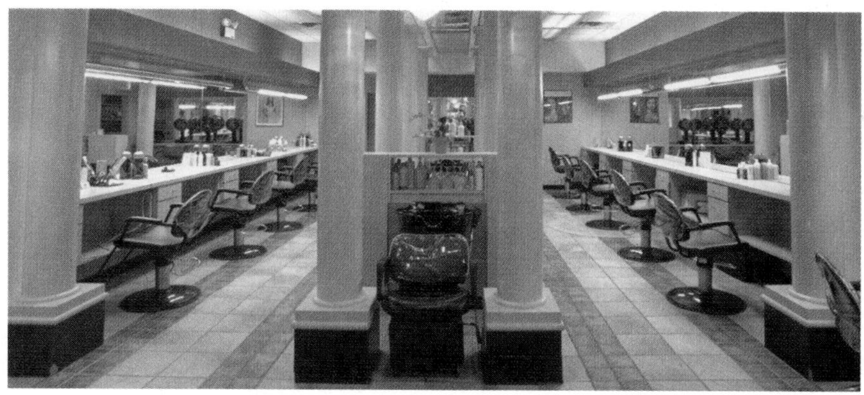

Figure 25-6 A high-end salon.

Booth Rental Establishments

Booth renting (also called chair rental) is possibly the least expensive way of owning one's own business. For a detailed discussion of booth rental, see Chapter 24. 3

Other Career Opportunities

Refer to Chapter 1 of this textbook to review other career paths that are open to licensed cosmetologists. These include platform artist, manufacturer's representative, state board inspector or examiner, state board member, technical specialist, educator, beauty industry journalist, chemist for beauty products, and business manager or owner.

Resume Development

Going into the job market without a resume is like going on a trip to another country without a passport. You will not get very far without one. A **resume** is a written summary of your education and work experience. It tells potential employers at a glance what your achievements and accomplishments are. Here are some basic guidelines to follow when preparing your professional resume.

- Keep it simple and to one page if at all possible.
- Print it on good-quality bond paper that is either white, buff, or gray.
- Include your name, address, phone number, and e-mail address on both the resume and your cover letter.
- List recent, relevant work experience.
- List relevant education and the name of the institution from which you graduated, as well as relevant courses attended.
- List your abilities and accomplishments.
- Focus on information that is relevant to the position you are seeking.

The average time a potential employer will spend scanning your resume to determine if you should be granted an interview is about 20 seconds. That means you must market yourself in such a manner that the reader will want to meet you. Never make the mistake of detailing your prior duties and responsibilities. Rather, focus on your achievements. Accomplishment statements should always enlarge on your basic duties and responsibilities. The best way to do that is to add numbers or percentages whenever possible. You might ask yourself the following questions.

- How many regular clients do I serve?
- How many clients do I serve weekly?
- What percentage of the clinic revenue that I generated in training came from chemical services I performed?
- What was my service ticket average?
- What was my client retention rate?
- What percentage of my clinic revenue came from retailing?
- What percentage of my clinic revenue came from color or texture services?

This type of questioning can help you develop accomplishment statements that will interest a potential employer. There is no better time for you to achieve significant accomplishments than while you are in school. Even though your experience may be minimal, you must still present evidence of your skills and accomplishments. This may seem a difficult task at this early stage in your working career, but by closely examining your training performance, extracurricular activities, and the full- or part-time jobs you have held, you should be able to create a good, attention-getting resume.

For example, did you receive any honors during your course of training? Were you ever selected "student of the month?" Did you receive special recognition for your attendance or academic progress? Did you win any cosmetology-related competitions while in school? What was your attendance average while in school? Did you work with the student body to organize any fund-raisers? What were the results? Answers to these types of questions may indicate your people skills, personal work habits, and personal commitment to success (Figure 25–7).

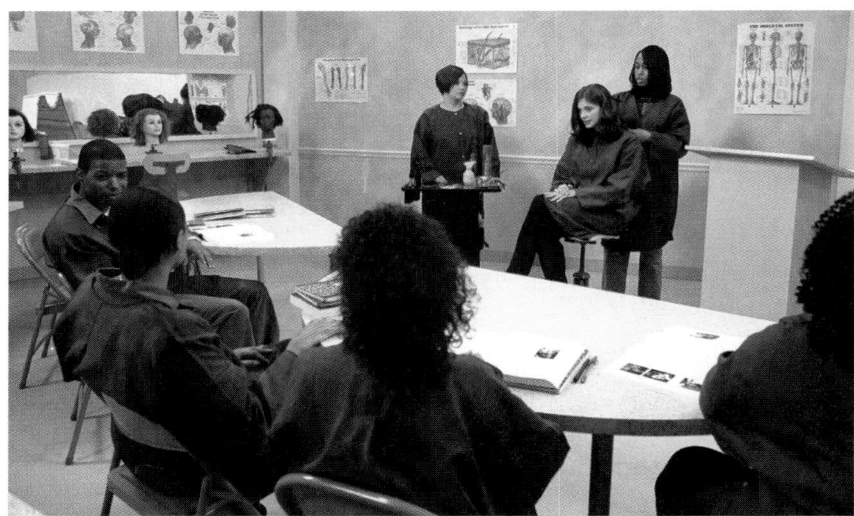

Figure 25-7 Excelling in school can help you build a good resume.

insights

Adam Broderick

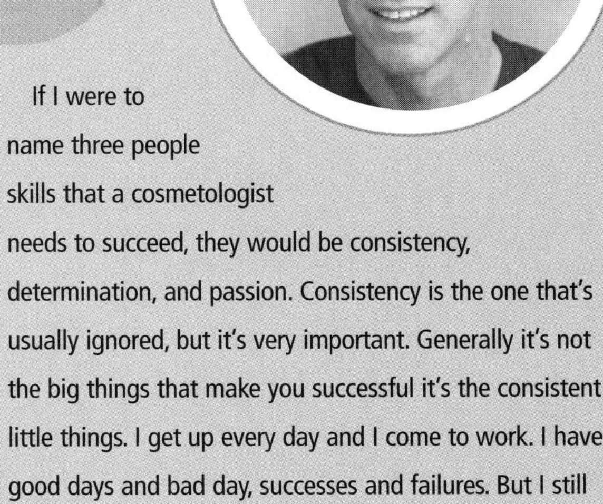

The owner of a high-end salon and spa in Connecticut, Adam Broderick came into cosmetology via an unusual route.

I wanted to be a veterinarian but didn't have the science and math, so I did dog grooming for a while. But I realized, while I was still very young, that it just wasn't right for me. I started to think about what my options were. I could have gone back to college, but I thought it might be cool to be a hairdresser. So I enrolled in beauty school. The first two days we learned basic haircutting. I went to the owner of the school and said, I don't like this. He said, Stay open-minded, and let me show you some things with color. That was what grabbed me. I loved chemistry in school, so I was intrigued with all the bottles and dyes. It was fascinating. From that day on, I wanted to be a haircolorist. That was 24 years ago.

What I love about cosmetology is how you can touch someone's self-esteem in a really profound way. To make someone look as good on the outside as they feel on the inside is very moving, and it happens to cosmetologists ten or fifteen times a day. On the other hand, you also have to realize that, because you're dealing with people's self-esteem, they can be very frightened. You need good communication skills and the ability to listen when you work in this field. People say, Oh, I have a bad haircut. You don't have a bad haircut; you usually have a haircut you didn't ask for or something you didn't expect. So most often it's not a technical issue; it's a communication issue.

If I were to name three people skills that a cosmetologist needs to succeed, they would be consistency, determination, and passion. Consistency is the one that's usually ignored, but it's very important. Generally it's not the big things that make you successful it's the consistent little things. I get up every day and I come to work. I have good days and bad day, successes and failures. But I still come in the next day to do it all over again. And over time, I've built up a clientele, a reputation, and a network of friends.

Students should be thinking about where they want to work while they're still in school. If you see people on the street with a look you admire, ask them where they got their hair cut or colored. Talk to other hairdressers about where they work. You can get incredible inside information that way. And make phone calls! One thing about the salon industry is that you can get almost anyone on the phone. We've all come up the ranks from beauty school—we know how hard it can be—and with very few exceptions, salon professionals are giving, compassionate people who are more than happy to share information with a student.

This is a fun industry. If you're good and work hard, you'll find employment wherever you want, particularly given the shortage of qualified employees these days. But what happens in the dynamics of a service is about so much more than just the service. It's about the interactions between people. So keep it light and fun!

Since you haven't completed your training yet, you still have the opportunity to make some of the examples listed above become a reality before you graduate. Positive developments of this nature while you are still in school can do much to improve your resume.

The Do's and Don'ts of Resumes

You will save yourself a lot of problems and disappointment right at the start of your job search if you keep a clear idea in your mind of what to do and not to do when it comes to creating a resume. Here are some of the do's.

- *Make it easy to read.* Use concise, clear sentences and avoid "overwriting" or flowery language.
- *Know your audience.* Use vocabulary and language that will be understood by your potential employer.
- *Keep it short.* Make sure the overall length does not exceed one or two pages.
- *Stress accomplishments.* Emphasize past accomplishments and the skills you used to achieve them.
- *Focus on career goals.* Highlight information that is relevant to your career goals and the position you are seeking.
- *Emphasize* **transferable skills.** These are the skills you have already mastered at other jobs that can be put to use in a new position.
- *Use action verbs.* Begin accomplishment statements with such action verbs as *achieved*, *coordinated*, *developed*, *increased*, *maintained*, and *strengthened* rather than with the word *I*.
- *Make it neat.* A poorly structured, badly typed resume does not reflect well on you.

And now for the don'ts to watch out for.

- *Avoid salary references.* Don't state your salary history or reason for leaving your former employment.
- *No photos.* Don't enclose a photograph (you may look like someone the reader dislikes!).
- *Don't stretch the truth.* Misinformation or untruthful statements usually catch up with you.
- *Don't include personal references.* Potential employers are really only interested in references who can speak about your professional ability.
- *Avoid the personal.* Don't make references to hobbies or memberships that are not business-related.
- *Don't expect too much.* Don't have unrealistic expectations of what your resume can accomplish. Review Figure 25–8, which represents an achievement-oriented resume for a recent graduate of a cosmetology course. But keep in mind that you are much more than the sum of your parts. It just may take a while before someone recognizes that.

MARY CURL
143 Fern Circle
Anytown, USA 12345
(123) 555-1234

A cosmetologist with honors in attendance and practical skills who is creative, artistic, and works well with people of all ages.

ACCOMPLISHMENTS/ABILITIES

Academics	Achieved an "A" average in theoretical requirements and excellent ratings in practical requirements; Exceeded the number of practical skills required for graduation.
Sales	Named "Student of the Month" for best attendance, best attitude, highest retail sales, and most clients served; Increased chemical services to 30 percent of my clinic volume by graduation. Achieved a client ticket average comparable to $33.00 in the area salon market. Increased retail sales of cosmetics by over 18 percent during part-time employment at local department store.
Client Retention	Developed and retained a personal client base of over 75 individuals of all ages, both male and female.
Image Consulting	Certified as an Image Consultant who aids in providing full salon services to all clientele.
Administration	Supervised a student "salon team" which developed a business plan for opening a twelve chair, full service salon; project earned an "A" and was recognized for thoroughness, accuracy and creativity. As President of the student council, organized fund raising activities including car washes, bake sales, and yard sales which generated enough funds to send 19 students to a hair show in El Paso.
Externship	Trained one day weekly at the salon for ten weeks under the state approved student externship program.
Special Projects	Reorganized school facial room for more efficiency and client comfort. Organized the school dispensary which increased inventory control and streamlined operations within the clinic. Catalogued the school's library of texts, books, videos and other periodicals by category and updated the library inventory list.

EXPERIENCE

Salon Etc.	Spring 2002 Student Extern in all Phases of Cosmetology
Dilberts	Summer 2002 Retail Sales, Cosmetics
Food Emporium	1999 - 2001 Cashier

EDUCATION

Graduate, New Alamo High School, 2000
Graduate, Milady Career Institute of Cosmetology, August 2002
Licensed as Cosmetologist, September 2002

Figure 25-8 An achievement-oriented resume.

Employment Portfolio

As you prepare to work in the field of cosmetology, an **employment portfolio** can be extremely useful. An employment portfolio is a collection, usually bound, of photos and documents that reflect your skills, accomplishments, and abilities in your chosen career field (Figure 25–9). While the actual contents of the portfolio will vary from graduate to graduate, there are certain items that have a place in any portfolio.

A powerful portfolio includes:

- diplomas, both high school and cosmetology school.
- awards and achievements received while a cosmetology student.
- current resume, focusing on accomplishments.
- letters of reference from former employers.
- summary of continuing education and/or copies of actual training certificates.
- statement of membership in industry and other professional organizations.
- statement of relevant civic affiliations and/or community activities.
- before and after photographs of services you have performed on clients or models.
- a brief statement about why you have chosen a career in cosmetology.
- any other information that you regard as relevant.

Once you have assembled your portfolio, ask yourself if it portrays you and your career skills as you hoped it would. If it does not, identify what needs to be changed. If you are not sure, run it by a totally disinterested party for feedback about how to make it more interesting and accurate. This kind of feedback is also useful when creating a resume. The portfolio, like the resume, should be prepared in a way that projects professionalism. Nothing should be handwritten. All summaries and letters should be typed. For ease of use, you may want to separate sections with tabs.

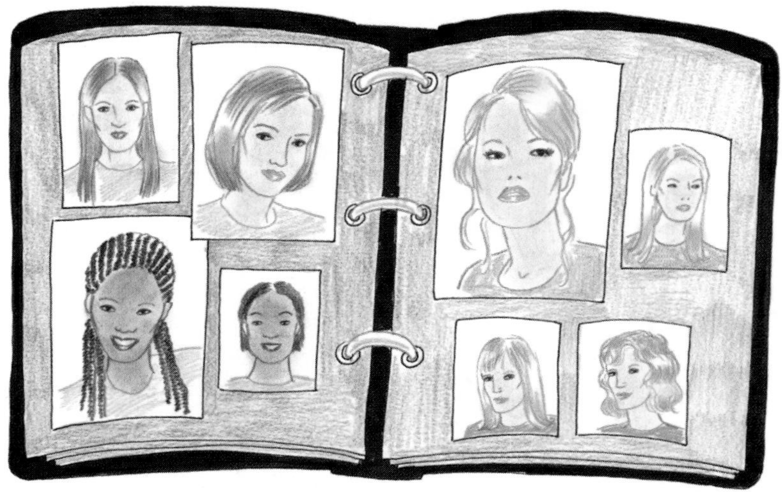

Figure 25-9 Before and after photos in an employment portfolio.

When writing your statement on why you chose a career in cosmetology, you might include:

- a statement that explains what you love about your new career.
- a description of your philosophy about the importance of teamwork and how you see yourself as a contributing team member.
- a description of methods you would try in an effort to increase clinic and retail revenue.

Targeting the Establishment

One of the most important steps in the process of job-hunting is narrowing your search. Here are some points to keep in mind about targeting potential employers.

- *Accept that you probably will not begin in your dream job.* Few people are so lucky.
- *Do not wait until graduation to begin your search.* If you do, you will probably take the first offer you receive, and that may not be the best situation for you.
- *Locate a salon that serves the type of clients you wish to serve.* You may not be starting exactly where you want to, but your experience there will be more beneficial if you can find aspects of the job that are related to your ultimate career goals.
- *Make a list of area salons or establishments.* The yellow pages in your local telephone book will be your best source for this. If you are considering relocating to another area, your local library will probably have out-of-state phone directories to help you compile your list. You may also find the Internet useful for this task.
- *Follow newspapers, television, and radio for salon advertising.* Get a feel for what market each salon is targeting.

Field Research

A great way to find out about jobs is to actually get out there and use your eyes, ears, and any other sense that can help you gather information. A highly effective technique you should learn is called networking. Networking allows you to establish contacts that may eventually lead to a job and that also help you gain valuable information about the workings of various establishments. If possible, make contact with salons while you are still a student in training. You might even make contact as a salon customer yourself. When you are ready to network, your first contact should be by telephone, and you should follow these guidelines:

1. Use your best telephone manner. Speak with confidence and self-assurance.
2. Ask to speak to the owner, manager, or personnel director.
3. State your name and explain that you are preparing to graduate from a cosmetology program.
4. Explain that you are researching the local salon market for potential positions and that you need just a few minutes to ask a few questions.

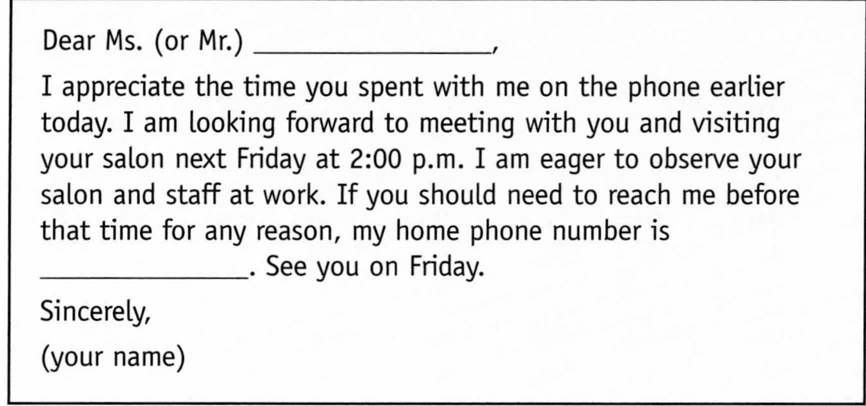
Dear Ms. (or Mr.) ________________,

I appreciate the time you spent with me on the phone earlier today. I am looking forward to meeting with you and visiting your salon next Friday at 2:00 p.m. I am eager to observe your salon and staff at work. If you should need to reach me before that time for any reason, my home phone number is ______________. See you on Friday.

Sincerely,

(your name)

Figure 25–10 A sample appointment confirmation note.

5. If the person with whom you are speaking is open to continuing the conversation, ask if the salon is in need of any new practitioners at this time and how many they currently employ.
6. Ask if you can make an appointment to visit the salon so that you might observe their operations sometime during the next few weeks.

If the salon is agreeable to your scheduled observation appointment, confirm the appointment with a typewritten or handwritten note on good quality paper (Figure 25–10).

Remember that a rejection is not a poor reflection on you. Many professionals are too busy to make time for this kind of networking, and, of course, there are those individuals who are not so generous with their time in general. The good news, however, is that you are bound to discover many genuinely kind people who remember what it was like when they started out and are willing to devote a bit of their time to helping others who are beginning their careers.

25

The Salon Visit

When you visit the salon, take along a checklist to ensure that you observe all the key areas that might ultimately affect your decision-making. The checklist will be similar to the one used for field trips you probably have taken to area salons while in school. Keep the checklist on file for future reference so that you can make informed comparisons between establishments (Figure 25–11).

After your visit, always remember to write a brief note thanking the salon representative for his time. Even if you did not like the salon or would never consider working there, it is important that you send a thank-you note. Never burn your bridges. Rather, build a network of contacts who have a favorable opinion of you (Figure 25–12 and Figure 25–13). 5

SALON VISIT CHECKLIST

When you visit a salon, observe the following areas and rate them from 1 to 5, with 5 considered being the best.

____ **SALON IMAGE:** Is the salon's image consistent and appropriate for your interests? Is the image pleasing and inviting? What is the decor and arrangement? If you are not comfortable or if you find it unattractive, it is likely that clients will also.

____**PROFESSIONALISM:** Do the employees present the appropriate professional appearance and behavior? Do they give their clients the appropriate levels of attention and personal service or do they act as if work is their time to socialize?

____**MANAGEMENT:** Does the salon show signs of being well managed? Is the phone answered promptly with professional telephone skills? Is the mood of the salon positive? Does everyone appear to work as a team?

____**CLIENT SERVICE:** Are clients greeted promptly and warmly when they enter the salon? Are they kept informed of the status of their appointment? Are they offered a magazine or beverage while they wait? Is there a comfortable reception area? Are there changing rooms, attractive smocks, or perhaps a complimentary hand treatment while clients wait?

____**PRICES:** Compare price for value. Are clients getting the money's worth? Do they pay the same price in one salon but get better service and attention in another? If possible, take home salon brochures and price lists.

____**RETAIL:** Is there a well-stocked retail display offering clients a variety of product lines and a range of prices? Do the stylists and receptionist (if applicable) promote retail sales?

____**IN-SALON MARKETING:** Are there posters or promotions throughout the salon? If so, are they tasteful and of good quality?

____**SERVICES:** Make a list of all services offered by each salon and the product lines they carry. This will help you decide what earning potential stylists have in each salon.

SALON NAME: ______________________________

SALON MANAGER: ______________________________

Figure 25–11 Salon Visit Checklist.

Arranging the Employment Interview

After you have graduated from your course of study and completed the first two steps in the process of securing employment—targeting and observing salons—you are ready to pursue employment more vigorously. The next step is to contact those establishments you are interested in by sending them a resume with a cover letter requesting an interview (Figure 25–14).

Dear Ms. (or Mr.) _______________,

I appreciate having had the opportunity to observe your salon/spa in operation last Friday. Thank you for the time you and your staff gave me. I was impressed by the efficient and courteous manner in which your stylists served their clients. The atmosphere was pleasant and the mood was positive. Should you ever have an opening for a professional with my skills and training, I would welcome the opportunity to apply. You can contact me at the address and phone number listed below. I hope we will meet again soon.

Sincerely,

(your name, address, telephone)

Figure 25–12 A sample thank-you note.

Dear Ms. (or Mr.) __________________,

I appreciate having had the opportunity to observe your salon in operation last Friday. I know how busy you and all your staff are and want to thank you for the time that you gave me. I realize that it can be somewhat disruptive to have visitors observing your activities. I hope my presence didn't interfere with the flow of your operations too much. I certainly appreciate the courtesies that were extended to me by you and your staff. I wish you and your salon continued success.

Sincerely,

(your name)

Figure 25–13 A thank-you note to a salon at which you do not expect to seek employment.

Mark your calendar for a time when it would be suitable to make a follow-up call to this letter. A week is generally sufficient. When you call, try to schedule an interview appointment. The salon may not have an opening and the owner, manager, or personnel director may not wish to schedule an interview at this time. If that is the case, be polite and ask them to keep your resume on file should an opening arise in the future. Be sure to thank them for their time and consideration.

Your Name
Your Address
Your Phone Number

Ms. (or Mr.) _______________
Salon Name
Salon Address

Dear Ms (or Mr.) __________________,

We met in August when you allowed me to observe your salon and staff while I was still in cosmetology training. Since that time, I have graduated and have received my license, which allows me to practice cosmetology. I have enclosed my resume for your review and consideration.

I would very much appreciate the opportunity to meet with you and discuss either current or future career opportunities at your salon. I was extremely impressed with your staff and business, and I would like to discuss with you how my skills and training might add to your salon's success.

I will call you next week to discuss a time that is convenient for us to meet. I look forward to meeting with you again soon.

Sincerely,
(your name)

Figure 25–14 A sample resume cover letter.

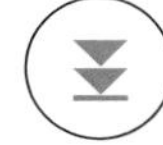

Here's a tip:

When you call a salon to make an appointment for an interview, you may be told they are not hiring at this time, but they would be happy to conduct an interview for future reference. Don't think to yourself that it would be a waste of time. Take advantage of the opportunity. Not only will it give you valuable interview experience, but who knows? There is such a thing as love at first sight!

Interview Preparation

When preparing for an interview, make sure you have all the necessary information and materials in place (use Figure 25–15 as a guide). These include the following items.

1. *Identification.*
   a. Social Security number
   b. Driver's license number
   c. Names, addresses, and phone numbers of former employers
   d. Name and phone number of the nearest relative not living with you

2. *Interview wardrobe.* Your appearance is crucial, especially since you are applying for a position in the image and beauty industry. It is recommended that you obtain one or two "interview outfits." You may be requested to return for a second interview, hence the need for the second outfit. Consider the following points.
   a. Is the outfit appropriate for the position?
   b. Is it well-fitted, comfortable, and flattering to your shape and personality?
   c. Is it clean and pressed?
   d. Are your shoes clean and in good repair?
   e. Is jewelry basic and minimal?
   f. Is your hairstyle current and appropriate for your face shape and features?
   g. Is your makeup current and appropriate for face shape and features (if female)?

PREPARING FOR THE INTERVIEW CHECKLIST

RESUME COMPOSITION

1. Does it present your abilities and what you have accomplished in your jobs and training?
2. Does it make the reader want to ask, "How did you accomplish that?"
3. Does it highlight accomplishments rather than detailing duties and responsibilities?
4. Is it easy to read, short, and does it stress past accomplishments and skills?
5. Does it focus on information that's relevant to your own career goals?
6. Is it complete and professionally prepared?

PORTFOLIO CHECKLIST

_____ Diploma, secondary and post-secondary
_____ Awards and achievements while in school
_____ Current resume focusing on accomplishments
_____ Letters of reference from former employers
_____ List of, or certificates from, trade shows attended while in training.
_____ Statement of professional affiliations (memberships in cosmetology organizations, etc.)
_____ Statement of civic affiliations and/or activities.
_____ Before and after photographs of technical skills services you have performed.
_____ Any other relevant information

Ask: Does my portfolio portray me and my career skills in the manner that I wish to be perceived? If not, what needs to be changed?

GENERAL INFORMATION

Describe specific methods or procedures you will employ in the salon to build your clientele.

Describe how you feel about retail sales in the salon and give specific methods you would use in the salon to generate sales.

State why you feel consumer protection and safety is so important in the field of cosmetology.

After careful thought, explain what you love about you new career. Describe your passion for cosmetology.

Figure 25-15 Preparing for the Interview Checklist.

h. Are you clean shaven or is your beard properly trimmed (if male)?
i. Is your perfume or cologne subtle, not too strong?
j. Carry a handbag or briefcase, never both (Figure 25–16).

3. *Supporting materials.*
   a. *Resume.* Even if you have already sent one, take another copy with you.
   b. *Facts and figures.* Have ready a list of names and dates of former employment, education, and references.
   c. *Employment portfolio.*
4. *Answers to anticipated questions.* Certain questions are typically asked during an interview. It would be a good idea to reflect on your answers ahead of time. You might even consider role-playing an interview situation with friends, family, or fellow students. Typical questions include the following.
   a. What did you like best about your training?
   b. Are you punctual and regular in attendance?
   c. Will your school director or instructor confirm that?
   d. What skills do you feel are your strongest?
   e. What areas do you consider to be less strong?
   f. Are you a team player? Please explain.
   g. Do you consider yourself flexible? Please explain.
   h. What are your career goals?
   i. What days and hours are you available for work?
   j. Do you have your own transportation?
   k. Are there any obstacles that would prevent you from keeping your commitment to full-time employment?
   l. What assets do you believe you would bring to this salon and his position?
   m. Who is the most interesting person you have met in your work and/or education experience and why?
   n. How would you handle a problem client?
   o. How do you feel about retailing?
   p. Would you be willing to attend our company training program?
   q. Describe ways in which you feel you provide excellent customer service.
   r. Please share an example of consultation questions that you might ask a client.
   s. What steps do you take to build your business and ensure clients return to see you?
5. *Preparing to perform a service.* Some salons require applicants to bring a model and perform a cut and style service as part of the interview. Be sure to confirm whether this is a requirement. If it is, make sure that your model is appropriately dressed and properly prepared for the experience.

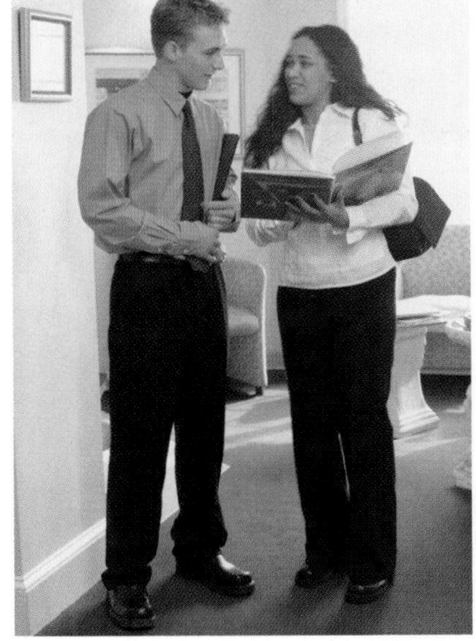

Figure 25-16 Dressed for an interview.

The Interview

On the day of the interview, try to make sure that nothing occurs that will keep you from completing the interview successfully. There are certain behaviors you should practice in connection with the interview itself.

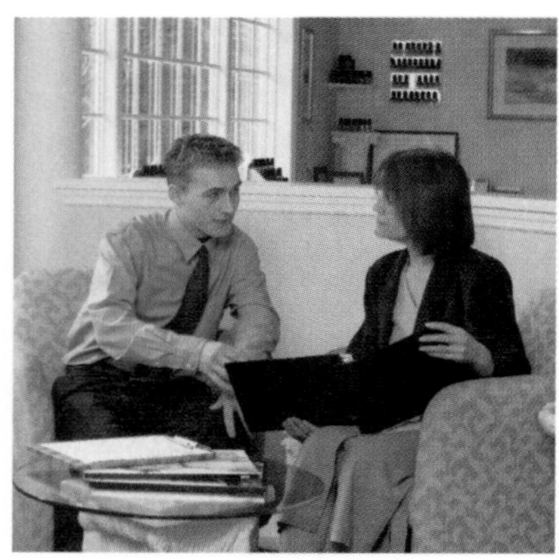

Figure 25-17 An interview in progress.

- Always be on time or, better yet, early. If you are unsure of the location, find it the day before so there will be no reason for delays.
- Project a warm, friendly smile. Smiling is the universal language.
- Walk, sit, and stand with good posture.
- Be polite and courteous.
- Do not sit until asked to do so or until it is obvious that you are expected to do so.
- Never smoke or chew gum, even if either is offered to you. Do not come to an interview with a cup of coffee, a soft drink, snacks, or anything else to eat or drink.
- Never lean on or touch the interviewer's desk. Some people do not like their personal space invaded without invitation.
- Try to project a positive first impression and to appear as confident and relaxed as you can (Figure 25–17).
- Speak clearly. The interviewer must be able to hear and understand you.
- Answer questions honestly. Think the question and answer through carefully. Do not speak before you are ready and not for more than two minutes at a time.
- Never criticize former employers.
- Always remember to thank the interviewer at the end of the interview.

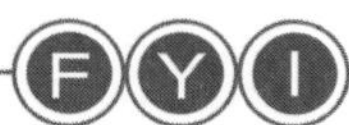

Many women find it difficult to afford the two or three outfits necessary to project a confident and professional image when going out into the workplace. Fortunately, several nonprofit organizations have been formed to address this need. These organizations receive donations of clean, beautiful clothes in good repair from individuals and manufacturers. These are then passed along to women who need them. For more information, visit Wardrobe for Opportunity at http://www.wardrobe.org and Dress for Success at http://www.dressforsuccess.org

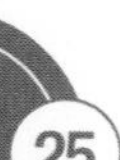

Another critical part of the interview comes when you are invited to ask the interviewer questions of your own. You should think about those questions ahead of time and bring a list if necessary. Doing so will show that you are organized and prepared. Some questions that you might consider include the following.

- Is there a job description, and may I review it?
- Is there a salon manual?
- How frequently does the salon advertise?
- How long do stylists typically work here?
- Are employees encouraged to grow in skills and responsibility? How so?
- Does the salon offer continuing education opportunities?
- Is there room for advancement?
- If so, what are the requirements for promotion?
- What benefits does the salon offer, such as paid vacations, personal days, and medical insurance?
- What is the form of compensation?
- When will the position be filled?
- Should I follow up on your decision, or will you contact me?

Do not feel that you have to ask all of your questions. The point is to create as much of a dialogue as possible. Be aware of the interviewer's reactions and make note of when you have asked enough questions. By obtaining the answers to at least some of your questions, you can compare the information you have gathered about other salons and then choose the one that offers the best package of income and career development.

Remember to write a thank-you note. It should simply thank the interviewer for the time she spent with you. Close with a positive statement that you want the job (if you do). If the interviewer's decision comes down to two or three possibilities, the one expressing the most desire may be offered the position. Also, if the interviewer suggests that you call to learn about the employment decision, then by all means do so.

Legal Aspects of the Employment Interview

Over the years, a number of issues have arisen about questions that may or may not be included in an employment application or interview. These include:

- *race, religion, and national origin.* Generally, there should not be questions in any of these categories.
- *age or date of birth.* It is permissible to ask the age of an applicant younger than 18. Age should not be relevant in most hiring decisions, so date-of-birth questions prior to employment are improper.
- *disabilities or physical traits.* The Americans with Disabilities Act prohibits general inquiries about health problems, disabilities, and medical conditions.
- *drug use or smoking.* Questions regarding drug or tobacco use are permitted. In fact, the employer may obtain the applicant's agreement to be bound by the employer's drug and smoking policies and to submit to drug testing.
- *citizenship.* Employers are not allowed to discriminate because an applicant is not a U.S. citizen.

It is important to recognize that not all potential employers will understand that they may be asking improper or illegal questions. If you are asked any of these, you may choose to answer the question or not. You

activity

Find a partner among your fellow students and role-play the employment interview. Each of you can take turns as the applicant and the employer. After each session, conduct a brief discussion regarding how it went: what worked and what didn't work. Discuss how the process could be further improved. Bear in mind that a role-play activity will never predict exactly what will occur in the real-life interview. However, the process will assist you in being better prepared for that important event in your employment search.

FYI

These are examples of illegal questions as compared to legal questions:

Illegal Questions

How old are you?

Please describe your medical history.

Are you a U.S. citizen?

What is your native tongue?

Legal Questions

Are you over the age of 18?

Are you able to perform this job?

Are you authorized to work in the U.S.?

In which languages are you fluent?

might simply respond that you believe the question is irrelevant to the position you are seeking and that you would like to focus on your qualities and skills that are suited to the job and the mission of the establishment.

The Employment Application

Any time you are applying for any position, you will be required to complete an application, even if your resume already contains much of the requested information. Your resume and the list you have prepared prior to the interview will assist you in completing the application quickly and accurately. You may want to fill out the sample form in Figure 25–18 in preparation for your employment interviews. The form each salon uses may be different, but it will probably request similar information. 6

YOU ARE ON YOUR WAY

Once you have gotten that highly desired first position, there are a few reminders that will help you make the most of it. It is important to remember that, as a new stylist, you may not always be fully booked and working with clients. How you use that "down time" can be critical in ensuring your future success on the job. When not serving clients, consider reading industry journals regarding the newest techniques and products. Offer to help your coworkers with shampooing, sweeping up hair, washing and folding towels, and so forth. Offer to assist the manager in doing anything that may be needed. Observe the more seasoned professionals as they perform the many services they offer. Learn from them and continue to improve your own skills.

Although going above and beyond the job requirements can be a big plus for you, recognize when you have given too much. Don't push yourself so hard trying to make a good impression that you begin to lose needed sleep or become so tired that you are less productive on the job. You must remain healthy and energetic if you are to serve your employer well. Make sure to include rest and relaxation in your work week. Try to exercise daily, get enough rest, wear well-fitting and comfortable shoes, drink plenty of water, and eat a balanced diet. Avoid tobacco and excess alcohol and remain drug-free. You will need every ounce of strength and stamina to get your new career off to a good start. Remember, both your body and mind can accomplish amazing things if you take proper care of them.

Remember, too, that becoming a part of a new organization's "family" can be stressful. Practice the people skills and communication skills that have been discussed throughout this book. If you receive criticism early in your employment, try not to take it too personally. Consider it from a professional perspective, determine if it is valid, and decide what you should do to improve. You might even ask the person making the comments how you can do better in that particular area. By responding with openness,

EMPLOYMENT APPLICATION

Applicants are considered for all positions, and employees are treated during employment without regard to race, color, religion, sex, national origin, age, marital or veteran status, medical condition or handicap.

PERSONAL INFORMATION

SS# ____________ Phone ________________ Date ______________

Last name ________________ First ______________ Middle ______________

Present street address City State Zip

Permanent street address City State Zip

If related to anyone employed here, state name: ______________________________

Referred to salon by: ______________________________

EMPLOYMENT DESIRED

Position ________________

Date you can start ____________ Salary Desired ________

Current Employer ______________________________

May we contact? ____________

Ever applied with this company before? ________ Where? ________ When? ________

EDUCATION

Name/location of School	Years Completed	Subjects Studied

Subject of special study or research work:

What foreign languages do you speak fluently?
Read fluently: ______________________
Write fluently: ______________________

US Military Service Rank Present Membership

In Nat'l Guard/Reserve

Figure 25-18 A typical job application form.

Activities (other than religious) Civic, Athletic, Fraternal, etc. (Exclude organizations for which the name or character might indicate race, creed, color or national origin of its members.)

FORMER EMPLOYMENT

List below last four employers, beginning with the most recent one first.

DATE: Month/Year	Name, Address of Employer	Salary	Position	Reason For Leaving
From: To:				
From: To:				
From: To:				
From: To:				

REFERENCES

Give below the names of three persons not related to you whom you have known at least one year.

Name	Address	Business	Years Known

PHYSICAL RECORD

25

Please list any defects in hearing, vision, or speech that might affect your job performance.

In case of emergency, please notify:

Name Address Telephone

I authorize investigation of all statements contained in this application. I understand that misrepresentation or omission of facts called for is cause for dismissal if hired.

Signature ______________________ Date ______________

Figure 25-18 *(continued)*

honesty, and a sincere interest in improving your performance, you will earn the respect and encouragement of your coworkers.

If you should find yourself on a team with coworkers who bicker and gossip, keep a positive attitude. In any business situation, attitudes can be contagious. You may begin your new job with a positive attitude and high hopes, then meet a "veteran" stylist who complains about everything from inconvenient staff parking to the way the manager dresses. Some people just live in a "black box" and want everyone else to join them there. They tend to gravitate toward newcomers because everyone who has been there for a while steers clear of these complainers. Do not let yourself get dragged down by such people. Remind yourself that your career is what you make of it. You can choose to be miserable or you can choose to be positive and upbeat. And since attitudes, even positive ones, are contagious, you might even bring the complainers around to your way of thinking (Figure 25–19).

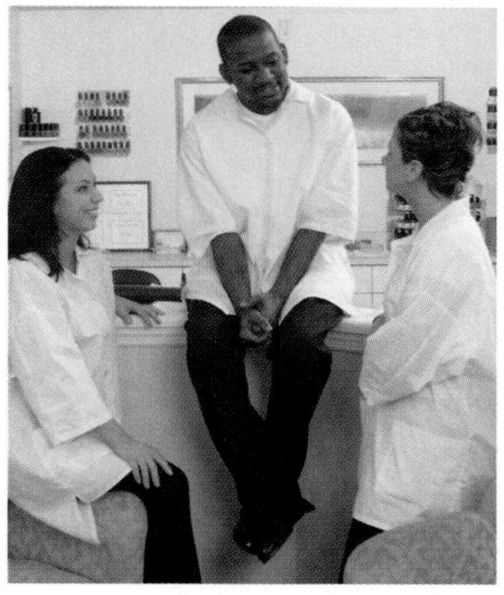

Figure 25-19 A positive attitude is contagious.

DOING IT RIGHT

You are ready to set out on your exciting new career as a professional cosmetologist. The right way to proceed is by learning those important study and test-taking skills early and applying them throughout your program. Think ahead to your employment opportunities and use your time in school to develop a record of interesting, noteworthy activities that will make your resume sizzle with excitement. When you compile a history that shows how you have achieved your goals, not only will your resume sizzle, but so will you. Your confidence will build and your ambitions will grow.

Remember to go step-by-step, however. Be sure to take the helpful preliminary steps we have discussed when preparing for employment. Develop a dynamic portfolio. Keep your materials, information, and questions organized in order to ensure a high-impact interview.

Once employed, take the necessary steps to learn all you can about your new position and the establishment you will be serving. Read all you can about the industry. Attend trade shows and take advantage of as much continuing education as you can manage. Become an active participant in making this great industry even better.

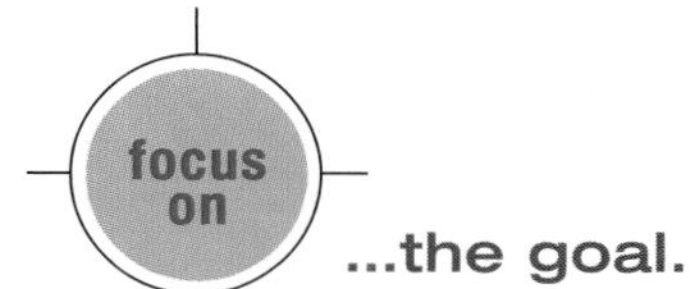

Baseball legend Lou Holtz once said, "Ability is what you're capable of doing. Motivation determines what you do. Attitude determines how well you do it." Those are wise words for anyone, but especially someone setting out on a new path. Success doesn't come to you: you create it!

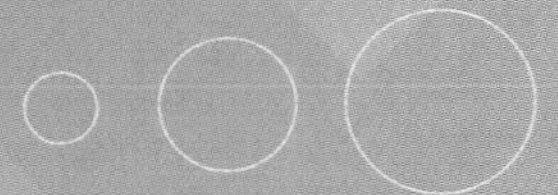

chapter glossary

deductive reasoning	process of reaching logical conclusions by employing logical reasoning
employment portfolio	collection, usually bound, of photos and documents that reflect your skills, accomplishments, and abilities in your chosen career field
resume	written summary of a person's education and work experience
test-wise	having a complete and thorough knowledge of the subject matter and understanding the strategies for taking tests successfully
transferable skills	skills mastered at other jobs that can be put to use in a new position
work ethic	belief that work is good and commitment to delivering worthy service for the value received from one's employer

review questions

1. What is the most important way a learner can do well on any test?
2. Explain deductive reasoning.
3. List eight steps learners should take prior to the actual examination to improve results.
4. List at least 12 strategies learners can use on the day of the actual examination for improved results.
5. When considering a statement on a true/false test, why are long statements more likely to be true than shorter statements?
6. Name and describe at least five types of salon businesses.
7. List up to eight strategies that you will find helpful when writing your resume.
8. List at least six things you should avoid when developing your resume.
9. List several items that should be included in your professional portfolio.
10. Briefly summarize the preliminary things you should consider before beginning your salon search.
11. In your own words, explain what can be accomplished by visiting a salon prior to an employment interview.
12. Why are thank-you notes important even if you visit a salon where you do not wish to become employed?
13. List twelve important interview behaviors that you should practice.

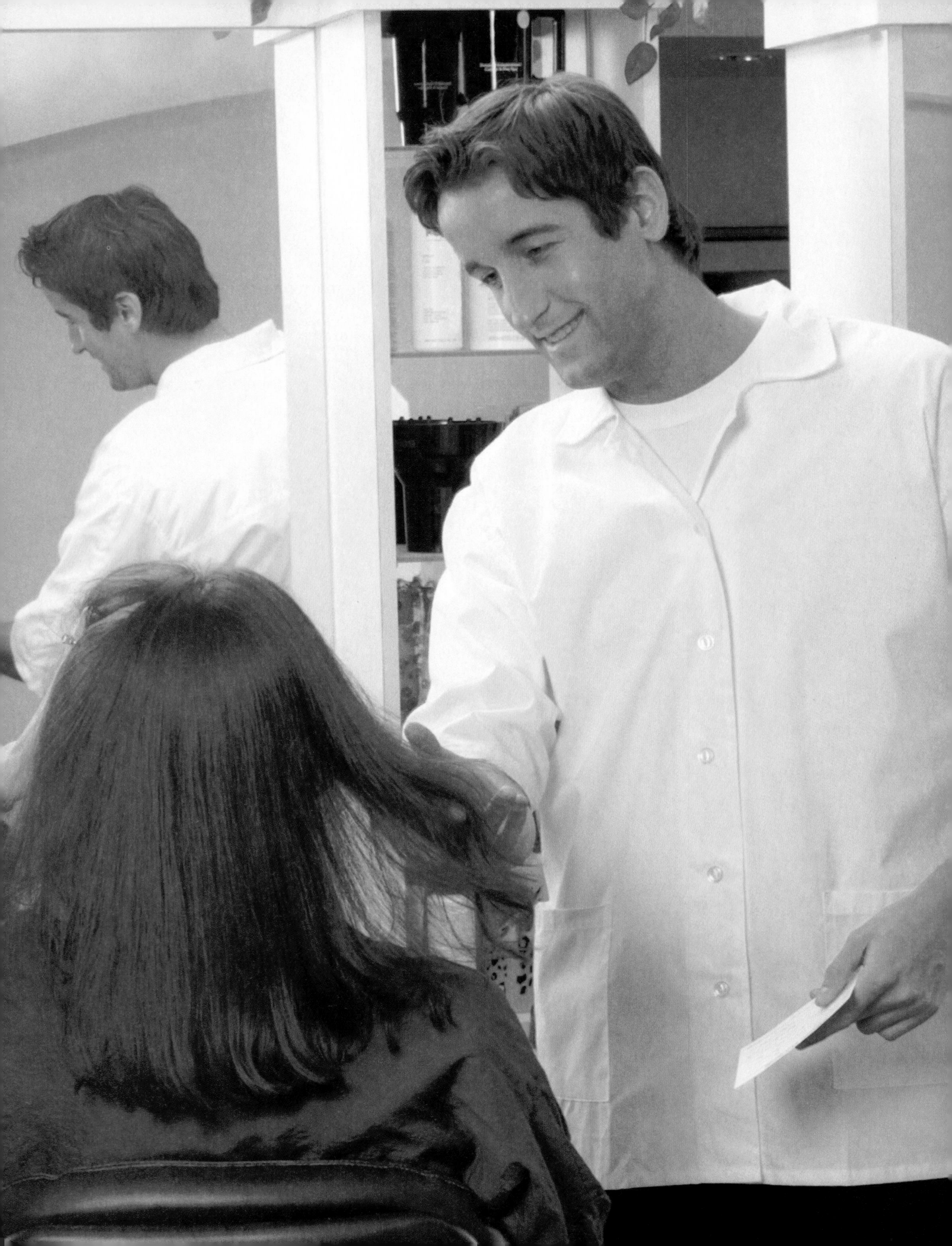

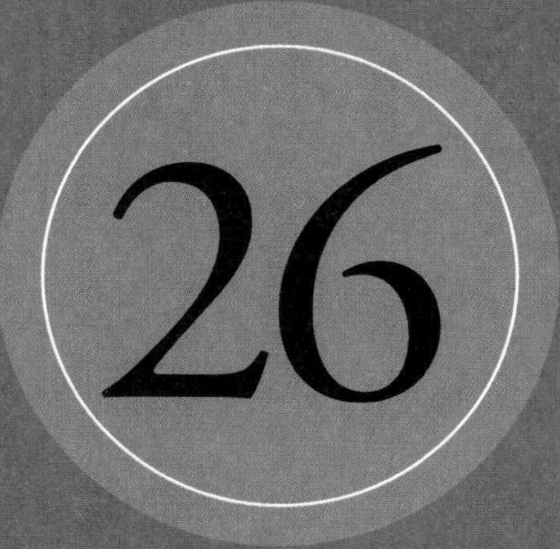

ON THE JOB

Catherine Frangie
BEAUTY INDUSTRY CONSULTANT

Chapter Outline

Learning Objectives:

After completing this chapter, you should be able to:

1. Describe the qualities that help a new employee succeed in a service profession.
2. List the habits of a good salon team player.
3. Explain the function of a job description.
4. Describe three different ways in which salon professionals are compensated.
5. Create a personal budget.
6. List the principles of selling products and services in the salon.
7. List the most effective ways to build a client base.

National Skill Standards

This chapter provides you with the necessary information to master these National Industry Skill Standards for Entry-Level Cosmetologists.

Interacting effectively with coworkers as part of a team.

Managing time to provide efficient client services.

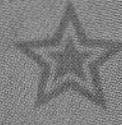
Taking the necessary steps to develop and retain clients.

Marketing professional salon products.

Maintaining business records on client development, income, and expenses.

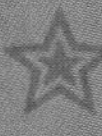
Participating in lifelong learning to stay current with trends, technology, and techniques pertaining to the cosmetology industry.

Key Terms

Page number indicates where in the chapter the term is used.

client base
pg. 907

commission
pg. 898

job description
pg. 895

retailing
pg. 904

ticket upgrading or upselling services
pg. 903

Congratulations! You have worked hard in cosmetology school, you have taken and passed your state's licensing exam, and you have successfully interviewed for and been offered your first job in the field. Now, more than ever, it is time to do some real, serious learning.

One of the first things you will want to learn is how to establish and prioritize your goals and how to create personal rules of conduct and behavior. These goals and rules can guide you throughout your career. If you let them do so, you can always expect to have work and to enjoy the freedom that your chosen profession can offer you (Figure 26–1).

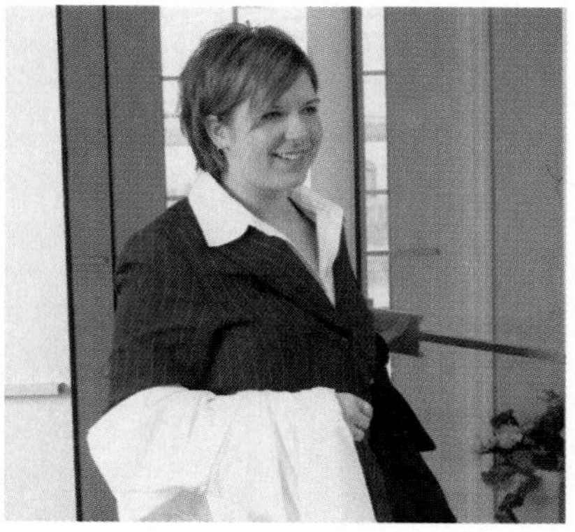

Figure 26-1 Getting off to a good start.

MOVING FROM SCHOOL TO WORK

Making the transition from school to work can be difficult. While you may be thrilled to have a job, working for a paycheck brings with it a number of duties and responsibilities that you may not have thought about.

Cosmetology school is a forgiving environment. You are given the chance to do a certain procedure over and over again until you get it right. Making and fixing mistakes is an accepted part of the process, and your instructors and mentors are there to help you. Schedules can be adjusted if necessary, and you are given some leeway in the matter of juggling your personal life with the demands of your schooling.

On the other hand, when you become the employee of a salon, you will be expected to put the needs of the salon and its clients ahead of your own. That means that you must always be on time for your scheduled shifts and be prepared to perform whatever services or functions are required of you, regardless of what is happening in your personal life at the moment. If someone comes to you with tickets for a concert on Saturday, you cannot just "take the day off." To do so may inconvenience your clients, who may even decide not to return to the salon. Or it may mean burdening your coworkers, who, if asked to take on your appointments, may feel resentful. In short, one stylist's selfish and immature decision can create problems for the entire salon.

Finding the Right Salon

In order to be successful on the job, it is important to seek out and accept a position at a salon that is right for you. You may think that any salon that

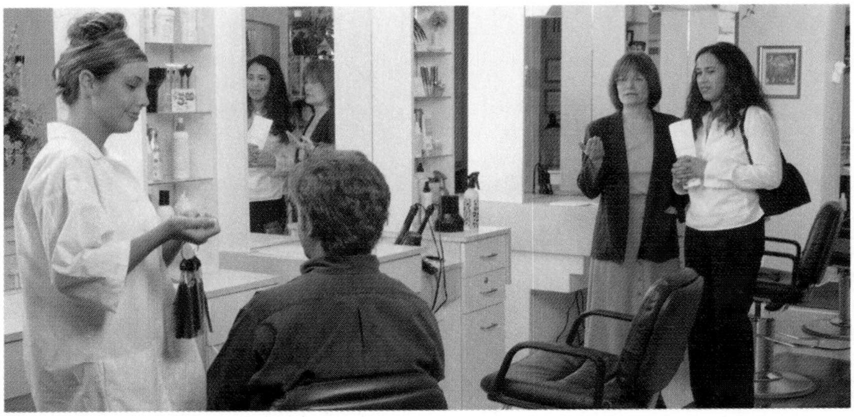

Figure 26-2 Don't be afraid to ask questions.

will give you an actual paycheck is the "right" salon, but that may not be so. You need to find a salon that matches your personal style and, to some extent, reflects your attitudes about life. Taking a job too quickly or without having done the right kind of research can get you into trouble.

Here are some questions to ask yourself when considering a new job.

- *What do you stand for?* What is really important to you? What are you really opposed to? What are the things you would never do, even if your job depended on it?
- *What are you committed to?* Are there certain times or days when you are committed to do something or be somewhere that might interfere with your work situation? You need to be as frank about these as possible. It is never a good idea to "deal with it later."
- *What are your educational goals?* What is your attitude about continuing education? Do you think school is "over" and you never have to learn again? What is your salon's attitude about continuing education? Will you get help if you need it?
- *What do you care about?* What are the issues that you care most deeply about? Does the salon feel the same way about these issues as you do? Is the salon tolerant of differing opinions and views? Does it feel like a comfortable environment for people of different cultures?

All these issues can be explored by asking questions of the salon manager and of the other stylists, especially the ones who have been working at the salon the longest (Figure 26–2).

OUT IN THE REAL WORLD

Many students believe that they should be rewarded with a full-time, high-paying job as soon as they graduate from cosmetology school, doing only the kinds of services they wish to do. Well, welcome to the world. It does not work out that way, at least not for most people. In a job, you will often be asked to do work that you may find boring or confusing or exhausting. You may be asked to create hairstyles that you feel are truly unattractive. The good news, however, is that when you are really working hard, "in the trenches," you are learning every moment, and there is no substitute for that kind of experience.

Depending on the type of salon you start in, you may first be asked to be an assistant before you become a full-service stylist. There is nothing demeaning about graduating from cosmetology school and taking a position as an assistant. In fact, many of today's most famous stylists began their careers as assistants or apprentices to more experienced stylists.

Another entry-level salon job is junior stylist. A junior stylist generally has a light schedule of servicing clients while also assisting experienced stylists. On the other hand, you may find yourself in a position where you take on a full workload of salon clients right from the start.

The important thing is to be honest with yourself as you evaluate your skills in order to best determine which type of position is right for you. If you need help and direction in sorting out the different issues around the different workplaces you are considering, ask your instructor for advice.

Thriving in a Service Profession

The number one thing to remember when you are in a service business is that your work revolves around serving your clients. Some people have a hard time with the idea of customer service because they feel it is demeaning in some way. While it is true that there will always be some clients who treat people badly, the majority of people you will encounter will truly appreciate the work you do for them. They will look forward to seeing you and will show their appreciation for your hard work with their loyalty. So do not let the negativity of a few discolor your overall outlook. Serving others in any capacity is something of which you can be proud.

Here are some points that will help guide you as you serve your clients.

- *Put others first.* You will have to quickly get used to putting your own feelings or desires aside and putting the needs of the salon and the client first. That means doing what is expected of you unless you are physically unable to do so.
- *Be true to your word.* Choose your words carefully and be honest. Be someone who can be counted on to tell the truth and to do what you say you will do.
- *Be punctual.* Scheduling is central to the salon business. Getting to work on time is respectful not only to your clients but also to your coworkers, who will have to handle your clients if you are late.
- *Be grateful.* Remember that it is an honor to have a job that will provide you and your family with financial stability, so be very grateful. If you become unhappy with your salon, look for another job and move on before you start acting out in an ungrateful, disrespectful manner.
- *Be a problem-solver.* No job or situation comes without its share of problems. Be someone who recognizes problems promptly and finds ways to resolve them constructively.

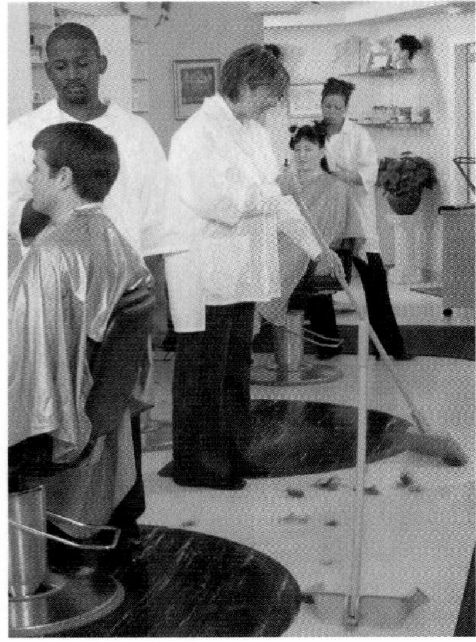

Figure 26–3 Pitch in wherever you're needed.

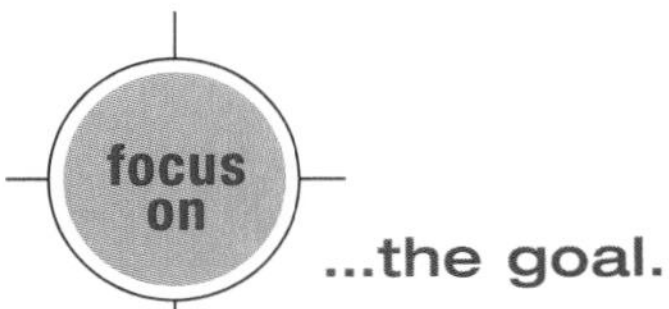

Always put the team first. While each individual may be concerned with getting ahead and being successful, a good teammate knows that no one can be successful alone. The only way you can truly be successful is for the entire salon to be successful!

26

- *Be respectful.* Although you may not like or agree with the salon manager or her rules, you must give her the benefit of the doubt. If you find that you really cannot come to terms with the salon's rules, then it might be time for you to find a new job before your anger takes over.
- *Be a lifelong learner.* A valued employee is one who intends to keep on learning. Thinking that you will never need to learn anything more once you are out of school is immature and limiting. Your career might go in all kinds of interesting directions depending on what new things you learn. This applies to everything in your life, not just learning new technical skills but also to new ways of behaving or dealing with people, problems, and issues. 1

Salon Teamwork

Working in a salon requires that you practice and perfect your people skills. A salon is very much a team environment, and to become a good team player you should do the following things.

- *Strive to help.* Be concerned not only with your own success, but also with the success of others. Stay a little later or come in a little earlier to help out a teammate.
- *Pitch in.* Be willing to help with whatever needs to be done in the salon—from folding towels to making appointments—when you are not busy servicing clients (Figure 26–3).
- *Share your knowledge.* Be willing to share what you know. This will make you a respected member of any team.
- *Remain positive.* Given the stress of a typical salon, there will be lots of opportunities for you to become negative or to have conflicts with your teammates. Resist all temptations to give in to maliciousness and gossip.
- *Become a relationship builder.* Just as there are different kinds of people in the world, there are different types of relationships within the world of the salon. You do not have to be someone's best friend in order to build a good working relationship with that person.
- *Be willing to resolve conflicts.* The most difficult part of being in a relationship is when conflict arises. A real teammate is someone who knows that conflict and tension are bad for the people who are in it, bad for the people who are around it, and bad for the salon as a whole. But conflict is also a natural part of life, and if you can work constructively toward resolving conflict, you will always be a valued member of the team.
- *Be willing to be subordinate.* No one starts at the top. Keep in mind that beginners almost always start out lower down in the pecking order.
- *Be sincerely loyal.* Loyalty is vital to the workings of a salon. Stylists need to be loyal to the salon and its management. Management needs to be loyal to the staff and to clients. Ideally, clients will be loyal to the stylist and the salon. As you work on all the team-building characteristics, you will start to feel a strong sense of loyalty building up within you (Figure 26–4). 2

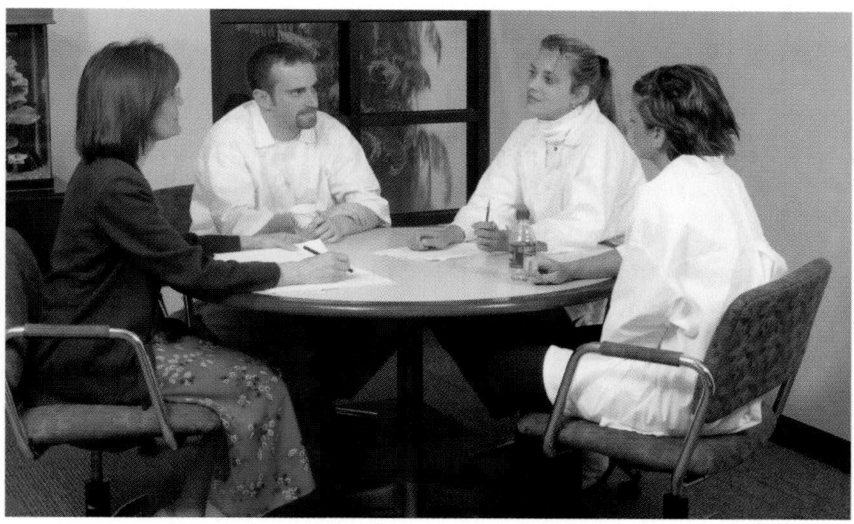

Figure 26-4 Staff meetings are essential for building a loyal team.

The Job Description

When you take a job, you will be expected to behave appropriately, to perform services asked of you, and to conduct your business professionally. In order to do this to the best of your abilities, you should be given a **job description**, a document that outlines all the duties and responsibilities of a particular position in a salon or spa. Many salons have a preprinted job description they can give you. If you find yourself at a salon that does not use job descriptions, you may want to write one for yourself. You can then present this to your salon manager so that you will both have a good understanding of what is expected of you.

Once you have your job description, be sure you understand it. While reading it over, make notes and jot down any questions you may want to ask your manager. When you assume your new position, you are agreeing to do everything as it is written down in the job description, so if you are unclear about something or need more information, it is your responsibility to ask. Remember, not only will you be expected to fulfill all of the different functions set forth in the job description, but also your future at the salon and your financial rewards will be based on how well you execute those duties.

In crafting a job description, the best salons cover all their bases. They make sure to outline not only the duties and responsibilities of the job, but also the attitudes they expect their employees to have and the opportunities that are available to them. Figure 26–5 shows some highlights from a well-written job description. This is just one example. Like the salons that generate them, job descriptions come in all sizes and shapes, and feature a variety of requirements, benefits, and incentives. 3

Compensation Plans

When you assess a job offer, your first concern will probably be around the issue of compensation, or what you are actually getting paid for your work. Different salons handle compensation in different ways. There are, however, three standard methods of compensation that you are likely to encounter: salary, commission, or salary plus commission.

Job Description: Assistant

Every assistant must have a cosmetology license as well as the determination to learn and grow on the job. As an assistant you must be willing to cooperate with coworkers in a team environment, which is most conducive to learning and to good morale among all employees. You must display a friendly yet professional attitude toward coworkers and clients alike.

Excellent time management is essential to the operation of a successful salon. An assistant should be aware of clients who are early and late or stylists who are running ahead or behind in their schedule. You should be prepared to assist in those situations and to change your routine if necessary. Keep the receptionist and stylists informed about clients who have entered the salon. Be prepared to stay up to an hour late when necessary. Keep in mind always that everyone needs to work together to get the job done.

The responsibilities of an assistant include:

1. Greeting clients by offering them a beverage, hanging up coats, and informing the receptionist and stylist that they have arrived.
2. Shampooing and conditioning clients.
3. Assisting stylists on the styling floor.
4. Assisting stylists in services that require extra help, such as dimensional coloring.
5. Cleaning stations and mirrors, including hand-held mirrors.
6. Keeping the styling stations and back bars well stocked with appropriate products.
7. Notifying the salon manager about items and supplies that need to be reordered.
8. Making sure the shampoo sink and drain are clean and free of hair.
9. Keeping the makeup display neat and clean.
10. Keeping the retail area neat and well stocked.
11. Keeping the bathroom and dressing room neat, clean, and stocked.
12. Performing housekeeping duties such as: emptying trash receptacles, cleaning haircolor from the floor, keeping the lunch room and dispensary neat and clean, helping with laundry, and dusting shelves.
13. Making fresh coffee when necessary.
14. Training new assistants.

Continuing Education

Your position as assistant is the first step toward becoming a successful stylist. In the beginning, your training will focus on the duties of an assistant. Once you have mastered those, your training will focus on the skills you will need as a stylist. As part of your continuing education in this salon you will be required to:

- attend all salon classes
- attend our special Sunday Seminars
- acquire all professional tools necessary for training at six weeks (shears, brushes, combs, clips, etc.)

Advancement

Upon successful completion of all required classes and seminars and your demonstration of the necessary skills and attitudes, you will have the opportunity to advance to the position of junior stylist. This advancement will always depend upon your performance as an assistant as well as the approval of management. Remember: how quickly you achieve your goals in this salon is up to you!

Figure 26-5 An example of a job description.

insights

Larry Walthers

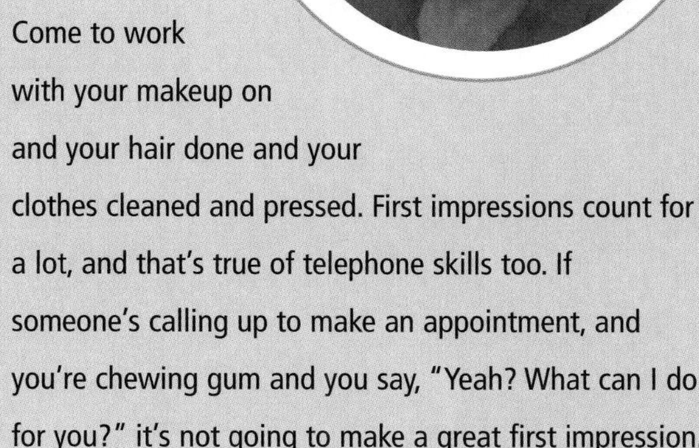

The owner of a salon-spa, Larry Walthers is also a past president of the National Interstate Council State Boards of Cosmetology (NIC).

I'll be blunt: I went into cosmetology for the money and the freedom. I was so tired of being poor. One day I looked at the barber on my block, who had a three-bedroom house and a new car in the driveway, and I said to myself, "I can do that." And I was right—I could and I did.

Cosmetology is all up to you. You get out of it what you put into it. It has allowed me to travel, to pick and choose my own hours, to take days off when I want to, and to decide whom I want to work with. In other words, it provides money and freedom—the two things that were so important to me. But it doesn't come without a lot of hard work.

You've got to keep in mind that it's all about customer service. You're dealing with the consumer and the consumer is always right, as far as I'm concerned. I'm very old-fashioned in that regard. Customer service is what makes all the difference in this field. There are lots of good haircutters out there, but it's the hairdresser who makes the customer feel special that gets the return visit.

As a cosmetologist, you've got to be a good listener. Your clients want to be pampered; they don't want to be pampering you. So have a smile on your face. I don't think we smile enough. Look professional. Come to work with your makeup on and your hair done and your clothes cleaned and pressed. First impressions count for a lot, and that's true of telephone skills too. If someone's calling up to make an appointment, and you're chewing gum and you say, "Yeah? What can I do for you?" it's not going to make a great first impression.

When I interview potential employees, I look for a nice smile and good hygiene to start out with. And a good printed resume. If I hire someone, I'm committed to that person, but they won't last long if I sense that they're lazy. When I first opened this new salon, I hired somebody I had great hopes for. Her second day she came to me and said, "I have to have a scheduled lunch hour every day, and I have to have a smoke break during the day." Needless to say, she didn't last long. In our business, we can't predict when you can take a smoke break. We just can't adjust for that. I have no problem with giving stylists a lunch hour, but it can't be a set time. If we're behind, then they have to help us get out from behind.

But it's such a great field. I have employees who come in at six in the morning and work till seven or eight at night, and they'll do this for three days a week, and I give them four days a week at home with their families. They're all in the $70,000-to-$100,000-a-year income bracket. Now, how are you going to beat that?

In addition to your regular salary, it is customary for salon professionals to receive tips or gratuities from satisfied clients. These must also be factored into your total compensation package and reported as income. It is important to keep good records and to honestly report all of your earnings.

Salary

To be compensated with a salary is usually the best way for a new salon professional to start out since that person will most likely not have an established clientele for a while. A salaried position is generally offered to a new stylist and is usually based on the minimum wage. Some salons offer a salary that is slightly higher than the minimum wage to encourage new stylists or assistants to take the job and stick with it. Regular taxes will be taken out of this salary, which can be paid in either a flat rate or on an hourly basis.

Being paid a flat rate means being paid the same amount of dollars no matter how many hours you actually work. There may be a minimum requirement for the salary, such as 40 hours per week, but you may work 42 hours and still be paid the same salary as if you were there for 40 hours. This may sound unfair, but you should keep in mind that there are high points and low points in salon work and a guaranteed salary will protect you during the slow periods.

With a salaried compensation, you may also be paid by the hour, with an hourly rate. For example, if your salary is $8 per hour and you work 40 hours, you will be paid $320 that week. If you work more hours, you will get more pay. Fewer hours means less pay.

Commission

A **commission**, a percentage of the money that the salon takes in from its sales, is usually offered to stylists once they have built up a loyal clientele. A commission payment structure is very different from salaried compensation in that any money you eventually are paid is a direct result of the total amount of service dollars you generate for the salon.

Commissions are paid on percentages of your total service dollars and can range anywhere from 25 percent to 60 or 70 percent, depending on your length of time at the salon and your performance levels. For example, at the end of the week, when you add up all the services you have performed, your total is $1,000. If you are at the 50 percent commission level, then you would be paid $500, less taxes. Keep in mind that until you have a year or so of servicing clients under your belt, you may not be able to make a living on straight commission compensation.

Salary Plus Commissions

A salary-plus-commissions structure is another common way to be compensated in the salon business. It basically means that you receive both a salary and a commission. This kind of structure is commonly used during the transition from junior stylist to full-time stylist and is often used to motivate stylists to perform more services, thereby increasing their

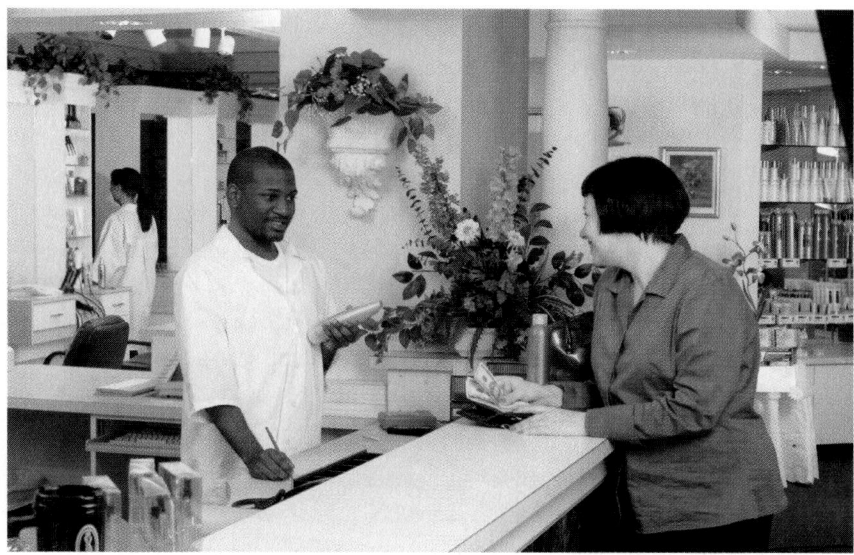

Figure 26-6 Commissions on retail sales boost income.

productivity. For example, imagine that you earn a salary of $300 per week and you perform about $600 worth of services every week. Your salon manager may offer you an additional commission of 25 percent on any services you perform over your usual $600 per week. Or perhaps you receive a straight salary but you can receive as much as 20 percent commission on all the retail products you sell. You can see how this kind of structure quickly leads to significantly increased compensation (Figure 26–6). 4

Tips

When you receive satisfactory service at a hotel or restaurant, you are likely to leave your server a tip. It has become customary for salon clients to acknowledge beauty professionals in this way, too. Some salons have a tipping policy and others have a no-tipping policy. This is determined by what the salon feels is appropriate for its clientele.

The usual amount to tip is 15 percent of the total service ticket. For example, if someone spends $50, then the tip might be 15 percent of that, or $7.50. Tips are income in addition to your regular compensation and must be tracked and accounted for as income. You must report all your earnings, including tips, for tax purposes. Reporting tips will be beneficial to you if you wish to take out a loan or mortgage and want your income to appear as strong as it really is.

As you can see, there are a number of ways to structure compensation for a salon professional. You will probably have the opportunity to try each of these methods at different points in your career. When deciding whether a certain compensation method is right for you, it is important to be aware of what your monthly expenses are and to have a personal financial budget and plan in place. We will address budget issues later in this chapter.

Employee Evaluation

The best way to keep tabs on your progress is to ask for and get feedback from your salon manager and from key and trusted coworkers. Most likely, your salon will have in place a structure for evaluation purposes. Commonly, evaluations are scheduled 90 days after hiring and then once a year after that. But you should feel free to ask for help and feedback when you need it. This feedback can help you to improve your technical abilities as well as your customer service skills.

Ask a senior stylist to sit in on one of your client consultations and to make note of areas where you can improve. Ask your manager to observe your technical skills and to point out ways in which you can perform your work more quickly and more efficiently. Have a trusted coworker watch and evaluate your skills when it comes to selling retail products. All of these kinds of evaluations will benefit your learning process enormously.

Find a Role Model

On of the best ways to improve your performance is to use as a role model someone who is having the kind of success you wish to have. Watch the other stylists in your salon. You will easily be able to identify who is really good and who is just coasting along. Focus in on the skills of the ones who are really good. What do they do? How do they treat their clients? How do they treat the salon staff and the salon manager? How do they book their appointments? How do they handle their continuing education? How do they hold their implements and tools? What process do they use when formulating color or deciding on product? What is their attitude toward their work? How do they handle crisis? Conflict?

Go to those persons for advice. Ask for a few minutes of their time but be willing to wait for it, for in a busy salon it may not be easy to find time to talk during the day. If you are having a problem, explain your situation and ask if they can help you to see things differently. Be prepared to listen and not argue your points. Remember that you asked for help, even if what they are saying is not what you want to hear. Thank them for their help and reflect on the advice you've been given.

A little help and direction from skilled, experienced coworkers will go a long way toward helping you to achieve your goals.

MANAGING YOUR MONEY

Although a career in the beauty industry is very artistic and creative, it is also a career that requires financial understanding and planning. Too many cosmetologists live for the moment and do not plan for their futures. They may wind up feeling cheated out of the benefits their friends and family in other careers are enjoying.

In a corporate structure, the human resources department of the corporation handles a great deal of the employee's financial planning for them. For example, health and dental insurance, retirement accounts, savings accounts, and many other items may be automatically deducted and paid out of the employee's salary. Most beauty professionals, however, must research and plan for all those things on their own. This may seem difficult, but in fact it is a small price to pay for the kind of freedom, financial reward, and job satisfaction a career in cosmetology can offer. And the good news is that managing money is something everyone can learn to do.

Meeting Financial Responsibilities

In addition to making money, responsible adults are also concerned with paying back their debts. Throughout your life and your career, you will undoubtedly incur debt in the form of car loans, housing loans or mortgages, or student loans. While it is easy for some people to merely ignore their responsibility involved in repaying these loans, it is extremely irresponsible and immature to take a loan and then to shrug off the debt. Not paying back your loans is called "defaulting" and it can have serious consequences regarding your personal and professional credit.

The best way to meet all of your financial responsibilities is to know precisely what you owe and what you earn so that you can make informed decisions about where your money goes.

A Personal Budget

It is amazing how many people work hard and earn very good salaries but never take the time to create a personal budget. Many people are afraid of the word "budget" because they think it will be too restrictive on their spending or because they think that they need to be mathematical geniuses in order to work with a budget. Thankfully, neither of these fears is rooted in reality.

You can create a personal budget that can range from extremely simple to extremely complex. It all depends on what your needs are. In the beginning of your career, a simple budget should be sufficient. To get started, take a look at the worksheet in Figure 26–7. It lists the standard monthly expenses for which most people have to budget. It also includes school loan repayment, savings, and payments into an individual retirement account (IRA).

Keeping track of where your money goes is one step toward making sure you always have enough. It also helps you plan ahead and save for bigger expenses such as a vacation or your own home. Even your own business. All in all, sticking to a budget is a good practice to follow faithfully for the rest of your life.

Giving Yourself a Raise

Once you have taken some time to create, use, and work with your personal budget, you may want to look at ways in which you can generate greater income for yourself. You might automatically jump to the most obvious sources, such as asking your employer for a raise or asking for a higher percentage of commission. While these tactics are certainly valid, you will also want to think about other ways to increase your income. These include the following points.

- *Spending less money.* Although it may be difficult to reduce your spending, it is certainly one way to increase the amount of money that is left over at the end of the month. These dollars can be used to invest or save.

Personal Budget Worksheet

A. Expenses

1. My monthly rent (or share of the rent) is $________
2. My monthly car payment is ________
3. My monthly car insurance payment is ________
4. My monthly auto fuel/upkeep expenses are ________
5. My monthly electric bill is ________
6. My monthly gas bill is ________
7. My monthly health insurance payment is ________
8. My monthly entertainment expense is ________
9. My monthly bank fees are ________
10. My monthly grocery expense is ________
11. My monthly dry cleaning expense is ________
12. My monthly personal grooming expense is ________
13. My monthly prescription/medical expense is ________
14. My monthly telephone is ________
15. My monthly student loan payment is ________
16. My IRA payment is ________
17. My savings account deposit is ________
18. Other expenses: ________

TOTAL EXPENSES $________

B. Income

1. My monthly take-home pay is ________
2. My monthly income from tips is ________
3. Other income: ________

TOTAL INCOME $________

C. Balance

Total Income (B) ________

Minus Total Expenses (A) ________

BALANCE $________

Figure 26-7 A budget worksheet.

- *Increasing service prices.* Although it will probably take some time before you are in a position to be able to increase your service prices, once you have fully mastered all the services you are performing and you have a loyal client base, there is nothing wrong with increasing your prices every year or two, as long as you do so by a reasonable amount. Do a little research to determine what your competitors are charging for similar services and increase your fees accordingly.

Seek Professional Advice

Just as you will want your clients to seek out your advice and services when it comes to their hair and beauty needs, sometimes it is important for you to seek out the advice of experts, especially when it comes to your finances. You can research and interview financial planners who will be able to give you advice on reducing your credit card debt, on how to invest your money, and on retirement options. You can speak to the officers at your local bank who may be able to suggest bank accounts that offer you greater returns or flexibility with your money, depending on what you need.

When seeking out advice from other professionals, be sure not to take anyone's advice without carefully considering whether or not the advice makes sense for your particular situation and needs. Before you buy into anything, be an informed consumer of other people's goods and services. 5

DISCOVER THE SELLING YOU

Another area that touches on the issue of you and money is selling. As a salon professional, you will have an enormous opportunity to sell retail products and to upgrade service tickets. **Ticket upgrading,** or **upselling**

26

activity

Go through the budget worksheet and fill in the amounts that apply to your current living and financial situation. If you are unsure of the amount of an expense, put in the amount you have averaged over the past three months, or give it your best guess. For your income, you may need to have three or four months of employment history in order to answer, but fill in what you can.

- How do your expenses compare to your income?
- What is your balance after all your expenses are paid?
- Were there any surprises for you in this exercise?
- Do you think that keeping a budget is a good way to manage money?
- Do you know of any other methods people use to manage money?

services, is the practice of recommending and selling additional services to your clients, which may be performed by you or by other practitioners (such as estheticians or nail technicians) in the salon (Figure 26–8). **Retailing** is the act of recommending and selling products to your clients for at-home hair, skin, and nail care. These two activities can make all the difference in your economic picture.

The following dialogue is an example of ticket upgrading. In this scene, Judy, the stylist, suggests an additional service to Ms. King, her client, who has just had her hair styled for a wedding she will be attending that evening. Read the script yourself and change the words to make them fit your personality. Then try it the next time you feel an additional service could help one of your clients.

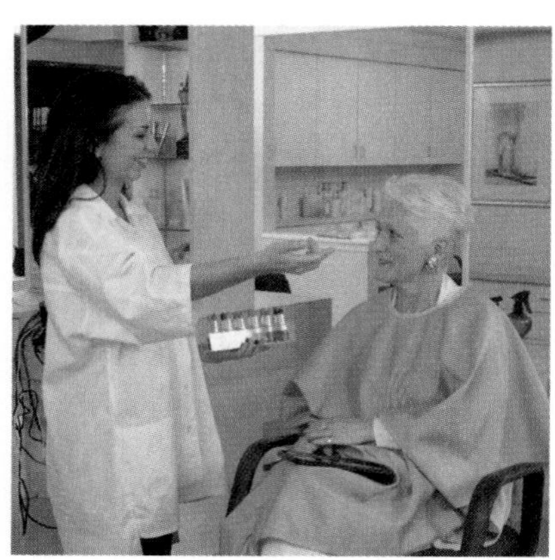

Figure 26-8 This client may wish a makeup service as well as hairstyling.

Judy: I'm really glad you like your hairstyle. It will be perfect with the dress you described. Don't you just love formal weddings?

Ms. King: I don't know. To tell you the truth, I don't get dressed up all that often, and putting the look together was harder than I thought it would be.

Judy: Yes, I know what you mean. Are you all set with your makeup for tonight, Ms. King? It would be a shame to have a beautiful new dress and this gorgeous hairstyle, and then have to worry about your makeup.

Ms. King: Well, actually, I was sort of wondering about that. I'm wearing this long black dress and I'm not really sure what's the best look for the occasion. Got any ideas?

Judy: Well, as you know, my specialty is hairstyling, but we have an excellent makeup artist right here on staff who's available for a consultation. You might want to make an appointment with her and she can do your makeup for you. I don't know if you've ever had a professional do it before, but it's a real treat, and it only costs $15. Plus they throw in a small lipstick to take with you. Shall I get her for you?

Ms. King: Definitely. That sounds terrific!

Principles of Selling

Some salon professionals shy away from sales. They think it is pushy or scary or beneath them. But a look at how selling works can set your mind at ease. Not only can you become very good at selling, if you understand the principles behind it, but also feel good about providing your clients with a valuable service.

To be successful in sales, you need ambition, determination, and a good personality. The first step in selling is to sell yourself. Clients must like and trust you before they will purchase beauty services, cosmetics, skin or nail care items, shampoos and conditioners, or other merchandise.

Remember, every client who enters the salon is a potential purchaser of additional services or merchandise. Recognizing the client's needs and preferences lays the foundation for successful selling.

To become a proficient salesperson, you must understand and be able to apply the following principles of selling.

- Be familiar with the merits and benefits of the various services and products you are trying to sell, and recommend only those that the client really needs.
- Adapt your approach and technique to meet the needs and personality of each client. Some clients may prefer a "soft sell," during which you inform the client about the product without stressing that they purchase it, while others are comfortable with a "hard sell" approach, which focuses emphatically on why a client should buy the product.
- Be self-confident when recommending products for sale. You become confident by knowing about the products you are selling and by believing that they are as good as you say they are.
- Generate interest and desire in the customer by asking questions that determine a need.
- Never misrepresent your service or product. Making unrealistic claims will only lead to your client's disappointment and will make it unlikely that you will ever be able to sell to that client again.
- Do not underestimate the client's intelligence or her knowledge of her own beauty regimen or particular needs.
- To sell a product or service, deliver your sales talk in a relaxed, friendly manner and, if possible, demonstrate use (Figure 26–9).
- Recognize the right psychological moment to close any sale. Once the client has offered to buy, quit selling. Do not oversell, except to praise the client for the purchase and to assure him that he will be happy with it. 6 ✓

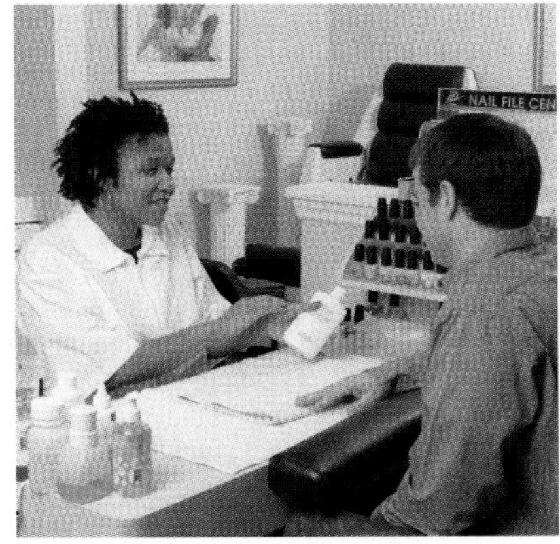

Figure 26-9 Demonstrate a product's benefits.

The Psychology of Selling

Most people have reasons for doing what they do, and when you are selling something, it is your job to figure out the reasons that might motivate a person to buy. When dealing with salon clients, you will find that their motives for buying salon products vary widely. Some may be concerned with issues of vanity (they want to look better). Some are seeking personal satisfaction (they want to feel better about themselves, or they want to look like someone they find beautiful, such as a movie actress or a singer). Others need to solve a problem that is bothersome (they want to spend less time untangling their hair).

Sometimes, a client may inquire about a product or service but may still be undecided or doubtful. In this type of situation, you can help the decision along by offering honest and sincere advice. For example, if a client is thinking about coloring her hair and she already has had a permanent, you might advise her about the extra care that is needed with both treatments.

When you explain a beauty service to a client, address the results and benefits of that service. Always keep in mind that the best interests of the client should be your first consideration. You will need to know exactly what your client's needs are, and you need to have a clear idea as to how those needs can be fulfilled. Refer to the sample dialogues in this section, one involving ticket upgrading (p. 904) and another involving retailing (p. 906), which demonstrate effective selling techniques.

Here are a few tips on how to get the conversation started on retailing products:

- ask every client what products they are using to shampoo, condition, and style their hair
- place products in the client's hands whenever possible, or have them in view (Figure 26–10)
- advise the client how the recommended service will benefit her (her hair will be easier to style or shinier, for instance)
- keep retail areas clean, well-lit, and appealing
- inform clients of any promotions and sales that are going on in the salon
- be informed about the merits of using a professional product as opposed to generic store brands

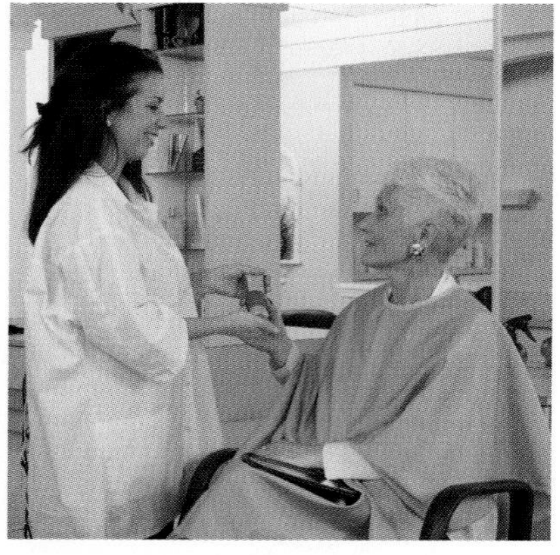

Figure 26-10 Place the product in the client's hands.

While you realize that retailing products is a service to your clients, you may not be sure how to go about it. Imagine the following scene and see how Lisa, the stylist, highlights the benefits and features of a product to her client, Ms. Steiner. Note that price is not necessarily the "bottom line."

Ms. Steiner: I just love the way you style my hair. How do you always get so much volume on top?

Lisa : Well, I run some styling lotion through it and I use this round brush when I'm blow-drying to get the movement. The lotion is really light but it gives a nice strong hold that lasts all day. And the good thing is you only need a little—a dollop about the size of a quarter does the trick. But what I really love about this styling lotion is that it doesn't contain anything that is drying to the hair, so it leaves it all pumped up and shiny. What do you use at home when you style your hair?

Ms. Steiner: Oh, I don't know . . . whatever. Some kind of mousse, I think.

Lisa: It doesn't sound like it performs as well as this lotion.

Ms. Steiner: Oh, it's probably just me. You stylists can make anything look good!

Lisa: Well, thanks for the compliment, but I have a lot of clients who are using this lotion at home, and they're styling their hair as beautifully as I can, every day.

Ms. Steiner: Really?

Lisa: Really. You may want to give it a try yourself and see how it works for you. It's available at the front when you check out. I'll grab you a bottle and you can look at it while I'm blowing your hair dry.

Ms. Steiner: Great!

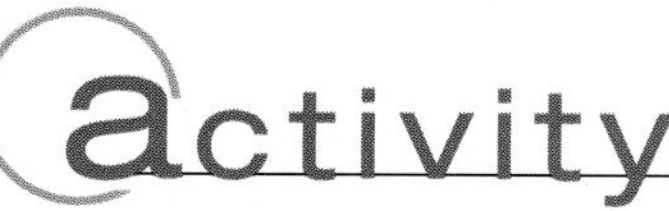

Pick a partner from class and role-play the dynamics of a sales situation. Take turns being the customer and the cosmetologist. Evaluate each other on how you did, with suggestions about where you can improve. Then try this exercise with someone else, as no two customers are the same!

Building a Client Base

In order to have a successful career in cosmetology, it is vital that you start, as soon as possible, to build a client base. A **client base** consists of the clients you serve on a regular basis, who return to you again and again for your services. The larger your client base, the larger your income, especially if you work on increasing the average ticket for each client through retailing and ticket upgrading.

Successfully building a client base depends mainly on your ability to build strong relationships with others. Here are some points to keep in mind as you begin to build your client base.

- *Provide good service.* It seems basic enough, but it is amazing how many professionals, once they have worked hard to get a client, will lose that client simply because they rush through a service and leave the client feeling that the quality of the service was inadequate. Providing good, quality service must always be your first concern.
- *Be reliable.* Always be courteous, thoughtful, and professional. Be at the salon when you say you will be there and don't keep clients waiting (refer to Chapter 4 for tips on how to handle the unavoidable times when you are running late). Give the client the style or service she asks for, not something else. Recommend a retail product only when you have tried it yourself and you know what it can and cannot do. Establish yourself as someone the client can trust.
- *Be respectful.* When you treat others with respect, then you become worthy of respect yourself. Being respectful means that you do not gossip or make fun of anyone or anything related to the salon. That goes for clients, coworkers, your salon manager, whomever. Negative energy brings everyone down, especially you.
- *Be positive.* Become one of those people who always sees the glass as half full. Look for the positive in every situation. No one enjoys being around a person who is always unhappy.
- *Be professional.* Sometimes, a client may try to make your relationship more personal than it ought to be. It is in your best interest, and your client's best interest, not to cross that line. Remember that your job is to be the client's beauty advisor, not a psychiatrist, a marriage counselor, or a buddy. The relationship you have with your client can be friendly and pleasant, but it is still a business relationship.

How to Expand Your Client Base

Once you have mastered the basics of good service, take a look at some marketing techniques that will keep your clients coming back to you for services. These are only a few suggestions; there are many, many others that may work for you. The best way to decide which techniques are most effective is to try several.

- *Birthday cards.* Ask the client for his birth date on the client consultation card and then use it as a tool to get him into the salon again. About one month prior to the client's birthday, send him a card with a special offer

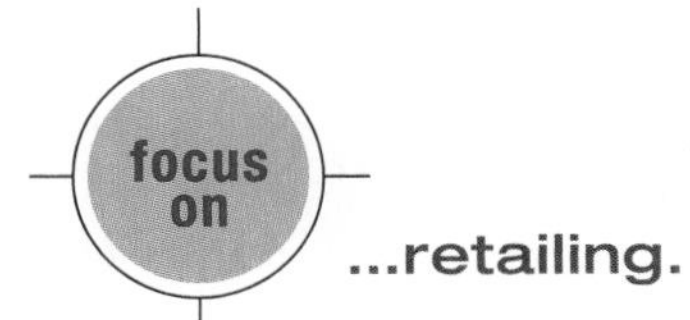

For quick reference, keep these five points in mind when selling.

1. Establish rapport with the client
2. Determine the client's needs.
3. Recommend products/services based on those needs.
4. Emphasize benefits.
5. Close the sale.

26

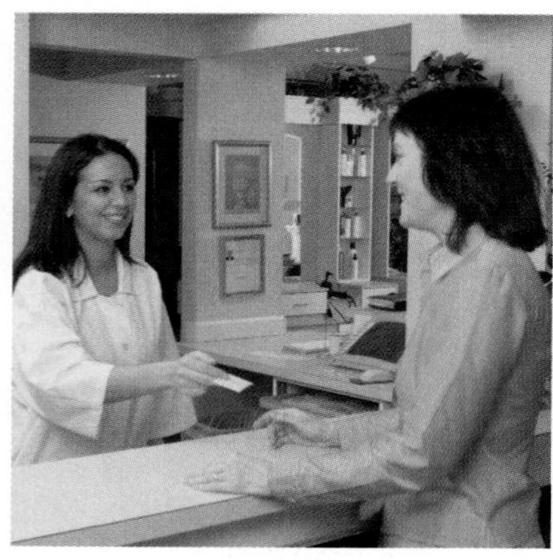

Figure 26–11 Referral cards help build your client base.

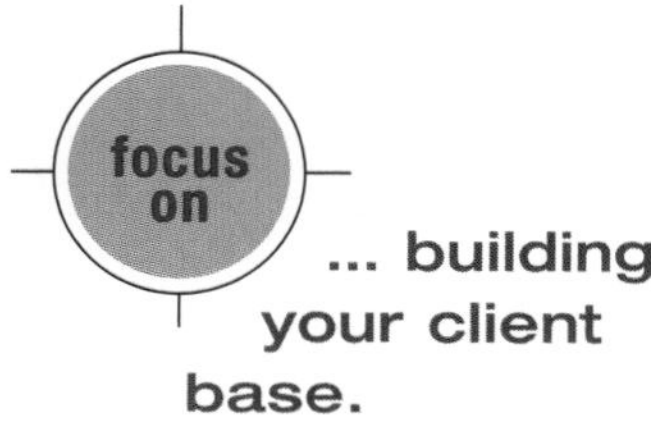

... building your client base.

Some professionals believe that the more time they spend with their clients performing services, the better the service will be. Not so! Your client should be in the salon only as long as is necessary for you to adequately complete a service.

Be aware of how much time it takes you to apply and process a color service, a wrap, a perm, and so on, and then schedule accordingly. As you become more and more experienced, you should see a reduction in the amount of time it takes you to perform these services. That means clients wait less, you can increase your number of services, and the increase in services naturally increases your income.

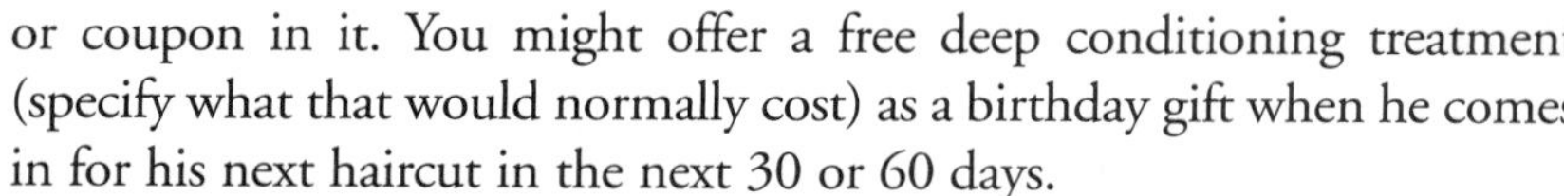
or coupon in it. You might offer a free deep conditioning treatment (specify what that would normally cost) as a birthday gift when he comes in for his next haircut in the next 30 or 60 days.

- *Business card referrals.* Make up a special business card with your information on it but leave room for a client to put her name on it is well. If your client is clearly pleased with your work, give her several cards and ask her to put her name on them and to refer her friends and associates to you. For every card you receive from a new customer with her name on it, give her 10 percent off her next color or perm service. This gives the client lots of motivation to recommend you to others, which in turn, helps you build up your clientele (Figure 26–11).
- *Local business referrals.* Another terrific way to build business is to work with other businesses in your area. Look for clothing stores, florists, gift and novelty shops, and other small businesses near your salon. Offer to have a card swap and commit to referring your clients to them when they are in the market for goods or services that your neighbors can provide, if they will do the same for you. This is a great way to build a feeling of community among local vendors and to reach new clients you may not be able to otherwise.
- *Public speaking.* Make yourself available to speak to local women's groups, the PTA, organizations for young men and women, and anywhere else that will put you in front of people in your community who are all potential clients. Put together a short program (20 to 30 minutes) in which, for example, you might discuss professional appearance such as how to style the hair, what kind of makeup to use, and other grooming tips for people looking for jobs or already employed. You might offer your services to local community groups or nursing homes. Always make sure to have lots of business cards, salon flyers, and anything else that will make people aware of the salon.

Rebooking Clients

The best time to think about getting your client back into the salon is while she is still in your chair. It may seem a little difficult to assure your client that you are concerned with her satisfaction on this visit while you are talking about her next visit, but, in fact, the two go together. The best way to encourage your client to book another appointment before she leaves is to simply talk with her, ask questions, and listen carefully to her answers.

During the time that you are working on a client's hair, for instance, talk about the condition of the hair, her grooming habits at home, and the benefits of regular or special salon maintenance. You might raise these issues in a number of ways.

1. "Mrs. Rivera, I had to cut a lot of your perm out today. It will probably take you longer to style your hair every morning. Shall I book a perm for your next visit?"
2. "It sounds like your vacation to Hawaii was terrific, but you want to be careful about how you handle your hair now after

being in the hot sun for two weeks. I think it would be a good idea to give you a couple of deep conditioning treatments before we do your color again. Since you usually color every two months, we should book a couple of treatments this month."

3. "Your son is getting married next month? How wonderful. Have you thought about how you'd like to wear your hair? Have you chosen your outfit? I'll check my schedule to make sure you get the appointment you need and that we have time for perm, cut, and styling for the big day. Would you like to come in the day before the wedding?"

Again, you will want to listen carefully to what your clients are telling you during their visit, because they will often give the careful listener many good clues as to what is happening in their lives. That will open the door to discussing their next appointment. 7

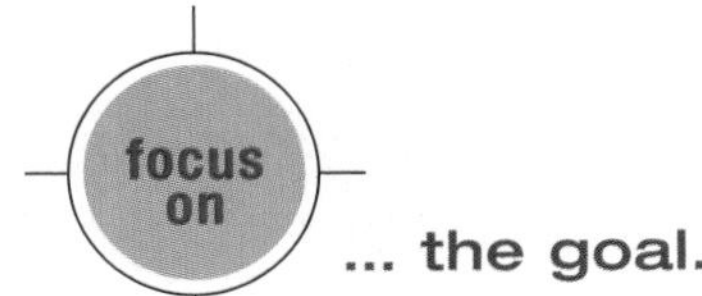

... the goal.

Always remember that success does not just come to you. You make it happen. How? By being a team player, having a positive attitude, and keeping a real sense of commitment to your work foremost in your mind.

ON YOUR WAY

Your first job in the beauty industry will most likely be your most difficult. Getting started in this business means being on a big learning curve for a while. You will be in the process of making the transition from the "school you" to the "professional you." Always remember that in your work life, as in everything else you do, practice makes perfect. You will not know everything you need to know right at the start, but be confident in the fact that you are graduating from cosmetology school with a solid base of knowledge. Make use of the many generous and experienced professionals you will encounter and let them teach you the tricks of the trade that they have learned over the years. Make the commitment to perfecting your technical skills and your customer service.

Above all, always be willing to learn. If you let the concepts you've learned in this book be your guide, you will enjoy your life and reap the amazing benefits of a career in cosmetology (Figure 26–12).

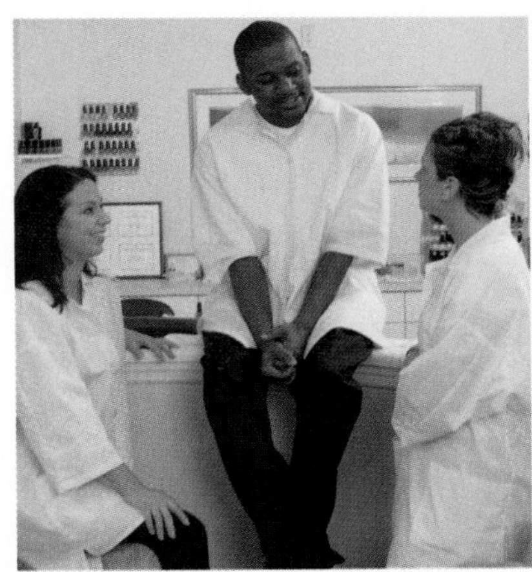

Figure 26-12 Make career satisfaction your goal.

chapter glossary

client base	those customers who are loyal to a particular cosmetologist
commission	a percentage of the money that a salon takes in from sales
job description	a document that outlines all the duties and responsibilities of a particular position in a salon or spa
retailing	the act of recommending and selling products to your clients for at-home hair, skin, and nail care
ticket upgrading or upselling services	the practice of recommending and selling additional services to clients

review questions

1. What should you look for in a salon to determine whether or not it is right for you?
2. List seven rules of conduct that help a new employee succeed in a service profession like cosmetology.

3. List six habits of a good team player.
4. Explain how a job description is used by the salon and by the employee.
5. What are the three most common methods of salon compensation?
6. Complete a personal budget and explain why managing your personal finances is important to your success.
7. Name at least six principles of selling retail products in the salon.
8. List the important personal characteristics that help you build a client base.
9. Explain at least three different activities you can undertake to expand your client base.

in closing

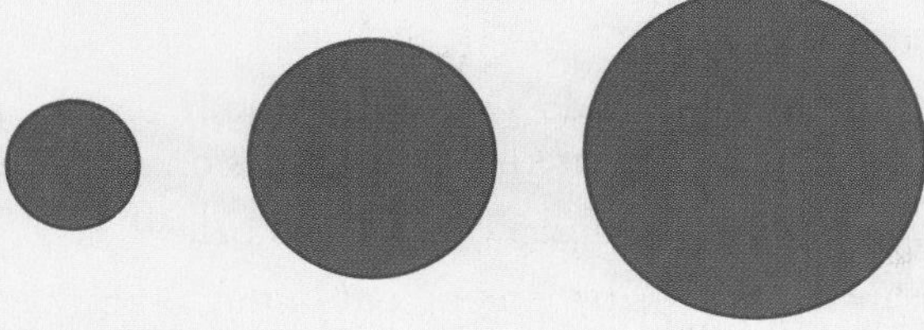

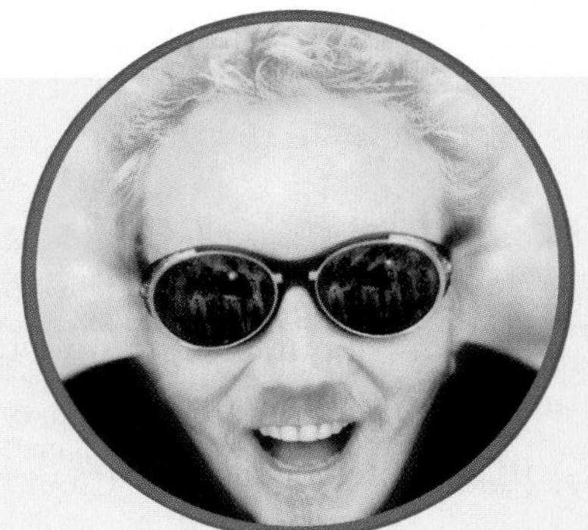

A Special Message from Robert Cromeans

The first thing I want to ask you is "Why?" Why do we want to be hairdressers? What was the first thing that inspired us to take that walk through the beauty school door, that first step into the industry? Many times we wonder if it's because of the way we look, or because we want a certain sense of freedom. Why did you want to be a hairdresser?

What It's All About

People often compare us to artists, who have a very unusual perspective on life. The only thing I hate about being called an artist is that it brings to mind the "starving artist." That's an old mentality. Hairdressing is truly a business, so for those of you who choose it for art and fun and expressiveness—yahoo! You're going to have a lot of fun. But one of the greatest factors of this industry today is the possibility to make money. Having fun and making money: that's what it's all truly about.

I once said to my mom on the phone, "Mom, I'm going to be a hairdresser." She paused for a few seconds and said, "Son, do you have something else to tell me?" I had to laugh because my mom thought I had made a career choice based on a stereotypical affluent lifestyle. When I told my dad, who is a dentist in Mississippi, he said, "Oh, son, you're not going to make any money. You would be better served to become an accountant." Well, that was not something that drove me, even though I do have a sense of numbers. I wanted to have fun. I wanted to travel the world. I wanted to do supermodels' hair and get tipped fifty bucks every time. I had a vision of what hairdressing could be. It was traveling around having fun, crazy with a purpose.

Use Your Time Wisely

Many times in school, all we're focused on is getting out. The reality is we need to focus every single day on making the right choices so that we can be the best hairdresser possible. One thing I remember from being a student is the idle time, the down time, and if there's anything I wish I had done differently, it's this: I wish I had done more hair. If there was an idle mannequin sitting there, if I had even just applied conditioner to it, pretending it was a foil highlight, that would have taken me closer to my goal of becoming a great hairdresser.

Vidal Sassoon, Trevor Sorbie, Irvine Rusk, Robert Lombetta—they're all my mentors, and they all have one thing in common. They all started at age fourteen, fifteen, sixteen, seventeen. Which means if you're twenty-four years old and reading this, Vidal Sassoon was already doing hair seven years before you ever started! Does that mean you can never be as great as he is? No. What you have to do is accelerate your learning. The more you do,

in closing

(continued)

the more you learn. It's not about sitting in the class; it's about doing simultaneous actions with your mind and hands. That is what truly defines us as professionals. But it's doing it every day. So instead of taking off till three o'clock and hanging and waiting for somebody to come in to teach you something, you have got to do hair, whether it's your neighbor's hair, your friend's, a mannequin's, people in the street. Get them in and do hair.

Form Good Habits

Many times we think that when we're in school, we can dress or act a certain way. But these are the first habits you're going to form in your new profession. So why not start forming habits now that will change your whole attitude when you get into the industry? Your professional life starts when you walk into school. From day one, you are a hairdresser. Think forward to the end result—you want to be a good hairdresser. You don't want to be mediocre. That means you dress up, you apply makeup, and if you don't like makeup, be a nurse. You're in the beauty business. Do not treat school like a backstage rehearsal. Treat school like you're on stage. Start being the person you want to be while you're in beauty school.

Seek Mentors

While I was in beauty school I picked a few mentors that helped me. The first was a company, Paul Mitchell, which may not sound like it's a mentorship, but the reality is, companies can give common knowledge to an industry. I think it's very important to use a company as a mentor for information and ideas. Being connected into something bigger is just smart business. The business values are the enterprise it operates on. So find a company to believe in by looking out in the industry to see what inspires you, what seems to make the most connection to you.

When I was in school, Jeanne Braa, who was Paul Mitchell's partner at the time, was to my mind the most incredible hairdresser in the world. I never touched hair until I was 24 years old. I had two left thumbs and my hands didn't move naturally. She had magical hands and could make stuff happen so quickly. As a hair mentor she was incredible—it was the greatest mentor experience I could ever have.

There are many mentors to focus on in the industry, people like Trevor Sorbie, Vidal Sassoon. As you go through your career, your mentors may change; maybe your dreams get a little bigger. There was a time when my beauty school teacher was my mentor. Later I had the audacity to look to Mr. Sassoon, who has been the great leader of the industry for three or four decades and is still the most highly regarded educator in the world. He's my focus right now because I want to be the next Vidal Sassoon.

Explore the Possibilities

I think the most important thing for young hairdressers after getting their license is to find the right salon environment to work in. Start today on your homework—targeting salons you want to work for. We want you to stay in the business. There are far too few hairdressers, and we want to keep each and every one of you and show you how to make it. There are many career paths you can choose. You can go for a team-based salary or a commission bracket, or for booth rental, where you become an independent

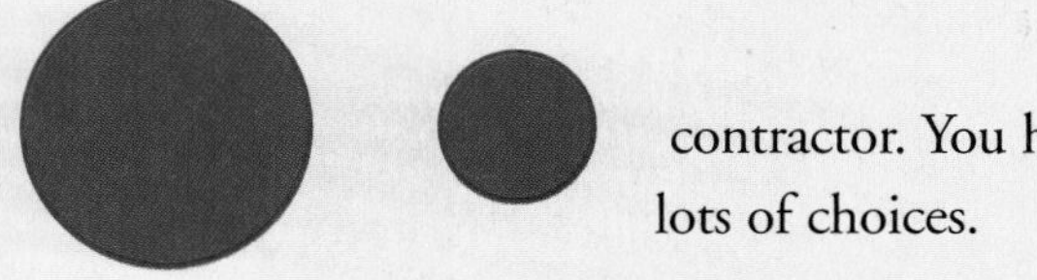

contractor. You have lots of choices.

Look into assistant programs.

Look at the top salons in your community. Look for a product line that identifies the highest-quality salons in the neighborhood. Those are the people you want to get the opportunity to assist. In my salon there are twenty-four hairdressers who work with every assistant throughout their program and training. Assistants learn from the stylist who can upgrade more people into color than anybody else in the salon. They learn from the geniuses who do updos, sometimes two thousand dollars a day of updos. These young kids watch it and they take it away.

Being an assistant is a noble job, as long as you understand you're not there to sweep hair. You're there to do as much hair as possible, and as you learn more, you get to do more. So look at an assistant program as an endorsement from me personally.

Look around and pick one or two salons you'd like to work in—not when you think you're going to take your license, not when you plan to graduate, but many months before. Many of these salons would like to meet you in advance. You could already be working in there after hours, not doing hair but just serving coffee and water. That way you can start to feel the vibe, start to see what hairdressing is truly about. Communication, connecting with people, is the key. Start while you're in school.

Young kids sometimes say to me, "I'm working through school. What do I do?" I tell them the best thing to do is wait tables, because waiting tables you get to blend with lots of different types of people, and you're there to serve them. It's very similar to hairdressing—not that we're waiters or waitresses; we're professionals, but with a human attitude. We're not working on mannequins. We're working on human beings, and our job is to make them feel beautiful inside and out. We're the healers of hearts and souls, not just split ends.

Learn the Business

Business may seem like the farthest thing from your mind while you're in school. I'm not talking about balancing your checkbook; I'm talking about starting to understand business as it applies to hairstyling—that somebody getting $9 a haircut can be making more money than somebody getting $25 a haircut, because often a $9 haircutter can do four an hour. The $25 haircutter does one an hour. Which one earns more?

Business skills can be learned, and the information is out there. It's on Web sites, it's in industry journals; even the large companies are a source. Remember, the point here is that we have to accelerate your education, and the way you accelerate is not by studying harder but by doing more. That will make a tremendous difference.

Continue to Learn

Advanced education is one of the most important things you can do, while in school and definitely when you're first beginning. Videos are a good way to learn because you can fast forward, stop and go back, or watch it again a day later and find those missing clues that didn't make sense the first time. Web sites like www.behindthechair.com are an incredible way to get information and ideas. A friend of mine, Winn Claybaugh, tapes interviews with

in closing

(continued)

successful cosmetologists and markets them as the Master Series. You want to sign up for those because the people he interviews will give you tons of working tools.

Distributors do some of the most important education for our industry. They're at the local level, so you don't have to be tied into a national program. Distributors are looking for people like you. My first connection with Paul Mitchell was via one of my distributors in Memphis, who started utilizing me for local classes while I was in beauty school. Make a point of getting to as many of their local events as you can. It's not a case of which company you love; anybody who is teaching at the level you're at right now will help you, either by showing you what to do or in some cases what not to do. Either way it's learning, and the quicker you can eliminate mistakes based on watching other people, the better.

There is so much going on, so get out and look around. Don't just look at the education you want; look at where in the world you haven't been yet. Find the education and make that your point of reference. You'll get to see other places, like the Italian streets, and it will make you think differently about style in America. Everybody in America has a certain way of thinking about Europe, and in Europe everybody wants everything American. Even in Japan they want a piece of America. You've taken on a license that gives you the language we all speak, the language of hair. So get a passport and get ready. It's all about education, travel, having fun, and making money.

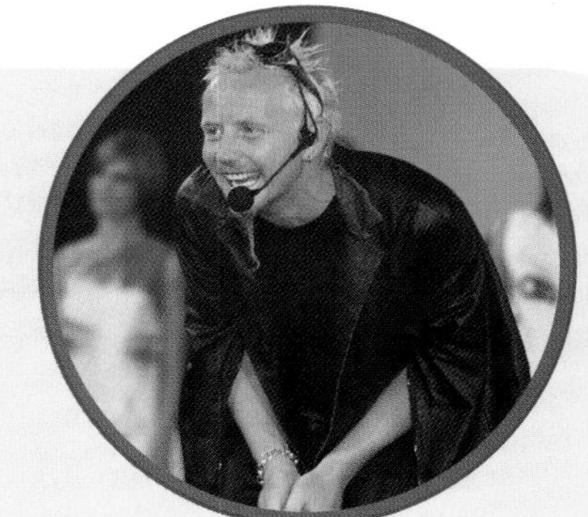

One of my greatest privileges in this industry is talking to and motivating thousands of young hairdressers just like you. I would like to extend this invitation: whenever you see our name or anybody synonymous with our companies in the neighborhood, please come and let us know that you caught us in beauty school and are already thinking of us. Come and see us at shows and say hello. Hang out with us. I know you'll have fun.

I want to be the first to congratulate you and welcome you into our incredible industry. You know the things we must do together to make things happen. Zig Zeigler, one of my favorite motivational speakers, said it the best: "If you do the things you ought to do when you ought to do it, the day comes when you get to do what you want to do when you want to do it."

So pick your mentors, pick a target, and start thinking of school as a place where you learn your skills and develop a good work ethic. Develop the habit of working hard in school; that will make things so easy when you become an employee of a hair salon because you'll fit right in. You'll already be up to speed. The thing about this industry that will blow your mind is how quickly you get to move closer to your goal. If you focus every day on taking a step in that direction, in no time at all you will realize your first goal—and then, my friends, you get to move on to the second one.

See you at a hair show soon!

APPENDIX A: RESOURCES
BOOKS FROM MILADY FOR THE STUDENT

Barber Styling

Milady's Professional Barber-Styling Workbook, 3E. 1-56253-367-3.

Scali-Sheehan, Maura T. *Milady's Standard Textbook of Professional Barber-Styling, 3E.* 1-56253-366-5.

State Exam Review for Professional Barber-Styling, 3E. 1-56253-370-3.

Basic Cosmetology

Hayden, Thomas, and James Williams. *Milady's Black Cosmetology.* 0-87350-3775.

Milady's Standard Cosmetologia. 1-4018-66085.

Basic Cosmetology Supplements

Barnes, Letha. *Milady's Standard: Cosmetology Study Guide – The Essential Companion.* 1-56253-888-8.

Beatty, Deborah. *Preparing for the Practical Exam: Cosmetology.* 1-4018-1532-4.

Guia de Estudios de Cosmetologia: La Acompanante Esencial. 1-4018-9286-8.

Libro de Ejercicios de Cosmetologia Teorico Revisado. 1-4018-1243-0

Libro de Ejericios de Cosmetologia Practico Revisado. 1-4018-1242-2.

Milady's Standard: Cosmetology Exam Review. 1-56253-892-6.

Milady's Standard: Cosmetology Fundamentals CD-ROM Student Version. 1-56253-893-4.

Milady's Standard: Cosmetology Study Summary for Chinese. 1-4018-1085-3.

Milady's Standard: Cosmetology Study Summary for Korean. 1-4018-1084-5.

Milady's Standard: Cosmetology Study Summary for Vietnamese. 1-4018-1083-7.

Milady's Standard: Cosmetology Theory Workbook. 1-56253-890-X.

Milady's Standard Practical Workbook. 1-56253-891-8.

Repaso del Examen de Cosmetologia. 1-4018-1241-4.

Business/Career

Bergant, Kathleen Ann. *Communication Skills for Cosmetologists.* 1-56253-087-9.

Capellini, Steve. *Massage Therapy Career Guide for Hands-on Success.* 1-56253-382-7.

Cotter, Louise and Francis London DuBose. *The Transition: How to Become a Salon Professional.* 1-56253-263-4.

Ducoff, Nancy and Nancy Flinn. *Fast Forward Salon & Spa Business Resource Book.* 0-9701028-0-1.

Edgerton, Leslie. *Managing Your Business: Milady's Guide to the Salon.* 1-56253-084-4.

Foley, Mark D. *The Motivated Salon.* 1-56253-320-7.

Gambino, Henry J. *Marketing and Advertising for the Salon.* 1-56353-262-2.

_____. *Salons and Computers: A Starter's Guide for Success.* 1-56253-354-1.

Hoffman, Lee. *Salon Dialogue for Successful Results.* 1-56253-3223.

Kilmer, Beverly. *Staffing Policies and Procedures.* 1-56253-314-2.

Maurer, Gretchen. *The Business of Bridal Beauty.* 1-56253-338-X.

Morehouse, Jayne. *Public Relations for the Salon.* 1-56253-271-5.

Oppenheim, Robert. *101 Salon Promotions.* 1-56253-358-4.

Phillips, Carol. *In the Bag: Selling in the Salon.* 1-56253-236-7.

Spear, J. Elaine. *Salon Client Care: How to Maximize Your Potential for Success.* 1-56253-349-5.

Tezak, Edward. *Successful Salon Management for Cosmetology Students, 5E.* 1-56253-679-6.

Ventura, Judy. *Salon Promotions: Creative Blueprints for Success.* 1-56253-350-9.

Wiggins, Joanne L. *Milady's Guide to Owning and Operating a Nail Salon.* 1-56253-201-4.

Esthetics

Bickmore, Helen. *Milady's Hair Removal Techniques: A Comprehensive Manual.* 1-4018-1555-3.

Deitz, Sallie. *The Esthetician's Guide to Succeeding in a Medical Office.* 1-4018-1788-2.

Gambino, Henry J. *Modern Esthetics: A Scientific Source for Estheticians.* 1-56253-043-7.

Gerson, Joel and Alison O'Neil. *Milady's Standard: Fundamentals for Estheticians, 9E.* 1-56253-836-5.

Lees, Mark. *Skin Care: Beyond the Basics, 2E.* 1-56253-625-7.

Milady's Standard: Comprehensive Training for Estheticians. 1-56253-805-5.

Milady's Standard: Esthetics Student CD-ROM. 1-56253-840-3.

Place, Stan Campbell. *The Art and Science of Professional Makeup.* 0-87350-361-9.

Poignard, Renee. *Milady's Waxing Made Easy: A Step-by-Step Guide.* 1-56253-171-9.

Rayner, Victoria. *Clinical Cosmetology: A Medical Approach to Esthetics Procedures.* 1-56253-056-9.

Skin Care: Beyond the Basics Workbook. 1-56253-626-5.

Thrower, Angelo P. *Black Skin Care for the Practicing Professional.* 1-56253-352-5.

Haircoloring

Rangl, Deb. *Milady's Standard Hair Coloring Manual and Activities Book.* 1-56253-356-8.

Warren, Roxy. *Haircoloring in Plain English.* 1-56253-357-6.

Haircutting/Hairstyling

Bailey, Diane Carol. *Natural Hair Care and Braiding.* 1-56253-316-9.

Cotter, Louise. *Mature Elegance: Styles and Techniques for Mature Clients.* 1-56253-339-8.

Jones, Jamie Rines. *Braids and Updos Made Easy.* 1-56253-318-5.

_____. *Long Hair System.* 0-8273-87-30-X.

Milady's Standard System of Salon Skills: Hairdressing, Student Package. 1-56253-398-3.

The Multicultural Client: Cuts, Styles, and Chemical Services. 1-56253-178-6.

Scali-Sheahan, Maura. *Milady's Standard Textbook of Professional Barber-Styling, 3E.* 1-56253-366-5.

Young, Kenneth. *Milady's 18 Men's Styles.* 1-56253-177-8.

_____. *Milady's 28 Black Styles.* 1-56253-042-9.

_____. *Milady's 28 Styles.* 1-56253-070-4.

_____. *Milady's Haircutting: Men's, Women's, and Children's Cuts.* 1-56253-103-4.

_____. *Milady's Hairstyling: Men's, Women's, and Children's Styles.* 1-56253-154-9.

_____. *Milady's Razor Cutting.* 1-56253-180-8.

Massage

Beck, Mark. *Milady's Theory and Practice of Therapeutic Massage, 3E, 1999.* 1-56253-404-1 (HC), 1-56253-536-6 (SC).

Nails

Anthony, Elizabeth. *Airbrushing for Nails.* 1-56253-270-7.

Beatty, Deborah. *Preparing for the Practical Exam: Nail Technology.* 1-4018-1757-2.

Bigan, Tammy. *Nail Art and Design.* 1-56253-118-2.

McCormick, Janet. *Spa Manicuring.* 1-56253-460-2.

Milady's Standard: Nail Technology State Exam Review. 1-56253-909-4.

Milady's Standard: Nail Technology Student Workbook. 1-56253-907-8.

Milady's Standard: Nail Technology Study Summary for Chinese. 1-4018-1187-6.

Milady's Standard: Nail Technology Study Summary for Korean. 1-4018-1186-8.

Milady's Standard: Nail Technology Study Summary for Vietnamese. 1-4018-1185-X.

Milady's Standard: Tecnologia de Unas. 1-56253-911-6.

Mix, Godfrey. *The Salon Professional's Guide to Foot Care.* 1-56253-332-0.

Peters, Vicki. *SalonOvations' Nail Q and A Book.* 1-56253-266-9.

Schoon, Douglas D. *Milady's Nail Structure and Product Chemistry.* 1-56253-239-1.

Schultes, Sue Ellen. *Milady's Standard: Nail Technology, 4E.* 1-56253-882-9.

Tecnologia de Unas – Libro de Ejercicios. 1-56253-912-4.

Videos

Beck, Mark. *Milady's Massage Fundamentals Video Series.* 1-56253-750-4.

Hair Structure and Chemistry Simplified Video. 1-4018-0868-9.

Jones, Jamie Rines. *Braids and Updos Video Series:*
Advanced Braiding Made Easy. 0-87350-241-8.
Braiding Made Easy. 0-87350-650-2.
French Braiding Made Easy. 0-87350-459-3.
More Updos Made Easy. 1-56253-379-7.
Ribbon Braiding Made Easy. 1-56253-377-0.
Updos Made Easy. 1-56253-378-9.

Nelson, Dennis. *Safety and Health in the Salon Training System.* 1-56253-709-1.

FOR THE INSTRUCTOR

Answers to Milady's Professional Barber-Styling Workbook, 3E. 1-56253-368-1.

Barnes, Letha. *Milady's Standard: Cosmetology Course Management Guide.* 1-56253-9035. CD-ROM 1-56253-904-3.

Barnes, Letha. *Milady's Standard: Cosmetology Study Guide – The Essential Companion Answer Key.* 1-56253-889-6.

Beatty, Deborah. *Preparing for the Practical Exam: Instructor's Manual.* 1-4018-1756-4.

Halal, John. *Hair Structure and Chemistry Simplified Course Management Guide.* 1-56253-632-X.

Milady's Professional Barber-Styling Lesson Plans, 3E. 1-56253-369-X.

Milady's Standard: Comprehensive Training for Estheticians Leader's Manual with CTB. 1-56253-808-X.

Milady's Standard: Cosmetology Fundamentals CD-ROM School/Networked Version. 1-56253-894-2.

Milady's Standard: Esthetics Course Management Guide, 9E. 1-56253-838-1.

Milady's Standard: Nail Technology Course Management Guide, 4E. 1-56253-910-8.

Milady's Standard System of Salon Skills: Hairdressing Image Library, CD-ROM. 1-56253-559-5.

Milady's Standard System of Salon Skills: Hairdressing Leader's Manual. 1-56253-399-1.

Milady's Standard System of Salon Skills Support Tools, CD-ROM. 1-56253-665-6.

Milady's Theory and Practice of Therapeutic Massage Course Management Guide. 1-56253-406-8.

Poignard, Renee. *Milady's Standard: Fundamentals for Estheticians Course Management Guide.* 1-56253-8381.

Skin Care: Beyond the Basics Answer Key. 1-56253-627-3.

Successful Salon Management for Cosmetology Students, 5E Answer Key. 1-56253-681-8.

VIDEOS/DVDs

Barnes, Letha. *Milady's Master Educator Program, 2002.* (Instructor's package) 1-56253-735-0.

Jones, Jamie Rines. *Braids & Updos Made Easy: The Long Hair System.* 0-82738-730-X.

_____. *Braids & Updos Made Easy: The Training Package.* 0-82738-729-6.

Milady's Standard: Comprehensive Training for Estheticians System. (Instructor's package) 1-4018-1259-7.

Milady's Standard: Cosmetology DVD Series. 1-56253-905-1.

Milady's Standard System of Salon Skills: Hairdressing. (Instructor's package) 1-56253-401-7.

Miller, Erica. *Facial Treatment Videotapes – Professional Education Series.* 1-56253-392-4.

Whitten, Cheryl. *Step-by-Step Makeup Videos and Course Management Guide.* 1-4018-0660-0.

FOR REFERENCE

Balhorn, Linda A. *The Professional Model's Handbook.* 0-87350-376-7.

Chesky, Sheldon R., Isabel Christina, and Richard B. Rosenberg. *Playing It Safe: Milady's Guide to Decontamination, Sterilization, and Personal Protection.* 1-56253-179-4.

Halal, John. *Milady's Hair Care Products Ingredients Dictionary.* 1-56253-919-1.

Hess, Shelley. *SalonOvations' Guide to Aromatherapy.* 1-56253-313-4.

_____. *The Professional's Reflexology Handbook.* 1-56253-334-7.

Levine, Karen. *A Survival Guide for Cosmetologists.* 1-4018-1545-6.

Michalun, Natalia. *Milady's Skin Care and Cosmetic Ingredients Dictionary, 2E.* 1-56253-660-5.

Milady's Illustrated Cosmetology Dictionary, 2E. 1-56253-667-2.

Miller, Erica. *Day Spa Operations.* 1-56253-255-3.

_____. *Day Spa Techniques.* 1-56253-261-8.

_____. *Shiatsu Massage.* 1-56253-264-2.

Nelson, Dennis. *Safety and Health in the Salon Training System.* 1-56253-709-1.

Schoon, Douglas. *HIV/AIDS and Hepatitis: Everything You Need to Know to Protect Yourself and Others.* 1-56253-175-1.

Ventura, Judy. *Milady's Salon Receptionist's Handbook.* 1-56253-044-5.

MAGAZINES

American Salon

Official publication of the National Cosmetology Association (NCA)

Subscriptions: (218) 723-9477

Beauty Store Business

Subscriptions: (800) 624-4196

PO Box 10751

Riverton, NJ 08076-0751

www.beautystorebusiness.com

Canadian Hairdresser

Subscriptions: (416) 923-1111
11 Spadina Road
Toronto, Ont.
Canada M5R 2S9
www.canhair.com

Day Spa

Subscriptions: (800) 624-4196
PO Box 10566
Riverton, NJ 08076-0566
www.dayspamag.com

Dermascope

Subscriptions: (972) 226-2309
2611 N. Beltline Rd., Suite 140
Sunnyvale, TX 75182
www.dermascope.com

Les Nouvelles Esthetiques

Subscriptions: (800) 471-0229
306 Alcazar Ave.
Coral Gables, FL 33134
www.lneonline.com

Modern Salon

Subscriptions: www.modernsalon.com
PO Box 1414
Lincolnshire, IL 60069

NailPro

Subscriptions: (800) 624-4196
PO Box 10534
Riverton, NJ 08076
www.nailpro.com

Nails

Subscriptions: (888) NAILS-44
PO Box 1067
Skokie, IL 60076

Salon News

Subscriptions: (800) 477-6411
PO Box 5035
Brentwood, TN 37024-5035

Salon Today

Subscriptions: (800) 808-2623 ext. 305
400 Knightsbridge Parkway
Palatine, IL 60069
www.modernsalon.com

Skin, Inc.

Subscriptions: (800) 469-7445
3625 S. Schmale Road
Carol Stream, IL 60188-2787

WEB SITES

www.beautynet.com
Virtual salon for hair, skin, and nail care.

www.beautytech.com
Trade show schedule, continuing education calendar, message center (to trade information), information specifically for nail technicians, cosmetologists, and salon owners.

www.beautyworks.com
Resource for skin and hair care, electrolysis, body massage, spas/salons, dermatologists, makeup, nails.

www.behindthechair.com
BTC Bookstore, up-to-date products and trends, find a job, post a job.

www.bworks.com/elec/
Information on electrolysis, electrologists online, schools, supplies, relaxation products.

www.cosmeticworld.com
Daily supplement to the leading weekly newsletter for cosmetics and fragrance industry.

www.hairnet.com
Beauty On-line, an online magazine; *American Salon,* inside look at the beauty business; list of salons in the U.S.; window shopping; more.

www.milady.com
Milady's Web site: information on books, audio, and video tapes, computer software programs, The Career Institute.

APPENDIX B: ASSOCIATIONS

Accrediting Commission of Career Schools and Colleges of Technology
2101 Wilson Blvd., Suite 302
Arlington, VA 22201
(703) 247-4212
www.accsct.org

Aesthetics International Association
PO Box 468
Kaufman, TX 75142
(877) 968-7539
www.beautyworks.com/aia/index.html

Allied Beauty Association (ABA)
450 Matheson Blvd. East, Units 46 & 47
Mississauga, Ont.
Canada L4Z 1R5
(905) 568-0158
www.abacanada.com

American Association of Cosmetology Schools (AACS)
15825 N. 71st St., Suite 100
Scottsdale, AZ 85254-1521
(800) 831-1086
www.beautyschools.org

American Beauty Association (ABA)
401 N. Michigan Ave.
Chicago, IL 60611-4267
(312) 245-1595
www.americanbeautyassociation.org

American Health & Beauty Aids Institute (AHBAI)
401 N. Michigan Ave., #2200
Chicago, IL 60611-4267
(312) 644-6610
www.proudlady.org

American Society of Esthetic Medicine (ASEM)
3901 Livingston Ave.
Columbus, OH 43227
(614) 239-9000
www.beautyworks.com/asem/index.html

Beauty and Barber Supply Institute (BBSI)
11811 N. Tatum Blvd., Suite 1085
Phoenix, AZ 85028
(800) 468-BBSI
www.oneroof.org

The Cosmetic, Toiletry, and Fragrance Association
1101 17th St. NW, Suite 300
Washington, DC 20036
(202) 331-1770
www.ctfa.org

Cosmetology Advancement Foundation (CAF)
PO Box 811
FDR Station
New York, NY 10150-0811
(212) 750-2412
www.cosmetology.org

Cosmetology Educators Association (CEA)
11811 N. Tatum Blvd., Suite 1085
Phoenix, AZ 85028-1625
(800) 831-1086
www.oneroof.org

Fashion and Beauty Internet Association
529 E. 85th St.
New York, NY 10028
www.fbia.com

Independent Cosmetic Manufacturers and Distributors (ICMAD)
1220 W. Northwest Highway
Palatine, IL 60067
(800) 334-2623
www.icmad.org

Intercoiffure
11 bis
rue Jean Goujon
75008 Paris
www.intercoiffure.com

International Guild of Professional Electrologists, Inc. (IGPE)
803 N. Main St.
High Point, NC 27262
(800) 830-3247
www.ipge.org

National Accrediting Commission of Cosmetology Arts & Sciences (NACCAS)
4401 Ford Ave., Suite 1300
Alexandria, VA 22302
(703) 527-7600
www.naccas.org

National Cosmetology Association (NCA)
401 N. Michigan Ave.
Chicago, IL 60611-4267
(312) 245-1595
www.salonprofessionals.org

National-Interstate Council of State Boards of Cosmetology
PO Box 11390
Columbia, SC 29211
www.nictestng.org/indx-main.html

The Salon Association
11811 N. Tatum Blvd., Suite 1085
Phoenix, AZ 85028
(800) 211-4TSA
www.salons.org/index2.html

Society of Permanent Cosmetic Professionals
(888) 584-7729
www.spcp.org

VICA (Vocational Industrial Clubs of America, Inc.)
PO Box 3000
Leesburg, VA 20177-0300
(703) 777-8810
www.sallsusa.org

Western Beauty Reps Association
31131 Via Collinas, #607
Westlake Village, CA 91362-3929
(818) 889-2201

GLOSSARY/INDEX

B

C

E

G

H

I

J

K

M

N

O

P

Q

R

S

Y

Z

WILDER BRANCH LIBRARY
7140 E. SEVEN MILE RD.
DETROIT, MI 48234